T0178164

Nutrition and Health

Series editors:
Adrianne Bendich, Ph.D., FACN, FASN
Wellington, FL, USA

Connie W. Bales, Ph.D., R.D.
Human Dev't, Ctr Aging Blue Zone Rm 2508
Duke Univ Med Ctr, Ctr Study of Aging
Durham, NC, USA

The Nutrition and Health series has an overriding mission in providing health professionals with texts that are considered essential since each is edited by the leading researchers in their respective fields. Each volume includes: 1) a synthesis of the state of the science, 2) timely, in-depth reviews, 3) extensive, up-to-date fully annotated reference lists, 4) a detailed index, 5) relevant tables and figures, 6) identification of paradigm shifts and consequences, 7) virtually no overlap of information between chapters, but targeted, inter-chapter referrals, 8) suggestions of areas for future research and 9) balanced, data driven answers to patient/health professionals questions which are based upon the totality of evidence rather than the findings of a single study. Nutrition and Health is a major resource of relevant, clinically based nutrition volumes for the professional that serve as a reliable source of data-driven reviews and practice guidelines.

More information about this series at http://www.springer.com/series/7659

Mark L. Dreher

Dietary Patterns and Whole Plant Foods in Aging and Disease

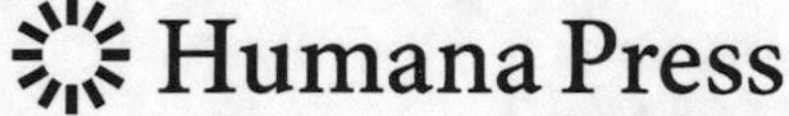

Mark L. Dreher
Chief Science Officer
Nutrition Science Solutions LLC
Wimberley, TX
USA

Nutrition and Health
ISBN 978-3-030-09641-0 ISBN 978-3-319-59180-3 (eBook)
https://doi.org/10.1007/978-3-319-59180-3

Printed on acid-free paper

This Humana Press imprint is published by Springer Nature
The registered company is Springer International Publishing AG
The registered company address is: Gewerbestrasse 11, 6330 Cham, Switzerland

Preface

For most people, aging and chronic diseases rates are not genetically predetermined. It is estimated that as much as 70–80% of aging and chronic disease rates are associated with lifestyle choices. Unhealthy aging and chronic disease rates are largely associated with excessive intake of Western energy dense, poor nutritional quality diets and sedentary lifestyles, which lead to overweight and obesity being the normal phenotype. Overweight and obesity lead to increased risk of cardiovascular diseases, type 2 diabetes, nonalcoholic fatty liver disease and chronic kidney disease, reduced healthy life expectancy, and premature mortality. Excessive body fat is not inert but accelerates metabolic dysfunction processes by stimulating increased systemic, organ and tissue inflammation. Healthy aging and lower chronic disease rates are largely associated with adherence to healthy dietary patterns, increasing physical activity most days of the week, achieving and maintaining lean body weight and waist circumference. Unhealthy aging and higher chronic disease rates are largely associated with adherence to Western dietary patterns, relatively sedentary or inactive lifestyles, and a positive energy balance leading to weight gain and central obesity. Among cancer survivors a study indicated that healthy diets are associated with a reduced mortality rate of 20% compared to an over 40% increased mortality rate for those consuming Western diets. Over the last 30–40 years, the expansion of the Western diet and sedentary lifestyle has led to pandemic levels of obesity, chronic disease rates, and unhealthy life expectancy in children and young and older adults, which is progressively moving toward a global healthcare and economic crisis, which is expected to be a critical global issue in the next 20 years. Over the last decade, dietary and nutrition science has advanced significantly with thousands of prospective cohort, case-control, and cross-sectional studies, and randomized controlled trials to identify dietary and specific healthy foods that can help healthcare professionals and government policy makers to limit this current and growing global health crisis, but it will require major changes in our food systems and polices and increased investment in high-quality food and nutrition research.

The objective of this book is to comprehensively review published research on the effects of dietary patterns and whole plant foods in aging and disease to help increase awareness of the thousands of studies in a comprehensive, condensed resource for health professionals to help them in addressing current global health issues associated with unhealthy diets and lifestyles. This book is divided into five parts focusing on the effects of dietary patterns and whole plant foods. The first part provides an overview of lifestyle and dietary factors associated with aging and chronic disease. The second part addresses specific effects of dietary patterns and especially fiber-rich diets on gastrointestinal tract health and disease. The third part examines the effects of dietary patterns and whole plant foods on body weight and composition regulation, type 2 diabetes, and nonalcoholic fatty liver disease. The fourth part provides an in-depth analysis of the effects of dietary patterns on coronary heart disease, hypertension, chronic kidney disease, stroke, and age-related cognitive decline and dementia. The fifth part comprehensively reviews the evidence related to dietary patterns, whole plant foods, nutrients, and phytochemicals on breast and colorectal cancer risk and survival. Figures are extensively used to highlight important findings. Tables provide summaries of many published observational and intervention trials and their meta-analyses to provide specific details on the health effects of dietary patterns and whole plant foods. This book is for dietitians, physicians, nurses, nutritionists, pharmacists, food industry scientists, academic researchers and educators, naturopathic doctors, health professionals, graduate and medical students, policy makers, and all others interested in the role of healthy plant-based diets and the benefits of individual foods in aging and disease risk.

Wimberley, TX Mark L. Dreher

Series Editor

The great success of the Nutrition and Health Series is the result of the consistent overriding mission of providing health professionals with texts that are essential because each includes (1) a synthesis of the state of the science, (2) timely, in-depth reviews by the leading researchers and clinicians in their respective fields, (3) extensive, up-to-date fully annotated reference lists, (4) a detailed index, (5) relevant tables and figures, (6) identification of paradigm shifts and the consequences, (7) virtually no overlap of information between chapters, but targeted, interchapter referrals, (8) suggestions of areas for future research, and (9) balanced, data-driven answers to patient as well as health professionals' questions that are based upon the totality of evidence rather than the findings of any single study.

The Series volumes are not the outcome of a symposium. Rather, each editor has the potential to examine a chosen area with a broad perspective, both in subject matter and in the choice of chapter authors. The international perspective, especially with regard to public health initiatives, is emphasized where appropriate. The editor(s), whose trainings are both research and practice oriented, have the opportunity to develop a primary objective for their book, define the scope and focus, and then invite the leading authorities from around the world to be part of their initiative. The authors are encouraged to provide an overview of the field, discuss their own research, and relate the research findings to potential human health consequences. Because each book is developed *de novo*, the chapters are coordinated so that the resulting volume imparts greater knowledge than the sum of the information contained in the individual chapters.

"Dietary Patterns and Whole Plant Foods in Aging and Disease," edited as well as written by Mark L. Dreher, Ph.D., is a very welcome addition to the **Nutrition and Health Series** and fully exemplifies the series' goals. This volume represents a critical, in-depth review of the recent developments in the studies of dietary patterns and their role in health and disease and concentrates on their role in affecting the health of seniors. Evaluations of the major dietary patterns that have been examined in large survey studies and in certain clinical trials are discussed in depth including, but not limited to, the Mediterranean diet, Dietary Approaches to Stop Hypertension (DASH), new Nordic, and vegetarian diets. The volume also examines the importance of whole plant foods in disease prevention and reduction in disease severity in the aging population. The volume is designed as an important resource for physicians in many clinical fields, nutritionists and dietitians, research and public health scientists, and related health professionals who treat senior adult patients. The volume provides objective and relevant information for professors and lecturers, advanced undergraduates and graduates, researchers and clinical investigators who require extensive, up-to-date literature reviews, instructive tables and figures, and excellent references on all aspects of diet and health as well as nutrition's role in treatments of the major chronic diseases affecting the aging population. This volume is especially relevant as the number of research papers and meta-analyses in the clinical nutrition arena increases every year and clients and patients are very interested in dietary components such as whole plant foods and their components for disease prevention. Certainly, the obesity epidemic remains a major concern especially as the comorbidities, such as the metabolic syndrome, type 2 diabetes, hypertension, and hyperlipidemia, are seen more frequently in older individuals whose diets contain lower than recommended levels of fiber-rich, whole plant foods.

Dr. Dreher, who has written every chapter in this volume, has made every effort to provide health professionals with the most up-to-date and comprehensive volume that highlights the key, well-accepted nutrition information available to date on the importance of plant-based dietary patterns for many aspects of health and wellness. Clear definitions and distinctions are made concerning commonly asked patient questions such as what are the differences between the various types of dietary patterns and how do these affect the risk of developing the major diseases including obesity, cardiovascular and cerebrovascular diseases, and cancers. Explanations are also provided for the numerous types of vegetable-based diets that are often questioned by clients and patients and discussed by health professionals even among themselves as there are many findings in this field of nutrition research that are complex.

The author of the volume, Dr. Mark L. Dreher, Ph.D., is an internationally recognized expert in the field of dietary fiber research. Currently, he serves as President and Chief Science Officer of Nutrition Science Solutions, LLC. He received his education in biochemistry and agricultural biochemistry and nutrition at UCLA and the University of Arizona. Dr. Dreher started his career as a research scientist in medical food product development at McGaw Laboratories in Irvine, California. Later, he served as Assistant Professor in Food and Nutrition at North Dakota State University leading research on sunflower seeds, dry edible beans, and emerging grains. During his subsequent 30+ year career in the food, agricultural, and pharmaceutical industries, he held key roles in over 150 new healthy product development projects and food-based clinical research trials. He has authored or coauthored over 50 research journal articles and book chapters. Dr. Dreher has authored and edited the impressive **2017** volume entitled **"Dietary Fiber in Health and Disease"** that is part of the **Nutrition and Health Series**. Earlier, he authored the *Handbook of Dietary Fiber* in 1987 and was an editor and contributor to the second edition of the *Handbook of Dietary Fiber* and the *Complex Carbohydrates in Foods* book. He served as the chair of the International Life Science Institute—North American Food, Nutrition and Safety and

Carbohydrate Committees and vice chair of the Functional Foods for Health Committee. Dr. Dreher was a member of the 1997 Joint FAO/WHO Expert Consultation on Carbohydrate and Human Nutrition. He was a Fellow in the National Center for Food and Agricultural Policy and Resources Leadership Program for the Future in Washington DC. Dr. Dreher is an active member of the American Society for Nutrition, American Heart Association, Academy of Nutrition and Dietetics, the Nutrition Society (UK), American Chemical Society, and Institute of Food Technology. Dr. Dreher is actively engaged in projects and research related to the role of healthy diets, whole foods, and phytochemicals in health, chronic disease prevention, and optimal aging.

Dr. Dreher provides extensive summaries and assessments of the major prospective cohort studies, randomized controlled trials, and relevant meta-analyses on the role of dietary patterns and lifestyles on the health and disease status in aging. All 20 chapters contain Key Points and Key Words as well as targeted references, useful tables and figures, and a listing of recommended readings. In addition, the volume contains an extensive index and helpful Appendices. The volume chapters are organized in a logical progression so that the reader can identify the areas most relevant for their needs. All chapters and the entire volume are available online and are downloadable. The book focuses on the effects of whole plant foods on the colonic microbiota, body weight regulation, and digestive health in the aging population. Diseases and syndromes reviewed include those of the digestive tract including irritable bowel syndrome, inflammatory bowel disease, and diverticular disease. The interactions between diet and metabolic diseases, coronary heart disease, hypertension, chronic kidney disease, nonalcoholic fatty liver disease, stroke as well as reduced cognitive functions, and cancers of the colon and breast are examined in individual chapters.

Part I: Overview of Aging and Disease

The three introductory chapters in the first part provide readers with a broad review of the major lifestyles and phenotypes of the aging population and then examine the most prevalent dietary patterns and whole plant foods that are consumed. Chapter 1 reviews the effects of aging on tissues, organs, and organ systems that increase vulnerability to disease and give rise to the characteristic manifestations of aging including, but not limited to, the loss of muscle (sarcopenia) and bone mass, a decline in reaction time, compromised hearing and vision, reduced kidney function, and elasticity of the skin. The chapter includes key tables that identify the aging processes that affect the mind and body. We also learn that the rate of aging varies by individual with 25–30% programmed by heredity factors and 70–75% due to external factors such as lifestyle factors and random events. Thus, it appears to be possible for individuals to significantly influence their rate of aging. However, data are reviewed that indicate that the gains in life expectancy seen during the twentieth century are decreasing globally due to the rapid rise in obesity and its related diseases as well as the increase in sedentary long-term work environments and non-exercise-related relaxation lifestyles. The chapter concludes with an in-depth examination of the components of healthy aging lifestyles and dietary patterns and includes 17 tables and figures and over 100 relevant references.

The second chapter provides up-to-date definitions of healthy aging, healthy diets, Western diets, and the role of each in reducing the risks of age-related chronic diseases. Healthy aging is the absence of premature chronic disease, lack of physical disability, and the presence of good social engagement and mental health. Of the lifestyle choices, the type of dietary pattern followed appears to have a significant effect on aging and longevity including a lower risk of obesity and overweight, cardiovascular disease, hypertension as well as type 2 diabetes, cognitive declines, and reductions in the risk of developing certain cancers. The chapter includes a discussion of the major health, environment, and lifestyle challenges that make meeting dietary recommendations difficult for the elderly. Some of the impediments to consuming healthy nutrient-dense diets include losses of the ability to taste and smell, loss of appetite, dental and chewing problems, less family support, and limitations in mobility for accessing high-quality fresh whole foods. The aging-related inefficiencies in essential nutrient absorption and utilization that result in increased nutrient requirements are reviewed. The major research studies are illustrated in the 21 tables and figures included in this comprehensive chapter that also contains over 80 targeted references.

Chapter 3 describes the role of whole plant foods in maintaining the health of aging populations. Overall, healthy dietary guidelines recommend eating 2 1/2 cups of a variety of vegetables/day; two cups of fruits, especially whole fruits/day; six servings of total grains at ≥3 servings of whole grains/day and ≤3 servings of refined grains/day, ≥4 weekly servings of legumes (dietary pulses or soy), and/or ≥5 weekly servings of nuts, all of which belong to the category of whole plant foods. The chapter describes in detail the functions of the macro- and micronutrients found in these foods and their major health effects. This comprehensive chapter includes 29 tables and figures, as well as extensive appendices and almost 200 excellent references that provide the reader with an extensive body of data from well-controlled and large survey studies that consistently point to the health value of whole plant foods for the aging population.

Part II: Gastrointestinal Tract

Part II contains three chapters that examine the critical issues of the importance of the human microbiome and its role in laxation and constipation, irritable bowel syndrome, inflammatory bowel disease, and diverticular disease. Chapter 4 reviews the key role of fiber in maintaining an optimal microbiome. Fiber is the primary dietary energy source of the microbiota bacteria that produce short chain fatty acids such as butyrate. Butyrate is the major energy source of normal colon cells and thus the microbiome is actively involved in maintaining the colonic barrier defenses associated with protecting the colon from bacterial infections such as *C. difficile*, decreasing the risk of inflammatory bowel disease, and reducing colon cancer risk. The chapter also reviews other critical functions of the microbiota including aiding the absorption of nutrients, the synthesis of certain vitamins, fermentation of fiber to metabolically active molecules linked to optimizing colonic and systemic immune function, and improving cardiometabolic health and glycemic control. References, tables, and figures provide the reader with summaries of key studies in aging populations. Chapter 5 provides more detailed descriptions of the fiber-rich dietary patterns associated with improved laxation and reduced constipation by increasing stool weight and bulk volume. Adequate intake of fiber from whole cereal, fruits (including dried fruits), and vegetables and common fiber-rich food ingredients including polydextrose, psyllium, konjac glucomannan, guar gum, and inulin are discussed with regard to providing constipation relief. The seven comprehensive tables and figures provide valuable data for the reader.

Irritable bowel syndrome (IBS), examined in Chap. 6, is the most common gastrointestinal disorder occurring in people younger than 45 years. IBS is a chronic and relapsing functional colonic disorder characterized by abdominal pain, bloating, distension, and other changes in bowel habits that lack visible structural or anatomic abnormalities. Emerging research shows that the colon of the IBS patient contains low-grade inflammation and neuronal hyperexcitability. Often, there is also reduced bacteria diversity including lower levels of butyrate producing bacteria and increased levels of pathogenic bacteria. Certain dietary patterns and foods can be triggers for IBS symptoms. Avoidance of certain food components, called FODMAP (fermentable oligosaccharides, disaccharides, monosaccharides, and polyols), may reduce acute IBS symptoms. Chapter 6 also examines the influence of dietary patterns, foods, and fiber on diverticular disease. Diverticulae or colonic submucosal herniated pouches, and/or diverticulosis' incidence increases with age affecting 5–10% of adults under 40 years, 30% by age 50 years, and 70% by the age of 85 years. The chapter summarizes the data from the intervention trials that looked at the effects of fiber-rich diets, foods, and/or supplements. Six RCTs showed beneficial effects of different fiber sources including fiber-rich diets, bran, bran crisps, psyllium, and methylcellulose on symptoms and/or bowel function. The chapter contains 144 relevant references and 16 tables and figures.

Part III: Weight Management and Related Diseases

The four chapters included in the third part review the roles of dietary patterns and whole plant foods as well as dietary fiber in affecting the risk of becoming overweight or obese during the aging process. Observational studies have consistently shown that from 50 years of age onward, healthy dietary patterns are inversely associated with weight gain and central obesity in both men and women and a small positive energy balance of 50 kcals/day can lead to an average increase in weight of 1 pound/year; at the same time, height and activity levels are decreasing adding further to the increased risk of becoming overweight or obese during the sixth, seventh, and eighth decades of life. We learn, in Chap. 7, that obesity is a complex multifactorial disease resulting from chronic increased energy intake and insufficient energy expenditure that is caused by many factors including, but not limited to, genetic, environmental, lifestyle, and emotional factors as well as age and sex of the individual. The chapter includes details of the major healthy diets including the Mediterranean diet, the DASH diet, the Healthy Eating Index (HEI), and other healthy eating diets and summary tables of studies utilizing these diets and others in which obese and overweight individuals consumed higher than their normal levels of fiber. In addition to the 21 informative tables and figures and over 140 references, the Appendix reviews the foods and portions used in each of the major healthy diets discussed in the chapter.

Chapter 8 concentrates on the composition of diets containing whole plant foods and their role in weight control. Whole plant foods are generally associated with lower energy density, reduced obesity, and decreased chronic disease risk than highly processed plant foods. However, these foods, including grains, fresh and dried fruits, vegetables, nuts, and pulses, vary widely in nutrient composition, energy density, and physical properties. Detailed analyses of whole plant foods and their effects on body composition are included. As examples, randomized control intervention studies indicate that whole grains are more effective in reducing body fat and waist circumference than in reducing body weight or body mass index. For fruits and vegetables, cohort studies found an association with a lower risk of weight, waist circumference, body fat gain, and obesity especially when diets included healthier varieties of fruits and vegetables. However, higher energy dense, lower fiber fruits and vegetables promoted weight gain. Eating lower energy dense, higher fiber and flavonoid rich fruits and vegetables was associated with lower risk of weight gain or modest weight loss, promoted additional weight loss in a hypocaloric diet, and helped support weight maintenance after weight loss. The chapter includes over 100 references, 14 tables and figures, and an informative appendix that describes the nutrient composition of the major categories of whole plant foods.

Chapter 9 looks at the data that link certain dietary patterns that emphasize whole plant foods reducing the risk of developing type 2 diabetes with beneficial effects in older individuals with type 2 diabetes. The emphasis of this chapter is on the senior population. The chapter reviews the prospective cohort studies that consistently show that increased intake of diet patterns identified as healthy that include higher than average intakes of whole foods and provided lower glycemic loads was effective in reducing diabetes risk. The emphasis on dietary patterns is due to their influence on various diabetes and cardiometabolic risk factors including controlling body weight, visceral fat, glucose-insulin homeostasis, oxidative stress, inflammation, and endothelial health, lipoprotein concentrations, and blood pressure. High-quality diets that lower diabetes and cardiovascular risks can help to control body weight and composition. The mechanisms of action include better control of whole body inflammatory responses that are linked to improved insulin sensitivity and vascular endothelial function, reduced risk of diabetes-related atherosclerosis, and other cardiovascular comorbidities. There are over 130 references, 21 tables and figures, and two additional appendices that help the reader understand the details of the major dietary patterns and nutrient content of important whole foods that are of value to patients at risk of/or with type 2 diabetes.

Chapter 10, containing seven relevant tables and figures and 84 references, provides an in-depth review of another chronic disease seen more frequently in older obese/overweight individuals. Nonalcoholic fatty liver disease (NAFLD) can progress to a more severe, related disease, nonalcoholic steatohepatitis (NASH), which is characterized by hepatocellular injury or hepatic steatosis and associated hepatocyte injury, inflammation, and fibrosis. Approximately two-thirds of obese adults have NAFLD and 20% have NASH. NASH occurs more frequently in older people especially those with sarcopenia. The primary clinical risk factors for NAFLD are excess body weight especially abdominal fatness, insulin resistance associated with both prediabetes and type 2 diabetes, and cardiovascular disease. Both NAFLD and NASH are also associated with the Western lifestyle and dietary patterns including high energy dense, low fiber and nutrient dense diets, and inactivity. The chapter includes a review of the nutrients and diets associated with reducing the risk of these liver diseases as well as improving treatment.

Part IV: Cardiovascular and Cerebrovascular Diseases and Age-Related Cognitive Function

The eight chapters in Part IV review the effects of dietary patterns and consumption of whole plant foods on the aging population's risk of developing cardiovascular and cerebrovascular diseases including coronary heart disease, hypertension, kidney disease, stroke, and cognitive decline. Chapter 11 emphasizes coronary heart disease, as this disease is most prevalent in individuals >50 years of age, and reviews the totality of the evidence that healthy dietary patterns with greater concentrations of whole plant foods are associated with decreased risk of coronary heart disease (CHD). These dietary patterns are characterized by greater intakes of vegetables, fruits, whole grains, low-fat dairy, and seafood, and limited intakes of red and processed meat, refined grains, and sugar-sweetened foods and beverages compared to the increased CHD risk associated with greater adherence to Western dietary patterns. These healthy dietary patterns, including the Elderly Dietary Index, are associated with CHD protective effects because they are reduced in energy density and higher in fiber, healthier fatty acid profiles, essential nutrients, antioxidants, and electrolytes, and are anti-inflammatory compared with Western diets. Chapter 12 examines the role of whole plant foods in the reduction of primary and secondary risks of CHD. The major causative agent of CHD is higher than recommended levels of cholesterol in the blood that has been implicated in the development of atherosclerotic plaques in coronary vessels. Lifestyle changes recommended for those with high cholesterol levels include adopting a diet low in saturated and *trans* fatty acids, incorporating fiber, antioxidants, plant sterols and stanols into the diet, exercising regularly, not smoking, and maintaining a healthy weight. The prospective cohort studies are reviewed and consistently show that higher intakes of whole and minimally processed plant foods (whole plant foods) including whole grains, fruit, vegetables, legumes, and nuts and seeds are associated with reduced CHD risk compared with lower intakes. Chapter 12 contains 12 important tables and figures and over 150 references.

There are strong links between hypertension (elevated blood pressure [BP]) and subsequent CHD that may be the result of high cholesterol levels seen in both conditions. Moreover, both conditions are also found in patients with excess body weight. Overweight and obesity are associated with increased activity of the renin-angiotensin-aldosterone system, insulin resistance, and reduced kidney function associated with salt-sensitive hypertension. Rates of hypertension are twice as likely to occur in obese (40%) vs. normal weight (20%) individuals. Chapter 13 looks at the data related to dietary patterns and hypertension and includes 12 tables and figures as well as 77 references. The major factors associated with elevated BP are aging, especially unhealthy aging associated with overweight and obesity, poor dietary habits, inactivity or lack of exercise, and ineffective stress management. Adherence to healthy dietary patterns, including the Dietary Approaches to Stop Hypertension (DASH), the Mediterranean (MedDiet), Nordic Diet, dietary guidelines-based, and vegetarian diets, is an effective strategy to help prevent elevated BP and important adjuncts in the treatment of hypertensive populations. Chapter 14 looks at the role of whole plant foods in controlling hypertension. The chapter examines foods and dietary constituents associated with hypertension and foods that are associated with risk reduction. Foods that are low in fiber density and high in energy density and contain a higher ratio of sodium to potassium, and have high saturated fat to polyunsaturated fat ratios are associated with increased prevalence of hypertension and prehypertension. In contrast, whole plant foods and minimally processed foods contain higher concentrations of fiber, potassium, magnesium, carotenoids, polyphenols, unsaturated fat, and plant proteins and are lower in sodium and sugar compared to highly processed plant foods; these food components are associated with normal blood pressures in older individuals as well as modestly reducing elevated blood pressures. The data are compiled in 11 tables and figures and the chapter includes over 130 references.

Hypertension and obesity are major risk factors for chronic kidney disease (CKD) that is discussed in Chap. 15. The chapter concentrates on patients with CKD and its stages and reviews the literature concerning the dietary patterns, foods, beverages, and specific nutrient needs of CKD patients including low phosphorus intakes. Relevant topics reviewed with regard to clinical data available include protein sources, fibers especially from whole grains and fruits and vegetables, minerals including sodium, phosphorous, and magnesium, and beverage data from studies on sugar-sweetened versus artificially sweetened sodas, alcohol, and coffee consumption.

The next two chapters concentrate on stroke risk. Strokes are caused by a disruption of the blood supply to the brain due to either vessel blockage as seen in almost 90% of strokes that are defined as ischemic strokes or rupture of a blood vessel that results in a hemorrhagic stroke. With regard to clinical data, most are based on findings from studies involving patients with ischemic stroke. Chapter 16 examines the dietary patterns associated with increasing the risk of stroke as well as the patterns associated with reducing its risk. Stroke risk is linked to poor diet, low physical activity, smoking, high systolic blood pressure, high body mass index and obesity, high fasting plasma glucose, and above normal total cholesterol. The chapter examines the data linking the American Heart Association's "Life's Simple 7" plan for ideal cardiovascular health and lower stroke risk that includes (1) nonsmoking or quit >1 year ago; (2) BMI < 25; (3) blood pressure (BP) <120/80 mmHg; (4) ≥ 150 min/week of physical activity; (5) healthy dietary pattern (high in fruits and vegetables, fish, fiber-rich whole grains), (6) low intake of sodium, and (7) limiting or avoiding sugar-sweetened beverages, and reduced risk of stroke seen in clinical studies. Specific healthy dietary patterns are also reviewed and findings are presented in 11 informative tables and figures; 75 references are included in this chapter. Chapter 17, with over 100 references, looks at the role of whole plant foods in reducing the risk of stroke. Whole plant foods contain a variety of macro- and micronutrients and phytochemicals including fibers, antioxidant vitamins, potassium, magnesium, carotenoids, flavonoids, and phytosterols that have been associated with reducing stroke risk in prospective as well as intervention studies that are reviewed and presented in 11 tables and figures. The mechanisms that have been postulated to reduce stroke risk include promoting vascular health by attenuating elevated blood pressure, lowering LDL-cholesterol levels and systemic inflammation associated with atherosclerosis, and promoting better insulin sensitivity, blood glucose control, weight control, and microbiota health compared to less healthy or highly processed plant foods.

Chapter 18 reviews the studies that have included dietary patterns, whole foods, and beverages and the risk of cognitive impairments including dementia and provides over 100 references and 14 tables and figures. The chapter includes data from systematic reviews, randomized, placebo-controlled trials, and prospective cohort studies that support the benefits of high polyphenolic fruits and vegetables, dairy (especially yogurt), 100% vegetable and fruit juices (polyphenol rich), coffee, tea, flavanol-rich cocoa beverages, and low-moderate wine consumption (1 glass/day) on improving age-related cognitive performance and reducing risk of dementia. In addition to diet, exercise is also linked to reduced risk of cognitive dysfunction as well as Alzheimer's disease; inversely, sedentary lifestyle and poor nutrient diets are associated with increased risk of cognitive decline and Alzheimer's disease.

Part V: Cancer Prevention and Survival

Chapters 19 and 20 provide objective, up-to-date reviews of the associations between dietary patterns, whole plant foods, and the nutrients and phytochemicals contained within these foods, on the risks associated with the development of precancerous colon adenomas and/or colorectal cancer (Chap. 19), and breast cancer (Chap. 20). The dietary risk factors for colorectal cancer reviewed in Chap. 19 include higher than recommended intakes of alcohol, total dietary fat, and red meat and lower intakes of dietary fiber, calcium and folate, isoflavones, flavonoids, antioxidant vitamins, carotenoids, magnesium, and selenium. The chapter examines the mechanisms by which soluble fibers may lower colorectal cancer risk including the ability of fermentable fiber to lower colonic pH and inhibit pathogenic bacteria, increase butyrogenic bacteria to promote healthy colonic mucosal cells, reduce colon inflammation, and inhibit cancer cell proliferation and facilitate apoptosis. Insoluble fiber may reduce the colon's exposure to carcinogens by bulking stools and binding carcinogens. The chapter, containing over 100 important references, tabulates the convincing evidence that higher intakes of calcium and fiber-rich foods reduce colorectal cancer risk and that lower intakes are associated with an increased risk of colorectal cancer. Data are organized in 14 informative tables and figures.

Chapter 20 looks at the studies linking dietary patterns and foods with breast cancer (BC) risk. Both positive and negative studies are included and tabulated in 23 relevant tables and figures. The chapter, with more than 130 references, examines the types of breast cancer and the genetics behind these differences, clinical studies on breast cancer primary prevention as well as secondary prevention of recurrence, and importantly, dietary management for the breast cancer patient. Dietary patterns associated with lower BC risk include diets with 45–65% energy from fiber-rich sources including whole grains, fruits, vegetables, and legumes; 10–35% energy from healthy dietary fats low in saturated fats; and 10–35% energy from protein sources which are very low or devoid of processed meats. Unhealthy dietary patterns and obesity, especially among postmenopausal women, are associated with negative changes in biomarkers such as insulin, lipoproteins, and estradiol, which are risk factors for BC. Biological mechanisms associated with dietary intake and increased risk of BC and breast cancer recurrence include exposure to heterocyclic amines, lipid peroxidation and systemic inflammation, and other causes of oxidative stress and low antioxidant status. These factors are reviewed as well as lifestyle indicators that are associated with increased breast cancer risk, recurrence, and mortality.

Conclusions

Of importance to physicians, nutritionists, dieticians, researchers, nurses, and allied health professionals who provide advice concerning diet, foods, nutrition, and clinical management of nutritionally related conditions and/or diseases is the identification of reputable sources of nutrition information. **"Dietary Patterns and Whole Plant Foods in Aging and Disease"** provides 20 valuable chapters that review and integrate these relevant and objective resources. The volume examines the major dietary patterns that have been identified as containing the components of a healthy diet and contrasts these with dietary patterns, such as Western diets and other patterns that are considered as unhealthy based upon a totality of the epidemiological evidence available to date. Moreover, the volume includes extensive reviews of the whole plant foods associated with the healthy dietary patterns, and each chapter contains detailed analyses of the nutrients and bioactive molecules contained within these foods.

This comprehensive volume examines patient-related topics including chapters on the major changes in lifestyle and dietary patterns, and organ functions during the aging process and the potential for whole plant foods to help reduce certain of the health risks associated with aging. Topics included in this comprehensive volume include the aging effects on the gastrointestinal tract including laxation and constipation and diseases of the colon including irritable bowel syndrome and diverticular disease and cancer. Weight management during aging often includes dealing with being overweight or obese and the resulting diabetes, heart, liver, and kidney diseases are reviewed in depth. The potential for dietary patterns to reduce the risks of cognitive decline and Alzheimer's disease is examined and studies are tabulated. Two cancers relevant to aging and dietary choices are reviewed in depth in individual chapters on breast and colon cancer.

The volume contains over 300 data-rich tables and figures and appendices as well as more than 2200 up-to-date references that give physicians and health providers important tools that can help to alter patient dietary habits that may be less than ideal, and chapters also review the many types of whole plant foods that may enhance their patients' and clients' diets and health. Patients and consumers are concerned about many claims that are made for common nutrients and fibers found in foods, such as juice drinks, soy products, novel fruits, and organically grown vegetables. The chapters in this volume examine these and other provocative areas of diet information. There are more than a dozen chapters that provide clinically relevant information on risk reduction of the major chronic diseases associated with the aging process. The 20 chapters within this valuable volume provide a wealth of timely information for health providers, medical students, graduate students, nurses, dietitians, and other related health professionals.

Dr. Mark L. Dreher is an internationally recognized leader in the field of human nutrition with more than 30 years of research in the importance of whole food intake for the reduction in risk of obesity and other critical clinical outcomes reviewed in this comprehensive volume. Dr. Dreher is a proven excellent communicator and has worked tirelessly to develop this volume that is destined to be the benchmark in the field of clinical nutrition because of its extensive coverage of the most important aspects of the complex interactions between diet, foods, nutrients, bioactive food components, and health and disease. Hallmarks of all of the chapters include complete definitions of terms with the abbreviations fully defined for the reader and consistent use of terms between chapters. Useful features of this comprehensive volume include the informative Key Points and Keywords that are at the beginning of each chapter and relevant references at the end of each chapter.

In conclusion, **"Dietary Patterns and Whole Plant Foods in Aging and Disease," edited as well as written by Mark L. Dreher, Ph.D.,** provides health professionals in many areas of research and practice with the most up-to-date, organized volume on the clinically researched and documented healthy dietary patterns that are linked to reducing the risks of the major chronic diseases associated with the aging process. Of great importance, these are also the major chronic diseases that are often discussed by patients with their healthcare providers. Thus, the data provided in this book enables the reader to answer their patient or client questions with the confidence that their answers are based upon the totality of the evidence from well-accepted, data-driven nutrition research. This volume serves the reader as the benchmark in this complex area of interrelationships between the major dietary patterns that have been associated with reducing the age-related risks of unhealthy body weight, type 2 diabetes, cancer, cardiovascular and cerebrovascular disease, diseases of the gastrointestinal tract, liver, and kidney, and reduced brain function. Dr. Dreher is applauded for his efforts to develop this volume with the firm conviction that nutrition research serves as an essential source of important data for all health professionals. This excellent text is a very welcome addition to the Nutrition and Health series.

Morristown, NJ Adrianne Bendich, Ph.D., FACN, FASN

About the Series Editors

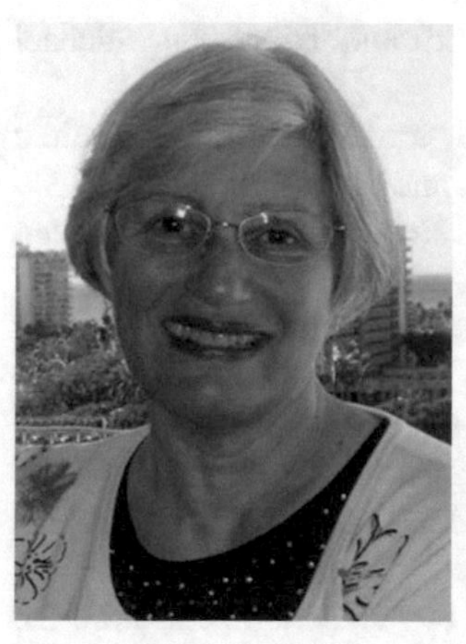

Adrianne Bendich, Ph.D., F.A.S.N., F.A.C.N., has served as the **"Nutrition and Health" Series Editor** for more than 20 years and has provided leadership and guidance to more than 200 editors that have developed the 80+ well-respected and highly recommended volumes in the series.

In addition to **"Dietary Patterns and Whole Plant Foods in Aging and Disease," edited as well as written by Mark L. Dreher, Ph.D.,** major new editions published in 2012–2017 include the following:

1. **Dietary Fiber in Health and Disease,** edited as well as written by Mark L. Dreher, Ph.D., 2017
2. **Clinical Aspects of Natural and Added Phosphorus in Foods**, edited by Orlando M. Gutierrez, Kamyar Kalantar-Zadeh, and Rajnish Mehrotra, 2017
3. **Nutrition and Fetal Programming**, edited by Rajendram Rajkumar, Victor R. Preedy, and Vinood B. Patel, 2017
4. **Nutrition and Diet in Maternal Diabetes**, edited by Rajendram Rajkumar, Victor R. Preedy, and Vinood B. Patel, 2017
5. **Nitrite and Nitrate in Human Health and Disease, Second Edition**, edited by Nathan S. Bryan and Joseph Loscalzo, 2017
6. **Nutrition in Lifestyle Medicine**, edited by James M. Rippe, 2017
7. **Nutrition Guide for Physicians and Related Healthcare Professionals, Second Edition**, edited by Norman J. Temple, Ted Wilson, and George A. Bray, 2016
8. **Clinical Aspects of Natural and Added Phosphorus in Foods**, edited by Orlando M. Gutiérrez, Kamyar Kalantar-Zadeh, and Rajnish Mehrotra, 2016
9. **L-Arginine in Clinical Nutrition**, edited by Vinood B. Patel, Victor R. Preedy, and Rajkumar Rajendram, 2016

10. **Mediterranean Diet: Impact on Health and Disease**, edited by Donato F. Romagnolo, Ph.D. and Ornella Selmin, Ph.D., 2016
11. **Nutrition Support for the Critically Ill**, edited by David S. Seres, MD, and Charles W. Van Way, III, MD, 2016
12. **Nutrition in Cystic Fibrosis: A Guide for Clinicians,** edited by Elizabeth H. Yen, M.D., and Amanda R. Leonard, MPH, RD, CDE, 2016
13. **Preventive Nutrition: The Comprehensive Guide For Health Professionals, Fifth Edition,** edited by Adrianne Bendich, Ph.D., and Richard J. Deckelbaum, M.D., 2016
14. **Glutamine in Clinical Nutrition,** edited by Rajkumar Rajendram, Victor R. Preedy, and Vinood B. Patel, 2015
15. **Nutrition and Bone Health, Second Edition,** edited by Michael F. Holick and Jeri W. Nieves, 2015
16. **Branched Chain Amino Acids in Clinical Nutrition, Volume 2,** edited by Rajkumar Rajendram, Victor R. Preedy, and Vinood B. Patel, 2015
17. **Branched Chain Amino Acids in Clinical Nutrition, Volume 1,** edited by Rajkumar Rajendram, Victor R. Preedy, and Vinood B. Patel, 2015
18. **Fructose, High Fructose Corn Syrup, Sucrose and Health,** edited by James M. Rippe, 2014
19. **Handbook of Clinical Nutrition and Aging, Third Edition,** edited by Connie Watkins Bales, Julie L. Locher, and Edward Saltzman, 2014
20. **Nutrition and Pediatric Pulmonary Disease,** edited by Dr. Youngran Chung and Dr. Robert Dumont, 2014
21. **Integrative Weight Management**, edited by Dr. Gerald E. Mullin, Dr. Lawrence J. Cheskin, and Dr. Laura E. Matarese, 2014
22. **Nutrition in Kidney Disease, Second Edition**, edited by Dr. Laura D. Byham-Gray, Dr. Jerrilynn D. Burrowes, and Dr. Glenn M. Chertow, 2014
23. **Handbook of Food Fortification and Health, Volume I**, edited by Dr. Victor R. Preedy, Dr. Rajaventhan Srirajaskanthan, and Dr. Vinood B. Patel, 2013
24. **Handbook of Food Fortification and Health, Volume II**, edited by Dr. Victor R. Preedy, Dr. Rajaventhan Srirajaskanthan, and Dr. Vinood B. Patel, 2013
25. **Diet Quality: An Evidence-Based Approach, Volume I**, edited by Dr. Victor R. Preedy, Dr. Lan-Ahn Hunter, and Dr. Vinood B. Patel, 2013
26. **Diet Quality: An Evidence-Based Approach, Volume II**, edited by Dr. Victor R. Preedy, Dr. Lan-Ahn Hunter, and Dr. Vinood B. Patel, 2013
27. **The Handbook of Clinical Nutrition and Stroke,** edited by Mandy L. Corrigan, MPH, RD, Arlene A. Escuro, MS, RD, and Donald F. Kirby, MD, FACP, FACN, FACG, 2013
28. **Nutrition in Infancy, Volume I**, edited by Dr. Ronald Ross Watson, Dr. George Grimble, Dr. Victor Preedy, and Dr. Sherma Zibadi, 2013
29. **Nutrition in Infancy, Volume II**, edited by Dr. Ronald Ross Watson, Dr. George Grimble, Dr. Victor Preedy, and Dr. Sherma Zibadi, 2013
30. **Carotenoids and Human Health**, edited by Dr. Sherry A. Tanumihardjo, 2013

31. **Bioactive Dietary Factors and Plant Extracts in Dermatology**, edited by Dr. Ronald Ross Watson and Dr. Sherma Zibadi, 2013
32. **Omega 6/3 Fatty Acids**, edited by Dr. Fabien De Meester, Dr. Ronald Ross Watson, and Dr. Sherma Zibadi, 2013
33. **Nutrition in Pediatric Pulmonary Disease,** edited by Dr. Robert Dumont and Dr. Youngran Chung, 2013
34. **Nutrition and Diet in Menopause,** edited by Dr. Caroline J. Hollins Martin, Dr. Ronald Ross Watson, and Dr. Victor R. Preedy, 2013.
35. **Magnesium and Health**, edited by Dr. Ronald Ross Watson and Dr. Victor R. Preedy, 2012.
36. **Alcohol, Nutrition and Health Consequences**, edited by Dr. Ronald Ross Watson, Dr. Victor R. Preedy, and Dr. Sherma Zibadi, 2012
37. **Nutritional Health, Strategies for Disease Prevention, Third Edition**, edited by Norman J. Temple, Ted Wilson, and David R. Jacobs, Jr., 2012
38. **Chocolate in Health and Nutrition**, edited by Dr. Ronald Ross Watson, Dr. Victor R. Preedy, and Dr. Sherma Zibadi, 2012
39. **Iron Physiology and Pathophysiology in Humans**, edited by Dr. Gregory J. Anderson and Dr. Gordon D. McLaren, 2012

Earlier books included **Vitamin D, Second Edition**, edited by Dr. Michael Holick; "**Dietary Components and Immune Function**" edited by Dr. Ronald Ross Watson, Dr. Sherma Zibadi, and Dr. Victor R. Preedy; "**Bioactive Compounds and Cancer**" edited by Dr. John A. Milner and Dr. Donato F. Romagnolo; "**Modern Dietary Fat Intakes in Disease Promotion**" edited by Dr. Fabien De Meester, Dr. Sherma Zibadi, and Dr. Ronald Ross Watson; "**Iron Deficiency and Overload**" edited by Dr. Shlomo Yehuda and Dr. David Mostofsky; "**Nutrition Guide for Physicians**" edited by Dr. Edward Wilson, Dr. George A. Bray, Dr. Norman Temple, and Dr. Mary Struble; "**Nutrition and Metabolism"** edited by Dr. Christos Mantzoros; and "**Fluid and Electrolytes in Pediatrics**" edited by Leonard Feld and Dr. Frederick Kaskel. Recent volumes include "**Handbook of Drug-Nutrient Interactions**" edited by Dr. Joseph Boullata and Dr. Vincent Armenti; "**Probiotics in Pediatric Medicine**" edited by Dr. Sonia Michail and Dr. Philip Sherman; "**Handbook of Nutrition and Pregnancy**" edited by Dr. Carol Lammi-Keefe, Dr. Sarah Couch, and Dr. Elliot Philipson; "**Nutrition and Rheumatic Disease**" edited by Dr. Laura Coleman; "**Nutrition and Kidney Disease**" edited by Dr. Laura Byham-Grey, Dr. Jerrilynn Burrowes, and Dr. Glenn Chertow; "**Nutrition and Health in Developing Countries**" edited by Dr. Richard Semba and Dr. Martin Bloem; "**Calcium in Human Health**" edited by Dr. Robert Heaney and Dr. Connie Weaver; and "**Nutrition and Bone Health**" edited by Dr. Michael Holick and Dr. Bess Dawson-Hughes.

Dr. Bendich is President of Consultants in Consumer Healthcare, LLC, and is the editor of ten books including "**Preventive Nutrition: The Comprehensive Guide for Health Professionals, Fifth Edition**," co-edited with Dr. Richard Deckelbaum (www.springer.com/series/7659). Dr. Bendich serves on the Editorial Boards of the *Journal of Nutrition in Gerontology and*

Geriatrics and *Antioxidants* and has served as Associate Editor for *Nutrition*, the International Journal; served on the Editorial Board of the *Journal of Women's Health and Gender-Based Medicine*; and served on the Board of Directors of the American College of Nutrition.

Dr. Bendich was Director of Medical Affairs at GlaxoSmithKline (GSK) Consumer Healthcare and provided medical leadership for many well-known brands including TUMS and Os-Cal. Dr. Bendich had primary responsibility for GSK's support for the Women's Health Initiative (WHI) intervention study. Prior to joining GSK, Dr. Bendich was at Roche Vitamins Inc. and was involved with the groundbreaking clinical studies showing that folic acid-containing multivitamins significantly reduced major classes of birth defects. Dr. Bendich has coauthored over 100 major clinical research studies in the area of preventive nutrition. She is recognized as a leading authority on antioxidants, nutrition and immunity and pregnancy outcomes, vitamin safety, and the cost-effectiveness of vitamin/mineral supplementation.

Dr. Bendich received the Roche Research Award, is a *Tribute to Women and Industry* Awardee, and was a recipient of the Burroughs Wellcome Visiting Professorship in Basic Medical Sciences. Dr. Bendich was given the Council for Responsible Nutrition (CRN) Apple Award in recognition of her many contributions to the scientific understanding of dietary supplements. In 2012, she was recognized for her contributions to the field of clinical nutrition by the American Society for Nutrition and was elected a Fellow of ASN. Dr. Bendich is Adjunct Professor at Rutgers University. She is listed in Who's Who in American Women.

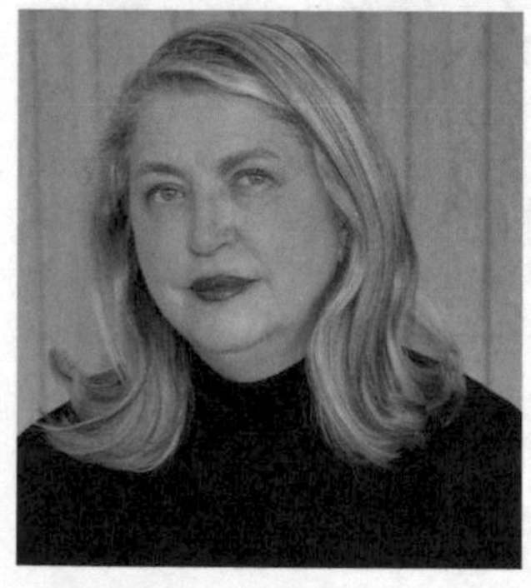

Connie W. Bales, Ph.D., R.D., is a Professor of Medicine in the Division of Geriatrics, Department of Medicine, at the Duke School of Medicine and Senior Fellow in the Center for the Study of Aging and Human Development at Duke University Medical Center. She is also Associate Director for Education/Evaluation of the Geriatrics Research, Education, and Clinical Center at the Durham VA Medical Center. Dr. Bales is a well-recognized expert in the field of nutrition, chronic disease, function, and aging. Over the past two decades, her laboratory at Duke has explored many different aspects of diet and activity as determinants of health during the latter half of the adult life course. Her current research focuses primarily on enhanced protein as a means of benefiting muscle quality, function, and other health indicators during geriatric obesity reduction and for improving perioperative outcomes in older patients. Dr. Bales has served on NIH and USDA grant review panels and is Past-Chair of the Medical Nutrition Council of the American Society for Nutrition. She has edited three editions of the *Handbook of Clinical Nutrition and Aging*, is Editor-in-Chief of the *Journal of Nutrition in Gerontology and Geriatrics*, and is a Deputy Editor of *Current Developments in Nutrition*.

Authors' Biography

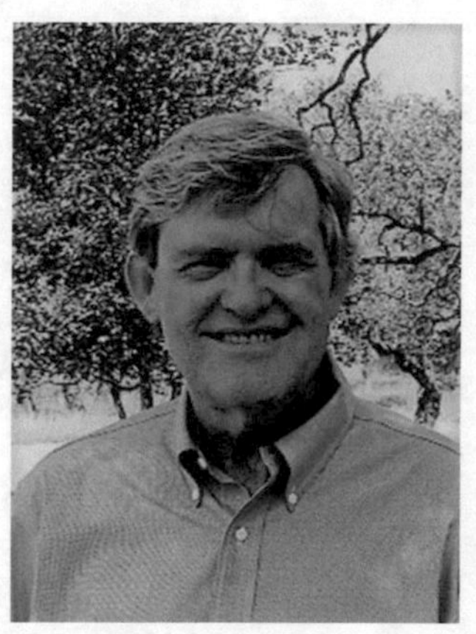

Mark L. Dreher, Ph.D., is president and chief science officer of Nutrition Science Solutions, LLC. He received his education in biochemistry and agricultural biochemistry and nutrition at UCLA and the University of Arizona. Dr. Dreher started his career as a research scientist in medical food product development at McGaw Laboratories in Irvine, California. Later, he served as assistant professor in food and nutrition at North Dakota State University, leading research on sunflower seeds, dry edible beans, and emerging grains. During his subsequent 30-plus-year career in the food, agricultural, and pharmaceutical industries, he held key roles in over 150 new healthy product development projects and food-based clinical research trials. He has authored or coauthored over 50 research journal articles and book chapters. Dr. Dreher has authored or coauthored two handbooks on dietary fiber, one book on complex carbohydrates and the 2017 Dietary Fiber in Health and Disease book. He served as the chair of the International Life Sciences Institute—North American Food, Nutrition and Safety, and Carbohydrate Committees—and vice chair of the Functional Foods for Health Committee. Dr. Dreher was a member of the 1997 Joint FAO/WHO Expert Consultation on Carbohydrate and Human Nutrition. He was a fellow in the National Center for Food and Agricultural Policy and Resources for the Future Leadership Program in Washington, DC. Dr. Dreher is involved in the American Society for Nutrition, American Heart Association, Academy of Nutrition and Dietetics, UK Nutrition Society, Institute of Food Technologists. American Chemical Society and the American Association for the Advancement of Science. Dr. Dreher is actively engaged in projects and research related to the role of healthy diets, whole foods, and phytochemicals in health, chronic disease prevention, and optimal aging.

Acknowledgments

I am profoundly appreciative to the hundreds of investigators who have studied and published on the effects of dietary patterns and whole plant foods in aging and chronic disease which made this book possible.

I want to thank Dr. Adrianne Bendich, editor of **Preventative Nutrition: The Comprehensive Guide for Health Professionals**, for her support, and critical guidance and insights that inspired me at each phase of this book project.

Finally, I am indebted to my wife Claudia, who provided love and support, constructive criticism and insights, and for space and time that was essential for completing this book.

Contents

Part I Overview of Aging and Disease

1 Major Lifestyles and Phenotypes in Aging and Disease 3

2 Dietary Patterns in Aging and Disease 29

3 Whole Plant Foods in Aging and Disease 59

Part II Gastrointestinal Tract

4 Fiber-Rich Dietary Patterns and Colonic Microbiota in Aging and Disease 119

5 Fiber-Rich Dietary Patterns and Foods in Laxation and Constipation 145

6 Dietary Patterns, Foods and Fiber in Irritable Bowel Syndrome and Diverticular Disease 165

Part III Weight Management and Related Diseases

7 Dietary Patterns and Fiber in Body Weight and Composition Regulation 195

8 Whole Plant Foods in Body Weight and Composition Regulation 233

9 Dietary Patterns and Whole Plant Foods in Type 2 Diabetes Prevention and Management 257

10 Dietary Patterns, Foods, Nutrients and Phytochemicals in Non-Alcoholic Fatty Liver Disease 291

Part IV Cardiovascular and Cerebrovascular Diseases, and Age-Related Cognitive Function

11 Dietary Patterns and Coronary Heart Disease............. 315

12 Whole Plant Foods and Coronary Heart Disease 337

13 **Dietary Patterns and Hypertension** 371

14 **Whole Plant Foods and Hypertension** 391

15 **Dietary Patterns, Foods and Beverages in Chronic Kidney Disease** 417

16 **Dietary Patterns and Stroke Risk** 435

17 **Whole Plant Foods and Stroke Risk** 451

18 **Dietary Patterns, Foods and Beverages in Age-Related Cognitive Performance and Dementia** 471

Part V Cancer Prevention and Survival

19 **Dietary Patterns, Whole Plant Foods, Nutrients and Phytochemicals in Colorectal Cancer Prevention and Management** 521

20 **Dietary Patterns, Whole Plant Foods, Nutrients and Phytochemicals in Breast Cancer Prevention and Management** 557

Index 611

Part I

Overview of Aging and Disease

1 Major Lifestyles and Phenotypes in Aging and Disease

Keywords
Healthy aging • Mortality • Healthy dietary patterns • Western diet • Obesity • Body mass index • Central obesity • Physical activity • Metabolic syndrome • Type 2 diabetes • Prediabetes • Sarcopenia

Key Points

- Since an estimated 70 to 80% of the rate of aging is related to lifestyle choices, it is possible for individuals to significantly influence their odds of healthy aging and longevity, even if healthy lifestyles are adopted later in life.
- Unhealthy or premature aging, which is largely associated with excessive intake of Western energy dense diets and sedentary lifestyles, involves a complex interplay between obesity and related metabolic dysfunctional effects leading to increased risk of chronic disease and mortality, and reduced healthy life expectancy.
- In general, obesity, especially central adiposity, represents a state of accelerated aging as adipose cells produce adipokines, which can lead to increased systemic and tissue inflammation and peripheral insulin resistance.
- Metabolic syndrome, type 2 diabetes and prediabetes, and sarcopenia are major unhealthy aging phenotypes, which can be prevented by appropriate lifestyle choices.
- The concept of healthy aging includes healthy life expectancy (e.g., absence or delay of chronic diseases and the maintenance of cognitive, physical, and other functions with limited dependence on family members or extended care assistant living) and longevity. Since a higher percentage of people worldwide are surviving to older ages, it is critical to promote optimal healthy aging lifestyle habits to assure quality of life for aging individuals and their families, and for sustainable healthcare cost management.
- The probability of healthy aging can be significantly increased by up to 80% by following a healthy lifestyle even if it is adopted in middle age adulthood or older. These lifestyle choices include: adhering to a healthy dietary pattern, increasing physical activity most days of the week, achieving and maintaining a healthy body weight and waist size, and smoking avoidance.

M.L. Dreher, *Dietary Patterns and Whole Plant Foods in Aging and Disease*, Nutrition and Health,
https://doi.org/10.1007/978-3-319-59180-3_1

1.1 Introduction

Aging is the biological progressive deterioration of physiological functions and metabolic processes leading to chronic diseases such as neurodegenerative disorders, cardiovascular disease (CVD), type 2 diabetes (diabetes) and cancer, and ultimately to death [1–3]. Aging is the accumulation of random damage to the body's DNA, structural and regulatory proteins such as hormones and enzymes, or from excessive metabolically dysfunctional adipose tissue, that begins early in life and eventually exceeds the body's self-repair capabilities [2, 3]. This damage gradually impairs the functioning of cells, tissues, organs, and organ systems, thereby increasing the risk of chronic diseases/frailty and quality of life markers of aging, such as loss of muscle and bone mass, a decline in reaction time, and reduced hearing, vision, and skin elasticity. However, aging processes are highly malleable and influenced by lifestyle factors that can improve the odds of healthy aging, even if they are adapted in mid- or older age [2]. Since the rate of aging varies by individual with 20–30% programmed by heredity factors (e.g., rate of cellular senescence), and 70–80% due to external factors such as lifestyle factors and random events, it is possible for individuals to significantly influence their rate of aging [1]. Aging is measured by: (1) chronological age (longevity, life expectancy), the absolute years a person lives and (2) biological age (health span or healthy life expectancy), the healthy quality of the aging process. Common physical and physiological changes associated with aging are summarized in Table 1.1 [1]. An overview of the gradual transition during aging from homeostasis to loss of function due to age-related diseases are presented in Table 1.2 [1–5]. Major biological processes linked to the rate of aging include: elevated oxidative and inflammatory stress, genomic instability, telomere attrition, epigenetic alterations, mitochondrial dysfunction, cellular senescence, stem cell exhaustion, progenitor cell dysfunction, and altered intercellular communication [5].

During the twentieth century, life expectancy at birth increased from 50 years to ≥80 years in countries such as Japan, Western Europe, the USA, Canada, Australia, and New Zealand [2, 6]. Much of the early improved life expectancy was due to reduced childhood mortality and treatments for infectious diseases. Since the mid-twentieth century, life expectancy gains have been due mainly to reduced mortality at birth, childhood and older age, cleaner drinking water, advances in health care (e.g., vaccines, antibiotics, preventive and therapeutic medicines, devices and surgeries), and better hygiene, nutrition, housing and education. With this increased life expectancy, the world population is expected to double from 6 billion people in 2000 to 11.5 billion people by 2100 with increasing aging demographic changes in every region and across most socioeconomic groups [7, 8]. The proportion of the population that is ≥65 years old has been rising and is projected to increase from 8% (550 million people) in 2010 to 21% (>1.5 billion people) by 2050. Increased rates of chronic disease, disability and frailty are common in this age group with unhealthy aging.

There is the potential for a significant global decline in life and healthy life expectancy with a major global health crisis expected by 2040 or sooner, as today's children and young adults develop pandemic rates of obesity, diabetes, chronic liver diseases, and other cardiometabolic diseases that normally occur later in life [1, 6–15]. The US annual rate of increased life expectancy is forecasted to decline by half between 2015 and 2040 [6, 7]. Currently, Americans have shorter and less healthy lives than their peer populations in most other high-income countries with the US ranked 32nd [14]. Worldwide, the primary chronic diseases are CVD (e.g., heart attacks and stroke), cancer, chronic respiratory disease and diabetes, which account for 80% of all chronic disease deaths and disability [11–15].

Ideal healthy life expectancy would be to delay for as long as possible chronic disease and physical or mental disability, which have detrimental effects on individual's and their family's quality of life, and adds burden and

Table 1.1 Common physical and physiological changes occurring during the aging process [1]

Category	Body function	Changes with aging
Physical capability	Strength, locomotion, balance and dexterity	– Physical capability declines progressively in later life with men performing better than women at all ages – Low performance on grip strength, walking speed, chair rise time and standing balance tests are associated with higher mortality rates
Physiological function	Lung function, body composition (including bone mass and skeletal muscle), cardiovascular (CV) function and glucose metabolism	– Beginning at about 25 years of age, forced expiratory volume declines at approximately 32 mL/year in men and 25 mL/year in women – Bone mass declines with age, and bone mass or density predicts risk for future fractures and mortality – Large waist size, greater BMI and weight-gain in middle age are all associated with higher mortality or poor health status – Declining skeletal muscle mass is associated with increased functional impairment and disability (sarcopenia) – Elevated blood pressure and blood lipids are the strongest predictors of CV morbidity and mortality – Diminished glucose homeostasis is associated with raised fasting blood glucose, CV events and mortality
Cognitive function	Memory, processing speed and executive function	– Executive function is affected by aging, with an inverted U-shape pattern across the lifespan – Processing speed declines progressively with age and is associated with greater mortality risk, and cardiovascular and respiratory diseases – Episodic memory is sensitive to brain aging and declines with mild cognitive impairment and neurodegenerative diseases – Higher blood pressure in midlife is associated with cognitive decline in senior years
Endocrine system function	Hypothalamic, pituitary, adrenal axis; thyroid, sex and growth hormones	– Decreases with aging: aldosterone, calcitonin, growth hormone, renin; in women estrogen and prolactin and in men testosterone – The pituitary gland gradually becomes smaller with aging – Thyroid hormone is often reduced especially in women – Increases with aging: follicle-stimulating hormones, luteinizing hormone, norepinephrine, and parathyroid hormone
Immune function	Immunosenescence	Aging is associated with increased systemic inflammatory cytokines (plasma concentrations of IL-6 and TNF-α), which are associated with lower grip strength and gait speed
Sensory function	Hearing, vision, smell, and pain	– Most sensory functions, with the exception of pain, decrease across the lifespan – Sensory changes may overlap with changes in cognitive and motor functions with loss of audition and vision being the most prominent – Smell acuity declines with age, especially in men, and is thought to be an indicator of brain integrity in older people as smell dysfunction is among the earliest signs of neurodegenerative diseases such as Alzheimer's disease and Parkinson's disease, and is associated with mortality

cost to health care systems and long-term care facilities [9, 16]. However, since the 1970s and 1980s, as a result of increased adherence to unhealthy lifestyles leading to excessive energy intake and sedentary habits (positive energy balance), the global obesity pandemic has been a primary cause of a significant reduction in the odds of healthy life expectancy. This global

Table 1.2 Overview of the gradual loss of function and transition to aging related diseases [1–5]

Diminishment of functions: Cardiometabolic dysfunction Extracellular and intracellular damage Oxidative DNA damage Degraded regenerative and cell proliferation ability Decrease or loss of beta-cell function Reduced immune function Increased fibrosis Loss of bone, muscle and physical degradation Age-related cognitive decline Weight and body composition changes Shorter telomeres and epigenetic changes	**Aging biochemical, physiological and pathology transition**	**Age-related diseases:** Atherosclerosis Stroke Cancer Diabetes Macular degeneration Arthritis Osteoporosis Alzheimer's disease Sarcopenia Metabolic syndrome Non-alcoholic fatty liver disease Chronic kidney disease

trend in excessive weight gain, especially when seen as central obesity, has been a major factor in the increased rates of chronic diseases and related disabilities not only just in older adults but also in children and young adults [8–20]. A 2016 systematic review (164 cohort studies; 5 to 36 years of follow-up) found consistent evidence that higher adherence to healthy behaviors such as healthy diets and recommended levels of physical activity were associated with successful aging and reduced disability, dementia and frailty in later life [13]. A Greek study of older adults (2663 adults aged 65–100 years) found an inverse association between high energy intake and successful aging [17]. Adipose cells are not inactive fat storehouses of excessive energy intake, but part of an active endocrine organ that can speed up the aging process [15, 18, 19]. The Merck Manual identified three primary strategies that might help people live healthier and longer lives including: body weight control, energy controlled healthy diets, and exercising most days of the week [20]. The objective of this chapter is to comprehensively review the association of lifestyle factors and related phenotypes on aging, disease and mortality risk.

1.2 Unhealthy Aging

Unhealthy or premature aging, which is largely associated with excessive intake of Western energy dense diets and sedentary lifestyles, involves a complex interplay between obesity and related metabolic dysfunctional adverse effects leading to increased risk of chronic disease and mortality risk, and reduced healthy life expectancy and is especially associated with several specific accelerated aging phenotypes including metabolic syndrome, diabetes and prediabetes, and sarcopenia [1–15].

1.2.1 Obesity

1.2.1.1 Metabolic Dysfunction

Metabolic dysfunction associated with the overweight and obesity pandemic is a major global concern now and if not addressed it will become a major global crisis by 2040 [1, 6–13]. It is estimated that in the US almost 40% of adults and 20% of children are obese [21]. In general, the excessive fat mass associated with obesity leads to a state of accelerated aging as adipose cells produce adipokine cell signaling messengers, such as leptin, adiponectin, IL-6, and TNF-α, which can influence systemic and tissue inflammation, oxidative stress, and insulin resistance [15, 18, 19, 22]. This metabolic stress can lead to cellular and systemic dysregulation associated with increased risk of developing insulin resistance, β-cell dysfunction, diabetes, atherosclerosis, tumorigenesis, or neurodegenerative disorders such as age related cognitive decline or Alzheimer's disease [1, 4, 5, 18, 19, 22]. A French prospective study (2,733 participants; baseline age range 45 to 60 years; 23 years of follow-up) found that increased body mass index (BMI) above normal levels was negatively associated with healthy aging [22]. Compared to normal BMI, individuals with obese BMIs in mid-life had a significantly 32% higher risk of unhealthy aging compared to 9% for those who were overweight at mid-life. Emerging research suggests that increased BMI in the obese range is associated with structural brain changes including reduction in gray matter and white matter alterations of the prefrontal regions, which could increase risk for cognitive decline during aging [23]. Also, several systematic reviews and meta-analyses have concluded that generally all obese individuals are at an increased risk of CVD compared with normal-weight healthy individuals, especially in studies with ≥10 years of follow-up [24–26]. Some studies suggest that there is an intermediate phenotype known as metabolically healthy obese, without metabolic syndrome and the CVD risk typically associated with metabolically unhealthy obese [27]. One potential mechanism associated with the "metabolically healthy obese" phenotype may be a lower fasting respiratory quotient, which may lower the risk of insulin resistance. However, a meta-analysis (8 cohort studies; 61,386 participants; 3988 CVD events) found that overweight and obese metabolically healthy individuals still had a 21–24% increased risk for CVD events compared with metabolically healthy normal-weight individuals [26]. Consequently, most obese individuals appear to be at increased risk for adverse long-term aging health outcomes.

1.2.1.2 All-Cause Mortality Risk

Body Mass Index (BMI)

The effect of BMI on mortality risk has been extensively evaluated in prospective cohort studies. Generally, BMIs at the extremes of underweight or obesity are associated with increased all-cause and disease specific mortality risk, with some variability in older age, ethnicity or timing of the weight gain or loss. A collaborative analysis (57 prospective studies; 894,576 participants; mostly in Western Europe and North America; 61% male; mean recruitment age 46 years; mean BMI 25; mean 13 years of follow-up with first 5 years excluded; 66,552 deaths) found that BMI and all-cause mortality risk followed a U-shaped curve with extreme leanness and obesity associated with increased mortality risk for both genders [28, 29]. Compared to the normal BMI (18.5–24.9), each increased 5 BMI units was on average associated with about 30% higher all-cause mortality with median survival age reduced for stage 1 obesity (BMI 30–34.9) by 2–4 years and stage 2–3 obesity (BMI >35) by 8–10 years. Several other meta-analyses have projected that an increase in 5 BMI units can significantly increase the risk of diabetes during early weight gain by 207% and later weight gain by 112% [30]. Also, an increase in 5 BMI units was associated with a 20% higher risk of prostate cancer death or recurrence by 20% [31]. Another meta-analysis (8 prospective studies published between 1999–2014; 5.8 million participants; 582,000 deaths) found for all-cause mortality rates for normal weight individuals (18.5–24.9 BMI) were higher than those who were overweight (25–29.9 BMI) or grade 1 obesity and as expected the highest significantly increased rates were observed for those with grades 2 and 3 obesity (35–40 plus BMI) [32]. This analysis has been critically reviewed by other investigators who suggest that there are possible methodological confounders in this analysis, especially related to smoking, reverse causation due to existing chronic disease, and non-specific loss of lean mass and function in the frail elderly [18, 32]. A systematic review and meta-analysis (230 cohort studies; 3.74 million deaths among 30.3 million participants) found a 15% increase in all-cause mortality for each 5-unit increase in BMI among never smokers [33]. Overall this analysis of cohort studies showed that both overweight and obesity increase the risk of all-cause mortality with a J shaped dose-response relation with the lowest risk at 23–24 BMI range among never smokers. The 2016 pooled analysis of the Nurses' Health Study (1980–2012) and Health Professionals Follow-up Study (1986–2012) (74,582 women and 39,284 men; up to 32 years of follow-up) found a U-shaped relation between BMI and premature mortality with the lowest all-cause mortality risk between a BMI of

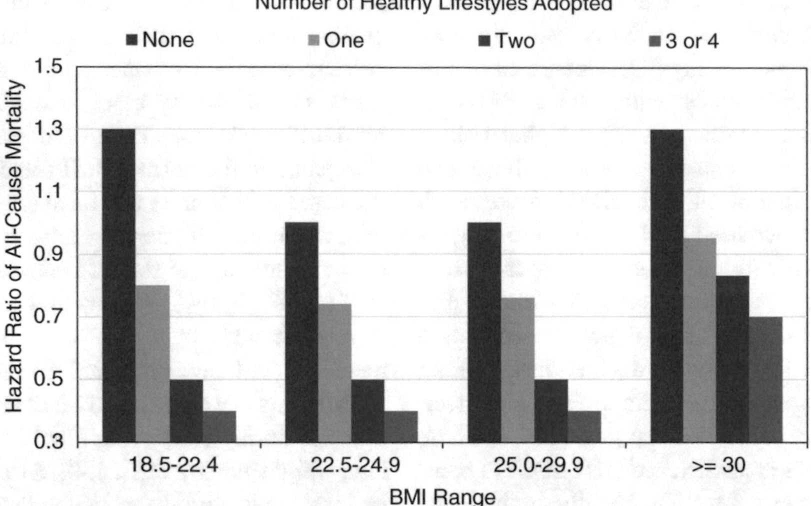

Fig. 1.1 Risk of all-cause mortality as a function of combined body mass index (BMI) and number of healthy lifestyle factors* from the pooled data of the Nurses' Health Study (1980–2012) and Health Professionals Follow-up Study (1986–2012) (adapted from [34]). *No smoking, exercise ≥30 min/day at moderate or vigorous intensity, healthy diet index, and low to moderate alcohol intake (5-15 g in women and 5–30 g in men)

22.5–27.4 [34]. The higher the number of low risk lifestyle behaviors adapted the greater the reduction of mortality risk across the BMI range (Fig. 1.1) [34]. This analysis found that those who were underweight or obese in mid-life had an increased risk of premature death over 10 to 30 years of follow-up. A 2014 meta-analysis of older adults (32 studies; 197,940 subjects; baseline age ≥ 65 years; average 12-year follow-up) demonstrated a U-shape curve for the effect of BMI on all-cause mortality risk with a relatively broad lower risk base of 24–30 BMI with the lowest risk between a BMI of 27.0–27.9 [35]. Also, BMIs of ≤20 had at least a 28% greater mortality risk than those at the reference BMI of 23.0–23.9. A 2017 UK cohort study (130,473 participants; mean baseline age 64 years and BMI 27; 52% women; mean follow-up 6.5 years) found that non-smokers with increased central adiposity and normal or overweight BMIs had an increased in mortality risk of 33% and 41%, respectively [36]. This study suggests that the paradoxical increase mortality risk in normal BMI participants later in life compared to overweight or moderately obese BMI participants observed in some studies may be largely attributed to increased central adiposity, which is not measured by BMI and not a result of some protective physiological benefit of higher body fat.

1.2.1.3 Body Composition

BMI can only estimate body composition and does not accurately reflect central abdominal fat mass or fat-free mass, which includes skeletal muscle mass [35, 36]. A high BMI reflects high fat free mass and fat mass in women but only high fat mass in men. Additionally, body composition and central obesity may affect mortality risk independently of BMI [19]. A loss of fat free mass significantly increases the risk of mortality in adults ≥65 years by 102% with greater effects in men than women [37]. The Women's Health Initiative (10,525 postmenopausal women; age 50–79 years; 13.6 years of follow-up) observed that evaluating body composition provides a more robust assessment of mortality risk among postmenopausal women than BMI [38]. Specifically, among women 50–59 years, higher fat mass increased risk of death by 144% and higher lean body mass reduced the risk of death by 59%, whereas this relationship begins

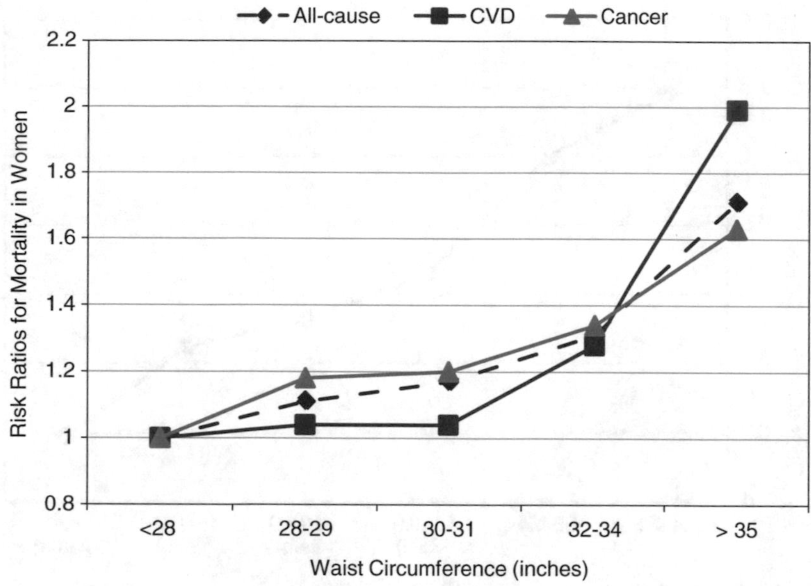

Fig. 1.2 Association between increasing waist circumference and mortality risk in women from the Nurses' Health Study (p-trend <0.001 for all; multivariate adjusted) (adapted from [39])

to be reversed in women >70 years with higher fat mass lowering mortality risk. The Nurses' Health Study (44,000 women; mean age 52 years; 16 years of follow-up; 3507 deaths) found that higher abdominal adiposity (waist circumference) was strongly and positively associated with all-cause, CVD, and cancer mortality independently of BMI (Fig. 1.2) [39]. Additionally, central obesity was a better indicator than BMI of increased risk of nonalcoholic fatty liver disease [40], aortic stiffness [41] and atrial fibrillation [42].

1.2.2 Unhealthy Life Expectancy

Elevated BMI or excessive abdominal fat during early and middle adulthood increases the odds of unhealthy life expectations with significant limitations or disability in older ages. The Nurses' Health Study (17,065 women who survived until at least the age of 70) found that weight gain after age 18 years, especially in early adulthood and middle age, was significantly associated with a linearly decreased probability of healthy survival at age ≥ 70, as defined by an absence of major chronic diseases and physical, cognitive, and mental limitations (Fig. 1.3) [43]. The Osteoarthritis Initiative study (2378 participants; mean age 68 years; 62% women; 6-year follow-up) observed that obese participants had worse physical activity scores, lower quality of life, and higher risk of disability than those who were overweight or normal weight [44]. A Finnish prospective study (6542 middle-aged Helsinki city employees; mean age 50 years; 32% of women and 46% of men were overweight and 15% of both women and men were obese; mean follow-up of 7.8 years) observed that obese employees had a significantly elevated risk for disability at retirement, especially for musculoskeletal causes of lowered physical functioning (Fig. 1.4) [45]. The Women's Health Initiative study (36,611 participants; mean age 72 years; follow-up 14–19 years) observed a significant increased risk of mobility disability in overweight women by 60% and obese women by 220–570% compared to normal weight women [46]. Other studies in adults age ≥ 60 years show that elevated waist circumference is associated with lower quality of life and a decline in

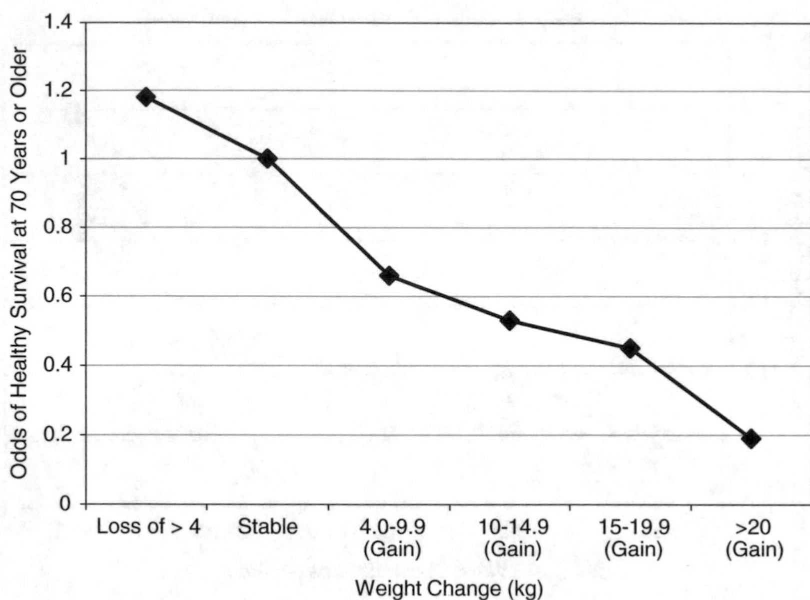

Fig. 1.3 Odds of healthy survival at age 70 years or older associated with weight change since age 18 years from the Nurses' Health Study (p-trend <0.001) (adapted from [43])

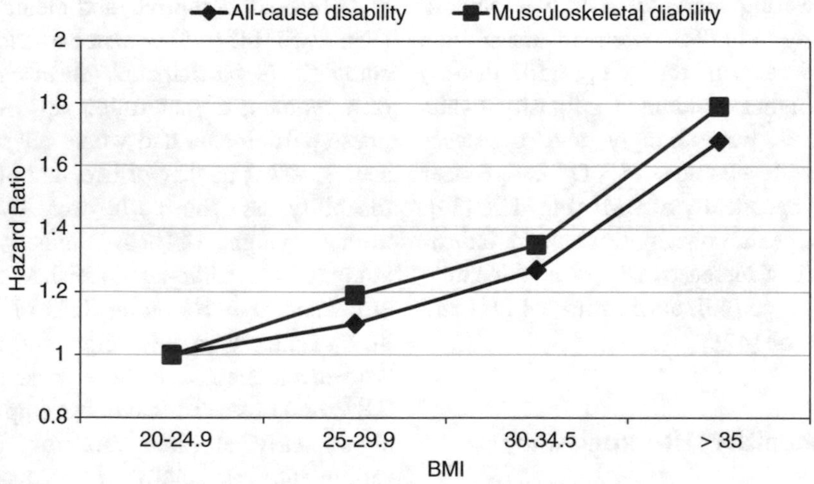

Fig. 1.4 Association between BMI and odds of disability at retirement (p-trend <0.01; multivariate adjusted) (adapted from [45])

physical function [47] and weight loss is associated with improved mobility [48]. Although obesity is associated with significant functional limitations in older adults, there have been concerns that weight loss diets could diminish muscle mass along with fat mass to increase frailty complications [49]. A randomized controlled trial (RCT) [67 obese adults; mean BMI 37; mean age 68 years; traditional vs. high protein (30 g per meal) weight loss regimen; 6-months] showed that both diets significantly reduced weight, but the protein group also significantly improved physical function by over twofold.

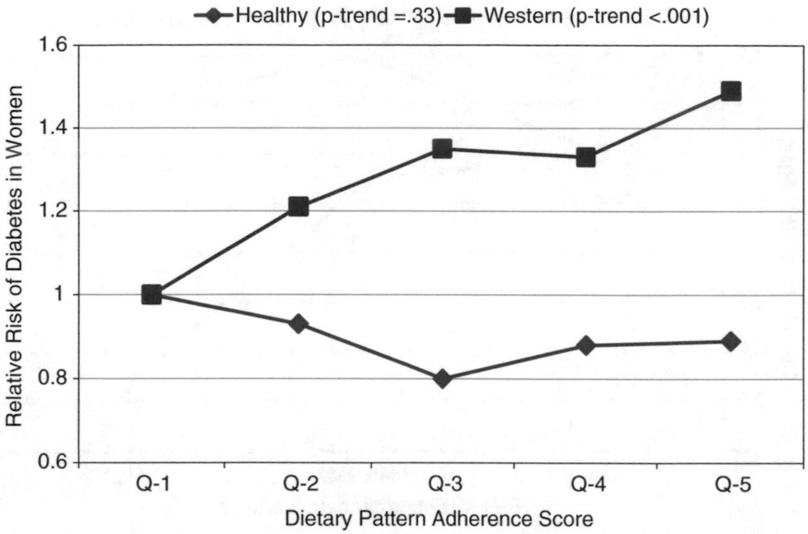

Fig. 1.5 Association between dietary pattern score and type 2 diabetes (diabetes) risk in women from the Nurses' Health Study, multivariate adjusted (adapted from [50])

1.2.3 Western Dietary Patterns

Several large prospective studies show that high adherence to Western dietary patterns, especially those with the lowest dietary fiber levels, increase the risk of weight gain, unhealthy aging and premature death especially when consumed during midlife and older years compared to healthy dietary patterns [50–53]. The Nurses' Health Study (69,554 women; age 38–63 years; 14 years of follow-up; 2699 incident cases of type 2 diabetes) found that high adherence to a Western pattern significantly increased risk of diabetes (Fig. 1.5) [50], and increased risk of cardiovascular disease, cancer, and all-cause mortality by 20% [51]. The British Whitehall II cohort study (5350 participants; mean age 51 years; 71% men; 16 years of follow-up) observed that high adherence to Western-type diets significantly lowered odds of ideal aging (a composite of cardiovascular, metabolic, musculoskeletal, respiratory, mental, and cognitive functions), independently of other health behaviors (Fig. 1.6) [52]. In the French SU.VI.MAX ((SUpplementation en Vitamines et Mineraux AntioXydants) study (2796 participants; mean age 52 years; mean 13.3 years of follow-up), Western diets produced a 20% lower odds of healthy aging compared to significantly improved odds of healthy aging by about 50% for moderately energy restricted healthy dietary patterns, after full multivariate adjustments [53]. Also, high adherence to a Western dietary pattern is associated with poorer cognitive outcomes such as lower processing speed and executive function and an overall increased rate of cognitive decline compared to diets rich in fruit, vegetables, and other plant-based food items which conferred cognitive benefits [54].

1.2.4 Sedentary Lifestyle

A sedentary lifestyle throughout adulthood is associated with an increased risk of obesity, chronic diseases, disability, frailty and premature death with aging [55–59]. A meta-analysis (6 cohort studies; 595,086 adults; mainly female, middle-aged or older adults from high-income countries; 2.8 to >8 years of follow-up; 29,162 deaths) found a non-linear association with sitting time and all-cause mortality risk with a 2% increase for each hour of daily sitting time up to 7 h/day and 5% increase for each 1-h increment in daily sitting above 7 h/day, after adjusting for the protective effects of physical activity [56]. A large Taiwan prospective cohort study (416,175 adults; 52% women; various ages; 8-year follow-up)

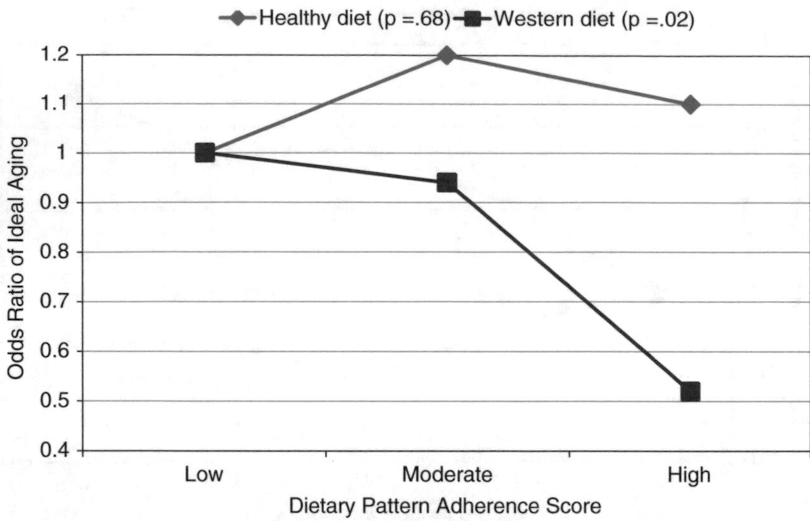

Fig. 1.6 Association between dietary pattern type and the odds of ideal aging from the British Whitehall II Study (multivariate adjusted) (adapted from [52])

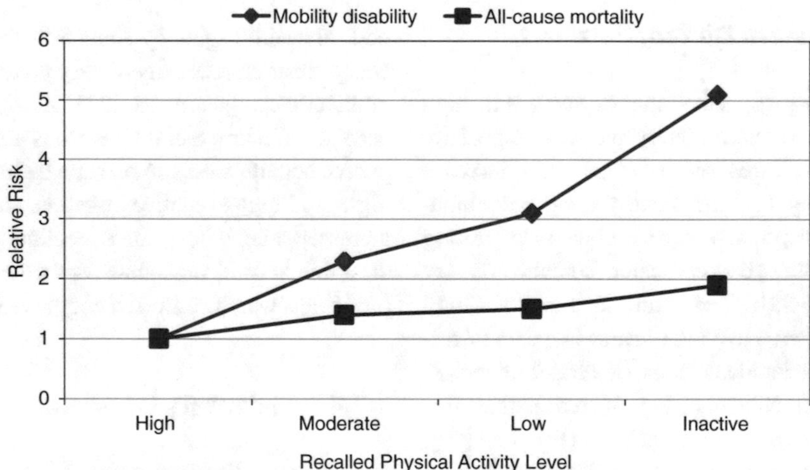

Fig. 1.7 Level of physical activity during early and middle adulthood and risk of mobility disability and all-cause mortality at 75 years of age (p > 0.01; multivariate adjusted) (adapted from [58])

found that individuals who were inactive had a 17% increased risk of all-cause mortality compared with individuals exercising for only 15 min/day [57]. The 2015 Finnish InCHIANTI study (1149 participants; mean age 75 years; 10 years of follow-up) observed that recalled physical inactivity during younger and middle adulthood was at age 75 years significantly associated with higher rates of mobility disability and premature death compared to those who had been physically active (Fig. 1.7) [58]. The Osteoarthritis Initiative (2252 participants; mean age 66–70 years; 6-year follow-up) found that more physical activity maintained healthy physical function through increased muscle strength in older adults with or at risk for osteoarthritis [59]. A meta-analysis (92,986 participants; approx. 90% men; mean age 51 years; mean 11.4 years of follow-up) demonstrated that unfit individuals had twice the mortality risk regardless of BMI as more fit participants [60]. Also, each 1 metabolic equivalent decrease in cardiorespiratory fitness increased mortality risk by 13%.

1.3 Major Unhealthy Aging Phenotypes

Three major phenotypes responsible for accelerated aging and premature death are: (1) the metabolic syndrome; in which excess abdominal body and ectopic fat drive cardiometabolic dysfunction, (2) type 2 diabetes (diabetes) and prediabetes due to relative insulin deficiency or impaired effectiveness of insulin action, and (3) sarcopenia or sarcopenia plus obesity; age-related loss of lean muscle mass due to inactivity and inadequate protein intake [61–67].

1.3.1 Metabolic Syndrome

Metabolic syndrome occurs in 20–40% of the worldwide adult population [64]. It is a major and escalating public-health challenge as a result of urbanization, surplus energy intake, increasing obesity, and sedentary life habits [68]. Metabolic syndrome causes a twofold increase in risk of CVD, CVD mortality, and stroke, and a 1.5-fold increase in risk of all-cause mortality over 5–10 years compared with those without the syndrome, regardless of a previous history of cardiovascular events [69]. Its features are central obesity and ectopic fat infiltration into the skeletal muscle, liver, heart, pancreas, and kidney; atherogenic dyslipidemia (elevated triglycerides, elevated apolipoprotein B and reduced high-density lipoprotein); elevated blood pressure; elevated glucose levels; and proinflammatory and pro-thrombotic states, which are strongly associated with the positive energy balance often found with the Western lifestyle [61, 69]. One of the defects associated with ectopic fat in metabolic syndrome is an excess production of reactive oxygen species generated by mitochondria, or from other sites within or outside the cell, causing damage to mitochondrial components and initiating degradative processes including increased inflammation. Metabolic syndrome is strongly related to unhealthy aging. Weight loss, exercise and healthy dietary patterns, including fiber-rich diets, have been shown to be effective in reducing the risk of metabolic syndrome [70, 71]. Metabolic syndrome is also associated with increased risk of non-alcoholic fatty liver disease which is another important factor associated with unhealthy aging.

1.3.2 Type 2 Diabetes and Prediabetes

The prevalence of prediabetes and diabetes has increased globally in parallel with the rising levels of obesity in adults and children, a phenomenon sometimes called diabesity [66, 67, 72]. If this global trend continues, by 2030 about one billion people will have prediabetes or diabetes. Diabetes is a threat to healthy aging as its prevalence increases during aging, with 26% of Americans 65 years or older having diabetes compared with about 9.0% in the general population. Diabetes is a major risk factor for premature onset of multiple age-related conditions, including renal dysfunction, cardiovascular disease, stroke, impaired wound healing, infection, depression, and cognitive decline [66]. Diabetes is preventable through the practice of a healthy lifestyle, including weight loss/control, regular exercise, and modification of an unhealthy to a healthy diet, but weight control offers the greatest benefit [67, 73, 74]. A meta-analysis of prospective cohort studies found that compared to healthy normal-weight adults, the risk for diabetes was increased by 300% to 800% depending on obesity classification or degree of metabolic dysfunction [75].

Individuals with prediabetes have blood glucose levels above normal but below the threshold for diabetes [66, 67]. Prediabetes is associated with subclinical transition to insulin resistance and β-cell dysfunction, and early complications associated with damage to kidney and nerves. For prediabetic individuals, identification and treatment with a healthy diet and physical activity to prevent weight gain or promote weight loss is the cornerstone of diabetes prevention. A 2017 meta-analysis (50 RCTs) found that adapting healthy lifestyle habits reduced the risk of progression from prediabetes to diabetes by 36% (range 28% to 43%) in interventions with durations lasting from 6 months to 6 years [76].

1.3.3 Sarcopenia

Adults, especially those who are inactive and consume inadequate protein, tend to have a 3–8% reduction in lean muscle mass per decade after the age of 30 years, [64, 77–81]. If this muscle mass loss progresses unchecked, sarcopenia (loss of muscle and function, body water, and bone density) develops in approximately 30% of individuals over 60 years of age and ≥50% of those over 80 years [79]. In the later stages, sarcopenia or sarcopenia obesity (fat replaces much of the muscle) results in accelerated aging including increased physical dependence, risk of chronic disease, inflammation, insulin resistance, and endocrine dysfunction [64, 77]. Even short term reductions in activity, such as a reduction of daily step counts from 6000 to 1500, over time can reduce insulin sensitivity and lean mass, and increase fat mass in both young and older adults within 2 weeks [79]. A minimum of 7000 steps/day and adequate protein intake is recommended to lower sarcopenia risk [80]. Although a high-quality protein supplementation of about 25 g divided between breakfast and lunch/day for 24 weeks in healthy older adults resulted in a positive (+0.6 kg) difference in lean tissue mass compared with an isoenergetic, non-protein control [80], 25–30 g of high quality protein per meal has been proposed to maximize muscle protein synthesis and lean body mass with aging [77, 78].

1.4 Healthy Aging

The concept of healthy aging includes healthy life expectancy (e.g., absence or delay of chronic diseases and the maintenance of cognitive, physical, and other functions with limited dependence on family members or extended care assisted living) and longevity [19]. Since older individuals are a growing portion of the worldwide population, it is critical to figure out how to promote guidance for healthy aging lifestyles in this population to assure better quality of life and to help control the expected surge in healthcare expenses. From a clinical and public health perspective, maintaining a healthy weight through diet and physical activity is the foundation of the prevention of chronic diseases and the promotion of healthy aging. In Western countries, such as the US, only a small fraction (< 10%) of the population is both at normal weight and practicing multiple healthy lifestyles (i.e., eating a healthy diet, exercising regularly, and not smoking) [19]. The adherence to healthy lifestyles throughout adulthood can promote healthy aging processes by helping to increase lean muscle mass, healthy mitochondrial biogenesis (e.g., in the liver and muscle cells) and genome stability. Age protective nutrition and phytochemical dietary quality are important in lowering diabetes and other metabolic, cardiovascular and neurological disease, and oxidative and inflammatory stress risks [82]. The Finnish nutritional guidelines emphasize that due to the impact of good nutrition on health and well-being in later life, nutrition among older people should be given more attention [83]. These guidelines emphasize the importance of adequate intake of energy, protein, fiber, other nutrients such as vitamin D supplementation and fluids plus regular physical activity. In addition, weight changes, oral health, and constipation should be monitored.

1.4.1 Healthy Body Weight

Prospective cohort studies generally demonstrate that maintaining normal body weight is important for healthy aging, but this can vary with age and body composition. A systematic review and meta-analysis (19 prospective studies; 1.5 million white adults; median age 58 years; median BMI 26; median 10-year follow-up; 160,087 deaths) demonstrated that all-cause mortality was lowest with a normal BMI range of 20.0–24.9 whereas overweight and obese BMI range individuals were associated with significantly increased death rates [84]. However, a meta-analysis of older adults (32 observational studies; 197,940 adults ≥65 years of age; average follow-up of 12 years) found that in older adults being overweight was not significantly associated with an increased risk of mortality [85]. Also, the risk of mortality increased in older people with a BMI <23.0, which suggests the importance of monitoring weight loss in older age groups as an indicator of some serious health issue or sarcopenia. Compared to a reference BMI of 23.0–23.9, there was a 12% higher mortality risk for individuals in the BMI range of 21.0–21.9 and a 19% greater risk for a range of 20.0–20.9. In the obesity range mortality risk began to increase for BMI ≥ 33 with only a slight attenuation after adjustment for intermediary factors. Exclusion of early deaths or preexisting disease did not markedly alter the associations. In a large, population-based California cohort study, the Leisure World Cohort Study (13,451 participants; average aged 73 years; women 64%; average 13 years of follow-up; 11,203 deaths) it was observed that compared to normal weight individuals those who were either underweight or obese had significantly higher all-cause mortality risk (Fig. 1.8) [86].

Maintaining normal weight in midlife (45–65 years) is an important predictor of healthy aging as obesity is one of the underlying causes of frailty. A prospective cohort study within the Honolulu Heart Program/Honolulu Asia Aging Study (5820 healthy Japanese-American men, mean age 54 years; 40 years of follow-up) showed that leaner men had greater odds of survival at age 85 years than those who were overweight or obese [87]. The Uppsala Longitudinal Study (2293 Swedish men; mean age 50 years; 4 decades of follow-up; 38% survived to age 85 years) observed that the maintenance of normal weight at age 50 significantly improved odds of survival by 20% and independent aging by 66% [88]. Similarly, the Nurses' Health Study (40,000 US women; mean age 58.5 years; 4-year follow-up) found weight maintenance and/or weight loss (5–20 lb) in overweight and obese women was associated with significantly improved physical function and vitality and reduced body pain [89]. The Helsinki Businessmen Study (1114 participants, mean age 47 years; 26 years of follow-up; 425 deaths) observed that men who were overweight or obese at a mean of 47 years had a significantly higher risk of developing frailty at 73 years of age compared with men at constant normal weight with

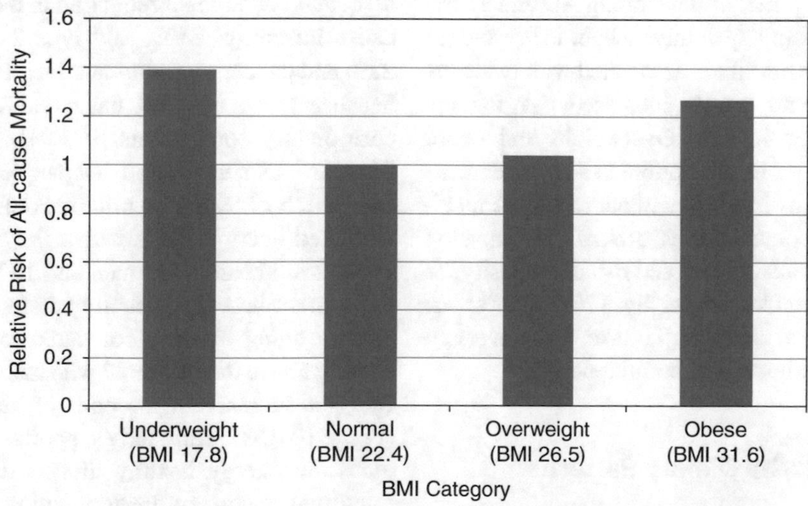

Fig. 1.8 Association between BMI and all-cause mortality risk over 23 years of follow-up from the California Leisure World Cohort Study of adults with a mean baseline age of 73 years (adapted from [86])

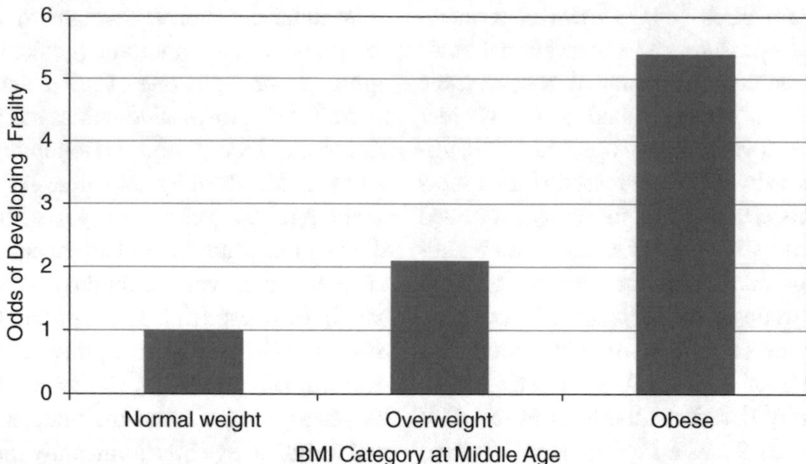

Fig. 1.9 Association between BMI in mid-life (mean age 47 years) and odds of developing frailty at age 73 years from the Helsinki Businessmen Study ($p < 0.001$; multivariate adjusted) (adapted from [90])

aging (Fig. 1.9) [90]. In this study, each 1% increase in body weight was associated with increased risk of developing both coronary artery disease and frailty by 16%. A meta-analysis (15 prospective studies; 25,624 participants; 3.2–36 years of follow-up) suggested a U-shaped relationship between midlife BMI and late-life risk of Alzheimer's disease (AD) with normal BMI in midlife having the lowest risk of AD and obese BMI in midlife having the highest risk [91]. Compared with midlife normal BMI, (1) overweight BMI in midlife is associated with 35% increased risk of developing AD and a 26% increased risk of any dementia later in life and (2) obese BMI in midlife is associated with twice the risk of AD and a 64% increased risk for any dementia later in life. Overweight and obese women were more susceptible to AD and dementia than were overweight and obese men. A meta-analysis (17 cohort studies; 563,277 participants) found a significantly reduced risk of adiposity for fruit or vegetables intake by 17% (highest vs. lowest intakes) and fruit intake was inversely associated with waist circumference [92].

1.4.2 Healthy Dietary Patterns

Prospective studies generally show a positive association between fiber-rich healthy dietary patterns (e.g., rich in vegetables, fruits, whole grains, low- or non-fat dairy, seafood, legumes, and nuts and low in red and processed meats, sugar-sweetened foods and drinks and refined grains), and healthy aging [93, 94]. Several meta- or pooled analyses report that higher adherence to any healthy dietary pattern, including the Healthy Eating Index (HEI)-2010, Alternative Healthy Eating Index (AHEI)-2010, Alternate Mediterranean Diet (aMED), and Dietary Approaches to Stop Hypertension (DASH) converge to have a similar inversely associated significant reduction in the risk of all-cause mortality, CVD, and type 2 diabetes by 22% and cancer mortality and incidence by 15% because these diets all have relatively similar core dietary components [93, 94]. The French SU.VI.MAX study found that people with adherence to a healthy diet in midlife combined with a regulated energy intake below the threshold of about 2500 kcal/day in men and 1820 kcals/day in women, had significantly improved odds of healthy aging by 46% compared to those consuming above the threshold who had an insignificant 7% increase in the odds of healthy aging (Fig. 1.10) [53]. This study supports a controlled, moderate energy healthy diet as a potentially important factor in healthy aging. A dietary mechanism related to healthy aging with the consumption of healthy diets such as the

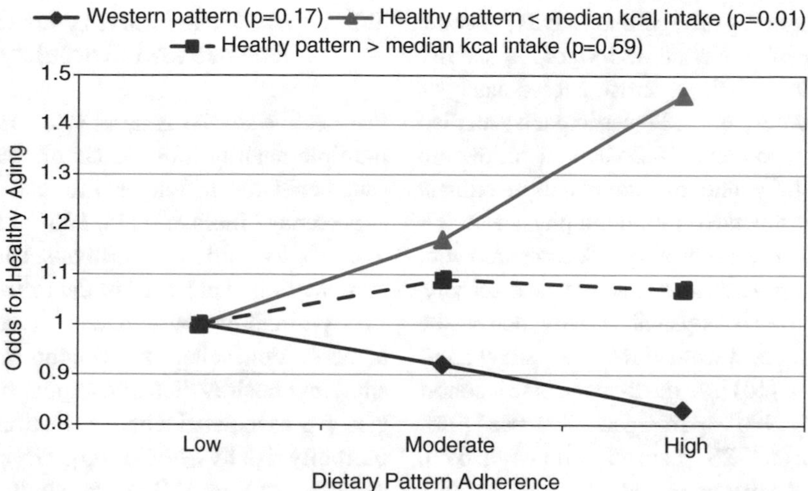

Fig. 1.10 Odds of healthy aging for healthy dietary pattern above and below the median energy level (median energy intake of 2500 kcal/day in men and 1820 kcals/day in women) and the Western dietary pattern (adapted from [53])

Mediterranean diet (MedDiet) or other healthy plant-based diets is that they appear to maintain or promote longer telomere length [95]. In contrast, the Western diet with high saturated fat, refined grains, meat and meat products, and sugar-sweetened beverages intake appears to be associated with shorter telomeres.

The World Health Organization (WHO) has formulated global guidelines for a healthy diet plan to prevent chronic diseases and premature death [96–98]. This plant based diet consists primarily of fruits, vegetables, legumes (e.g. lentils, beans), nuts and whole grains (e.g. unprocessed maize, millet, oats, wheat, brown rice) and specific dietary guidance including: (1) at least 400 g (5 portions) of fruits and vegetables a day (excluding potatoes, sweet potatoes, cassava and other starchy roots); (2) less than 10% of total energy intake from free sugars, which is equivalent to 50 g (or around 12 level teaspoons) per daily 2000 calories; (3) healthy fats (e.g. found in fish, avocados, nuts, sunflower, canola and olive oils) being preferable to saturated fats (e.g. found in fatty meat, butter, palm and coconut oil, cream, cheese, ghee and lard); (4) avoidance of industrial trans fats found in processed food, fast food, snack food, fried food, frozen pizza, pies, cookies, margarines and spreads; and (5) <5 g of salt is allowed (equivalent to 1 teaspoon) per day (as iodized salt) [93]. Several analyses have evaluated the effect of the WHO diet on longevity and cardiovascular disease mortality in adults >60 years. The first pooled analysis of cohort studies (11studies; 400,000 participants; 42% women) estimated that greater adherence to the WHO guidelines increased life expectancy by at least 2 years in European and United States men and women >60 years old [97]. The second WHO pooled analysis (10 cohort studies; 280,000 men and women; aged >60 years) found that higher adherence to the WHO dietary guidelines was inversely associated with CVD mortality observed in older populations in southern Europe and the United States but significant reductions were not observed across other European regions [98].

1.4.3 Physically Active Lifestyle

The role of physical activity in promoting healthy life expectancy (e.g., chronic disease risk reduction) and reducing premature mortality is well established [99–103]. Over 5 decades of systematic epidemiological and intervention research supports the US and WHO minimum physical activity guidelines of 150 min of moderate activity, 75 minutes of vigorous activity, or some combination of moderate and vigorous activity per week [99, 100]. A 2015 pooled analysis (6 cohort studies; 661,137 participants; median aged 62 years; median 14.2 years of follow-up; 116,686 deaths) found that individuals meeting at least the recommended minimum physical activity had a 31% lower mortality risk compared with those reporting no leisure time physical activity, whereas increased physical activity above the recommended level yielded relatively small additional benefits [101]. A meta-analysis (33 cohort studies; 102,980 participants; mean age 37–57 years; 1.1–26 years of follow-up; 6910 deaths) showed that an increased aerobic activity of 15 minutes/day or 90 minutes/week extended life expectancy by an average of 3 years [102]. A dose response meta-analysis (80 prospective studies; 1,338,143 participants; 85% US/EU,15% Asian; median age 56 years; median 10.7 years of follow-up; 118,121 deaths) found that higher levels of total and specific types of physical activity were associated with reduced all-cause mortality with the largest reductions observed with vigorous activity, supporting the message that 'some is good; more is better' (Fig. 1.11) [103]. The beneficial effects of physical activity on all-cause mortality risk tends to be independent of other lifestyle risk factors such as BMI [104].

1.5 Multiple Healthy Lifestyles Factors and Mortality Risk

Prospective studies generally find that following multiple healthy lifestyle factors has accumulative benefits for longer life and healthy life expectancy (Table 1.3) [34, 105–111]. A systematic review and meta-analysis showed that a combination of at least 4 of the following healthy lifestyle habits: low-moderate consumption of alcohol; not being overweight or obese, not smoking; healthy diet; and regular physical exercise was associated with a reduction of all-cause mortality risk by ≥66% [105]. The pooled analysis of the Nurses' Health Study and Health Professionals Follow-up Study with over 100,000 men and women evaluated over 26 to 32 years showed that an increased number of healthy lifestyle factors significantly reduced all-cause mortality rate in normal, overweight and obese populations (Fig. 1.1) [34]. A combination of at least 3 low risk lifestyle factors and BMI between 18.5 and 22.4 was associated with the lowest risk of all-cause mortality by 71%. The Physicians' Health Study (1163 men with type 2 diabetes; average baseline age 69 years; mean 9 years of follow-up) found an inverse association between the number of healthy lifestyle factors and total mortality risk with a

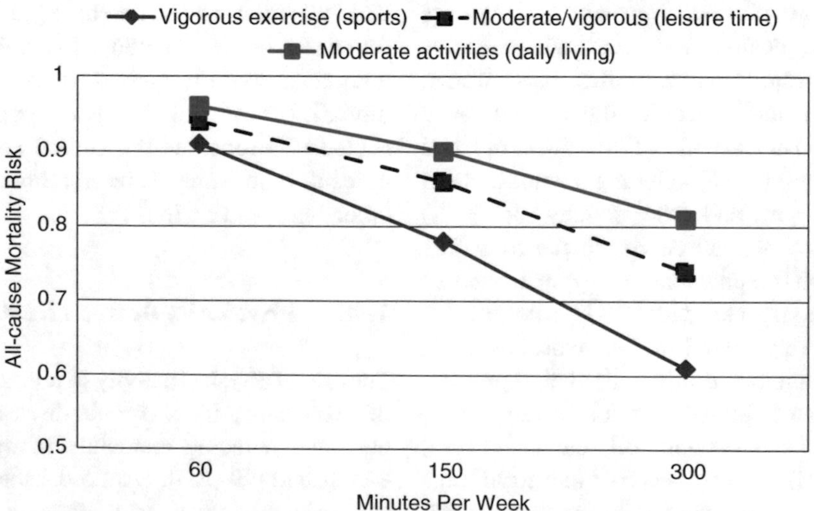

Fig. 1.11 Association between type and intensity of physical activity and all-cause mortality risk (multivariate adjusted) (adapted from [103])

Table 1.3 Summaries of studies on adherence to multiple healthy lifestyle behavior and all-cause and disease mortality

Objective	Study details	Results
Meta-analysis		
Loef et al. (2012) Investigate combined effects of lifestyle behaviors on all-cause mortality (German) [105]	15 cohort studies; 531,804 people; mean follow-up of 13 years	A combination of at least 4 healthy lifestyle factors including: low-moderate consumption of alcohol; not being overweight or obese; not smoking; healthy diet; and regular physical exercise is associated with a reduction of the all-cause mortality risk by 66%
Prospective cohort studies		
Veronese et al. (2016) Evaluate the combined associations of diet, physical activity, moderate alcohol consumption, and smoking with body weight on risk of all cause and cause specific mortality (Nurses' Health Study and Health Professionals Follow-up Study; US) [34]	74,582 women and 39,284 men; up to 32 years of follow-up; 30,013 deaths (including10,808 from cancer and 7189 from Cardiovascular disease); lifestyle factors included body mass index (BMI), score on the alternate healthy eating index, level of physical activity, smoking habits, and alcohol drinking	In each of the four categories of BMI studied (18.5–22.4, 22.5–24.9, 25–29.9, ≥30), people with one or more healthy lifestyle factors had a significantly lower risk of total mortality (Fig. 1.1), and cardiovascular and cancer mortality than individuals with no low risk lifestyle factors. A combination of at least 3 low risk lifestyle factors and BMI between 18.5–22.4 was associated with the lowest risk of all-cause mortality by 71%
Patel et al. (2016) Examine the association of healthy lifestyle factors on mortality in people with type 2 diabetes (Physicians Health Study; US) [106]	1163 men with type 2 diabetes; average baseline age 69 years; mean 9 years of follow-up; lifestyle factors consisted of currently not smoking, moderate drinking (1–2 drinks/day), vigorous exercise (1+/week), BMI < 25 kg/m^2, and being in the top 2 quintiles of the alternate healthy eating index-2010 (AHEI-2010)	An inverse relationship was found between the number of healthy lifestyle factors and total mortality; compared with participants who had ≤1 healthy lifestyle factor, the risk of death was 42% lower for those with 2 healthy lifestyle factors, 41% lower for those with 3, and 44% lower for those with 4 or more healthy lifestyle factors
Prinelli et al. (2015) Evaluate the association of the Mediterranean diet (MedDiet), smoking habits and physical activity with all-cause mortality (Italian) [107]	974 Italian completers; 51% women; mean age 56 years; mean BMI 27; median 17.4 years of follow-up; 193 deaths	A high adherence to the MedDiet, non-smoking and physical activity were strongly associated with a reduced risk of all-cause mortality in healthy subjects after long-term follow-up (Fig. 1.12). All-mortality risk was reduced with high adherence to the MedDiet Score by 38%, non-smokers by 29% and physically active subjects by 45%. Each point increase in the MedDiet score was associated with a significant 5% reduction of death risk. The average risk of death was significantly reduced for 1, 2 or 3 healthy lifestyle behaviors by 39%, 56%, and 73%, respectively

(continued)

Table 1.3 (continued)

Objective	Study details	Results
May et al. (2015) Assess the effect of several healthy behaviors on disability-adjusted life years (DALYs) (EPIC-Netherland cohort) [108]	33,066 participants; mean age 50 years; 12 years of follow-up; 6647 disease incidences and 1482 deaths	Non-smoking, maintaining a lean BMI (<25 kg/m^2), being physically active, and consuming a MedDiet were all associated with a significantly lower disease burden. Individuals adhering to all four healthy lifestyle factors lived a minimum of 2 years longer in good health than those not following any healthy lifestyles. Due to challenges in follow-up, the total number of DALYs, and consequently the estimates, are underestimated. Therefore, true lifetime health benefits of a healthy lifestyle were under reported
Petersen et al. (2015) Investigate the combined impact of adherence to five lifestyle factors (smoking, alcohol intake, physical activity, waist circumference and diet) on all-cause, cancer and cardiovascular (CV) mortality based on health recommendations (Denmark) [109]	51,521 subjects (27,256 women and 24,265 men); mean baseline age 55 years; 14 years follow-up; 6768 deaths (3941 men and 2827 women); of these, 43% of men and 51% of women died due to cancer, and 20% of men and 12% of women died due to CVD	Among men, adherence to one additional health recommendation was associated with an adjusted mortality risk reduction for all-cause by 27%, for cancer by 26% and for CV by 30%. Among women, the adjusted risk was reduction for all-cause by 28%, cancer by 24% and CV by 37%. Figs. 1.13 and 1.14 summarizes the effects of the number of healthy lifestyle choices on all-cause, cancer and CV mortality risk in men and women
Behrens et al. (2013) Determine the effect of healthy lifestyle behaviors on mortality risk in older US adults (National Institutes of Health-AARP Diet and Health Study; US) [110]	170,000 participants; age 51–71 years; mean 13 years of follow-up; 20,903 deaths	Adherence to all 4 low risk lifestyle factors, including achieving healthy waist size, recommended physical activity guidelines, non-smoking, and adherence to a healthy diet significantly reduced mortality risk by 73% vs. following none of these risk factors
Van den Brandt et al. (2011) Investigate the association between adherence to the Mediterranean diet (MedDiet) and total mortality and estimate the overall impact of a combined healthy lifestyle on premature death (The Netherlands) [111]	120,852 men and women; baseline age 55–69 years; 10 years of follow-up; 18,091 deaths	Adherence to the MedDiet was significantly related to lower mortality in women but not in men. The healthy lifestyle score was strongly inversely related to mortality in women and men. The least-healthy compared to the healthiest lifestyle scores increased premature death in women by 4.1-fold and in men by 2.6-fold (p-trend = 0.001)

reduction of up to 41–44% depending on the number of healthy lifestyle factors [106]. In an Italian cohort (974 completers; 51% women; mean age 56 years; mean BMI 27; median 17.4 years of follow-up) high adherence to the MedDiet and physical activity were significantly associated with reduced all-cause mortality in middle aged healthy adults over 17 years of follow-up (Fig. 1.12) [107]. The Rotterdam Study (5974 participants from the general population;

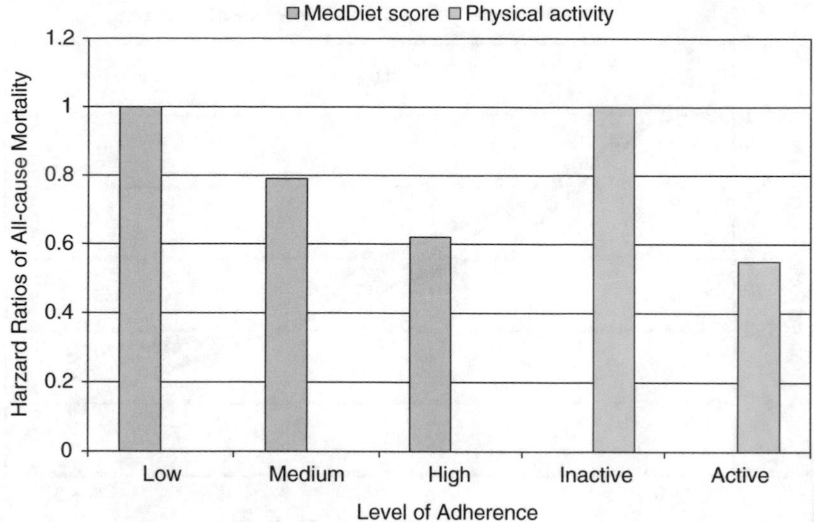

Fig. 1.12 Association between the Mediterranean diet (MedDiet) Score and physical activity on all-cause mortality (multivariate adjusted) (adapted from [107])

average age 69 years; 595 women; mean 15.1 years of follow-up; 3174 deaths) observed that smoking status (pack-years), energy intake, blood pressure, BMI, waist size, C-reactive protein level, total cholesterol, bone mineral density of the femoral neck, aortic calcification, diabetes, cardiac diseases, cancer and cognitive function were independent indicators of mortality risk [108]. A Danish cohort analysis (51,521 subjects; mean baseline age 55 years; 14-year follow-up) found that the adherence to multiple healthy lifestyle factors significantly lowered all-cause, cancer and cardiovascular mortality by up to about 80% compared to no healthy lifestyle factors in men (Fig. 1.13) and women (Fig. 1.14) [109]. The US National Institutes of Health-AARP study (170,000 subjects; 13 years of follow-up) observed a 73% lower morality risk in subjects adhering to all four low risk lifestyle factors of healthy waist circumference, recommended physical activity, adherence to healthy diets and non-smoking compared to subjects adhering to none of these healthy lifestyles [110]. A Dutch cohort analysis found that the least-healthy vs. the healthiest lifestyle scores increased premature death in women by 4-fold and in men by 2.6-fold [111]. Lifestyle factors can influence aging related DNA methylation related epigenetics affecting genomic maintenance and functional factors, which may influence aging mortality risk [112]. A meta-analysis (4 cohorts; 4658 subjects; 662 deaths; mean baseline ages range from 66–79 years) found that a 5-year higher DNA methylation age than chronological age was associated with a 16% higher mortality risk [113].

Conclusions

Aging is the biological progressive deterioration of physiological functions and metabolic processes that can lead to chronic diseases such as neurodegenerative disorders, CHD, type 2 diabetes and cancer, and ultimately to death. Since it is estimated that 70 to 80% of the rate of aging is related to external factors such as lifestyle choices, it is possible for individuals to significantly influence their odds of healthy aging and longevity, even if healthy lifestyles are adopted later in life. Unhealthy or premature aging, which is largely associated with excessive intake of Western energy dense diets and sedentary lifestyles, involves a complex interplay between obesity and related metabolic dysfunctional effects leading to increased risk of chronic disease and mortality, and reduced healthy life

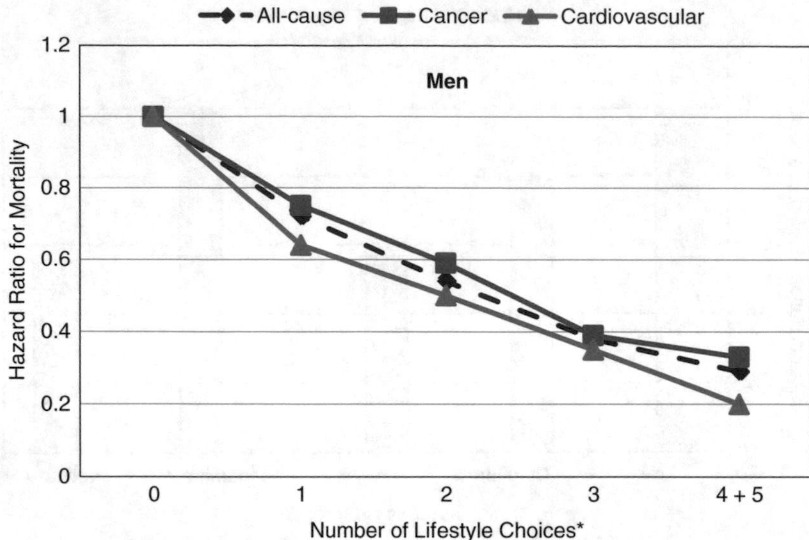

Fig. 1.13 Association between number of healthy lifestyle choices adopted and all-cause mortality in men (mean age 55 years; followed for 14 years; p-trend <0.001; multivariate adjusted) (adapted from [109]). *Healthy lifestyle: smoking cessation, limited alcohol intake, physically active, healthy waist circumference, and healthy diet

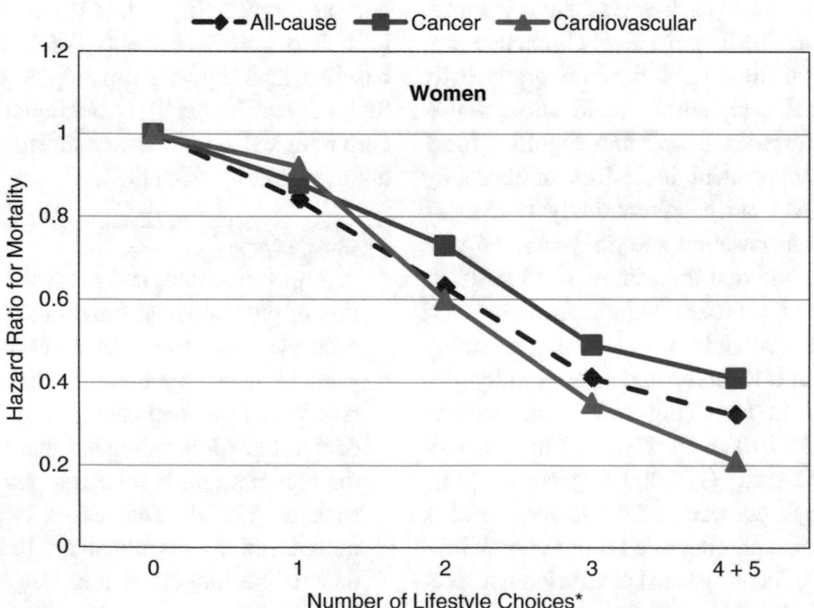

Fig. 1.14 Association between number of healthy lifestyle choices adopted and all-cause mortality in women (mean age 56 years; followed for 14 years; p-trend <0.001; multivariate adjusted) (adapted from [109]). *Healthy lifestyle: smoking cessation, limited alcohol intake, physically active, healthy waist circumference, and healthy diet

expectancy. In general, obesity, especially central adiposity represents a state of accelerated aging as adipose cells produce adipokines, which can lead to increased systemic and tissue inflammation and peripheral insulin resistance. Metabolic syndrome, type 2 diabetes and prediabetes, and sarcopenia are major unhealthy aging phenotypes, which can be prevented by adapting healthy lifestyle choices. The concept of healthy aging includes healthy life expectancy (e.g., absence or delay of chronic diseases and the maintenance of cognitive, physical, and other functions with limited dependence on family members or extended care assisted living) and longevity. Since a higher percentage of people worldwide are surviving to older ages, it is critical to promote optimal healthy aging lifestyle habits to assure quality of life for aging individuals and their families and for sustainable healthcare cost management. The odds of healthy aging can be significantly increased by following a healthy lifestyle even if it is adopted in middle age adulthood or older. These lifestyle choices include; adhering to a healthy dietary pattern, increasing physical activity most days of the week, achieving and maintaining a healthy body weight and waist size, and smoking avoidance.

References

1. Mathers JC. Impact of nutrition on the ageing process. Br J Nutr. 2015;113:S18–22.
2. Olshansky SJ, Hayflick L, Carnes BA. No truth to the fountain of youth. Sci Am. 2008;14:98–102.
3. Kirkwood TBL. Why and how are we living longer? Exp Physiol. 2017;102(9):1067–74.
4. Zhavoronkov A, Bhupinder B. Classifying aging as a disease in the context of ICD-11. Front Genet. 2015;6(3262):1–8.
5. Lopez-Otin C, Blasco MA, Partridge L, et al. The hallmarks of aging. Cell. 2013;153:1194–217.
6. Olshansky SJ. Has the rate of human aging already been modified? Cold Spring Harb Perspect Med. 2015;5(12). https://doi.org/10.1101/cshperspect.a025965.
7. Olshansky SJ, Passaro DJ, Hershow RC, et al. A potential decline in life expectancy in the United States in the 21st century. N Engl J Med. 2005;352(11):1138–45.
8. Global Burden of Disease Study (GBD). Mortality and Causes of Death Collaborators. Global, regional, and national age-sex specific all-cause and cause-specific mortality for 240 causes of death, 1990-2013: a systematic analysis for the Global Burden of Disease Study. 2013. Lancet. 2015;385(9963):117–71.
9. Beltran-Sanchez H, Soneji S, Crimmins EM. Past, present, and future of healthy life expectancy. Cold Spring Harb Perspect Med 2015;5(11). doi: https://doi.org/10.1101/cshperspect.a025957.
10. Murray CJ, Vos T, Lozano R, Naghavi M, et al. Disability-adjusted life years (DALYs) for 291 diseases and injuries in 21 regions, 1990–2010: a systematic analysis for the Global Burden of Disease Study 2010. Lancet. 2013;380:2197–223.
11. World Health Organization. WHO global status report on noncommunicable diseases. Geneva: World Health Organization Press; 2010. p. 2010.
12. Murray CJ, Lopez AD. Measuring the global burden of disease. N Engl J Med. 2013;369(5):448–57.
13. Lafortune L, Martin S, Kelly S, et al. Behavioural risk factors in mid-life associated with successful aging, disability, dementia and frailty in later life: a rapid systematic review. PLOS ONE. 2016:11(2):e0144405.
14. Avendano M, Kawachi I. Why do Americans have shorter life expectancy and worse health than people in other high-income countries? Annu Rev Public Health. 2014;35:307–25.
15. Nevalainen T, Kananen L, Marttila, et al. Obesity accelerates epigenetic aging in middle-aged but not in elderly individuals. Clin Epigenetics. 2017; 9:20.
16. Lunenfeld B, Stratton P. The clinical consequences of an ageing world and preventive strategies. Best Pract Res Clin Obstet Gynaecol. 2013;27(5): 643–59.
17. Tyrovolas S, Haro JM, Mariolis A, et al. The role of energy balance in successful aging among elderly individuals: The Multinational MEDIS Study. J Aging Health. 2015;27(8):1375–91.
18. Fontana L, Hu FB. Optimal body weight for health and longevity: bridging basic, clinical, and population research. Aging Cell. 2014;13:391–400.
19. Newman AB. Is the onset of obesity the same as aging? PNAS. 2015. doi-https://doi.org/10.1073/pnas.1515367112.
20. Beers MH. The Merck manual of health & aging. Whitehouse Station: Merck Laboratories; 2004. p. 2.
21. Ogden CL, Carroll MD, Fryar CD, Flegal KM. Prevalence of obesity among adults and youth: United States, 2011–2014. NCHS Data Brief. 2015;219:1–7.
22. Verdile G, Keane KN, Cruzat VF, et al. Inflammation and oxidative stress: the molecular connectivity

between insulin resistance, obesity, and Alzheimer's disease. Mediators Inflamm. 2015;2015:105828. https://doi.org/10.1155/2015/105828.

23. Kullmann S, Callaghan MF, Heni M, et al. Specific white matter tissue microstructure changes associated with obesity. Neuroimage. 2016;125:36–44.
24. Eckel N, Meidtner K, Kalle-Uhlmann T, et al. Metabolically healthy obesity and cardiovascular events: a systematic review and meta-analysis. Eur J Prev Cardiol. 2016;23(9):956–66. https://doi.org/10.1177/2047487315623884.
25. Roberson LL, Aneni EC, Maziak W, et al. Beyond BMI: the "metabolically healthy obese" phenotype & its association with clinical/subclinical cardiovascular disease and all-cause mortality—a systematic review. BMC Public Health. 2014. https://doi.org/10.1186/1471-2458-14-14.
26. Kramer CK, Zinman B, Retnakaran R. Are metabolically healthy overweight and obesity benign conditions? A systematic review and meta-analysis. Ann Intern Med. 2013;159:758–69.
27. Pujia A, Gazzaruso C, Ferro Y, et al. Individuals with metabolically healthy overweight/obesity have higher fat utilization than metabolically unhealthy individuals. Forum Nutr. 2016;8:2. https://doi.org/10.3390/nu8010002.
28. Whitlock G, Lewington S, Sherliker P, et al. Body-mass index and cause-specific mortality in 900,000 adults: collaborative analyses of 57 prospective studies. Lancet. 2009;373:1083–96.
29. Lorenzini A. How much should we weigh for a long and healthy life span? The need to reconcile caloric restriction versus longevity with body mass index versus mortality data. Front Endocrinol. 2014;5(121):1–8. https://doi.org/10.3389/fendo.2014.00121.
30. Kodama S, Horikawa C, Fujihara K, et al. Quantitative relationship between body weight gain in adulthood and incident type 2 diabetes: a meta-analysis. Obes Rev. 2014;15(3):202–14.
31. Cao Y, Ma J. Body mass index, prostate cancer–specific mortality, and biochemical recurrence: a systematic review and meta-analysis. Cancer Prev Res. 2011;4(4):486–501.
32. Flegal KM, Kit BK, Orpana H, Graubard BI. Association of all-cause mortality with overweight and obesity using standard body mass index categories: a systematic review and meta-analysis. JAMA. 2013;309:71–82.
33. Aune D, Sen A, Prasad M, et al. BMI and all-cause mortality: systematic review and non-linear dose-response meta-analysis of 230 cohort studies with 3.74 million deaths among 30.3 million participants. BMJ. 2016;353:i2156. https://doi.org/10.1136/bmj.i2156.
34. Veronese N, Li Y, Manson JE, et al. Combined associations of body weight and lifestyle factors with all cause and cause specific mortality in men and women: prospective cohort study. BMJ. 2016;355:i5855. doi.org/10.1136/bmj.i5855.
35. Winter JE, MacInnis RJ, Wattanapenpaiboon N, Nowson CABMI. All-cause mortality in older adults: a meta-analysis. Am J Clin Nutr. 2014;99:875–90.
36. Bowman K, Atkins JL, Delgado J, et al. Central adiposity and the overweight risk in aging: follow-up of 130,473 UK Biobank participants. Am J Clin Nutr. 2017;106:130–5.
37. Graf CE, Herrmann FR, Spoerri A, et al. Impact of body composition changes on risk of all-cause mortality in older adults. Clin Nutr 2016; 35(6):1499–1505. doihttps://doi.org/10.1016/j.clnu.2016.04.003.
38. Bea JW, Thomson CA, Wertheim BC, et al. Risk of mortality according to body mass index and body composition among postmenopausal women. Am J Epidemiol. 2015;182(7):585–96.
39. Zhang C, Rexrode KM, van Dam RM, et al. Abdominal obesity and the risk of all-cause, cardiovascular, and cancer mortality: a sixteen years of follow-up in US women. Circulation. 2008;117:1658–67.
40. Pang Q, Zhang J-Y, Song S-D, et al. Central obesity and nonalcoholic fatty liver disease risk after adjusting for body mass index. World J Gastroenterol. 2015;21(5):1650–62.
41. Wohlfahrt P, Somers VK, Cifkova R, et al. Relationship between measures of central and general adiposity with aortic stiffness in the general population. Atherosclerosis. 2014;235(2):625–31. https://doi.org/10.1016/j.atherosclerosis.2014.05.958.
42. Aronis KN, Wang N, Phillips CL, et al. Associations of obesity and body fat distribution with incident atrial fibrillation in the biracial health aging and body composition cohort of older adults. Am Heart J. 2015;170(3):498–505.
43. Sun Q, Townsend MK, Okereke OI, et al. Adiposity and weight change in mid-life in relation to healthy survival after age 70 in women: prospective cohort study. BMJ. 2009;339. https://doi.org/10.1136/bmj.b3796.
44. Batsis JA, Zbehlik AJ, Barre LK, et al. Impact of obesity on disability, function, and physical activity: data from the Osteoarthritis Initiative. Scand J Rheumatol. 2015;44(6):495–502.
45. Roos E, Laaksonen M, Rahkonen O, et al. Relative weight and disability retirement: a prospective cohort study. Scand J Work Environ Health. 2013;39(3):259–67.
46. Rillamas-Sun E, LaCroix AZ, Waring ME, et al. Obesity and survival to age 85 years without major disease or disability in older women. JAMA Intern Med. 2014;174(1):98–106.
47. Batsis JA, Zbehlik AJ, Barre LK, et al. The impact of waist circumference on function and physical activity in older adults: longitudinal observational data from the osteoarthritis initiative. Nutr J. 2014;13:81. https://doi.org/10.1186/1475-2891-13-81.
48. Beavers KM, Beavers DP, Nesbit BA, et al. Effect of an 18-month physical activity and weight loss

intervention on body composition in overweight and obese older adults. Obesity (Silver Spring). 2014;22(2):325–31.

49. Porter Starr KN, Pieper CF, Orenduff MC, et al. Improved function with enhanced protein intake per meal: a pilot study of weight reduction in frail, obese older adults. J Gerontol A Biol Sci Med Sci. 2016;71(10):1369–75. https://doi.org/10.1093/gerona/glv210.
50. Fung TT, Schulze M, Manson JE, et al. Dietary patterns, meat intake, and the risk of type 2 diabetes in women. Arch Intern Med. 2004;164:2235–40.
51. Heidemann C, Schulze MB, Franco OH, et al. Dietary patterns and risk of mortality from cardiovascular disease, cancer, and all causes in a prospective cohort of women. Circulation. 2008;118:230–7.
52. Akbaraly T, Sabia S, Hagger-Johnson G, et al. Does overall diet in midlife predict future aging phenotypes? A cohort study. Am J Med. 2013;126:411–9.
53. Assmann KE, Lassale C, Andreeva VA, et al. A healthy dietary pattern at midlife, combined with a regulated energy intake, is related to increased odds for healthy aging. J Nutr. 2015;145:2139–45.
54. Ashby-Mitchell K, Peeters A, Anstey KJ. Role of dietary pattern analysis in determining cognitive status in elderly Australian adults. Forum Nutr. 2015;7:1052–67.
55. Bouchard C, Blair SN, Katzmarzyk PT. Less sitting, more physical activity, or higher fitness? Mayo Clin Proc. 2015;90(11):1533–40.
56. Chau JY, Grunseit AC, Chey T, et al. Daily sitting time and all-cause mortality: a meta-analysis. PLoS One 2013; 8(11):e80000. doi: https://doi.org/10.1371/journal.pone.0080000.
57. Wen CP, Wai JPM, Tsai MK, et al. Minimum amount of physical activity for reduced mortality and extended life expectancy: a prospective cohort study. Lancet. 2011;378:1244–53.
58. Stenholm S, Koster A, Valkeinen H, et al. Association of physical activity history with physical function and mortality in old age. J Gerontol A Biol Sci Med Sci. 2016;71(4):496–501. https://doi.org/10.1093/gerona/glv111.
59. Batsis JA, Germain CM, Vasquez E, et al. Physical activity predicts higher physical function in older adults: The Osteoarthritis Initiative. J Phys Act Health. 2016;13(1):6–16. https://doi.org/10.1123/jpah.2014-0531.
60. Barry VW, Baruth M, Beets MW, et al. Fitness vs. fatness on all-cause mortality: a meta-analysis. Prog Cardiovasc Dis. 2014;56:382–90.
61. Bonomini F, Rodella LF, Rezzani R. Metabolic syndrome, aging and involvement of oxidative stress. Aging Dis. 2015;6(2):109–20.
62. Rossi AP, Fantin F, Bertassello P, et al. Chapter 13. Visceral fat predicts ectopic fat accumulation mechanisms and health consequences. Nutrition in the prevention and treatment of abdominal. Obesity. 2014:141–50.
63. Weiss EP, Fontana L. Caloric restriction: powerful protection for the aging heart and vasculature. Am J Physiol Heart Circ Physiol. 2011;301:H1205–19.
64. Ribeiro SML, Kehayias JJ. Sarcopenia and the analysis of body composition. Adv Nutr. 2014;5:260–7. https://doi.org/10.3945/an.113.005256.
65. Grundy SM. Adipose tissue and metabolic syndrome: too much, too little or neither. Eur J Clin Invest. 2015;45(11):1209–17.
66. Ley SH, Hamdy O, Mahan V, Prevention HFB. Management of type 2 diabetes: dietary components and nutritional strategies. Lancet. 2014;383:1999–2007.
67. Tabák AG, Herder C, Rathmann W, et al. Prediabetes: a high-risk state for developing diabetes. Lancet. 2012;379(9833):2279–90.
68. Kaur J. A comprehensive review on metabolic syndrome. Cardio Res Pract. 2014;2014:943162. https://doi.org/10.1155/2014/943162.
69. Mottillo S, Filion KBJ, Genest J, et al. The metabolic syndrome and cardiovascular risk: a systematic review and meta-analysis. J Am Coll Cardiol. 2010;56:1113–32.
70. Ma Y, Olendzki BC, Wang J, et al. Single-component versus multicomponent dietary goals for the metabolic syndrome. A randomized trial. Ann Intern Med. 2015;162:248–57.
71. Esposito K, Marfella R, Ciotola M, et al. Effect of a Mediterranean-style diet on endothelial dysfunction and markers of vascular inflammation in the metabolic syndrome. A randomized trial. JAMA. 2004;292:1440–6.
72. Murray MT. Diabetes mellitus (Chapter 161). In: Pizzorno JE, Murray MT, editors. Textbook of natural medicine. 4th ed. Philadelphia: Elsevier; 2013. p. 1320–48.
73. FB H, Manson E, Stampfer MJ. Diet, lifestyle and the risk of type 2 diabetes mellitus in women. N Engl J Med. 2001;345(11):790–7.
74. Alhazmi A, Stojanovski E, McEvoy M, Garg ML. The association between dietary patterns and type 2 diabetes: a systematic review and meta-analysis of cohort studies. J Hum Nutr Diet. 2014;27:251–60.
75. Bell JA, Kivimaki M, Hamer M. Metabolically healthy obesity and risk of incident type 2 diabetes: a meta-analysis of prospective cohort studies. Obes Rev. 2014;15:504–15.
76. Barry E, Roberts S, Oke J, et al. Efficacy and effectiveness of screen and treat policies in prevention of type 2 diabetes: systematic review and meta-analysis of screening tests and interventions. BMJ. 2017; 356:i6538. doi: org/https://doi.org/10.1136/bmj.i6538.
77. Jackman RW, Kandarian SC. The molecular basis of skeletal muscle atrophy. Am J Physiol Cell Physiol. 2004;287:C834–43.

78. Paddon-Jones D, Rasmussen BB. Dietary protein recommendations and the prevention of sarcopenia: protein, amino acid metabolism and therapy. Opin Clin Nutr Metab Care. 2009;12(1):86–90.
79. Moore DR. Keeping older muscle "young" through dietary protein and physical activity. Adv Nutr. 2014;5(5):599S–607S.
80. von Haehling S, Morley JE, Anker SD. From muscle wasting to sarcopenia and myopenia: update 2012. J Cachexia Sarcopenia Muscle. 2012;3:213–7.
81. Norton C, Toomey C, McCormack WG, et al. Protein supplementation at breakfast and lunch for 24 weeks beyond habitual intake increases whole-body lean tissue mass in healthy older adults. J Nutr. 2016;146(1):65–9. https://doi.org/10.3945/jn.115.219022.
82. North BJ, Sinclair DA. The intersection between aging and cardiovascular disease. Circ Res. 2012;110:1097–108.
83. Suominen MH, Jyvakorpi SK, Pitkala KH, et al. Nutritional guidelines for older people in Finland. J Nutr Health Aging. 2014;18(10):861–7.
84. de Gonzalez AB, Hartge P, Cerhan JR, et al. Body-mass index and mortality among 1.46 million white adults. N Engl J Med. 2010;363(23):2211–9.
85. Winter JE, MacInnis RJ, Wattanapenpaiboon N, Nowson CABMI. All-cause mortality in older adults: a meta-analysis. Am J Clin Nutr. 2014;99:875–90.
86. Corrada MM, Kawas CH, Mozaffar F, Paganini-Hill A. Association of body mass index and weight change with all-cause mortality in the elderly. Am J Epidemiol. 2006;163(10):938–49.
87. Willcox BJ, He Q, Chen R, et al. Midlife risk factors and healthy survival in men. JAMA. 2006;296:2343–50.
88. Franzon K, Zethelius B, Cederholm T, Kilander L. Modifiable midlife risk factors, independent aging, and survival in older men: report on long-term follow-up of the Uppsala longitudinal study of adult men cohort. J Am Geriatr Soc. 2015;63(5):877–85.
89. Fine JT, Colditz GA, Coakley EH, et al. A prospective study of weight change and health -related quality of life in women. JAMA. 1999;282:2136–42.
90. Strandberg TE, Sirola J, Pitkata KH, et al. Association of midlife obesity and cardiovascular risk with old age frailty: a 26-year follow-up of initially healthy men. Int Obes (Lond). 2012;36(9):1153–7.
91. Anstey KJ, Cherbuin N, Budge M, et al. Body mass index in midlife and late-life as a risk factor for dementia: a meta-analysis of prospective studies. Obes Rev. 2012;12:e426–37.
92. Schwingshackl L, Hoffmann G, Kalle-Uhlmann T, et al. Fruit and vegetable consumption and changes in anthropometric variables in adult populations: a systematic review and meta-analysis of prospective cohort studies. PLoS One. 2015;10(10). https://doi.org/10.1371/journal.pone.0140846.
93. Harmon BE, Boushey CJ, Shvetsov YB, et al. Associations of key diet-quality indexes with mortality in the multiethnic cohort: the dietary patterns methods project. Am J Clin Nutr. 2015;101:587–97.
94. Schwingshackl L, Hoffmann G. Diet quality as assessed by the Healthy Eating Index, the Alternate Healthy Eating Index, the Dietary Approaches to Stop Hypertension score, and health outcomes: a systematic review and meta-analysis of cohort studies. J Acad Nutr Diet. 2015;15(5):780–800.e5. https://doi.org/10.1016/j.jand.2014.12.009.
95. Freitas-Simoes TM, Ros E, Sala-Vila A. Nutrients, foods, dietary patterns and telomere length: update of epidemiological studies and randomized trials. Metabolism. 2016;65(4):406–15.
96. WHO. Healthy diet. 2015; http://www.who.int/mediacentre/factsheets/fs394/en. Accessed 10.27.2015.
97. Jankovic N, Geelen A, Streppel MT, et al. Adherence to a healthy diet according to the World Health Organization guidelines and all-cause mortality in elderly adults from Europe and the United States. Am J Epidemiol. 2014;180(10):978–88.
98. Jankovic N, Geelen A, Streppel MT, et al. WHO guidelines for a healthy diet and mortality from cardiovascular disease in European and American elderly: the CHANCES project. Am J Clin Nutr. 2015;102:745–56.
99. US Department of Health and Human Services. 2008 Physical activity guidelines for Americans. Washington, DC: US Dept of Health and Human Services; 2008.
100. World Health Organization. Global recommendations on physical activity for health. World Health Organization website. 2010; http://www.who.int/dietphysicalactivity/publications/9789241599979/en/. accessed November 23, 2015.
101. Arem H, Moore SC, Patel A, et al. Leisure time physical activity and mortality: a detailed pooled analysis of the dose-response relationship. JAMA Intern Med. 2015;175(6):959–67.
102. Kodama S, Saito K, Tanaka S, et al. Cardiorespiratory fitness as a quantitative predictor of all-cause mortality and cardiovascular events in healthy men and women: a meta-analysis. JAMA. 2009;301(19):2024–35.
103. Samitz G, Egger M, Zwahlen M. Domains of physical activity and all-cause mortality: systematic review and dose-response meta-analysis of cohort studies. Int J Epidemiol. 2011;40:1382–400.
104. Katzmarzyk PT, Janssen I, Ardern CI. Physical inactivity, excess adiposity and premature mortality. Obes Rev. 2003;4(4):257–90.
105. Loef M, Walach H. The combined effects of healthy lifestyle behaviors on all-cause mortality: a systematic review and meta-analysis. Prev Med. 2012;55:163–70.
106. Patel YR, Gadiraju TV, Gaziano JM, Djoussé L. Adherence to healthy lifestyle factors and risk of death in men with diabetes mellitus: The Physicians' Health Study. Clin Nutr. 2016; doi: 10.1016/j.clnu.2016.11.003.

107. Prinelli F, Yannakoulia M, Anastasiou CA, et al. Mediterranean diet and other lifestyle factors in relation to 20-year all-cause mortality: a cohort study in an Italian population. Br J Nutr. 2015;113(6):1003–11.
108. May AM, Struijk EA, Fransen HP, et al. The impact of a healthy lifestyle on disability-adjusted life years: a prospective cohort study. BMC Med. 2015;13:39. https://doi.org/10.1186/s12916-015-0287-6.
109. Petersen KEN, Johnsen NF, Olsen A, et al. The combined impact of adherence to five lifestyle factors on all-cause, cancer and cardiovascular mortality: a prospective cohort study among Danish men and women. Br J Nutr. 2015;113(5):849–58.
110. Behrens G, Fischer B, Kohler S, et al. Healthy lifestyle behaviors and decreased risk of mortality in a large prospective study of U.S. women and men. Eur J Epidemiol. 2013;28(5):361372. https://doi.org/10.1007/s10654-013-9796-9.
111. van den Brandt PA. The impact of a Mediterranean diet and healthy lifestyle on premature mortality in men and women. Am J Clin Nutr. 2011;94:913–20.
112. Walter S, Mackenbach J, Vokó Z, et al. Genetic, physiological, and lifestyle predictors of mortality in the general population. Am J Public Health. 2012;102:e3–e10.
113. Marioni RE, Shah S, McRae AF, et al. DNA methylation age of blood predicts all-cause mortality in later life. Genome Biol. 2015;16:25. https://doi.org/10.1186/s13059-015-0584-6.

2 Dietary Patterns in Aging and Disease

Keywords
Aging • All-cause mortality • Disease-specific mortality • Chronic disease • Cardiovascular disease • Cancer • Cognitive function • Alzheimer's disease • Dietary patterns • Healthy diets • Western diets • Mediterranean diet • Telomeres

Key Points

- Dietary pattern habits have a significant effect on aging, chronic disease risk, and longevity but in developed countries like the US mean diet quality scores are only about half of the optimal healthy eating diet score. Healthy dietary patterns include adequate whole-grain cereals, legumes, fruits, vegetables, and nuts, and lower intakes of red and processed meats and sugar-sweetened beverages.
- Prospective cohort studies with middle and older age adults consistently show that high adherence to Western dietary patterns increases cardiovascular disease (CVD), diabetes and cancer, and premature death risk whereas high adherence to healthy/plant-based dietary patterns lowers CVD, diabetes and cancer, and premature mortality risks.
- Among cancer survivors, healthy diets are associated with reduced overall mortality risk by 20% and Western diets are associated with increased risk by over 40%.
- For older adults, higher adherence to healthy dietary patterns reduces the odds of unhealthy aging and frailty whereas higher adherence to Western diets increases the odds. Simple dietary rules for healthy aging are to limit the intake of energy dense, low nutrient quality foods, red and processed meats and added salt and sugar, and increase the intake of fiber, and nutrient and phytochemical-rich whole or minimally processed plant foods.
- Healthy dietary patterns, especially the Mediterranean diet, are associated with reduced risk of age-related decline in cognitive performance and Alzheimer's disease, and longer telomere length compared to Western diets.
- High adherence to healthy dietary patterns supports healthy aging and reduces chronic disease and mortality risk through beneficial effects on body weight regulation and adiposity, energy metabolism, lipoprotein concentrations and function, blood pressure, glucose-insulin homeostasis, oxidative stress, inflammation, endothelial health, hepatic function, cardiac and cognitive function, telomere length, and the microbiota ecosystem.

M.L. Dreher, *Dietary Patterns and Whole Plant Foods in Aging and Disease*, Nutrition and Health,
https://doi.org/10.1007/978-3-319-59180-3_2

2.1 Introduction

By 2050, the world's aging population (≥60 years) is forecasted to double to two billion making up 21% of the population and exceeding the number of young children for the first time [1, 2]. The growing aging population will increasingly stress health care systems and present challenging economic implications with major effects on the labor force, health, social security and family support systems. It has been estimated that poor lifestyle choices account for about 70–80% of the risk of chronic diseases in later life and the quality of aging, successful vs. premature [1–6]. Globally, the high rates of Western diets and sedentary lifestyle choices, especially since the 1980s have resulted in pandemic rates of obesity, metabolic syndrome, type 2 diabetes (diabetes) and other related health conditions leading to sub-optional aging [5–11]. Healthy aging is the absence of premature chronic disease, lack of physical disability, and the presence of good social engagement and mental health [3]. Of the lifestyle choices, the type of dietary pattern followed appears to have one of the most significant effects on aging and longevity but in developed countries like the US the mean dietary quality score is only about half of the optimal diet score (53 vs. 100) [3–13]. Older adults often have major health, environment and lifestyle challenges that make meeting dietary recommendations difficult [1]. Some of the impediments to consuming healthy nutrient-dense diets include changes in taste and smell, loss of appetite, dental and chewing problems, less family support and limitations in mobility for accessing high-quality fresh whole foods. Also, aging-related inefficiencies in essential nutrient absorption and utilization tends to increase nutrient requirements, which leads older adults to commonly fall below recommendations for intake of a number of nutrients, including protein, omega-3 fatty acids, dietary fiber, carotenoids (vitamin A precursors), calcium, magnesium, potassium, and vitamins B-6, B-12, D, and E, the lack of which are related to elevated health risk. Healthy dietary patterns, containing adequate whole-grain cereals, legumes, fruits, vegetables, and nuts, and lower intakes of red and processed meats and sugar-sweetened beverages, generally promote healthy aging and lower of risk premature chronic disease and mortality [7, 8]. For example, these healthy diets reduce risk of common age-related diseases such as cardiovascular disease, dementia, and cancers by increasing dietary levels of major shortfall nutrients such as dietary fiber (fiber), calcium, vitamin D and potassium. Healthy diets also reduce intake of cholesterol raising saturated and trans fats, sodium and refined carbohydrates, which are of public health concern because of their association in the scientific literature to adverse health outcomes, unhealthy aging and premature death rates [5–13]. The objective of this chapter is to comprehensively review the effects of dietary patterns on aging and chronic disease risk.

2.2 Dietary Patterns in Aging and Disease

Suboptimal dietary patterns, with poor nutrition quality and/or excess energy intake, are a leading risk factor leading to unhealthy aging, increased chronic disease risk, and premature death in the US and worldwide [14]. Overconsumption of unhealthy foods and under-consumption of healthier foods remains a major global public health challenge. Western dietary patterns, especially those with excess calories, contribute to unhealthy levels of saturated fat, added sugars, high sodium foods, red and processed meats, refined grains, and energy dense desserts and beverages, which are associated with an increased risk for overweight, obesity, chronic disease, such as hypertension, dyslipidemia, insulin resistance and colorectal cancer, disability, and premature death [14]. Table 2.1 provides a list of food category substitutes for a Western dietary pattern to achieve a healthy dietary pattern, which can help in the maintenance of a healthy body weight and help to avoid the development of unhealthy aging and chronic disease [14, 15]. In that context, under consumption of whole grains, vegetables, fruits, and nonfat and low-fat dairy by the vast majority of the population in developed countries has resulted in inadequate intakes of dietary

Table 2.1 Diet modifications to change from a Western to a healthy dietary pattern (adapted from [14, 15])

Western dietary pattern (foods to discourage)	Healthy dietary pattern (foods to encourage)
Vegetables mixed with sauces or fried	Vegetables (e.g., fresh, frozen, dried with low to no salt; roasted, microwaved, stir-fried in healthy oils or steamed)
Fruit pies, jams, jellies or fruit juices with added sugar	Whole or minimally processed fruits (fresh/frozen/dried/canned without added sweetener, canned in natural juice)
Refined-grains (e.g., white bread or rice, cookies, granola bars, crackers, sugar rich cereals, donuts, cakes) with added sugar and solid fats or little to no fiber.	Whole grains and grains high in dietary fiber
French fries, hash brown potatoes or white rice	Legumes (beans, peas), sweet potatoes
Salted or candy-coated nuts or chips	Unsalted nuts and seeds; cut vegetables or fruit; baked, low-sodium chips; unsalted popcorn; low sodium dried seaweed
Full-fat dairy	Low-fat and nonfat milk, dairy products, calcium-fortified nondairy milks
Poultry with skin or fried	Poultry (skinless; grilled/baked/broiled)
Fish (battered and fried)	Fish and seafood (grilled with unsaturated oils/baked/broiled)
Processed meats (e.g., sausage and hot dogs)	Lean meat
Sugar sweetened beverages (soda, sweet teas, fruit drinks, sports drinks or energy drinks	Water and beverages without added sugars

fiber (current intakes are only half the recommended (28–30 g/day), potassium, calcium, and vitamin D, all considered major shortfall nutrients of global public health concern. An overweight and obesity epidemic currently affects the majority of the US population, including an estimated 33% of all US children. There are many reasons for poor adherence to healthy dietary recommendations: (1) inadequate knowledge or priority focus on nutrition guidance, cost factors, or lack of motivation to change; and (2) lack of access to or availability of healthy foods, and easy access to unhealthy foods are common, especially in certain geographic areas. Also, healthcare providers typically lack financial incentive, interest, knowledge, and office visit time to discuss health dietary and other lifestyle guidance with their patients [15]. A comparison of the foods and nutrient content of the Western and common healthy dietary patterns is found in Appendix A.

Over the last two decades, the critical importance of nutrition science in health management has been elevated by a significant increase in more rigorous evidence from well-designed prospective cohort studies and randomized controlled trials (RCTs) [14]. It is now evident that dietary habits have a strong direct metabolic influence on aging and chronic disease risk factors, including; obesity, lipoprotein concentrations and function, blood pressure, glucose-insulin homeostasis, oxidative stress, inflammation, endothelial health, hepatic function, adipocyte metabolism, cardiac function, metabolic expenditure, pathways of weight regulation, visceral adiposity, and the microbiota ecosystem. Worldwide, chronic diseases are forecasted to cause an estimated $17 trillion of cumulative economic loss between 2011 and 2030 from healthcare expenditures, reduced productivity, and other economic losses.

Human research on the effects of dietary patterns on health and longevity has increased several fold over the past decade or so. Some of these findings show that simple dietary rules can help promote healthy aging including limiting the intake of energy dense, low nutrient quality foods, red and processed meats and added salt and sugar, and increasing the intake of fiber, nutrient and phytochemical -rich whole or minimally processed plant foods [2, 5, 7, 8, 16]. Important differences between the Western diet and healthy dietary patterns including those based on the US Dietary Guidelines, Dietary Approaches to Stop

Hypertension (DASH), Mediterranean diet (MedDiet), lacto-ovovegetarian or healthy vegan diets are summarized in Appendix A. All of these dietary patterns meet or exceed the US adequate intake of fiber (≥28–30 g/day compared to the usual diet which contributes about half of the adequate fiber intake) and other major shortfall nutrients including potassium and calcium by increasing intake of whole or minimally processed plant foods (e.g., fruits, vegetables, wholegrains, legumes and nuts/seeds), reducing levels of energy dense food, and limiting levels of refined carbohydrates and saturated fats found in the Western diet. These healthy dietary patterns are associated with healthier aging quality of life, physical function and cognitive function [2] and lower chronic disease risk and premature death [14]. The effect of dietary patterns will now be assessed based on mortality risk, chronic disease risk, effects on healthy aging and physical function, age-related cognitive function and dementia, and telomere length (cellular senescence).

2.2.1 Mortality Risk

Twenty-five prospective cohort studies or their meta- or pooled analyses on dietary patterns and mortality risk include three 2017 meta- or pooled analyses [17–19] and 22 meta-or pooled analyses and cohort studies from 2016 or earlier and are summarized in Table 2.2 [20–41].

2.2.1.1 Meta-analyses and Pooled Data

Ten meta-analyses and pooled prospective data analyses provide strong evidence that healthy dietary patterns reduce the odds of premature mortality [17–26]. A 2017 meta-analysis (225 cohort studies) found that the optimal intake of healthy foods (e.g., whole grains, fruits, vegetables, legumes, nuts, and fish) significantly reduced all-cause mortality by 56% compared to a 2-fold increased risk with the high intake of unhealthy foods (e.g., red and processed meats and sugar-sweetened beverages along with low intake of healthy foods) [17]. Another 2017 meta-analysis (12 cohort studies) showed that the highest adherence to the Healthy Eating Indices significantly lowered all-cause and CVD mortality by 23% and cancer mortality by 17% [18]. A 2017 pooled analysis of the Nurses' Health Study and Health Professionals Follow-up study found that a 20% improvement in diet quality was significantly associated with lower all-cause mortality by 8 to 17% and CVD mortality by 7 to 15% compared to no change in diet quality [19]. A 2016 meta-analysis of cancer survivors (117 cohort studies; 209,597 subjects) found adherence to healthy dietary patterns to be inversely associated with overall mortality, whereas a Western dietary pattern was positively associated with overall mortality (Fig. 2.1) [20]. A 2015 meta-analysis (13 cohorts; 338,787 participants) demonstrated that healthy dietary patterns significantly lowered mortality risk for all-cause mortality by 24% and cardiovascular disease (CVD) mortality by 19% whereas the Western dietary pattern insignificantly increased the risk of all-cause, CVD and stroke mortality risk by 1–7% [21]. A meta-analysis of a number of healthy dietary patterns (15 cohorts; 1,020,642 participants) showed that subjects with the highest adherence to the Healthy Eating Index (HEI), the Alternate Healthy Eating Index (AHEI), and the Dietary Approaches to Stop Hypertension (DASH) had similar significantly lowered risk for all-cause mortality by 22%, CVD mortality by 22%, and cancer mortality by 15% compared to the lowest adherence scores [22]. The Consortium on Health and Ageing: Network of Cohorts in Europe and the US (CHANCES) pooled analysis (10 cohorts; 281,874 adults ≥60 years; 5–15+ years of follow-up) showed lowered CVD mortality risk in Southern Europeans by 13% and US participants by 15% with higher adherence to the WHO dietary guidelines [23]. A second CHANCES pooled analysis (11 cohorts; 396,391 adults ≥60 years; 5–15 years of follow-up) found significantly reduced all-cause mortality by about 10% (or an average of 2 years increased longevity) for each 10-point improvement in adherence to the WHO dietary guidelines [25]. A meta-analysis of vegetarian diets (7 cohort studies; 124,706 adults) showed that vegetarian diets lowered risk for mortality for all-cause by 9%, CVD by 16%, ischemic heart disease by 29% and stroke by 12%, and overall cancer incidence by18% compared to nonvegetarians

Table 2.2 Summary of dietary pattern prospective cohort studies on all-cause and chronic disease mortality risk

Objective	Study details	Results
Systematic reviews and meta-analyses or large pooled data sets		
Schwedhelm et al. (2016) Investigate the association between dietary patterns and overall mortality among cancer survivors [20].	117 cohort studies; 209,597 cancer survivors; 60,134 deaths.	In cancer survivors, adherence to a high-quality diet index and a prudent/healthy dietary pattern is inversely associated with overall mortality, whereas a Western dietary pattern is positively associated with overall mortality (Fig. 2.1).
Li et al. (2015) Assess the effects of adherence to dietary patterns on all-cause, CVD, and stroke mortality risk [21].	13 cohort studies; 338,787 participants.	Healthy dietary patterns were significantly inversely associated with reduced mortality risk for all-cause by 24% and CVD by 19%, whereas stroke mortality risk was insignificantly reduced by 11% (for highest vs. lowest adherence). Western diets insignificantly increased all-cause, CVD, and stroke mortality risk by 1–7%.
Schwingshackl and Hoffmann (2015) Examine the associations of diet healthy dietary quality score and mortality risk [22].	15 cohort studies; 1,020,642 subjects; healthy dietary patterns including the Healthy Eating Index (HEI), Alternate Healthy Eating Index (AHEI), and DASH diets.	Diets that scored highly on the HEI, AHEI, and DASH were associated with a significant reduction in mortality risk for all-cause by 22%, CVD by 22%, and cancer by 15%.
Jankovic et al. (2015) Examine the effects of WHO dietary guidelines on CVD mortality in persons aged ≥60 years (Consortium on Health and Ageing: Network of Cohorts (CHANCES) in EU and US) [23].	10 prospective cohort studies; 281,874 healthy men and women aged ≥60 years; WHO healthy dietary guidelines; median follow-up of 5 to 15 years.	Greater adherence to the WHO dietary guidelines was insignificantly associated with reduced CVD mortality risk by 6%, after multivariable adjustments. However, the results varied by region with significant inverse CVD associations observed in southern Europe by 13% and the US by 15%.
Huang et al. (2012) Estimate the effect of vegetarian dietary patterns on CVD mortality and cancer incidence [24].	7 cohort studies; 124,706 individuals.	Vegetarians had significantly lower ischemic heart disease mortality risk by 29% and overall cancer incidence by18% than nonvegetarians.
Jankovic et al. (2014) Investigate the association between the adherence to WHO dietary guidelines, and all-cause mortality in men and women ≥60 years of age from Europe and the US (CHANCES) [25].	11 cohort studies; 396,391 participants; 42% women; baseline age ≥ 60 years; WHO healthy dietary guidelines; median follow-up of 5 to 15 years.	Greater adherence to the WHO guidelines was associated with greater longevity in older men and women in Europe and the US with an average lower risk of premature death for men by 10% and women by 11% for each 10-point increase in adherence score, after multivariable adjustments. These estimates translate to an increased mean life expectancy of 2 years after age ≥ 60 years.
Sofi et al. (2010) Assess the effect of adherence to the Mediterranean diet (MedDiet) on disease incidence [26].	18 cohorts; 2,190,627 follow-up of 4 to 20 years.	A 2-point increase in adherence to the MedDiet was associated with a significant reduced mortality risk from all-causes by 8%, CVD by 10% and from cancer by 6%.
Prospective cohort studies		
Gopinath et al. (2016) Examine the relationship between overall diet quality (reflecting adherence to dietary guidelines) and mortality and successful aging in older adults (Blue Mountains Eye Study; Australia) [27].	1609 healthy adults; baseline age ≥ 49 years; 10-year follow-up; 610 (37.9%) died; 249 (15.5%) aged successfully.	Higher adherence to dietary guidelines had 20% lower odds of premature death after 10 years compared to poor adherence to guidelines. Adherence to recommended dietary guidelines significantly increases the probability of reaching old age disease free and fully functional.

(continued)

Table 2.2 (continued)

Objective	Study details	Results
Yang et al. (2015) Explore the effect of diet on prostate mortality risk (Physicians' Health Study I or II; US) [28]	22,071 male physicians; baseline age 40–84 years; mean diagnosis age 68 years; 926 men diagnosed with non-metastatic prostate cancer, 333 men died, 17% of prostate cancer mortality; median 9.9-years of follow-up.	Comparing men in the highest versus the lowest quartile of the Western pattern, there was a significant 150% increased risk for prostate cancer-specific mortality and 67% for all-cause mortality. The healthy pattern was associated with a significantly lower post diagnosis all-cause mortality by 36%.
Harmon et al. (2015) Assess the effect of 4 healthy diet quality indices On risk of mortality from all causes, CVD, and cancer in men and women (Multiethnic Cohort; US) [29].	215,782 participants; mean baseline age 59 years; mean age death 75 years; Healthy Eating Index-2010 (HEI-2010), the Alternative HEI-2010 (AHEI-2010), the alternate Mediterranean diet score (aMED), DASH diets; 13–18 years of follow-up; 34,430 deaths, 11,919 deaths were from CVD, and 10,883 deaths were from cancer.	All healthy indices were significantly associated with reduced risk of mortality from all causes, CVD, and cancer in both men and women (Fig. 2.2). The highest vs. lowest adherence of these healthy diets lowered risk of mortality from all causes, CVD, or cancer for men by 17–26%, and women by 11–24%.
Reedy et al. (2015) Examine the effects of major healthy dietary patterns on mortality risk (NIH-AARP Diet and Health Study, the Multiethnic Cohort, and the Women's Health Initiative Observational Study; US) [30].	492,823 participants; mean baseline age 62 years; dietary patterns including HEI-2010, AHEI-2010, aMed, and DASH diet scores; 15-year follow-up; 86,419 deaths, including 23,502 CVD and 29,415 cancer-specific deaths, on all-cause, CVD, and cancer mortality.	Higher diet quality adherence scores were significantly and consistently associated with a significantly reduced risk of death due to all causes, CVD, and cancer compared with the lowest adherence, independent of known confounders. In men, mortality risk was reduced for all cause by 17–24%, CVD by 15–26%, and cancer by 18–24%. In women, mortality was reduced for all-cause by 22–24%, for CVD by 21–28% and for cancer by 12–21%.
Liese et al. (2015) Evaluate the relationships between 4 diet quality indices and all cause, CVD, and cancer mortality (Dietary Patterns Methods Project/ NIH-AARP Diet and Health Study; US) [31].	492,823 participants; mean baseline age early 60s; dietary pattern score - HEI-2010, AHEI-2010, aMED, and DASH; 15 years of follow-up.	In women, a high diet quality score was associated with a lower risk of all-cause mortality by 18–26%, CVD mortality by 19–28%, and cancer mortality by 11–23%. In men, high diet quality score was associated with a lower risk of all-cause mortality by 17–25%, CVD mortality by 14–26%, and cancer mortality by 19–24%.
Shi et al. (2015) Estimate the effects of food habits, lifestyle factors and all-cause mortality in elderly adults (Chinese Longitudinal Healthy Longevity Survey) [32].	8959 participants; baseline age > 80 years; follow-up home visits over 6.5 years for men and 12 years for women; 6626 deaths.	Fruit and vegetable intakes were inversely associated with mortality risk with a 15% reduction for fruit and 26% reduction for vegetables. However, the intake of salt-preserved vegetables increased premature death risk 10%.
George et al. (2014) Study the relationships between 4 diet quality indices and all cause, CVD, and cancer mortality among postmenopausal women (Women's Health Initiative Observational Study; US) [33].	64,000 participants; mean baseline age 63 years; dietary pattern scores -HEI-2010, AHEI-2010, aMED, and DASH 12.9 years of follow-up; 5692 deaths, including 1483 from CVD and 2384 from cancer.	Across indices and after adjustment for multiple covariates, having high diet quality scores was significantly associated with a 18%–26% lower all-cause and CVD mortality risk. Higher HEI, aMED, and DASH (but not AHEI) scores were associated with a significant reduction in risk of cancer mortality by approx. 20%.

Table 2.2 (continued)

Objective	Study details	Results
Zazpe et al. (2014) Evaluate the effect of dietary patterns on all-cause mortality (Seguimiento Universidad de Navarra Project; Spain) [34].	16,008 middle-aged Spanish University graduates; mean baseline age 38 years; 60% women, 12.9 years of follow-up.	The traditional Mediterranean diet was associated with a significant reduction in the risk of all-cause mortality among middle-aged adults by 47% whereas the Western diet was not significantly associated with all-cause mortality.
Yu et al. (2014) Assess the effect of adherence to the Chinese Food Pagoda on total and cause-specific mortality (Shanghai Men's Health Study and Shanghai Women's Health Study) [35].	61,239 men and 73,216 women; mean baseline age early to mid-50s; 2954 deaths in men and 4348 deaths in women; mean follow-ups of 6.5 and 12.0 years.	A higher pagoda score was associated with significantly lower total mortality with multivariable-adjusted risk in men by 33% and in women by 13% (high vs. low adherence. Significant lower risks for CVD, cancer, and diabetes mortality, particularly in men were associated with higher pagoda scores.
Martinez-Gonzalez et al. (2014) Examine the effect of a pro-vegetarian dietary pattern on all-cause mortality risk (Prevencion con Dieta Mediterranea (PREDIMED) sub-study; Spain [36].	7216 high CVD risk participants, 57% women; mean baseline age 67 years; median 4.8 years of follow-up; 323 deaths.	Among omnivorous subjects those with food patterns that emphasized whole plant-derived foods (pro-vegetarian) were associated with a 41% reduced risk of all-cause mortality.
Orlich et al. (2013) Evaluate the effect of vegetarian dietary patterns on mortality (Adventist Health Study 2; US) [37].	96,500 Seventh-day Adventist men and women; mean follow-up of 5.8 years; 2570 deaths.	The adjusted all-cause mortality risk was significantly reduced for all vegetarians combined by 12% vs. non-vegetarians. The adjusted risk for all-cause mortality was reduced for vegans by 15%, lacto-ovo–vegetarians by 9%, pesco-vegetarians by 19%, and in semi-vegetarians by 8% vs. nonvegetarians.
Akbaraly et al. (2011) Examine the effects of adherence to the Alternate Healthy Eating Index (AHEI) on all-cause and cause-specific mortality in a British working population (Whitehall II Study; UK) [38].	7319 participants; mean baseline age 49.5 years; 30% women; follow-up of 18 years.	Higher adherence to the AHEI was significantly associated with 25% lower all-cause mortality, 40% lower CVD mortality and an insignificant 20% lower cancer mortality.
Anderson et al. (2011) Assess the effect of dietary patterns in older adults on survival (The Health, Aging, and Body Composition Study; US) [39].	3075 adults; mean baseline age 74 years; approx. 40% men; follow-up of 10 years.	High-fat dairy, sweets and desserts dietary intake was associated with a 1.4-fold higher risk of mortality compared to a healthy foods cluster, characterized by higher intake of low-fat dairy products, fruit, whole grains, poultry, fish, and vegetables.
Buckland et al. (2011) Explore the effects of adherence to the MedDiet on mortality risk (EPIC-Spain) [40].	40,622 adults; mean baseline age 48 years; mean BMI 28; 38% males; mean follow-up of 13.4 years; 1855 deaths.	A high MedDiet score compared with a low score was associated with a significant reduction in mortality from all causes by 21%, from CVD by 34%, but not from overall cancer by 8%. A 2-unit increase in MedDiet score was associated with a significant 6% lower risk of all-cause mortality.

(continued)

Table 2.2 (continued)

Objective	Study details	Results
Heidemann et al. (2008) Evaluate the effect of healthy vs. Western dietary patterns on the mortality risk of women (The Nurses' Health Study; US) [41].	72,000 women; mean baseline age of 50 years; 18-years of follow-up.	Higher adherence to a healthy dietary pattern significantly lowered mortality risk of all-cause by 17% and CVD by 28% vs. higher adherence to a Western dietary pattern which significantly increased risk of mortality from all causes by 21%, CVD by 22%, and cancer by 16% (Fig. 2.3).
Barnia et al. (2007) Investigate the effect of dietary patterns on overall survival of older Europeans (EU EPIC-Elderly cohort) [42].	74,607 adults; baseline age ≥ 60 years; 3–21 years of follow-up.	Higher adherence to a plant-based diet was associated with a significant lower overall mortality by 14% per one standard deviation increment.

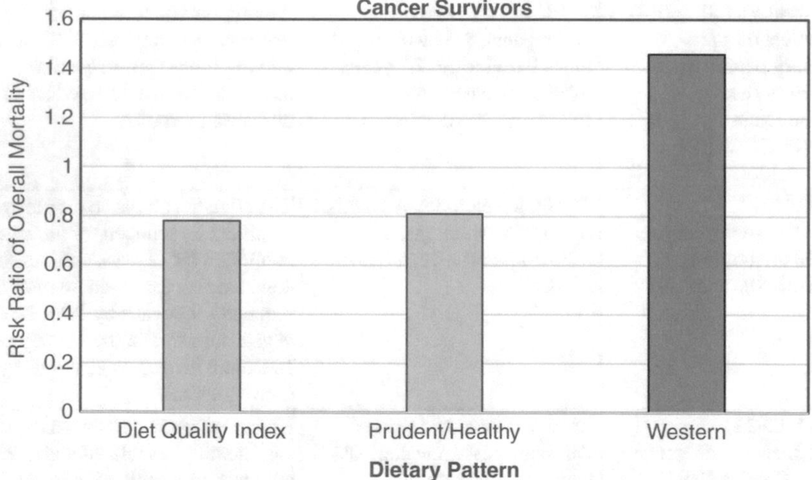

Fig. 2.1 Association between the type of dietary pattern consumed and overall mortality in cancer survivors (adapted from [20])

[24]. For the Mediterranean diet (MedDiet), a meta-analysis (18 cohorts; 2,190,627 subjects) showed that higher adherence significantly reduced mortality from all-causes, CVD, and cancer by 6–10% for each 2-point increase in adherence [26].

2.2.1.2 Specific Cohort Studies

Fourteen prospective studies report consistent beneficial effects of high adherence to healthy dietary patterns on all-cause and disease specific mortality risk [27–41].

Western Dietary Patterns

Studies consistently show that high adherence to the Western dietary pattern has adverse effects on mortality risk. In the Physicians' Health Study (22,071 men; mean age at diagnosis 68 years; 9.9-year follow-up) the Western diet was shown to significantly increase prostate cancer mortality by 150% and all-cause death by 67% compared to a 36% lower risk of all-cause mortality after diagnosis for healthy patterns [28]. In a prospective study of older US adults (3075; mean age of 74 years at baseline; 10 years of follow-up), high-fat dairy, sweets and desserts dietary intake was associated with a 1.4-fold higher multivariate risk of mortality compared to a healthy foods, characterized by higher intake of low-fat dairy products, fruit, whole grains, poultry, fish, and vegetables [39].

Healthy Dietary Patterns

Non-US Cohorts. A number of prospective cohort studies from Australia, the EU and China consistently show that high adherence to a variety of healthy dietary patterns significantly reduced mortality risk or promoted longevity [27, 32, 34, 35, 37, 40, 41]. The Australian Blue Mountains Eye Study (1609 participants; ≥ 49 years; 10 years of follow-up) observed that higher adherence to healthy dietary patterns reduced risk of mortality by 20% [27]. The Chinese Longitudinal Healthy Longevity Survey (8959 participants; ≥80 years; follow-up of 6.5 years for men and 12 years for women) reported that fruit and vegetable intake was inversely associated with all-cause mortality [32]. Also, the Shanghai Women and Men Health Studies (61,239 men and 73,216 women; age early to mid-50s; 6.5 and 12 years of follow-up for men and women, respectively) found that a higher adherence to the Chinese (Healthy) Food Pagoda lowered total mortality by 33% in men and 13% in women along with lower CVD, cancer and diabetes mortality [35]. Three EU studies observed that the consumption of healthy dietary patterns in mid-life (45–65 years) significantly reduced all-cause mortality in both men and women, which was primarily as a result of lower CVD mortality [38, 40, 42]. In the British Whitehall II Study (7319 mid-age adults, 30% women; 18 years of follow-up) higher adherence to the AHEI dietary pattern (rich in fruit, vegetables, nuts, soy, white meat, fiber, polyunsaturated fat and multivitamin use and lower in red meat, saturated and trans-fat, and alcohol) lowered mortality risk from all-cause by 25% and CVD by 40% [38]. A 2011 European Prospective Investigation into Cancer and Nutrition (EPIC)-Spanish cohort (40,622 middle-aged adults, mean follow-up of 13.4 years) found that a higher MedDiet score was associated with a significant reduction in mortality from all causes by 21% and from CVD by 34% compared to a low score [40]. A 2-unit increase in MedDiet score was associated with a significant 6% lower risk of all-cause mortality. A 2007 EPIC study of a cohort of older adults age ≥60 years observed that each one standard deviation increase in plant foods in combination with the avoidance of margarine, sugar-sweet beverages and potatoes, was associated with a significant 14% lower all-cause mortality [42]. A Prevencion con Dieta Mediterranea (PREDIMED) sub-study demonstrated that among omnivorous older adults with high CVD risk, those with food patterns rich in whole plant foods had a 41% reduced all-cause mortality risk compared to those consuming diets low in whole plant foods [36].

US Cohorts. Several large cohort studies show that higher adherence to healthy dietary patterns, including the HEI-2010, AHEI-2010, the alternate Mediterranean Diet (aMedDiet), and DASH diets have similar effects on all-cause and disease specific mortality because all these patterns have similar core dietary components such as emphasizing whole plant foods with limits on red and processed meats, refined grains and sugar sweetened beverages [29–31]. The US Multiethnic Cohort (215,782; mean age 58 years; followed for 13–18 years) found that high adherence to all of the healthy dietary patterns lowered all-cause mortality in men by 19–25% and in women by 20–22% (Fig. 2.2) [29]. These healthy dietary patterns also decreased disease specific mortality for CVD in men by 17–26% and in women by 19–24%, and for cancer in men by 17–24% and in women by 11–15%. The 2015 NIH-AARP Diet and Health Study found that high adherence to major healthy dietary patterns significantly reduced premature death by 12–28% [30]. In women, mortality was reduced for all-cause by 22–24%, for CVD by 21–28%, and for cancer by 12–21%. In men, mortality was reduced for all-cause by 17–24%, for CVD by 15–26%, and for cancer by 18–24%. Similar findings were observed in the Dietary Patterns Methods/NIH-AARP and the Women's Health Initiative Observational Study [30, 31, 33]. The Adventist Health Study II observed that all-cause mortality was reduced for vegans by 15%, lacto-ovovegetarian by 9%, pesto-vegetarians by 19%, and semi-vegetarians by 8% vs. nonvegetarians [37]. The Nurses' Health study (72,113 women; mean age of 50 years; 18 years of follow-up) observed that total mortality risk, especially CVD mortality, was reduced with adherence to a healthy diets and significantly increased with adherence to Western diets (Fig. 2.3) [41].

2.2.2 Chronic Disease Risk

Chronic diseases such as CVD, stroke, and type 2 diabetes become more common with aging and the rates of these chronic diseases are increasing

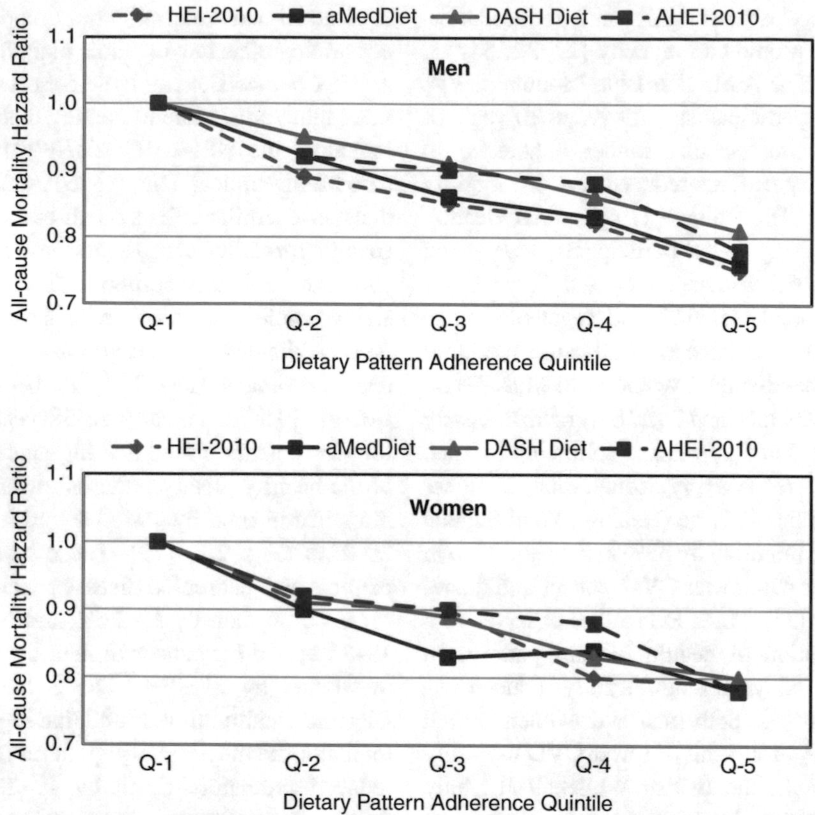

Fig. 2.2 Association between dietary pattern adherence and all-cause mortality risk among US middle-aged men and women during 18 years of follow-up ($p < 0.001$ for all; multivariate adjusted) (adapted from [29])

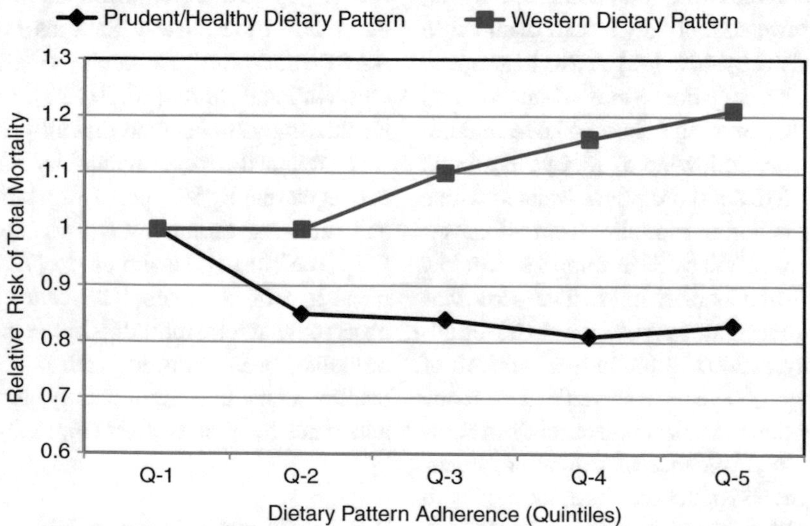

Fig. 2.3 Association between adherence to dietary patterns and total mortality risk in women (p-trend <0.001 for all diets; multivariate adjusted) (adapted from [41])

in mid-age because of the global increased intake of Western diets, sedentary lifestyles and the obesity pandemic effects on accelerating the aging processes [1, 14]. Eight systematic reviews and meta- and pooled analyses of observational studies, and RCTs evaluating the effects of dietary patterns on chronic disease risk are summarized in Table 2.3 [22, 26, 43–48].

2.2.2.1 Healthy vs. Western Dietary Patterns

Four meta-analyses comparing the effects of healthy and unhealthy (Western) dietary patterns found that high adherence to healthy diets reduces risk of major chronic disease and Western diets increased this risk [44–47]. A meta-analysis of colorectal cancer (CRC) studies

Table 2.3 Summary of systematic reviews, meta- and pooled analyses of prospective studies and randomized controlled trials (RCTs) on dietary patterns and chronic disease risk

Objective	Study details	Results
Ndanuko et al. (2016) Assess the effect of healthy dietary patterns on blood pressure (BP) in adults [43].	17 RCTs; 5014 adults; average mid-age or older; duration 6 weeks to 2 years; 13 RCTs allowed use of BP meds.	The pool results of the 4 healthy diets, DASH, Nordic diet, MedDiet, and Tibetan diet significantly lowered systolic BP by 4.3 mm Hg and diastolic BP by 2.4 mm Hg. The specific BP lowering effects are summarized in Fig. 2.7.
Feng et al. (2016) Identify the association between dietary patterns and the risk of colorectal cancer (CRC) [44].	40 studies; 22 cohorts, 17 case-controls and 1 cross-sectional; mean subject age mid-age or older.	For the highest vs. lowest adherence: 'healthy' dietary patterns decreased CRC risk by 25% ($p < .00001$]; Western style dietary patterns increased CRC risk by 40% ($p < .00001$); alcohol-consumption pattern is characterized by high consumption of beers, wines, and white spirits increased CRC risk by 44% ($p = .003$) (Fig. 2.4).
Maghsoudi et al. (2015) Review cohort studies about the association between dietary patterns and type 2 diabetes incidence [45].	10 cohort studies; 404,528 subjects.	For highest vs. lowest adherence: (1) 'healthy' dietary patterns significantly lowered diabetes risk by 14% (no difference between men and women) and (2) 'unhealthy' western dietary patterns increased diabetes risk by 30% (men were more significantly affected than women). Subgroup analysis showed that unhealthy dietary patterns containing foods with high phytochemical content insignificantly increased risk by 6% (Fig. 2.5).
Rodriguez-Monforte et al. (2015) Estimate the association between empirically derived dietary patterns and cardiovascular disease (CVD), coronary heart disease (CHD) and stroke risk [46].	19 cohort studies; number of cases ranged from 449 to 74,942.	Comparing the highest vs. the lowest category: (1) healthy dietary patterns reduced risk of CVD, CHD and stroke and unhealthy/Western diets slightly increased risk for these vascular chronic diseases (Fig. 2.6).
Schwingshackl and Hoffmann (2015) Examine the effects of diet quality scores on aging health outcomes [22].	15 cohort studies; 1,020,642 subjects; healthy dietary patterns including the Healthy Eating Index (HEI), the Alternate Healthy Eating Index (AHEI), and DASH diets.	Higher healthy diet scores were associated with a significantly reduced risk of CVD and type 2 diabetes by 22% and cancer by 15%, but the effects for neurodegenerative diseases were insignificant.
Hou et al. (2015) Evaluate the effects of dietary patterns on CHD risk [47].	12 cohort studies; 409,780 subjects; 4.6–13 years of follow-up; 6298 CHD cases.	There was an inverse association between healthy dietary patterns and CHD risk with a 20% lower risk for highest vs. lowest adherence. The Western diet globally resulted in a 5% increased CHD risk but in the US cohorts there was a significant 45% increase in CHD risk.

(continued)

Table 2.3 (continued)

Objective	Study details	Results
Sofi et al. (2010) Assess the effect of adherence to the Mediterranean diet (MedDiet) on incidence of chronic diseases [26].	18 cohorts; 2,190,627; follow-up 4 to 20 years.	A 2-point increased adherence to a MedDiet was associated with significant reduction in incidence of CVD by 10% and cancer by 6%.
Chiuve et al. (2012) Evaluate the association between the Alternative Healthy Eating Index-2010 (AHEI-2010) and risk of major chronic diseases (Nurses' Health Study and Health Professionals Follow-Up Study; US) [48].	71,495 women, 26,759 chronic disease events, 24 years of follow-up; 41,029 men. 15,558 chronic disease events, 22 years of follow-up.	The AHEI-2010, which emphasizes high intakes of whole grains, PUFA, nuts, and fish and reductions in red and processed meats, refined grains, and sugar-sweetened beverages, was associated with significantly multivariate lower risk of a composite of major chronic diseases by 19% (p < .001). Risk reduction for specific disease is summarized in Fig. 2.8.

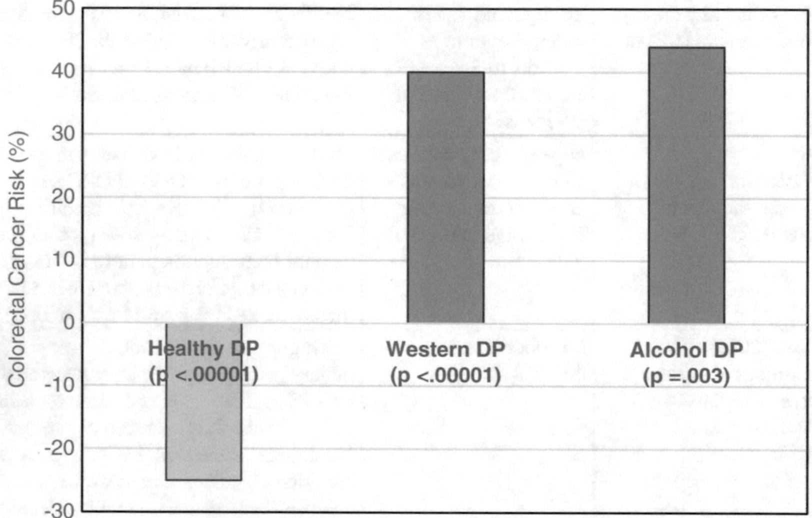

Fig. 2.4 Association between high adherence to dietary pattern (DP) types and colorectal cancer risk from meta-analysis of 40 observational studies (adapted from [44])

(40 studies; 22 cohorts, 17 case-controls and 1 cross-sectional) found that higher adherence to healthy dietary patterns significantly reduced CRC risk by 25% whereas adherence to unhealthy/Western diets increased risk by 40% (both p < .0001; Fig. 2.4) [44]. A meta-analysis (10 cohort studies; 404,528 subjects) showed that high adherence to healthy dietary patterns lowered type 2 diabetes (diabetes) risk by 14% and unhealthy/Western diets increased risk by 30% (Fig. 2.5) [45]. However, subjects that enriched their Western dietary pattern with high phytochemical-rich plant foods reduced their increased diabetes risk from 30 to 6% [45]. For vascular diseases, a meta-analysis (19 cohorts) found that high adherence to healthy dietary patterns reduced incidence of CVD, coronary heart disease (CHD) and stroke compared to Western dietary patterns (Fig. 2.6) [46]. Another meta-analysis (12 cohort studies; 409,780 subjects) reported that healthy patterns lowered CHD risk by 20% and Western patterns increased CHD risk by 5% globally but US participants with the highest adherence to the Western diet had a significant 45% increase in CHD risk [47]. The Reasons for Geographic and Racial Differences in Stroke (REGARDS) prospective study (17,418 subjects; national, population-based, longitudinal study of adults aged ≥45 years; median follow-up of 5.8 years) found that high adherence to

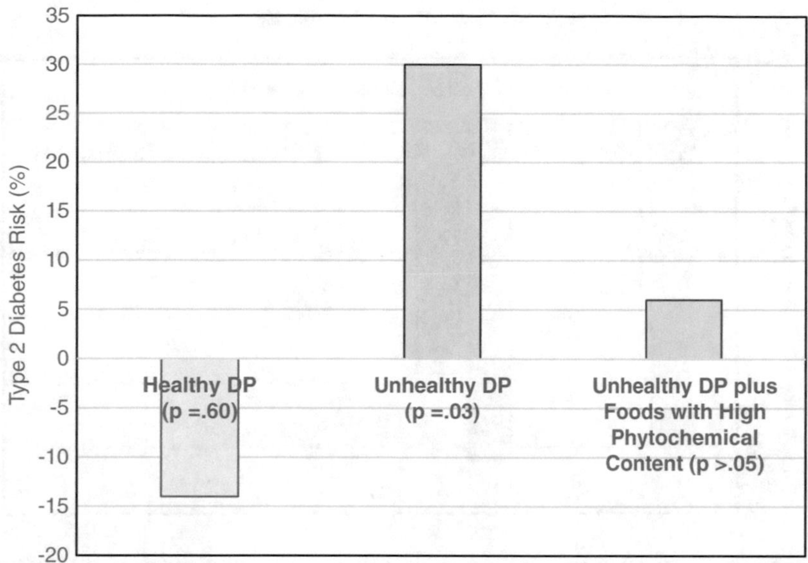

Fig. 2.5 Association between high adherence to dietary patterns (DP) and type 2 diabetes risk from meta-analysis of 10 cohort studies (adapted from [45])

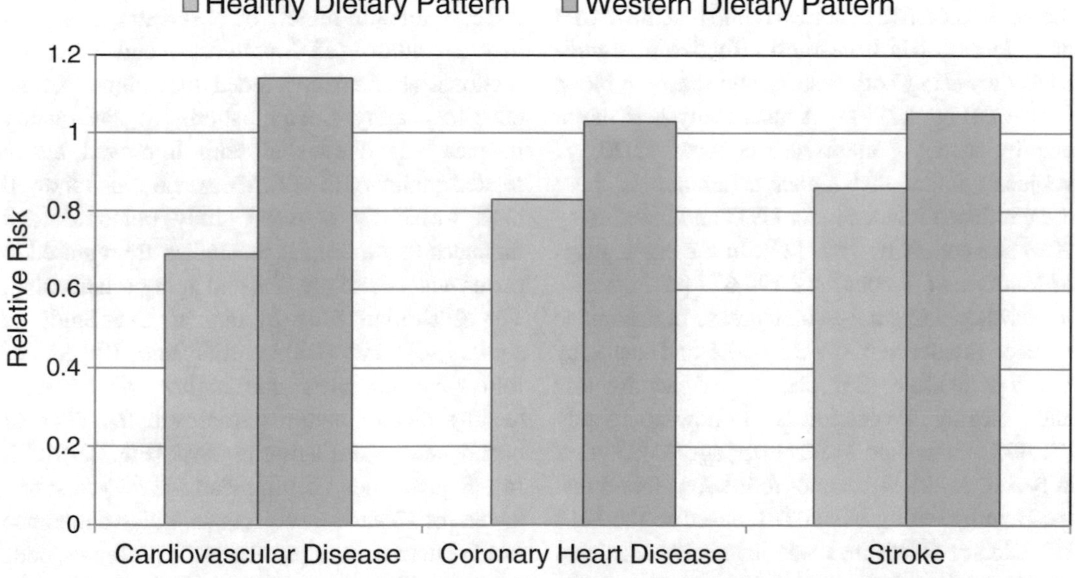

Fig. 2.6 Association between dietary patterns quality and vascular chronic disease incidence risk from a meta-analysis of 19 cohort studies (adapted from [46]

the US Southern dietary pattern (characterized by added fats, fried food, eggs, organ and processed meats, and sugar-sweetened beverages) significantly increased risk of acute CHD by 36% compared to low adherence (or a healthier diet) [49].

2.2.2.2 Healthy Dietary Patterns Adherence

Four meta-analyses consistently found that increased adherence to a range of healthy dietary patterns significantly reduced incidence rates of CVD, coronary heart disease (CHD) and cancer

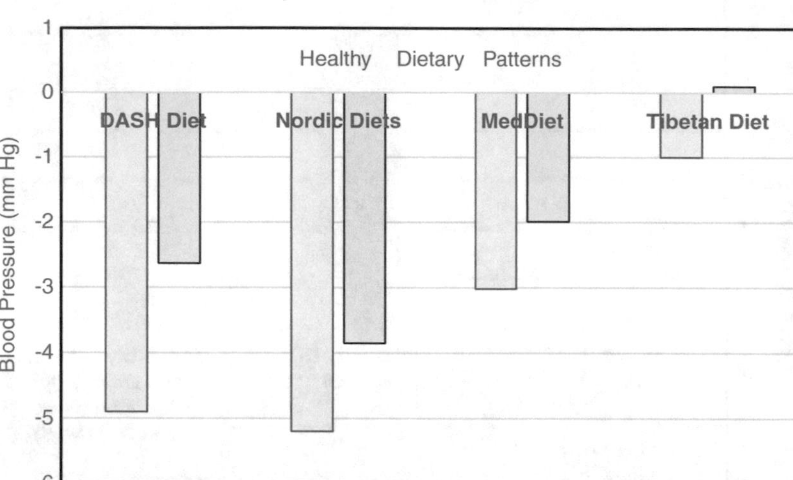

Fig. 2.7 Effect of dietary pattern (DP) type on lowering blood pressure from a meta-analysis of 17 RCTs (adapted from [43])

[22, 26, 43, 48]. A meta-analysis on four healthy diets (17 RCTs; 5014 adults) found that the DASH and Nordic diets were most effective in significantly lowering both systolic and diastolic blood pressure (Fig. 2.7) [43]. A meta-analysis of major healthy dietary patterns (15 cohorts; 1,020,642 subjects) found that higher adherence to these diets reduced incidence for CVD and diabetes by 22% and cancer by 15% [22]. In a meta-analysis of MedDiets (18 cohorts; 2,190,627 participants), it was shown that a 2-point increase in adherence reduced incidence of CVD by 10% and cancer by 6% (9 point scale) [26]. The Nurses' Health Study and Health Professionals Follow-up Study (71,495 women and 41,029 men; age 30–75 years at baseline; 22–24 years of follow-up) found that the Healthy Eating Index-2010 based on the 2010 US Dietary Guidelines was inversely associated with the risk of CVD, stroke, diabetes, and cancer (Fig. 2.8) [48].

2.2.3 Healthy Aging and Physical Function (Frailty)

One systematic review of observational studies and seven cohort studies on the effects of dietary patterns on general health and physical function are summarized in Table 2.4 [2, 27, 50–55]. A 2016 systematic review of observational studies in older adults (23 longitudinal and 11 cross-sectional studies) concluded that higher adherence to healthy dietary patterns or diet quality indexes was associated with improved health related quality of life [2]. This review also showed high variability between study outcomes and indicated that more, larger studies are required to better understand the diet and aging relationship. The Australian Blue Mountains Eye Study in adults ≥49 years (1609 participants; 10 years of follow-up) observed that higher adherence to healthy dietary patterns improved the odds of healthy/successful aging by 58% (Fig. 2.9) [27]. In a French study (2796; mean age 52 years; followed for 13 years), subjects with high adherence to a Western dietary pattern had 17% higher odds for unhealthy aging compared to significantly better healthy aging odds by 46% for a moderate energy healthy dietary pattern (Fig. 2.10) [52]. In a study of older adults (1872 subjects; mean age 69 years; 3.5 years of follow-up), those consuming a healthy dietary pattern had an inverse relationship with the risk of frailty and those consuming a Westernized pattern had an increased frailty risk by 61% (Fig. 2.11) [53]. The British Whitehall II study (5350 adults; mean age at

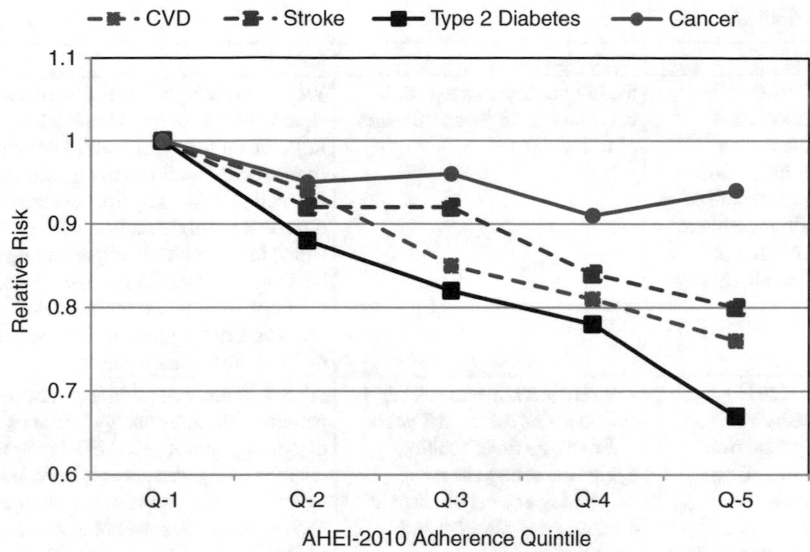

Fig. 2.8 Association between 2010 Alternative Healthy Eating Index (AHEI-2010) and chronic disease risk from the pooled analysis of the Nurses' Health Study and Health Professionals Follow-Up Study (p-trend <.001; for all except cancer with p-trend = .003; multivariate adjusted) (adapted from [48])

Table 2.4 Summary of dietary patterns studies on healthy aging and physical function (frailty)

Objective	Study details	Results
Systematic reviews		
Milte et al. (2016) Examine dietary patterns and quality of life, physical function, cognitive function and mental health among older adults [2].	11 cross-sectional and 23 longitudinal studies.	In older adults, this analysis found that higher adherence to healthy dietary patterns or diet quality indexes was associated with improved health related quality of life. This review also showed high variability between study outcomes and indicated that more larger studies are required to better understand the diet and aging relationship.
Prospective studies		
Pilleron et al. (2017) Analyze the association of dietary patterns and frailty in community-dwelling elderly (France) [50].	972 initially non-frail and nondemented participants; 336 men and 636 women; average baseline age 73 years; 12-year follow-up; 78 men and 221 women became frail.	Men in the 'pasta' pattern and women in the 'biscuits and snacking' pattern had a significant 2-fold higher risk of frailty compared to those in the 'healthy' pattern (p = .09 for men and p = 1.3 for women). Men had a 3-fold greater risk for muscle weakness with the 'biscuit and snacking' pattern vs. the healthy pattern (p = .003).
Gopinath et al. (2016) Examine the relationship between overall diet quality (reflecting adherence to dietary guidelines) and mortality and successful aging in older adults (Blue Mountains Eye Study; Australia) [27].	1609 healthy adults; baseline aged ≥49 years; 10 years of follow-up; 610 (37.9%) died; 249 (15.5%) aged successfully.	High adherence to healthy dietary guidelines resulted in 58% higher odds of successful aging after 10 years compared to poor adherence to guidelines (Fig. 2.9). Adherence to recommended dietary guidelines significantly increases the probability of reaching old age disease free and fully functional.

(continued)

Table 2.4 (continued)

Objective	Study details	Results
Hagan et al. (2016) Examine the association between the Alternative Healthy Eating Index-2010 (AHEI-2010), a measure of diet quality, with impairment in physical function with aging (Nurses' Health Study; US) [51].	54,762 healthy women; mean baseline age 56 years; 18 years of follow-up.	Women with higher AHEI-2010 scores were significantly13% less likely to have physical impairment than those with low scores (multivariable-adjusted). Further, significantly reduced physical impairments were also observed for higher intake of vegetables and fruits; lower intake of sugar sweetened beverages and sodium intake. The strongest relations were found for increased intake of oranges, orange juice, apples and pears, romaine or leaf lettuce, and walnuts.
Assmann et al. (2015) Investigate healthy vs. Western dietary patterns in midlife on healthy aging (SUpplementation en Vitamines et Mineraux AntioXydants Study; France) [52].	2796 subjects; mean baseline age 52 years; mean 13.2 years of follow-up time; healthy aging was defined as not developing any major chronic disease, good physical and cognitive function, no limitations in activities of daily living, no depressive symptoms, no health-related limitations in social life, good overall self-perceived health, and no function-limiting pain over 13 years of follow-up.	High adherence at midlife to a healthy dietary pattern with lower energy intake (≤ 2500 kcal/day in men and ≤1820 kcal/day in women) resulted in significantly higher odds of healthy aging by 46% compared to those consuming above the energy thresholds who had only an insignificant 7% improved odds of healthy aging (Fig. 2.10). Those consuming a Western diet in midlife had 17% lower odds of healthy aging (highest vs. lowest adherence), which was insignificant after adjusting for potential confounders.
Leon-Munoz et al. (2015) Study the association of healthy vs. Western dietary patterns on frailty risk in older adults (Spanish Seniors-ENRICA cohort) [53].	1872 free-living adults; mean baseline age 70 years; 50% women; 3.5 years of follow-up.	High adherence to a healthy dietary pattern had significantly lower risk of frailty by 60% compared to high adherence to a Western pattern, which increased risk by 61% (Fig. 2.11).
Samieri et al. (2013) Explore the relation of dietary patterns in midlife to the prevalence of healthy aging; no major chronic diseases or cognitive, physical function or mental health impairments (Nurses' Health Study; US) [54].	10,670 women; median baseline age 59 years; Alternative Healthy Eating Index-2010 (AHEI-2010) and Alternate MedDiet scores; average 15 years of follow-up; healthy aging was based on survival to 70+ years.	Higher midlife adherence to healthy dietary patterns significantly improved the multivariate odds for healthy aging: AHEI-2010 improved odds by 34% and the alternative MedDiet improved odds by 46%.
Akbaraly et al. (2013) Assess the effects of the healthy (Alternative healthy eating index [AHEI]) pattern vs. the Western pattern on healthy aging (Whitehall II study; UK) [55].	5350 healthy adults; mean baseline age 51 years; 29% women; mean 16 years of follow-up; participants were screened every 5 years for ideal aging, composite of metabolic, cardiovascular, musculoskeletal, respiratory, mental, and cognitive functions.	Subjects adhering to the Western pattern (characterized by high intakes of fried and sweet food, processed food and red meat, refined grains, and high-fat dairy products) had a significant 42% lower odds of ideal aging (for top vs. bottom tertile), independently of other health behaviors. The healthy diet improved trend for ideal aging odds by 8% (Fig. 2.12).

51 years; 29% women; mean 16 years of follow-up) showed that high adherence to a Western pattern at mid-life significantly lowered the odds of ideal aging by 42% and high adherence to a healthy pattern directionally improved the odds of ideal aging by 7% (Fig. 2.12) [55]. Two Nurses' Health Studies showed that high adherence to healthy dietary patterns in midlife significantly

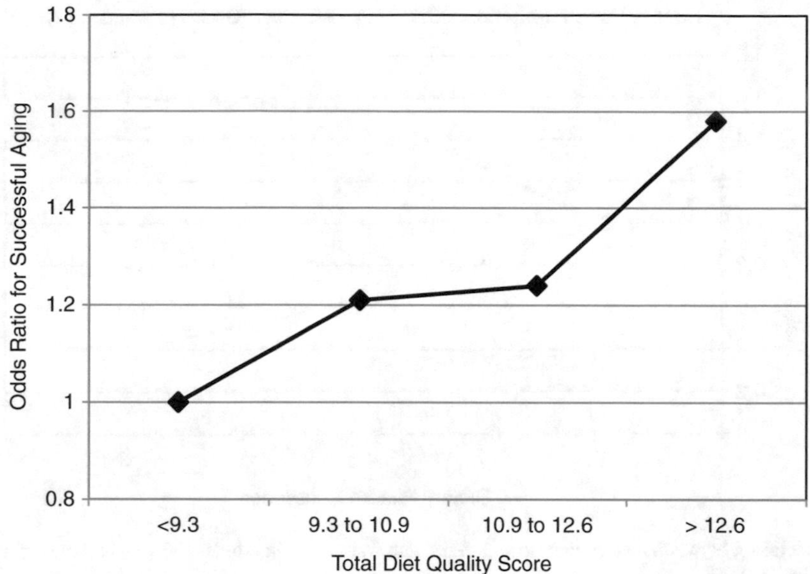

Fig. 2.9 Association between total diet quality score on odds of successful aging (adapted from [27])

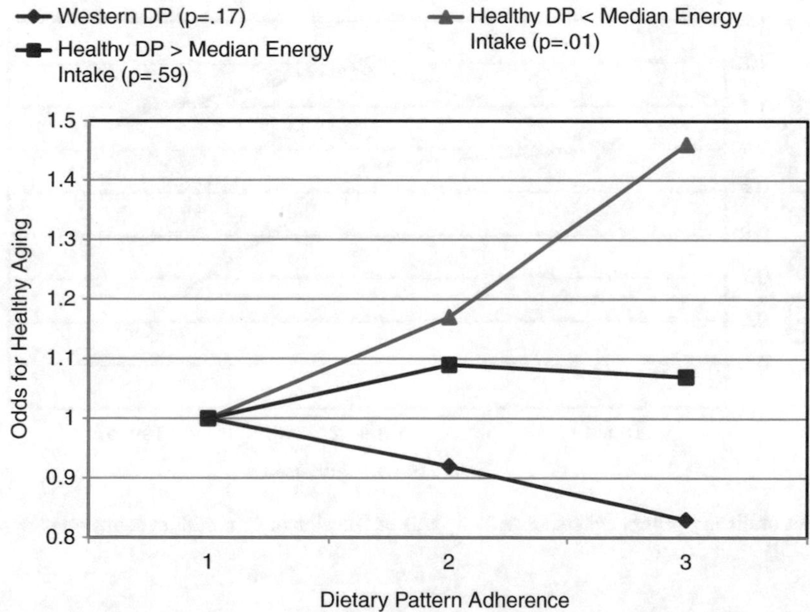

Fig. 2.10 Association between healthy dietary patterns (DP), stratified by energy median intake level, compared to a Western DP and the odds for healthy aging (multivariate adjusted; median energy intake 2500 kcal/day for men and 1820 kcal for women) (adapted from [52])

reduced multivariate risk of physical impairment by 13% (with increased fruits and vegetables being beneficial and increased sugar sweetened beverage and sodium being detrimental) [51] and significantly improved the multivariate odds for overall healthy aging by 34–46% [54]. A 2017 French cohort (972 healthy subjects (336 men and 636 women); mean baseline age 73 years; 12 years of follow-up) found that a dietary pattern characterized as high biscuits and snacking

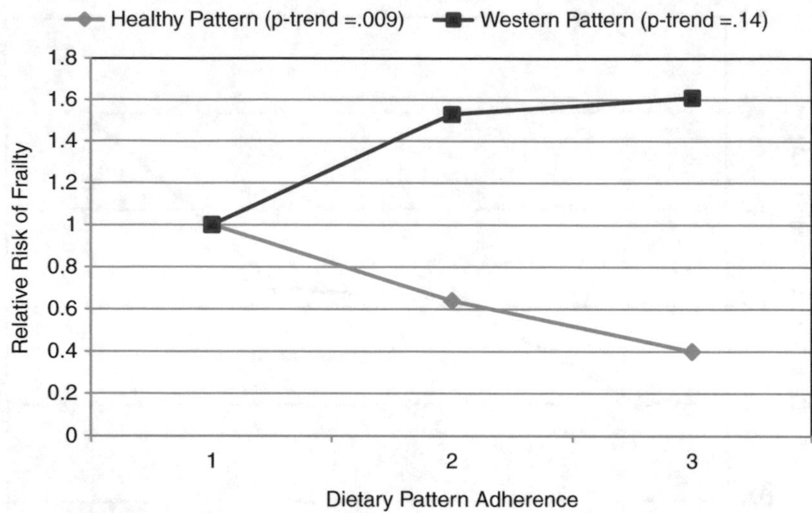

Fig. 2.11 Association between dietary pattern adherence and frailty risk in adults ≥60 years after a 3.5 years of follow-up (adapted from [53])

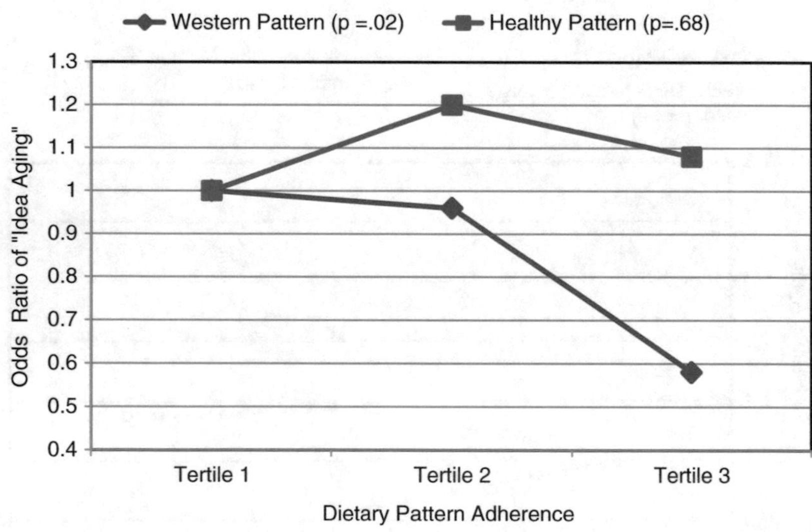

Fig. 2.12 Effect of dietary pattern adherence and the odds of "ideal aging" in midlife adults after 13-year follow-up (adapted from [55])

increased the risk of becoming frail by twofold in men and women and significantly increased the risk of muscle weakness in men [50].

2.2.4 Age-Related Cognitive Function and Dementia

Three meta-analyses, eight cohort studies, one large cross-sectional study and two RCTs provide important insights on the effects of dietary patterns and age-related cognitive performance and Alzheimer's disease (Table 2.5) [26, 56–68].

2.2.4.1 Mediterranean Diet (MedDiet)

The protective effects of the MedDiet on age-related cognitive decline and Alzheimer disease risk have been extensively investigated [26, 56–59, 64, 67, 68]. Three meta-analyses concluded that the high adherence to a MedDiet can significantly improve age-related cognitive performance and reduce Alzheimer's disease risk

Table 2.5 Summary of dietary pattern studies on age-related cognitive performance and Alzheimer's disease risk

Objective	Study details	Results
Systematic reviews and meta-analyses		
Wu and Sun (2017) Evaluate the association and dose-response of the MedDiet on cognitive function [56].	9 cohort studies; 34,168 participants; baseline age ≥ 45 years (45–98 years); 2–12 years of follow-up.	Compared with the lowest category, the pooled analysis showed that the highest MedDiet scores were inversely associated with the developing of cognitive disorders by 21%. Subgroup analysis showed that the MedDiet was inversely associated with mild cognitive impairment by 17% and Alzheimer's disease by 40% (Fig. 2.13).
Singh et al. (2014) Determine whether there is an association between the Mediterranean diet (MedDiet) and risk of cognitive impairment (57).	6 cohorts; 8019 subjects, mean baseline age mid-70s; cognitively normal; follow-up of 4–8 years.	Subjects in the highest MedDiet tertile had significantly lower adjusted risk of cognitive impairment by 33% as compared to the lowest tertile. Among cognitively normal individuals, higher adherence to the MedDiet was associated with significantly reduced risk of mild cognitive impairment by 27% and Alzheimer's disease by 36%.
Sofi et al. (2010) Assess the effect of adherence to the MedDiet on neurodegenerative diseases [26].	18 cohorts; 2,190,627 follow-up of 4 to 20 years.	A 2-point increase in adherence to the MedDiet was associated with a significant reduction in neurodegenerative diseases by 13%.
Prospective studies		
Haring et al. (2016) Determine the effect of dietary patterns on cognitive function in older women (Women's Health Initiative Memory Study; Germany) [58].	6425 postmenopausal women; baseline age 65 to 79 years; alternate MedDiet score, HEI-2010), the AHEI-2010, or DASH diet score; median follow-up of 9.1 years; 499 cases of mild cognitive impairment and 390 probable dementia cases.	There was no significant relationship between the adherence to a healthy dietary pattern and cognitive function, especially in women with hypertension.
Galbete et al. (2015) Evaluate the effect of adherence to the MedDiet on cognitive function (Spanish) [59].	823 participants; mean age 62 years; 6 to 8 years of follow-up.	Although high MedDiet adherence was associated with a small decline (−0.6 units) in cognitive function, there was a significantly slower rate of cognitive decline compared to those with low or moderate MedDiet adherence.
Jacka et al. (2015) Examine the association between dietary patterns and hippocampal volume in humans (Personality and Total Health Through Life project; Australian) [60].	255 healthy adults; mean baseline age 63 years; follow-up of 4 years.	Increased adherence to a healthy dietary pattern was associated with a larger left hippocampal volume, while higher adherence to an unhealthy Western dietary pattern was (independently) associated with a smaller left hippocampal volume (Fig. 2.14). These relationships were independent of covariates including age, gender, education, labor-force status, depressive symptoms and medication, physical activity, smoking, hypertension and diabetes.

(continued)

Table 2.5 (continued)

Objective	Study details	Results
Shakersaina et al. (2015) Assess the association between dietary patterns and cognitive changes with aging (Swedish National study on Aging and Care-Kungsholmen) [61].	2223 healthy participants; mean baseline age 71 years; 39% men; 6-years of follow-up.	Higher adherence to the Western dietary pattern was associated with a higher mini-mental state examination (cognitive) decline than the lowest adherence to this pattern. In contrast, higher adherence to a healthy dietary pattern was inversely associated with cognitive decline.
Tsai (2015) Examine the effect of dietary patterns on cognitive decline in older Taiwanese (Taiwan Longitudinal Study of Aging [62].	1926 Chinese men and 1744 Chinese women; baseline age > 65 years; 8 years of follow-up.	A Western dietary pattern was positively associated with an 8-fold increased risk of cognitive decline over 8 years (adjusted), whereas traditional and healthy dietary patterns were not. Diets rich in meats and infrequent consumption of fish, beans/legumes, vegetables and fruits may adversely affect cognitive function in older Taiwanese.
Gardener (2015) Investigate the association of three well-recognised dietary patterns with cognitive change (Australian Imaging, Biomarkers and Lifestyle study of Ageing) [63].	527 subjects; mean baseline age 69 years; 40% male; 3 years of follow-up.	Of the diets, higher adherence to the MedDiet was significantly associated after 36 months with better performance in the executive function in apolipoprotein E (APOE) ε4 allele carriers compared to higher Western diet adherence, which was significantly associated with greater cognitive decline.
Tangney et al. (2014) Estimate the effects of DASH and MedDiet on age-related cognitive function (US Memory and Aging Project) [64].	826 participants; mean baseline age 81.5 years; 26% men; 4.1 years of follow-up.	The subject mean global cognitive score at baseline was 0.08 units. Adherence to the DASH and MedDiets significantly slowed the rate of global cognitive decline by 0.002 to 0.007 units, which is equivalent to between 1.3 and 4.4 years of younger brain age.
Ozawa et al. (2013). Investigate the effect of dietary patterns on risk of dementia in older Japanese (Hisayama Study) [65].	1006 healthy community-dwelling Japanese subjects; baseline age 60–79 years; median follow-up of 15 years; 144 Alzheimer disease cases, 88 vascular dementia cases.	A dietary pattern with high intakes of soybeans and soybean products, vegetables, seaweed, milk and dairy products and a low intake of rice was associated with 35% lower risk of Alzheimer's disease and a 55% lower risk of vascular dementia.
Cross-sectional study		
Pearson et al. (2016) Evaluate associations between empirically derived dietary patterns and cognitive function in the Southeast USA known as the stroke belt. (Reasons for Geographic and Racial Differences in Stroke (REGARDS) cohort; US) [66].	18,080 black and white subjects; baseline age ≥ 49 years.	Dietary patterns including plant-based foods were associated with higher cognitive scores and reduced risk of cognitive impairment, and a pattern including fried food and processed meat typical of a southern diet was associated with lower scores and significantly increased risk of cognitive impairment (Fig. 2.15).

Table 2.5 (continued)

Objective	Study details	Results
RCTs		
Valls-Pedret et al. (2015) Investigate the effect of MedDiet on the decline of cognitive function in older adults (PREDIMED trial; Spain) [67].	**Parallel RCT:** 447 cognitively healthy volunteers with high CVD risk; mean baseline age 67 years; 51% women; randomly assigned to a MedDiet supplemented with extra-virgin olive oil (1 L/week) or mixed nuts (30 g/day) vs. a control diet (advice to reduce dietary fat); median of 4.1 years.	The MedDiet supplemented with olive oil or mixed nuts was associated with significantly improved cognitive function. Compared with the low-fat control diets, MedDiet + nuts improved memory (p = 0.04) and MedDiet + olive oil improved frontal and global cognition.
Martinez-Lapiscina et al. (2013) Assess effects of MedDiets on cognitive function (PREDIMED-NAVARRA; Spain) [68].	**Parallel RCT:** 522 participants at high vascular risk; mean baseline age 75 years; 45% men; randomly assigned to a MedDiet supplemented with extra-virgin olive oil (1 L/week) or mixed nuts (30 g/day) vs. a control diet (advice to reduce dietary fat); 6.5 years of follow-up.	The MedDiet supplemented with olive oil or mixed nuts significantly enhanced cognitive function as measured by mini-mental state exam and clock draw test vs. a low-fat diet.

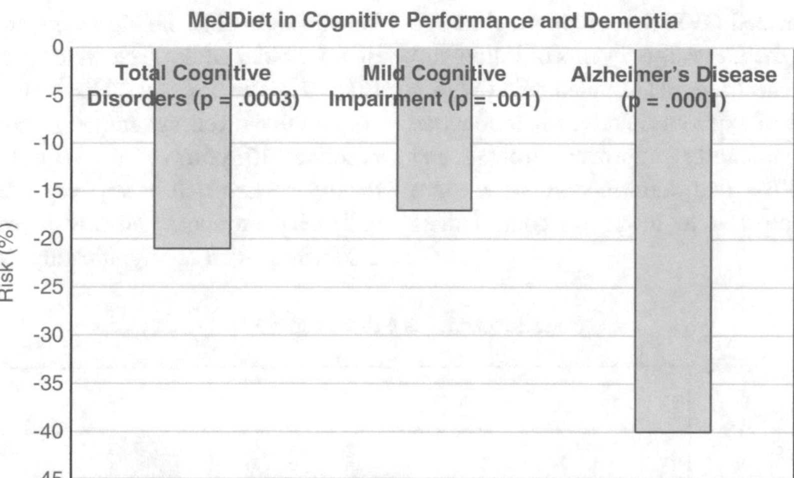

Fig. 2.13 Association between high adherence to the Mediterranean diet (MedDiet) and risk of developing cognitive disorders in adults (≥45 years) from a meta-analysis of 9 cohort studies (adapted from [56])

[56–58]. A 2017 meta-analysis (9 cohort studies; 34,169 subjects; baseline age >45 years; 2–12 years of follow-up) found that high adherence to a MedDiet significantly lowered multivariate age-related mild cognitive impairment by 17% and risk of Alzheimer's disease by 40% (Fig. 2.13) [56]. Also, a 2014 meta-analysis (6 cohorts; 8019 subjects; 4–8 years of follow-up) showed that high adherence to the MedDiet significantly reduced multivariate age-related cognitive decline by 27% and Alzheimer's disease risk by 36% [57]. A 2010 meta-analysis (18 cohorts; 2,190,627 subjects; 4 to 20 years of follow-up) demonstrated a 13% reduction in neurodegenerative diseases for each 2-point improved adherence to the MedDiet [26]. The effect of the MedDiet on cognitive performance appears to vary with the type of MedDiet guidance and/or traditional dietary culture and food availability; as the German Women's Health Initiative Memory Study (6425 postmenopausal women; baseline age 65–79 years; 9.1 years of follow-up) found no significant effect of the aMedDiet on slowing cognitive decline, especially in women with hypertension [58] compared to Spanish prospective cohort (823 subjects; mean baseline age 62 year, 6–8 years follow-up) which showed a high adherence to a more traditional MedDiet and culture resulted in a significantly slower rate of cognitive decline compared to low or moderate adherence [59]. The US Memory and Aging Project cohort of elderly adults (826 participants; mean baseline age 81.5 years; 4.1 years of follow-up) demonstrated that high adherence to the DASH or MedDiets significantly slowed the rate of cognitive decline by 1.3–4.4 years [64]. Two Spanish PREDIMED trials in older adults (447–522 subjects with elevated CVD risk; mean baseline age 67–75 years; median 4.1–6.5 years of follow-up) showed that the MedDiet supplemented with a liter per week of extra virgin olive oil or 30 g tree nuts/day significantly improved frontal and global cognitive and mini-mental state exam measures compared to lower fat control diets [67, 68].

2.2.4.2 Western vs. Healthy Diets

Six observational studies consistently support the adverse effects of Western dietary patterns and the beneficial effects of healthy or traditional dietary patterns in protecting against age related cognitive decline [60–63, 65, 66]. An Australian longitudinal investigation of older adults (255 subjects; aged 60–64 years at baseline; 4 years of follow-up) showed that persons with a high adherence to unhealthy diets or moderate adherence to healthy diets had significantly smaller left hippocampal volumes than those with high adherence to healthy diets (Fig. 2.14) [60]. Another Australian study (527 subjects with apolipoprotein E (APOE) ε4 allele; mean baseline age 69 years; 3 years of follow-up) suggested that high adherence to the MedDiet significantly improved cognitive performance compared to high adherence to the Western dietary pattern [63]. Two cohort studies from Sweden and Taiwan show that the high adherence to Western diets by older adults accelerates cognitive decline [61, 62]. The Japanese Hisayama Study (1006 community-dwelling subjects; 60–79 years at baseline; 15 years of follow-up) found that a dietary pattern rich in soy, vegetables, seaweed, and dairy products and low in white rice was associated with a significantly lower risk of

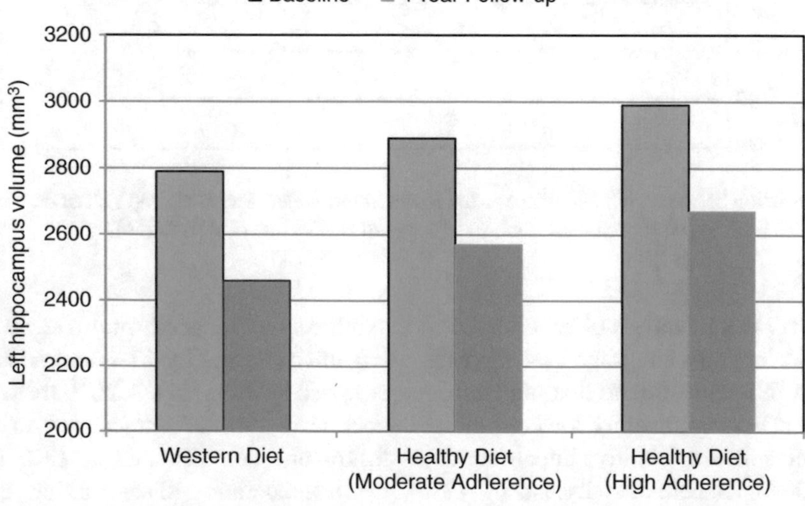

Fig. 2.14 Association between dietary pattern and left hippocampus volume in adults aged 60–64 years at baseline ($p = 0.008$ high healthy diet adherence vs. other diets) (adapted from [60])

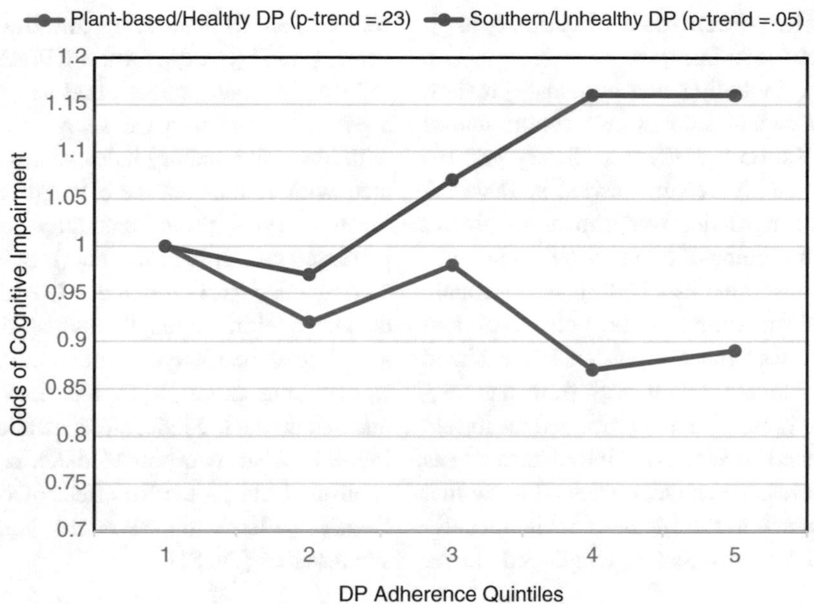

Fig. 2.15 Association between dietary pattern (DP) type and odds of cognitive impairment from the Reasons for Geographic and Racial Differences in Stroke (REGARDS) cohort (adapted from [66])

Alzheimer's disease by 35% and vascular dementia by 55% [65]. A large cross-sectional analysis of the US REGARDS cohort (18,080 black and white subjects; age $\geq$ 49 years) showed that high adherence to a healthy plant based diet improved cognitive function, and Southern diets rich in fried foods and processed meats, lowered cognitive function (Fig. 2.15) [66].

2.2.5 Telomere Length (Cellular Senescence)

2.2.5.1 Overview of Telomere Length and Aging

The shortening of telomeres destabilizes the genome, leading to cell senescence, accelerated aging and potential increased chronic disease risk [16]. Telomere length is independent of chronological age as it appears to be influenced by modifiable factors, such as lifestyle variables including diet, adiposity, and physical exercise. There is some limited human evidence that diet can influence telomere length with antioxidant and fiber-rich, plant based diets and whole foods helping to maintain telomere length compared to the intake of saturated fat, refined flour cereals, meat and meat products, and sugar-sweetened beverages which are associated with shorter telomeres. Being overweight and obese appears to accelerate the telomere shortening process whereas weight loss or maintaining a healthy weight slows the telomere shortening process [69–71]. Individuals from two Danish prospective cohort studies: The Copenhagen City Heart Study and the Copenhagen General Population Study found that short telomeres in peripheral blood leukocytes were associated with increased mortality risk by 40% for individuals in the shortest vs. the longest decile of telomere length [72]. A meta-analysis (24 studies; 43,725 participants) found a 54% increased CHD risk for those subjects with the shortest versus the longest leukocyte telomere lengths in the general population, independently of conventional vascular risk factors [73]. A meta-analysis of three prospective studies found that shorter leukocyte telomere length is independently associated with an increased pooled risk of diabetes incidence by 31% [74].

2.2.5.2 Dietary Patterns and Leukocyte Telomere Length

Nine studies, including one systematic review, four cross-sectional studies, two cohort studies and two RCTs, on the effect of dietary patterns on telomere length are summarized in Table 2.6 [75–83]. The MedDiet was shown to protect against the shortening of telomere length in seven of nine of these studies [77–82]. A systematic review (17 observational studies) concluded that the MedDiet was most consistently associated with longer telomere length with fruits and vegetables being protective and processed meats and sugar sweetened beverages having adverse effects [75]. Three cross-sectional studies all show that higher adherence to the MedDiet is significantly protective of longer telomere length and slower cellular senescence during mid-life and elderly years [76–78]. A Spanish PREDIMED cohort (520 participants; mean baseline age 67 years; 5 years of follow-up) observed that MedDiets with low inflammatory index scores were associated with longer telomere length compared to Western type proinflammatory diets, which increased risk of telomere shorting by 80% [80]. Two Spanish RCTs found that MedDiets are protective of telomere length compared to lower fat and higher carbohydrate diets, especially in women, but more RCTs are needed to better understand the MedDiet effect on telomere length [82, 83]. Also, two non-MedDiet cohort studies confirmed the protective effect of other healthy dietary patterns on telomere length vs. the Western diet [79, 81].

Table 2.6 Summary of studies on dietary patterns and telomere length (TL)

Objective	Study details	Results
Systematic review		
Rafie et al. (2017) Evaluate the effect of dietary pattern and foods on TL [75].	1 cohort, 3 case-control, and 13 cross-sectional studies; 56 to 5862 subjects.	This review concluded that high MedDiet adherence was associated with longer TL. Fruit and vegetable intake was more positively associated with TL than other dietary factors. Also, processed meat and sugar-sweetened beverages appear to be associated with shorter TL.
Cross-sectional studies		
Gu et al. (2015) Examine the relation between MedDiet and leukocyte TL (The Washington Heights-Inwood Community Aging Project study; US) [76].	1743 multi-ethnic community residents of New York; mean age 78 years; 68% female.	In elderly subjects, higher adherence to a MedDiet was associated with longer leukocyte TL among whites compared to blacks and Hispanics.
Crous-Bou et al. (2014) Examine whether adherence to the MedDiet was associated with longer TL, a biomarker of aging (Nurses' Health Study; US) [77].	4676 healthy middle aged and older women; mean age 59 years.	Greater adherence to the MedDiet was associated with longer telomeres after adjustment for potential confounders. Least squares mean TL z scores were −0.038 for the lowest MedDiet score groups and 0.072 for the highest score group (p-trend = 0.004).
Boccardi et al. (2013) Assess the effect of adherence to the MedDiet on TL and telomerase activity (Sothern Italy) [78].	217 elderly subjects; mean 78 years; stratified according to MedDiet score in low adherence, medium adherence and high adherence groups.	The high adherence MedDiet group was associated with significantly longer leukocyte TL, and higher telomerase activity compared to lower adherence.

Table 2.6 (continued)

Objective	Study details	Results
Sun et al. (2012). Examine healthy lifestyle practices on leukocyte TL (US Nurses' Health Study) [79].	5862 women; mean age 57 years.	High adherence to a healthy lifestyle, such as healthy diet and physical activity, was associated with longer TL in leukocytes.
Prospective studies		
Garcia-Calzon et al. (2015) Examine if inflammation is associated with telomere attrition rate (PREDIMED-NAVARRA; Spain) [80].	520 participants at high CVD risk; mean baseline age 67 years; 45% males; 5 years of follow-up.	MedDiets with low dietary inflammatory index scores were inversely associated with leukocyte TL in older adults at high risk of CVD. Less healthy high proinflammatory diets were associated with an 80% higher risk of shorter TL.
Lee et al. (2015). Determine the association between dietary patterns or consumption of specific foods and leukocyte TL in adults (Korean Genome Epidemiology Study) [81].	1958 subjects; baseline age 40 to >60 years; 10 years of follow-up.	Healthy dietary patterns including whole grains, seafood, legumes, vegetables and seaweed were associated with longer leukocyte TL. In contrast, Western dietary patterns, especially rich in red meat or processed meat and sweetened carbonated beverages, were associated with shorter TL.
RCTs		
Garcia-Calzon et al. (2016). Assess the effect of MedDiets on TL in older adults at increased risk of CVD (Spain- PREDIMED-NAVARRA trial) [82].	**Parallel RCT:** 520 participants; mean age 67 years; 55% women; randomly assigned to 3 diets: a low-fat control or one of 2 MedDiets, one supplemented with extra virgin olive oil and the other with mixed nuts; 5 years.	Better adherence to MedDiets was associated with significantly longer basal telomeres in women but not in men.
Marin et al. (2012). Evaluate the effect of dietary patterns on cellular senescence (Spain) [83].	**Crossover RCT** 20 subjects; ≥ 65 years; 10 males and 10 females; saturated fatty acid diet, a lower-fat diet, higher-carbohydrate diets, and MedDiet; each for 4 weeks.	MedDiet significantly protected against endothelial cell senescence as shown by lower intracellular oxidative stress, less shortening of telomeres, and lower apoptosis compared to lower-fat and higher-carbohydrate diets.

Conclusions

In the US and worldwide, high rates of Western diets and sedentary lifestyle habits, especially since the 1980s have led to pandemic rates of obesity, non-alcoholic fatty liver disease, metabolic syndrome, type-2 diabetes, chronic kidney disease, and other related health conditions associated with unhealthy aging. Dietary pattern habits have a significant effect on aging, chronic disease risk, and longevity but in developed countries like the US mean diet quality scores are only about half of the optimal healthy eating diet score. Healthy dietary patterns include adequate whole-grain cereals, legumes, fruits, vegetables, and nuts, and lower intakes of red and processed meats and sugar-sweetened beverages. Prospective cohort studies with middle and older age adults consistently show that high adherence to Western dietary patterns increases CVD, diabetes and cancer, and premature death risks whereas high adherence to healthy/plant-based dietary patterns lower CVD, diabetes and cancer risk, and premature mortality risk. Among cancer survivors, healthy diets are associated with reduced overall mortality risk by 20% and Western diets are associated with increased risk by over 40%. For older adults, higher adherence to healthy dietary patterns reduces the odds of unhealthy aging and frailty whereas higher adherence to Western diets increases the odds. Simple dietary rules for healthy aging are to limit the intake of energy dense, low nutrient quality foods, red and processed meats and added salt and sugar, and increase the intake of fiber, and nutrient and phytochemical-rich whole or minimally processed plant foods. Healthy dietary patterns, especially the Mediterranean diet, are associated with reduced age-related decline in cognitive performance and Alzheimer's disease, and longer telomere length compared to Western diets. High adherence to healthy dietary patterns support healthy aging and reduce chronic disease and mortality risk through beneficial effects on body weight regulation and adiposity metabolism, lipoprotein concentrations and function, blood pressure, glucose-insulin homeostasis, oxidative stress, inflammation, endothelial health, hepatic function, cardiac and cognitive function, telomere length, and the microbiota ecosystem.

Appendix A: Comparison of Western and Healthy Dietary Patterns per 2000 kcal (Approximated Values)

Components	Western dietary pattern (US)	USDA Base pattern	DASH diet pattern	Healthy Mediterranean pattern	Healthy vegetarian pattern (Lact-ovo based)	Vegan pattern
Emphasizes	Refined grains, low fiber foods, red meats, sweets and solid fats	Vegetables, fruit, whole-grain, and low-fat milk	Potassium rich vegetables, fruits, and low fat milk products	Whole grains, vegetables, fruit, dairy products, olive oil, and moderate wine	Vegetables, fruit, whole-grains, legumes, nuts, seeds, milk products, and soy foods	Plant foods: Vegetables, fruits, whole grains, nuts, seeds, and soy foods
Includes	Processed meats, sugar sweetened beverages, and fast foods	Enriched grains, lean meat, fish, nuts, seeds, and vegetable oils	Whole-grain, poultry, fish, nuts, and seeds	Fish, nuts, seeds, and pulses	Eggs, non-dairy milk alternatives, and vegetable oils	Non-dairy milk alternatives
Limits	Fruits and vegetables, and whole-grains	Solid fats and added sugars	Red meats, sweets, and sugar-sweetened beverages	Red meats, refined grains, and sweets	No red or white meats, or fish; limited sweets	No animal products
Estimated nutrients/components						
Carbohydrates (% Total kcal)	51	51	55	50	54	57
Protein (% Total kcal)	16	17	18	16	14	13
Total fat (% Total kcal)	33	32	27	34	32	30

(continued)

Components	Western dietary pattern (US)	USDA Base pattern	DASH diet pattern	Healthy Mediterranean pattern	Healthy vegetarian pattern (Lact-ovo based)	Vegan pattern
Saturated fat (% Total kcal)	11	8	6	8	8	7
Unsat. Fat (% Total kcal)	22	25	21	24	26	25
Fiber (g)	16	31	29+	31	35+	40+
Potassium (mg)	2800	3350	4400	3350	3300	3650
Vegetable oils (g)	19	27	25	27	19–27	18–27
Sodium (mg)	3600	1790	1100	1690	1400	1225
Added sugar (g)	79 (20 tsp.)	32 (8 tsp.)	12 (3 tsp.)	32 (8 tsp.)	32 (8 tsp.)	32 (8 tsp.)
Plant food groups						
Fruit (cup)	≤ 1.0	2.0	2.5	2.5	2.0	2.0
Vegetables (cup)	≤ 1.5	2.5	2.1	2.5	2.5	2.5
Whole-grains (oz.)	0.6	3.0	4.0	3.0	3.0	3.0
Legumes (oz.)	–	1.5	0.5	1.5	3.0	3.0+
Nuts/seeds (oz.)	0.5	0.6	1.0	0.6	1.0	2.0
Soy products (oz.)	0.0	0.5	–	–	1.1	1.5

U.S. Department of Agriculture, Agriculture Research Service, Nutrient Data Laboratory. 2014. USDA National Nutrient Database for Standard Reference, Release 27. https://www.ars.usda.gov/nutrientdata. Accessed Feb 17, 2015
Dietary Guidelines Advisory Committee. Scientific Report. Advisory Report to the Secretary of Health and Human Services and the Secretary of Agriculture. Appendix E-3.7: Developing vegetarian and Mediterranean-style food patterns. 2015;1–9
U.S. Department of Agriculture and U.S. Department of Health and Human Services. Dietary Guidelines for Americans, 2010. 7th Edition, Washington, DC: U.S. Government Printing Office. 2010; Table B2.4; http://www.choosemyplate.gov/. Accessed Aug 22, 2015

References

1. Shlisky J, Bloom DE, Beaudreault AR, et al. Nutritional considerations for healthy aging and reduction in age-related chronic disease. Adv Nutr. 2017;8:17–26. https://doi.org/10.3945/n116.3474.
2. Milte CM, McNaughton SA. Dietary patterns and successful ageing: a systematic review. Eur J Nutr. 2016;55:423–50. https://doi.org/10.1007/s00394-015-1123-7.
3. Rowe JW, Kahn RL. Human aging: usual and successful. Science. 1987;237:143–9.
4. Beers MH, et al. The Merck manual of health & aging. Whitehouse Station: Merck Laboratories; 2004. p. 2.
5. Fontana L, Optimal HFB. Body weight for health and longevity: bridging basic, clinical, and population research. Aging Cell. 2014;13:391–400.
6. Péter S, Saris WHM, Mathers JC, et al. Nutrient status assessment in individuals and populations for healthy aging - statement from an expert workshop. Forum Nutr. 2015;7:10491–500.
7. Dietary Guidelines Advisory Committee. Scientific report. Advisory Report to the Secretary of Health and Human Services and the Secretary of Agriculture. Part D. Chapter 1: Food and nutrient intakes, and health: current status and trends. 2015. p. 1–78.
8. Dietary Guidelines Advisory Committee (DGAC). Scientific report. Advisory report to the Secretary of Health and Human Services and the Secretary of Agriculture. Part D. Chapter 2: Dietary patterns, foods and nutrients and health outcomes. 2015. p. 1–35.
9. World Health Organization. WHO global status report on noncommunicable diseases, vol. 2010. Geneva: World Health Organization Press; 2010.
10. WHO/FAO. Joint Expert Consultation on Diet. Nutrition and the prevention of chronic diseases. WHO Technical Series. 2003. p. 916.
11. http://health.gov/dietaryguidelines/2015/guidelines/message. Accessed January 17, 2016.
12. Avendano M, Kawachi I. Why do Americans have shorter life expectancy and worse health than people in other high-income countries? Annual Rev Public Health. 2014;35:307–25.
13. Millen BE, Abrams S, Adams-Campbell L, et al. The 2015 Dietary Guidelines Advisory Committee Scientific Report: development and major conclusions. Adv Nutr. 2016;7:438–44.

14. Mozaffarian D. Dietary and policy priorities for cardiovascular disease, diabetes, and obesity a comprehensive review. Circulation. 2017;133(2):187–225. https://doi.org/10.1161/CIRCULATIONAHA.11519.018585.
15. Van Horn L, Carson JA, Appel LJ, et al. Recommended dietary pattern to achieve adherence to the American Heart Association/American College of Cardiology Guidelines: A Scientific Statement from the American Heart Association. Circulation. 2016;134(22):505–29.
16. Freitas-Simoes TMF, Ros E, Sala-Vila A. Nutrients, foods, dietary patterns and telomere length: update of epidemiological studies and randomized trials. Metabolism. 2016;65(4):406–15.
17. Schwingshackl L, Schwedhelm C, Hoffmann G, et al. Food groups and risk of all-cause mortality: a systematic review and meta-analysis of prospective studies. Am J Clin Nutr. 2017;105:1462–73.
18. Onvani S, Haghighatdoost F, Surkan PJ, et al. Adherence to the Healthy Eating Index and Alternative Healthy Eating Index patterns and mortality from all-causes, cardiovascular disease and cancer: a meta-analysis of observational studies. J Hum Nutr Diet. 2017;30(2):216–26.
19. Sotos-Pieto M, Bhupathiraju SN, Mattei J, et al. Association of changes in diet quality with total and cause-specific mortality. N Engl J Med. 2017; 377(2):143–53.
20. Schwedhelm C, Boeing H, Hoffmann G, et al. Effect of diet on mortality and cancer recurrence among cancer survivors: a systematic review and meta-analysis of cohort studies. Nutr Rev. 2016;74(12):737–48.
21. Li F, Hou L, Chen W, et al. Associations of dietary patterns with the risk of all-cause, CVD and stroke mortality: a meta-analysis of prospective cohort studies. Br J Nutr. 2015;113:16–24.
22. Schwingshackl L, Hoffmann G. Diet quality as assessed by the healthy eating index, the alternate healthy eating index, the dietary approaches to stop hypertension score, and health outcomes: a systematic review and meta-analysis of cohort studies. J Acad Nutr Diet. 2015;115:780–800.
23. Jankovic N, Geelen A, Streppel MT, et al. WHO guidelines for a healthy diet and mortality from cardiovascular disease in European and American elderly: the CHANCES project. Am J Clin Nutr. 2015;102:745–56.
24. Huang T, Yang B, Zheng J, et al. Cardiovascular disease mortality and cancer incidence in vegetarians: a meta-analysis and systematic review. Ann Nutr Metab. 2012;60:233–40.
25. Jankovic N, Geelen A, Streppel MT, et al. Adherence to a healthy diet according to the World Health Organization guidelines and all-cause mortality in elderly adults from Europe and the United States. Am J Epidemiol. 2014;180(10):978–88.
26. Sofi F, Abbate R, Gensini GF, Cesari F. Accruing evidence on benefits of adherence to the Mediterranean diet on health: an updated systematic review and meta-analysis. Am J Clin Nutr. 2010;92:1189–96.
27. Gopinath B, Russell J, Kifley A, et al. Adherence to dietary guidelines and successful aging over 10 years. J Gerontol A Biol Sci Med Sci. 2016;71(3):349–55.
28. Yang M, Kenfield SA, Van Blarigan EL, et al. Dietary patterns after prostate cancer diagnosis in relation to disease-specific and total mortality. Cancer Prev Res (Phila). 2015;8(6):545–51.
29. Harmon BE, Boushey CJ, Shvetsov YB, et al. Associations of key diet-quality indexes with mortality in the Multiethnic Cohort: the Dietary Patterns Methods Project. Am J Clin Nutr. 2015;101:587–97.
30. Reedy J, Krebs-Smith SM, Miller PE, et al. Higher diet quality is associated with decreased risk of all-cause, cardiovascular disease, and cancer mortality among older adults. J Nutr. 2014;144:881–9.
31. Liese AD, Krebs-Smith SM, Subar AF, et al. The dietary patterns methods project: synthesis of findings across cohorts and relevance to dietary guidance. J Nutr. 2015;145:393–402.
32. Shi Z, Zhang T, Byles J, et al. Food habits, lifestyle factors and mortality among oldest old Chinese: The Chinese Longitudinal Healthy Longevity Survey (CLHLS). Forum Nutr. 2015;7:7562–79.
33. George SM, Ballard-Barbash R, Manson JE, et al. Comparing indices of diet quality with chronic disease mortality risk in postmenopausal women in the Women's Health Initiative Observational Study: evidence to inform national dietary guidance. Am J Epidemiol. 2014;180(6):616–25.
34. Zazpe I, Sánchez-Tainta A, Toledo E, et al. Dietary patterns and total mortality in a Mediterranean cohort: The SUN Project. J Acad Nutr Diet. 2014;114: 37–47.
35. Yu D, Zhang X, Xiang Y-B, et al. Adherence to dietary guidelines and mortality: a report from prospective cohort studies of 134,000 Chinese adults in urban Shanghai. Am J Clin Nutr. 2014;100:693–700.
36. Martınez-Gonzalez MA, Sanchez-Tainta A, Corella D, et al. A provegetarian food pattern and reduction in total mortality in the Prevencion con Dieta Mediterranea (PREDIMED) study. Am J Clin Nutr. 2014;100(suppl):320S–8S.
37. Orlich MJ, Singh PN, Sabate J, et al. Vegetarian dietary patterns and mortality in the Adventist Health Study 2. JAMA Intern Med. 2013;173(13):1230–8.
38. Akbaraly TN, Ferrie JE, Berr C, et al. Alternative healthy eating index and mortality over 18 y of follow-up: results from the Whitehall II cohort. Am J Clin Nutr. 2011;94:247–53.
39. Anderson AL, Harris TB, Tylavsky FA, et al. Dietary patterns and survival of older adults. J Am Diet Assoc. 2011;111(1):84–91.
40. Buckland G, Agudo A, Travier N, et al. Adherence to the Mediterranean diet reduces mortality in the Spanish cohort of the European Prospective Investigation into Cancer and Nutrition (EPIC-Spain). Br J Nutr. 2011;106:1581–91.
41. Heidemann C, Schulze MB, Franco OH, et al. Dietary patterns and risk of mortality from cardiovascular disease, cancer, and all causes in a prospective cohort of women. Circulation. 2008;118:230–7.

42. Bamia C, Trichopoulos D, Ferrari P, et al. Dietary patterns and survival of older Europeans: The EPIC-Elderly Study (European Prospective Investigation into Cancer and Nutrition). Public Health Nutr. 2007;10(6):590–8.
43. Ndanuko RN, Tapsell LC, Charlton KE, et al. Dietary patterns and blood pressure in adults: a systematic review and meta-analysis of randomized controlled trials. Adv Nutr. 2016;7:76–89. https://doi.org/10.3945/an.115.009753.
44. Feng YL, Shu L, Zheng PF, et al. Dietary patterns and colorectal cancer risk: a meta-analysis. Eur J Cancer Prev. 2017;26(3):201–11. https://doi.org/10.1097/CEJ.0000000000000245.
45. Maghsoudi Z, Ghiasvand R, Solehi-Abargouei A. Empirically derived dietary patterns and incident type 2 diabetes mellitus: a systematic review and meta-analysis on prospective observational studies. Public Health Nutr. 2015;19(2):230–41.
46. Rodríguez-Monforte M, Flores-Mateo G, Sánchez E. Dietary patterns and CVD: a systematic review and meta-analysis of observational studies. Br J Nutr. 2015;114(9):1341–59. https://doi.org/10.1017/S0007114515003177.
47. Hou L, Li F, Wang Y, Ou Z. Association. Between dietary patterns and coronary heart disease: a meta-analysis of prospective cohort studies. Int J Clin Exp Med. 2015;8(1):781–90.
48. Chiuve SE, Fung TT, Rimm EB, et al. Alternative dietary indices both strongly predict risk of chronic disease. J Nutr. 2012;142:1009–18.
49. Shikany JM, Safford MM, Newby P, et al. Southern dietary pattern is associated with hazard of acute coronary heart disease in the Reasons for Geographic and Racial Differences in Stroke (REGARDS) Study. Circulation. 2015;132:804–14. https://doi.org/10.1161/CIRCULATIONAHA. 114.014421.
50. Pilleron S, Ajana S, Juland MA, et al. Dietary patterns and 12-year risk of frailty: results from the three-city Bordeaux study. J Am Med Dir Assoc. 2017;18(2):169–75. https://doi.org/10.1016/j.jamda.2016.09.014.
51. Hagan K, Chiuve SE, Stampfer MJ, et al. Greater adherence to the Alternative Healthy Eating Index is associated with lower incidence of physical function impairment in the Nurses' Health Study. J Nutr. 2016;146(7):1341–7. https://doi.org/10.3945/jn.115.227900.
52. Assmann KE, Lassale C, Andreeva VA, et al. A healthy dietary pattern at midlife, combined with a regulated energy intake, is related to increased odds for healthy aging. J Nutr. 2015;145(9):2139–1245. https://doi.org/10.3945/jn.115.210740.
53. León-Muñoz LM, García-Esquinas E, López-García E, et al. Major dietary patterns and risk of frailty in older adults: a prospective cohort study. BMC Med. 2015;13:11. https://doi.org/10.1186/s12916-014-0255-6.
54. Samieri C, Sun Q, Townsend MK, et al. The relation of midlife diet to healthy aging: a cohort study. Ann Intern Med. 2013;159(9):584–91.
55. Akbaraly TN, Sabia S, Hagger-Johnson G, et al. Does overall diet in midlife predict future aging phenotypes? A cohort study. Am J Med. 2013;126:411–9.
56. Wu L, Sun D. Adherence to Mediterranean diet and risk of developing cognitive disorders: an updated systematic review and meta-analysis of prospective cohort studies. Sci Rep. 2017;7:41317. https://doi.org/10.1038/srep41317.
57. Singh B, Parsaik AK, Mielke MM, et al. Association of Mediterranean diet with mild cognitive impairment and Alzheimer's disease: a systematic review and meta-analysis. J Alzheimers Dis. 2014;39(2): 271–82.
58. Haring B, Wu C, Mossavar-Rahmani Y, et al. No association between dietary patterns and risk for cognitive decline in older women with 9-year follow-up: data from the Women's Health Initiative Memory Study. J Acad Nutr Diet. 2016;116:921–30.
59. Galbete C, Toledo E, Toledo JB, et al. Mediterranean diet and cognitive function: the SUN project. J Nutr Health Age. 2015;19(3):305–12.
60. Jacka FN, Cherbuin N, Anstey KJ, et al. Western diet is associated with a smaller hippocampus: a longitudinal investigation. BMC Med. 2015;13:215. https://doi.org/10.1186/s12916-015-0461-x.
61. Shakersaina B, Santonia G, Larssonb SC, et al. Prudent diet may attenuate the adverse effects of western diet on cognitive decline. Alzheimer's. Dementia. 2016;12(2):100–9. https://doi.org/10.1016/j.jalz.2015.08.002.
62. Tsai HJ. Dietary patterns and cognition decline in Taiwanese aged 65 years and older. Int J Geriatr Psychiatry. 2015;30(5):523–30.
63. Gardener SL, Rainey-Smith SR, Barnes MB, et al. Dietary patterns and cognitive decline in an Australian study of ageing. Mol Psychiatry. 2015;20(7):860–6.
64. Tangney CC, Li H, Wang Y, et al. Relation of DASH- and Mediterranean-like dietary patterns to cognitive decline in older persons. Neurology. 2014;83:1410–6.
65. Ozawa M, Ninomiya T, Ohara T, et al. Dietary patterns and risk of dementia in an elderly Japanese population: The Hisayama Study. Am J Clin Nutr. 2013;97:1076–82.
66. Pearson KE, Wadley VG, McClure LA, et al. Dietary patterns are associated with cognitive function in the REasons for Geographic And Racial Differences in Stroke (REGARDS) cohort. J Nutr Sci. 2016;5:e38. https://doi.org/10.1017/jns.2016.27.
67. Valls-Pedret C, Sala-Vila A, Serra-Mir M, et al. Mediterranean diet and age-related cognitive decline. A randomized clinical trial. JAMA Intern Med. 2015;175(7):1094–103.
68. Martinez-Lapiscina EH, Clavero P, Toledo R, et al. Mediterranean diet improves cognition: the PREDIMED-NAVARRA randomized trial. J Neurol Neurosurg Psychiatry. 2013;84(12):1318–25.
69. Garcia-Calzon S, Gea A, Razquin C, et al. Longitudinal association of telomere length and obesity indices in an intervention study with a Mediterranean diet: the PREDIMED-NAVARRA trial. Int J Obes (London). 2014;38:177–82.

70. Garcia-Calzon S, Moleres A, Marcos A, et al. Telomere length as a biomarker for adiposity changes after a multidisciplinary intervention in overweight adolescents: The EVASYON Study. PLoS One. 2014;9(2):e89828. https://doi.org/10.1371/journal.pone.0089828.
71. Kim S, Parks CG, DeRoo LA, et al. Obesity and weight gain in adulthood and telomere length. Cancer Epidemiol Biomark Prev. 2009;18(3):816–25.
72. Rode L, Nordestgaard BG, Bojesen SE. Peripheral blood leukocyte telomere length and mortality among 64,637 individuals in the general population. J Natl Cancer Inst. 2015;107(6). https://doi.org/10.1093/jnci/djv074.
73. Haycock PC, Heydon EE, Kaptoge S, et al. Leukocyte telomere length and risk of cardiovascular disease: systematic review and meta-analysis. BMJ. 2014;349:g4227. https://doi.org/10.1136/bmj.g4227.
74. Willeit P, Raschenberger J, Heydon EE, et al. Leukocyte telomere length and risk of type 2 diabetes mellitus: new prospective cohort study and literature-based meta-analysis. PLoS One. 2014;9(11):e112483. https://doi.org/10.1371/journal.pone.0112483.
75. Rafie N, Hamedani SG, Barak F, et al. Dietary patterns, food groups and telomere length: a systematic review of current studies. Eur J Clin Nutr. 2017;71:151–8. https://doi.org/10.1038/ejcn.2016.149.
76. Gu Y, Honig LS, Schupf N, et al. Mediterranean diet and leukocyte telomere length in a multi-ethnic elderly population. Age. 2015;37:24. https://doi.org/10.1007/s11357-015-9758-0.
77. Crous-Bou M, Fung TT, Prescott J, et al. Mediterranean diet and telomere length in Nurses' Health Study: population based cohort study. BMJ. 2014;349:g6674. https://doi.org/10.1136/bmj.g6674.
78. Boccardi V, Esposito A, Rizzo MR, et al. Mediterranean diet, telomere maintenance and health status among elderly. PLoS One. 2013;8(4):e62781. https://doi.org/10.1371/journal.pone.0062781.
79. Sun Q, Shi L, Prescott J, et al. Healthy lifestyle and leukocyte telomere length in U.S. women. PLoS One. 2012;7(5):e38374. https://doi.org/10.1371/journal.pone.0038374.
80. García-Calzón S, Zalba G, Ruiz-Canela M, et al. Dietary inflammatory index and telomere length in subjects with a high cardiovascular disease risk from the PREDIMED-Navarra study: cross-sectional and longitudinal analyses over 5 y. Am J Clin Nutr. 2015;102:897–904.
81. Lee J-Y, Jun N-R, Yoon D, et al. Association between dietary patterns in the remote past and telomere length. Eur J Clin Nutr. 2015;69(9):1048–52. https://doi.org/10.1038/ejcn.2015.58.
82. Garcia-Calzon S, Martinez-Gonzalez MA, Razquin C, et al. Mediterranean diet and telomere length in high cardiovascular risk subjects from the PREDIMED-NAVARRA study. Clin Nutr. 2016;35(6):1399–405. https://doi.org/10.1016/j.clnu.2016.03.013.
83. Marin C, Delgado-Lista J, Ramirez R, et al. Mediterranean diet reduces senescence-associated stress in endothelial cells. Age. 2012;34:1309–16. https://doi.org/10.1007/s11357-011-9305-6.

3 Whole Plant Foods in Aging and Disease

Keywords
Whole-plant foods • Healthy aging • Mortality risk • Cardiovascular disease • Cancer • Type 2 diabetes • Cognitive performance • Lipoproteins • Blood pressure • Cancer • Stroke • Telomeres • Whole-grains • Fruits • Vegetables • Legumes • Soybeans • Nuts

Key Points

- The rate and quality of the aging processes can be modified by consuming healthy diets overall and specific types of uniquely healthy foods.
- Healthy dietary guidelines generally recommend eating: 2 1/2 cups of a variety of vegetables/day; 2 cups of fruits, especially whole fruits/day; 6 servings of total grains at ≥3 servings of whole grains/day and ≤3 servings of refined grains/day, ≥4 weekly servings of legumes (dietary pulses or soy), and/or ≥5 weekly servings of nuts, and limiting consumption of red or processed meats, added saturated and trans-fat, sugar or sodium for improved odds for healthy aging and reduced chronic disease and premature mortality risk.
- Whole plant foods range widely in their health effects because of their variation in level and type of fiber, nutrients and phytochemicals, which can have differential effects on aging, chronic disease risk, cognitive function and longevity by their impact on weight regulation, lipoprotein concentrations and function, blood pressure, glucose-insulin homeostasis, oxidative stress, inflammation, endothelial health, hepatic function, adipocyte metabolism, visceral adiposity, brain neurochemistry and the microbiota ecosystem.
- For whole-grains, β-glucan-rich oats and barley lower total and LDL-cholesterol better than other cereal grains and whole-grain bread tends to be more beneficial than white bread in controlling weight gain and abdominal fat.
- For fruits and non-starchy vegetables, low energy dense and flavonoid and/or carotenoid rich varieties including apples, pears, berries, citrus fruits, cruciferous vegetables, and green leafy vegetables are especially associated with improved odds of healthy aging, cognitive performance and weight control, and reduced risk of chronic disease and premature death. Legumes (dietary pulses or soy) are associated with reduced weight gain, chronic disease and mortality risks.
- All nuts tend to have similar effects on managing body weight, and glycemic, lipoprotein

M.L. Dreher, *Dietary Patterns and Whole Plant Foods in Aging and Disease*, Nutrition and Health,
https://doi.org/10.1007/978-3-319-59180-3_3

and inflammatory profiles, but among nuts walnuts appear to be uniquely effective in promoting better vascular endothelial function such as flow mediated dilation, which helps to reduce the rate of vascular aging.

3.1 Introduction

The global adoption of the Western lifestyle, especially since the 1980s, has resulted in a pandemic of sub-optimal aging with increased rates of obesity, metabolic syndrome, type 2 diabetes and other related health conditions in both adults and children [1–7]. US adults have shorter and less healthy lives than populations in 32 other high-income countries [8]. As a result, population longevity forecasts suggest a stagnation or decline in life expectancy over the next 25 years [4–8]. The aging process rate and quality is only partly genetically pre-determined as it can be modified by lifestyle habits including dietary patterns, level of activity or exercise, personal habits or risk-taking, and psychosocial and stress management factors [9]. The habitual consumption of recommended levels of whole and minimally processed plant foods (whole plant foods) and avoiding excess energy intake are among the most important lifestyle factors associated with healthy aging and reduced chronic disease and premature mortality risk [9–26] but only a small fraction (<10%) of western populations consume adequate whole foods [10, 11]. According to the 2015 US Dietary Guidelines, ≥3/4 of the population consume very low levels of whole-grains, vegetables and fruits, legumes and nuts [11].

Healthy dietary consumption guidelines, such as the 2015 US dietary guidelines, primarily focus on increasing intake of whole plant foods with general recommendations for eating: 2 1/2 cups of a variety of vegetables/day; 2 cups of fruits, especially whole fruits/day; 6 servings of total grains at ≥3 servings of whole grains/day and ≤3 servings of refined grains/day; alternatives to animal protein including legumes (beans and peas), and nuts, seeds, and soy products including ≥4 weekly servings of legumes (dietary pulses or soy), and/or ≥5 weekly servings of nuts, along with limited consumption of red or processed meats, added saturated/trans-fat, sugar or sodium [11]. These healthy whole plant food diets both directly add healthy nutrients and phytochemicals to the diet and also displace a portion of high energy, low fiber, high added sugar, sodium, and saturated and trans-fat rich-foods typical of the Western diet. Adherence to this type of healthy dietary pattern would significantly improve the odds of healthy aging and reduce risk of weight gain, obesity, chronic diseases, and premature mortality compared to Western dietary patterns [11, 12]. The nutrient and phytochemical compositions of whole plant foods are summarized in Appendix A. Whole plant foods tend to be lower in energy density and higher in nutrient quality than more highly refined foods; they are lower in saturated and trans-fatty acids, sodium, and added sugars and richer in essential nutrients and phytochemicals like potassium and antioxidants such as vitamin C and E, carotenoids, and polyphenols [13–17]. Whole plant foods influence a range of healthy biological mechanisms including the improvement of weight regulation, lipoprotein concentrations and function, blood pressure, glucose-insulin homeostasis, oxidative stress, systemic inflammation, endothelial health, hepatic function, adipocyte metabolism, visceral adiposity, brain neurochemistry and the microbiota ecosystem, which can help to attenuate the risk of obesity, cardiovascular diseases (CVD), metabolic syndrome, type 2 diabetes (diabetes), certain cancers and cognitive dysfunction [18–21]. However, there are a spectrum of whole plant foods that range from healthy to less healthy options which is illustrated by the following example; a pooled analysis of three US prospective cohort studies (69,949 women from the Nurses' Health Study, 90,239 women from the Nurses' Health Study 2, and 40,539 men from the Health Professionals Follow-Up Study) showed that the consumption of a plant-based (vegetarian) diet that emphasized specifically healthy whole plant foods was associated with a decrease in diabetes risk by 34%, while consumption of a plant-based diet high in less healthy processed and refined plant foods was associated with a 16% increased diabetes risk (Fig. 3.1) [21]. The objective of this chapter is to comprehensively assess the effects of whole (minimally processed) plant foods in general and specific uniquely effective options on promoting healthy aging and reducing the risk of chronic disease and premature deaths.

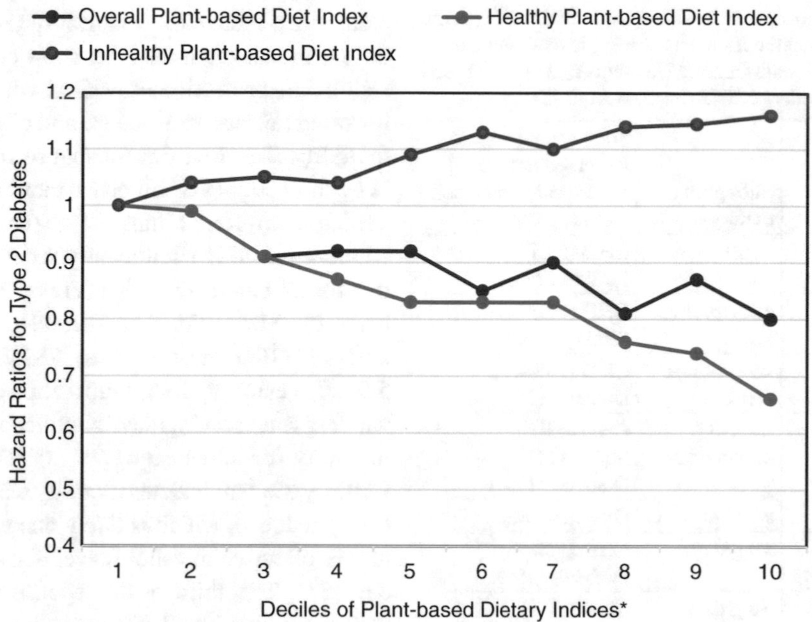

Fig. 3.1 Association between plant-based diet indices and type 2 diabetes risk from the pooled analysis of Nurses' Health Studies and Health Professionals Follow-Up Study with approx. 20 years of follow-up; baseline age 35–55 years ($p < 0.001$ for all) (adapted from [21]).
*Plant-based diet index, where healthy plant foods (whole grains, fruits, vegetables, nuts, legumes, vegetable oils, tea/coffee) received positive scores, while less healthy plant foods (fruit juices, sweetened beverages, refined grains, potatoes, sweets/desserts) and animal foods received reverse scores

3.2 Whole Plant Foods in Aging and Disease

The US National Center for Health Statistics estimates that about 45% of cardiometabolic deaths are associated with suboptimal intake of ten dietary factors including low intakes of fruits, vegetables, nuts and seeds, whole-grains, and seafood omega 3 and other polyunsaturated (PUFA) fats, and excessive intake of red and processed meats, sugar sweetened beverages, and sodium (Table 3.1) [22]. The optimal intake of these dietary factors is at least 300 g of non-juice fruit/day, 400 g vegetables including legumes/day, 5 weekly servings of nuts, 2.5–3 servings of whole-grains/day, 11% kcal from PUFA as a replacement for carbohydrate and saturated fat kcal, and 250 mg of seafood omega-3 fat, to limit red meat to 100 g/week and sodium to 2000 mg/day, and to avoid or rarely consume processed meat or sugar sweetened beverages.

3.2.1 Whole-Grains

3.2.1.1 Background

Whole-grains consist of the intact, ground, cracked or flaked kernel after removal of the inedible parts such as the husk and hull, and includes the starchy endosperm, germ and bran fiber in similar proportions that are found in the intact kernel compared to refined grains which consist primarily of the starchy endosperm with low amounts of fiber, vitamins, minerals and phytonutrients. Common examples of whole-grain foods and ingredients include brown rice, oatmeal, whole oats, bulgur (cracked wheat), popcorn, whole rye, graham flour, and whole wheat. Reviews of whole-grain human studies recommend that dietary patterns containing ≥3 servings of whole-grains and ≤3 serving of refined grains, without significant added saturated/trans-fat, sugar or sodium, are associated with healthy aging and reduced chronic disease risk [11, 23–25].

Table 3.1 Association of sub-optimal intake of specific food groups on annual increased specific cardiometabolic disease related deaths among US adults (≥25 years) based on 702,308 deaths in 2012 (adapted from [22])

Food group	Suboptimal dietary intake	Total annual disease increased number of related cardiometabolic disease deaths (%)
Fruit	<300 g/day	CHD (6%) Stroke (22%)
Vegetables	<400 g/day	CHD (7%) Stroke (22%)
Nuts and Seeds	<5 servings/ week	CHD (15%) Diabetes (7%)
Whole-grains	<2.5–3 serving/day	CHD (4%) Stroke (11%) Diabetes (17%)
Red meats	>100 g/week	Diabetes (4%)
Processed meats	>0 g/day	CHD (12%) Diabetes (18%)
Sugar sweetened beverages	>0 g/day	CHD (11%) Stroke (1%) Diabetes (15%)
PUFA as a replacement for carbohydrates and saturated fat	<11% kcal/ day	CHD (4%)
Seafood omega 3 fat	<250 mg/day	CHD (15%)
Sodium	>2000 mg/ day	CHD (10%) Stroke (11%)

However, only about 1% of Americans follow the recommendation for whole-grain intake as the average American intake is <1 serving of whole grains/day and ≥70% exceed the recommended intake for refined grains [11, 26, 27].

3.2.1.2 Mortality Risk

Five systematic reviews and meta-analyses of prospective cohort studies and five representative cohort studies assessing the effects of whole-grains intake on all-cause and disease specific mortality are summarized in Table 3.2 [28–37].

Meta-analyses

All five of these meta-analyses of prospective studies published in 2016 strongly support the protective effects of a daily intake of ≥3 servings of whole-grains in reducing all-cause, cardiovascular disease and cancer mortality [28–32]. Three dose response meta-analyses show consistent and significant protective effects of whole-grains in lowering premature all-cause and disease specific mortality. The first dose-response meta-analysis (11 cohort studies on all-cause mortality; 705,253 participants) found that 90 g (or 3 servings) whole-grains/day significantly reduced mortality risk for all-cause by 17%, CVD by 29% and diabetes by 51% [28]. The second dose-response analysis (10 cohort studies; 782,751 subjects; 5.5–26 years of follow-up) showed that one whole-grain serving/day significantly reduced mortality for all-cause by 7%, CVD by 5% and CHD by 8% but diabetes morality was not significantly reduced, which is likely due to requiring a higher effective threshold level above 1 serving/day [31]. The third dose-response analysis (20 cohort studies; 2,282,603 subjects; follow-up of 5.5–26 years) found that the daily consumption of three servings (90 g) whole-grains significantly reduced risk of all-cause mortality by 17% and reduced CVD mortality by 25% and total cancer mortality by 10% [32]. Two other non-dose-response meta-analyses provide similar significant supporting evidence for the protective effect of ≥3 whole grain servings/day in lowering the risk of premature mortality [29, 30].

Specific Prospective Cohort Studies

Five large prospective studies demonstrate that increased whole-grain intake significantly reduced all-cause and disease specific mortality [33–37]. For ready to eat cereal (RTEC) intake, the National Institutes of Health (NIH)-AARP Diet and Health Study (367,442 subjects; average 14-year follow-up) found that participants who consumed high RTEC with whole-grain or high cereal fiber had a significant 15% lower risk of all-cause mortality and 10–30% lower risk of specific chronic diseases compared to non-consumers [33]. The US Nurses' Health and the Health Professionals Follow-Up studies (118,000; mean age 50–53 years; 25 years of follow-up) showed that whole-grain intake was inversely associated with total and CVD mortality (Fig. 3.2) [34]. Each serving of whole grains (28 g/day) was significantly inversely

Table 3.2 Summary of whole-grain prospective cohort studies on all-cause and disease specific mortality risk

Objective	Study details	Results
Systematic Reviews and Meta-Analyses		
Aune et al. (2016). Quantify the dose-response relation between consumption of whole grain or specific types of grains and all cause and cause specific mortality [28].	11 cohort studies; whole grain bread, whole grain breakfast cereals, and added bran; 705,253 participants; 100,726 deaths.	A 90 g/day increase in whole grain intake equivalent to 3 servings (for example, two slices of bread and one bowl of cereal or one and a half pieces of pita bread made from whole grains) significantly reduced risk of mortality from all causes by 17%, CVD by 29%, and diabetes by 51%. Reductions in risk were observed up to an intake of 225 g whole-grain products (7.5 servings/day)/day.
Wei et al. (2016). Determine the effects of whole-grain consumption and the risk of all-cause, CVD and cancer mortality [29].	11 prospective studies; total of 816,599 subjects; 89,251 deaths.	On the basis of the highest vs. the lowest categories of intake, whole grains were associated with a lower risk of mortality from all causes by 13%, CVD by 19%. and all cancers by 11%. For each 3 servings/day increase in whole-grain intake, there was a 19% reduction in the risk of all-cause mortality, a 26% reduction in CVD mortality and a 9% reduction in cancer mortality.
Zong et al. (2016). Evaluate the effect of whole-grain intake on mortality from all-cause, CVD and cancer [30].	14 cohort studies plus unpublished results from National Health and Nutrition Examination Survey (NHANES) III and NHANES 1999–2004; 786,076 participants, 97,867 deaths.	Comparing highest vs. lowest intake of whole-grain intake there was a significant reduced risk for total mortality by 16%, for CVD by 18%, and for cancer by 12%. For each 16-g/day increase in whole-grains intake morality risk reductions were 7% for total, 9% for CVD, and 5% for cancer.
Li et al. (2016) Investigate the dose–response correlation between consumption of whole grains and the risk of all-cause, CVD, and diabetes-specific mortality [31].	10 cohort studies; 782,751 subjects; 92,647 deaths; 5.5–26 years of follow-up.	Per increment of 1 serving (30 g) a day of whole grain intake, mortality risk was significantly reduced for all-cause by 7%, CVD by 5% and CHD by 8%. Higher consumption of whole grains was not appreciably associated with risk of mortality from stroke and diabetes.
Benisi-Kohansal et al. (2016) conduct a meta-analysis of prospective cohort studies to summarize the relation between whole-grain intake and risk of mortality from all-causes, CVD and total and specific cancers [32].	9 cohort studies on total whole-grain intake and 11 cohort studies on specific whole-grain food intake; 2,282,603 subjects; follow-up of 5.5–26 years; 191,979 deaths (25,595 from CVD, 32,746 from total cancers, and 2671 from specific cancers).	For an increase of 3 servings total whole grains/d (90 g/d), there was a significantly reduced risk of all-cause mortality by 17%. Also, each additional daily 3 servings total whole grains reduced CVD mortality by 25% and total cancer mortality by 10%.
Prospective Cohort Studies		
Xu et al. (2016). Assess the associations of ready to eat cereal (RTEC) intakes on all causes and disease-specific mortality risk (US National Institutes of Health (NIH)-AARP Diet and Health Study) [33].	367,442 participants; average 14 years of follow-up; 46,067 deaths (multivariate adjusted).	In multivariate models, participants in the highest intake of RTEC, compared to non-consumers of RTEC, had a 15% lower risk of all-cause mortality and 10%–30% lower risk of disease specific mortality. Within RTEC consumers, total fiber intakes were associated with reduced risk of mortality from all-cause mortality and deaths from CVD, all cancers, and respiratory disease (all p- trend <0.005).

(continued)

Table 3.2 (continued)

Objective	Study details	Results
Wu et al. (2015). Examine the association between dietary whole grain consumption and risk of mortality (US Nurses' Health and the Health Professionals Follow-Up studies) [34].	74,341women and 43,744 men; mean age 50–53 years; followed for 24–26 years; 26,920 deaths (multivariate adjusted).	Whole-grains were inversely associated with total and CVD mortality (Fig. 3.2). Every serving (28 g/day) of whole grain was associated with a 5% lower total mortality or a 9% lower CVD mortality, whereas the same intake level was non-significantly associated with lower cancer mortality.
Huang et al. (2015). Assess the association of whole grains and cereal fiber intake with all causes and cause-specific mortality (US NIH-AARP Diet and Health Study) [35].	367,442 participants; average 14 years of follow-up; 46,067 deaths (multivariate adjusted).	On the basis of highest to lowest intake, whole grains showed significant reduction in mortality risk for all-cause by 17% and 11–48% lower risk of disease-specific mortality. The highest intake of cereal fiber had a 19% lower risk of all-cause mortality and 15–34% lower risk of disease-specific mortality (all $p < 0.05$).
Johnsen et al. (2015). Investigate the association of whole-grain intake and all-cause and cause-specific mortality (Scandinavian HELGA cohort; Norwegian Women and Cancer Study, the Northern Sweden Health and Disease Study, and the Danish Diet Cancer and Health Study) [36].	120,010 adults; median age 52 years; mean BMI 25; 11–17 years of follow-up (multivariate adjusted).	Whole-grain products were associated with a significantly lower all-cause mortality of 11% (highest vs. lowest intake) with the strongest associations being for breakfast cereals and non-white bread, especially whole-grain oat, wheat and rye.
He et al. (2010). Investigate whole grain and its components cereal fiber, bran, and germ in relation to all-cause and CVD-specific mortality in patients with type 2 diabetes mellitus (US Nurses' Health Study) [37].	7822 US women with type 2 diabetes mellitus; mean age 47 years; mean BMI 30; 26 years of follow-up; 852 all-cause deaths and 295 CVD deaths (multivariate adjusted).	For the highest versus the lowest intakes, lower all-cause mortality risk for whole grain was reduced by 11%, cereal fiber by 19%, bran by 25%, and germ by 5%. Only the association for bran intake was significant. Whole-grain and with bran intakes were associated with a significant lowering in CVD-specific mortality in women with diabetes.

associated with all-cause mortality by 5% and CVD mortality by 9%. The US NIH-AARP Diet and Health Study (367,442; mean age 62 years; 14 years of follow-up) observed that higher intake of whole-grains significantly reduced the risk of all-cause mortality by 17% and mortality risk from diabetes by 48%, CVD by 17% and cancer by 15% [35]. The large Scandinavian HELGA cohort (120,010; median age 52 years; mean BMI 25; 11–17 years of follow-up) found that whole-grain products were associated with a significantly lower all-cause mortality of 11% (highest vs. lowest intake) with the strongest associations observed for breakfast cereals and non-white bread, especially whole-grain oat, wheat and rye [36]. A Nurses' Health Study evaluation of women with type 2 diabetes (7822 women; mean 47 years at baseline; 26-year follow-up) showed that the intake of whole-grain was inversely associated with all-cause and CVD-specific mortality [37]. In each of these studies, the mortality protective effects of whole-grains were primarily due to its bran (fiber) component.

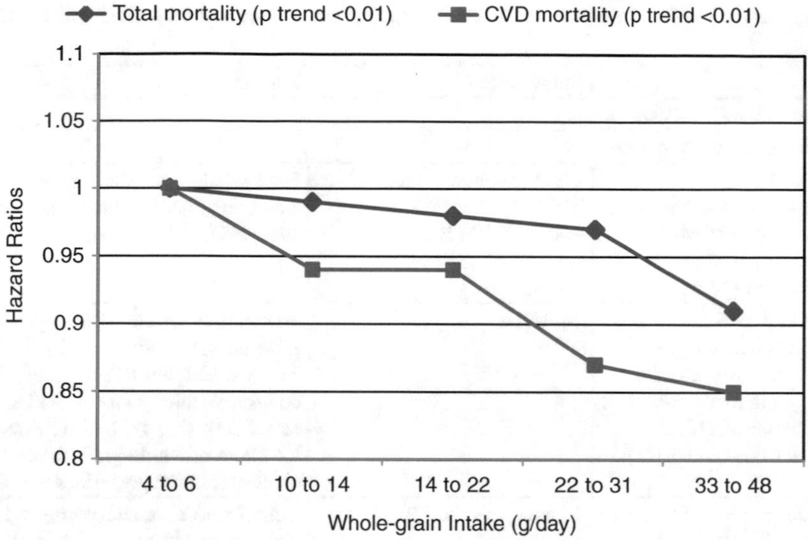

Fig. 3.2 Effects of whole-grain foods intake on mortality risk of US men and women approx. 50 years of age at baseline and followed for 24–26 years (adapted from [34])

3.2.1.3 Chronic Disease Risk

Whole-grain systematic reviews and meta-analyses, and individual prospective cohort studies and RCTs on chronic disease risk and risk biomarkers are summarized in Table 3.3 [28, 38–53].

Cardiovascular Diseases (CVD)

Five systematic reviews and meta analyses support the protective effects of ≥3 daily servings of whole-grains in lowering the risk of developing CVD or biomarkers [28, 38–41]. A dose-response meta-analysis (17 cohort studies; 1 million participants; 33,300 cases) found that three daily whole grain servings (90 g) significantly reduced risk for CVD by 22% and CHD by19% [28]. A systematic review of 24 RCTs found that increased intake of whole oats was primarily responsible for most of the total and LDL cholesterol lowering effects of whole grains (Fig. 3.3) [38]. Another meta-analysis (45 prospective cohort studies and 21 RCTs) found in cohort that 48–80 g whole-grains/day significantly lowered CVD risk by 21% compared to never or very low intake and RCTs showed that higher whole-grain intake significantly lowered mean fasting glucose, and total and LDL cholesterol compared to refined-grains [39]. A 2007 Cochrane systematic review of RCTs (10 RCTs with 8 of these on whole oats; 4–8 week durations) showed that oatmeal accounted for virtually all the total and LDL-cholesterol lowering effects of whole-grains [40].

Hypertension/Blood Pressure (BP)

One cohort study [41] and two RCTs [42, 43] support the protective effects of ≥3 daily whole-grain servings in reducing the risk of elevated BP or hypertension. The Health Professionals Follow-up Study (31,684 men; baseline age range 45–75; 18 years of follow-up) reported that men with higher whole-grain and bran intake had significantly lower risk of hypertension by 19% (multivariate adjusted) [41]. A double-blind, crossover RCT (40 overweight/obese men and women; mean age 39 years; mix of whole grains vs. refined grains at 50 g/1000 kcal; 8 weeks) found that the whole grain supplemented diet significantly lowered diastolic BP by 4.2 mm Hg more than a similar diet supplemented with refined grains [42]. A second RCT (233 adults; mean age 52 years; 12 weeks) demonstrated that three daily servings of mixed whole-grain foods significantly lowered systolic BP compared to diets with refined grain foods (Fig. 3.4) [43].

Table 3.3 Summary of whole-grain prospective cohort studies and randomized controlled trials (RCTs) on chronic disease risk

Objective	Study details	Results
Cardiovascular Disease (CVD)		
Systematic Reviews and Meta-Analyses		
Aune et al. (2016). Quantify the dose-response relation between consumption of whole grain or specific types of grains and the risk of CHD and CVD [28].	CHD (7 cohort studies; 316,491 subjects; 7068 cases); CVD (10 cohort studies; 704,317 subjects; 26,243 cases).	Per 3 whole-grain daily servings (90 g), there was a significant reduced risk for CHD by 19% and CVD by 22%.
Hollænder et al. (2015). Assess the effect of whole-grain compared with non–whole-grain foods on changes in total cholesterol (TC), LDL cholesterol, HDL cholesterol, and triglycerides [38].	24 RCTs.	Specifically, overall whole -grains significantly lowered LDL cholesterol by 0.09 mmol/L and TC by 0.12 mmol/L compared with the control. Whole-grain oats had the greatest effect, lowering TC by 0.17 mmol/L Fig. 3.3). No effect of whole-grain foods on HDL cholesterol or triglycerides was found.
Ye et al. (2012). Systematically examine human studies investigating whole-grain and fiber intake and CVD risk [39].	45 cohort studies; 21 RCTs.	Cohort studies, which compared never/rare consumers of whole-grains with those consuming 48–80 g whole grain/day showed lower risk of CVD by 21% for the whole-grain consumers. In RCTs, whole-grains significantly lowered TC by 0.83 mmol/L and LDL-cholesterol by 0.72 mmol/L vs. control diets (multivariate adjusted).
Kelly et al. (2007). Assess the effects of whole-grain intake on CHD risk factors in participants previously diagnosed with CHD or with existing risk factors for CHD (Cochrane Systematic Review) [40].	10 RCTs with 8 of these testing whole-grain oats; ranged in duration from 4 to 8 weeks.	Whole-grain oats significantly lowered TC by 0.20 mmol/L and LDL cholesterol by 0.18 mmol/L (all, $p < 0.0001$) vs. control diets. However, there was a lack of evidence for significant lowering effects for other non-oat whole grains.
Hypertension/Blood Pressure		
Prospective Cohort Study		
Flint et al. (2009) Evaluate the association between whole-grain intake (g/day) and risk of hypertension in men (The Health Professionals Follow-up Study; US) [41].	31,684 men free of hypertension, cancer, stroke, or coronary heart disease; baseline age 45–75 years; 18 years of follow-up (multivariate adjusted).	In multivariate-adjusted analyses, whole-grain intake was inversely associated with risk of hypertension by 19% (highest vs. lowest quintile; p-trend <0.0001). A similar inverse association was shown for total bran with a risk reduction of 15% (p-trend =0.002).
RCTs		
Kirwan et al. (2016). Evaluate the efficacy of whole grains compared with refined grains on body composition, hypertension, and related mediators of CVD in overweight and obese adults (US) [42].	**Double-blind, Crossover RCT**: 40 overweight or obese men and women; mean age 39 years with no known history of CVD; whole-grain and refined-grain (control) diets (50 g/1000 kcal in each diet); 8-week periods; 10-week washout.	The whole-grain supplemented diet significantly lowered diastolic blood pressure (BP) by 4.2 mm Hg more than the refined grain control diet ($p = 0.01$). This decreased whole-grain diastolic BP was correlated with higher circulating adiponectin levels ($r = 0.35$, $p = 0.04$).

Table 3.3 (continued)

Objective	Study details	Results
Tighe et al. (2010). Assess the effects of the intake of 3 daily portions of whole-grain foods (provided as only wheat or a mixture of wheat and oats) on markers of CVD risk in relatively high-risk individuals (UK) [43].	**Parallel RCT**: 233 middle age healthy subjects; mean age 52 years; after a 4-week run-in period with a refined grain diet, subjects were randomly allocated to a control (refined grain diet); 3 daily portions wheat, or combined wheat and oats; 12 weeks.	After 6 weeks of the intervention, the wheat and oats group systolic BP was significantly lowered by 3.7 mmHg more than the refined grain group. By 12 weeks, the decrease in systolic BP was significantly lowered in both whole-grain groups compared to the refined grain group (P = 0.01; Fig. 3.4).
Ischemic Stroke		
Systematic Reviews and Meta-analyses		
Chen et al. (2016). Evaluate the effect of whole and refined grains on stroke risk [44].	7 cohort studies; 446,451 subjects; 5892 stroke events.	High intake of whole grains was inversely associated with ischemic stroke risk by 25% vs. low whole-grain intake. Consumption of refined grains was not associated with risk of stroke or its subtypes.
Fang et al. (2015). Examine the association between whole-grain intake and stroke risk [45].	6 cohort studies; 247,487 subjects; 1635 stroke events.	Highest whole grain intake vs. lowest intake was significantly associated with reduced risk of total stroke by 14%. In subgroup analysis inverse stroke associations were also found in the American population by 19% and in women by 22%.
Prospective Cohort Study		
Liu et al. (2000). Examine the relationship between whole-grain intake and the risk of ischemic stroke in women (Nurses' Health Study; US) [46].	75,521 women; baseline age 38–63 years; 12 years of follow-up; 352 cases of ischemic stroke (multivariate adjusted).	For the highest vs. lowest whole-grain intake, the risk of ischemic stroke was significantly reduced by 31% and for never smokers the risk was reduced by 50%.
Type 2 Diabetes (Diabetes)		
Systematic Reviews and Meta-analyses		
Chanson-Rolle et al. (2015). Quantitative evaluation of the relationship between whole grain intake and diabetes risk [47].	8 observational studies; 7 cohort studies; 316,051 participants; 15,573 diabetes cases.	The daily consumption of 45 g of whole grains significantly reduced diabetes risk by 20% compared to the daily intake of 7.5 g.
Aune et al. (2013). Assess the dose–response relationship between whole grain intake and diabetes risk [48].	16 cohorts; whole grain (10 cohorts; 385,868 participants 19,829 cases); refined grain (6 cohorts; 258,078 participants; 9545 cases).	Per 3 daily whole grain servings diabetes risk was reduced by 32% and for refined grain the diabetes risk was reduced by 5%. A significant nonlinear association was observed for whole grains but not for refined grains. Fig. 3.5 summarizes the diabetes risk lowering effects of specific whole grain foods.
Specific Prospective Studies		
Sun et al. (2010). Examine the effects of white and brown rice on US men and women (Nurses' Health Studies 1 and II and the Health Professionals Follow-up Study) [49].	39,765 men and 157,463 women; baseline age range 26–87 years; 14–22 years of follow-up; 2359–5500 diabetes cases (multivariate adjusted).	Replacing 50 g/day (cooked, equivalent to 1/3 serving/day) of white rice with the same amount of brown rice was associated with a 16% lower risk of diabetes, whereas the same replacement with other types whole grains lowered diabetes risk by 36%.

(continued)

Table 3.3 (continued)

Objective	Study details	Results
de Munter et al. (2007). Evaluate intakes of whole grain, bran, and germ in relation to risk of diabetes in prospective cohort studies (Nurses' Health Studies plus a meta-analysis) [50].	161,737 women; baseline age 26–65 years; 12–18 years of follow-up; 6486 diabetes cases. 6 cohort studies; 286,125 participants; 10,944 diabetes cases (multivariate adjusted).	The daily intake of 31–40 g vs. about 5 g whole-grains significantly lowered diabetes risk by 14–25% with the largest risk reduction in the older women. Associations for bran intake were similar to those for total whole grain intake, whereas no significant association was observed for germ intake after adjustment for bran. In the meta-analysis, 2 daily whole grain servings were associated with a 21% decrease in diabetes risk after adjustment for potential confounders and BMI.
Colorectal Cancer (CRC)		
Systematic Reviews and Meta-analyses		
Aune et al. (2011). Assess the whole-grain dose-response effect on CRC risk [51].	6 cohorts	This dose-response analysis found that CRC risk per 3 whole-grain increment servings daily was reduced by 17%.
Haas et al. (2009). Evaluate the effectiveness of whole- grain in preventing CRC [52].	11 cohort studies, 1,719,590 participants; baseline age 25–76 years; 6–16 years of follow-up; 7745 colorectal cancer cases.	In the multivariate analysis, the highest quintile of whole-grain intake was associated with 6% lower risk of CRC. A sub-analysis by tumor location showed reduced risk in the colon by 7% and rectum by 11%.
Prospective Cohort Study		
Kyro et al. (2013). Assess the dose-response association between whole-grain intake and CRC risk (Scandinavian cohort HELGA consisting of Danish, Swedish, and Norwegian persons [53].	108,000 participants; median baseline age mid-50s; median 11 years of follow-up; 1123 colorectal cancer cases (multivariate adjusted).	Intake of whole-grain products was associated with a lower incidence of CRC per 50-g increment by 6%. Intake of whole-grain wheat (highest vs. lowest quartile) was associated with a lower incidence of colorectal cancer by 34% but the effect was non-linear.

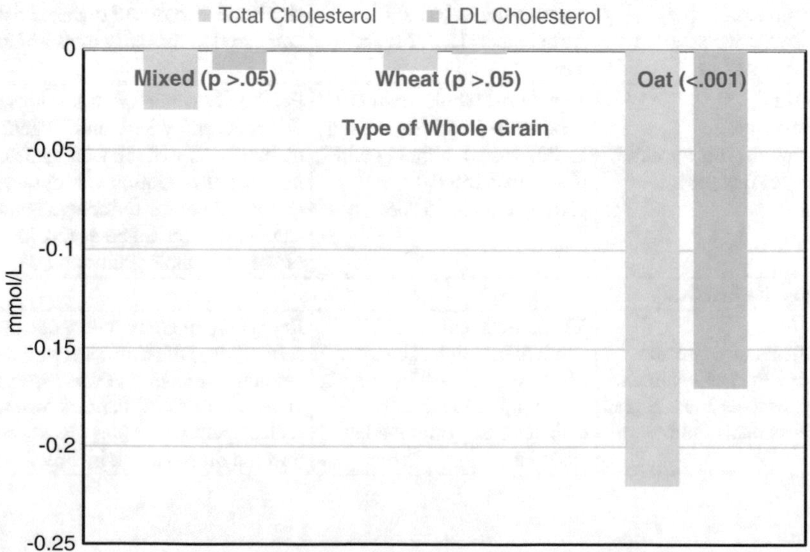

Fig. 3.3 Association between wheat, oats and a mixture of the two whole-grains on total and LDL-cholesterol from a meta-analysis of 24 RCTs (adapted from [38])

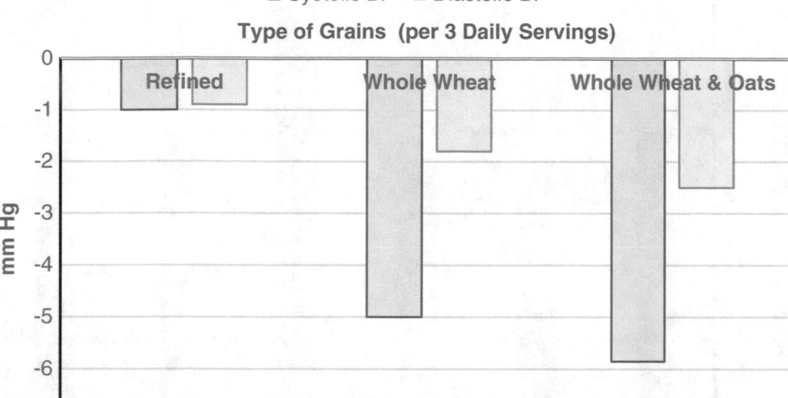

Fig. 3.4 Effect of type of grains consumed on blood pressure (BP) in 233 UK men and women with mean age of 52 years and BMI of 28 (adapted from [43])

Ischemic Stroke

Two meta-analyses of prospective cohort studies [44, 45] and one representative cohort study example [46] provide support evidence for the protective effects of ≥3 daily whole-grain servings on reducing the risk of ischemic stroke. A 2016 meta-analysis (7 cohort studies; 446,451 subjects) found that higher whole-grain intake reduced ischemic stroke risk by 25% whereas refined grains were not associated with lower stroke risk [44]. A 2015 meta-analysis (6 cohort studies; 247,487 subjects) reported that higher intake of whole-grains reduced total stroke risk by 14% in the total population and by 22% when only women were analyzed [45]. The Nurses' Health Study (75,521 women; baseline age range 38–63; 12 years of follow-up) showed that higher whole-grain intake significantly lowered ischemic stroke risk in all women by 31% and in non-smoking women by 50% (highest vs. lowest quintile of intake; multivariate adjusted) [46].

Type 2 Diabetes (Diabetes)

Three meta-analyses of cohort studies [47, 48, 50] and one representative large pooled cohort study [49] support the protective effects of ≥3 daily whole-grain servings on reducing the risk of diabetes. A systematic review and meta-analysis (7 prospective studies and 1 case control study; 316,051 adults; 15,573 diabetes cases) showed a significant linear inverse relationship between whole grain intake and diabetes incidence; 45 g of whole grains/day significantly reduced diabetes risk by 20% compared to consuming 7.5 g of whole grains/day [47]. In a dose-response meta-analysis (16 cohort studies), 3 servings of whole-grains significantly reduced diabetes risk by 32% whereas the same number of servings of refined grains slightly reduced risk by 5% [48]. The effects of various grain foods on diabetes risk are summarized in Fig. 3.5. A systematic review (6 cohort studies; 286,125 participants; 10,944 diabetes cases) found that two servings per day of whole-grains was associated with a 21% lower risk of diabetes, after adjusting for potential confounders including BMI [50]. The 2010 pooled data from the Nurses' Health Study I and II and Health Professionals Follow-up Study (39,765 men and 157,463 women; baseline age range 26–87 years; 14–22 years follow-up) showed that replacing 50 g/day cooked white rice with the same portion of brown rice was associated with a 16% reduced risk of diabetes, whereas the same portion of a variety of whole grains further lowered diabetes risk by 36% [49].

Colorectal Cancer (CRC)

Two meta-analyses of cohort studies [51, 52] and a representative cohort study [53] support the protective effects of ≥3 daily whole-grain

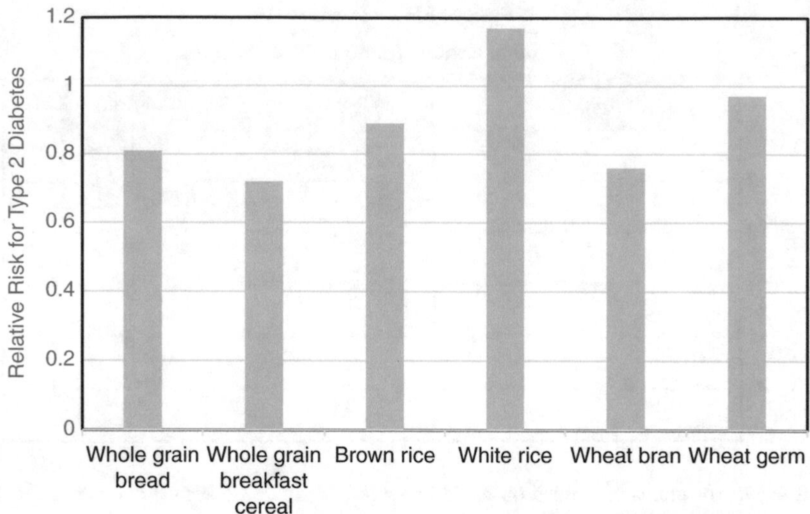

Fig. 3.5 Subtypes of grains on type 2 diabetes risk from meta-analysis of 16 cohort studies (adapted from [48])

servings in reducing the risk of colorectal cancer. A meta-analysis (6 cohort studies) showed that 3 daily servings of whole-grains significantly reduced colorectal cancer risk by 17% [51]. Another meta-analysis (11 cohort studies; 1,719,590 subjects) found that higher whole-grain intake reduced colorectal cancer risk by 6% [52]. The Scandinavian HELGA cohort study (108,000 adults; age 52 years at baseline; 11 years of follow-up) observed that whole-grain intake was associated with a lower incidence of colorectal cancer risk for total whole grains by 6% per 25 g intake [53].

3.2.1.4 Aging

Elevated levels of proinflammatory cytokines and acute phase proteins, such as interleukin (Il)-6, tumor necrosis factor (TNF)-α, and C-reactive protein (CRP) have been associated with suboptimal aging, known as inflammaging, and associated with increased chronic disease risk [54–57]. A review of observational studies suggests that there is an inverse association between diets high in whole-grains and CRP concentrations [58]. Higher intake of fiber-rich whole-grains may promote healthy aging by modulating systemic inflammation and helping to (1) maintain a healthy colonic microbiota ecosystem which promotes colon barrier defenses against pathogenic bacteria and their endotoxins reducing chronic systemic and acute episodes of colonic inflammation, (2) reduce the risk of excessive levels of visceral fat, a known source of systemic inflammation, and (3) protect against periodontitis, a source of increased systematic inflammation with aging. In adults >65 years higher IL-6 and CRP levels are especially associated with poorer cognitive and/or functional performance, and a higher risk of mortality [59].

Microbiota Ecosystem

A healthy microbiota is an important barrier to inflammaging processes and helps to promote healthy aging and reduced chronic disease risk and progression to frailty in later life [60–65]. Whole-grains provide a major source of fiber, which is the main energy source for colonic bacteria and resulting fermentation products, which among other functions, are important in maintaining low systemic inflammation. In contrast, refined grain products are processed to remove most of their fiber and other bioactive components [66, 67]. Increased intake of fiber-rich whole-grain foods can increase the relative numbers of bifidobacteria and lactobacilli bacteria, and fecal butyrate concentration and lower colonic pH, which promote colon barrier defenses against pathogenic bacteria and their endotoxins to reduce chronic systemic inflammation, aid in healthier aging, and reduce chronic disease risk. Three RCTs demonstrate the beneficial effects of whole-grains on the microbiota and inflammatory markers [68–70]. One parallel RCT (49 men and 32 postmenopausal women; age range 40–65 years; 6 weeks) found that diets with whole grains (16 g whole grain/1000 kcal) significantly increased butyrate producing bacteria, total fecal short chain fatty acids (SCFAs) concentrations and acute innate immune response, and reduced colonic pro-inflammatory Enterobacteriaceae bacteria levels compared to refined grain diets [68]. A crossover RCT (28 healthy adults; daily dose of 60 g whole grain barley, brown rice or mixture of the two; 4 weeks) showed improvements in the colonic microbiota ecosystem that coincided with significantly reduced plasma IL-6 and peak postprandial blood glucose [69]. A parallel, single blind RCT (79 healthy; mean age 52 years, mean BMI 29; 3 daily whole-grain or refined grain servings in the form of bread and breakfast cereal added into habitual diets; 4 weeks) demonstrated that the whole-grain diet significantly lowered plasma CRP levels [70].

Visceral Fat

Unhealthy aging is often associated with inflammaging, characterized by a relative increase in visceral fat and loss of peripheral subcutaneous fat, which is associated with increased systemic free fatty acid and inflammatory biomarkers such as CRP [58, 71]. People consuming the recommended levels of whole-and refined-grains have lower odds of central obesity, including visceral fat and waist circumference gains [26, 72–76]. A meta-analysis (26 RCTs, ≤16 weeks) found that increased intake of whole-grains was shown to modestly but significantly lower percentage of body fat by 0.48% compared with a refined grain control (in a relatively short time-frame) [73]. A 2015 systemic review of observational studies and intervention trials concluded that whole-grain bread was more beneficial than white bread in controlling weight gain and abdominal fat and there was a possible relationship between high white bread intake and excess abdominal fat [74]. Also, this review summarized a 2013 PREvencion con DIeta MEDiterranea (PREDIMED) trial on 4 year changes in adiposity, which found that subjects with the highest white bread intake gained 0.8 kg more weight and increased waist circumference by 1.3 cm more than those with the lowest intake, which impaired weight control by reducing their odds of losing weight by 33% and waist circumference by 36%. In the Framingham Heart Study (2834 adults; mean age 51 years; 49% women), increasing whole-grain intake was associated with lower visceral adipose tissue volumes whereas higher intakes of refined grains were associated with higher visceral fat levels (Fig. 3.6) [75]. A 2017 RCT (81 adults; age range 40–65 years; 6 weeks) found that subjects on a whole-grain rich diet (207 g/day) had a significantly higher net daily energy loss by 92 kcal/day compared to those on a refined-grain diet (0 g whole-grains/day), which provides mechanistic support for whole-grain observational findings for lower risk of weight and fat gain via increased resting metabolic rate and metabolizable energy excretion in the stool [76].

Periodontal Disease

Periodontal disease is a set of inflammatory diseases affecting the tissues that surround and support the teeth [77]. Approximately half of adults age ≥30 years in the US have mild, moderate or severe periodontal disease [78]. The risk of periodontal disease increases with age and is more common in men than women. Periodontal disease and CVD share a common etiology of chronic inflammation. NHANES analyses from 2009–2010 and 2011–2012 (6052 US adults; age ≥30 years) found an inverse relation between fiber intake and periodontal disease among US adults [78]. Also, periodontal disease was associated with low whole-grain intake but not with low fruit and vegetable intake. The Health Professionals Follow-up Study (34,160 men; age range 45–75 years; 14 years of follow-up) showed that men with a median intake of >3.4 daily servings of whole grains had 23% lower odds of developing periodontal disease than those who consumed <0.3 servings (multivariate; p-trend <0.001) [79]. In contrast, refined-grain intake was associated

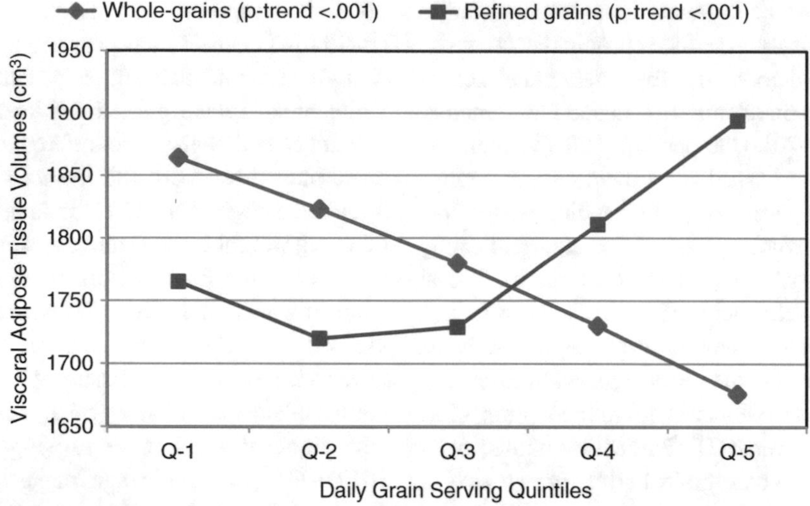

Fig. 3.6 Association between increasing whole and refined grains and visceral adipose tissue volume in US adults (whole grain: Q-5 [3 servings]; refined grains: Q-5 [4 servings]) (adapted from [75])

with an insignificant 4% increased odds of periodontal disease (multivariate; p-trend = 0.37).

3.2.2 Fruit and Vegetables

3.2.2.1 Background

The 1990 World Health Organization (WHO) report recommended a minimum daily intake of five daily servings of fruits and vegetables, which provide aging and chronic disease protective levels of micro and macronutrients, and phytochemicals such as flavonoids and carotenoids [80]. However, globally only a small fraction of populations consume recommended intake of fruit and vegetables; for example, >85% of the US population falls short of meeting the daily recommendations [10, 11]. Most Americans consume less than one cup of fruit and less than two cups of vegetables daily, with the primary contributors consisting of juice and processed potatoes, compared to the current recommendations of 2 cups of fruit and 2.5 cups of vegetables per day [11, 81]. A 2016 pooled analysis of 124,086 US men and women suggests that consuming high flavonoid fruits and vegetables, such as apples, pears, berries, and peppers, may be especially helpful in preventing weight gain and obesity compared to other types of fruits and vegetables [81]. The USDA MyPlate educational concept, devotes one-half the plate to fruit and vegetables as a displacement of other foods of higher energy density from the diet. This promotes healthy aging, weight control and the prevention of chronic disease risk and premature mortality, especially if the fruits and vegetables consumed are rich in flavonoids and fiber.

3.2.2.2 Mortality Risk

It is estimated that the global intake of < 500g/day of fruit and vegetables was associated with 5.4 million premature deaths, including 710,000 CHD deaths, 1.5 million stroke deaths, and 560,000 cancer deaths [82]. Table 3.4 summarizes the findings from one meta-analysis of cohort studies and six representative cohort studies on the effects of fruits and vegetables on all-cause and disease specific mortality [82–89]. A 2017 systematic review and dose-response meta-analysis (94 cohort studies; 2,123,415 participants) found significant reduced all-cause mortality risk for combined fruit and vegetable intake by 10%, for fruit intake by 15% and vegetable intake by 13% per 200 g/day [82]. Also, there was evidence that high vs. low intake of apples, pears, berries, citrus fruits, 100% fruit juice, cooked vegetables,

Table 3.4 Summary of fruit and vegetable prospective studies on mortality risk

Reference/Objective	Methods/Subjects	Results
Systematic Review and Meta-Analysis		
Aune et al. (2017) Assess the effects of total fruits and vegetables and specific types on all-cause mortality risk [82].	94 cohort studies; 2,123,415 participants.	Per 200 g/day, there was a significant reduced risk of all-cause mortality for combined fruit and vegetable intake by 10%, for fruit intake by 15% and vegetable intake by 13%. There was evidence that high vs. low intake of apples/pears, berries, citrus fruits, 100% fruit juice, cooked vegetables, cruciferous vegetables, potatoes and green leafy vegetables/salads were inversely associated with all-cause mortality and canned fruits increased risk. Also, a dose-response analysis found that 100% fruit juice, cruciferous vegetables and green leafy vegetables/salads were significantly associated with reduced all-cause risk (Fig. 3.7).
Wang et al. (2014). Examine and quantify the potential dose-response relation between fruit and vegetable consumption and risk of mortality from all-cause, CVD, and cancer [83].	16 cohorts up to August 2013; 833,234; 4.6–26 years of follow-up; 56,423 deaths.	Higher consumption of fruit and vegetables is associated with a reduced risk of all-cause mortality with an average 5% reduced risk per additional daily serving (Fig. 3.8). There was a threshold at 5 servings/day, after which the risk of mortality did not reduce further. There was a significant inverse association for CVD mortality by 4% for each added serving. However, there was no appreciable association with cancer mortality.
Prospective Cohort Studies		
Bellavia et al. (2016). Determine the effect of fruit and vegetable intake on red meat mortality risk (the Swedish Mammography Cohort and the Cohort of Swedish Men) [84].	74,645 men and women; baseline age 45–83 years; 16 years of follow-up; 17,909 deaths occurred in the cohort (mortality resulting from CVD-related death 5495 and 4426 cancer deaths (multivariate adjusted).	In high red meat consumers, increased fruit and vegetable intake did not affect the increased mortality risk of all-cause by 21% or CVD mortality by 29%. This study found no detectable affect of fruit and vegetables lowering the elevated mortality risk in people with a high intake of red meat.
Nguyen et al. (2016). Examine the association between intake of vegetables and fruits, and raw vs. cooked vegetables consumption on the risk of all-cause mortality (Australia) [85].	150,969 adults; mean baseline age 60 years; 55% women; average follow-up 6.2 years; 6038 all cause deaths (multivariate adjusted).	The consumption of ≥7 servings/ day of total fruit and vegetables reduced all-cause mortality risk by 10% (p for trend =0.002; high vs. low quartile). Fruit intake was inversely associated with all-cause mortality with a 16% risk reduction (p-trend ≤0.001; high vs. low intake). Consumption of total and cooked vegetables, significantly reduced risk by 7% and 13%, respectively (p-trend <0.05) but raw vegetables reduced risk by 6% (p-trend =0.79).
Oyebode et al. (2014). Examine the association between fruit and vegetable consumption and all-cause, cancer and cardiovascular mortality (Health Surveys for England) [86].	65,226 participants; baseline age 35+ years; median 7.7 years of follow-up (multivariate adjusted).	High daily fruit and vegetables intake (≥ 7 daily serving) was associated with a significant 33% lower multivariate all-cause mortality risk, which was lowered to 48% lower risk after excluding deaths during the first year of the study. Also, high fruit and vegetable intake was associated with reduced cancer mortality by 25% and CVD mortality by 31%. The effects of specific fruits and vegetables on all-mortality risk are summarized in Fig. 3.9.

(continued)

Table 3.4 (continued)

Reference/Objective	Methods/Subjects	Results
Leenders et al. (2013). Evaluate the association between fruit and vegetables intake and risk of mortality (European Prospective Investigation into Cancer and Nutrition [EPIC]) [87].	451,151 participants; range of 10–18 years of follow-up (multivariate adjusted).	Higher fruit and vegetables intake was significantly associated with lower mortality risk for all-cause by 10% and for CVD by 15% (daily intake of >570 g of fruit and vegetables vs. <250 g). Stronger inverse associations with both cancer and CVD mortality were seen for raw vegetables than for cooked vegetables.
Bellavia et al. (2013). Examine the dose-response relation between fruit and vegetable intake and mortality, in terms of both time and rate (The Swedish Mammography Cohort and the Cohort of Swedish Men) [88].	71,706 participants, 38,221 men and 33,485 women; mean baseline age 60 years;13 years of follow-up; 11,439 deaths, 6803 men and 4636 women (multivariate adjusted).	Those who rarely or never consumed fruit and vegetables lived shorter lives by 3 years and had a 53% higher mortality rate than those who consumed ≥5 servings fruit and vegetables/day.
Zhang et al. (2011). Investigate the associations of cruciferous vegetables, non-cruciferous vegetables, total vegetables, and total fruit intake with risk of all-cause and cause-specific mortality (Shanghai Women's Health Study and the Shanghai Men's Health Study) [89].	134,796 Chinese adults; mean follow-up of 4.6–10 years; 3442 deaths among women; and 1951 deaths among men (multivariate adjusted).	Fruit and vegetable intake was inversely associated with risk of total mortality in both women and men. A significant dose-response was observed for cruciferous vegetable intake with a significant reduction in total morality risk by 22% (high vs. low quintiles) and 16% for total vegetables. Similar risk reduction was observed for CVD mortality but not for cancer mortality.

cruciferous vegetables, and green leafy vegetables/salads were inversely associated with all-cause mortality and 100% fruit juice, cruciferous vegetables and green leafy vegetables/salads were significantly associated with reduced mortality risk per 100 g intake (Fig. 3.7). Another large dose-response meta-analysis (16 cohort studies; 833,234; 4.6–26 years of follow-up) found that total fruit and vegetable intake was inversely associated with all-cause mortality risk by 5% per daily serving (6% for fruits and 5% for vegetables) until a threshold of 5 servings/day was reached (Fig. 3.8) [83]. Similar findings were observed for CVD mortality, but not cancer mortality. A Swedish cohort study (74,645 adults; age range 45–83 years; 16 years of follow-up) observed that high intakes of red meat (120–300 g/day), especially processed meats, were associated with a higher risk of mortality from all-causes by 21% and CVD by 29% [84]. The increased risks were consistently observed in participants with low, medium, and high fruit intake suggesting no beneficial interaction between high red meat and increased fruit and vegetable intake. A large Australian study (150,969 adults; mean baseline age 60 years; 55% women; average follow-up 6.2 years) observed that the consumption of ≥7 servings/day of total fruit and vegetables reduced all-cause mortality risk by 10% (p for trend = .002; high vs. low quartile) [85]. Also, increased fruit intake was inversely associated with all-cause mortality by a significant 16% risk reduction (fully adjusted; high vs. low intake) and higher intake of total and cooked vegetables in the fully adjusted models significantly reduced risk by 7% and 13%, respectively, but higher raw vegetables insignificantly reduced risk by 6%. In English Health Surveys (65,226; aged 35+ years; median follow-up of 7.7 years) the consumption of vegetables, salad, and fresh and dried fruit were associated with significantly lower all-cause mortality whereas the consumption of frozen or canned fruit was associated with a significantly increased risk and 100% fruit juice was not

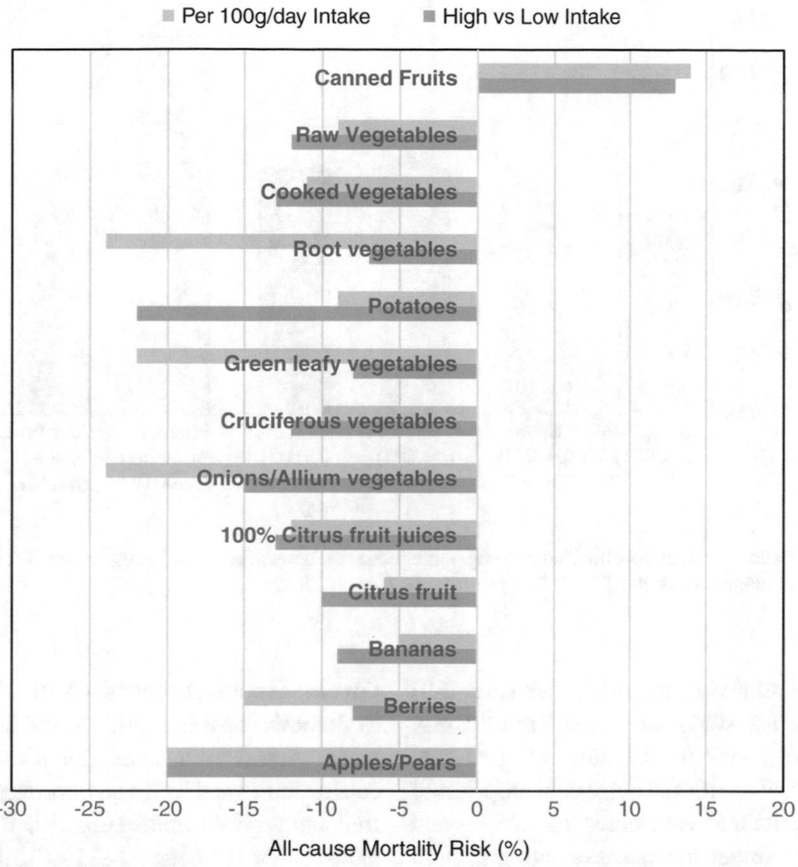

Fig. 3.7 Association between subtype of fruits and vegetables and all-cause mortality risk from a meta-analysis of 94 cohort studies (adapted from [82])

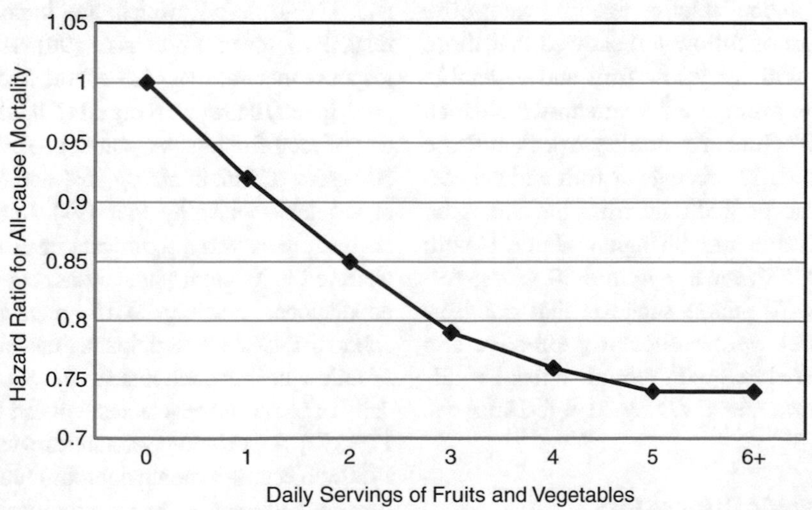

Fig. 3.8 Frequency of daily fruit and vegetables consumption and the risk of all-cause mortality from a meta-analysis of 16 cohort studies ($p < 0.001$) (adapted from [83])

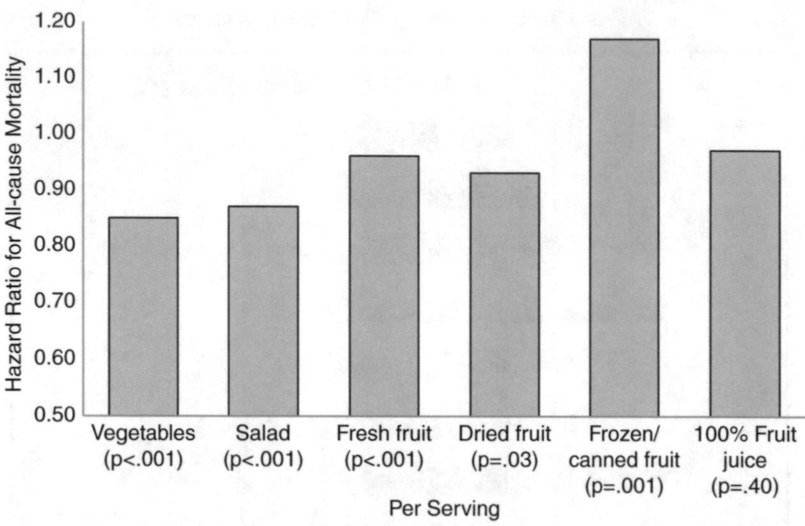

Fig. 3.9 Association between specific fruit and vegetable foods and beverages and all-cause mortality risk in UK adults aged ≥35 years (adapted from [86])

significantly related to mortality risk (Fig. 3.9) [86]. An EPIC study observed significantly lower mortality risk for all cause by 10% and for CVD by 15% with the daily consumption of >570 g of fruits and vegetables vs. <250 g and there was a stronger inverse association in both cancer and CVD mortality seen for raw vegetables than for cooked vegetables [87]. A large Swedish dose-response cohort study (71,706 participants; mean baseline age 60 years; 60% men; 13 years of follow-up) showed that those participants with very low fruit and vegetable intake had on average a 3-year shorter lifespan and had a 53% higher mortality risk than those consuming 5 daily servings of fruit and vegetables [88]. The pooled data from the Shanghai Women's Health and Shanghai Men's Health studies (134,796; mean age mid-50 years; follow-up of 5–10 years) suggests that cruciferous vegetables were particularly effective and inversely associated with mortality risk for all-causes by 22% and CVD by 31% (>166 g vs. <34 g/day) [89].

3.2.2.3 Chronic Disease Risk

Table 3.5 [90–117] summarizes the protective effect of fruits and vegetables on chronic disease from cohort studies and RCTs.

Cardiovascular Diseases (CVD)

Systematic Reviews and Meta-Analyses. Four meta-analyses summarize the pooled data from cohort studies and RCTs on the effects of increased fruit and vegetable intake on CVD risk [90–93]. A meta-analysis of berries (22 RCTs; 1251 subjects; 2–24 weeks) found that increased intake of berries significantly attenuated LDL cholesterol, systolic blood pressure (BP), fasting blood glucose, BMI and TNF-α levels, which are important factors related to lower CVD risk [90]. A 2015 dose response meta-analysis (23 cohort studies; 937,665 participants) showed a reduced CHD risk for 477 g/day of total fruit and vegetable intake by 12%, for 300 g/day of fruit intake by 16% and for 400 g/day of vegetable intake by 18% [91]. In the subgroup analysis, there was a significant inverse association observed in Western populations, but not in Asian populations. Another 2015 meta-analysis (38 cohorts; 1,498,909 participants; median 10.5 years of follow-up) reported that those consuming 800 g daily of fruits and vegetables reduced CVD risk by 17% [92]. A Cochrane systematic review (10 RCTs; 1730 subjects; ≥3-month duration) found increased fruit and vegetables intake significantly lowered systolic and diastolic BP and LDL-cholesterol [93].

Specific Studies. Three cohort studies and one large RCT provide important insights on the effects

Table 3.5 Summary of fruit and vegetables prospective studies and randomized controlled trials (RCTs) on chronic disease risk

Objective	Study details	Results
Cardiovascular Disease (CVD)		
Systematic Reviews and Meta-analyses		
Huang et al. (2016). Estimate the effect of berries consumption on CVD risk factors [90].	22 RCTs; 1251 subjects; 2–24 weeks.	The pooled results showed that berries intake significantly lowered LDL-cholesterol by 0.21 mmol/L, systolic blood pressure by 2.7 mmHg, fasting glucose by 0.10 mmol/L, BMI by 0.36 kg/m^2, HbA1c by 0.20% and TNF-α by 0.99 ρg/mL vs. control diets. Berries consumption appears to be effective in prevention and control of CHD and CVD risk.
Gan et al. (2015). Evaluate the dose-response relationship of fruit and vegetable intake with CHD risk and quantify the dose–response relationship [91].	23 cohort studies; 937,665 participants; 18,047 patients with CHD.	A dose–response analysis found a reduced CHD risk of 12% per 477 g/day of total fruit and vegetable intake; 16% per 300 g/day of fruit intake; and 18% per 400 g/day of vegetable consumption. A significant nonlinear association of CHD risk and fruit or vegetable consumption was found (p - nonlinearity <0.001). In the subgroup analysis, there was a significant inverse association observed in Western populations, but not in Asian populations.
Zhan et al. (2015). Examine the dose-response relation between fruit and vegetable intake and CVD risk [92].	38 cohort studies; 1,498,909 participants; median follow-up of 10.5 years; 44,013 CVD events.	For the highest versus lowest intake, pooled CVD risk was reduced for total fruits and vegetables by 17%, fruits by 16%, and vegetables by 13%. Dose-response analysis showed that those eating 800 g per day of fruits and vegetables had the lowest CVD risk
Hartley et al. (2013). Evaluate the effects of increased fruit and vegetable intake on the primary prevention of CVD (Cochrane Systematic Reviews) [93].	10 RCTs; 1730 subjects; ≥ 3 months of duration.	None of the trials reported clinical events or showed strong evidence for lowering CVD risk factors, but trials were heterogeneous and short term. Increased fruit or vegetable intake showed beneficial lowering effects on systolic blood pressure (BP) mean lowering by 3.0 mmHg, diastolic BP mean lowering by 0.90 mmHg. Two studies showed significantly lower LDL cholesterol.
Prospective Cohort Studies		
Larsson, Wolk (2016). Examine the association between potato consumption and risk of total and specific CVD events (Cohort of Swedish Men and the Swedish Mammography Cohort) [94].	69,313 healthy men and women; mean baseline age approx. 60 years; 13 years of follow-up; 10,147 major CVD events (multivariate adjusted).	3 to 7 servings/week of total potato consumption (boiled potatoes, fried potatoes, and French fries) had no effect on CVD events, heart failure or myocardial infarction (Fig. 3.10).
Miedema et al. (2015). Assess the relationship between intake of fruits and vegetables during young adulthood and coronary atherosclerosis later in life (Coronary Artery Risk Development in Young Adults [CARDIA] Study; US) [95].	2506 participants; 63% women; baseline age 25 years; 20 years of follow-up (multivariate adjusted).	Higher intake of fruits and vegetables was associated with a lower prevalence of coronary artery calcium by 26% (p-trend <0.001) in middle-aged adulthood, which was attenuated after adjustment for other dietary variables to a lower risk of 8%, but the trend remained significant (p-value for trend <0.002). This reinforces the importance of establishing a high fruit and vegetable intake early in life for CVD health.

(continued)

Table 3.5 (continued)

Objective	Study details	Results
Bhupathiraju et al. (2013). Examine the independent roles of quantity and variety in fruit and vegetable intake in relation to CHD incidence (Nurses' Health Study and Health Professionals Follow-Up Study) [96].	71,141 women and 42,135 men; mean baseline age approx. 50 years; 24 and 22 years of follow-up; 2582 CHD cases among women and 3607 CHD cases among men (multivariate adjusted).	Participants in the highest quintile of fruit and vegetable intake had a 17% lower CHD risk. A higher consumption of citrus fruit, green leafy vegetables, and β-carotene– and vitamin C–rich fruit and vegetables was associated with a lower CHD risk (Fig. 3.11).
RCT		
CVD Prevention		
Buil-Cosiales et al. (2016). Investigate the association of fiber, fruit, vegetable and whole-grain consumption with CVD in a Mediterranean cohort of elderly adults at high cardiovascular risk (PREvención con DIeta MEDiterránea (PREDIMED) trial; Spain) [97].	**Parallel RCT:** 7216 elderly men and women with high CVD risk; mean baseline age 67 years; up to 7-years follow-up; 342 confirmed cases of CVD; yearly repeated measurements of diet (multivariate adjusted).	This RCT found a significant inverse association with CVD incidence and total daily fruit and vegetable consumption. Those Subjects consuming ≥9 servings/day of fruits and vegetables had a 40% lower CVD risk vs. those consuming <5 servings/ day.
Hypertension/Blood Pressure		
Systematic Review and Meta-analyses		
Li et al. (2016). Assess the hypertension risk for highest vs. lowest fruit and vegetable consumption [98].	3 cohort, 2 case-control and 20 cross-sectional studies; 334,468 subjects; 41,713 hypertension cases.	Comparing the highest with the lowest consumption, the pooled hypertension risk was reduced by 19% for total fruits and vegetables, 27% for fruit, and 3% for vegetables. A significantly inverse association between fruit consumption and hypertension risk by 30% was found in Asian studies.
Wu et al. (2016). Evaluate dose-response association between the intake of fruit and/or vegetables and the risk of developing hypertension [99].	9 cohorts; 185,676 participants.	The risk of hypertension was decreased by 1.9% for each daily fruit serving, and by 1.2% for each daily serving of total fruit and vegetables. For highest vs. lowest intake, there was an inverse association with hypertension risk for fruit by 13%, vegetables by 12% and total fruit and vegetables by 10%.
Prospective Cohort Studies		
Borgi et al. (2016). Examine the independent association of whole fruit (excluding juices) and vegetable intake, as well as the change in consumption of whole fruits and vegetables with hypertension incidence (Nurses' Health Study, Nurses' Health Study II, and Health Professionals Follow-up Study; US) [100].	187,453 participants; baseline age range 43–55 years; >20 years of follow-up; 77,373 hypertension cases (multivariate adjusted).	Compared with participants whose consumption was ≤4 servings/week, the pooled hypertension risk among those whose intake was ≥4 servings/ day was reduced by 8% for total whole fruit intake and 5% for total vegetable intake. Analyses of individual fruits and vegetables consumption levels of ≥4 servings/week (as opposed to <1 serving/month) showed broccoli, carrots, avocado, tofu or soybeans, raisins, and apples or pears were associated with lower hypertension risk (Fig. 3.12).

Table 3.5 (continued)

Objective	Study details	Results
Borgi et al. (2016). Determine whether higher intake of baked or boiled potatoes, French fries, or potato chips is associated with incidence of hypertension (Nurses' Health Study, Nurses' Health Study II, and Health Professionals Follow-up Study; US) [101].	187,453 participants; baseline age range 43–55 years; >20 years of follow-up; 77,726 hypertension cases (multivariate adjusted).	Compared with the intake of <1 serving a month, the pooled hypertension risk for ≥4 servings a week was increased for baked or mashed potatoes by 11% (p trend =0.05), French fries by 17% (p-trend =0.001) and there was an insignificant risk reduction for potato chips by 3% (p- trend =0.98) (Fig. 3.13). In substitution analyses, replacing 1 daily serving of baked, boiled, or mashed potatoes with one serving a day of non-starchy vegetables was associated with decreased risk of hypertension by 7%.
RCT		
Appel et al. (1997). Examine the clinical effects of increased fruits and vegetables on blood pressure (US) [102].	**Parallel RCT:** 154 subjects in each group; mean age approx. 45 years; mean systolic and diastolic blood pressures were 131 and 85 mm Hg; 8 weeks.	A high fruit and vegetable diet with 8.5 daily servings reduced systolic BP by 2.8 mm Hg ($p < 0.001$) and diastolic BP by 1.1 mm Hg ($p = 0.07$) more than the control diet with 3.6 daily fruit and vegetable servings.
Ischemic Stroke		
Systematic Review and Meta-analysis		
Hu et al. (2014). Summarize evidence from prospective cohort studies on the association of fruits and vegetables consumption and stroke risk [103].	20 cohort studies; 760,629 participants; mean follow-up ranged from 3 to 37 years; 16,981 stroke events.	For highest vs. lowest intake, stroke risk was reduced for total fruits and vegetables by 21%, for fruits by 23%, and vegetables by 14%. Citrus fruits, apples, pears, and leafy vegetables especially contributed to the protection. The linear dose–response relationship showed that the risk of stroke decreased for fruits by 32% and vegetables by 11% per 200 g/day intake increment.
Prospective Cohort Studies		
Cassidy et al. (2016). Examine the relation between habitual anthocyanin and flavanone intake and coronary artery disease and stroke (Health Professionals Follow-Up Study) [104].	43,880 healthy men; mean baseline age 53 years; 24 years of follow-up; 4046 myocardial infarction and 1572 stroke cases (multivariate adjusted).	Higher intakes of flavonoids-rich fruits such as oranges, limes, lemons, apples and pears were associated with a lower risk of ischemic stroke in men by 22% (p-trend =0.059), with the greatest effects in participants aged ≥65 years (p-interaction =0.04).
Oude Griep et al. (2011). Examine associations between consumption of fruit and vegetable color groups with 10-year stroke incidence (Monitoring Project on Risk Factors and Chronic Diseases in the Netherlands [MORGEN Study] [105].	20,069 men and women; baseline average age 42 years; 10 years of follow-up; 233 stroke cases (multivariate adjusted).	Green, orange/yellow, and red/purple fruits and vegetables were not related to stroke incidence. Higher intake of white fruits and vegetables (e.g., apples, pears, apple juice and sauce, bananas, cauliflower, chicory, cucumbers, and mushrooms) were inversely associated with incident stroke (171 vs. 78 g/day) by 52%. Each 25-g/day increase in white fruit and vegetable consumption was associated with a 9% lower risk of stroke. Apples and pears were the most commonly consumed white fruit and vegetables (55%).

(continued)

Table 3.5 (continued)

Objective	Study details	Results
Joshipura et al. (1999). Evaluate the associations between fruit and vegetable intake and ischemic stroke risk (Nurses' Health Study and Health Professionals Follow-up Study; US) [106].	75,596 women; baseline age range 34–59 years; 14 years of follow-up; 366 ischemic stroke cases; and 38,683 men; baseline age range 40–75 years; 8 years of follow-up; 204 ischemic stroke cases (multivariate adjusted).	Higher fruit and vegetable intake (5.1 servings for men and 5.8 servings for women) reduced ischemic stroke risk by 31% vs. the lowest intake. An increase in 1 serving of fruits and vegetables significantly reduced risk by 6% (p = 0.01). Citrus fruit including juice, cruciferous vegetables, and green leafy vegetables contributed the most to lower ischemic stroke risk. Potatoes and legumes were not associated with stroke risk.
Type 2 Diabetes (Diabetes)		
Systematic Reviews and Meta-analyses		
Wang et al. (2016). Evaluate the effects of higher fruit and vegetables intake on diabetes risk [107].	23 cohort articles; baseline age range 25–79 years; 4–24 years of follow-up.	For the highest vs. lowest intake, the pooled lower multivariate diabetes risk was reduced for total fruits by 9%, blueberries by 25%, green leafy vegetables by 13%, yellow vegetables by 28%, and cruciferous vegetables by 18% for follow-ups of ≥10 years (Fig. 3.14).
Li et al. (2014). Clarify and quantify the potential dose-response association between the intake of fruit and vegetables and diabetes risk [108].	10 cohort studies, 434,342 participants; 24,013 diabetes cases.	Evidence of a curve-a-linear association was seen between fruit and green leafy vegetables intake and diabetes risk, without heterogeneity between studies. Each daily serving reduced diabetes risk for fruit by 7% and for vegetables by 10%. For green leafy vegetables, each 0.2 serving consumed/day reduced diabetes risk by 13%.
Xi et al. (2014). Estimate the association between sweetened and 100% fruit juice intake and diabetes risk [109].	4 sugar sweetened fruit juice cohort studies; 191,686 participants; and 4100% fruit juice cohort studies; 137,663 participants; follow-up ranged from 5.7 to 25 years.	Higher intake of sweetened fruit juice was significantly associated with increased diabetes risk by 28% (p = 0.02), whereas intake of 100% fruit juice was not associated with diabetes risk (p = 0.62).
Prospective Cohort Studies		
Mamluk et al. (2017). Assess the relationship between fruit and vegetable intake and diabetes risk (Consortium on Health and Aging Network of Cohorts in Europe and the United States [CHANCES]) [110].	NIH-AARP 401,909 subjects; mean baseline age 62 years; mean follow-up of 10.6 years; 22,782 diabetes cases; EPIC elderly 20,629 subjects; mean baseline age 63 years; mean follow-up of 11.8 years; 1567 diabetes cases (multivariate adjusted).	Comparing highest vs. lowest intake, fruit, vegetables or green leafy vegetable intake showed no association with diabetes risk for the overall study. However, independent results from the NIH-AARP study showed significant lower diabetes risk for fruit by 5% and for green leafy vegetables by 13%.
Muraki et al. (2016). Determine the effect of potato intake on diabetes risk (Nurses' Health Study, Nurses' Health Study II, and Health Professionals Follow-up Study; US) [111].	87,739 women and 40,669 men; >20 years of follow-up; 15,362 diabetes cases (multivariate adjusted).	Increased intake of French fries was positively associated with subsequent diabetes risk. Per each 3 weekly servings diabetes risk was increased for baked, boiled, or mashed potatoes by 4% and for French fries by 19%, independent of demographic, lifestyle, dietary factors, and BMI.

Table 3.5 (continued)

Objective	Study details	Results
Colorectal Cancer (CRC)		
Systematic Review and Meta-analysis		
Aune et al. (2011). Summarize the evidence for fruit and vegetable intake and CRC risk from cohort studies [112].	19 cohort studies.	For highest vs. the lowest intake, CRC risk was lowered for fruits and vegetables combined by 8%, fruit by 10%, and vegetables by 9%. This analysis showed a non-linear association between fruit and vegetable intake and lower CRC risk. For fruit, most of the risk reduction occurred during the first 100 g/day with higher intakes more modestly decreasing risk up to 600 g/day. For vegetables, the greatest risk reduction was between 100 and 200 g/day with modest lowering up to 500 g/day.
Prospective Cohort Studies		
Kunzmann et al. (2016). Evaluate the association between fruit and vegetable intake and CRC development by evaluating the risk of incident and recurrent colorectal adenoma and CRC (Prostate, Lung, Colorectal and Ovarian Cancer Screening Trial; US) [113].	57,774 subjects; mean baseline age 63 years; mean 12.1 years of follow-up; 733 CRC cases (multivariate adjusted).	Higher total fruit and vegetable intake was not associated with reduced incident or recurrent adenoma risk overall, but a protective association was observed for lower risk of multiple adenomas by 62%. Higher fruit and vegetable intakes were associated with a borderline reduced risk of CRC by 18%, which reached significance among individuals with high processed meat intakes with a 26% lower CRC risk.
Leenders et al. (2015). Examine the effect of separate subtypes and variety of fruits and vegetables in the diet on risk of colon and rectal cancer (EPIC; EU) [114].	442,961 participants from 10 EU countries; average of 13 years of follow-up; 3370 participants were diagnosed with colon or rectal cancer (multivariate adjusted).	For highest vs. lowest intake, a lower risk of colon cancer was observed with higher self-reported consumption of fruits and vegetables combined by 13% (p-trend =0.02), but no consistent association was observed for separate consumption of fruits and vegetables. No associations with risk of rectal cancer were observed.
Breast Cancer		
Systematic Reviews and Meta-analyses		
Hui et al. (2013). Summarize the association between flavonoids and its sub-classes (common in fruits and vegetables) and breast cancer (BC) risk [115].	6 cohort studies and 6 case-control studies; 190,000 subjects; 9513 cases.	BC was significantly reduced with high intake of flavonols by 12% and flavones by 17%. When the data was stratified by menopausal status, higher flavonols and flavones intake was associated with a significant reduced risk of BC in post-menopausal women but not in pre-menopausal women.
Aune et al. (2012). Summarize the evidence for an association between fruit and vegetable intake and BC [116].	15 cohort studies.	For the highest vs. lowest intake, BC risk was reduced for fruit and vegetables combined by 11%, fruits by 8%, and vegetables by 1%. A dose-response analysis found a lower BC risk per 200 g/day for fruit by 5%, fruit and vegetables combined by 4% and no lowering for vegetables.
Aune et al. (2012). Summarize the evidence of dietary intake and blood concentrations of carotenoids and BC risk [117].	25 cohort studies.	For dietary intake studies, only intake of β-carotene was significantly associated with a reduced BC risk by 5% per 5000 μg/day. However, blood concentrations of carotenoids showed more robust BC risk reductions: total carotenoids reduced risk by 22% per 100 μg total carotenoids/dL; β-carotene reduced risk by 26% per 50 μg β-carotene/dL; α-carotene by 18% per 10 μg α-carotene/dL, and lutein reduced risk by 32% per 25 μg lutein/dL (Fig. 3.15). Blood concentrations of carotenoids are more strongly associated with reduced BC risk than are carotenoids assessed by dietary questionnaires.

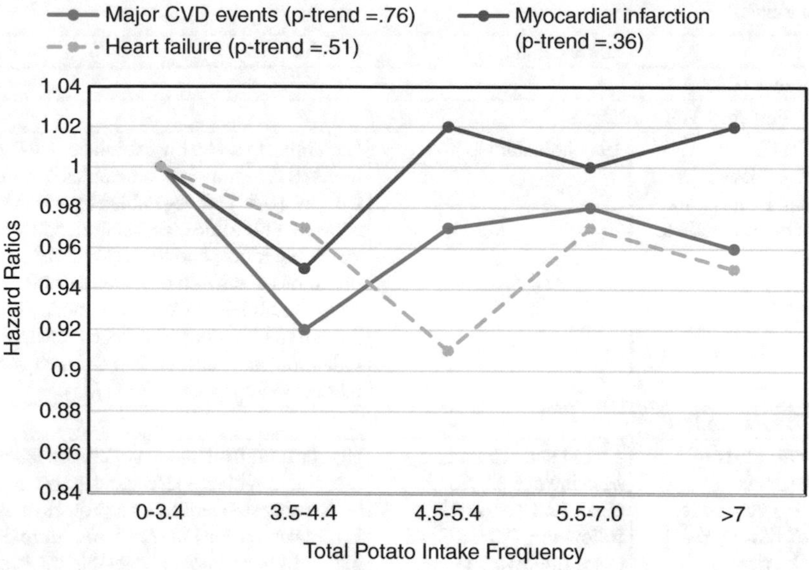

Fig. 3.10 Weekly potato servings and risk major and specific cardiovascular events (adapted from [94])

of specific fruits and vegetables on CHD and CVD risk [94–97]. A Swedish cohort study (69,313 adults, mean age 60 years; 13-years of follow-up) found that the consumption of 3 to 7 weekly servings of potatoes boiled, fried or French fries had no significant adverse effects on CVD events, heart failure or myocardial infarction (Fig. 3.10) [94]. The US CARDIA Study (2506 adults, mean baseline age 25 years; 20 years of follow-up) demonstrated that subjects with a higher intake of fruits and vegetables as young adults had significantly reduced coronary artery calcium in middle-age adulthood [95]. The pooled analysis of the Nurses' Health and Health Professionals Follow-Up Studies (113,000 men and women; mean baseline age 50 years; 22–24 years of follow-up) observed that participants in the highest intake quintile of fruits and vegetables (excluding potatoes, legumes, and fruit juices) had a 17% lower adjusted CHD risk [96]. Specifically, the consumption of 1–1.5 servings/day of green leafy vegetables, and β-carotene and vitamin C rich fruits and vegetables was associated with a significant 15–22% lower adjusted CHD risk (Fig. 3.11). The PREDIMED trial (7216 elderly men and women with high CVD risk; mean baseline age 67 years; up to 7-years follow-up) found a significant inverse association with CVD incidence and total daily fruit and vegetable consumption [97]. Subjects who consumed ≥9 servings/day of fruits and vegetables had a 40% lower multivariate CVD risk in comparison with those consuming <5 servings/day.

Hypertension and Blood Pressure (BP)

Meta-analyses. Two meta-analyses summarize the findings from observational studies on the effect of increased fruit and vegetables intake on hypertension risk [98, 99]. A meta-analysis comparing highest vs. lowest fruit and vegetable intake (3 cohort, 2 case-control, and 20 cross-sectional studies; 334,468 subjects) found a lower risk of hypertension for total fruits and vegetables by 19%, for fruits by 27%, and for vegetables by 3% [98]. A dose response meta-analysis (9 cohorts; 185,676 subjects) found that the risk of hypertension was decreased by 1.9% for each daily fruit serving and by 1.2% for each daily serving of total fruits and vegetables [99]. Also, high intake was associated with a lower risk of hypertension for fruits by 13% and vegetables by 12%.

Specific Studies. Several prospective studies and one RCT show the effects of increased fruits and vegetables on hypertension and blood pressure risk [100–102]. Two pooled analyses from

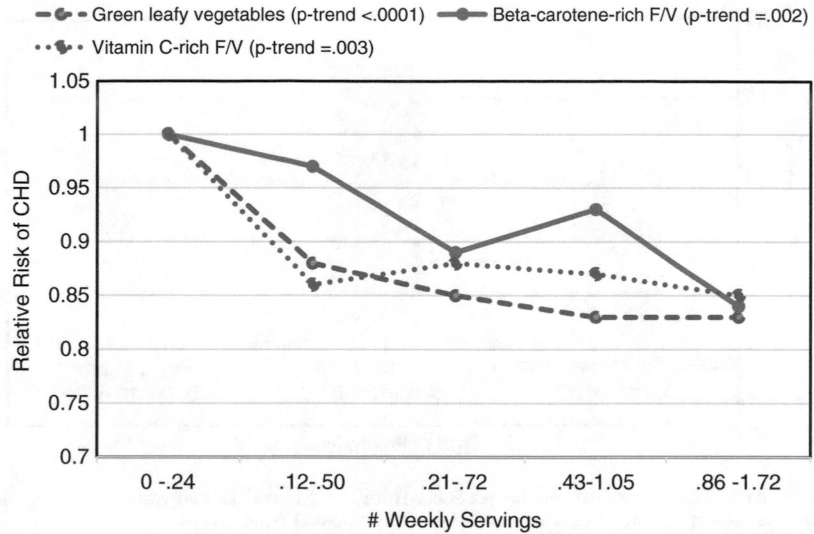

Fig. 3.11 Risk of coronary heart disease (CHD) by fruit and vegetable (F/V) variety and number of weekly servings based on multivariate pooled data from the Nurses' Health Study and Health Professionals Follow-up Study (adapted from [96])

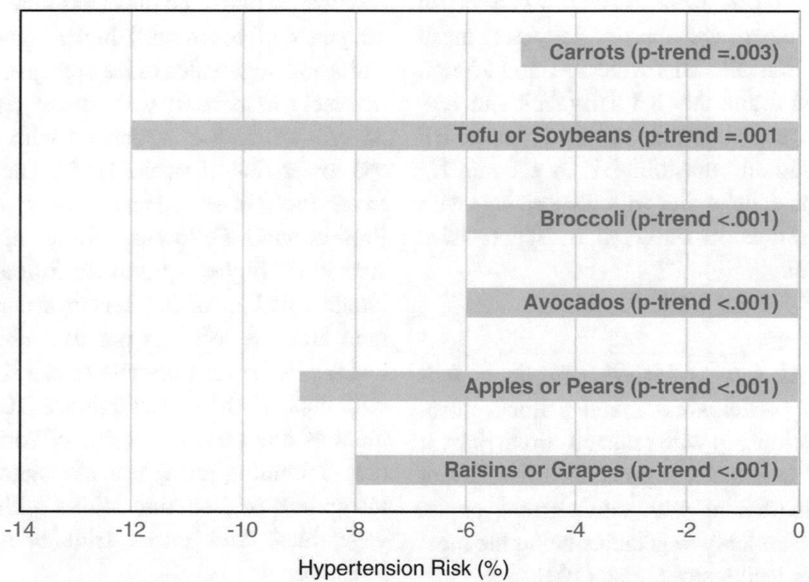

Fig. 3.12 Pooled hypertension risk reduction for individual fruits and vegetables from the Nurses' Health Study and Health Professionals Follow-up Study (≥ 4 weekly servings vs. ≤ 1 monthly serving) (adapted from [100])

the US Nurses' Health Studies and Health Professionals Follow-up Study (187,453 participants; mean baseline age range 43–55 years; >20 years of follow-up) observed that higher intake (≥4 weekly servings) lowered hypertension risk for fruits by 8% and vegetables by 5% [100, 101]. Also, higher intake (≥4 weekly servings) of broccoli, carrots, avocado, tofu or soybean, apples, pears and raisins significantly lowered hypertension risk (Fig. 3.12) [100]. Potato products significantly increased hypertension risk for baked or mashed potatoes by 11%

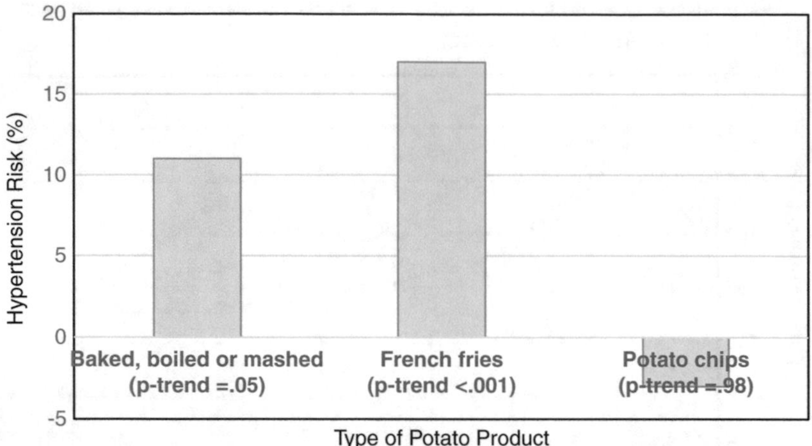

Fig. 3.13 Pooled hypertension risk for potato products from the Nurses' Health Study and Health Professionals Follow-up Study (≥4 weekly servings vs. ≤1 monthly serving) (adapted from 101])

and French fries by 17% whereas potato chips did not increase the risk for hypertension (Fig. 3.13) [101]. A 1997 RCT (154 subjects in each group; mean age approx. 45 years; mean systolic and diastolic BPs were 131 and 85 mm Hg; 8-weeks) found that 8.5 daily fruit and vegetable servings significantly reduced systolic BP by 2.8 mm Hg and diastolic BP by 1.1 mm Hg more than the control diet with 3.6 servings with greater BP reduction observed in hypertensive subjects [102].

Ischemic Stroke

Meta-analysis. A meta-analysis (20 cohort studies; 760,629 participants) found a linear dose-response relationship with reduced stroke risk for fruits by 32% and for vegetables by 11% per 200 g/day increment with citrus fruits, apple, pears, and green leafy vegetables being the most effective in reducing stroke risk [103].

Specific Studies. Three cohort studies provide specific insights on the effect of fruits and vegetables on ischemic stroke risk [104–106]. The Health Professionals Follow-up Study (43,880 men; mean baseline age 53 years; 24-year follow-up) found that men with the highest intake of flavonoid-rich fruits, such as oranges, limes, lemons, apples and pears, had significantly reduced multivariate ischemic stroke risk in mean by 22%, especially in men >65 years of age compared to men with the lowest intake [104]. In a Dutch population cohort (20,069 participants; mean baseline age 42 years; 10 years of follow-up) higher intake of white fruits and vegetables (55% apples and pears) was inversely associated with stroke risk with each 25 g/day increase associated with a significant 9% lower risk of stroke [105]. The pooled data from the Nurses' Health Study and Health Professionals Follow-up Study found that persons in the highest quintile of fruit and vegetable intake (median of 5.1 servings per day among men and 5.8 servings per day among women) had a 31% lower ischemic stroke risk compared with those in the lowest quintile [106]. An increment of one serving per day of fruits or vegetables (including juice) was associated with a 6% lower risk of ischemic stroke with cruciferous vegetables, and citrus fruit being the most effective.

Diabetes

Meta-analyses. Three meta-analyses of cohort studies summarize the effects of increased intake of fruits and vegetables on diabetes risk [107–109]. A 2016 meta-analysis (23 cohort studies; 4–24 years of follow-up) found that cohorts with ≥10 years of follow-up had significantly lower multivariate diabetes risk for total fruit, blueberries, green leafy, yellow and cruciferous vegetables intake

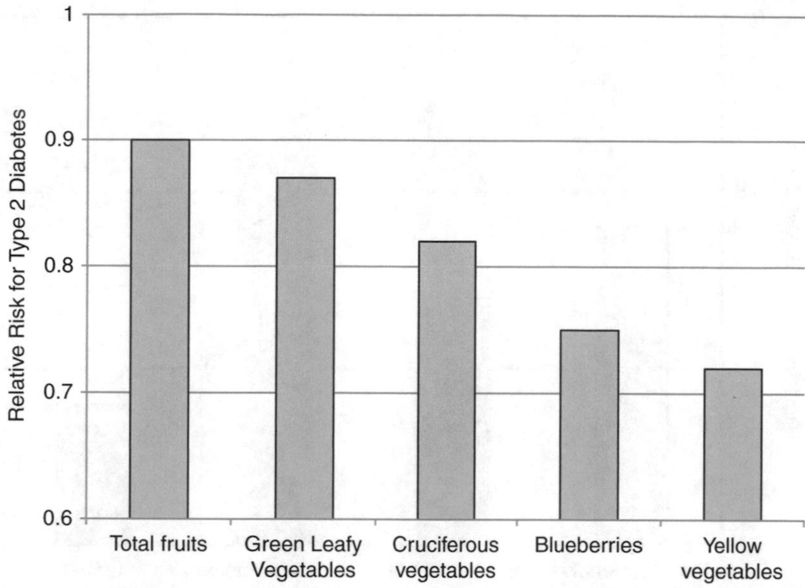

Fig. 3.14 Association between specific fruit and vegetables and type 2 diabetes risk based on data from a meta-analysis of cohort studies with follow-up of ≥10 years (adapted from [107])

(Fig. 3.14) [107]. A dose-response meta-analysis (10 cohort studies; 434,342 participants) showed a curve-a-linear association for total fruit and green leafy vegetables and diabetes with a daily serving of fruit lowering risk by 7% and 0.2 serving of green leafy vegetables lowering risk by 13%. A meta-analysis of fruit juice (8 cohort studies; 4 on sweetened juices; 4 on 100% juices; 191,686 participants) showed that sweetened fruit juice significantly increased diabetes risk by 28% whereas 100% fruit juices were not associated with diabetes risk (p = 0.62) [109].

Specific Studies. Two pooled cohort studies provide important insights on specific vegetables and diabetes risk [110, 111]. The US NIH-AARP cohort (401,909 participants; mean baseline age 62 years; 10.6 years of follow-up) found a significant lower diabetes risk for fruit by 5% and green leafy vegetables by 13% [110]. The pooled data from US Nurses' Health Studies and Health Professionals Follow-up Study (87,739 women and 40,669 men; >20 years of follow-up) found that 3 weekly servings of French fries significantly increased diabetes risk by 19% compared to a 4% increased risk for baked, boiled or mashed potatoes [111].

Cancer

Colorectal cancer (CRC). One meta-analysis of cohort studies and two specific cohort studies assessed the effect of increased intake of fruits and vegetables on CRC risk [112–114]. The meta-analysis (19 cohort studies) found modest but significant reductions in CRC risk for fruits and vegetables by 8–10%, for highest vs. lowest intake [112]. This analysis showed a non-linear association between fruit and vegetable intake and CRC risk. For fruits, most of the risk reduction occurred during the first 100 g/day with higher intakes more modestly decreasing risk up to 600 g/day. For vegetables, the greatest risk reduction was between 100 and 200 g/day with modest lowering up to 500 g/day. An analysis of the US Prostate, Lung, Colorectal and Ovarian Cancer Screening Trial (57,774 subjects; mean baseline age 63 years; mean 12.1 years of follow-up) showed that higher fruit and vegetable intake significantly reduced the risk of multiple adenomas by 62% and CRC risk among individuals with high intake of processed meat by 26% [113]. The 2015 EPIC analysis (442,961 participants; 13 years of follow-up) observed that the participants with the highest intake of total fruits and

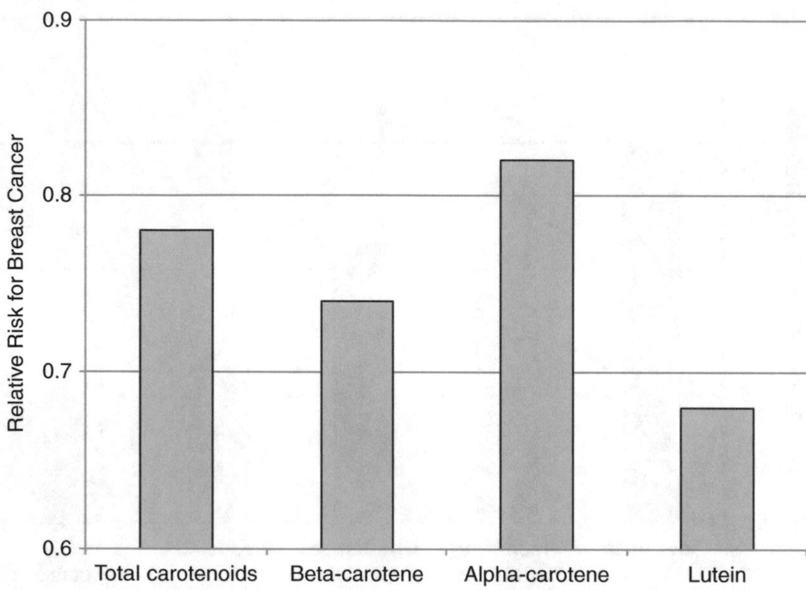

Fig. 3.15 Association between carotenoids blood concentrations and breast cancer risk based on data from a meta-analysis of 14 prospective studies (per total carotenoid 100 μg/dL; β-carotene 50 μg/dL; α-carotene 10 μg/dL; and lutein 25 μg/dL) (adapted from [117])

vegetables significantly reduced colon cancer risk by 13% [114].

Breast cancer (BC). Three meta-analyses, primarily from cohort studies, summarize the effects of increased fruit and vegetable intake on BC risk [115–117]. A meta-analysis of flavonoids and its subclasses common in fruits and vegetables (6 cohort and 6 case-control studies; 190,000 subjects) found that BC risk was significantly reduced with high intake of flavonols by 12% and flavones by 17% [115]. When the data was stratified by menopausal status, higher flavonols and flavones intake was associated with a significant reduced risk of BC in post-menopausal women but not in pre-menopausal women. A dose-response meta-analysis (15 cohort studies) showed a lower BC risk per 200 g/day of fruits by 5% and fruits and vegetables combined by 4% but no effect for vegetables alone [116]. A meta-analysis comparing dietary intake vs. blood concentration of carotenoids, a common phytochemical in fruits and vegetables (25 cohort studies), reported that higher blood levels of carotenoids were associated with lower BC risk by 18–32%, and were a better indicator of BC risk than dietary carotenoid intake (Fig. 3.15) [117].

3.2.2.4 Healthy Aging

Table 3.6 summarizes the evidence from studies on the effects of increased fruit and vegetable intake on healthy aging with a focus on slowing age-related cognitive performance and delaying general aging indicators and frailty [118–127].

Age-Related Cognitive Performance

The contribution of increased fruits and vegetables to the daily dietary intake of nutrient and phytochemical antioxidants may attenuate brain oxidative or inflammatory stress or elevate serum levels of brain-derived neurotrophic factor (BDNF) for possible protective effects on cognitive performance [118–123].

Systematic reviews. Several reviews have analyzed the protective effect of fruit and vegetable intake on age related cognitive function [118, 119]. A 2014 systematic review found statistically significant benefits of fruits, vegetables, or 100% juice consumption for improved cognitive function in older adults reported in 17 of 19

Table 3.6 Summary of fruit and vegetable prospective studies and randomized controlled trials (RCTs) on age related cognitive performance and frailty risk.

Objective	Study details	Results
Cognitive Function Performance		
Systematic Reviews		
Lamport et al. (2014). Summarize the association between polyphenol intake from fruit, vegetable, and juice consumption and cognition [118].	19 observational studies and 6 intervention studies.	17 observational studies and 3 intervention studies reported significant benefits of fruit, vegetable, or juice consumption on cognitive performance. The data suggest that chronic intake of fruits, vegetables, and juices are beneficial for cognition in healthy older adults. However, there was a high degree of variability in cognitive effects depending on the type of fruit, vegetable or juice consumed.
Loef and Walach (2012). Summarize the effects of fruit and vegetable intake on age related cognitive function [119].	6 cohort studies on fruits and vegetables with a follow-up of 6 months or longer.	Five of the 6 studies that analyzed fruit and vegetable consumption separately found that higher consumption of vegetables, but not fruit, was associated with a decreased risk of cognitive decline or dementia. In these studies, the vegetables most associated with slower cognitive decline included cruciferous vegetables, legumes, and green leafy vegetables, particularly cabbage, zucchini, squash, broccoli, and lettuce, at a daily intake of 3 servings (200 g) a day. The authors suggest that these beneficial effects might be due to higher intake of flavonoids or antioxidants in both fruits and vegetables, or increased vitamin E in vegetables, compared to fruits, which have more vitamin C. Furthermore, people frequently consume vegetables with added fats (e.g., oils) which may aid in absorption of nutrients/ phytochemicals.
RCTs		
Neshatdousta et al. (2016). investigate the link between changes in serum brain-derived neurotrophic factor (BDNF) and changes in human cognitive performance following fruit and vegetable flavonoid intake (UK) [120].	**Dose-response Parallel RCT:** 154 men and women; aged 26–70 years; intervention diet averaged 3 portions of fruit and vegetables per day to deliver high-flavonoid (>15 mg/100 g) or low-flavonoid (<5 mg/100 g). Intake was increased by 2 portions every 6 weeks; control was habitual diet; 18-week duration. Incrementally, 2, 4 and 6 portions of fruit and vegetable intake delivered 3, 6 and 7 mg/d (low-flavonoid intervention) and 49, 121 and 198 mg/d (high flavonoid intervention) total flavonoids.	High-flavonoid intake from fruit and vegetables intake induced significant improvements in cognitive performance and increases in serum brain-derived neurotrophic factor (BDNF) levels ($p = <0.001$) compared to low flavonoid fruits and vegetables and habitual diets. (Fig. 3.16 and 3.17). Flavonoid rich fruits and vegetables include: apples, pears, berries, oranges, peppers, broccoli, onions, cabbage.

(continued)

Table 3.6 (continued)

Objective	Study details	Results
Kean et al. (2015). Investigate the effects of flavonoid rich orange juice on cognitive function (US) [121].	**Double-blind, Crossover RCT:** 37 healthy older adults; mean age 67 years; high-flavanoid (305 mg) 100% orange juice and an equicaloric low-flavanoid (37 mg) orange-flavored drink (500 mL) were consumed daily; 8 weeks/4-week washout.	In healthy older adults, the daily consumption of flavanoid-rich 100 orange juice significantly improved global cognitive and executive function compared to a low-flavanoid control orange juice after 8 weeks.
Prospective Cohort Studies		
Nooyens et al. (2011). Evaluate the effect of habitual fruit and vegetable intake during mid-age on cognitive function (Doetinchem Cohort Study; The Netherlands) [122].	2613 men and women; baseline age 43–70 years (mean 55 years); examined for cognitive function twice, with a 5-year time interval (multivariate adjusted).	Higher vegetable intake was associated with smaller decline in information processing speed ($p < 0.01$) and global cognitive function ($p = 0.02$) over 5 years. High intakes of some subgroups of vegetables (i.e. cabbage and root vegetables such as carrots, red beets, mushrooms) were associated with smaller decline in cognitive function. Total intakes of fruits, legumes and juices were not associated with change in cognitive function.
Peneau et al. (2011). Examine the association between fruit and vegetable intake and cognitive performance in a sample of adults (Supplementation with Antioxidant Vitamins and Minerals 2; France) [123].	2533 subjects; baseline age 45–60 years; mean age at evaluation 66 years; 13 years of follow-up (multivariate adjusted).	Higher intakes of fruit and vitamin C–rich fruits and vegetables were associated with better verbal memory. In contrast, higher intakes of vegetables, and β-carotene-rich fruits and vegetables were associated with poorer executive function. Further research is required to better understand the complex associations between different groups of fruits and vegetables and specific areas of age related cognitive decline.
General Aging and Frailty		
RCTs from the Ageing and Dietary Intervention Trial (UK)		
Neville et al. (2013). Examine the effect of increased fruit and vegetable intake on measures of muscle strength and physical function among healthy, free-living older adults [124].	**Parallel RCT:** 83 participants habitually consuming ≤2 portions of fruits and vegetables/day; aged 65–85 years (mean age 71 years); usual diet (≤2 portions/day) vs. ≥5 fruit and vegetable portions/day; 16 weeks.	Subjects consuming ≥5 servings of fruits and vegetables had significantly higher biomarkers of micronutrient status. At 16 weeks, there was a trend towards a greater improvement in grip strength in the ≥5 portions/day to 2 kg vs. 0.1 kg for usual diet group ($p = 0.06$). Although increasing F/Vs. intake to ≥5 portions/day did not significantly improve lower-extremity physical function, it is possibly due to the study's relatively short duration.
Gibson et al. (2012). Determined whether increased fruit and vegetable intake improves measures of immune function [125].	**Parallel RCT:** 83 participants habitually consuming ≤2 fruit and vegetable portions/day; aged 65–85 years (mean age 71 years); usual diet (≤2 portions/day) vs. ≥5 fruit and vegetable portions/day; 16 weeks.	Antibody binding to pneumococcal capsular polysaccharides (total IgG) increased more in the 5-fruit and vegetable portion/day group than in the 2-portion/day group with geometric mean ratio of 3.1 vs. 1.7 ($p = 0.005$).

Table 3.6 (continued)

Objective	Study details	Results
Observational studies		
Ribeiro et al. (2016). Investigate the effect of fruit and vegetable intake on different progressive aging disabilities (Longitudinal study) [126].	432 late middle age African Americans; 6-year follow-up (multivariate adjusted).	Vegetables other than carrots, salads and potatoes were associated with improved grip strength and lower frailty whereas high sugar sweetened fruit juices worsened grip strength and frailty.
Lian et al. (2015). Examine the potential effect of dietary factors on the association between telomere length and hypertension risk (community-based case-control study; China) [127].	271 hypertensive patients and 455 normotensive controls; aged 40–70 years (mean age 57 years) habitually consuming ≤2 portions of fruits and vegetables/day (multivariate adjusted).	Subjects with longer age-adjusted peripheral leucocyte relative telomere length were associated with higher vegetable intake ($p = 0.01$). Individuals with longer age-adjusted median relative telomere length were 30% less likely to have hypertension.

observational studies and 3 of 6 intervention trials [118]. However, there was a high degree of variability in cognitive effects depending on the type of fruit, vegetable or juice consumed. A 2012 systematic review (six cohort studies; ≥6 months of follow-up) showed in five of six studies that higher consumption of vegetables, but not fruit, was associated with a decreased risk of cognitive decline or dementia [119]. In these studies, the vegetables most associated with slower cognitive decline included cruciferous vegetables, legumes, and green leafy vegetables; particularly cabbage, zucchini, squash, broccoli, and lettuce, at a daily intake of three servings (200 g) a day. The effect of vegetables may be associated with the fact that people frequently consume vegetables with added healthy oils, which aid in absorption of fat soluble antioxidants such as vitamins A and E, and carotenoids.

Specific Studies. Four studies are representative of the effects of increased fruit and vegetable intake on cognitive function [120–123]. Two RCTs on flavonoid-rich fruits and vegetables or their juices show them to improve cognitive performance in aging subjects [120, 121]. One parallel RCT (154 adults; aged 20–70 years; 18 weeks) found that high flavonoid fruits and vegetables such as berries, oranges, apples, pears, peppers, or broccoli significantly improved cognitive performance and BDNF compared to the usual low fruit and vegetable diet or low flavonoid fruits and vegetables (Figs. 3.16 and 3.17) [120]. A cross-over RCT (37 healthy adults; mean age 67 years; 8 weeks) showed significantly improved global cognitive and executive function with high flavonoid orange juice (305 mg) compared with low flavonoid orange juice (37 mg) [121]. Two European cohort studies showed somewhat inconsistent findings for fruits and vegetables on cognitive performance [122, 123]. The Dutch Doetinchem Cohort Study (2613 adults; mean age 55 years; 5 years of follow-up) reported that higher vegetable intake, especially from root vegetables, such as carrots, red beets and mushrooms, significantly slowed the decline in information processing speed and global cognitive function [122]. A French cohort study (2533 subjects; mean age at evaluation 66 years; 13 years of follow-up) found that higher intake of fruit and vitamin C rich fruits and vegetables was associated with better verbal memory whereas higher intake of vegetables and β-carotene rich fruits and vegetables was associated with poorer executive function [123].

General Aging Indicators

Two RCTs and two observational studies provide representative insights on the effects of

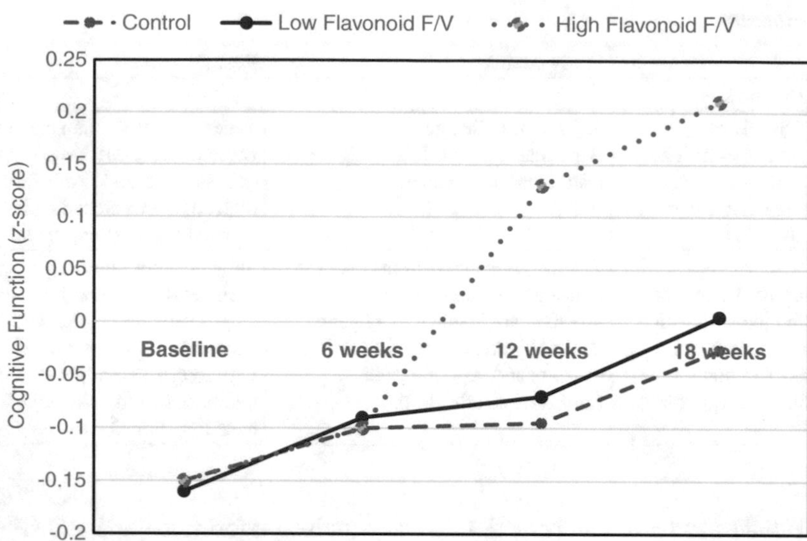

Fig. 3.16 Effect of fruits and vegetables (F/V) flavonoid level on cognitive function after 18 weeks from a randomized controlled trial with 154 adults ($p < 0.001$ for high flavonoid F/V at 12 and 18 weeks) (adapted from [120])

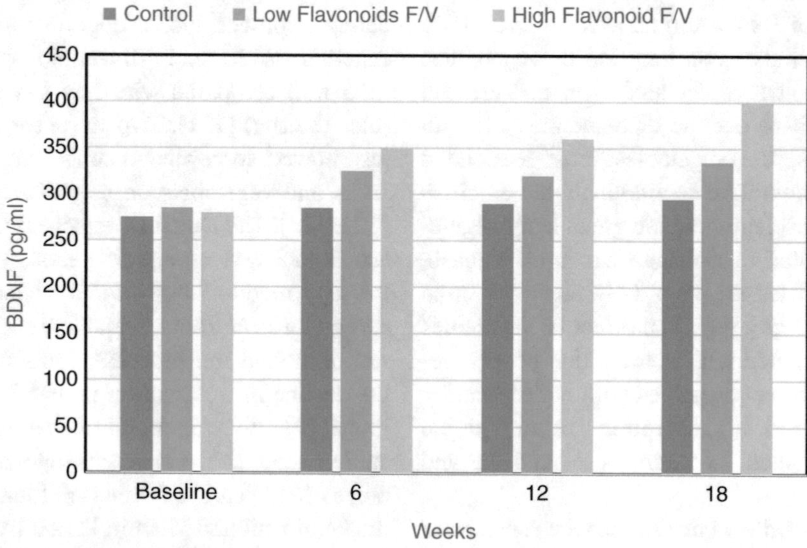

Fig. 3.17 Effect of fruits and vegetables (F/V) flavonoid level on serum brain-derived neurotrophic factor (BDNF) concentration over 18 weeks from a randomized controlled trial with 154 adults ($p < 0.001$ for high flavonoid F/V after 18 weeks) (adapted from [120])

increased fruit and vegetable intake on general aging indicators [124–127]. Two publications analyzing the British Ageing and Dietary RCT (84 subjects; mean age 71 years; 16 weeks) found that subjects consuming ≥5 fruit and vegetable portions daily showed directionally improved grip strength ($p = .06$) [124] and significantly improved antibody binding to pneumococcal capsular polysaccharides compared to the intake of ≤2 portions [125]. A longitudinal study (432 late middle age African Americans; 6-year follow-up) showed that the increased intake of vegetables (exclusive of carrots, salads and potatoes) was associated with improved grip strength and lower frailty whereas increased sugar sweetened fruit juices decreased grip strength and increased frailty [126]. A Chinese community-based case-control study (272 hypertensive patients and 455 normotensive controls; mean age 57 years) observed that subjects with higher vegetable intake had significantly longer leucocyte telomere length and a 30% lower risk of hypertension [127].

3.2.3 Legumes

3.2.3.1 Background

Legumes, including pulses (e.g., pinto beans, split peas, lentils, chickpeas) and soybeans, are rich in fiber, protein, B vitamins, iron, calcium and potassium and bioactive phytochemicals such as phenolics, saponins, and isoflavones, which are especially concentrated in soy foods [16, 128]. Legumes are often consumed as a lower energy dense, lower saturated fat, and higher fiber meat or milk replacer. Their intake has been in decline with the global shift to Western-style diets [129]. Legumes are infrequently consumed by North Americans and northern Europeans, with <8% of Americans consuming them on any given day. Also, between the 1960s and 1990s, legume intake decreased by 40% in India and by 24% in Mexico. Table 3.7 summarizes the effects of increased intake of legumes, both dietary pulses and soy, on mortality, chronic disease and age-related cognitive function [130–154].

3.2.3.2 Mortality Risk

Legumes have been associated with longevity and are important traditional food staples in many countries known for healthier diets; soy, tofu, natto, and miso in Japan, brown beans and peas in Sweden, and lentils, chickpeas and white beans in the Mediterranean countries [129]. Three prospective studies frame-up the effects of high legume intake on reduced mortality risk [130–132]. The Iranian Golestan Cohort Study (42,403 adults; 11 years of follow-up) found that increased legume intake significantly reduced total cancer mortality risk by 28% [130]. A Taiwanese cohort study (2820 men and 2950 women; 6.5 years of follow-up) showed that a bean-free diet significantly increased the risk of all-cause mortality by 98% in women [131]. The 2004 Food Habits in Later Life Study longitudinal study (785 adults from Japan, Sweden, Greece and Australia; aged 70+ years; 7 years of follow-up) found that higher legume intake was the most protective dietary predictor of survival for the elderly subjects, regardless of their ethnicity [132]. Specifically, there was a 7–8% lower risk of all-cause mortality for each 20 g/day of legumes consumed, independent of other mortality risk factors.

3.2.3.3 Chronic Diseases

Cardiovascular Disease (CVD) and Stroke

Systematic Reviews and Meta-analyses. Six meta-analyses of prospective cohort studies and RCTs summarize the effects of increased legume intake from soy, dietary pulses, and soy protein on CVD, ischemic heart disease (IHD), blood lipid profiles and stroke risk [133–138]. A 2017 meta-analysis (11 cohort studies; 367,000 subjects) found that increased legume intake reduced the risk of both CVD and CHD by 10% but had no substantial effect on stroke [133]. Also, a 2014 meta-analysis (5 IHD cohort studies, 199,000 subjects; and 6 stroke studies, 255,000 subjects) showed that 4 weekly servings of legumes reduced IHD risk by 14% but had no effect on stroke risk [136]. A 2015 meta-analysis of soy foods (35 RCTs; 2670 subjects; 4 weeks to 1 year) demonstrated that increased intake of soy products significantly reduced total and LDL cholesterol, and triglycerides, and increased HDL cholesterol [134]. The LDL cholesterol lower effects were greater in hypercholesterolemic patients by 7.5 mg/dL compared to 3.0 mg/dL in healthy subjects. Also, the LDL cholesterol lowering effects were stronger for soy food products such as soy milk, soy beans or nuts than for soy extract supplements. A 2011 meta-analysis of soy protein (43 RCTs) found that 30 g of soy protein/day significantly lowered LDL cholesterol by up to 5.5% and triglycerides by 10.7%, and increased HDL cholesterol by 3.2% [138]. A 2014 meta-analysis of dietary pulses (26 RCTs; 1037 subjects; ≥3 weeks)

Table 3.7 Summary of legume (including soy) prospective studies and randomized controlled trial (RCTs) on mortality and chronic disease risk, age-related cognitive function, and telomere length.

Objective	Study details	Results
Mortality Risk		
Prospective Cohort Studies		
Farvid et al. (2017). Evaluate the effect of dietary protein source on mortality risk (The Golestan Cohort Study; Iran) [130].	42,403 participants; 11 years of follow-up; 3291 deaths (multivariate adjusted).	The highest vs. lowest quintile of legume intake was associated with a reduced total cancer risk of 28% (p-trend =0.004) and gastrointestinal cancer risk by 24% (p-trend =0.05).
Chang et al. (2011). Evaluate the associations of all-cause mortality and a bean-free diets in adults (Taiwan) [131].	2820 men and 2950 women; average baseline mid-40 years; average follow-up of 6.5 years, 225 all-cause deaths (multivariate adjusted).	A bean-free diet significantly increased adjusted (1) metabolic syndrome risk by 83% in men and 45% in women and (2) significantly increased adjusted all-cause mortality among women by 98% but insignificantly in men by 28%.
Darmadi-Blackberry et al. (2004). Assess protective dietary predictors associated with long-lived elderly (Food Habits in Later Life Study) [132].	785 elderly; 5 cohort studies from Japan, Sweden, Greece and Australia; up to 7 years of follow-up (multivariate adjusted).	The legume food group showed 7% reduction in mortality risk for every 20 g increase in daily intake. Other food groups were not found to significantly predict survival among these cohorts.
Cardiovascular Disease (CVD) and Stroke Risk		
Systematic Reviews and Meta-analyses		
Marventano et al. (2017). Summarize the association between dietary legume consumption and CVD risk, including CHD and stroke [133].	11 cohorts; 367,000 subjects; 18,475 cases of CVD (7451 CHD and 6336 stroke cases); 4.9–26 years of follow-up; intake <1 serving/d to 3–4 weekly servings.	Compared with lower legume consumption, the highest category of intake was associated with a decreased risk of 10% in both CVD and CHD with no or little evidence of heterogeneity and no publication bias. There was no significant effect of increased legume intake on stroke risk.
Tokede et al. (2015). Examine the effects of soy consumption on the lipid profiles using published RCTs [134].	35 RCTs (50 comparisons);; 2670 subjects (aged 28–83 years and 82% women); average intake of soya protein was 30 g/day (range:14–50 g/day); 4 weeks to 1 year.	Intake of soy products resulted in a significant reduction in total cholesterol by 5.3 mg/dL, LDL-cholesterol (LDL) concentration by 4.8 mg/dL, triglycerides by 4.9 mg/dL. There was also a significant increase in serum HDL-cholesterol (HDL) by 1.4 mg/dL. LDL reductions were greater in hypercholesterolemic patients by 7.5 mg/dL than in healthy subjects (3.0 mg/dL). LDL lowering was stronger for whole soy products (soy milk, soybeans and nuts) by 11.1 mg/dL compared to processed soy extracts (3.2 mg/dL).
Ha et al. (2014). Assess the effect of dietary pulse intake on established therapeutic lipid targets for CVD risk reduction [135].	26 RCTs; 1037 subjects; ≥3 weeks duration.	Diets emphasizing dietary pulse intake at a median dose of 130 g/day (about 1 serving daily) significantly lowered LDL by a mean of 0.17 mmol/L compared with the control.
Afshin et al. (2014). Investigate and quantify associations of legume intake with ischemic heart disease (IHD) and stroke [136].	IHD: 5 cohort studies; 198,904 participants; 6514 events. Stroke: 6 cohort studies; 254,628 participants; 6690 events.	Four weekly 100-g servings of legumes were associated with a 14% lower risk of IHD. Four weekly 100-g servings of legume intake were not significantly associated with total stroke or stroke subtypes,

Table 3.7 (continued)

Objective	Study details	Results
Bazzano et al. (2011). Summarize RCTs evaluating the effects of non-soy legume consumption on blood lipids [137].	10 RCTs compared a non-soy legume diet to control; 268 participants; ≥ 3-week duration.	Compared to control diets, pooled mean net reduction in total cholesterol was 11.8 mg/dL and mean lowering of LDL was 8.0 mg/dL These results indicate that a diet rich in legumes other than soy decreases total and LDL cholesterol.
Anderson et al. (2011). Assess the effect of soy protein on serum lipoproteins and CHD risk [138].	20 parallel and 23 crossover RCTs.	Compared to control, 30 g/day soy protein reduced LDL by 5.5% in parallel trials and by 4.2% in crossover studies. In parallel trials soy increased HDL by 3.2% ($p < 0.007$) and lowered fasting triglycerides by 10.7% ($p < 0.006$).
RCTs		
Liu et al. (2013). Examine effects of soy protein with isoflavones or isoflavones alone on blood pressure (BP) (China) [139].	**Double-blind, Parallel RCT:** 180 post-menopausal Chinese women; 3-arms: 15 g soy protein and 100 mg isoflavones (Soy group), or 15 g milk protein and 100 mg isoflavones (Iso group), or 15 g milk protein (placebo group); 6 months.	Subgroup analysis among 130 pre- and hypertensive women suggested that soy protein and isoflavones significantly reduced systolic BP by 4.25% ($p = 0.02$).
Pittaway et al. (2008). Evaluate the effects of chickpea supplementation on ad libitum nutrient intake, body weight, serum lipids, lipoproteins, and other metabolic changes (Australia) [140].	**Parallel RCT:** 45 free-living adults; 728 g chickpeas weekly (4 cans) as part of their habitual diet for 12 weeks (chickpea phase), followed by 4 weeks of habitual diet without chickpeas (usual phase).	Serum total cholesterol and LDL cholesterol were 7.7 mg/dL and 7.3 mg/dL lower, respectively, after the chickpea phase ($p \leq 0.01$), fasting insulin was 0.75 μIU/mL lower ($p = 0.045$), and the homeostasis assessment model of insulin resistance (HOMA-IR) was 0.21 lower ($p = 0.01$). In the chickpea phase, mean dietary fiber intake was 6.8 g/day more and mean polyunsaturated fatty acid consumption was 2.7% higher.
He et al. (2005). Examine the effect of soybean protein intake on BP (China) [141].	**Double-blind Parallel RCT:** 302 adults; aged 35–64 years; mean baseline systolic BP 135 mm Hg and diastolic BP 85 mm Hg; 40 g isolated soybean protein daily; 12 weeks.	Compared to control, soy protein significantly reduced systolic BP by 4.3 mm Hg ($p < 0.001$) and diastolic BP by 2.8 mm Hg ($p < 0.001$). For subjects with hypertension the net reduced systolic and diastolic BP changes were 7.9 and 5.3 mm Hg, respectively. For normotensive subjects, the BP changes were more modestly reduced by 2.3 and 1.3 mm Hg.
Cardiometabolic and Type 2 Diabetes Risk Management		
Systematic Reviews and Meta-analyses		
Afshin et al. (2014). Investigate and quantify the associations between legume intake and diabetes risk [136].	2 cohort studies; 100,179 participants.	When these studies were pooled, legume consumption insignificantly reduced diabetes risk by 22%.
Liu et al. (2011). Evaluate the effects of soy intake on measures of glycemic control [142].	24 RCTs; 1518 subjects; 4–52 weeks; ≤ 40 g soy protein/ day.	Soy consumption did not significantly affect measures of glycemic control with a mean lowering of fasting glucose by 0.7 mg/dL ($p = 0.16$) and of fasting insulin by 0.2 mg/dL ($p = 0.50$). There was significant heterogeneity in the results of fasting insulin levels and HOMA-IR.

(continued)

Table 3.7 (continued)

Objective	Study details	Results
Sievenpiper et al. (2009). Assess the clinical effects of dietary pulses on glycemic control [143].	41 RCTs; 1674 participants; ≥7 days.	Pulses modestly improved glycemic control through a possible insulin-sparing mechanism; intake of chickpeas was most effective for individuals with diabetes with a study duration of >4 weeks.
Prospective Cohort Studies		
Ding et al. (2016). Evaluate the effect of soy food and isoflavones intake on diabetes risk in US adults (Nurses' Health Study I and II and the Health Professionals Follow-Up Study [144].	142,176 women and 21,781 men; >20 years of follow-up 9185 diabetes cases (multivariate adjusted).	Compared to non-consumers of soy foods, those consuming >1 serving weekly had a trend for reduced diabetes risk by 7% (p-trend =0.14) and high intake of total isoflavones significantly reduced diabetes risk by 11% (p- trend =0.009).
Villegas et al. (2008). Examine the association between legume and soy food consumption and diabetes risk (Shanghai Women's Health Study; China) [145].	64,227 healthy women; mean baseline age 49 years; average 4.6 years of follow-up (multivariate adjusted).	Consumption of legumes, especially soybeans, was inversely associated with the risk of diabetes (Fig. 3.18).
RCT		
Jenkins et al. (2012). Evaluate the effect of low-glycemic index (GI) diets and CVD risk in people with type 2 diabetes, with a focus on dietary pulses (e.g., beans, chickpeas or lentils) and whole-grain (Canada) [146].	**Parallel RCT:** 121 adults with diabetes; mean age 60 years; approx. 50/50 men and women; low-GI pulse diet: ≥ 1 cup dietary pulses daily vs. increased insoluble fiber rich whole wheat products; 3 months.	The dietary pulse supplemented diet lowered HbA1c levels by 0.2% more than the whole-grain wheat supplement diet ($p < 0.001$). Also, dietary pulses significantly lowered the absolute 10-year CHD risk vs. the whole grain wheat diet, primarily because of a greater effect on lowering of systolic and diastolic BP ($p < 0.001$).
Colorectal Cancer (CRC)		
Systematic Reviews and Meta-analyses		
Yu et al. (2016). Assess the association between soy foods isoflavone intake and CRC risk [147].	17 observational studies (13 case-control and 4 cohort studies); foods included soy, soy foods, soybeans, tofu, soy protein, miso, and natto.	Higher intake of soy isoflavone reduced CRC risk by 22% ($p = 0.024$). Based on subgroup analyses, a significant CRC protective effect was observed with soy foods and in Asian populations both by 21%.
Zhu et al. (2015). Investigate the association between dietary legume consumption and risk of CRC [148].	14 cohort studies; 1,903,459 participants; 12,261 cases; beans and soybeans.	Higher legume consumption was associated with a decreased risk of CRC by 9%. Subgroup analyses suggested that higher legume consumption was inversely associated with CRC risk in Asians by 18% and soybean intake was associated with a decreased risk of CRC by 15%.
Prospective Cohort Study		
Yang et al. (2009). Investigate the effect of soy food intake on CRC risk (Shanghai Women's Health Study; China) [149].	68,412 women; mean baseline age 52 years; mean follow-up of 6.4 years; 321 CRC cases (multivariate adjusted).	Each 5-g/day increment intake of soy foods as assessed by dry weight [equivalent to 1 oz. (28.35 g) tofu/day] was associated with an 8% lower CRC risk. Women in the highest tertile of intake had a risk reduction by 33% compared with those in the lowest tertile (p-trend =0.008) (Fig. 3.19). This inverse association was primarily for postmenopausal women. Similar results were also found for intakes of soy protein and isoflavones.

Table 3.7 (continued)

Objective	Study details	Results
Breast Cancer (BC)		
Systematic Reviews and Meta-analyses		
Chen et al. (2014). Systematically explore the association between soy isoflavone from soy food and protein intake and BC risk for pre- and post-menopausal women [150].	10 cohort studies (4 studies in Asian countries and 6 studies in Western countries) and 21 case-control studies (13 studies in Asia, and 8 studies in Western countries).	Pooled data from Asian country studies found soy isoflavones lowered BC risk in both pre- and post-menopausal women by 41%. However, data on post-menopausal women from Western countries suggested that soy isoflavone intake had a marginally significant protective effect by 8%.
Xie et al. (2013). Examine the association between soy isoflavones intake and BC risk by meta-analysis [151].	22 studies (7 cohort and 15 case-control designs); menopausal status in 14 studies; 9 studies from Asian populations and 5 studies from Western populations.	Higher soy isoflavone intake significantly reduced the BC risk in Asian women by 32% compared to an insignificant reduction of 2% in Western women. Further analysis found that the intake of isoflavones reduced BC risk by 54% in postmenopausal Asian women and 37% in premenopausal women. The lack of significant effects in the studies of Western women appears to be related to their relatively lower intake of soy products and isoflavones.
Age-related Cognitive Function		
Prospective Study		
Chen et al. (2012). Investigate the association between dietary habits and declines in cognitive function (Chinese Longitudinal Health Longevity Study) [152].	Population-based, prospective nested case-control study; 6911 illiterate subjects; 76% women; mean baseline age 83 years; 3 years of follow-up (multivariate adjusted).	There was an inverse association with cognitive decline in subjects frequently eating vegetables by 34% or legumes by 22% ($p < 0.0001$ for both).
RCTs		
St John et al. (2014). Determine associations of soy protein and urine excretion of isoflavonoids with cognitive performance (Women's Isoflavone Soy Health Clinical trial; US) [153].	**Double-blind, Parallel RCT:** 350 healthy postmenopausal women; mean age 61 years, daily 25 g of isoflavone-rich soy protein or milk protein-matched placebo; 2.5 years.	After 2.5 years, there was no significant difference in global cognition performance compared to milk protein control ($p = 0.39$). A secondary analysis, indicated that soy isoflavones decreased general intelligence by >4 age-associated years compared to the milk control group.
Kreijkamp-Kaspers et al. (2004). Investigate whether soy protein with isoflavones improves cognitive function, bone mineral density, and plasma lipids in postmenopausal women (The Netherlands) [154].	**Double-blind, Parallel RCT:** 202 healthy postmenopausal women; mean baseline age 67 years; 25.6 g of soy protein containing 99 mg of isoflavones vs. milk protein daily; 1 year.	After 1 year, cognitive function, bone mineral density, or plasma lipids did not differ significantly between the groups.

found that each daily serving of pulses significantly lowered LDL cholesterol by 0.17 mmol/L vs. control food [135]. A 2011 meta-analysis of non-soy legumes (10 RCTs; 268 participants; ≥3 weeks) showed similar total and LDL cholesterol lowering effects as seen for soy products [137].

Specific RCTs. Three RCTs summarize cardiometabolic protective effects for soy products and protein and chickpeas [139–141]. The lipoprotein lowering effects of soy products is well established [134, 138], and two double-blind RCTs demonstrated that soy products and protein are also effective in reducing systolic and diastolic BP, especially for hypertensive patients over ≥12 weeks [139, 141]. The consumption of chickpeas (4 cans per week) was shown to significantly lower total and LDL cholesterol, fasting insulin and insulin resistance (HOMA-IR) over 12 weeks [140].

Diabetes Risk and Management

Meta-analyses. Several meta-analyses of prospective studies and RCTs show beneficial effects for legumes on reducing diabetes risk and managing diabetes related health effects [136, 142, 143]. A 2014 meta-analysis of legumes (4 cohort studies; 100,179 participants; 4 weekly100-g servings) showed high total legume intake lowered diabetes risk by 22%, which did not reach statistical significance after multivariate adjustments [136]. Two meta-analyses of RCTs showed that pulses and soy food intake have relatively modest effects on lowering fasting blood glucose and insulin, and insulin resistance (HOMA-IR) compared to control diets [142, 143].

Prospective Cohort Studies. Two cohort studies in the US and China and one RCT provide insights on the effects of legumes (dietary pulses and soy) on diabetes risk [144–146]. The pooled data from a 2016 Nurses' Health Studies and Health Professionals Follow-up Study (142,176 women and 21,781 men; >20 years of follow-up) showed that the high consumption of soy foods such as tofu or soy milk insignificantly lowered diabetes risk by 7%, but higher intake of isoflavones significantly lowered risk by 11% [144]. The 2008 Shanghai Women's Health Study (64,227; 4.6 years of follow-up) found that Chinese women with a high intake of pulses (e.g., beans, lentils, and peas), soybeans and soymilk had significantly lower diabetes risk (Fig. 3.18) [145]. A 2012 Canadian RCT (121 people with diabetes; mean age 60 years; 3 months) found that dietary pulses diets (≥1 cup daily of beans, chickpeas or lentils) significantly reduced HbA1c values by 0.2% and lowered absolute 10-year CHD risk, and systolic and diastolic BP compared to high wheat fiber diets [146].

Cancer

Four meta-analyses and one large cohort study provide insights on the effects of legumes on colorectal cancer (CRC) and breast cancer (BC) risk [147–151].

Colorectal Cancer (CRC) Risk. Two meta-analyses evaluated the effects of soy foods/isoflavone intake and total legumes on CRC risk and a Chinese cohort study provided insights on the effects of legumes on CRC risk [147–149].

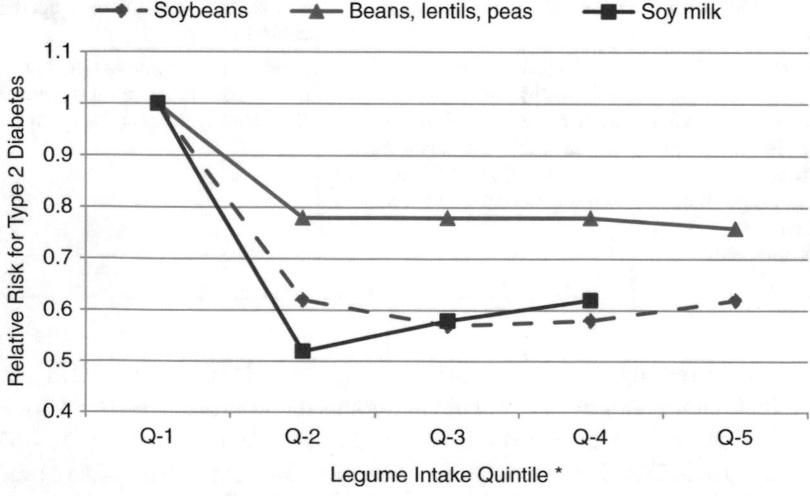

Fig. 3.18 Association between legumes and soy milk intake and type 2 diabetes risk in Chinese women from the Shanghai Women's Health Study ($p < 0.0001$ for all) (adapted from [145]). *Quintile 5: Beans, lentils and peas (37.1 g/day) and soybeans (32 g/day); Quintile 4: soy milk (214 mL/day).

A 2016 meta-analysis (13 case-control and 4 cohort studies) found that higher soy foods/isoflavones intake was associated with a significant 22% lower CRC risk [147]. A 2015 meta-analysis of total legume intake (14 cohort studies; 1,903,459 participants) found that increased legume intake lowered CRC risk by 9%; subgroup analysis showed a doubling of the CRC risk lowering to 18% in Asians populations and for soybean intake [148]. The Shanghai Women's Health Study (68,412 women; mean baseline age 52 years; mean 6.4 years of follow-up) found that each daily 1 ounce intake of tofu reduced CRC risk by 8% and higher soy products intake lowered CRC risk in postmenopausal women by 33% (Fig. 3.19) [149].

Breast Cancer (BC) risk. Two meta-analyses provide insights on the effects of soy foods or protein sources on BC risk and recurrence in BC survivors [150, 151]. A 2014 meta-analysis (10 cohort studies and 20 case-control or cross-sectional studies) found that increased isoflavones from soy foods or proteins lowered BC risk in both pre- and post-menopausal Asian women by 41% whereas in Western women there was a marginally significant reduction by 8% [150]. A 2013 meta-analysis (7 cohort and 15 case-control designs) showed that higher soy isoflavone intake significantly reduced BC risk in all Asian women by 32% compared to an insignificant reduction of 2% in Western women [151]. Further analysis found that the higher intake of soy isoflavones reduced BC risk in Asian postmenopausal women by 54%. This apparent discrepancy between Asian and Western women is most likely the result of an overall lower soy intake and frequency of consumption in Western women compared to Asian women.

3.2.3.4 Age-Related Cognitive Function

The effect of increased total legume and soy intake on age-related cognitive function is summarized by one cohort study and two RCTs in postmenopausal women [152–154]. The Chinese Longitudinal Health Longevity Study (6911 illiterate older adults; mean baseline age 83 years; 76% women; 3 years of follow-up) observed that frequent consumption of legumes significantly reduced cognitive decline by 22% [152]. In postmenopausal women, two large double-blind RCTs (202–350 women; mean baseline age 61–67 years; isoflavone rich soy protein vs. milk protein; 1–2.5 years of duration) found that the long-term intake of isoflavonoid rich soy protein

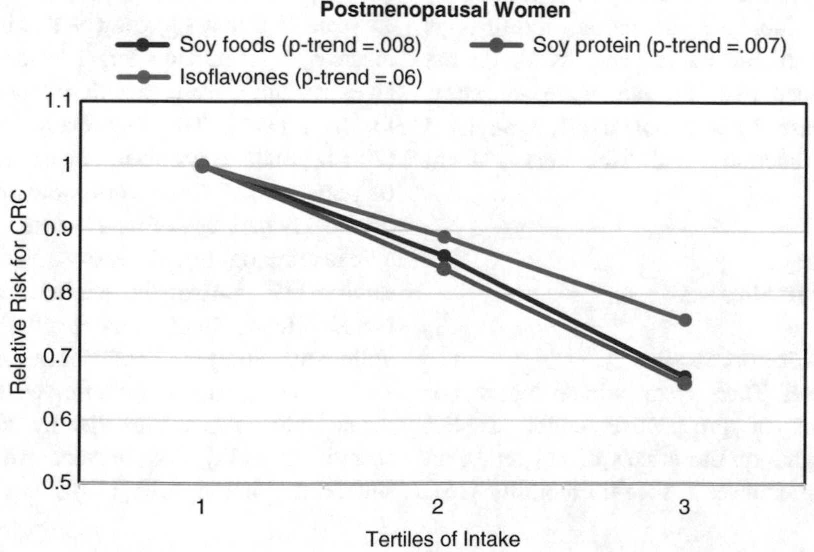

Fig. 3.19 Soy intake and colorectal cancer (CRC) risk from the Shanghai Women's Health Study (adapted from [149])

did not improve cognitive performance compared to milk protein [153, 154].

3.2.4 Nuts

3.2.4.1 Background

The consumption of a daily handful of nuts (approx. 45–60 g/day) can help to prevent or reduce weight gain, cardiometabolic dysfunction and related chronic diseases, especially if eaten as a replacement for unhealthful foods and snacks [155, 156]. Nuts are compositionally low in saturated fat and sugar, rich in unsaturated fats, protein and fiber, and contain a variety of healthy vitamins, minerals, and phytonutrients including carotenoids, polyphenols, and phytosterols [157]. Although nuts are energy dense (6 kcal/g), many nuts such as almonds have 25% lower metabolizable energy than estimated energy values used for nutrition labeling, which is one of the main reasons that nuts are not associated with the weight gain risk concern of other energy dense foods [158]. In the US >60% of men and women do not consume any nuts on a given day and 14% of men and 12% of women consume ≥1.5 ounces of nuts/daily [159]. Frequent nut consumption has been consistently associated with lower mortality, CVD or weight gain risk and normal blood lipids profiles, which are all important for healthy aging [160]. Table 3.8 summarizes the findings from observational studies and RCTs on the effects of increased nut intake on mortality, chronic disease risk and biomarkers, age-related cognitive function and telomere length [161–194].

3.2.4.2 Mortality Risk

Prospective Cohort Studies

Meta-analyses. Three systematic reviews and/or meta-analyses of prospective cohort studies provide insights on the effects of nut intake on all-cause and/or disease specific morality [161, 162, 166]. A 2016 dose-response meta-analysis (20 cohort studies; 819,448 participants) found per daily 28 g nut intake reduced mortality risk for all-cause by 22%, respiratory disease by 52%, and diabetes by 39% [161]. This analysis also estimated that >4 million global deaths are attributable to daily nut intake below 20 g. Another 2016 meta-analysis (20 cohort studies; 467,389 participants; primarily from North America and Europe) showed that 4 weekly servings of nuts reduced mortality risk from all-cause by 19%, CVD by 28% and sudden cardiac death by 75% [162]. A 2015 meta-analysis (4 cohort studies) found that each daily serving of nuts reduced all-cause mortality by 17% [166].

Specific Cohort Studies. Five specific cohort studies provide examples of the effect of increased nut intake on all-cause and disease specific mortality risk [168–175]. The Health Professionals Follow-up Study observed that the consumption of ≥5 weekly nut servings reduced after diagnosis prostate cancer mortality risk by 34% [168]. A large study of primarily peanut consuming Southern Americans and Shanghai Chinese (71,764 participants; 5.4–12.2 years of follow-up) found that total mortality risk was significantly reduced in the Americans by 21% and in Chinese by 17%, which was mainly due to lower CVD mortality [170]. A 2015 Australian cohort study (2893 participants; baseline age > 49 years; 15 years of follow-up) showed that increased nut intake by women had a larger lowering effect on all-cause and disease specific mortality risk than for men [171]. The Physicians Health Study (20,742 male physicians; mean baseline age 67 years; mean 9.6 years of follow-up) found that ≥5 weekly servings of nuts lowered multivariate all-cause mortality risk by 26% vs. <1 monthly serving [172]. Also, the pooled data from the Nurses' Health Studies and Health Professionals Follow-up Study (120,000 men and women; 24–30 years of follow-up) observed that daily nut intake reduced total mortality by 20%. Disease specific mortality risk preventative effects are summarized in Fig. 3.20 [173].

Table 3.8 Summary of nut prospective studies and randomized controlled trials (RCTs) on mortality, chronic disease risk and biomarkers, and age-related cognitive function.

Objective	Study details	Results
Mortality and Chronic Disease Risk		
Systematic Reviews and Meta-Analyses		
Aune et al. (2016). Conduct a systematic review and dose-response meta-analysis of nut consumption and risk of CVD, stroke, total cancer, and all-cause and cause-specific mortality [161].	20 cohort studies (29 publications); 819,448 participants; 12,331 CHD cases, 9272 stroke cases, 18,655 CV disease cases, 18,490 cancer cases, and 85,870 deaths.	Per 28 g/day nut intake, there was reduced risk for CHD by 29%, stroke by 7%, CVD by 21%, total cancer by 15%, mortality for all-cause by 22%, respiratory disease by 52% and diabetes by 39%. The results were similar for tree nuts and peanuts. An estimated 4.4 million annual premature deaths in America, Europe, Southeast Asia, and the Western Pacific may be attributable to a nut intake below 20 g/day.
Mayhew et al. (2016). Systematically review the literature and quantify associations between nut consumption and CVD/CHD outcomes and all-cause mortality [162].	20 cohort studies; 467,389 participants; 13,226 CVD outcomes including 10,120 deaths from CVD; primarily based on North American and European studies.	High nut intake significantly lowered risk of mortality for all-cause by 19%, total CVD by 27%, CHD by 30% and sudden cardiac death by 47%, as well as a lower disease risk for total CVD by 44% and CHD by 34% vs. low nut intake. Also, 4 weekly servings of nut intake (similar to the DASH diet) was associated with significantly lower risk for all-cause mortality by 19% and sudden cardiac death by 75%; plus, lower risk of total CVD by 28% and non-fatal CHD by 19%.
Wu et al. (2015) Clarify the association between nut consumption and risk of cancer or diabetes [163].	36 observational studies, 30,708 patients; 4.6–30 years of follow-up.	High nut intake significantly decreased risk for total cancer by 15%. colorectal cancer by 24%, endometrial cancer by 42%, and pancreatic cancer by 32% vs. very low or no nut intake. No significant association was found with other cancers or diabetes.
Guo et al. (2015). Assess the effect of the intake of nuts on hypertension and diabetes risk [164].	9 cohort studies (3 hypertension and 6 diabetes).	Compared to never/rare consumers, the consumption of >2 weekly servings of nuts significantly lowered hypertension risk by 8% but there was an insignificant reduction of diabetes risk by 2%.
Zhang et al. (2015). Evaluate the effect of nuts on stroke risk [165].	6 cohort studies; 476,181 participants.	High nut intake reduced stroke risk by 10% (insignificant trend), but a subgroup analysis showed a significant 12% lower stroke risk in women,
Luo et al. 2014). Assess the relation between nut intake and incidence of diabetes, CVD, and all-cause mortality [166].	18 cohort studies; 12,655 diabetes, 8862 CVD, 6623 ischemic heart disease, 6487 stroke, and 48,818 mortality cases.	Each incremental serving of nuts/day reduced risk for ischemic heart disease by 28%, CVD by 29%, and all-cause mortality by 17%. The reduction in diabetes risk was insignificant after adjusting for BMI.

(continued)

Table 3.8 (continued)

Objective	Study details	Results
Zhou et al. (2014). Investigate the association between nut consumption and risk of coronary artery disease, stroke, hypertension, and diabetes [167].	23 prospective cohort studies; 744,830 participants.	The consumption of each 1 serving of nuts/day was significantly associated with lower coronary artery disease by 19%, and hypertension by 34%. However, there was no association between the intake of each 1 serving of nuts/day and the risk of stroke or diabetes.
Prospective Cohort Studies		
Wang et al. (2016). Evaluate the association between nut intake and prostate cancer incidence and survivorship (Health Professionals Follow-up Study; US) [168].	47,299 men; 6810 incidences of prostate cancer; 26 years of follow-up (multivariate adjusted).	There was no association between nut intake and prostate cancer incidence. However, patients who consumed ≥5 servings of nuts weekly after diagnosis had a 34% lower rate of mortality than those who infrequently consumed nuts (<1 serving monthly).
Yang et al. (2016). Evaluate the association of long-term nut intake on colorectal cancer (CRC) risk (Nurses' Health Study II; US) [169].	75,680 women; mid-age at baseline; >20 years of follow-up; 1503 CRC cases (multivariate adjusted).	Women consuming ≥2 servings nuts weekly vs. those who rarely consumed nuts had a 13% lower risk of CRC (p-trend =0.06). There was no association with peanut butter.
Luu et al. (2015). Examine the association of nut consumption with total and cause-specific mortality in Americans of African and European descent who were predominantly of low socioeconomic status and in Chinese individuals in Shanghai, China (Southeastern US -Southern Community Cohort Study, Shanghai Women's Health Study and the Shanghai Men's Health Study) [170].	71,764 participants; median follow-up of 5.4 years in the US and 6.5–12.2 years in China; 14,440 deaths were identified; peanuts were the primary nut consumed in this study (multivariate adjusted).	Higher nut intake was significantly inversely associated with risk of total mortality in all 3 cohorts with lower risk in the US cohort by 21% and the Shanghai cohort by 17% (highest vs. lowest quintiles). This inverse association was predominantly driven by CVD mortality. There was significantly reduced ischemic heart disease in the US cohort by 38% and in the Shanghai cohort by 30% and stroke risk by 23% in both populations (highest vs. lowest quintile).
Gopinath et al. (2015). Assess the association between nut intake and risk of total mortality and mortality from CVD (Australia) [171].	2893 participants; baseline age ≥ 49 years; 15 years of follow-up; 1004 deaths (multivariate adjusted).	Higher nut consumption significantly reduced mortality risk for all-cause by 24%, for CVD by 24% and IHD by 23%. Associations were more marked in women compared to men. Women with higher nut intake had reduced risk of death from all causes by 27%, CVD by 39%, IHD by 34% and stroke mortality by 49%.
Hshieh et al. (2015). Test the hypothesis that nut consumption is inversely associated with the risk of all-cause mortality (Physicians Health Study; US) [172].	20,742 male physicians; mean age 67 years; mean 9.6 years of follow-up; 2732 deaths (multivariate adjusted).	Compared to <1 serving nuts/month, ≥5 servings nuts/week reduced all-cause mortality risk by 26% after adjustment for age, BMI, alcohol use, smoking, exercise, prevalent diabetes and hypertension, and intakes of energy, saturated fat, fruit and vegetables, and red meat. In a secondary analysis, higher nut intake was suggestive for lower CVD mortality and insignificant for CHD and cancer mortality.

Table 3.8 (continued)

Objective	Study details	Results
Bao et al. (2013). Examine the association between nut consumption and subsequent total and cause-specific mortality (Nurses' Health Study and Health Professionals Follow-up Study; US) [173].	76,464 women, 30 years of follow-up, 16,200 women died; 42,498 men, 24 years of follow-up, 11,229 men died (multivariate adjusted).	Compared with those who did not consume nuts, those who ate ≥7 nut servings/week had a significantly 20% lower total mortality risk. Significant inverse associations were also observed between nut consumption and deaths due to cancer, heart disease, and respiratory disease (Fig. 3.20).
Bao et al. (2013). Investigate the association between nut consumption and risk of pancreatic cancer in a large cohort of women (Nurses' Health Study; US) [174].	75,680 women; 30 years of follow-up; 466 confirmed cases of pancreatic cancer (multivariate adjusted).	28 g serving of nuts 2 times week significantly lowered risk of pancreatic cancer by 35% (p-trend = 0.007) vs. rarely or non-nut consumers. The results did not appreciably change after further adjustment for BMI and history of diabetes or adjustments for physical activity, smoking, and intakes of red meat, fruits, and vegetables.
Jenab et al. (2004) Determine the effects of nut and seed intake on CRC risk (European Prospective Investigation into Cancer and Nutrition (EPIC) Study; EU) [175].	478,040 subjects (141,988 men, 336,052 women); mean 4.8 years of follow-up (multivariate adjusted).	There was no significant association between higher intake of nuts and seeds and risk of colon cancer in men and women combined, but a subgroup analysis showed that women with high nut intake had significantly lower colon cancer risk by 31%.
RCTs		
Mortality Risk		
Guasch-Ferre et al. (2013). Investigate the association between frequency of nut consumption and mortality in individuals at high CVD risk (PREDIMED; Spain) [176].	**Parallel RCT:** 7216 men and women; mean baseline age 67 years; MedDiets supplemented with extra virgin olive oil or nuts vs. lower fat control diet; median follow-up of 4.8 years; 323 total deaths, 81 CVD deaths and 130 cancer deaths (multivariate adjusted).	Increased nut intake was associated with a significantly reduced risk of all-cause mortality (p-trend <0.05). Compared to non-consumers, subjects consuming nuts >3 servings/week had a 39% lower mortality risk. A similar protective effect against cardiovascular and cancer mortality was observed. Participants consuming more nuts at baseline and allocated to a MedDiet supplemented with nuts showed a significantly reduced total mortality risk by 63%.
Chronic Disease Risk		
Toledo et al. (2015). Examine the effect of MedDiet on primary prevention of breast cancer (BC) (PREDIMED; Spain) [177].	**Parallel RCT:** 7216 men and women with high CVD risk; mean baseline age 68 years; MedDiets supplemented with extra virgin olive oil or tree nuts vs. low-fat guidance control; median follow-up of 4.8 years (multivariate adjusted).	Compared to the lower fat control, the MedDiet plus extra virgin olive oil group significantly reduced BC risk by 68% and the MedDiet plus nuts group insignificantly lowered BC risk by 41%.
Salas-Salvado et al. (2014). Assess the effect of the MedDiet for the primary prevention of diabetes (PREDIMED; Spain) [178].	**Parallel RCT:** 7216 men and women with increased CVD risk; mean baseline age 67 years; MedDiets supplemented with extra virgin olive oil or tree nuts vs. lower fat control diet; median follow-up of 4.1 years (multivariate adjusted).	Compared with the lower fat control group, diabetes risk was significantly reduced in the MedDiet plus extra virgin olive oil group was significant reduced diabetes risk by 40% vs. an insignificantly lowered risk in the MedDiet plus tree nuts group by 18%.

(continued)

Table 3.8 (continued)

Objective	Study details	Results
Estruch et al. (2013). Evaluate the effects of MedDiets supplemented with tree nuts or extra virgin olive oil vs. lower fat diets on the primary prevention of CVD (PREDIMED; Spain) [179].	**Parallel RCT:** 7216 men and women with increased CVD risk; mean baseline age 67 years; MedDiets supplemented with nuts or extra virgin olive oil vs. lower fat control diet; median follow-up of 4.8 years; 288 primary CVD events (multivariate adjusted).	Compared to the lower fat control, risk of primary CVD events was significantly reduced by MedDiets plus tree nuts by 28% ($p = 0.02$) and MedDiets plus extra virgin olive oil by 30% ($p = 0.009$).
Cardiometabolic Disease and Type 2 Diabetes Biomarkers		
Systematic Reviews and Meta-Analyses of RCTs		
Musa-Veloso et al. (2016). Determine the effects of almond consumption on blood lipid levels [180].	18 RCT publications; 27 strata; approx. 1000 subjects; average daily intake of almonds ranged from 20 to 113 g; 4 weeks to 18 months.	Compared to control diets, almond supplemented diets significantly reduced total cholesterol by 0.153 mmol/L, LDL-cholesterol by 0.124 mmol/L, and triglycerides by 0.067 mmol/L, whereas HDL-C was insignificantly lowered by 0.017 mmol/L.
Del Gobbo et al. (2015). Evaluate the effects of tree nuts on blood lipids, lipoproteins and other cardiometabolic outcomes in adults aged ≥18 years without CVD [181].	61 RCTs; 2582 subjects; dose-standardized to one 1-oz. (28.4 g) serving/day walnuts, pistachios, macadamia nuts, pecans, cashews, almonds, hazelnuts, and Brazil nuts; 3–26 weeks.	Each daily nuts serving significantly lowered the following pooled mean values: total cholesterol by 4.7 mg/dL, LDL cholesterol by 4.8 mg/dL, ApoB by 3.7 mg/dL; and triglycerides by 2.2 mg/dL. The dose-response between nut intake and total cholesterol and LDL cholesterol was nonlinear (p-nonlinearity <0.001 all) with stronger effects observed for ≥60 g nuts/day. Significant heterogeneity was not observed by nut type. There were insignificant effects of tree nuts on HDL cholesterol, systolic or diastolic blood pressure, and inflammation such as C-reactive protein (CRP).
Mohammadifard et al. (2015). Estimate the effect of nut consumption on blood pressure (BP) [182].	21 RCTs; 1652 adults; baseline age 18–86 years; 2–16 weeks.	This analysis indicates that nut intake leads to a very modest but significant reduction in systolic BP in participants without diabetes by 1.3 mm Hg ($p = 0.02$). Sub-group analyses of different nut types suggest that pistachios were the only nut that significantly reduced systolic BP by 1.8 mm Hg ($p = 0.002$).
Blanco Mejia et al. (2014). Assess effect of tree nuts on metabolic syndrome criteria [183].	49 RCTs; 2226 subjects healthy or with dyslipidemia, metabolic syndrome criteria or diabetes; median nut intake approx. 50 g; median duration 8 weeks.	Tree nut diets modestly lowered triglycerides by 0.06 mmol/L and fasting blood glucose by 0.08 mmol/L compared with control diets. There was no effect of nuts on HDL cholesterol or blood pressure although there was a trend toward lower waist circumference.

Table 3.8 (continued)

Objective	Study details	Results
Banel and Hu (2009). Estimate the effect of walnuts on blood lipids [184].	13 RCTs; 365 subjects; walnuts 10–24% of energy; 4–24 weeks.	Compared with control diets, diets supplemented with walnuts resulted in a significantly greater decrease in total cholesterol by 10 mg/dL and LDL-cholesterol by 9.2 mg/dL ($p = 0.001$ for both) whereas there were insignificant decreases in HDL cholesterol by 0.2 mg/dL and triglycerides by 3.9 mg/dL. Other results show that walnuts provided significant benefits for antioxidant capacity and inflammatory markers and had insignificant effects on body weight and BMI.
Viguiliouk et al. (2014). Assess the effects of tree nuts on markers of glycemic control in individuals with diabetes [185].	12 RCTs; 450 subjects.	Compared to control diets, diets emphasizing tree nuts at a median dose of 56 g/day significantly lowered HbA1c by 0.07% ($p = 0.0003$) and fasting glucose by 0.15 mmol/L ($p = 0.03$). Insignificant lowering effects were observed for fasting insulin and HOMA-IR with the consumption of tree nuts.
Flores-Mateo et al. (2013). Evaluate the effect of nut intake on adiposity measures [186].	28 RCTs, 1806 subjects.	Pooled results indicated a nonsignificant lowering of body weight by 0.47 kg, BMI by 0.40, and waist circumference by 1.25 cm. from diets including nuts compared with control diets.
Xiao et al. (2017). Assess the effect of nut consumption on vascular endothelial function [187]	10 RCTs; 374 subjects	Increased nut consumption significantly improved flow mediated dilation ($p = 0.001$) but subgroup analyses indicated that the benefit was limited to walnuts.
Intervention Trials		
Gulati et al. (2017). Evaluate the effects of almonds on cardiometabolic and diabetes disease management biomarkers in Asian Indians with type 2 diabetes (India) [188].	**Open Label Trial:** 50 diabetic subjects; 27 men and 23 women; mean age 46 years; mean BMI 29; 20% of energy intake from almonds vs. nut free phase; 24 weeks.	Almonds significantly improved waist circumference, waist-to-height ratio, total and LDL-cholesterol, serum triglycerides, glycosylated hemoglobin, and hs-CRP in Indian diabetic subjects. This study supports the incorporation of almonds in a well-balanced healthy diet for multiple beneficial effects on the management of glycemic and CVD risk factors in Asian Indian patients with diabetes.
Njike et al. (2015). Assess the effects of walnut intake in subjects at risk for diabetes on cardiometabolic health and assess body composition in persons consuming walnuts (US) [189].	**Parallel RCT:** 112 subjects at risk for diabetes; walnut-included diet with daily 56 g (366 kcal) of walnuts and a walnut-excluded diet; 6 months.	The walnut diet significantly improved diet quality as measured by the Healthy Eating Index 2010, endothelial function, total and LDL cholesterol without significantly changing BMI, percent body fat, visceral fat, fasting glucose, glycated hemoglobin, and blood pressure compared with a walnut-excluded diet.

(continued)

Table 3.8 (continued)

Objective	Study details	Results
Sauder et al. (2015). Examine the effects of daily pistachio consumption on the lipid/lipoprotein profile, glycemic control, markers of inflammation, and endothelial function in adults with type 2 diabetes (US) [190].	**Crossover, Controlled Feeding RCT:** 30 adults with type 2 diabetes (mean glycated hemoglobin 6.2%); mean age 56 years; 50% women; pistachios 20% of energy vs. nut free control; 4 weeks on each diet; washout 2 weeks.	Pistachios supplemented diets significantly improved total cholesterol and the ratio of total to HDL cholesterol and lowered triglycerides and fructosamine compared to the control diet. However, pistachio supplemented diets did not significantly improve fasting glucose and insulin or inflammatory markers and endothelial function.
Age-related Cognitive Function		
Prospective Cohort Studies		
Valls-Pedret et al. (2015). Examine the effect of MedDiets supplemented with nuts or olive oil vs. lower fat diets on age-related cognitive decline (PREDIMED; Spain) [191]	447 cognitively healthy adults with increased CVD risk; mean baseline age 67 years; median follow-up 4.1 years (multivariate adjusted).	MedDiet plus nuts improved performance above the baseline in memory test ($p = 0.04$) whereas the subjects on MedDiet plus extra virgin olive oil performed better in tests of frontal ($p < 0.003$) and global cognition ($p < 0.005$). All cognitive tests on the lower fat control diets were significantly decreased ($p < 0.05$).
O'Brien et al. (2014). Examine the effects of long-term nuts intake on cognition in older women (The Nurses' Health Study; US) [192].	16,010 women; mean baseline age 74 years; 6 years of follow-up (multivariate adjusted).	Women consuming ≥5 servings of nuts/week had higher cognitive scores than non-consumers with a mean improvement by 0.08 standard units (p-trend = 0.003). This mean difference of 0.08 is equivalent to a mean 2-year improved cognitive age.
RCT		
Sanchez-Villegas et al. (2011). Assess the role of a MedDiet on plasma brain-derived neurotrophic factor (BDNF) levels (PREDIMED; Spain) [193].	**Parallel RCT:** 243 adults with increased CVD risk; mean baseline age 67 years from the Navarra center; 3 dietary interventions: control (low-fat) diet, MedDiet supplemented with extra virgin olive oil, or MedDiet supplemented with tree nuts. Plasma BDNF levels were measured after 3 years of intervention.	Participants assigned to MeDiet plus nuts showed a significant lower risk of low plasma BDNF values (<13 μg/mL) by 78% as compared to the low-fat control group. Among participants with prevalent depression at baseline, significantly higher BDNF levels were found for those assigned to the MedDiet supplemented with nuts.
Telomere Length		
Prospective Cohort Study		
Lee et al. (2015). Determine the association between dietary patterns or consumption of specific foods and leukocyte telomere length (LTL) (Korean) [194].	1958 middle-aged and older Korean adults from a population-based cohort; semi-quantitative food frequency questionnaire; 10 years of follow-up (multivariate adjusted).	Higher intake of legumes, nuts, seaweed, fruits and dairy products and lower consumption of red meat or processed meat and sweetened carbonated beverages were associated with longer LTL (Fig. 3.21).

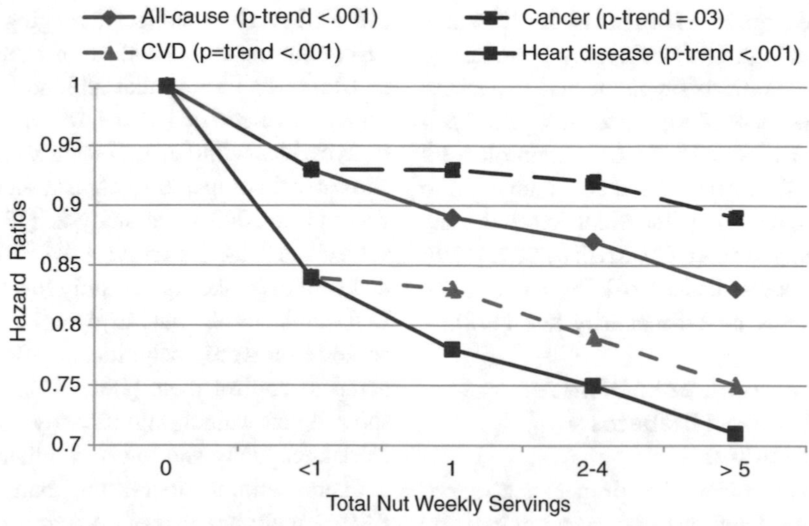

Fig. 3.20 Association between frequency of total nut intake (tree nuts and peanuts) on all-cause and disease specific mortality risk in US men and women (mean baseline age 60 years; 24–30 years of follow-up) (adapted from [173])

Randomized Controlled Trial (RCT)

The PREDIMED trial (7216 adults; mean age 67 years; high CVD risk; MedDiets supplemented with 30 g mixed nuts (15 g walnuts, 7.5 g hazelnuts, and 7.5 g almonds); median follow-up of 4.8 years) found that consuming >3 weekly nut servings resulted in significantly reduced all-cause mortality risk by 39% with similar effects for CVD and cancer mortality risks [176].

3.2.4.3 Chronic Disease Risk

Prospective Cohort Studies

Meta-analyses. Seven systematic reviews and/or meta-analyses of prospective cohort studies provide insights on the effects of increased nut intake on chronic disease risk [161–167]. A 2016 meta-analysis (20 cohort studies; 467,389 participants) found that each daily 28 g nut intake reduced risk for total CVD by 21%, CHD by 29%, stroke by 7%, and total cancer by 15% [161]. A second 2016 meta-analysis (20 cohort studies; 819,448 participants) showed 4 weekly nut servings reduced risk for CVD by 28% and CHD by 19%, primarily based on North American and European studies [162]. The overall findings from five meta-analyses concluded that: (1) higher nut intake insignificantly lowered diabetes risk vs. lower nut consumption [163–167]; (2) each additional nut serving significantly lowered coronary artery disease (CAD) by 19%, hypertension by 34%, and IHD by 28% [165, 166]; (3) higher nut intake significantly lowered colorectal cancer (CRC) by 24% [163]; (4) >2 weekly servings significantly lowered hypertension by 8% [164]; and (5) higher nut intake significantly lowered stroke risk by 12% in women [165].

Prospective Studies. Four cohort studies provide insights on the effects of increased nut intake on cancer risk [168, 169, 174, 175]. Two cohort studies support a protective effect of nuts on CRC risk. The 2016 Nurses' Health Study showed that consuming ≥2 weekly nut servings lowered CRC risk by 13% in women but there was no CRC protective effect with the consumption of peanut butter [169]. A 2004 EPIC study found that higher intake of nuts reduced CRC risk by 31% in women but there was no effect for men [175]. For prostate cancer, the Health Professionals Follow-up Study (47,299 men; 6810 cases; 26 years of follow-up) showed that increased nut intake did not reduce prostate cancer incidence but prostate cancer patients consuming ≥5 weekly servings of nuts after diagnosis had a 34% lower mortality risk [168]. For pancreatic cancer, the Nurses' Health Study found that 2 weekly servings of nuts significantly lowered multivariate adjusted risk by 35% [174].

RCTs. Three large PREDIMED trials (7216 men and women at high CVD risk; mean baseline age 67–68 years; MedDiets supplemented 30 g mixed nuts (15 g walnuts, 7.5 g hazelnuts, and 7.5 g almonds) or 1 L weekly of extra virgin olive oil vs. a lower fat control) found that compared to the lower fat control diet, the MedDiets with nuts: (1) significantly lowered CVD risk by 28% [179]; (2) lowered breast cancer risk by 41% [177]; and (3) lowered type 2 diabetes by 18% [178].

3.2.4.4 Cardiometabolic Disease and Type 2 Diabetes Biomarkers

Eight systematic reviews and/or meta-analyses of RCTs [180–187] and three intervention trials on almonds, walnuts and pistachios [188–190] provide insights on the effects of increased nut intake on cardiometabolic disease biomarkers.

Systematic Reviews and Meta-Analyses

Eight systematic reviews and/or meta-analyses summarize the effects of increased tree nut intake on cardiovascular 'biomarkers' [180–187]. A 2015 dose-response meta-analysis of tree nuts (61 RCTs, 2582 subjects; 3–24 weeks) found that a one ounce (28.4 g) serving had significant lowering effects for tree total and LDL cholesterol, ApoB and triglycerides compared to control diets [181]. This analysis showed the total and LDL cholesterol lowering effects of tree nuts was significantly non-linear with stronger lowering effects demonstrated for intake >60 g/day. In general, all types of tree nuts had similar lowering effects on blood lipid profiles. There were no significant effects from tree nut intake on HDL cholesterol, systolic or diastolic blood pressure, and CRP. Another 2015 meta-analysis (21 RCTs; 1652 subjects) showed that tree nuts modestly but significantly lowered mean systolic BP by1.3 mmHg with pistachios having the best systolic BP lowering by 1.8 mmHg vs. control diets [182]. A 2014 meta-analysis (49 RCTs; 2226 subjects) reported that median tree nut intake of 50 g/day modestly improved metabolic syndrome factors including triglycerides, blood glucose and waist circumference but not HDL cholesterol or BP compared to control diets [183]. For almonds, a 2016 meta-analysis (18 RCTs; 1000 subjects; ranging from 20 to 113 g/day; approx. 10–20% of energy; 4 weeks to 18 months) found that almond intake significantly lowered total and LDL-cholesterol, and triglycerides without significantly reducing HDL cholesterol compared to control diets [180]. For walnuts, a 2009 meta-analysis (13 RCTs; 365 subjects; 10–24% energy; 4–24 weeks) showed that walnut intake significantly lowered total and LDL-cholesterol, but triglycerides and HDL cholesterol were insignificantly lowered compared to control diets [184]. This analysis also showed that walnuts significantly improved antioxidant capacity and lowered inflammatory biomarkers without increasing body weight or BMI. A meta-analysis of diabetic individuals (12 RCTs; 450 patients) showed that diets with a median daily intake of 56 g of tree nuts significantly lowered HbA1c and fasting blood glucose compared to control diets [185]. Another meta-analysis (28 RCTs; 1806 subjects) found that diets that included tree nuts insignificantly lowered body weight, BMI and waist circumference vs. control nut free diets [186]. For vascular endothelial function, a 2017 systematic review and meta-analysis (10 RCTs; 374 subjects) found that increased nut consumption significantly improved flow mediated dilation but subgroup analyses indicated that the benefit was limited to walnuts [187]. This analysis suggests that walnuts are more effective in reducing the rate of vascular aging than other tree nuts.

Specific Intervention Trials

Three intervention trials on almonds, walnuts and pistachios provide insights on their effects on cardiometabolic and diabetes biomarkers [188–190]. For almonds, a 2017 intervention trial (50 type 2 diabetes subjects; 27 men and 23 women; mean age 46 years; mean BMI 29; 24 weeks) showed that a diet with 20% of the energy intake from almonds significantly improved waist circumference, waist-to-height ratio, total and LDL-cholesterol, serum triglycerides, glycosylated hemoglobin, and hs-CRP [188]. For walnuts, a 2015 RCT (112 subjects; mean age 55 years; 31 men and 81 women; 6 months) compared a walnut-excluded diet with a walnut-included (56 g walnuts (366 kcal)/day) diet, and showed that the walnut diet significantly improved diet quality as measured by the Healthy Eating Index 2010, endothelial function, and total and LDL cholesterol without significantly changing BMI, percent body fat, visceral fat, fasting glucose, glycated hemoglobin, and BP [189]. For pistachios, a 2015 cross-over RCT (30 adults with type 2 diabetes; mean age 56 years; 50% women; 4 weeks) found that a diet with 20% of energy from pistachios significantly improved total cholesterol and the ratio of total to HDL cholesterol and lowered triglycerides compared to the control diet [190]. However, pistachio supplemented diets did not significantly improve fasting glucose and insulin or inflammatory markers and endothelial function, although they did significantly lower fructosamine (a measure of long-term glycemic control in people with diabetes) compared to the control.

3.2.4.5 Age Related Cognitive Performance

One prospective cohort study and two RCTs provide indications that increased nut intake helps to protect against age related cognitive decline [191–193]. The Nurses' Health Study (15,467 women; mean age of 74 years; 15–21 years of follow-up) found that higher total nut intake was associated with better average cognitive status for all cognitive attributes measured [192]. Women consuming ≥5 servings of nuts/week had significantly higher cognitive scores equivalent to a 2-year improved cognitive age vs. non-consumers. Two PREDIMED RCTs show that MedDiets supplemented with nuts consumed by older men and women with high CVD risk showed subjects had improvements in memory and increased levels of plasma brain derived neurotrophic factor (BDNF), known to improve brain function, compared to lower fat control diets [191, 193].

3.2.4.6 Telomeres

A Korean prospective study (1958 subject; age 40 to >60; 10 years) observed that healthy dietary patterns including nuts, whole grains, seafood, legumes, vegetables and seaweed were associated with longer leukocyte telomere length [194]. This study suggests that nuts are uniquely associated with longer telomere length compared to other healthy food sources (Fig. 3.21). In contrast, higher consumption of red meat or processed meat and sweetened carbonated beverages, which are common in the Western dietary pattern, were associated with shorter telomere length.

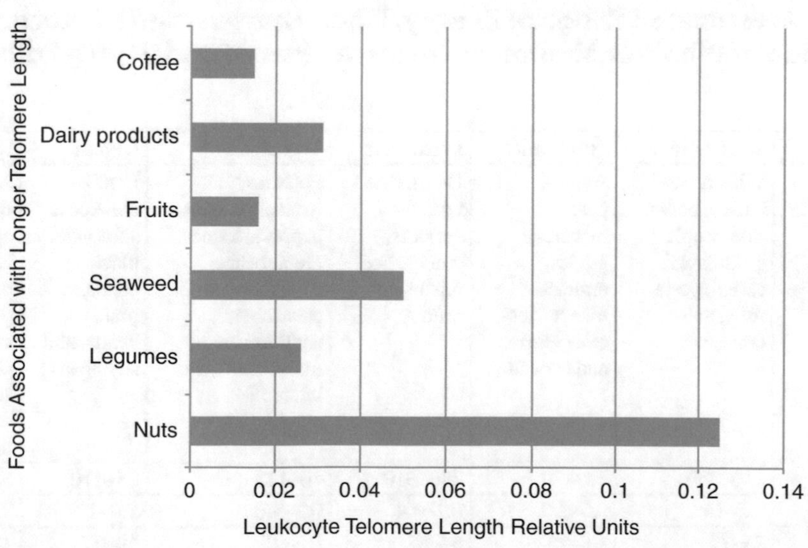

Fig. 3.21 Association between consumption of specific "healthy" foods and leukocyte telomere length in middle-aged and older adults from a Korean population-based cohort followed for 10 years (adapted from [194])

Conclusions

The rate and quality of the aging processes is only partly influenced by genetic and it can be modified by consuming healthy diets overall and specific types of uniquely healthy foods. Healthy dietary guidelines generally recommend eating: 2 1/2 cups of a variety of vegetables/day; 2 cups of fruits, especially whole fruits/day; 6 servings of total grains at ≥3 servings of whole grains/day and ≤3 servings of refined grains/day, ≥4 weekly servings of legumes (dietary pulses or soy), and/or ≥5 weekly servings of nuts, and limiting consumption of red or processed meats, added saturated and trans-fat, sugar or sodium for improved odds for healthy aging and reduced chronic disease and premature mortality risk. Whole plant foods range widely in their health effects because of their variation in level and type of fiber, nutrients and phytochemicals, which can have differential effects on aging, chronic disease risk, cognitive function and longevity by their impact on weight regulation, lipoprotein concentrations and function, blood pressure, glucose-insulin homeostasis, oxidative stress, inflammation, endothelial health, hepatic function, adipocyte metabolism, visceral adiposity, brain neurochemistry and the microbiota ecosystem. For whole-grains, β-glucan-rich oats and barley lower total and LDL-cholesterol better than other cereal grains and whole-grain bread tends to be more beneficial than white bread in controlling weight gain and abdominal fat. For fruits and non-starchy vegetables, low energy dense and flavonoid and/or carotenoid rich varieties including apples, pears, berries, citrus fruits, cruciferous vegetables, and green le afy vegetables are especially associated with improved odds of healthy aging, cognitive performance and weight control, and reduced risk of chronic disease and premature death. Legumes (dietary pulses or soy) are associated with reduced weight gain, chronic disease, and mortality risks. All nuts tend to have similar effects on managing body weight, and glycemic, lipoprotein and inflammatory profiles, but among nuts walnuts appear to be uniquely effective in promoting better vascular endothelial function such as flow mediated dilation.

Appendix A: Estimated Range of Energy, Fiber, Nutrient and Phytochemical Composition of Whole or Minimally Processed Plant Foods/100 g Edible Portion

Components	Whole-grains	Fresh fruit	Dried fruit	Vegetables	Legumes	Nuts/seeds
Nutrients and phytochemicals	Wheat, oats, barley, brown rice, whole grain bread, cereal, pasta, rolls, and crackers	Apples, pears, bananas, grapes, oranges, blueberries, strawberries, and avocados	Dates, dried figs, apricots, cranberries, raisins and prunes	Potatoes, spinach, carrots, peppers, lettuce, green beans, cabbage, onions, cucumber, cauliflower, mushrooms, and broccoli	Lentils, chickpeas, split peas, black beans, pinto beans, and soy beans	Almonds, Brazil nuts, cashews, hazelnuts, macadamias, pecans, walnuts, peanuts, sunflower seeds, and flaxseed
Energy (kcal)	110–350	30–170	240–310	10–115	85–170	520–700
Protein (g)	2.5–16	0.5–2.0	0.1–3.4	0.2–5.0	5.0–17	7.8–24
Available Carbohydrate (g)	23–77	1.0–25	64–82	0.2–25	10–27	12–33

Components	Whole-grains	Fresh fruit	Dried fruit	Vegetables	Legumes	Nuts/seeds
Fiber (g)	3.5–18	2.0–7.0	5.7–10	1.2–9.5	5.0–11	3.0–27
Total fat (g)	0.9–6.5	0.0–15	0.4–1.4	0.2–1.5	0.2–9.0	46–76
SFA[a] (g)	0.2–1.0	0.0–2.1	0.0	0.0–0.1	0.1–1.3	4.0–12
MUFA[a] (g)	0.2–2.0	0.0–9.8	0.0–0.2	0.1–1.0	0.1–2.0	9.0–60
PUFA[a] (g)	0.3–2.5	0.0–1.8	0.0–0.7	0.0.0.4	0.1–5.0	1.5–47
Folate (μg)	4.0–44	<5.0–61	2–20	8.0–160	50–210	10–230
Tocopherols (mg)	0.1–3.0	0.1–1.0	0.1–4.5	0.0–1.7	0.0–1.0	1.0–35
Potassium (mg)	40–720	60–500	40–1160	100–680	200–520	360–1050
Calcium (mg)	7.0–50	3.0–25	10–160	5.0–200	20–100	20–265
Magnesium (mg)	40–160	3.0–30	5.0–70	3.0–80	40–90	120–400
Phytosterols (mg)	30–90	1.0–83	—	1.0–54	110–120	70–215
Polyphenols (mg)	70–100	50–800	—	24–1250	120–6500	130–1820
Carotenoids (μg)	—	25–6600	0.6–2160	10–20,000	50–600	0.0–1200

U.S. Department of Agriculture, Agriculture Research Service, Nutrient Data Laboratory. 2014. USDA National Nutrient Database for Standard Reference, Release 27.
https://www.ars.usda.gov/nutrientdata. Accessed 17 February 2015
Dietary Guidelines Advisory Committee. Scientific Report. Advisory Report to the Secretary of Health and Human Services and the Secretary of Agriculture. Part D. Chapter 1: Food and nutrient intakes, and health: current status and trends. 2015;1–78
Ros E, Hu FB. Consumption of plant seeds and cardiovascular health epidemiological and clinical trial evidence. Circulation. 2013;128:553–565
USDA. What we eat in America, NHANES 2011–2012, individuals 2 years and over (excluding breast-fed children). Available: www.ars.usda.gov/nea/bhnrc/fsrg
Slavin JL, Lloyd B. Health benefits of fruits and vegetables. Adv Nutr. 2012;3:506–516
Rebello CJ, Greenway FL, Finley JW. A review of the nutritional value of legumes and their effects on obesity and its related co-morbidities. Obes Rev. 2014;15:392–407
Gebhardt SE, Thomas RG. Nutritive Value of Foods. 2002; U.S. Department of Agriculture, Agricultural Research Service, Home and Garden Bulletin 72
Holden JM, Eldridge AL, Beecher GR, et al. Carotenoid content of U.S. foods: an update of the database. J Food Comp An. 1999;12:169–196
Lu Q-Y, Zhang Y, Wang Y, et al. California Hass avocado: profiling of carotenoids, tocopherol, fatty acid, and fat content during maturation and from different growing areas. J Agric Food Chem. 2009;57(21):10,408–10,413
Wu X, Beecher GR, Holden JM, et al. Lipophilic and hydrophilic antioxidant capacities of common foods in the United States. J Agric Food Chem. 2004;52:4026–4037
Dahl WJ, Steward ML. Position of the Academy of Nutrition and Dietetics: health implication of dietary fiber. J Acad Nutr Diet. 2015;115(11):1861–1870
U.S. Department of Agriculture and U.S. Department of Health and Human Services. Dietary Guidelines for Americans, 2010. 7th Edition, Washington, DC: U.S. Government Printing Office. 2010; Table B2.4; http://www.choosemyplate.gov/ Accessed 8.22.2015
http://wholegrainscouncil.org/whole-grains-101/what-counts-as-a-serving. Accessed 12.26.2015
[a]SFA (saturated fat), MUFA (monounsaturated fat) and PUFA (polyunsaturated fat)

References

1. Olshansky SJ. Has the rate of human aging already been modified? Cold Spring Harb Perspect Med. 2015;5. https://doi.org/10.1101/cshperspect.a025965.
2. Olshansky SJ, Hayflick L, Carnes BA. No truth to the fountain of youth. Sci Am. 2008;14:98–102.
3. WHO/FAO. Joint Expert Consultation on Diet, Nutrition and the Prevention of Chronic Diseases. Diet. Nutrition and the Prevention of Chronic Diseases. WHO Technical Series. 2003:916.
4. Fontana L, Hu FB. Optimal body weight for health and longevity: bridging basic, clinical, and population research. Aging Cell. 2014;13:391–400.

5. Newman AB. Is the onset of obesity the same as aging? Proc Natl Acad U S A. 2015;112(52):E7163. https://doi.org/10.1073/pnas. 1515367112.
6. Beltran-Sanchez H, Soneji S, Crimmins EM. Past, present, and future of healthy life expectancy. Cold Spring Harb Perspect Med. 2015;5. https://doi.org/10.1101/cshperspect.a025957.
7. World Health Organization. WHO global status report on noncommunicable diseases 2010. Geneva: World Health Organization Press; 2010.
8. Avendano M, Kawachi I. Why do Americans have shorter life expectancy and worse health than people in other high-income countries? Annu Rev Public Health. 2014;35:307–25.
9. Rowe JW, Kahn RL. Human aging: usual and successful. Science. 1987;237:143–9. https://doi.org/10.1126/science.3299702.
10. Micha R, Khatibzadeh S, Shi P, et al. Global, regional and national consumption of major food groups in 1990 and 2010: a systematic analysis including 266 country-specific nutrition surveys worldwide. BMJ Open. 2015;5(9):e008705. https://doi.org/10.1136/bmjopen-2015-008705.
11. Dietary Guidelines Advisory Committee. Scientific Report. Advisory Report to the Secretary of Health and Human Services and the Secretary of Agriculture. Part D. Chapter 1: Food and nutrient intakes, and health: current status and trends 2015. p. 1–78.
12. http://health.gov/dietaryguidelines/2015/guidelines/appendix-3/ Accessed June 21, 2016.
13. Wu X, Beecher GR, Holden JM, et al. Lipophilic and hydrophilic antioxidant capacities of common foods in the United States. J Agric Food Chem. 2004;52:4026–37.
14. Ros E, Hu FB. Consumption of plant seeds and cardiovascular health epidemiological and clinical trial evidence. Circulation. 2013;128:553–65.
15. Slavin JL, Lloyd B. Health benefits of fruits and vegetables. Adv Nutr. 2012;3:506–16.
16. Rebello CJ, Greenway FL, Finley JW. A review of the nutritional value of legumes and their effects on obesity and its related co-morbidities. Obes Rev. 2014;15:392–407.
17. Gebhardt SE, Thomas R. Nutritive value of foods. Home and Garden Bulletin, Agriculture Research Service, United States Department of Agriculture, 2002,72:36–68
18. Dietary Guidelines Advisory Committee (DGAC). Scientific Report. Advisory Report to the Secretary of Health and Human Services and the Secretary of Agriculture. Part D. Chapter 2: Dietary patterns, foods and nutrients and health outcomes 2015. p. 1–35.
19. Mozaffarian D. Dietary and policy priorities for cardiovascular disease, diabetes, and obesity. A comprehensive review. Circulation. 2017;133(2):187–225. https://doi.org/10.1161/CIRCULATIONAHA.11519.018585.
20. Palmer AK, Tchkonia T, LeBrasseur NK, et al. Cellular senescence in type 2 diabetes: a therapeutic opportunity. Diabetes. 2015;64:2289–98.
21. Satija A, Bhupathiraju SN, Rimm EB, et al. Plant-based dietary patterns and incidence of type 2 diabetes in US men and women: results from three prospective cohort studies. PLoS Med. 2016;13(6):e1002039. https://doi.org/10.1371/journal.pmed.1002039.
22. Micha R, Peñalvo JL, Cudhea F, et al. Association between dietary factors and mortality from heart disease, stroke, and type 2 diabetes in the United States. JAMA. 2017;317(9):912–24. https://doi.org/10.1001/jama.2017.0947.
23. William PG. Evaluation of the evidence between consumption of refined grains and health outcomes. Nutr Rev. 2012;70(2):80–99.
24. Seal CJ, Brownlee IA. Whole-grain foods and chronic disease: evidence from epidemiological and intervention studies. Proc Nutr Soc. 2015;74:313–9.
25. Slavin J. Why whole grains are protective: biological mechanisms. Proc Nutr Soc. 2003;62:129–34.
26. Cho SS, Qi L, Fahey Jr GC, Klurfeld DM. Consumption of cereal fiber, mixtures of whole grains and bran, and whole grains and risk reduction in type 2 diabetes, obesity, and cardiovascular disease. Am J Clin Nutr 2013;98: 594–619.
27. McGill CR, Fulgoni VL III, Devareddy L. Ten-year trends in fiber and whole grain intakes and food sources for the United States population: National Health and Nutrition Examination Survey 2001-2010. Forum Nutr. 2015;7:1119–30.
28. Aune D, Keum N, Giovannucci E, et al. Whole grain consumption and risk of cardiovascular disease, cancer, and all cause and cause specific mortality: systematic review and dose-response meta-analysis of prospective studies. BMJ. 2016;353:i2716. https://doi.org/10.1136/bmj.i2716.
29. Wei H, Gao Z, Liang R, et al. Whole-grain consumption and the risk of all-cause, CVD and cancer mortality: a meta-analysis of prospective cohort studies. Br J Nutr. 2016;116(3):514–25. https://doi.org/10.1017/S0007114516001975.
30. Zong G, Gao A, FB H, Sun Q. Whole grain intake and mortality from all causes, cardiovascular disease, and cancer a meta-analysis of prospective cohort studies. Circulation. 2016;133:2370–80.
31. Li B, Zhang G, Tan M, et al. Consumption of whole grains in relation to mortality from all causes, cardiovascular disease, and diabetes. Dose–response meta-analysis of prospective cohort studies. Medicine. 2016;95:33(e4229); doi: org/10.1097/MD.00000000000429.
32. Benisi-Kohansal S, Saneei P, Salehi-Marzijarani M, et al. Whole-grain intake and mortality from all causes, cardiovascular disease, and cancer: a systematic review and dose-response meta-analysis of prospective cohort studies. Adv Nutr. 2016;7:1052–65. https://doi.org/10.3945/an.11615.
33. Xu M, Huang T, Lee AM, et al. Ready-to-eat cereal consumption with total and cause -specific mortality: prospective analysis of 367,442 individuals. J Am Coll Nutr. 2016;35(3):217–23.

34. Wu H, Flint AJ, Qi Q. Association between dietary whole grain intake and risk of mortality: two large prospective studies in US men and women. JAMA Intern Med. 2015;175(3):373–84.
35. Huang T, Xu M, Lee A, et al. Consumption of whole grains and cereal fiber and total and cause-specific mortality: prospective analysis of 367,442 individuals. BMC Med. 2015;13:59. https://doi.org/10.1186/s12916-015-0338-z.
36. Johnsen NF, Frederiksen K, Christensen J, et al. Whole-grain products and whole-grain types are associated with lower all-cause and cause-specific mortality in the Scandinavian HELGA cohort. Br J Nutr. 2015;114:608–23.
37. He M, van Dam RM, Rimm E, et al. Whole grain, cereal fiber, bran, and germ intake and the risks of all-cause and CVD-specific mortality among women with type 2 diabetes. Circulation. 2010;121(20):2162–8.
38. Hollænder PLB, Ross AB, Kristensen M. Whole-grain and blood lipid changes in apparently healthy adults: a systematic review and meta-analysis of randomized controlled studies. Am J Clin Nutr. 2015;102(3):556–72. https://doi.org/10.3945/ajcn.115.109165.
39. Ye EQ, Chacko SA, Chou EL, et al. Greater whole-grain intake is associated with lower risk of type 2 diabetes, cardiovascular disease, and weight gain. J Nutr. 2012;142:1304–13.
40. Kelly SAM, Summerbell CD, Brynes A, et al. Wholegrain cereals for coronary heart disease. Cochrane Database Syst Rev. 2007; 2:CD005051; doi:10.1002/14651858.CD005051.pub2.
41. Flint AJ, FB H, Glynn RJ, et al. Whole grains and incident hypertension in men. Am J Clin Nutr. 2009;90:493–8.
42. Kirwan JP, Malin SK, Scelsi AR, et al. Whole-grain diet reduces cardiovascular risk factors in overweight and obese adults: a randomized controlled trial. J Nutr. 2016;146:2244–51.
43. Tighe P, Duthie G, Vaughan N, et al. Effect of increased consumption of whole-grain foods on blood pressure and other cardiovascular risk markers in healthy middle-aged persons: a randomized controlled trial. Am J Clin Nutr. 2010;92:733–40.
44. Chen J, Huang Q, Shi W, et al. Meta-analysis of the association between whole and refined grain consumption and stroke risk based on prospective cohort studies, Asia Pacific. J Public Health. 2016;28(7):563–75.
45. Fang L, Li W, Zhang W, et al. Association between whole grain intake and stroke risk: evidence from meta-analysis. Int J Clin Exp Med. 2015;8(9):16978–83.
46. Liu S, Manson JE, Stampfer MJ, et al. Whole grain consumption and risk of ischemic stroke in women. JAMA. 2000;284(12):1534–40.
47. Aune D, Norat T, Romundstad P, Vatten LJ. Whole grain and refined grain consumption and the risk of type 2 diabetes: a systematic review and dose-response meta-analysis of cohort studies. Eur J Epidemiol. 2013;28:845–58. https://doi.org/10.1007/s10654-013-9852-5.
48. Chanson-Rolle A, Meynier A, Aubin F, et al. Systematic review and meta-analysis of human studies to support a quantitative recommendation for whole grain intake in relation to type 2 diabetes. PLoS One. 2015;10(6):e0131377. https://doi.org/10.1371/journal.pone.0131377.
49. Sun Q, Spiegelman D, van Dam RM, et al. White rice, brown rice and risk of type 2 diabetes in US men and women. Arch Intern Med. 2010;170(11):961–9.
50. de Munter JSL, Hu FB, Spiegelman D, et al. Whole grain, bran, and germ intake and risk of type 2 diabetes: a prospective cohort study and systematic review. PLoS Med. 2007;4(8):e261. https://doi.org/10.1371/journal.pmed.0040261.
51. Aune D, Chan DSM, Lau R, et al. Dietary fibre, whole grains, and risk of colorectal cancer: systematic review and dose-response meta-analysis of prospective studies. BMJ. 2011;343:d6617. https://doi.org/10.1136/bmj.d6617.
52. Haas P, Machado MJ, Anton AA, et al. Effectiveness of whole grain consumption in the prevention of colorectal cancer: meta-analysis of cohort studies. Int J Food Sci Nutr. 2009;60(Suppl 6):1–13.
53. Kyrø C, Skeie G, Loft S, et al. Intake of whole grains from different cereal and food sources and incidence of colorectal cancer in the Scandinavian HELGA Cohort. Cancer Causes Control. 2013;24:1363–74. https://doi.org/10.1007/s10552-013-0215-z.
54. Milani C, Ferrario C, Turroni F, et al. The human gut microbiota and its interactive connections to diet. J Hum Nutr Diet. 2016;29(5):539–46. https://doi.org/10.1111/jhn.12371.
55. De Angelis M, Montemurno E, Vannini L, et al. Effect of whole-grain barley on the human fecal microbiota and metabolome. Appl Environ Microbiol. 2015;81:7945–56.
56. vel Szic KS, Declerck K, Vidaković M, Vanden Berghe W. From inflammaging to healthy aging by dietary lifestyle choices: is epigenetics the key to personalized nutrition? Clin Epigenetics. 2015; 7:33. doi: 10.1186/s13148-015-0068-2.
57. de Heredia FP, Gomez-Martınez S, Marcos A. Chronic and degenerative diseases, obesity, inflammation and the immune system. Proc Nutr Soc. 2012;71:332–8.
58. Lefevre M, Jonnalagadda S. Effect of whole grains on markers of subclinical inflammation. Nutr Rev. 2012;70(7):387–96.
59. Puzianowska-Kuźnicka M, Owczarz M, Wieczorowska-Tobis K, et al. Interleukin-6 and C-reactive protein, successful aging, and mortality: The PolSenior Study. Immun Ageing. 2016;13:21. https://doi.org/10.1186/s12979-016-0076-x.
60. Jeffery IB, O'Toole PW. Diet-microbiota interactions and their implications for healthy living. Forum Nutr. 2013;5:234–52.
61. Arora T, Backhed F. The gut microbiota and metabolic disease: current understanding and future

perspectives. J Intern Med. 2016;280(4):339–49. https://doi.org/10.1111/joim.12508.
62. Keenan MJ, Marco ML, Ingram DK, Martin RJ. Improving health span via changes in gut microbiota and fermentation. Age. 2015;37(5):98.
63. O'Toole PWO, Jeffery IB. Gut microbiota and aging. Science. 2015;350(6265):1214–5.
64. Zapata HJ, Quagliarello VJ. The microbiota and microbiome in aging: potential implications in health and age-related diseases. J Am Geriatr Soc. 2015;63(4):776–81.
65. Claesson MJ, Jeffery IB, Conde S. Gut microbiota composition correlates with diet and health in the elderly. Nature. 2012;488:178–85.
66. Tuohy KM, Conterno L, Gasperotti M, Viola R. Up-regulating the human intestinal microbiome using whole plant foods, polyphenols, and/or fiber. J Agric Food Chem. 2012;60:8776–82.
67. Tap J, Furet JP, Bensaada M, et al. Gut microbiota richness promotes its stability upon increased dietary fibre intake in healthy adults. Environ Microbiol. 2015;17(12):4954–64.
68. Vanegas SM, Meydani M, Barnett JB, et al. Substituting whole grains for refined grains in a 6-wk randomized trial has a modest effect on gut microbiota and immune and inflammatory markers of healthy adults. Am J Clin Nutr. 2017;105(3): 653–0. https://doi.org/10.3945/ajcn.116.146928.
69. Martınez I, Lattimer JM, Hubach KL, et al. Gut microbiome composition is linked to whole grain-induced immunological improvements. ISME J. 2013;7:269–80.
70. Price RK, Wallace JMW, Hamill LL, et al. Evaluation of the effect of wheat aleurone-rich foods on markers of antioxidant status, inflammation and endothelial function in apparently healthy men and women. Br J Nutr. 2012;108:1644–51.
71. Sepe A, Tchkonia T, Thomou T, et al. Aging and regional differences in fat cell progenitors - a mini-review. Gerontology. 2011;57:66–75. https://doi.org/10.1159/000279755.
72. Karl JP, Saltzman E. The role of whole grains in body weight regulation. Adv Nutr. 2012;3:697–707.
73. Pol K, Christensen R, Bartels EM, et al. Whole grain and body weight changes in apparently healthy adults: a systematic review and meta-analysis of randomized controlled studies. Am J Clin Nutr. 2013;98:872–84.
74. Serra-Majem L, Bautista-Castaño I. Relationship between bread and obesity. Br J Nutr. 2015;113:S29–35. https://doi.org/10.1017/S0007114514003249.
75. McKeown M, Troy LM, Jacques PF, et al. Whole- and refined-grain intakes are differentially associated with abdominal visceral and subcutaneous adiposity in healthy adults: the Framingham Heart Study. Am J Clin Nutr. 2010;92:1165–71.
76. Karl JP, Meydani M, Barnett JB, et al. Substituting whole grains for refined grains in a 6-wk randomized trial favorably affects energy-balance metrics in healthy men and postmenopausal women. Am J Clin Nutr. 2017;105(3):589–99. https://doi.org/10.3945/ajcn.116.139683.
77. Alfakry H, Malle E, Koyani CN, et al. Neutrophil proteolytic activation cascades: a possible mechanistic link between chronic periodontitis and coronary heart disease. Innate Immun. 2016;22(1):85–99. https://doi.org/10.1177/1753425915617521.
78. Nielsen SJ, Trak-Fellermeier MA, Joshipura K, Dye BA. Dietary fiber intake is inversely associated with periodontal disease among US adults. J Nutr. 2016;146:2530–6. https://doi.org/10.3945/jn.116.237065.
79. Merchant AT, Pitiphat W, Franz M, Joshipura KJ. Whole-grain and fiber intakes and periodontitis risk in men. Am J Clin Nutr. 2006;83:1395–400.
80. World Health Organization. Diet, nutrition, and the prevention of chronic diseases. Geneva: World Health Organization; 1990. http://www.who.int/nutrition/publications/obesity/WHO_TRS_797/en/index.html. Accessed 16 April 2015
81. Bertoia ML, Rimm EB, Mukamal KJ, et al. Dietary flavonoid intake and weight maintenance: three prospective cohorts of 124,086 US men and women followed for up to 24 years. BMJ. 2016;352:i17. doi.org/10.1136/bmj.i17
82. Aune D, Giovannucci E, Boffetta P, et al. Fruit and vegetable intake and the risk of cardiovascular disease, total cancer and all-cause mortality-a systematic review and dose response meta-analysis of prospective studies. Int J Epidemiol. 2017:1–28. https://doi.org/10.1093/ije/dyw319.
83. Wang X, Ouyang Y, Liu J. Fruit and vegetable consumption and mortality from all causes, cardiovascular disease, and cancer: systematic review and dose-response meta-analysis of prospective cohort studies. BMJ. 2014;349:g4490. https://doi.org/10.1136/bmj.g4490.
84. Bellavia A, Stilling F, Wolk A. High red meat intake and all-cause cardiovascular and cancer mortality: is the risk modified by fruit and vegetable intake? Am J Clin Nutr. 2016;104:1137–43.
85. Nguyen B, Bauman A, Gale E, et al. Fruit and vegetable consumption and all-cause mortality: evidence from a large Australian cohort study. Int J Behav Nutr Phys Act. 2016;13:9. https://doi.org/10.1186/s12966-016-0334-S.
86. Oyebode O, Gordon-Dseagu V, Walker A, Mindell JS. Fruit and vegetable consumption and all-cause, cancer and CVD mortality: analysis of health survey for England data. J Epidemiol Community Health. 2014;68:856–62.
87. Leenders M, Sluijs I, Ros MM, et al. Fruit and vegetable consumption and mortality European Prospective Investigation into Cancer and Nutrition. Am J Epidemiol. 2013;178(4):590–602.
88. Bellavia A, Larsson SC, Bottai M, et al. Fruit and vegetable consumption and all-cause mortality: a dose response analysis. Am J Clin Nutr. 2013;98:454–9.

89. Zhang X, Shu X-O, Xiang Y-B, et al. Cruciferous vegetable consumption is associated with a reduced risk of total and cardiovascular disease mortality. Am J Clin Nutr. 2011;94:240–6.
90. Huang H, Chen G, Liao D, et al. Effects of berries consumption on cardiovascular risk factors: a meta-analysis with trial sequential analysis of randomized controlled trials. Sci Rep. 2016;6:23625. https://doi.org/10.1038/srep23625.
91. Gan Y, Tong X, Li L, et al. Consumption of fruit and vegetable and risk of coronary heart disease: a meta-analysis of prospective cohort studies. Int J Cardiol. 2015;183:129–37.
92. Zhan J, Liu Y-J, Cai L-B, et al. Fruit and vegetable consumption and risk of cardiovascular disease: a meta-analysis of prospective cohort studies. Crit Rev Food Sci Nutr. 2015. https://doi.org/10.1080/10408398.2015.1008980.
93. Hartley L, Igbinedion E, Holmes J, et al. Increased consumption of fruit and vegetables for the primary prevention of cardiovascular diseases. Cochrane Database Systematic Rev. 2013;6:CD009874; doi: 10.1002/14651858.CD009874.pub2.
94. Larsson SC, Wolk A. Potato consumption and risk of cardiovascular disease: 2 prospective cohort studies. Am J Clin Nutr. 2016;104:1245–53.
95. Miedema MD, Andrew Petrone A, Shikany JM, et al. Association of fruit and vegetable consumption during early adulthood with the prevalence of coronary artery calcium after 20 years of follow-up. The Coronary Artery Risk Development in Young Adults (CARDIA) Study. Circulation. 2015;132: 1990–8.
96. Bhupathiraju SN, Wedick NM, Pan A, et al. Quantity and variety in fruit and vegetable intake and risk of coronary heart disease. Am J Clin Nutr. 2013;98:1514–23.
97. Buil-Cosiales P, Toledo E, Salas-Salvadó J, et al. Association between dietary fibre intake and fruit, vegetable or whole-grain consumption and the risk of CVD: results from the PREvención con Dieta MEDiterránea (PREDIMED) trial. Br J Nutr. 2016;116(3):534–46. https://doi.org/10.1017/S0007114516002099.
98. Li B, Wang L, Zhang D. Fruit and vegetable consumption and risk of hypertension: a meta-analysis. J Clin Hypertens (Greenwich). 2016;18(5): 468–76.
99. Wu L, Sun D, He Y. Fruit and vegetable consumption and incident hypertension: dose-response meta-analysis of prospective cohort studies. J Hum Hypertens. 2016;30(10):573–80. https://doi.org/10.1038/jhh.2016.44.
100. Borgi L, Muraki I, Satija A, et al. Fruit and vegetable consumption and the incidence of hypertension in three prospective cohort studies. Hypertension. 2016;67:288–93.
101. Borgi L, Rimm EB, Willett WC, Forman JP. Potato intake and incidence of hypertension from three prospective US cohort studies. BMJ. 2016;353:i2351. https://doi.org/10.1136/bmj.i2351.
102. Appel LJ, Moore TJ, Obarzanek E, et al. A clinical trial of the effects of dietary patterns on blood pressure. N Engl J Med. 1997;336:1117–24.
103. Hu D, Huang J, Wang Y, et al. Fruits and vegetables consumption and risk of stroke. A meta-analysis of prospective cohort studies. Stroke. 2014;45:1613–9.
104. Cassidy A, Bertoia M, Chiuve S, et al. Habitual intake of anthocyanins and flavanones and risk of cardiovascular disease in men. Am J Clin Nutr. 2016;104:587–94.
105. Oude Griep LM, Verschuren WMM, Kromhout D, et al. Colors of fruit and vegetables and 10-year incidence of stroke. Stroke. 2011;42:3190–5.
106. Joshipura KJ, Ascherio A, Manson JE, et al. Fruit and vegetable intake in relation to risk of ischemic stroke. JAMA. 1999;282:1233–9.
107. Wang P-Y, Fang J-C, Gao Z-H, et al. Higher intake of fruits, vegetables or their fiber reduces the risk of type 2 diabetes: a meta-analysis. J Diabetes Investig. 2016;7:56–69. https://doi.org/10.1111/di.12376.
108. Li M, Fan Y, Zhang X, et al. Fruit and vegetable intake and risk of type 2 diabetes mellitus: meta-analysis of prospective cohort studies. BMJ Open. 2014;4(11):e005497. https://doi.org/10.1136/bmjopen-2014-005497.
109. Xi B, Li S, Liu Z, et al. Intake of fruit juice and incidence of type 2 diabetes: a systematic review and meta-analysis. PLoS One. 2014;9(3). https://doi.org/10.1371/journal.pone.0093471.
110. Mamluk L, O'Doherty MG, Orfanos P, et al. Fruit and vegetable intake and risk of incident of type 2 diabetes: results from the consortium on health and ageing network of cohorts in Europe and the United States (CHANCES). Eur J Clin Nutr. 2016;71:83–91. https://doi.org/10.1038/ejcn.2016.143.
111. Muraki I, Rimm EB, Willett WC, et al. Potato consumption and risk of type 2 diabetes: results from three prospective cohort studies. Diabetes Care. 2016;39:376–84. https://doi.org/10.2337/dc15-0547.
112. Aune D, Lau R, Chan DSM, et al. Nonlinear reduction in risk for colorectal cancer by fruit and vegetable intake based on meta-analysis of prospective studies. Gastroenterology. 2011;141:106–18.
113. Kunzmann AT, Coleman HG, Huang W-Y, et al. Fruit and vegetable intakes and risk of colorectal cancer and incident and recurrent adenomas in the PLCO cancer screening trial. Int J Cancer. 2016;138:1851–61.
114. Leenders M, Siersema PD, Overvad K, et al. Subtypes of fruit and vegetables, variety in consumption and risk of colon and rectal cancer in the European Prospective Investigation into Cancer and Nutrition. Int J Cancer. 2015;137(11):2705–14. https://doi.org/10.1002/ijc.29640.
115. Hui C, Qi X, Qianyong Z, Xiaoli P, et al. Flavonoids, flavonoid subclasses and breast cancer risk: a meta-analysis of epidemiologic studies. PLoS One. 2013;8(1):e54318. https://doi.org/10.1371/journal.pone.0054318.

116. Aune D, Chan DS, Vieira AR, et al. Fruits, vegetables and breast cancer risk: a systematic review and meta-analysis of prospective studies. Breast Cancer Res Treat. 2012;134(2):479–93. https://doi.org/10.1007/s10549-012-2118-1.
117. Aune D, Chan DS, Vieira AR, et al. Dietary compared with blood concentration of carotenoids and breast cancer risk: a systematic review and meta-analysis of prospective studies. Am J Clin Nutr. 2012;96:356–73.
118. Lamport DJ, Saunders C, Butler LT, Spencer JPR. Fruits, vegetables, 100% juices, and cognitive function. Nutr Rev. 2014;2(12):774–89.
119. Loef M, Walach H. Fruit, vegetable and prevention of cognitive decline or dementia: a systematic review of cohort studies. J Nutr Health Aging. 2012;16(7):625–30.
120. Neshatdousta S, Saunders C, Castle SM, et al. High-flavonoid intake induces cognitive improvements linked to changes in serum brain-derived neurotrophic factor: two randomised, controlled trials. Nutr Healthy Aging. 2016;4:81–93. https://doi.org/10.3233/NHA-1615.
121. Kean RJ, Lamport DJ, Dodd GF, et al. Chronic consumption of flavanone-rich orange juice is associated with cognitive benefits: an 8-wk, randomized, double-blind, placebo-controlled trial in healthy older adults. Am J Clin Nutr. 2015;101:506–14.
122. Nooyens ACJ, Bueno-de-Mesquita HB, van Boxtel MPJ. Fruit and vegetable intake and cognitive decline in middle-aged men and women: the Doetinchem Cohort Study. Br J Nutr. 2011;106:752–61.
123. Peneau S, Galan P, Jeandel C, et al. Fruit and vegetable intake and cognitive function in the SU.VI.MAX 2 prospective study. Am J Clin Nutr. 2011;94:1295–303.
124. Neville CE, Young IS, Gilchrist SECM, et al. Effect of increased fruit and vegetable consumption on physical function and muscle strength in older adults. Age. 2013;35:2409–22. https://doi.org/10.1007/s11357-013-9530-2.
125. Gibson A, Edgar JD, Neville CE, et al. Effect of fruit and vegetable consumption on immune function in older people: a randomized controlled trial. Am J Clin Nutr. 2012;96:1429–36.
126. Ribeiro SM, Morley JE, Malmstrom TK, Miller DK. Fruit and vegetable intake and physical activity as predictors of disability risk factors in African-American middle-aged individuals. J Nutr Health Aging. 2016;20(9):891–6. https://doi.org/10.1007/s12603-016-0780-4.
127. Lian F, Wang J, Huang X, et al. Effect of vegetable consumption on the association between peripheral leucocyte telomere length and hypertension: a case–control study. BMJ Open. 2015;5:e009305. https://doi.org/10.1136/bmjopen-2015-009305.
128. McCrory MA, Hamaker BR, Lovejoy JC, Eichelsdoerfer PE. Pulse consumption, satiety, and weight management. Adv Nutr. 2010;1:17–30.
129. Messina V. Nutritional and health benefits of dried beans. Am J Clin Nutr. 2014;100(suppl):437S–42S.
130. Farvid MS, Malekshah AF, Pourshams A, et al. Dietary protein sources and all-cause and cause-specific mortality: The Golestan Cohort Study in Iran. Am J Prev Med. 2017;52(2):237–48. https://doi.org/10.1016/j.amepre.2016.10.041.
131. Chang W-C, Wahlqvist ML, Chang H-Y, et al. A bean-free diet increases the risk of all-cause mortality among Taiwanese women: the role of the metabolic syndrome. Public Health Nutr. 2011;15(4):663–72. https://doi.org/10.1017/S1366890011002151.
132. Darmadi-Blackberry I, Wahlqvist ML, Kouris-Blazos A, et al. Legumes: the most important dietary predictor of survival in older people of different ethnicities. Asia Pac J Clin Nutr. 2004;13:217–20.
133. Marventano S, Pulido MI, Sánchez-González C, et al. Legume consumption and CVD risk: a systematic review and meta-analysis. Public Health Nutr. 2017;20(2):245–54.
134. Tokede OA, Onabanjo TA, Yansane A, et al. Soya products and serum lipids: a meta-analysis of randomised controlled trials. Br J Nutr. 2015;114:831–43.
135. Ha V, John L, Sievenpiper JL, et al. Effect of dietary pulse intake on established therapeutic lipid targets for cardiovascular risk reduction: a systematic review and meta-analysis of randomized controlled trials. CMAJ. 2014;186(8):252–62.
136. Afshin A, Micha R, Khatibzadeh S, Mozaffarian D. Consumption of nuts and legumes and risk of incident ischemic heart disease, stroke, and diabetes: a systematic review and meta-analysis. Am J Clin Nutr. 2014;100:278–88.
137. Bazzano LA, Thompson AM, Tees MT, et al. Non-soy legume consumption lowers cholesterol levels: a meta-analysis of randomized controlled trials. Nutr Metab Cardiovasc Dis. 2011;21(2):94–103.
138. Anderson JW, Bush HM. Soy protein effects on serum lipoproteins: a quality assessment and meta-analysis of randomized, controlled studies. J Am Coll Nutr. 2011;30(2):79–91.
139. Liua Z-M, Hob SC, Chen Y-M, Woo J. Effect of soy protein and isoflavones on blood pressure and endothelial cytokines: a 6-month randomized controlled trial among postmenopausal women. J Hypertens. 2013;31(2):384–92. https://doi.org/10.1097/HJH.0b013e32835c0905.
140. Pittaway JK, Robertson IK, Ball MJ. Chickpeas may influence fatty acid and fiber intake in an ad libitum diet, leading to small improvements in serum lipid profile and glycemic control. J Am Diet Assoc. 2008;108:1009–13.
141. He J, Gu D, Wu X, et al. Effect of soybean protein on blood pressure. A randomized, controlled trial. Ann Intern Med. 2005;143(1):1–9.
142. Liu ZM, Chen YM, Ho SC. Effects of soy intake on glycemic control: a meta-analysis of randomized controlled trials. Am J Clin Nutr. 2011;93:1092–101.
143. Sievenpiper JL, Kendall CW, Esfahani A, et al. Effect of non-oil-seed pulses on glycaemic control: a systematic review and meta-analysis of randomised

controlled experimental trials in people with and without diabetes. Diabetologia. 2009;52:1479–95.
144. Ding M, Pan A, Manson JE, et al. Consumption of soy foods and isoflavones and risk of type 2 diabetes: a pooled analysis of three US cohorts. Eur J Clin Nutr. 2016;70(12):1381–7. https://doi.org/10.1038/ejcn.2016.117.
145. Villegas R, Gao YT, Yang G, et al. Legume and soy food intake and the incidence of type 2 diabetes in the Shanghai Women's Health Study. Am J Clin Nutr. 2008;87:162–7.
146. Jenkins DJA, Kendall WC, Augustin LSA, et al. Effect of legumes as part of a low glycemic index diet on glycemic control and cardiovascular risk factors in type 2 diabetes mellitus. A randomized controlled trial. Arch Intern Med. 2012;172(21):1653–60.
147. Yu Y, Jing X, Li H, et al. Soy isoflavone consumption and colorectal cancer risk: a systematic review and meta-analysis. Sci Rep. 2016;6:25939. https://doi.org/10.1038/srep25939.
148. Zhu B, Sun Y, Qi L, et al. Dietary legume consumption reduces risk of colorectal cancer: evidence from a meta-analysis of cohort studies. Sci Rep. 2015;5:8797. https://doi.org/10.1038/srep08797.
149. Yang G, Shu X-O, Li H, et al. Prospective cohort study of soy food intake and colorectal cancer risk in women. Am J Clin Nutr. 2009;89:577–83.
150. Chen M, Rao Y, Zheng Y, et al. Association between soy isoflavone intake and breast cancer risk for pre- and postmenopausal women: a meta-analysis of epidemiological studies. PLoS One. 2014;9(2):e89288. https://doi.org/10.1371/journal.pone.0089288.
151. Xie Q, Chen M-L, Qin Y, et al. Isoflavone consumption and risk of breast cancer: a dose-response meta-analysis of observational studies. Asia Pac J Clin Nutr. 2013;22(1):118–27. https://doi.org/10.6133/apjcn.2013.22.1.16.
152. Chen X, Huang Y, Cheng HG. Lower intake of vegetables and legumes associated with cognitive decline among illiterate elderly Chinese: a 3-year cohort study. J Nutr Health Aging. 2012;16(6):548–52.
153. St. John JA, Henderson VW, Hodis HN, et al. Associations of urine excretion of isoflavonoids with cognition in postmenopausal women in the Women's Isoflavone Soy Health Clinical Trial. J Am Geriatr Soc. 2014;62(4):629–35. https://doi.org/10.1111/jgs.12752.
154. Kreijkamp-Kaspers S, Kok L, Gobbee DE, et al. Effect of soy protein containing isoflavones on cognitive function, bone mineral density, and plasma lipids in postmenopausal women a randomized controlled trial. JAMA. 2004;292:65–74.
155. Jackson CL, Hu FB. Long-term associations of nut consumption with body weight and obesity. Am J Clin Nutr. 2014;100(suppl):408S–11S.
156. Kris-Etherton PM, Hu FB, Ros E, Sabaté J. The role of tree nuts and peanuts in the prevention of coronary heart disease: multiple potential mechanisms. J Nutr. 2008;138(9):1746S–51S.
157. Brown RC, Tey SL, Gray AR, et al. Nut consumption is associated with better nutrient intakes: results from the 2008/09 New Zealand Adult Nutrition Survey. Br J Nutr. 2016;115:105–12.
158. Novotny JA, Gebauer SK, Baer DJ. Discrepancy between the Atwater factor predicted and empirically measured energy values of almonds in human diets. Am J Clin Nutr. 2012;96:296–301.
159. Nielsen SJ, Kit BK, Ogden CL. Nut consumption among U.S. adults, 2009-2010. NCHS data brief, no 176. Hyattsville, MD: National Center for Health Statistics 2014.
160. Grosso G, Estruch R. Nut consumption and age-related disease. Maturitas. 2015;84:11–6.
161. Aune D, Keum NN, Giovannucci E, et al. Nut consumption and risk of cardiovascular disease, total cancer, all-cause and cause specific mortality: a systematic review and dose-response meta-analysis of prospective studies. BMC Med. 2016;14:207. https://doi.org/10.1186/s12916-016-0730-3.
162. Mayhew AJ, de Souza RJ, Meyre D, et al. A systematic review and meta-analysis of nut consumption and incident risk of CVD and all-cause mortality. Br J Nutr. 2016;115:212–25.
163. Wu L, Wang Z, Zhu J, et al. Nut consumption and risk of cancer and type 2 diabetes: a systematic review and meta-analysis. Nutr Rev. 2015;73(7):409–25.
164. Guo K, Zhou Z, Jiang Y, et al. Meta-analysis of prospective studies on the effects of nut consumption on hypertension and type 2 diabetes mellitus. J Diabetes. 2015;7(2):202–12; doi: 1111/1753-0407.12173.
165. Zhang Z, Xu G, Wei Y, et al. Nut consumption and risk of stroke. Eur J Epidemiol. 2015;30(3):189–96. https://doi.org/10.1007/s10654-015-9999-3.
166. Luo C, Zhang Y, Ding Y, et al. Nut consumption and risk of type 2 diabetes, cardiovascular disease, and all-cause mortality: a systematic review and meta-analysis. Am J Clin Nutr. 2014;100:256–69.
167. Zhou D, Yu H, He F, et al. Nut consumption in relation to cardiovascular disease risk and type 2 diabetes: a systematic review and meta-analysis of prospective studies. Am J Clin Nutr. 2014;100:270–7.
168. Wang W, Yang M, Kenfield SA, et al. Nut consumption and prostate cancer risk and mortality. Br J Cancer. 2016;115(3):371–4. https://doi.org/10.1038/bjc.2016.181.
169. Yang M, FB H, Giovannucci E, et al. nut consumption and risk of colorectal cancer in women. Eur J Clin Nutr. 2016;70(3):333–7. https://doi.org/10.1038/ejcn.2015.66.
170. Luu HN, Blot WJ, Xiang Y-B, et al. Prospective evaluation of the association of nut/peanut consumption with total and cause-specific mortality. JAMA Intern Med. 2015;175(5):755–66.
171. Gopinath B, Flood VM, Burlutksy G, Mitchell P. Consumption of nuts and risk of total and cause-specific mortality over 15 years. Nutr Metab Cardiovasc Dis. 2015;25(12):1125–31.
172. Hshieh TT, Petrone AB, Gaziano JM, Djousse L. Nut consumption and risk of mortality in the Physicians' Health Study. Am J Clin Nutr. 2015;101(2):407–12.

173. Bao Y, Han J, FB H, et al. Association of nut consumption with total and cause-specific mortality. N Engl J Med. 2013;369(21):2001–11.
174. Bao Y, FB H, Giovannucci EL, et al. Nut consumption and risk of pancreatic cancer in women. Br J Cancer. 2013;109:2911–6.
175. Jenab M, Ferrari P, Slimani N, et al. Association of nut and seed intake with colorectal cancer risk in the European Prospective Investigation into Cancer and Nutrition. Cancer Epidemiol Biomarkers Prev. 2004;13:1595–603.
176. Guasch-Ferré M, Bulló M, Martínez-González MA, et al. Frequency of nut consumption and mortality risk in the PREDIMED nutrition intervention trial. BMC Med. 2013;11:164. https://doi.org/10.1186/1741-7015-11-164.
177. Toledo E, Salas-Salvado J, Donat-Vargas D, et al. Mediterranean diet and invasive breast cancer risk among women at high cardiovascular risk in the PREDIMED trial. A randomized clinical trial. JAMA Intern Med. 2015;175(11):1752–60. https://doi.org/10.1001/jamainternalmed2015.48.38.
178. Salas-Salvado J, Bullo M, Estruch R, et al. Prevention of diabetes with Mediterranean diets. Ann Intern Ned. 2014;160:1–10.
179. Estruch R, Ros E, Salas-Salvadó J, et al. Primary prevention of cardiovascular disease with a Mediterranean diet. N Engl J Med. 2013;368(14):1279–90.
180. Musa-Veloso K, Paulionis L, Poon T, Lee HY. The effects of almond consumption on fasting blood lipid levels: a systematic review and meta-analysis of randomised controlled trials. J Nutr Sci. 2016;5:e34. https://doi.org/10.1017/jns.2016.19.
181. Del Gobbo LC, Falk MC, Feldman R, et al. Effects of tree nuts on blood lipids, apolipoproteins, and blood pressure: systematic review, meta-analysis, and dose-response of 61 controlled intervention trials. Am J Clin Nutr. 2015;102:1347–56.
182. Mohammadifard N, Salehi-Abargouei A, Salas-Salvadó J, et al. The effect of tree nut, peanut, and soy nut consumption on blood pressure: a systematic review and meta-analysis of randomized controlled clinical trials. Am J Clin Nutr. 2015;101:966–82.
183. Viguiliouk E, Kendall CWC, Mejia SB, et al. Effect of tree nuts on glycemic control in diabetes: a systematic review and meta-analysis of randomized controlled dietary trials. PLoS One. 2014;9(7). https://doi.org/10.1371/journal.pone.0103376.
184. Banel DK, Hu FB. Effects of walnut consumption on blood lipids and other cardiovascular risk factors: a meta-analysis and systematic review. Am J Clin Nutr. 2009;90:56–63.
185. Blanco Mejia S, Kendall CWC, Viguiliouk E, et al. Effect of tree nuts on metabolic syndrome criteria: a systematic review and meta-analysis of randomised controlled trials. BMJ Open. 2014;4(7):e004660. https://doi.org/10.1136/bmjopen-2013-004660.
186. Flores-Mateo G, Rojas-Rueda D, Basora J, et al. Nut intake and adiposity: meta-analysis of clinical trials. Am J Clin Nutr. 2013;97:1346–55.
187. Xiao Y, Huang W, Peng C, et al. Effect of nut consumption on vascular endothelial function: A systematic review and meta-analysis of randomized controlled trials. Clin Nutr. 2017. https://doi.org/10.1016/j.clnu.2017.04.011.
188. Gulati S, Misra A, Pandey RM. Effect of almond supplementation on glycemia and cardiovascular risk factors in Asian Indians in North India with type 2 diabetes mellitus: a 24-week study. Metab Syndr Relat Disord. 2017;15(2):98–105. https://doi.org/10.1089/met.2016.0066.
189. Njike VY, Ayettey R, Petraro P, et al. Walnut ingestion in adults at risk for diabetes: effects on body composition, diet quality, and cardiac risk measures. BMJ Open Diabetes Res Care. 2015;3:e000115. https://doi.org/10.1136/bmjdrc-2015-000115.
190. Sauder KA, McCrea CE, Ulbrecht JS, et al. Effects of pistachios on the lipid/lipoprotein profile, glycemic control, inflammation, and endothelial function in type 2 diabetes: a randomized trial. Metabolism. 2015;64(11):1521–9. https://doi.org/10.1016/j.metabol.2015.07.021.
191. Valls-Pedret C, Sala-Vila A, Serra-Mir M, et al. Mediterranean diet and age-related cognitive decline a randomized clinical trial. JAMA Intern Med. 2015;175(7):1094–103. https://doi.org/10.1001/jamaiternmed.2015.1668.
192. O'Brien J, Okereke O, Devore E, et al. Long-term intake of nuts in relation to cognitive function in older women. J Nutr Health Aging. 2014;18(5):496–502.
193. Sánchez-Villegas A, Galbete C, Martinez-González MA. The effect of the Mediterranean diet on plasma brain-derived neurotrophic factor (BDNF) levels: The PREDIMED-NAVARRA Randomized Trial. Nutr Neurosci. 2011;14(5):195–201.
194. Lee J-Y, Jun N-R, Yoon D, et al. Association between dietary patterns in the remote past and telomere length. Eur J Clin Nutr. 2015;69(9):1048–52. https://doi.org/10.1038/ejcn.2015.58.

Part II

Gastrointestinal Tract

Fiber-Rich Dietary Patterns and Colonic Microbiota in Aging and Disease

4

Keywords

Dietary fiber • Dietary patterns • Microbiota • Short chain fatty acids Butyrate • Symbionts • Pathobionts • *C. difficile* • Inflammatory bowel disease • Colorectal cancer • Obesity • Type 2 diabetes • Metabolic syndrome • Aging • Frailty • Centenarians • Mortality

Key Points

- Over the course of human evolution, a symbiotic relationship was formed between fiber-rich diets, the colonic microbiota and human health homeostasis. However, the emergence of the Western low fiber diet as a dominant global dietary pattern has disrupted this symbiotic relationship leading to an increased population risk for unhealthy aging, chronic diseases and premature death.
- Fiber, a critical dietary factor in the maintenance of a healthy microbiota ecosystem, has emerged in recent decades for its importance in promoting colonic health, healthy aging, and reducing the risk of cardiometabolic chronic disease and premature death.
- Fiber is the primary dietary energy source of the microbiota bacteria and the breakdown products of the resulting fiber fermentation include short chain fatty acids such as butyrate which is the main energy source needed for healthy colonocytes and optimization of colonic barrier defenses.
- Daily adequate fiber intake supports colonic microbiota health by increasing probiotic and decreasing pathogenic bacteria, lowering risk of endotoxemia and reducing colonic pH and bowel transit time, and contributing to greater stool bulk to dilute potential toxic or carcinogenic compounds or metabolites.
- Fiber-rich healthy dietary patterns support the health of colonic microbiota and their action in protecting the colon from infections such as *C difficile*, inflammatory bowel disease and colorectal cancer; slowing the aging process by decreasing the risk of weight gain and obesity, type 2 diabetes, and metabolic syndrome; and reducing the risk of frailty and premature death.
- In the elderly, high-fiber diets play an important role in establishing a healthy colonic microbiota associated with lower risk of frailty and longer life expectancy due in part to higher butyrate production and lower risk of inflammaging.

M.L. Dreher, *Dietary Patterns and Whole Plant Foods in Aging and Disease*, Nutrition and Health,
https://doi.org/10.1007/978-3-319-59180-3_4

4.1 Introduction

Over the last decade, there has been increased human observational and clinical evidence supporting a strong relationship between the intake of dietary patterns with adequate dietary fiber (fiber) for healthy microbiota and colonic function, which in turn supports the prevention of chronic disease risk (e.g., cardiovascular diseases, type 2 diabetes, cancer), and weight gain, and supports healthy aging and a longer life expectancy with less frailty compared to results found with high adherence to Western low fiber dietary patterns [1–17]. The colonic microbiota serves a number of important human biological functions including aiding in the absorption of nutrients, synthesis of vitamins, fermentation fiber to metabolically bioactive short chain fatty acids (SCFAs), promoting barriers against pathogens, optimizing colonic and systemic immune function, and improving cardiometabolic health and glycemic control [17–22]. The symbiotic relationship between fiber-rich diets, microbiota and human health developed over the course of human evolution [23–28].

There is a balance between microbiota health and dysbiosis that depends on the level of fiber in the diet. Fiber is the primary source of microbiota-accessible carbohydrates for energy and fermentation to metabolites such as SCFAs, primarily butyrate, acetate, and propionate, which are crucially involved in promoting a healthy microbiota ecosystem [28]. The equilibrium between dietary fiber, gut microbiota and SCFAs levels, especially butyrate are important in maintaining a healthy colon (e.g., healthy colonic structure and acidic pH). Acetate and propionate tend to be rapidly absorbed into circulation in exchange for bicarbonate with a consequent rise in colonic pH. With an adequate fiber intake, there is more likely to be higher levels of butyrate-producing bacteria (e.g., *Roseburia* spp., *F. prausnitzii*, *Eubacterium rectale*), which help maintain an acidic colon at 5.5 pH as butyrate tends to maintain a presence in the colon [6]. Butyrate is also an important energy source for colonocytes and involved in the regulation of cell proliferation and differentiation to reinforcement of the colonic barrier to support colonic anti-inflammatory functions. When fiber becomes limiting, the colon pH increases to 6.5, which coincides with a reduction of butyrate-producing bacteria and an increase in acetate- and propionate-producing Bacteroides-related bacteria. With the higher pH, there is an increased opportunity for expansion of Proteobacteria, which includes a wide variety of pathogens, such as Escherichia, Salmonella, Vibrio and increased endotoxemia risk [21, 28]. Proteobacteria is emerging as a marker of chronic diseases risk (Fig. 4.1) [21]. The interplay between the level of fiber intake and colonic microbiota health, including a balance between symbionts (bacteria with health-promoting functions) and pathobionts (bacteria that potentially induce pathology), and the increased colonic concentration of fermentation metabolites such as butyrate and their effects on healthy aging and frailty are summarized in Fig. 4.2 [28–31]. The objective of this chapter is to comprehensively assess the effects of fiber-rich dietary patterns and colonic microbiota on healthy aging and chronic disease.

4.2 Fiber-Rich Dietary Patterns in Microbiota and Colonic Health

It has been hypothesized that individuals with high adherence to the Western diet and sedentary lifestyles are at increased risk of having colonic microbiota dysbiosis (e.g., low bacterial gene count diversity, a higher pathogenic to healthy bacteria level, colonic and systemic inflammation) and unhealthy phenotype (e.g., overweight/obesity, metabolic syndrome, elevated cardiometabolic risk biomarkers or prediabetes/diabetes) [9, 10, 23–31]. An overview of healthy dietary patterns providing adequate fiber or 14 g per 1000 kcal, a Western dietary pattern which provides approximately half the adequate fiber level and a list of the top 50 fiber rich foods are summarized in Appendices A and B. It is estimated that healthy fiber-rich dietary patterns generally contain 50–70% fermentable fiber available to help maintain a healthy microbiota ecosystem [28–32].

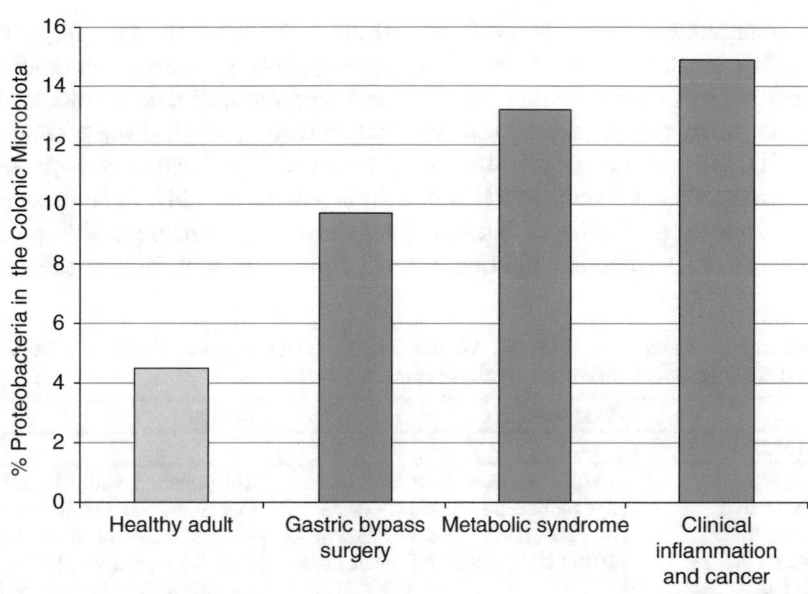

Fig. 4.1 Effect of health condition on the level of Proteobacteria in the colonic microbiota (adapted from [21])

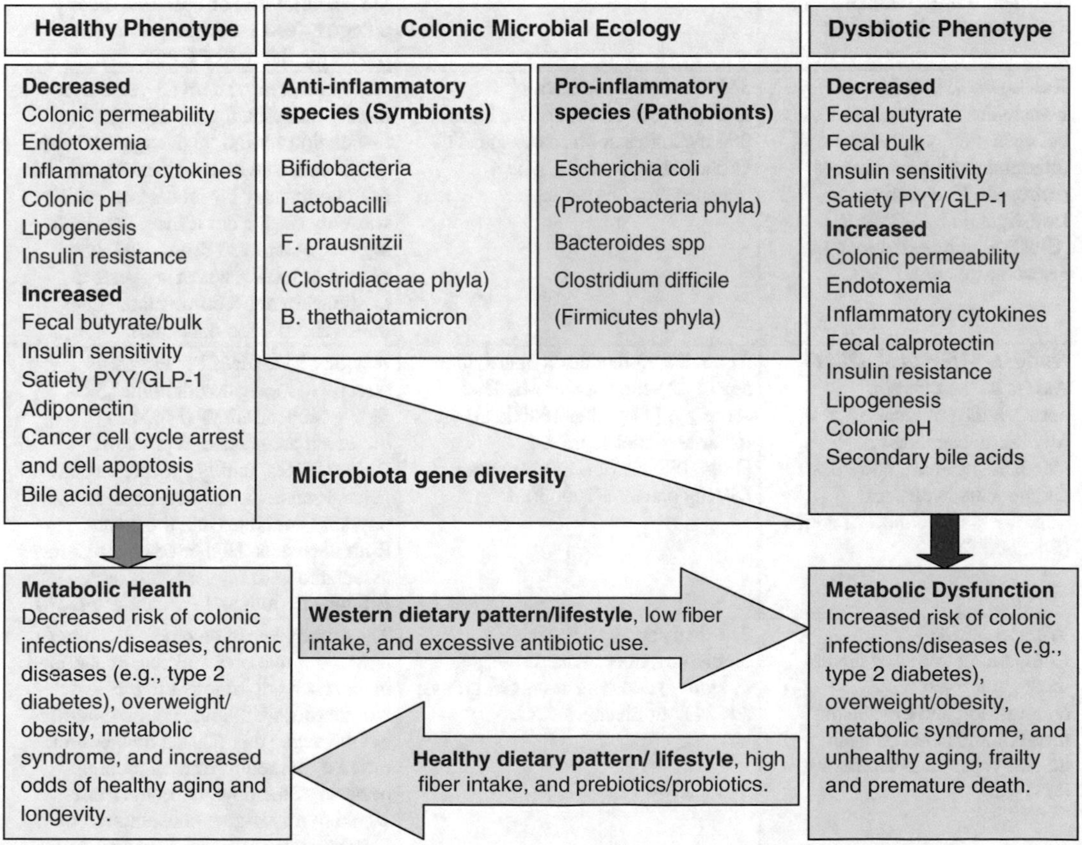

Healthy Phenotype

Decreased
Colonic permeability
Endotoxemia
Inflammatory cytokines
Colonic pH
Lipogenesis
Insulin resistance

Increased
Fecal butyrate/bulk
Insulin sensitivity
Satiety PYY/GLP-1
Adiponectin
Cancer cell cycle arrest and cell apoptosis
Bile acid deconjugation

Colonic Microbial Ecology

Anti-inflammatory species (Symbionts)
Bifidobacteria
Lactobacilli
F. prausnitzii
(Clostridiaceae phyla)
B. thethaiotamicron

Pro-inflammatory species (Pathobionts)
Escherichia coli
(Proteobacteria phyla)
Bacteroides spp
Clostridium difficile
(Firmicutes phyla)

Microbiota gene diversity

Dysbiotic Phenotype

Decreased
Fecal butyrate
Fecal bulk
Insulin sensitivity
Satiety PYY/GLP-1

Increased
Colonic permeability
Endotoxemia
Inflammatory cytokines
Fecal calprotectin
Insulin resistance
Lipogenesis
Colonic pH
Secondary bile acids

Metabolic Health
Decreased risk of colonic infections/diseases, chronic diseases (e.g., type 2 diabetes), overweight/obesity, metabolic syndrome, and increased odds of healthy aging and longevity.

Western dietary pattern/lifestyle, low fiber intake, and excessive antibiotic use.

Healthy dietary pattern/ lifestyle, high fiber intake, and prebiotics/probiotics.

Metabolic Dysfunction
Increased risk of colonic infections/diseases (e.g., type 2 diabetes), overweight/obesity, metabolic syndrome, and unhealthy aging, frailty and premature death.

Fig. 4.2 Overview of the effect of fiber intake and other lifestyle factors on human microbiota and metabolic and immune health, chronic disease, aging and frailty (adapted from [28–31])

Table 4.1 summarizes major observational studies and RCTs on the effects of fiber-rich dietary patterns in improving colonic microbiota health and reducing risk of major intestinal diseases [33–51]. Two large cohort studies, pooled data from the Nurses' Health and Health Professionals Follow-up Studies, and the European Prospective Investigation into Cancer (EPIC) Study show that high adherence to healthy dietary patterns rich in fiber are associated with reduced risk of colorectal cancer and inflammatory bowel disease compared to high adherence to a Western or high sugar and soft drink pattern [33, 34]. Eight observational studies show varying degrees of improved microbiota ecosystem with higher adherence to plant

Table 4.1 Summary of healthy fiber-rich vs. Western dietary patterns observational studies and randomized controlled trials (RCTs) on colonic microbiota health in aging and disease.

Objective	Study details	Results
Observational Studies		
Mehta et al. (2017). Examine the association between fiber rich prudent/ healthy vs. Western dietary patterns on colorectal cancer (CRC) risk in presence of intestinal F. nucleatum in tumor tissue (Nurses' Health Study and Health Professionals Follow-up Study; US) [33]	137,217 subjects; 35% male; mean age for men 54 years and women 46 years; 26–32 years of follow-up; 1019 CRC cases with F. nucleatum.	The prudent/healthy dietary pattern (rich in whole-grain and fiber) significantly lowered the multivariate risk of F. nucleatum positive CRC by 54% (p-trend = .003; highest vs. lowest diet score) but not F. nucleatum negative CRC, with insignificant lower risk by 5% (p-trend =.47). This study supports the potential role of fiber-rich dietary pattern effects on the microbiota in mediating the risk of CRC.
Racine et al. (2016). Investigate the association between dietary pattern and inflammatory bowel disease (European Prospective Investigation into Cancer (EPIC) study; nested matched case-control study) [34].	366,351 participants with inflammatory bowel disease data; 256 ulcerative colitis cases and 117 Crohn's disease cases, with 4 matched controls per case.	After excluding the first 2 years after dietary analysis, there was a positive association for the 'high sugar and soft drink' pattern with a 68% increased risk of inflammatory bowel disease, which was only significant if there was both high sugar and soft drink and low vegetable intake, which suggests a relationship between vegetable fiber intake and microbiota health.
Gutierrez-Diaz et al. (2016). Assess the association between the adherence to a Mediterranean dietary (MedDiet) pattern, and its components, with fecal microbiota in a cohort of adults (Spanish) [35].	31 adults; 23 females/8 males; mean age of 42 years; higher MedDiet score ≥ 4 [14 g fiber/1000 kcal] vs. lower MedDiet score < 4 [11 g/1000 kcal]; all diets contained 850 mg phenolic/1000 kcal.	A higher MedDiet fiber level was directly associated with higher fecal SCFA concentrations (Fig. 4.3), increased abundance of phylum Bacteroidetes, family Prevotellaceae and genus Prevotella and decreased levels of phylum Firmicutes and the genus Ruminococcus. Higher cereal intake was associated with higher levels of Bifidobacterium and Faecalibacterium.
Wu et al. (2016). Compare measures of dietary intake, gut microbiota composition and the plasma metabolome between healthy human vegans and omnivores (US) [36].	21 urban adults;15 vegans/6 omnivores; fiber intake for vegans (35 g/day) and omnivores (18 g/day); 3 × 24 hour dietary recalls.	The differences in colonic microbiota between omnivores and vegans sampled in an urban environment in the Northeastern USA were quite modest but the vegan diet plasma metabolome differed markedly from omnivores because of the phytonutrients from whole foods. Higher consumption of fiber by vegans was not associated with significantly higher levels of fecal SCFAs.

Table 4.1 (continued)

Objective	Study details	Results
De Filippis et al. (2015). Evaluate the association between the MedDiet, and the microbiota and its metabolites (Italian) [37].	153 healthy adults; vegans, vegetarians and omnivores had high MedDiet adherence; 7-day weighed food diary; fecal and urinary samples.	Subjects with good adherence to the MedDiet with higher fiber, fruits, vegetables, and legumes intake had higher levels of fecal SCFAs, Prevotella and some fiber degrading Firmicutes compared to those with lower adherence to the MedDiet. Western omnivore diets with adequate fiber intake are not necessarily detrimental to microbiota. Low adherence to the MedDiet was associated with higher urinary trimethylamine oxide levels.
Matijasic et al. (2014). Examine the association between omnivore vs. lacto-vegetarian and vegan dietary patterns on fecal microbiota composition (Slovenia) [38].	60 adults; 31 vegetarians (11 lacto-vegetarians, 20 vegans); 29 omnivores.	Vegetarian diets were associated with higher levels of Bacteroides-Prevotella, Bacteroides thetaiotaomicron, Clostridium clostridioforme and Faecalibacterium prausnitzii compared to omnivores.
Ou et al. (2013). Examine if the influence of diet on colon cancer risk is mediated by the microbiota through their metabolites (African American vs. Native African) [39].	12 healthy African Americans, urban Western diets; 12 native Africans, rural traditional diet; age- and sex-matched; mean age 58 years.	In their usual diets, African Americans consumed twice the protein, 3 times the dietary fat and less fiber than the native Africans. The African Americans and native African adults had fundamentally different predominance of core microbiota; Bacteroides vs. Prevotella, respectively. The native Africans had significantly higher total bacteria and fecal SCFAs than the African Americans. Stool butyrate concentrations were significantly correlated with the abundance of the butyrate producers Clostridium cluster IV and Clostridium cluster XIVa in the native Africans. Fecal secondary bile acid concentrations were higher in African Americans.
Zimmer et al. (2012). Assess the effects of vegetarian vs. omnivorous diets on microbiota composition (German) [40].	249 vegetarians or vegans; 249 control omnivores; matched for age and gender; mean age 52 years.	Subjects on a vegan or vegetarian diet showed significantly lower stool pH, and counts of E. coli and Enterobacteriaceae than those on the omnivorous diet suggesting a healthy microbiota environment (Fig. 4.4).
Kabeerdoss et al. (2012). Compare effects of lacto-vegetarian and omnivorous diets on the fecal microbiota of young women (Southern India) [41].	32 lacto-vegetarians and 24 omnivorous women from a similar social and economic background; median age 19 years; median BMI 21; macronutrient intake and anthropometric data were collected.	Omnivores had an increased relative abundance of Clostridium cluster XIVa bacteria, specifically Roseburia–E. rectale and butyryl-CoA-transferase gene, associated with microbial butyrate production, compared with vegetarians. Both diets had same median crude fiber intake. The relative proportions of other microbial communities were similar in both groups.

(continued)

Table 4.1 (continued)

Objective	Study details	Results
Wu et al. (2011). Investigate dietary pattern quality and its association with colonic microbiota profiles (US) [42].	98 healthy volunteers; collected diet information using two food frequency questionnaires that queried recent diet and habitual long-term diet.	The Bacteroides enterotype was highly associated with animal protein, a variety of amino acids, and saturated fats, which suggests a high level of meat intake (Western diet). In contrast, the Prevotella enterotype was associated with a higher carbohydrates/fiber based diet more typical of agrarian societies or a vegetarian diet.
Randomized Controlled Trials (RCTs)		
Tap et al. (2015). Assess the short-term effects of increased fiber intake on the microbial composition (France) [43].	**Crossover RCT:** 19 healthy normal weight adults; 10 females/9 males; age 19–25 years; basal diet supplemented with 40 or 10 g fiber/day; 5 days; 15-day washout period.	Higher fiber diets increased microbiota diversity, stability and promoted a higher Prevotella: Bacteroides ratio, increased fecal SCFAs and modulated the expression of microbiota metabolic pathways such as glycan metabolism, with genes encoding carbohydrate-active enzymes for fiber, compared to the low fiber diets, within 5 days. This was particularly true when subjects switched from their 10-g fiber diet to the 40-g fiber/day diet.
O'Keefe et al. (2015). Evaluate the acute effects on colonic microbiota after switching diets of African Americans (high colon cancer risk) and rural Africans (low colon cancer risk) (US and South Africans) [44].	**Crossover RCT:** 20 healthy middle aged African Americans and 20 rural South Africans; first 2 weeks in their own home environment, eating their usual food, and then again in-house they switched diets so the African Americans were fed a high-fiber, low-fat African-style diet, and rural Africans a high-fat low-fiber Western-style diet under close supervision for 2 weeks.	The food content of fiber and fat had substantial effects on the subject's colonic microbiota and metabolome within 2 weeks, which was associated with significant changes in mucosal inflammation and proliferation associated with potential colon cancer risk. Diets with higher animal protein and fat and lower fiber consumption resulted in higher colonic secondary bile acids, lower colonic short chain fatty acid quantities and higher mucosal proliferative biomarkers of cancer risk in the South Africans whereas higher fiber and lower fat diets increased fecal butyrate concentration and suppressed secondary bile acid synthesis in the African Americans.
David et al. (2014). Compare the effects of plant vs. animal based diets on microbiota (US) [45].	**Crossover RCT:** 10 US adults; 6 men and 4 women; ages 21–33 years; BMI range from 19–32; 2 diets: a plant-based diet (rich in whole-grains, legumes, fruits, and vegetables; 26 g fiber/1000 kcal); and an animal-based diet (consisting of meats, eggs, and cheeses; 0 g fiber/day); 5 days with a 6-day washout.	Plant based diets increased saccharolytic bacteria and SCFAs fecal content whereas animal-food based diets increased total count of bile-tolerant microorganisms, decreased the levels of Firmicutes able to ferment plant polysaccharides, and increased levels of the products of amino acid fermentation and Bilophila wadsworthia, known to elevate the risk of inflammatory bowel disease. This study suggests that microbiota can rapidly respond to large changes in diet composition.

Table 4.1 (continued)

Objective	Study details	Results
Fruits and Vegetables		
Klinder et al. (2016). Assess the impact of fruit and vegetable intake on gut microbiota (UK) [46].	**Dose-response, Parallel RCT:** 122 UK participants; 60% female; mean age 50 years; mean BMI 28; high-flavonoid and low flavonoid fruit and vegetable intervention groups consumed 2, 4 and 6 portions vs. habitual control diet; 6 weeks.	There was a dose effect for fruit and vegetable intake on increasing C. leptum-R. bromii/flavefaciens while a trend was reported for Bifidobacterium ($p = .090$) and Bacteroides/Prevotella ($p = .070$). Increased intake of fruit and vegetable portions high in flavonoids were protective against the growth of potentially pathogenic clostridia with a negative correlation of ($r = -0.145$) and higher fiber intake was weakly positively correlated with Bacteroides/ Prevotella ($r = .091$).
Whole-Grains		
Heinritz et al. (2016). Examine the effect of 2 diets with different levels of fiber and fat on microbial composition and metabolites (Netherlands) [47].	**Pig-Human Model Parallel RCT:** 8 pigs were equally allotted to 2 treatments, either fed a low-fat/ high-fiber (whole wheat-grain type), or a high-fat/low-fiber diet; 7 weeks; feces were sampled weekly.	Significantly higher numbers of lactobacilli, bifidobacteria and Faecalibacterium prausnitzii were found in the feces of the whole-wheat grain type (low-fat/high-fiber) diet fed pigs, while pathogenic type Enterobacteriaceae were significantly increased in the high-fat/low-fiber diet fed pigs. Significantly higher total and individual fecal SCFAs levels, especially butyrate, were found with whole-wheat grain type diets vs. the low fiber diets (Fig. 4.5).
Wang et al. (2016). Evaluate the effect of β-glucan enriched breakfast cereals on microbiota composition and cardiovascular disease (CVD) risk factors (Canada) [48].	**Single Blind, Crossover RCT:** 30 hyperlipidemic adults; American Heart Association (AHA) diet plus 4 breakfasts containing 3 g high molecular weight (MW) β-glucan, 3 g and 5 g low MW β-glucan, vs. refined wheat and rice (control); 5-week study period; 4-week washout.	The high MW β-glucan significantly increased Bacteroidetes and decreased Firmicutes abundance compared to control. At the genus level, consumption of 3 g/day high MW β-glucan increased Bacteroides, tended to increase Prevotella but decreased Dorea, whereas neither of the low MW β-glucan diets altered the microbiota composition. The high MW β-glucan changes in microbiota composition were significantly correlated with shifts of CVD risk factors, including reduced BMI, waist circumference, blood pressure, as well as triglyceride levels. This study suggests the microbiota health effects of high MW β-glucan.
Martinez et al. (2013). Assess the effect of whole-grains on both the colonic microbiome and human physiology (US) [49].	**Crossover RCT:** 28 healthy subjects; 11 males and 17 females; mean age 26 years; mean BMI 25; daily dose of 60 g of whole-grain barley (19 g fiber), brown rice (4.4 g fiber), or an equal mixture of the two (11.5 g fiber); 4-week treatments with 2-week washout; fecal and blood samples were taken at baseline and after each treatment period.	The barley whole-grain foods increased overall microbiota diversity and specifically Roseburia, Bifidobacterium and Dialister, and the species Eubacterium rectale, Roseburia faecis and Roseburia intestinalis. Additionally, whole grain barley reduced IL-6 associated with increased Dialister and decreased Coriobacteriaceae in the microbiota. No significant differences were detected in fecal SCFAs but this was bccausc of colonic absorption.

(continued)

Table 4.1 (continued)

Objective	Study details	Results
Carvalho-Wells et al. (2010). Evaluate the effects of maize-whole grain and refined breakfast cereal on the microbiota (UK) [50].	**Double Blind Crossover RCT:** 32 subjects; 20 females/12 males; mean age 32 years; mean BMI 23; 48 g/day maize-whole grain breakfast cereal or refined grain cereal placebo; 3-week trial periods; 3-week washout.	Maize-whole grain breakfast cereal significantly increased levels of fecal bifidobacteria compared with the control cereal, which returned to baseline levels after the washout period. There were no statistically significant changes in fecal SCFAs, bowel habit data, fasted lipids/ glucose, blood pressure, BMI and waist circumference.
Costabile et al. (2008). Compare the effects of whole grain wheat breakfast cereal to wheat bran on the human microbiota (UK) [51].	**Double Blind Crossover RCT:** 31 volunteers; average age 25 years; 16 females/15 males; BMI 20–30; 2 groups consuming daily either 48 g of whole grain wheat or wheat bran breakfast cereals; 3-week study periods, 2-week washouts.	Whole grain wheat cereals significantly increased the numbers of fecal bifidobacteria and lactobacilli compared with wheat bran cereal. Ingestion of both breakfast cereals resulted in a significant increase in ferulic acid concentrations in the blood but no discernible difference in feces or urine. No significant differences in fecal SCFAs, fasting blood glucose, insulin, total cholesterol, triglycerides or HDL-C were observed upon ingestion of whole grain wheat compared with wheat bran breakfast cereals.

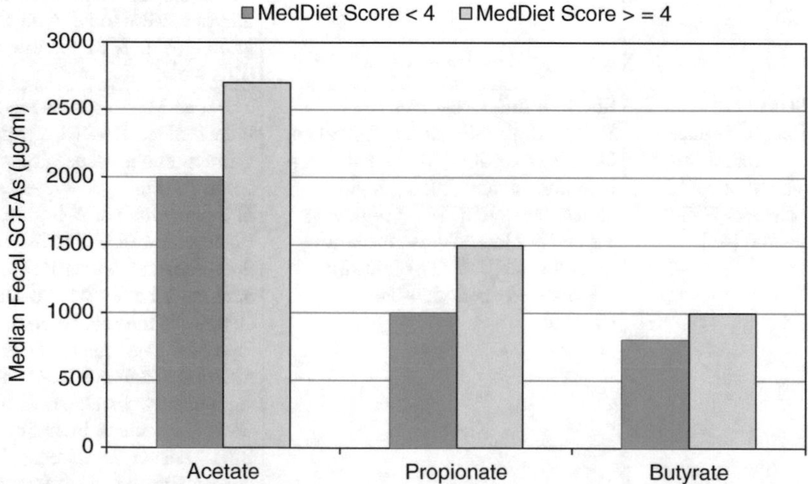

Fig. 4.3 Effect of Mediterranean diet (MedDiet) score on fecal short-chain fatty acids (SCFAs) concentrations (adapted from [35])

based diets compared to Western diets [35–42]. A fiber-rich Mediterranean diet (MedDiet) promotes a higher ratio of probiotic to pathogenic bacteria which functions by increasing fecal concentrations of SCFAs (Fig. 4.3) [35]. Vegan and vegetarian diets promote a higher ratio of probiotic to pathogenic bacteria compared to a Western omnivore dietary pattern (Fig. 4.4) [40]. Nine RCTs strongly and consistently support beneficial microbiota effects within 5 days to 7 weeks of consuming fiber-rich healthy dietary patterns compared to lower fiber Western diets [43–51]. A French crossover RCT (19 adults; 40 g vs. 10 g fiber/day dietary

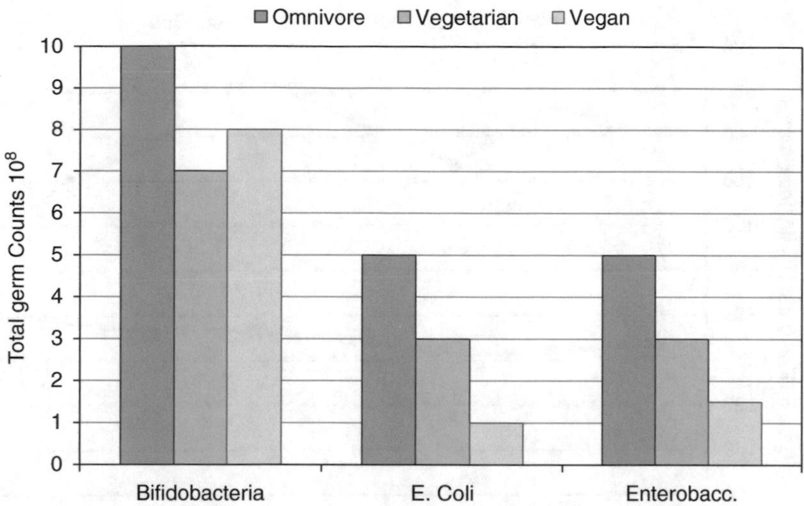

Fig. 4.4 Effect of vegetarian vs. omnivore dietary patterns on colonic microbiota bacteria composition (adapted from [40])

patterns) showed that the 40-g fiber diets increased microbiota diversity with a higher ratio of probiotic to pathogenic bacteria and increased SCFAs concentrations compared to 10-g fiber diets within 5 days [43]. A US and South African crossover RCT (20 healthy middle aged African Americans and 20 rural South Africans; diets were switched and African Americans consumed high fiber and low fat diets and rural Africans consumed high fat and low fiber diets for 2 weeks) found that after 2 weeks the African Americans had increased fecal butyrate concentrations and suppressed secondary bile acids synthesis and rural Africans had decreased butyrate concentrations and increased secondary bile acids synthesis [44]. A UK fruit and vegetable dose response RCT (122 participants mean age 50 years; 2, 4, and 6 servings daily vs. habitual control diet; 6 weeks) demonstrated that higher intake of fruits and vegetables, especially associated with higher fiber and flavonoid intake, had dose response type effects on promoting healthier microbiota bacteria profiles, lower inflammation, and greater protection from pathogenic bacteria [46]. A pig-human colonic model RCT (8 pigs; high fiber whole-grains and low fat diet vs. low fiber and high fat diet; 7 weeks) showed that a higher whole-grain fiber diet significantly increased fecal SCFAs, especially butyrate, compared to a low fiber diet (Fig. 4.5) [47].

4.3 Fiber-Rich Dietary Patterns in Aging and Disease

During the last few decades, there have been numerous human studies showing a high degree of synergy between dietary patterns with adequate fiber intake and healthy colonic microbiota with major beneficial effects on promoting colonic health, weight control, healthy aging, and lowering the risk of chronic disease and frailty.

4.3.1 Colonic Health

4.3.1.1 *Clostridium difficile* Infections

Unnecessary use of antibiotics and excessive hygienic precautions together with the Western diet have contributed to a decrease in adult colonic microbiota bacterial diversity [52, 53]. Over the past several decades, the growing aging populations, increase in antibiotics usage and resistance, high consumption of unhealthy low fiber Western diets, and growing prevalence of inflammatory bowel diseases and obesity has

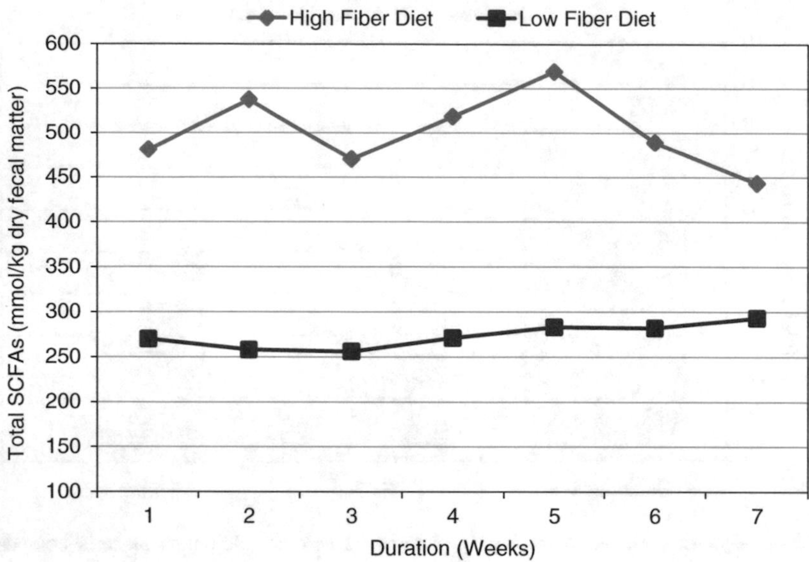

Fig. 4.5 Effect of fiber from wheat bran and cellulose on fecal short chain fatty acids (SCFAs) concentrations in pig model study over 7 weeks (p = .002) (adapted from [47])

been correlated with recurrent *Clostridium difficile (C. difficile)* infections. *C. difficile* colonic infections and associated gastrointestinal distress and prolonged diarrhea rates are increasing in both hospitals and communities worldwide, especially in elderly populations. *C. difficile* is an anaerobic, spore-forming bacterium with infection symptoms varying among patients, ranging from mild to severe diarrhea (>15 bowel movements/day) to death in severe cases [52]. *C. difficile* transmission is a major problem in hospitals across the developed world, as its spores are highly resistant to routine cleaning agents, including alcohol-based hand washes and can survive for months on aerobic surfaces (*e.g.*, hospital walls, doors, surgical tools, cell phones, *etc.*) in spore form. When ingested, the multiple layers of the spore help protect it from stomach acids and digestive enzymes but in the colon the spores can be germinated into active cells by taurine-conjugated bile acid and colonize within the gut microbiota to induce toxin associated intestinal damage and inflammation.

Low fiber diets and chronic antibiotic use are commonly associated with *C. difficile* infected patients, as both can lead to colonic microbiota dysbiosis, resulting in low butyrate production [54, 55]. Healthy fiber rich dietary patterns and/or prebiotic fiber can improve microbiotia biodiversity, especially healthy probiotic bacteria, and increase fecal butyrate concentrations to help protect against *C. difficile* associated diseases, colonic and systemic inflammatory and obesity-related metabolic syndromes [53]. Two prebiotic fibers, fructo-oligosaccharides and polydextrose, have been shown to actively re-establish indigenous microbiota, particularly those bacteria yielding large amounts of SCFAs, and decrease gut pH, which can contribute to the prevention of growth and toxin release by *C. difficile* [56]. Also, the combination of prebiotic fiber with antibiotics appears to have a synergist effect in fighting *C. difficile* infections [57].

4.3.1.2 Inflammatory Bowel Disease (IBD)

IBD, including Crohn's disease and ulcerative colitis, are chronic, life-long conditions that can be treated but not cured and most cases are diagnosed in genetically susceptible individuals due to colonic microbiota dysbiosis and related inflammatory responses usually before age 35 [34, 58]. A 2016 EPIC nested match case-control analysis (256 ulcerative colitis cases; 117 Crohns disease cases) observed that Western dietary patterns rich in sugar and soft drinks increased risk of ulcerative colitis by 68% especially with low vegetable intake [34]. A 2015 meta-analysis (2 cohort studies, 1 nested case-control study, and

5 case-control studies) indicated a significant inverse association between higher fiber intake and Crohn's disease risk by 56% and a marginally significant inverse association between higher fiber intake and ulcerative colitis risk by 20% [59]. In addition, a significant dose-response relationship was observed between fiber intake and Crohn's disease risk with a 13% lower risk per 10 g of fiber intake. Mechanisms by which increased fiber intake may help in lowering the risk of IBD include: improving colonic microbiota health, which has a regulatory influence on the colon immune response and maintenance of immunological homeostasis; and effecting aryl hydrocarbon receptor linking, a specific stimulus to protect against IBD pathogenesis [59]. IBD is associated with decreased colonic microbiota diversity, reduced proportions of Firmicutes and increased levels of *Proteobacteria* and *Actinobacteria* [58]. Specifically , with IBD proinflammatory bacteria (e.g., *Escherichia* and *Fusobacterium*) are increased and anti-inflammatory bacteria (e.g., *Faecalibacterium* and *Roseburia*) are decreased. The MedDiet has shown promise in improving IBD sysmptoms by promoting strong immunomodulatory and epigenetic effects that appear to normalize microbiota in IBD patients by increasing DNA methylation in genes coding for inflammation [58]. A 2016 EPIC nested match case-control analysis (256 ulcerative colitis cases; 117 Crohns disease cases) observed that Western dietary patterns rich in sugar and soft drinks increased risk of ulcerative colitis by 68% especially with low vegetable intake [34].

4.3.1.3 Colorectal Cancer (CRC)

The potential importance of fiber and the colonic microbiota in protecting against colorectal cancer was first hypothesized in the early 1970s by Dr. Burkitt, who observed lower rates of CRC among Africans who consumed a diet high in fiber [60]. Now, there are a number of strong biological mechanisms associated with adequate fiber intake and a lower risk of CRC. For example, the fiber colon microbiota fermentation metabolite butyrate, a histone deacetylase (HDAC) inhibitor that can suppress the viability and progressive growth of CRC cells [61, 62]. In 2011, a dose-response meta-analysis (16 cohort studies) showed each 10-g fiber increase in intake lowered risk of CRC by 10% [63]. Also, the World Cancer Research Fund and American Institute of Cancer Research continuous update concluded that there was convincing evidence that increased fiber intake was protective against CRC risk [64]. A prospective assessment of the Prostate, Lung, Colorectal, and Ovarian Cancer Screening Trial (57,774 colorectal cancers, 16,980 adenomas, and 1667 recurrent adenoma cases; mean baseline age 63 years; flexible sigmoidoscopy at baseline; 3 or 5 years of follow-up) found that participants consuming the

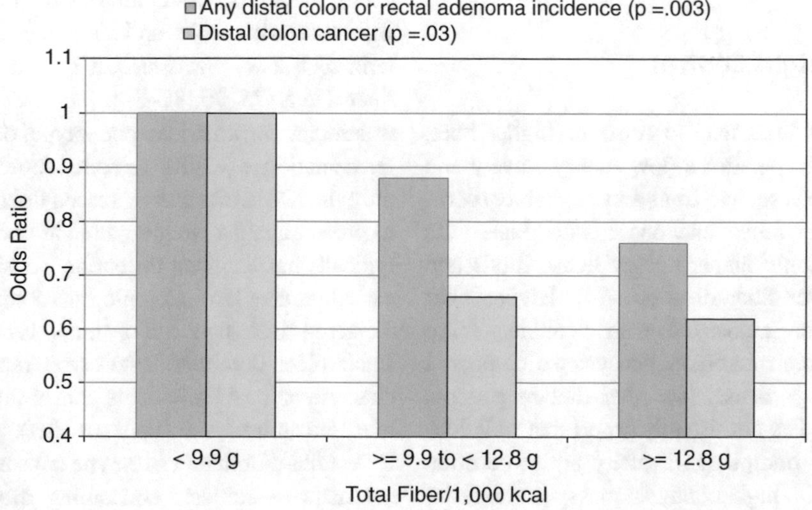

Fig. 4.6 Association between total fiber density and distal colon or rectal adenoma or distal colon cancer risk (adapted from [65])

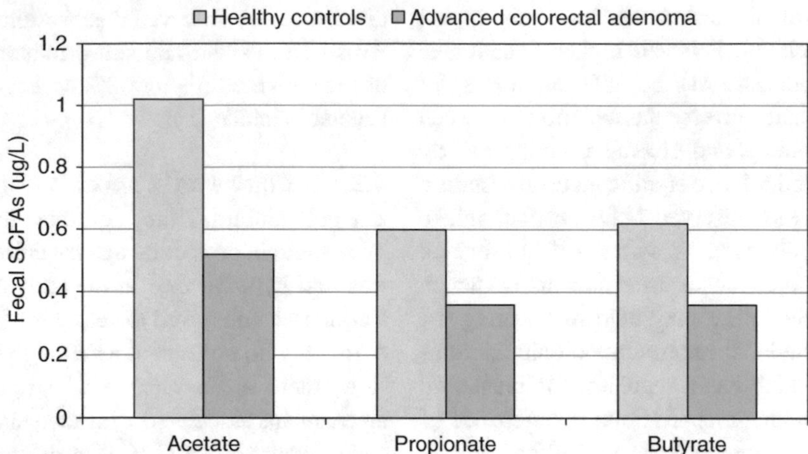

Fig. 4.7 Relationship between fecal short chain fatty acids (SCFAs) concentration in healthy subjects compared to advanced colorectal adenoma subjects ($p < .05$) (adapted from [66])

highest fiber levels, especially cereal and fruit fiber, had significantly reduced risk of colorectal adenoma and distal colon cancer (Fig. 4.6) [65]. In a cross-sectional design study (688 subjects eligible; 50% female; age > 50 years; healthy control vs. advanced colorectal adenoma groups), it was observed that a high-fiber diet, higher fecal SCFAs and healthy gut microbiota were associated with a reduced risk of advanced colorectal adenomas [66]. Healthy individuals with high fiber intake had significantly higher levels of fecal butyrate than either healthy individuals with low fiber intake or those individuals with advanced colorectal adenomas (Fig. 4.7).

4.3.2 Weight Control

Leaner individuals tend to consume higher fiber, healthier dietary patterns (low energy density and fiber-rich foods such as fruits and vegetables) compared to overweight and obese individuals who tend to consume higher energy dense foods and Western lower fiber diets [67–74]. Higher fiber diets are also associated with healthier, more diverse colonic microbiota ecosystems compared to high energy dense, low fiber dietary patterns [28–52]. Studies consistently report that individuals with low microbiota diversity are more often associated with higher body fat mass, insulin resistance, dyslipidemia, and low-grade systemic inflammation compared to individuals with higher microbiome diversity [75–81]. The overweight and obese phenotype is characterized by: more efficient capacity for extracting metabolizable energy from food; decreased abundance of butyrate-producing bacteria, in particular *F. prausnitzii*; increased pro-inflammatory functions such as mucus degradation and production of endotoxins such as lipopolysaccharides (LPS) from gram negative endobacterium; and more up-regulated genes to manage oxidative stress, which are suggestive of increased weight gain, inflammation, insulin resistance and metabolic disease risk [76–83]. In contrast, the lean, metabolically healthy phenotype is characterized by: more diverse microbiota bacterial gene functions; and increased abundance of Bifidobacteria species and butyrate-producing bacteria such as *F. prausnitzii*, a marker of a healthy microbiota [75, 76, 82–88]. Increased fiber intake is associated with a lean phenotype, despite fiber's fermentation to SCFAs (an added source of energy), the evidence shows that increased fiber intake helps to protect against weight gain and obesity, as fiber typically has only half the energy density of refined carbohydrates [85]. Colonic microbiota tend to be clustered into two major enterotypes with the Bacteroides-dominate enterotype reported to be characteristic of individuals consuming more protein and animal fat (Western diet), whereas the Prevotella-dominate enterotype appears to be characteristic of subjects consuming more fiber-rich whole plant foods [86]. A 2017 RCT (62 subjects with elevated waist size; ad libitum New Nordic

Diet high in fiber/wholegrain (43.3 g fiber) vs the Average Danish Diet (28.6 g fiber); approx. 65% women; mean age approx 45 years; 26 weeks duration) found individuals with a higher Prevotella spp. to Bacteroides spp. (P/B ratio) had effective body fat loss on a diet rich in fiber and whole grain compared to the body fat loss observed in individuals with a low P/B ratio [86]. Specifically, among individuals with high P/B the New Nordic Diet resulted in a significant 3.15 kg larger body fat loss compared to an average Danish diet. Among individuals with low P/B ratio the New Nordic Diet resulted in an insignificant 0.88 kg larger body fat loss compared to an average Danish diet. Individuals with high P/B ratio were more susceptible to lose body fat on diets high in fiber diet by 2.27 kg than subjects with a low P/B ratio. Potential mechanisms associated with the abundance of Prevotella could include: differences in fiber-utilization capacity and ratio of SCFAs produced, the secretion of gastrointestinal hormones affecting appetite, and post-prandial blood glucose and insulin responses [86]. Fiber directly or by its SCFA metabolites can modify some gut hormones that regulate satiety and energy intake, thus also affecting lipid metabolism and energy expenditure. Increased fiber intake may affect gut hormones such as ghrelin, glucagon-like peptide 1, peptide YY, and cholecystokinin. Dietary fiber is also known to affect adipose tissue expression and secretion of a variety of adipocytokines, including adiponectin, leptin, tumor necrosis factor-α, and interleukin-6, which can influence obesity, insulin resistance, and hyperlipidemia. SCFAs, especially butyrate and propionate, can act to promote a lean phenotype by: acting as ligands for free fatty acids receptors, which increases expression and secretion of satiety hormones glucagon-like-peptide 1 or peptide YY and leptin from adipocytes to reduce hunger and promote higher adiponectin and lower insulin resistance [89–92].

4.3.3 Type 2 Diabetes (Diabetes)

Diabetes, a consequence of elevated blood glucose and a deficit in the secretion and action of insulin, increases the risk for other chronic illnesses such as cardiovascular and renal disease, tuberculosis, and serious health complications such as retinopathy, neuropathy, shorter life expectancy, and causes higher medical costs [93, 94]. Growing evidence suggests that colonic microbiota may play a role in the pathogenesis of both type 1 and 2 diabetes [95–97]. Overweight and obesity are initiating factors for diabetes risk because of increased low grade inflammation, which reaches tissues involved in energy metabolism regulation, such as the liver, adipose tissue, and muscles and interferes with cellular insulin signals leading to insulin resistance. This low-grade inflammation and insulin resistance is known to be intimately linked to dysbiosis of the colonic microbiota [97]. Proteobacteria have been shown to be significantly higher in diabetic individuals compared to healthy persons and positively correlated with plasma glucose [98]. Two other studies also showed that diabetic subjects were characterized by a reduction in the number of Clostridiales bacteria (*Roseburia* species and *Faecalibacterium prausnitzii*), which produce butyrate [89, 99]. Adequate fiber intake may help to protect against the adverse effects of microbiota dysbiosis on insulin resistance associated with increased systemic inflammation related to colonic permeability of lipopolysaccharides (LPS) from gram-negative pathogenic bacteria, low incretin secretion and fecal butyrate production, and macrophage influx into visceral fat tissue, and activation of hepatic Kupffer macrophage cells [28–31, 89, 95]. Dietary fiber's effects on the microbiota plays a significant role in reducing colonic mucosa permeability and regulation of energy homeostasis, thereby reducing the risk of metabolic endotoxemia or persistent low-grade inflammatory response, insulin resistance associated with diabetes or metabolic syndrome [100]. Four RCTs provide insights for the actions of fiber-rich dietary patterns such as vegetarian diets [101, 102] and diets rich in resistant starch in promoting a healthy microbiota ecosystem and controlling diabetes risk [103, 104].

4.3.4 Metabolic Syndrome

Metabolic syndrome, which is associated with combinations of elevated blood pressure, dyslipidemia (defined by increased triglycerides and reduced high-density lipoprotein cholesterol), high fasting glucose and/or central obesity, occurs in 20–40% of the worldwide adult population [105]. The colonic microbiota can have a major influence on the pathogenesis of metabolic syndrome, which can increase the rate of unhealthy aging [106]. Prospective studies suggest that Western dietary patterns, rich in processed meats, snacks, baked desserts and sugar sweetened beverages are associated with higher metabolic syndrome risk, whereas healthy dietary patterns rich in vegetables, fruits, whole-grains, nuts and fish are associated with a reduced risk of metabolic syndrome [107]. Several RCTs suggest that a fiber-rich dietary pattern and healthy microbiota ecosystem can protect against metabolic syndrome [108–112]. For example, an Italian RCT (54 adults with metabolic syndrome; 31 females/23 males; mean age 58 years; mean BMI 31.5; whole-grain group with 29 g cereal fiber/day vs. control group with 12 g cereal fiber/day; 12 weeks) found that the whole-grain diet increased fasting plasma propionate, which correlated with lower postprandial insulin concentrations [108]. Another study suggests that the absorption of colonic propionate helps to prevent body weight gain and intra-abdominal fat accretion in overweight adults by stimulating release of the satiety gut hormones peptide YY and glucagon like peptide-1 [109]. Although the pathogenesis of the metabolic syndrome is complex and not fully understood, adherence to fiber-rich dietary patterns can help to reduce the risk of developing metabolic syndrome by promoting a healthy colonic microbiota, preventing central obesity, and promoting healthier systemic lipoprotein, inflammatory and blood pressure profiles and increasing insulin sensitivity [112].

4.3.5 Healthy Aging and Longevity

The adherence to healthy fiber-rich dietary patterns and/or prebiotic fiber supplementation supports a healthy microbiota, which can have a major effect on the body's age processes, to promote healthy aging and prevent premature death [113–118]. Healthy aging may be defined as the absence of chronic disease, lack of physical disability, good mental health, and good social engagement [117]. Adequate fiber intake is associated with a healthier microbiota diversity, including symbionts such as Prevotella, Lactobacillales, Christensenellaceae, Bifidobacteria groups and the butyrate-producing bacteria such as Roseburia spp., *F. prausnitzii*, and *Akkermansia muciniphila* [28–31, 115, 119]. This increased fiber intake provides the colon with the butyrate and lower pH needed to maintain a strong barrier to fight pathobionts and inflammaging; compared to a low fiber intake, which supports lower bacterial gene count diversity, fewer butyrate-producing bacteria, increased acetate- and propionate-producing Bacteroides-related bacteria, and optimal colonic pH levels. Several studies show that individuals with a low microbiota diversity are characterized by higher risk of weight gain or central adiposity, insulin resistance, dyslipidemia and inflammation when compared with high bacterial diversity individuals [78, 79]. Increased fiber intake from the regular diet has been shown to be directly associated with healthier microbiota profiles in comparison to lower fiber diets, regardless of a person's age [119]. A meta-analysis including 14 RCTs showed that an increase of 8 g/day of fiber compared with lower fiber control diets significantly reduced systemic C-reactive protein by 0.5 mg/L [120]. A 1999–2010 US National Health and Nutrition Examination Survey (NHANES) analysis observed that increasing levels of fiber intake were found to significantly reduce the risk of elevated CRP levels and to reduce the risk of metabolic syndrome and obesity, two microbiota related health conditions associated with accelerated inflammaging (Fig. 4.8) [121]. A cross-sectional analysis of the Nurses' Health Study (2284 women; mean age 59 years; mean BMI 26; 87% postmenopausal) showed fiber was positively associated with leukocyte telomere length with a significant increase in telomere length by 0.19 units between the extremes of fiber intake, after multivariate adjustment [122]. A Canadian cost -of-illness analysis estimated that each additional 1 g fiber/day resulted in an annual $3–51 million in savings in type 2 diabetes care and $5–92 million in cardiovascular disease care [123]. A meta-analysis (25 cohort studies; 1,752,848 midlife individuals; average 12.4 years of follow-up) suggests that fiber is inversely associated with mortality risk (Fig. 4.9) [124]. The large US National Institutes of Health (NIH)-AARP Diet and Health Study (567,169 men and women; mean age 62; mean BMI 27; 9-years follow-up; 20,126 deaths in men and 11,330 deaths in women) found that increased fiber intake by 15 g/day significantly reduced all-cause mortality rates by 22% in both men and women, and CVD mortality in men by 24% and women by 34% (multivariate adjusted) [125]. An EPIC prospective study (452,717 men and women; mean age 51 years; mean BMI 25.5; mean 12.7 years of follow-up) found an inverse association with total mortality and circulatory morality risk of 10% reduction per 10 g fiber increased intake [126]. Fiber-rich foods such as whole-grains, fruits, and vegetables have been consistently shown to reduce all-cause mortality risk [127, 128].

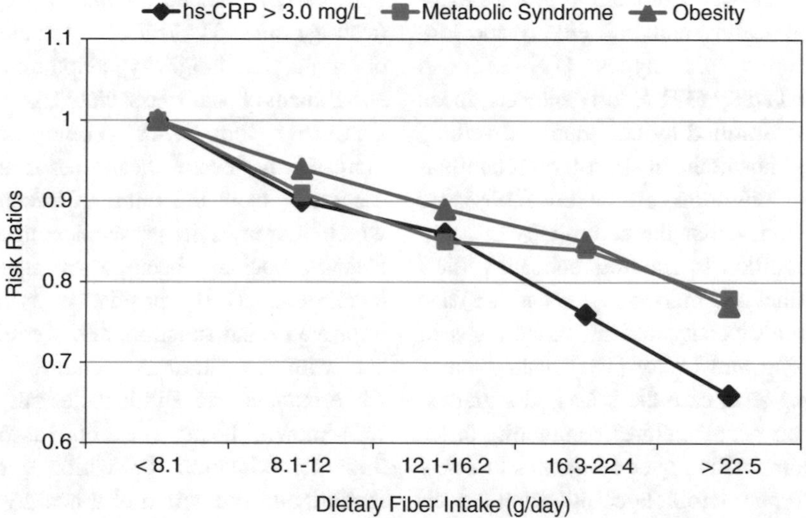

Fig. 4.8 Association between increasing fiber intake on risk of elevated hs-C-reactive protein (hs-CRP) levels and risk of metabolic syndrome and obesity from the 1999–2010 US National Health and Nutrition Examination Survey (p-trend <.001; multivariate adjusted) (adapted from [121])

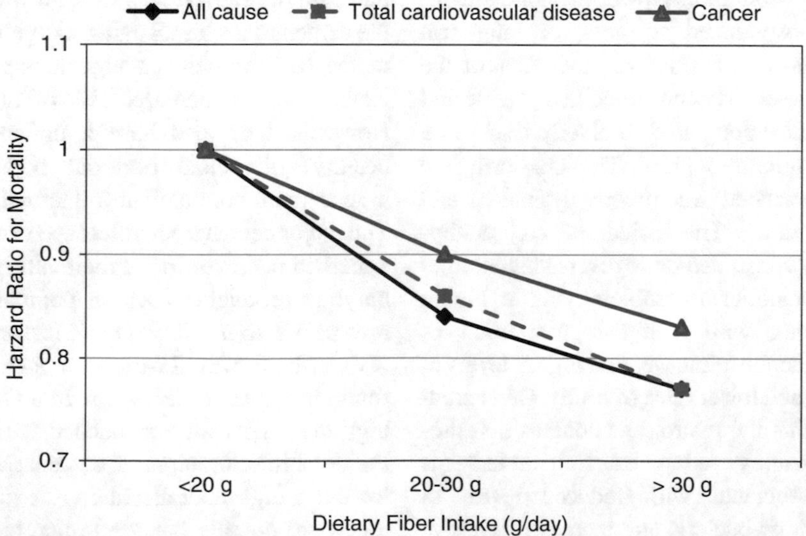

Fig. 4.9 Association between level of dietary fiber intake and all-cause, cardiovascular disease, and total cancer specific mortality risks based on a meta-analysis of 25 prospective cohort studies (adapted from [124])

4.4 Frailty and Longevity

In elderly adults, a fiber-rich dietary pattern, especially in long-stay care facilities, is important to reduce the risk of frailty by avoiding the adverse effects of standardized low fiber meals, which can subsequently reduce microbiota diversity and increase dysbiosis associated accelerated inflammaging related frailty [129, 130]. Table 4.2 summarizes the findings from nine cross-sectional studies on microbiota composition profiles associated with unhealthy and frail elderly and longevity/centenarian phenotypes [131–137]. A cross-sectional study (371 elderly subjects; mean age 78 years; stratified by community-dwelling, outpatient day hospitals, in short-term rehabilitation care or in long-term care facilities) observed that elderly from either the community or long-term care facilities consuming unhealthy diets (e.g., low in fiber and high in sugars and fats) had low microbiota diversity and increased signs of biological aging and frailty [131]. Additionally, elderly in long-term care facilities had a gradual change in their core healthier community-based microbiota composition over 18 months to a new core elderly type microbiota composition associated with colonic microbiota dysbiosis and frailty (in part due to lower fiber standardized diets). In another cross-sectional study (178 elderly adults; mean age 78 years; stratified by their current living situation: community-dwelling, outpatients, short-term hospitalized subjects, or long-term care residents) it was observed that 83% of the long-term care elderly consumed less diverse and lower fiber diets compared to elderly living in a residential community [129]. The long-term care elderly experienced microbiota dysbiosis, and accelerated frailty. The residential community-living elderly consumed more diverse/higher fiber diets, had healthier microbiota with a higher diversity index with a higher proportion of Firmicutes/Lachnospiraceae, and higher levels of fecal SCFAs and lower rates of frailty. Other studies indicate that the microbiota composition profile of unhealthy aging or frail elderly is generally associated with reduced levels of healthy probiotic bacteria and increased levels of pathogenic bacteria; such as marked reductions in lactobacilli, Bacteroides-Prevotella or *F. prausnitzii*, increases in Enterobacteriaceae and a major shift from Firmicutes to Bacteroidetes phyla [130, 135–137].

The centenarian phenotype has a unique and complex microbiota composition, which counterbalances inflammaging processes and is necessary to establish a microbiota ecosystem for exceptionally healthy longevity. A cross-sectional study (24 semi-supercentenarians, average age 106 years, 18 females, 6 males); 15 young adults (average age 31 years, 8 females, 7 males) observed that longevity adaptation involves an enrichment of health-associated microbiota [132]. Extremely long-living people experience an increase in several health-associated bacteria, especially from the family Christensenellaceae, which increases in prevalence in centenarians. Health-associated bacteria are inversely correlated with BMI, positively associated with improved renal function, and significantly interact with the human genome. Additionally, Akkermansia and Bifidobacterium, which have well-known health benefits associated with immunomodulation, protection against inflammation, and promotion of a healthy metabolism, are increased in centenarian's microbiota. An Italian cross-sectional study observed that centenarians had a unique microbiota species pattern that significantly differed from the typical adult-like pattern [134]. In this study, it was shown that the centenarians, as all aging individuals, have an increased microbiota pathogenic population associated with an increased risk of inflammaging. However, they also have a uniquely effective healthy microbiota bacterial population with higher than normal anti-inflammatory activity. The major centenarian difference was found to be a marked restructuring of their anti-inflammatory butyrate producing bacteria population from *F. prauznitzii* to *E. limosum* (Clostridium cluster XV), which was 15-times higher than levels found in typical older adults. In a Chinese study, high-fiber diets were associated with changes in the colonic microbiota of centenarians, suggesting that a high-fiber diet has a role in establishing a new structurally balanced microbiota that may benefit the health of centenarians [133].

Table 4.2 Summary of cross-sectional studies on microbiota composition and frailty in elderly individuals

Reference/Objective	Cohort/Method	Results
Jeffery et al. (2016). Identify dietary intervention and bacteriotherapy strategies for promoting health in older people (Ireland) [131].	371 elderly subjects; mean age 78 years; ranging from 64 to 102 years; community-dwelling, attending outpatient day hospitals, in short-term rehabilitation care (< 6 weeks) or in long-term care facilities.	Elderly from either the community or long-term care facilities consuming unhealthy diets (e.g., low in fiber and high in sugars and fats) had low microbiota diversity and increased signs of biological aging and frailty. Elderly in long-term care facilities had a gradual change in their core community-based microbiota composition over approximately18 months to a new core elderly type microbiota composition associated with dysbiosis and frailty. Elderly living in the community had more antibiotic associated microbiota loss but also more recovery following antibiotic treatment than long-term care elderly.
Biagi et al. (2016). Assess the microbiota associated with extreme longevity (Italy) [132].	24 supercentenarians (average age 106 years,18 females, 6 males); 15 young adults (average age 31 years, 8 females, 7 males).	Longevity adaptation appears to involve enriched health-associated microbiota. Extremely long-living people experience a parallel increase in several health-associated bacteria especially from the family Christensenellaceae, which is increased in terms of both relative abundance and prevalence in centenarians as health-associated bacteria inversely correlated with BMI, positively associated with improved renal function and with significant human genome interaction. A characteristic of centenarian's microbiota are increased levels of Akkermansia and Bifidobacterium, which have well-known health benefits associated with immunomodulation, protection against inflammation, and promotion of healthy metabolic homeostasis.
Wang et al. (2015). Examine the factors associated with the microbiota composition of centenarians (China) [133].	24 subjects, 8 aged 100–108 years, 8 aged rural elderly 85–99 years, and 8 urban elderlies, aged 80–92 years.	This study suggests that high-fiber diets can establish a new structurally balanced colonic microbiota architecture that may benefit the health of centenarians. The abundance of Bacteroidales and Lachnospiraceae was lower, but Ruminococcaceae was higher with high-fiber diet intake.
Claesson et al. (2012). Assess the relationship between diet, microbiota and health status in elderly subjects (Ireland) [129].	178 elderly adults; mean age 78 years; stratified by their current living situation: community-dwelling, outpatients, short-term hospitalized subjects and long-term care residents, community-dwelling elderly showed significantly healthier microbiota composition than long-term care residents; 98% of community and day hospital subjects consumed low fat/high fiber diets and 83% long-stay subjects consumed high fat/low fiber diets.	Elderly in long-term care facilities had significantly higher frailty test scores compared to elderly living in a residential community. The long-term care elderly consumed less diverse/lower fiber diets, had microbiota dysbiosis (higher proportion of Bacteroidetes and lower fecal SCFAs), and accelerated frailty. The residential community-living elderly consumed more diversity/higher fiber diets, had healthier microbiota (higher diversity index with a higher proportion of Firmicutes/Lachnospiraceae, and high levels of fecal SCFAs) and lower rates of frailty.

(continued)

Table 4.2 (continued)

Reference/Objective	Cohort/Method	Results
Claesson et al. (2011). Examine the composition, variability, and temporal stability of the colonic microbiota of the elderly (Ireland) [130].	161 subjects aged ≥65 years, approx. equal females and males; 9 healthy younger control subjects, 5 female/4 males, with ages between 28 and 46 years.	The microbiota of each individual constituted a unique profile that was separable from all others. In 68% of the elderly individuals, the microbiota was dominated by phylum Bacteroides. The proportions of some phyla and genera associated with disease or health also varied dramatically, including Proteobacteria, Actinobacteria, and Faecalibacteria. The core microbiota of elderly subjects was distinct from that previously established for younger adults, with a greater proportion of Bacteroides spp. and distinct abundance patterns of pathobiontic Clostridium groups.
Biagi et al. (2010) Determine differences in the microbiota of adults with increasing age (Italy) [134].	84 subjects belonging to different age groups; 21 centenarians (20 women, 1 man; average 101 years); 22 elderlies (11 women, 11 men; average 73 years; genetically unrelated to the centenarians); 21 elderly people (10 women, 11 men; average 68 years; offspring of the centenarians); 20 young adults (9 women, 11 men; average 31 years).	Young (30 years old) and older adults (70 years old) had very similar overall colonic microbiota composition, dominated by Bacteroidetes and Firmicutes (95% of the microbiota), and smaller fractions of Actinobacteria, and Proteobacteria. Although centenarians' microbiota was dominated by Bacteroidetes and Firmicutes (93% of microbiota), the specific microbiota species pattern significantly differed from the typical adult-like pattern. Some of the key differences from typical adults are: lower diversity in terms of species composition, a rearrangement in the Firmicutes population, an enrichment in facultative anaerobes, notably pathobionts associated with increased systemic inflammatory markers (inflammaging), marked decrease in the anti-inflammatory F. prauznitzii and different types of butyrate producers such as E. limosum (Clostridium cluster XV), which is approximately 15-fold higher, which may be a primary anti-inflammatory longevity bacteria. Centenarians have a unique and complex microbiota composition which counterbalances inflammaging processes and is necessary to establish a microbiota ecosystem for exceptional healthy longevity.
Mariat et al. (2009). Evaluate changes in human microbiota Firmicutes and Bacteroidetes ratio with aging (France) [135].	21 adults (25–45 years old); 21 infants (3 weeks to 10 months old); 20 elderly subjects (70–90 years old).	The ratio of Firmicutes to Bacteroidetes evolves during different life stages with mean ratios for infants, adults and elderly being 0.4, 11 and 0.6, respectively. Elderly subjects exhibited higher levels of E. coli and Bacteroidetes.
Van Tongeren et al. (2005). Examine the relationship between fecal microbiota composition and frailty in the elderly (The Netherlands) [136].	23 elderly subjects; median age 86 years; 83% females; living in the same long-term care center and receiving the same diet; 2 groups low frailty vs. high frailty score; no antibiotics for 4 weeks.	Fecal samples from elderly with high frailty scores showed a significant reduction in the number of lactobacilli by 26-fold, Bacteroides/ Prevotella by 3-fold and the Faecalibacterium prausnitzii by4-fold whereas the number of Enterobacteriaceae pathogenic bacteria was significantly higher by 7-fold.

Table 4.2 (continued)

Reference/Objective	Cohort/Method	Results
Bartosch et al. (2004). Characterize bacterial communities in feces from healthy elderly volunteers and hospitalized elderly patients (UK) [137].	35 healthy elderly subjects (mean age 71 years; all females; living in the local community); 38 elderly hospitalized patients (mean age 81 years; 60% males); 21 elderly hospitalized patients receiving antibiotic treatment (mean age 81 years; 79% males).	The primary difference between healthy community living elderly and both patient cohorts was a marked reduction in the Bacteroides-Prevotella group following hospitalization. Reductions in bifidobacteria, Desulfovibrio spp., Clostridium clostridiiforme, and Faecalibacterium prausnitzii were also found in the hospitalized patients. Antibiotic treatment resulted in further reductions in the numbers of bacteria and their prevalence with complete elimination of certain bacterial communities in some patients. Enterobacteria counts increased in the hospitalized patients who did not receive antibiotics and Enterococcus faecalis proliferated in antibiotic treated patients. Total bacteria counts were lower in the stool samples of the two groups of hospitalized patients compared to the community living elderly.

Conclusions

The colonic microbiota provides a number of important human biological functions including aiding in nutrient absorption, synthesis of vitamins, fermentation of fiber to SCFAs, and promoting barriers against pathogenic bacteria, secondary bile acid transformation, and inflammation. The colonic microbiota also defends against colonic tumor initiation and progression, and promotes cardiometabolic health (e.g., increased insulin sensitivity and satiety hormones, and lower cardiometabolic risk factors). Over the course of human evolution, a symbiotic relationship was formed between fiber-rich diets, the colonic microbiota and human health homeostasis. However, the emergence of the Western low fiber diet as a dominant global dietary pattern has disrupted this symbiotic relationship leading to an increased population risk for unhealthy aging, chronic diseases and premature death. Fiber, a critical dietary factor in the maintenance of a healthy microbiota ecosystem, has emerged in recent decades for its importance in promoting colonic health, healthy aging, and reducing the risk of cardiometabolic chronic disease and premature death. Fiber is the primary dietary energy source of the microbiota bacteria and the breakdown products of the resulting fiber fermentation include short chain fatty acids such as butyrate which is the main energy source needed for healthy colonocytes and optimization of colonic barrier defenses. Daily adequate fiber intake supports colonic microbiota health by increasing probiotic and decreasing pathogenic bacteria, lowering risk of endotoxemia and reducing colonic pH and bowel transit time, and contributing to greater stool bulk to dilute potential toxic or carcinogenic compounds or metabolites. Fiber-rich healthy dietary patterns supports colonic microbiota health and their action in protecting the colon from infections such as *C difficile*, inflammatory bowel disease and colorectal cancer; slowing the aging process by decreasing the risk of weight gain and obesity, type 2 diabetes, and metabolic syndrome; and reducing the risk of frailty and premature death. In the elderly, high-fiber diets play an important role in establishing a healthy colonic microbiota associated with lower risk of frailty and longer life expectancy due in part to higher butyrate production and lower risk of inflammaging.

Appendix A

Comparison of Western and Healthy Dietary Patterns per 2000 kcal (Approximated Values)

Components	Western dietary pattern (US)	USDA base pattern	DASH diet pattern	Healthy Mediterranean pattern	Healthy vegetarian pattern (Lact-ovo based)	Vegan pattern
Emphasizes	Refined grains, low fiber foods, red meats sweets, and solid fats	Vegetables, fruit, whole-grain, and low-fat milk	Potassium rich vegetables, fruits, and low-fat milk products	Whole grains, vegetables, fruit, dairy products, olive oil, and moderate wine	Vegetables, fruit, whole-grains, legumes, nuts, seeds, milk products, and soy foods	Plant foods: vegetables, fruits, whole grains, nuts, seeds, and soy foods
Includes	Processed meats, sugar sweetened beverages, and fast foods	Enriched grains, lean meat, fish, nuts, seeds, and vegetable oils	Whole-grain, poultry, fish, nuts, and seeds	Fish, nuts, seeds, and pulses	Eggs, non-dairy milk alternatives, and vegetable oils	Non-dairy milk alternatives
Limits	Fruits and vegetables, whole-grains	Solid fats and added sugars	Red meats, sweets, and sugar-sweetened beverages	Red meats, refined grains, and sweets	No red or white meats, or fish; limited sweets	No animal products
Estimated Nutrients/Components						
Carbohydrates (% Total kcal)	51	51	55	50	54	57
Protein (% Total kcal)	16	17	18	16	14	13
Total fat (% Total kcal)	33	32	27	34	32	30
Saturated fat (% Total kcal)	11	8	6	8	8	7
Unsat. fat (% Total kcal)	22	25	21	24	26	25
Fiber (g)	16	31	29+	31	35+	40+
Potassium (mg)	2800	3350	4400	3350	3300	3650
Vegetable oils (g)	19	27	25	27	19–27	18–27
Sodium (mg)	3600	1790	1100	1690	1400	1225
Added sugar (g)	79 (20 tsp.)	32 (8 tsp.)	12 (3 tsp.)	32 (8 tsp.)	32 (8 tsp.)	32 (8 tsp.)
Plant Food Groups						
Fruit (cup)	≤1.0	2.0	2.5	2.5	2.0	2.0
Vegetables (cup)	≤1.5	2.5	2.1	2.5	2.5	2.5
Whole-grains (oz.)	0.6	3.0	4.0	3.0	3.0	3.0
Legumes (oz.)	–	1.5	0.5	1.5	3.0	3.0+
Nuts/Seeds (oz.)	0.5	0.6	1.0	0.6	1.0	2.0
Soy products (oz.)	0.0	0.5	–	–	1.1	1.5

U.S. Department of Agriculture, Agriculture Research Service, Nutrient Data Laboratory. 2014. USDA National Nutrient Database for Standard Reference, Release 27. https://www.ars.usda.gov/nutrientdata. Accessed 17 February 2015.

Dietary Guidelines Advisory Committee. Scientific Report. Advisory Report to the Secretary of Health and Human Services and the Secretary of Agriculture. Appendix E-3.7: Developing vegetarian and Mediterranean-style food patterns. 2015;1–9.

U.S. Department of Agriculture and U.S. Department of Health and Human Services. Dietary Guidelines for Americans, 2010. 7th Edition, Washington, DC: U.S. Government Printing Office. 2010; Table B2.4; http://www.choosemyplate.gov/ Accessed 8.22.2015.

Appendix B

Fifty High Fiber Whole or Minimally Processed Plant Foods Ranked by Amount of Fiber per Standard Food Portion Size

Food	Standard portion size	Dietary fiber (g)	Calories (kcal)	Energy density (calories/g)
High fiber bran ready-to-eat-cereal	1/3–3/4 cup (30 g)	9.1–14.3	60–80	2.0–2.6
Navy beans, cooked	1/2 cup cooked (90 g)	9.6	127	1.4
Small white beans, cooked	1/2 cup (90 g)	9.3	127	1.4
Shredded wheat ready-to-eat cereal	1–1 1/4 cup (50–60 g)	5.0–9.0	155–220	3.2–3.7
Black bean soup, canned	1/2 cup (130 g)	8.8	117	0.9
French beans, cooked	1/2 cup (90 g)	8.3	114	1.3
Split peas, cooked	1/2 cup (100 g)	8.2	114	1.1
Chickpeas (Garbanzo) beans, canned	1/2 cup (120 g)	8.1	176	1.4
Lentils, cooked	1/2 cup (100 g)	7.8	115	1.2
Pinto beans, cooked	1/2 cup (90 g)	7.7	122	1.4
Black beans, cooked	1/2 cup (90 g)	7.5	114	1.3
Artichoke, global or French, cooked	1/2 cup (84 g)	7.2	45	0.5
Lima beans, cooked	1/2 cup (90 g)	6.6	108	1.2
White beans, canned	1/2 cup (130 g)	6.3	149	1.1
Wheat bran flakes ready-to-eat cereal	3/4 cup (30 g)	4.9–5.5	90–98	3.0–3.3
Pear with skin	1 medium (180 g)	5.5	100	0.6
Pumpkin seeds. Whole, roasted	1 ounce (about 28 g)	5.3	126	4.5
Baked beans, canned, plain	1/2 cup (125 g)	5.2	120	0.9
Soybeans, cooked	1/2 cup (90 g)	5.2	150	1.7
Plain rye wafer crackers	2 wafers (22 g)	5.0	73	3.3
Avocado, Hass	1/2 fruit (68 g)	4.6	114	1.7
Apple, with skin	1 medium (180 g)	4.4	95	0.5
Green peas, cooked (fresh, frozen, canned)	1/2 cup (80 g)	3.5–4.4	59–67	0.7–0.8
Refried beans, canned	1/2 cup (120 g)	4.4	107	0.9
Mixed vegetables, cooked from frozen	1/2 cup (45 g)	4.0	59	1.3
Raspberries	1/2 cup (65 g)	3.8	32	0.5
Blackberries	1/2 cup (65 g)	3.8	31	0.4
Collards, cooked	1/2 cup (95 g)	3.8	32	0.3
Soybeans, green, cooked	1/2 cup (75 g)	3.8	127	1.4
Prunes, pitted, stewed	1/2 cup (125 g)	3.8	133	1.1
Sweet potato, baked	1 medium (114 g)	3.8	103	0.9
Multi-grain bread	2 slices regular (52 g)	3.8	140	2.7
Figs, dried	1/4 cup (about 38 g)	3.7	93	2.5
Potato baked, with skin	1 medium (173 g)	3.6	163	0.9
Popcorn, air-popped	3 cups (24 g)	3.5	93	3.9
Almonds	1 ounce (about 28 g)	3.5	164	5.8
Whole wheat spaghetti, cooked	1/2 cup (70 g)	3.2	87	1.2
Sunflower seed kernels, dry roasted	1 ounce (about 28 g)	3.1	165	5.8
Orange	1 medium (130 g)	3.1	69	0.5
Banana	1 medium (118 g)	3.1	105	0.9
Oat bran muffin	1 small (66 g)	3.0	178	2.7
Vegetable soup	1 cup (245 g)	2.9	91	0.4

Food	Standard portion size	Dietary fiber (g)	Calories (kcal)	Energy density (calories/g)
Dates	1/4 cup (about 38 g)	2.9	104	2.8
Pistachios, dry roasted	1 ounce (about 28 g)	2.8	161	5.7
Hazelnuts or filberts	1 ounce (about 28 g)	2.7	178	6.3
Peanuts, oil roasted	1 ounce (about 28 g)	2.7	170	6.0
Quinoa, cooked	1/2 cup (90 g)	2.7	92	1.0
Broccoli, cooked	1/2 cup (78 g)	2.6	27	0.3
Potato baked, without skin	1 medium (145 g)	2.3	145	1.0
Baby spinach leaves	3 ounces (90 g)	2.1	20	0.2
Blueberries	1/2 cup (74 g)	1.8	42	0.6
Carrot, raw or cooked	1 medium (60 g)	1.7	25	0.4

Dahl WJ, Stewart ML. Position of the Academy of Nutrition and Dietetics: health implications of dietary fiber. J Acad Nutr Diet. 2015;115:1861–1870.

Dietary Guidelines Advisory Committee. Scientific Report. Advisory Report to the Secretary of Health and Human Services and the Secretary of Agriculture. Part D. Chapter 1: Food and nutrient intakes, and health: current status and trends. 2015;97, 98; Table D1.8.

Slavin, J.L. Position of the American Dietetic Association: Health implications of dietary fiber. J. Am. Diet. Assoc. 2008;108:1716–1731.

U.S. Department of Agriculture and U.S. Department of Health and Human Services. Dietary Guidelines for Americans, 2010. 7th Edition, Washington, DC: U.S. Government Printing Office. 2010; Table B2.4; http://www.choosemyplate.gov/ Accessed 8.22.2015.

References

1. Arora T, Backhed F. The gut microbiota and metabolic disease: current understanding and future perspectives. J Intern Med. 2016;280(4):339–49. https://doi.org/10.1111/joim.12508.
2. Keenan MJ, Marco ML, Ingram DK, Martin RJ. Improving healthspan via changes in gut microbiota and fermentation. Age (Dordr). 2015;37(5):98. https://doi.org/10.1007/s11357-015-9817-6.
3. El Enshasy H, Malik K, Malek RA, et al. Anaerobic probiotics: the key microbes for human health. Adv Biochem Eng Biotechnol. 2016;156:397–431. https://doi.org/10.1007/10-2015-5008.
4. Oozeer R, van Limpt K, Ludwig T, et al. Intestinal microbiology in early life: specific prebiotics can have similar functionalities as human-milk oligosaccharides. Am J Clin Nutr. 2013;98(suppl):561S–71S.
5. Nicholson JK, Holmes E, Kinross J, et al. Host-gut microbiota metabolic interactions. Science. 2012;336:1262–7.
6. Koh A, De Vadder F, Kovatcheva-Datchary P, Backhed F. From dietary fiber to host physiology: short-chain fatty acids as key bacterial metabolites. Cell. 2016;165:1332–45.
7. Jia W, Li H, Zhao L, Nicholson JK. Gut microbiota: a potential new territory for drug targeting. Nat Rev Drug Disord. 2008;7(2):123–9.
8. Mazidi M, Rezaie P, Kengne AP, et al. Gut microbiome and metabolic syndrome. Diabetes Metab Syndr. 2016;10(2 Suppl 1):S150–7. https://doi.org/10.1016/j.dsx.2016.01.024.
9. Sonnenburg ED, Sonnenburg JL. Starving our microbial self: the deleterious consequences of a diet deficient in microbiota-accessible carbohydrates. Cell Metab. 2014;20:779–86.
10. Sonnenburg ED, Smits SA, Tikhonov M, et al. Diet-induced extinctions in the gut microbiota compound over generations. Nature. 2016;529(7585):212–5.
11. Zhang C, Zhang M, Wang S, et al. Interactions between gut microbiota, host genetics and diet relevant to development of metabolic syndromes in mice. ISME J. 2010;4:232–41.
12. Ley RE, Turnbaugh P, Klein S, Gordon JI. Microbial ecology: human gut microbes associated with obesity. Nature. 2006;444:1022–3.
13. Woodmansey EJ. Intestinal bacteria and ageing. J Appl Microbiol. 2007;102:1178–86.
14. Tuohy KM, Fava F, Viola R. The way to a man's heart is through his gut microbiota'—dietary pro- and prebiotics for the management of cardiovascular risk. Proc Nutr Soc. 2014;73:172–85.
15. Albenberg LG, Wu GD. Diet and the intestinal microbiome: associations, functions, and implications for health and disease. Gastroenterology. 2014;146(6):1564–72.
16. Logan AC, Jacka FN, Prescott SL. Immune–microbiota interactions: dysbiosis as a global health issue. Curr Allergy Asthma Rep. 2016;16:13. https://doi.org/10.1007/s11882-015-0590-5.
17. Zeng H, Lazarova DL, Bordonaro M. Mechanisms linking dietary fiber, gut microbiota and colon cancer prevention. World J Gastrointest Oncol. 2014;6(2):41–51.

18. Hamer HM, Jonkers D, Venema K, et al. Review article: the role of butyrate on colonic function. Aliment Pharmacol Ther. 2008;27:104–19.
19. Meijer K, de Vos P, Priebe MG. Butyrate and other short-chain fatty acids as modulators of immunity: What relevance for health? Curr Opin Clin Nutr Metab Care. 2010;13(6):715–21.
20. Titgemeyer EC, Bourquin LD, Fahey GC, Garleb KA. Fermentability of various fiber sources by human fecal bacteria in vitro. Am J Clin Nutr. 1991;53:1418–24.
21. Shin NR, Whon TW, Bae JW. Proteobacteria: microbial signature of dysbiosis in gut microbiota. Trends Biotechnol. 2015;33(9):496–503.
22. Marchesi JR, Adams DH, Fava F, et al. The gut microbiota and host health: a new clinical frontier. Gut. 2015;65(2):330–9.
23. Deehan C, Walter J. The fiber gap and the disappearing gut microbiome: implications for human nutrition. Trends Endocrinol Metab. 2016;27(5):239–41.
24. Blaser MJ, Falkow S. What are the consequences of the disappearing human microbiota? Nat Rev Microbiol. 2009;7:887–94.
25. Jew S, Abumweis SS, Jones PJ. Evolution of the human diet: linking our ancestral diet to modern functional foods as a means of chronic disease prevention. J Med Food. 2009;12(5):925–34.
26. Dominianni C, Sinha R, Goedert JJ, et al. Sex, body mass index, and dietary fiber intake influence the human gut microbiome. PLoS One. 2015;10(4):e0124599. https://doi.org/10.1371/journal.pone.0124599.
27. IOM (Institute of Medicine). Dietary reference intakes for energy, carbohydrate, fiber, fat, fatty acids, cholesterol, protein, and amino acids. 2002/2005. National Academies Press, Washington DC.
28. Milani C, Ferrario C, Turron F, et al. The human gut microbiota and its interactive connections to diet. J Hum Nutr Diet. 2016;29(5):539–46. https://doi.org/10.1111/jhn.12371.
29. Parekh PJ, Balart LA, Johnson DA. The influence of the gut microbiome on obesity, metabolic syndrome and gastrointestinal disease. Clin Transl Gastroenterol. 2015;6:e91. https://doi.org/10.1038/ctg.2015.16.
30. Furusawa Y, Obata Y, Fukuda S, et al. Commensal microbe derived butyrate induces the differentiation of colonic regulatory T cells. Nature. 2013;504:446–50.
31. Conlon MA, Bird AR. The impact of diet and lifestyle on gut microbiota and human health. Forum Nutr. 2015;7:17–44.
32. Cummings JH, Englyst HN. Fermentation in the human large intestine and the available substrates. Am J Clin Nutr. 1987;45(5 suppl):1243–55.
33. Mehta RS, Nishihara R, Cao Y, et al. Association of dietary patterns with risk of colorectal cancer subtypes classified by Fusobacterium nucleatum in tumor tissue. JAMA Oncol. 2017. https://doi.org/10.1001/jamaoncol.2016.6374.
34. Racine A, Carbonnel F, Chan SS, et al. Dietary patterns and risk of inflammatory bowel disease in Europe: results from the EPIC study. Inflamm Bowel Dis. 2016;2292:345–54. https://doi.org/10.1097/MIB.0000000000000638.
35. Gutiérrez-Díaz I, Fernández-Navarro T, Sánchez B, et al. Mediterranean diet and faecal microbiota: a transversal study. Food Funct. 2016;;7(5):2347-56. https://doi.org/10.1039/c6fo00105j.
36. GD W, Compher C, Chen EZ, et al. Comparative metabolomics in vegans and omnivores reveal constraints on diet-dependent gut microbiota metabolite production. Gut. 2016;65(1):63–72.
37. De Filippis F, Pellegrini N, Vannini L, et al. High-level adherence to a Mediterranean diet beneficially impacts the gut microbiota and associated metabolome. Gut. 2015;65(11):1812–21. https://doi.org/10.1136/gutjnl-2015-309957.
38. Matijasic BB, Obermajer T, Lipoglavsek L, et al. Association of dietary type with fecal microbiota in vegetarians and omnivores in Slovenia. Eur J Nutr. 2014;53(4):1051–64.
39. Ou J, Carbonero F, Zoetendal EG, et al. Diet, microbiota, and microbial metabolites in colon cancer risk in rural Africans and African Americans. Am J Clin Nutr. 2013;98:111–20.
40. Zimmer J, Lange B, Frick J-S, et al. A vegan or vegetarian diet substantially alters the human colonic faecal microbiota. Eur J Clin Nutr. 2012;66(1):53–60.
41. Kabeerdoss J, Devi RS, Mary RR, et al. Faecal microbiota composition in vegetarians: comparison with omnivores in a cohort of young women in southern India. Br J Nutr. 2012;108:9544.
42. GD W, Chen J, Hoffmann C, et al. Linking long-term dietary patterns with gut microbial enterotypes. Science. 2011;334(6052):105–8. https://doi.org/10.1126/science.1208344.3-957.
43. Tap J, Furet JP, Bensaada M, et al. Gut microbiota richness promotes its stability upon increased dietary fibre intake in healthy adults. Environ Microbiol. 2015;17(12):4954–64.
44. O'Keefe JD, Li JV, Lahti L, et al. Fat, fiber and cancer risk in African Americans and rural Africans. Nat Commun. 2015;6:6342. https://doi.org/10.1038/ncomms7342.
45. David LA, Maurice CF, Carmody RN, et al. Diet rapidly and reproducibly alters the human gut microbiome. Nature. 2014;505:559–63.
46. Klinder A, Shen Q, Heppel S, et al. Impact of increasing fruit and vegetables and flavonoid intake on the human gut microbiota. Food Funct. 2016;7:1788–96.
47. Heinritz SN, Weiss E, Eklund M, et al. Intestinal microbiota and microbial metabolites are changed in a pig model fed a high-fat/low-fiber or a low-fat/high-fiber diet. PLoS One. 2016;11(4):e0154329. https://doi.org/10.1371/journal.pone.0154329.

48. Wang Y, Ames NP, Tun HM, et al. High molecular weight barley β-glucan alters gut microbiota toward reduced cardiovascular disease risk. Front Microbiol. 2016;7:129. https://doi.org/10.3389/fmicb.2016.00129.
49. Martinez I, Lattimer JM, Hubach KL, et al. Gut microbiome composition is linked to whole grain-induced immunological improvements. The. ISME J. 2013;7:269–80.
50. Carvalho-Wells AL, Helmolz K, Nodet C, et al. Determination of the in vivo prebiotic potential of a maize-based whole grain breakfast cereal: a human feeding study. Br J Nutr. 2010;104:1353–6.
51. Costabile A, Klinder A, Fava F, et al. Whole-grain wheat breakfast cereal has a prebiotic effect on the human gut microbiota: a double-blind, placebo-controlled, crossover study. Br J Nutr. 2008;99:110–20.
52. Reveles KR, Lee GC, Boyd NK, Frei CR. The rise in Clostridium difficile infection incidence among hospitalized adults in the United States: 2001-2010. Am J Infect Control. 2014;42:1028–32.
53. Van den Abbeele P, Verstraete W, Aidy SE, et al. Prebiotics, faecal transplants and microbial network units to stimulate biodiversity of the human gut microbiome. J Microbial Biotechnol. 2013;6(4):335–40. https://doi.org/10.1111/1751-7915.12049.
54. Zhang I, Dong D, Jiang C, et al. Insight into alteration of gut microbiota in Clostridium difficile infection and asymptomatic C. difficile colonization. Anaerobe. 2015;34:1–7. https://doi.org/10.1016/j.anaerobe.2015.03.008.
55. May T, Mackie RI, Fahey GC, et al. Effect of fiber source on short-chain fatty acid production and on the growth and toxin production by Clostridium difficile. Scand J Gastroenterol. 1994;29(10):916–22.
56. Forssten SD, Roytio H, Ashley A, et al. The effect of polydextrose and probiotic lactobacilli in a Clostridium difficile infected human colonic model. Microb Ecol Health Dis. 2015;26:27988. https://doi.org/10.3402/mehd.v26.27988.
57. Johnson LP, Walton GE, Psichas A, et al. Prebiotics modulate the effects of antibiotics on gut microbial diversity and functioning *in vitro*. Forum Nutr. 2015;7:4480–97.
58. Aleksandrova K, Romero-Mosquera B, Hernandez V. Diet, gut microbiome and epigenetics: emerging links with inflammatory bowel diseases and prospects for management and prevention, Nutrients. 2017;9:962.
59. Liu X, Wu Y, Li F, Zhang D. Dietary fiber intake reduces risk of inflammatory bowel disease: result from a meta-analysis. Nutr Res. 2016;2292:345–54; doi: 20.1097/MIB0000000000000638.
60. Burkitt DP. Possible relationships between bowel cancer and dietary habits. Proc R Soc Med. 1971;64:964–5.
61. Bultman SJ. The microbiome and its potential as a cancer preventive intervention. Semin Oncol. 2016;43(1):97–106. https://doi.org/10.1053/j.seminoncol.2015.09.001.
62. Bultman SJ. Interplay between diet, gut microbiota, epigenetic events, and colorectal cancer. Mol Nutr Food Res. 2017; 61(1); doi: 10.1002/mnfr.201500902.
63. Aune D, Chan DSM, Lau R, et al. Dietary fibre, whole grains, and risk of colorectal cancer: systematic review and dose-response meta-analysis of prospective studies. BMJ. 2011;343:d6617. https://doi.org/10.1136/bmj.d6617.
64. World Cancer Research Fund, American Institute of Cancer Research. Continuous Update Project. Colorectal Cancer 2011 Report. Food, Nutrition, Physical Activity, and the Prevention of Colorectal Cancer. London; 2011.
65. Kunzmann AT, Coleman HG, Huang W-Y, et al. Dietary fiber intake and risk of colorectal cancer and incident and recurrent adenoma in the Prostate, Lung, Colorectal, and Ovarian Cancer Screening Trial. Am J Clin Nutr. 2015;102:881–90.
66. Chen HM, Y-N Y, Wang J-L, et al. Decreased dietary fiber intake and structural alteration of gut microbiota in patients with advanced colorectal adenoma. Am J Clin Nutr. 2013;97:1044–52.
67. Miller WC, Niederpruem MG, Wallace JP, Lindeman AK. Dietary fat, sugar, and fiber predict body fat content. J Am Diet Assoc. 1994;94:612–5.
68. Epstein LH, Gordy CC, Raynor HA, et al. Increasing fruit and vegetable intake and decreasing fat and sugar intake in families at risk for childhood obesity. Obes Res. 2001;9:171–8.
69. Epstein LH, Paluch RA, Beecher MD, Roemmich JN. Increasing healthy eating vs. reducing high energy-dense foods to treat pediatric obesity. Obesity (Silver Spring). 2008;16(2):318–26.
70. Davis JN, Hodges VA, Gillham B. Normal-weight adults consume more fiber and fruit than their age- and height-matched overweight/obese counterparts. J Am Diet Assoc. 2006;106:833–40.
71. Davis JN, Alexander KE, Ventura EE, et al. Inverse relation between dietary fiber intake and visceral adiposity in overweight Latino youth. Am J Clin Nutr. 2009;90:1160–6.
72. Center for Disease Control and Prevention (CDC). Eat more weigh less? How to manage your weight without being hungry. http://www.cdc.gov/nccdphp/dnpa/nutrition/pdf/Energy_Density.pdf. Accessed May 21, 2016.
73. Savage JS, Marini M, Birch LL. Dietary energy density predicts women's weight change over 6 years. Am J Clin Nutr. 2008;88(3):677–84.
74. Bertoia ML, Mukamal KJ, Cahill LE, et al. Changes in intake of fruits and vegetables and weight change in United States men and women followed for up to 24 years: analysis from three prospective cohort studies. PLoS Med. 2015;12(9):e1001878. https://doi.org/10.1371/journalpmed.1001878.
75. Barczynska B, Bandurska K, Slizewska K, et al. Intestinal microbiota, obesity and prebiotics. Polish. J Microbiol. 2015;64(2):93–100.
76. Brahe LK, Astrup A, Larsen LH. Can we prevent obesity-related metabolic diseases by dietary

modulation of the gut microbiota? Adv Nutr. 2016;7:90–101. https://doi.org/10.3945/an.115.010587.

77. Turnbaugh PJ, Hamady M, Yatsunenko T, et al. A core gut microbiome in obese and lean twins. Nature. 2009;457:480–4.
78. Cotillard A, Kennedy SP, Kong LC, et al. Dietary intervention impact on gut microbial gene richness. Nature. 2013;500(7464):585–8.
79. Le Chatelier E, Nielsen T, Qin J, et al. Richness of human gut microbiome correlates with metabolic markers. Nature. 2013;500(7464):541–6.
80. Lozupone CA, Stombaugh JI, Gordon JI, et al. Diversity, stability and resilience of the human gut microbiota. Nature. 2012;489:220–30.
81. Miquel S, Martín R, Rossi O, et al. Faecalibacterium prausnitzii and human intestinal health. Curr Opin Microbiol. 2013;16:255–61.
82. Geurts L, Neyrinck AM, Delzenne NM, et al. Gut microbiota controls adipose tissue expansion, gut barrier and glucose metabolism: novel insights into molecular targets and interventions using prebiotics. Benefic Microbes. 2014;5(1):3–17.
83. Karlsson FH, Tremaroli V, Nookaew I, et al. Gut metagenome in European women with normal, impaired and diabetic glucose control. Nature. 2013;498:99–103.
84. Furet JP, Kong LC, Tap J, et al. Differential adaptation of human gut microbiota to bariatric surgery-induced weight loss: links with metabolic and low-grade inflammation markers. Diabetes. 2010;59:3049–57.
85. Sánchez D, Miguel M, Aleixandre A. Dietary fiber, gut peptides, and adipocytokines. J Med Food. 2012;15(3):223–30. https://doi.org/10.1089/jmf.2011.0072.
86. Hjorth MF, Roager HM, Larsen TM, et al. Pre-tretment microbial Prevotella-to-Bacteroides ratio, determeines body fat loss success during 6-month randomized controlled diet intervention. Int J Obes. 2017; doi:10.1038/ijo.2017.220.
87. Million M, Maraninchi M, Henry M, et al. Obesity-associated gut microbiota is enriched in Lactobacillus reuteri and depleted in Bifidobacterium animalis and Methanobrevibacter smithii. Int J Obes (Lond). 2012;36:817–25.
88. Kalliomäki M, Collado MC, Salminen S, Isolauri E. Early differences in fecal microbiota composition in children may predict overweight. Am J Clin Nutr. 2008;87:534–8.
89. Moreno-Indias I, Cardona F, Tinahones FJ, Queipo-Ortuño MI. Impact of the gut microbiota on the development of obesity and type 2 diabetes mellitus. Front Microbiol. 2014;5(190):1–10.
90. Fernandes J, Su W, Rahat-Rozenbloom S, et al. Adiposity, gut microbiota and faecal short chain fatty acids are linked in adult humans. Nutr Diabetes. 2014;4:e121. https://doi.org/10.1038/nutd.2014.23.
91. Blaut M. Gut microbiota and energy balance: role in obesity. Proc Nutr Soc. 2015;74:227–34; doi: 10.1017/S0029665114001700.
92. Chambers ES, Morrison DJ, Frost G. Control of appetite and energy intake by SCFA: what are the potential underlying mechanisms? Proc Nutr Soc. 2015;74:328–336; doi: 10.1017/S0029665114001657.
93. Ley SH, Hamdy O, Mahan V, Prevention HFB. management of type 2 diabetes: dietary components and nutritional strategies. Lancet. 2014;383:1999–2007.
94. Tabák AG, Herder C, Rathmann W, et al. Prediabetes: A high-risk state for developing diabetes. Lancet. 2012;379(9833):2279–90.
95. Everard A, Cani PD. Diabetes, obesity and gut microbiota. Best Pract Res Clin Gastroenterol. 2013;27:73–83.
96. Murri M, Leiva I, Gomez-Zumaquero JM, et al. Gut microbiota in children with type 1 diabetes differs from that in healthy children: a case–control study. BMC Med. 2013;11:46.
97. Serino M, Fernandez-Real JM, Garcıa Fuentes E, et al. The gut microbiota profile is associated with insulin action in humans. Acta Diabetol. 2013;50:753–61.
98. Larsen N, Vogensen FK, van den Berg FW, et al. Gut microbiota in human adults with type 2 diabetes differs from non-diabetic adults. PLoS One. 2010;5:e9085. https://doi.org/10.1371/journal.pone.0009085.
99. Qin J, Li Y, Cai Z, et al. A metagenome-wide association study of gut microbiota in type 2 diabetes. Nature. 2012;490:55–60.
100. Nagpal R, Kumar M, Yadav AK, et al. Gut microbiota in health and dsiease: an overview focused on metabolic inflammation. Benef Microbes. 2016; 7(2):181–94.
101. Kim MS, Hwang SS, Park EJ, Bae JW. Strict vegetarian diet improves the risk factors associated with metabolic diseases by modulating gut microbiota and reducing intestinal inflammation. Environ Microbiol Rep. 2013;5:765–75.
102. Fallucca F, Fontana L, Fallucca S, Pianesi M. Gut microbiota and Ma-Pi 2 macrobiotic diet in the treatment of type 2 diabetes. World J Diabetes. 2015;6(3):403–11.
103. Karimi P, Farhangi MA, Sarmadi B, et al. The therapeutic potential of resistant starch in modulation of insulin resistance, endotoxemia, oxidative stress and antioxidant biomarkers in women with type 2 diabetes: a randomized controlled clinical trial. Ann Nutr Metab. 2016;68(2):85–93.
104. Bodinham CL, Smith L, Thomas EL, et al. Efficacy of increased resistant starch consumption in human type 2 diabetes. Endocr Connect. 2014;3:75–84.
105. Grundy SM. Metabolic syndrome pandemic. Arterioscler Thromb Vasc Biol. 2008;28:629–36.
106. Festi D, Schiumerini R, Eusebi LH, et al. Gut microbiota and metabolic syndrome. World J Gastroenterol. 2014;20(43):16079–94.
107. Martinez-Gonzalez MA, Martin-Calvo N. The major European dietary pattern and metabolic syndrome. Rev Endocr Metab Disord. 2013;14(3):265–71.

108. Vetrani C, Costabile G, Luongo D, et al. Effects of whole-grain cereal foods on plasma short chain fatty acid concentrations in individuals with the metabolic syndrome. Nutrition. 2016;32:217–21.
109. Chambers ES, Viardot A, Psichas A, et al. Effects of targeted delivery of propionate to the human colon on appetite regulation, body weight maintenance and adiposity in overweight adults. Gut. 2015;64(11):1744–54.
110. Yoon NR, Yoon S, Lee S-M. Rice cakes containing dietary fiber supplemented with or without Artemisia annua and Gynura procumbens Merr. alleviated the risk factors of metabolic syndrome. Clin Nutr Res. 2016;5:79–88.
111. Brahe LK, Le Chatelier E, Prifti E. Specific gut microbiota features and metabolic markers in postmenopausal women with obesity. Nutr Diabetes. 2015; e159. doi: https://doi.org/10.1038/nutd.2015.9.
112. Galisteo M, Duarte J, Zarzuelo A. Effects of dietary fibers on disturbances clustered in the metabolic syndrome. J Nutr Biol. 2008;19:71–84.
113. Rehman T. Role of the gut microbiota in age-related chronic inflammation. Endocr Metab Immune Disord Drug Targets. 2012;12:361–7.
114. Brüssow H. Microbiota and healthy ageing: observational and nutritional intervention studies. Microbial Biotechnol. 2013;6:326–34.
115. O'Toole PWO, Jeffery IB. Gut microbiota and aging. Science. 2015;350(6265):1214–5.
116. Zapata HJ, Quagliarello VJ. The microbiota and microbiome in aging: potential implications in health and age-related diseases. J Am Geriatr Soc. 2015;63(4):776–81.
117. Rowe JW, Kahn RL. Human aging: usual and successful. Science. 1987;237:143–9. https://doi.org/10.1126/science.3299702.
118. Stenman LK, Burcelin R, Lahtinen S. Establishing a causal link between gut microbes, body weight gain and glucose metabolism in humans -towards treatment with probiotics. Benefic Microbes. 2015;7(1):11–22.
119. Cuervo A, Salazar N, Ruas-Madiedob P, et al. Fiber from a regular diet is directly associated with fecal short-chain fatty acid concentrations in the elderly. Nutr Res. 2013;33:811–6.
120. Jiao J, J-Y X, Zhang W, et al. Effect of dietary fiber on circulating C-reactive protein in overweight and obese adults: a meta-analysis of randomized controlled trials. Int J Food Sci Nutr. 2015;66(1):114–9.
121. Grooms KN, Ommerborn MJ, Quyen D, et al. Dietary fiber intake and cardiometabolic risk among US adults, NHANES 1999-2010. Am J Med. 2013;126(12):1059–67.
122. Cassidy A, De Vivo I, Liu Y, et al. Associations between diet, lifestyle factors, and telomere length in women. Am J Clin Nutr. 2010;91:1273–83.
123. Abdullah MM, Gyles CL, Marinangeli CP, et al. Cost-of-illness analysis reveals potential healthcare savings with reductions in type 2 diabetes and cardiovascular disease following recommended intakes of dietary fiber in Canada. Front Pharmacol. 2015;6:167. https://doi.org/10.3389/fphar.2015.00167.
124. Liu L, Wang S, Liu J. Fiber consumption and all-cause, cardiovascular, and cancer mortalities: A systematic review and meta-analysis of cohort studies. Mol Nutr Food Res. 2015;59:139–46.
125. Park Y, Subar AF, Hollenbeck A, et al. Dietary fiber intake and mortality in the NIH-AARP Diet and Health Study. Arch Intern Med. 2011;171(12):1061–8.
126. Chuang S-C, Norat T, Murphy N, et al. Fiber intake and total and cause-specific mortality in the European Prospective Investigation into Cancer and Nutrition cohort. Am J Clin Nutr. 2012;96:164–74.
127. Wei H, Gao Z, Liang R, et al. Whole-grain consumption and the risk of all-cause, CVD and cancer mortality: a meta-analysis of prospective cohort studies. Br J Nutr. 2016;116(3):514–25. https://doi.org/10.1017/S0007114516001975.
128. Nguyen B, Bauman A, Gale J, et al. Fruit and vegetable consumption and all-cause mortality: evidence from a large Australian cohort study. Int J Behav Nutr Phys Act. 2016;13:9. https://doi.org/10.1186/s12966-016-0334-5.
129. Claesson MJ, Jeffery IB, Conde S. Gut microbiota composition correlates with diet and health in the elderly. Nature. 2012;488:178–85.
130. Claesson MJ, Cusack S, O'Sullivan O, et al. Composition, variability, and temporal stability of the intestinal microbiota of the elderly. Proc Natl Acad Sci U S A. 2011;108(suppl. 1):4586–91.
131. Jeffery IB, Lynch DB, O'Toole PW. Composition and temporal stability of the gut microbiota in older persons. ISME J. 2016;10:170–82.
132. Biagi E, Franceschi C. Rampelli S, et al. Curr Bio: Gut microbiota and extreme longevity; 2016. https://doi.org/10.1016/j.cub.2016.04.016
133. Wang F, Yu T, Huang G, Cai D. Gut microbiota community and its assembly associated with age and diet in Chinese centenarians. J Microbiol Biotechnol. 2015;25(8):1195–204.
134. Biagi E, Nylund L, Candela M, et al. Through ageing, and beyond: gut microbiota and inflammatory status in seniors and centenarians. PLoS One. 2010;5(5):e10667. https://doi.org/10.1371/journal.pone.0010667.
135. Mariat D, Firmesse O, Levenez F, et al. The Firmicutes/Bacteroidetes ratio of the human microbiota changes with age. BMC Microbiol. 2009;9:123. https://doi.org/10.1186/1471-2180-9-123.
136. van Tongeren SP, Slaets JP, Harmsen HJ, Welling GW. Fecal microbiota composition and frailty. Appl Environ Microbiol. 2005;71:6438–42.
137. Bartosch S, Fite A, Macfarlane GT, McMurdo ME. Characterization of bacterial communities in feces from healthy elderly volunteers and hospitalized elderly patients by using real-time PCR and effects of antibiotic treatment on the fecal microbiota. Appl Environ Microbiol. 2004;70:3575–81.

Fiber-Rich Dietary Patterns and Foods in Laxation and Constipation

5

Keywords
Fiber-rich foods • Laxation • Bowel movement • Functional constipation • Chronic constipation • Colon health • Wheat bran • Oat bran • Prunes • Kiwi fruit • Polydextrose • Psyllium • Chicory inulin • Prebiotics • Symbiotics

Key Points

- The consumption of healthy dietary patterns with adequate dietary fiber (>25 g/day), recommended fluid intake, and regular physical activity, are especially beneficial in preventing and alleviating constipation.
- Fiber mechanisms associated with improved laxation and alleviated constipation include: increasing stool weight and bulk volume (through fiber and microbiota physical volume and water holding capacity), and gas volume trapped in the stool to increase bowel movement frequency and quality, especially in constipated individuals.
- Adequate intake of fiber from cereal, fruits, vegetables and common fiber-rich food ingredients including polydextrose, psyllium, chicory inulin and prebiotics or symbiotics have the potential to increase population-wide levels of regularity and provide constipation relief.
- In general, less fermentable dietary fiber tends to increase fecal weight to a greater amount than more fermentable fibers. Wheat bran is the most widely studied fiber; when baseline transit time was >48 h, each extra g/day of wheat bran significantly increased total stool weight by 3.7 g and reduced transit time by 45 min.
- Increased fiber intake did not change transit time in individuals with an initial time of <48 h. However, in people with an initial transit time ≥48 h, transit time was reduced by approximately 30 min per gram of cereal, fruit or vegetable fiber, regardless of fermentability.
- Several RCTs suggest that daily intake of prunes (dried plums) and/or kiwi fruit can help in relieving constipation symptoms similarly to psyllium.

5.1 Introduction

Constipation symptoms vary from person to person but are usually described as infrequent bowel movements, straining, passage of hard stools,

M.L. Dreher, *Dietary Patterns and Whole Plant Foods in Aging and Disease*, Nutrition and Health,
https://doi.org/10.1007/978-3-319-59180-3_5

and/or difficulty in passing stools, which effects most people at some time in their lives [1–3]. In Western countries, about 30% of the general adult population experiences problems with constipation during their life time, with elderly people and women being most affected. However, many people experience constipation that is more than a minor annoyance, and can be chronic, sometimes severe, and have significant and often debilitating effects on their quality of life. Physicians frequently define constipation as fewer than three bowel movements/week and most people have bowel movement frequency between 3 per day and 3 per week [4]. Chronic constipation is more commonly diagnosed in female patients at 2–3 times the rate of males. Individuals with constipation rarely report it to anyone or seek medical treatments [5, 6]. By 80 years of age, the prevalence of chronic constipation is about 34% in women and 26% in men [1]. The prevalence of childhood constipation is challenging to estimate but worldwide about 16% of mothers of toddlers report some degree of constipation in their children [7, 8]. Constipation can be acute lasting for a day or two, or chronic lasting for weeks, months, or years, as a result of a variety of potential factors including low dietary fiber (fiber) diets, inadequate fluid intake, inactivity or certain medicines such as opiates used to control pain [1–3, 9, 10]. Diet and lifestyle modifications, including adequate dietary fiber (>25 g/day; especially from whole plant foods) plus water intake and regular physical activity may especially represent an effective, inexpensive, and feasible therapeutic way to prevent and alleviate constipation [11, 12]. Fiber increases colonic stool volume and water content directly, or stimulates motility leading to shortened colonic transit and decreased water absorption [1–3]. Also, fiber supplements, or other types of laxatives plus fluids are frequently considered to effectively manage constipation. The objective of this chapter is to comprehensively review the role of fiber-rich diets and foods in promoting laxation and alleviating constipation.

5.2 Overview of Fiber, Laxation and Constipation

There are a number of health professional organizations recommending the intake of adequate dietary fiber (>25g/day or 14 g/1,000 kcal) to prevent constipation [9, 10, 13–16]. The American Medical Association recommends the consumption of adequate fiber intake of at least 25 g/day as a first step that may improve or eliminate constipation by increasing the intake of fiber containing fruit, vegetables, wholegrains (e.g., wheat bran breakfast cereals), legumes, and nuts and seeds or appropriate fiber supplement products such as psyllium [9, 10]. The American College of Gastroenterology suggests that fiber supplements, especially from soluble fibers such as psyllium, may be effective in the management of chronic constipation in adults [13]. The Academy of Nutrition and Dietetics recommends the adequate amounts of fiber from a variety of plant foods to support laxation by increasing fecal biomass, increasing stool frequency, and reducing intestinal transit time [14]. The European Food Safety Authority (EFSA) panel recommended that the consumption of at least 25 g fiber/day from food was adequate for normal laxation in adults [15]. The American Academy of Pediatrics recommends a fiber intake of 0.5 g/kg/day for all children, or alternatively for children older than age 2 years, fiber amount equivalent to their age in years plus 5 g/day (to a maximum of 35 g/day for older children or adolescents) as low fiber intake may be a risk factor for chronic constipation [16]. These organizations generally recommend introducing dietary fiber gradually to minimize bloating, distension, flatulence, and cramping, which could limit compliance and effectiveness [9, 10, 13].

Adequate intake of healthy fiber-rich dietary patterns, especially whole foods, minimally processed foods, or foods enriched with fiber-rich ingredients, such as with wheat bran or psyllium, along with adequate fluid intake and physical activity are the primary lifestyle factors for regularity in laxation [11, 12, 17–21]. Low fiber intake is often associated with constipation in epidemiologic studies [11, 12, 21]. The Nurses' Health Study (62,036 women; age range 36 to 61 years; 3327 reported bowel movement frequency every 3rd day or less) observed that women with a median intake of about 20 g fiber daily had a 36% lower prevalence of constipation compared with women who consumed about 7 g of fiber daily (Fig. 5.1) [11]. For physical activity and fiber, this study found that women in the highest quintile of physical activity (2–3 times/week) and fiber intake had a multivariate lower prevalence of constipation by 68% compared with those in the lowest quintile of physical activity (<1 time per week) and fiber intake; higher physical activity reduced constipation risk by 44% and higher fiber intake reduced risk by 36%. Adequate water intake is important for fiber laxation mechanisms to work optimally and low water intake may increase the prevalence of constipation [17, 18]. An intervention trial with chronically constipated individuals (117 subjects; mean age 39 years; 64% women; 10 g fiber/1000 kcals vs. 7 g fiber/1000 kcal; 2 months) showed that just increasing fiber intake by 3 g/1000 kcal plus 2 L of liquids/day was significantly more effective at increasing stool frequency and decreasing laxative use than consuming only 1 L of fluid/day (Fig. 5.2) [19]. For physical activity and fiber, the Nurses' Health Study (62,036 women; aged 36–61 years; 5.4% were classified as constipated defined as ≤2 bowel movements weekly; median daily fiber intake 20 g vs. 7 g) found that women in the highest quintile of physical activity (2–3 times/week) and fiber intake had a multivariate lower prevalence of constipation by 68% compared with those in the lowest quintile of physical activity (<1 time weekly) and fiber intake [11]. In these women, higher physical activity reduced constipation risk by 44% and higher fiber intake reduced risk by 36%. A 2015 study of Canadian adults found that each 1 g/day increase in dietary fiber from foods was projected to reduce constipation rates by about 2% [22]. Similarly, in the US, it was estimated that if fiber intake was increased by 9 g/day from bran (equivalent to one serving of high fiber breakfast cereal/day), there could be a billion dollars in annual savings in medical costs due to decreased constipation [23]. A meta-analysis (5 randomized controlled trials [RCTs]) found that increased fiber intake to the adequate intake range significantly improved stool frequency by 19% ($p < .05$) compared to the placebo [24].

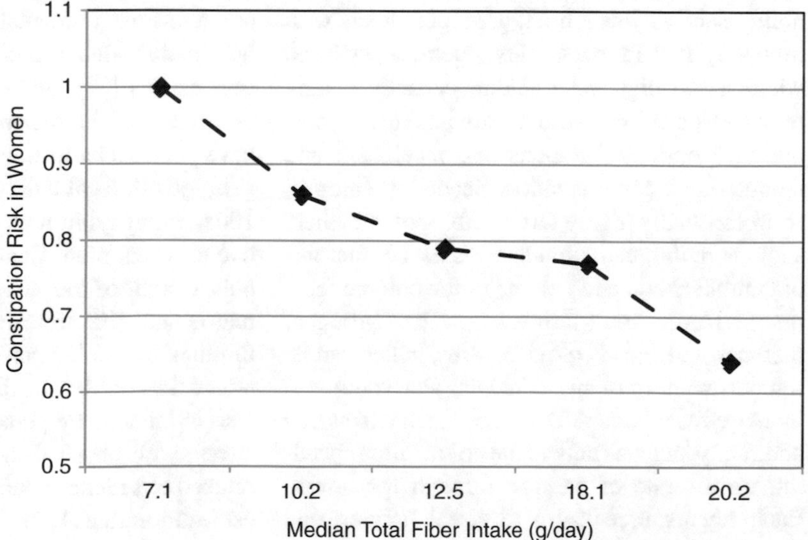

Fig. 5.1 Association between level of fiber intake and risk of constipation in women ($p < .0001$; multivariate adjusted) (adapted from [11])

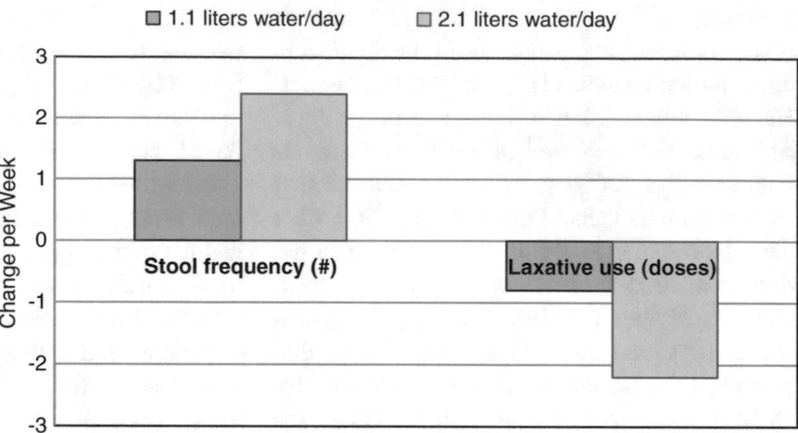

Fig. 5.2 Effect of level of water intake with a standard diet providing 25 g fiber/day on stool frequency and laxative usage in 117 patients with chronic functional constipation ($p < .001$) (adapted from [19])

However, there was no significant difference in stool consistency and painful defecation between the two groups.

5.3 Fiber Related Laxation Mechanisms

The way in which fiber affects bowel habit cannot be explained on the basis of one simple hypothesis [25]. There are several ways by which fiber increases laxation. First, plant cell walls especially rich in lignin with moderate water holding capacity and low to moderate fermentability such as wheat bran; or soluble fibers with relatively low fermentability, such as psyllium, which have a high water holding capacity leading to increased colonic volume, are among the most effective options for increasing fecal bulk and stimulating colonic laxation. Second, prebiotics, from especially highly fermentable soluble fibers such as inulin, can stimulate increased microbiota numbers and add volume to the colonic fecal mass. Third, fiber fermentation to hydrogen, methane and carbon dioxide gases, which can be trapped within colonic contents, add volume to increase fecal bulk. All of these mechanisms can additively increase bulk in the colon, often speeding up the rate of passage through the bowel. Each fiber source has a different bulking and fermentation capacity. There is a fecal bulking index for standardized measurement of the relative colonic bulking efficacy of foods relative to a typical edible serving size of wheat bran [26–28]. Table 5.1 provides an estimation of the fecal bulking capacity of whole and processed plant foods relative to wheat bran from a validated model system [28]. The fecal bulking index values for whole-grains breads or wheat bran enriched breakfast cereals range from about 12 to 50. Wheat bran and other fibers are fairly resistant to fermentation in the large bowel so the retained 3-dimensional fiber structure has a water binding capacity of 5 to 6 g water/g fiber in the distal colon. More fermentable fibers provide some bulk mainly due to increased bacterial mass and trapped gas [27]. Some soluble fiber, fermentation-resistant ingredients or supplements, can have polysaccharides with high water binding or gelling with fecal bulking capacities in excess of 100x, with psyllium having a value of 500x relative to wheat bran. Generally, the greater the wet bulk weight of the stool from fiber and the food matrix and the more rapid the rate of passage through the colon and the better the laxative effect. In addition to dietary effects, laxation is also influenced by personality type, and level of stress and physical activity with introverted, relaxed or sedentary individuals having the slowest laxation rates [29].

Table 5.1 Fecal bulking index and total fiber content per 100 g of plant foods [28].

Food	Fecal bulking index (%)	Total fiber content (g/100 g)
Ingredients		
Wheat bran	100	44
Wheat germ	37	16
Rye flour	21	12
Pea flour	11	16
Soy flour	9	18
Oat bran	8	11
Corn meal	2	7
Breakfast Cereals		
All-bran	51	30
Bran flakes	26	19
Muesli	17	7
Rolled oats	17	9
Puffed wheat	8	8
Special K	8	4
Wheat Chex	3	2
Puffed rice	−0.4	6
Cornflakes	−2	3
Bakery Products		
Ryvita crisp bread	23	14
Whole wheat bread	12	6
Multi-grain bread	4	6
White bread	1	3
Vegetables/Pulses		
Lentils, boiled	9	2
Green peas, boiled	7	6
Spinach, cooked	6	2
Cabbage, boiled	4	2
Carrots, cooked	3	3
Fruit		
Pear, dried	27	7
Apricot, dried	3	3

5.4 Laxation Effects of Fiber-Rich Diets, and Specific Foods and Supplements

Although the beneficial effects of whole-grain and wheat bran on laxation were known since Hippocrates in 370 BC, the advancement of the dietary fiber hypothesis refocused interest on the effects of dietary fiber and digestive health in a wider range of diets and foods [30]. Meta-analyses and specific representative RCTs on the laxative and constipation alleviating effects of fiber-rich diets and foods are summarized in Table 5.2 [24, 27, 31–57]. Appendix A provides a list of the top 50 fiber rich whole (minimally processed) plant foods.

5.4.1 Systematic Reviews and Meta-Analyses

Eight systematic reviews and meta-analyses provide an important overview of the best fiber-rich foods for laxation and alleviation of constipation [24, 31–34, 39, 41, 51]. These systematic reviews suggest that adequate intake of fiber from cereal, fruits, vegetables and common fiber-rich food ingredients including polydextrose, psyllium and chicory inulin have the potential to increase population-wide levels of regularity and may play a role in providing constipation relief.

5.4.1.1 Cereal, Fruit and Vegetable Sources

A 2016 systematic review of intervention trials on cereal, fruit and vegetable fibers (136 experimental studies; healthy subjects) found that cereal and vegetable fiber resulted in similarly increased fecal weight with fruit fiber being less effective [32]. Less fermentable food fibers increased fecal weight to a greater amount than more fermentable fibers. Fiber did not change transit time in individuals with an initial time of <48 h. In those with an initial transit time ≥48 h, transit time was reduced by approximately 30 min per gram of cereal, fruit or vegetable fiber, regardless of fermentability. This analysis indicates that slow transit time (≥48 h) may be normalized by increasing fiber, regardless of the type consumed.

5.4.1.2 Cereal Sources

Four specific systematic reviews and/or meta-analyses have evaluated the effects of cereal fiber-rich food sources on bowel function [24, 33, 34, 39]. A 2015 systematic review of cereal fiber intervention in studies with healthy subjects (65 trials; 90% wheat bran) found that wheat bran

Table 5.2 Summary of fiber-rich foods, food ingredient, dietary supplement intervention trials in laxation and constipation.

Objective	Study details	Results
Systematic Reviews and Meta-analyses of Intervention Trials		
Yu et al. (2017) Determine the effects of prebiotics and symbiotics on adults with functional constipation [31].	Prebiotics:5 RCTs; 199 patients. Symbiotics: 8 RCTs; 825 patients.	Prebiotics increased weekly stool frequency by 1 bowel movement/week and improved stool consistency. Subgroup analysis showed specific effects for galacto-oligosaccharides on stool frequency, consistency, ease of defecation and abdominal pain. Symbiotics significantly improved stool frequency by 1.15 bowel movements/ week, improved consistency and reduced whole-gut transit time by 13.5 h in patients with functional constipation. Subgroup analysis showed specific effects for fructo-oligosaccharides and probiotic combinations on stool frequency, consistency, straining defecation and bloating.
DeVries et al. (2016) Summarize the effects of cereal, vegetable and fruit fiber on fecal weight and transit time [32].	136 experimental studies; in healthy subjects.	Cereal and vegetable fiber had similar effects on fecal weight whereas fruit fibers were less effective. Lower fermentable fibers increased fecal weight to a greater degree than more fermentable fibers. Fiber did not change transit time in those with an initial time of <48 h. In those with an initial transit time ≥48 h, transit time was reduced by 30 min per gram of cereal, fruit or vegetable fibers, regardless of fermentability.
DeVries et al. (2015) Review and quantitatively examine the effects of cereal fiber-rich foods and ingredients on bowel function [33].	65 intervention studies; among generally healthy populations.	Each extra g/day of wheat fiber increased total stool weight by 3.7 g ($p < .0001$), dry stool weight by 0.75 g ($p < .0001$), and stool frequency by 0.004 times ($p = .0346$). Transit time decreased by 0.78 h per additional g/day ($p < .0001$) of wheat fiber among those with initial transit times >48 h.
Thies et al. (2014) Systematically review intervention studies on the effects of oats or oat bran on bowel function [39].	14 intervention trials.	Trials in healthy subjects suggest that oats or oat bran can significantly increase stool weight and decrease constipation. Oat consumption significantly increased wet and dry stool weight in 6 out of 9 studies (from 15 to 88% increase) and 5 out of 6 studies (from 15 to 101% increase), respectively. Stool frequency did not change significantly in 5 studies, improved in 2 studies and reduced in 1 study relative to wheat-bran and rice-bran interventions. Transit time decreased significantly by 17% in only 1 out of 4 studies.
Lever et al. (2014) Assess the effect of prunes on stool frequency and consistency [43].	4 RCTs; one in constipated subjects and three in non-constipated subjects.	In one trial with constipated subjects, 3 weeks of prune consumption (100 g/day) improved stool frequency (3.5 vs. 2.8 per week ($p = .006$) and stool consistency (3.2 vs. 2.8 on Bristol stool form scale, $p = .02$) compared with psyllium (22 g/day) as a positive control. In the 3 trials with non-constipated subjects, prunes softened stool consistency and increased stool weight (628 g vs. 514 g/72-h wet weight, $p = .001$) compared with control.

Table 5.2 (continued)

Objective	Study details	Results
Yang et al. (2012) Investigate the effects of dietary fiber on stool weight and transit time [24].	5 placebo controlled, double-blinded RCTs; limited to bran and glucomannan primarily.	Increasing fiber resulted in significantly increased mean stool frequency by 19% vs. placebo ($p < .05$) but there was no significant difference in stool consistency, laxative use and painful defecation between the two groups. Improved stool frequency was reported by all 5 RCTs, with either a trend or a significant improvement for the fiber group vs. control.
Suares and Ford (2011) Assess in systematic review the efficacy of soluble and insoluble fiber supplementation in the management of chronic idiopathic constipation [51].	6 RCTs (3 psyllium, 1 bran, 1 rye bread and 1 inulin).	Compared with placebo, psyllium improved global symptoms (86% vs. 47%), straining (56% vs. 29%), pain on defecation, stool consistency, increase in the mean number of stools per week (3.8 stools per week after therapy compared with 2.9 stools per week at baseline), and a reduction in the number of days between stools. Evidence for any benefit of insoluble fiber was inconsistent. Formal meta-analysis was not undertaken due to concern about methodological quality of identified studies.
Muller-Lissner et al. (1988) Investigate the effects of wheat bran on stool weight and transit [34].	20 RCTs.	Bran increased the stool weight and decreased the transit time in each study in healthy controls and in patients with irritable bowel syndrome, with diverticula, and with chronic constipation. However, bran was shown to be only partially effective in restoring normal stool weight and transit time in constipated subjects.
Mixtures of Fiber-Rich Plant Foods		
Wisten and Messner (2005) Study the effects of daily consumption of a fruit- and fiber-rich porridge on stool frequency, perceived wellbeing and laxative usage, when compared with traditional treatment with laxatives, in geriatric patients (Sweden) [41].	**Parallel RCT:** 20 patients in secondary geriatric hospitals; porridge (flaxseed, chopped prunes and apricots, raisins, rolled oats and oat bran) vs. control standard diet without porridge; 1-week run-in and 2-week study.	Patients in the porridge group had a daily defecation without laxatives on average 76% of the time compared with 23% of the time in the non-porridge group ($p = .003$). The discomfort was less in the porridge group (2.5 vs. 6.5 on a 10-degree visual analogue scale ($p = .008$) when compared with the control group. The cost for laxatives was lower in the porridge group by 93%.
Haack et al. (1998) Determine the responses of healthy adult men to increased intakes of fiber-rich foods, <15, 30, and 45 g/day (US) [35].	**Crossover RCT:** 9 healthy, young men; consumed constant diets with 3 amounts of fiber provided by a mixture of fruit, vegetables, and grains which contained 16, 30, and 42 g total fiber/day, of which 2.9, 4.8, and 7.7 g were soluble; 1 month each diet.	Fiber provided by a mixed-food diet: (1) increases stool weight as effectively as cereal bran; (2) even high amounts of fiber do not change transit time or defecation frequency if subjects already have between 1 to 3 daily bowel movements; (3) food patterns containing legumes and whole grains are necessary to achieve recommended fiber intakes of 14 g/1000 kcal; and (4) mixed-food fiber has little effect on calcium balance when calcium intakes are high (≥1.5 g/day).

(continued)

Table 5.2 (continued)

Objective	Study details	Results
Cereal Brans		
Lawton et al. (2013) Investigate the effect of wheat bran on subjective perception of bowel function and digestion, feelings and general well-being (UK) [36].	**Open Label Trial:** 153 low fiber consumers (baseline <15 g/day); one bowl of ready-to-eat breakfast cereal containing at least 5.4 g fiber (3.5 g from wheat bran); 14 days; completed a daily symptom diary.	The inclusion of 1 bowel of bran cereal /daily over two weeks, significantly improved subjective perception of: (1) bowel function (e.g., ease of defecation) and digestive feelings (less bloating, constipation, feeling sluggish and digestive discomfort) and (2) general wellbeing (feeling less fat, more mentally alert, slim, happy and energetic whilst experiencing less stress, mental and physical tiredness, difficulty concentrating and fewer headaches).
Sturtzel et al. (2009) Determine effects of adding oat-bran to a low fiber habitual diet on use of laxatives, well-being and body weight of the inhabitants of a long-term-care facility (Austria) [40].	**Single-blind Parallel RCT:** 30 frail inhabitants of a geriatric hospital; aged 57–100 years with laxative use; 15 subjects received 7-8 g oat-bran/day (fiber group) mixed up in the daily common diet of the ward and 15 received no oat bran (control group); 12 weeks.	Laxatives were successfully discontinued by 59% ($p < .001$) in the fiber-group; in the control-group there was an increase of 8% ($p = 0.218$). Body weight remained constant in the fiber-group and decreased in the control-group ($p = .002$). The oat-fiber supplementation was well tolerated.
Vuksan et al. (2008) Assess the effects of increasing fiber intake on bowel habits and gastrointestinal tolerance in healthy persons consuming a typical Canadian or US diet (Canada) [37].	**Crossover RCT:** 23 free-living participants; baseline diet 35% fat and 12 g fiber/day; received 25 to 29 g added fiber/day from each of 5 breakfast cereals: All-bran (AB), bran buds with corn (BBC), bran buds with psyllium (BBP), BBC with viscous fiber blend (VFB), or a low-fiber control; 3 weeks, with each study arm separated by a washout of ≥1 week; 7-day stool collections and a symptom diary were obtained during the last week of each study arm.	Compared to the low fiber control, all study cereals induced significant ($p < .05$) increases in fecal bulk from the control diet; less intestinal transit time; and significantly ($p < .05$) greater bowel movement frequency, while maintaining a good level of tolerance. Bran buds with psyllium was more effective than other cereals in terms of increasing fecal wet weight ($p < .05$).
Hongisto et al. (2006) Investigate the effects of fiber-rich rye bread and yogurt containing lactobacillus GG (LGG) on intestinal transit time and bowel function (Finland) [38].	**2-by-2 RCT:** 59 healthy women with self-reported constipation: 4 diet groups: (1) rye bread plus LGG yogurt, (2) rye bread, (3) LGG yogurt, and (4) control; 3 weeks.	The rye bread group had shortened total intestinal transit time by 0.7 days ($p = .007$), increased fecal frequency by 0.3 per day ($<.001$), softened feces by 0.3 units ($p < .001$) had easier defecation by 0.4 units ($p < .001$) and gastrointestinal symptoms score was increased by 1.6 units ($p < .001$) compared to the low-fiber toast consumed in the LGG and control groups. There were fewer gastrointestinal symptoms in the rye bread plus LGG group compared to the rye bread group by 1.3 units ($p = .027$).

Table 5.2 (continued)

Objective	Study details	Results
Jenkins et al. (1999) Test the effects of wheat bran particle size on colonic function (Canada) [27].	**Crossover RCT:** In healthy subjects, 2 studies, each with 3 phases: (1) 23 subjects; 19 g/day fiber from wheat bran with mean particle size (MPS) 50 mm or 758 mm in bread or a control low fiber bread and (2) 24 healthy subjects; breakfast cereal (*ad libitum*) with wheat bran MPS 692 mm and 1158 mm and the control was low fiber. 1 month metabolic ward; fecal collections last week of each diet.	In both studies, wheat bran supplements significantly increased fecal bulk compared to the control ($p < .004$), with no significant differences between brans of different particle size and no differences in fecal water content. However, higher fecal butyrate concentrations ($p < .007$), and breath CH_4 levels ($p = .025$) were seen on the smaller MPS wheat bran compared to the other two treatments, suggesting increased bacterial fermentation. Fine MPS wheat bran is an effective fecal bulking agent and may have added advantages in promoting colonic microbiota health.
Whole Fruits and Vegetables vs. Fruit and Vegetable Juices		
Kelsay et al. (1978) Assess the effect of high fiber vs. low fiber fruits and vegetables on bowel function (US) [42].	**Crossover RCT:** 12 men; age range 37–58 years; weight range 68–95 kg; high fiber fruit and vegetable diet vs. a low fiber diet containing fruit and vegetable juices; 26 days; no washout.	High fiber fruits and vegetables vs. low fiber fruit and vegetable juice intake significantly reduced fecal transit time (38 vs. 52 h), increased the number of daily bowel movements (1.4 vs. 1), and increased daily wet fecal weight (208 g vs. 90 g).
Prunes (Dried Plums)		
Attaluri et al. (2011) Assess and compare the effects of dried plums and psyllium in patients with chronic constipation (US) [44].	**Single-blind, Crossover RCT:** 40 constipated subjects; 37- females; mean age 38 years; 50 g dried plums or 11 g psyllium twice daily (6 g fiber/day); 3 weeks with a 1 week washout period.	The number of complete spontaneous bowel movements per week and stool consistency scores improved significantly ($p < 0.05$) with dried plums when compared to psyllium (Fig. 5.3). Straining and global constipation symptoms did not differ significantly between treatments ($p > .05$). Dried plums and psyllium were rated as equally palatable and both were safe and well tolerated.
Kiwi Fruit		
Chang et al. (2010) Examine the impact of kiwi fruit intake on bowel function in patients diagnosed with constipated irritable bowel syndrome (IBS-C) patients (Taiwan) [47].	**Parallel RCT:** 54 patients with IBS-C and 16 healthy adults; 41 IBS-C patients and 16 healthy subjects consumed 2 Hayward green kiwi fruits and 13 IBS-C patients in the control group took two placebo capsules/day; 4 weeks.	The intake of kiwi fruit significantly improved weekly defecation frequency ($p < .05$) and decreased colon transit time ($p = .026$) in the IBS-C group. This study indicates that kiwi fruit improves bowel function in adults diagnosed with IBS-C.
Chan et al. (2007) Investigate the effect of increased kiwi fruit intake on Chinese constipated patients (China) [46].	**Open Label Trial:** 33 constipated patients and 20 healthy volunteers; kiwi fruit twice daily; 4 weeks.	Responder rate was 54.5% in the constipated group. The mean complete spontaneous bowel movements per week increased after treatment from 2.2 to 4.4 ($p = .013$) and transit time improved ($p = .003$). There was also significant improvement in the scores for bothersomeness of constipation, and satisfaction of bowel habit, and decrease in days of laxative used.

(continued)

Table 5.2 (continued)

Objective	Study details	Results
Rush et al. (2002) Evaluate the effect of regular kiwi fruit intake on laxation in elderly people (New Zealand) [45].	**Crossover RCT:** 38 healthy adults of age > 60 years consumed their normal diet, one kiwi fruit per 30 kg bodyweight vs. no kiwi fruit; 3 weeks, followed by a 3-week crossover period; daily records were taken on frequency of defecation and characteristics of the stools.	Kiwi fruit consumption was associated with a significant increase in frequency of defecation ($p = .012$), stool bulk produced ($p = .002$) and softness of stools ($p < .0001$).
Polydextrose and Soluble Corn Fiber		
Shimada et al. (2015) Evaluate the effects of polydextrose on constipated dialysis patients (Japan) [50].	**Triple-blind RCT:** 50 constipated dialysis patients; 51–79 years of age; laxative for >3 months and dialysis >6 months; food products containing 10 g polydextrose vs. 0 polydextrose control; 8 weeks.	The polydextrose group showed significant improvement in stool frequency from 3.0 to 7.5 times weekly; there were no laxation problems such as abdominal distension, cramps or diarrhea ($p < .001$) (Fig. 5.5).
Timm et al. (2013) Compare the laxative effects of polydextrose and soluble corn fiber (SCF) compared to a low fiber control eaten daily as a muffin and cereal (US) [48].	**Double-blind, Crossover RCT:** 36 healthy men and women; 10-g polydextrose/day and 10-g SCF/ day vs. low fiber (LF) control (about 14 g fiber/day) control diet; 10-day treatment with a 2-week washout period; collected fecal samples during the last 5 days of each treatment and completed food diaries and gastrointestinal tolerance questionnaires on day 1, 2, and 10.	5-day fecal wet weight was higher after the polydextrose and SCF treatments vs. . LF control ($p \leq .0007$). The number of stools per day and daily fecal output also were significantly greater during the polydextrose period compared with the LF control (Fig. 5.4). The whole gut transit time did not differ among treatments. The polydextrose treatment resulted in a softer stool ($p = .002$) than the SCF and LF control. Fecal pH was lowered by the polydextrose treatment ($p = .02$), whereas SCF tended to lower it compared with the LF control ($p = .07$). Polydextrose and SCF subjects reported significantly more flatulence compared with when they consumed the LF control.
Vester Boler et al. (2011) Evaluate digestive effects of polydextrose and soluble maize fiber in healthy adults (US) [49].	**Crossover RCT:** 21 healthy adult men; 21 g/day polydextrose or soluble maize fiber (SCF) vs. no supplemental fiber (NFC) in a snack bar; 21 days with fecal collection during the last 5 days.	Fecal wet weight was highest ($p = .03$) when subjects consumed SCF compared with NFC. Fecal dry weight tended to be greater ($p = .07$) when subjects consumed polydextrose compared with NFC. Bifidobacterium spp. concentrations were greater ($p < .05$) when subjects consumed SCF compared with NFC. All tolerance scores were low (<2.5), indicating only slight discomfort; although flatulence ($p = .001$) and distention ($p = .07$) were increased by polydextrose and SCF vs. NFC. Faecal pH was lower ($p < .01$) when subjects consumed SCF compared with NFC, while polydextrose was intermediate. These functional fibers appear to be beneficial to gut health while leading to minimal GI-upset.

Table 5.2 (continued)

Objective	Study details	Results
Psyllium		
Nunes et al. (2005) Evaluate the effects of psyllium laxatives in adults with chronic constipation (Brazil) [52].	**Double-blind RCT:** 60 adults; 65% women; 10 g psyllium daily; 2 weeks.	87% of individuals receiving psyllium vs. only 30% of those in the placebo group had normal bowel movement frequency ($p < 0.001$). Psyllium was shown to be effective in relieving chronic constipation.
McRorie et al. (1998) Compare the effects of psyllium and docusate sodium on chronic constipation (US) [53].	**Double-blind RCT:** 170 adults; mean age 37 years; 90% women; 5.1 g psyllium twice daily; 2 weeks.	Psyllium was superior to docusate sodium for softening stools by increasing water content and improving overall laxative efficacy.
Ashraf et al. (1995) Evaluate the effects of psyllium therapy on stool characteristics and colon transit in chronic constipation (US) [54].	**Double-blind RCT:** 22 adults; 14 females; 5 g psyllium twice daily; 8 weeks.	In individuals with chronic constipation, psyllium increased stool frequency compared with placebo and improved stool consistency, reduced pain on defecation, lessened straining and increased sense of complete evacuation compared to baseline.
Stevens et al. (1988) Compare the effects of psyllium and wheat bran on colonic transit time and stool characteristics (US) [55].	**Parallel RCT:** 12 subjects; psyllium, wheat bran or low fiber diet; 2 weeks.	Both fiber sources decreased transit time, and increased the daily number of defecations and wet and dry weight of stools. Bran increased transit time greater than psyllium and psyllium had a greater effect on stool weight and % bound water. The fiber sources reduced the subjective ratings of hard stools by 40% compared to the control low fiber group.
Fenn (1986) Assess the effect of psyllium on chronic constipation (UK) [56].	**Single-blind RCT:** 201 subjects; 150 females; primary outcome improvement in global symptoms; 2-weeks.	87% of subjects allocated to psyllium trial reported an improvement in global symptoms compared with 47% of subjects receiving placebo ($p < 0.001$). Also, psyllium significantly reduced abdominal pain and straining on defecation. Psyllium was twice as effective in reducing chronic constipation symptoms compared to the placebo.
Chicory Inulin		
Micka et al. (2017) Determine the effect of chicory inulin on stool frequency in healthy constipated subjects (German) [57].	**Double blind, Crossover RCT:** 44 healthy constipated subjects; 75% women; mean age 47 years; 12 g/day inulin from chicory or 12 g/day maltodextrin; 4 weeks.	Consumption of chicory inulin significantly increased stool frequency compared to placebo (median 4.0 vs. 3.0 stools/week; $p = .038$); stools were softer and there was a trend toward higher satisfaction vs. placebo ($p = .059$).

improved measures of bowel function [33]. Specifically, when baseline transit time was >48 h, each extra g/day of wheat bran significantly increased total stool weight by 3.7 g and reduced transit time by 45 min. A meta-analysis of wheat bran trials (20 RCTs; healthy and constipated subjects) showed that bran increased the stool weight and decreased the transit time in healthy controls and in individuals with chronic constipation but in constipated individuals their stool weight and transit time were not completely restored to normal [34]. A systematic review of oats products intervention studies (14 trials) suggests that in healthy subjects oats or oat bran can significantly increase stool weight and decrease constipation [39]. Oat consumption significantly increased wet stool weight in six out of nine studies (from 15 to 88% increase) and dry stool weight in five out of six studies (from 15 to 101% increase). Stool frequency did not change significantly in five studies, improved in two studies and reduced in one study relative to wheat-bran and rice-bran interventions. Transit time decreased significantly by 17% in only one out of four studies. A meta-analysis (five double blind RCTs; primarily bran and glucomannan) demonstrated that increased fiber intake significantly improved stool frequency by 19% ($p < .05$) but there was no significant improvement in stool consistency or painful defecations [24].

5.4.1.3 Prunes (Dried Plums)

A systematic review of prunes and gastrointestinal function (4 RCTs;165 participants; mean age 36–54 years; 73% women; three studies in healthy and one in constipated subjects; duration 2 weeks to 3 months; 84–100 g prunes/day; controls included grape juice, dried apples, cookies, psyllium plus water) found that in constipated subjects prunes were similar to psyllium in increasing stool frequency and improving stool consistency and in non-constipated subjects prunes softened stool consistency and increased stool weight [43].

5.4.1.4 Psyllium

A systematic review of the efficacy of soluble and insoluble fiber supplementation in the management of chronic idiopathic constipation (6 RCTs including 3 psyllium, 1 bran, 1 rye bread and 1 inulin trials) determined that psyllium was the most effective fiber in promoting bowel function [51]. Compared with placebo, psyllium reduced global symptoms (86% vs. 47%), straining (56% vs. 29%), pain on defecation, improved stool consistency, and increased mean number of stools per week (3.8 stools per week after therapy compared with 2.9 stools per week at baseline).

5.4.1.5 Prebiotics and Symbiotics

A 2017 meta-analysis (prebiotics: 5 RCTs; 199 patients; symbiotics: 8 RCTs; 825 patients) found that: (1) prebiotics, especially galacto-oligosaccharides, increased weekly stool frequency by one bowel movement/week and improved stool consistency, ease of defecation and abdominal pain and (2) symbiotics, especially fructo-oligosaccharides and probiotic combinations, significantly improved stool frequency by 1.15 bowel movements/week and consistency, and reduced gut transit time by 13.5 hours, straining defecation and bloating in patients with functional constipation [31].

5.4.2 Specific Intervention Trials

5.4.2.1 Mixed Fiber-Rich Diets

Two RCTs provide important insights on the beneficial effects of fiber-rich diets on bowel function in both regular and low caloric diets [35, 41].

5.4.2.2 Dose-Response

A US crossover, dose response RCT (9 healthy, young male students; 16, 30, and 42 g fiber/day from a mixture of fruits, vegetables and cereal grains; duration 1 month for each dose with a 15-day washout) found that mean daily stool weights increased with the amount of fiber intake; wet fecal mass was 109, 156 and 195 g for 16, 30, and 42 g fiber intake, respectively [35]. Increasing dietary fiber intake from 16 to 30 g/day increased mean stool frequency from 0.7 to about 1 per day but increasing fiber intake from 30 to 42 g/day did not further increase stool frequency. Increasing fiber intake from a mixture of plant sources tended to be as effective as consuming cereal bran but there was no improvement in stool frequency if the baseline stool frequency rate was already between 1 and 3 times per day.

5.4.2.3 Pajala Porridge

Pajala porridge containing rolled oats, oat bran, flax seeds, chopped prunes, apricots and raisins has been shown to be a well-tolerated fiber food option for elderly residents in long-term care facilities to aid in the alleviation of constipation [41]. A parallel RCT (20 adults age >65 years; breakfast porridge with 7.5 g fiber vs. breakfast without porridge; 1-week run-in; 2 weeks) demonstrated that fiber-rich porridge was effective, well-liked and tolerated and reduced the need for laxatives in geriatric patients. Specifically, the porridge group significantly improved the number of bowel movements without laxatives compared to the control group (76% vs. 23% of the time) and bowel movement discomfort was significantly 40% lower in the porridge vs. the control group.

5.4.2.4 Cereal Bran-Rich Foods

Six intervention trials assessed the effects of cereal bran-rich foods in five publications [27, 36–38, 40].

Breakfast Cereals

Three intervention trials evaluated the effect of increased wheat bran in breakfast cereal [27, 36, 37]. An open label trial (153 subjects; 81 females and 72 males; mean age 34 years; mean baseline total fiber intake 10.5 g/day; one bowel of wheat bran-containing ready-to-eat-breakfast cereal with 5.4 g/day fiber (3.5 g from wheat bran); 14 days) found significant improvements in subjective perception of bowel function (e.g., ease of defecation), digestive feelings (less bloating, constipation, feeling sluggish and digestive discomfort) and general wellbeing (feeling less fat, more mentally alert, slim, happy and energetic; while experiencing less stress, mental and physical tiredness, difficulty concentrating and fewer headaches) [36]. A parallel RCT (23 subjects; mean age 35 years; 12 women and 11 men; 4 different fiber rich breakfast cereals including All Bran or Bran Buds with fiber blends of corn and psyllium at 2.5 servings/day to provide about 25 g fiber/day added to the habitual Western diet with 12 g fiber/day; 3 weeks; 1 week washout) showed that all the fiber enriched breakfast cereals significantly improved fecal wet bulk (199 vs. 128 g/day), reduced transit times (29 hrs vs. 41 hrs), and increased bowel movement frequency (1.2/day vs. 0.97/day) compared to the low fiber control diet, while maintaining a good level of tolerance [37]. Bran cereal with psyllium was more effective than the other breakfast cereals in increasing stool wet weight for softer consistency. A 3-phase crossover RCT evaluating the effect of bran particle size (24 healthy subjects; 12 females and 12 males; mean age 36 years; breakfast cereal with 19 g fiber from wheat bran/day made from medium and coarse particle size bran vs. a low fiber cereals control; 1 month metabolic ward) showed that both medium and coarse wheat bran breakfast cereals similarly increased daily wet stool bulk compared to the low fiber breakfast cereal [27]. Smaller particle size bran fiber did not adversely affect stool bulking or frequency of bowel movements.

Breads

Two RCTs evaluated the effects of bran enriched bread on bowel function [27, 38]. A 3-phase metabolic, crossover RCT (23 healthy subjects; 12 women and 11 men; mean age 58 years; bread with 19 g fiber/day from very fine or medium wheat bran vs. a low fiber control bread; 2 weeks) found that both fine and medium wheat bran particle size enriched bread significantly increased fecal bulk by 58 to 68 g/day compared to the low fiber bread [27]. There was a small but significantly increased bowel movement frequency for the medium bran fiber bread (1.5/day) compared to the fine bran fiber bread (1.4/day) and to low fiber bread (1.3/day). This study confirms the effectiveness of bread with fine wheat bran in improving fecal bulk and laxation and also found that the fine ground wheat bran was significantly fermented to produce a significantly higher fecal butyrate concentration, a contributor to colonic microbiota health, compared to the medium ground bran. A parallel RCT (59 women with constipation; mean age 41 years; 4 diets: (1) whole rye bread (30 g fiber/day), (2) whole rye bread plus *Lactobacillus rhamnosus* GG (LGG) enriched yogurt, (3) LGG enriched yogurt, and (4) a control low fiber bread; 3 weeks) found that rye bread shortened total intestinal transit time by 17 hours, increased fecal frequency by 0.3 per day, softened feces by 0.3 units and made defecation easier by 0.4 units, but also increased gastrointestinal symptoms score (higher bloating and flatulence) by 1.6 units compared to the low-fiber toast consumed in the LGG and control groups [38]. There were fewer gastrointestinal symptoms in the rye bread plus LGG group compared to the rye bread group by 1.3 units.

5.4.2.5 Oat Bran in Soups and Desserts

A blinded parallel RCT (30 assisted living subjects; mean age 85 years; 5.1 g oat bran fiber/day vs. 0 fiber control; 12 weeks) found that oat bran blended into the daily lunch soup or dessert served in a standard diet, or incorporated into the afternoon cake significantly reduced laxative usage by 59% whereas the control group slightly increased laxative use by 8% [40]. The oat bran was well tolerated.

5.4.2.6 Fruits and Vegetables

Fruit and Vegetables: Whole vs. Juice

A crossover RCT (12 men; age range 37–58 years; weight range 68–95 kg; high fiber fruit and vegetable diet vs. a low fiber diet containing fruit and vegetable juices; 26 days; no washout) showed that the higher fiber intake from fruits and vegetables vs. low fiber juice intake significantly reduced fecal transit time (38 vs. 52 h), increased the number of daily bowel movements (1.4 vs. 1), and increased daily wet fecal weight (208 g vs. 90 g) [42].

Prunes (Dried Plums)

A crossover RCT comparing prunes vs. psyllium (40 constipated subjects; 92% women; mean age 38 years; 50 g prunes or 11 g psyllium twice daily; 3 weeks; 1-week washout) found that prunes significantly improved constipation symptoms as reflected by a significant increase in the number of complete and spontaneous bowel movements/week (Fig. 5.3) and improved stool consistency (softer stools) compared with a psyllium fiber supplement [44]. This study showed that psyllium was also useful in improving bowel symptoms in individuals with mild to moderate constipation and affirmed prior studies on psyllium in chronic constipation. The laxative effects of prunes (dried plums) are most likely due to a combination of sorbitol (14.7 g per 100 g) and dietary fiber (6 g per 100 g).

Kiwi Fruit

Three RCTs assess the effects of kiwi fruit intake on bowel laxative function. Kiwi fruit cell walls have unique viscous polysaccharides with exceptionally high swell or water binding capacity and have fecal bulking and stool softening properties similar to that of psyllium [45–47]. A 2002 crossover RCT with elderly adults (38 healthy, overweight subjects; mean age 73 years; 25 females and 13 males; 2 kiwi fruit/day vs. no kiwi fruit; 3-week duration with a 3-week washout) showed that kiwi fruit significantly enhanced laxation, including bulkier and softer stools, increased ease of defecation, and more frequent bowel movements [45]. A second RCT in constipated Chinese subjects (33 constipated

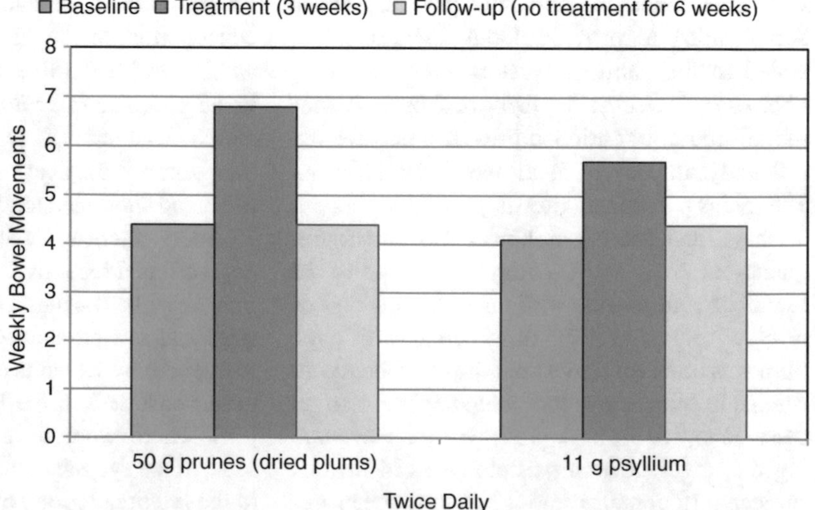

Fig. 5.3 Effect of dried prunes vs. psyllium supplement on bowel movements/week (p = .002) (adapted from [44])

subjects; mean age 50 years; 24 females; 20 healthy subjects with regular bowel movements; mean age 51 years; 16 females; kiwi fruit twice daily; 4 weeks) found that kiwi fruit significantly doubled complete spontaneous bowel movements from 2 to 4 times per week along with significantly improving transit time and satisfaction with bowel habits [46]. However, in the subjects with normal regularity, kiwi fruit resulted in no significant changes in normal bowel function. In a third RCT, subjects with a combination of irritable bowel syndrome and constipation (IBS-C) (54 subjects; 49 females; 2 kiwi fruit/day; 4 weeks) reported that kiwi fruit consumption significantly shortened colon transit time, increased defecation frequency and improved overall bowel function [47]. This study suggests that kiwi fruit (taken as a routine dietary constituent) appears to be a safe and effective natural laxative for individuals with IBS-C.

5.4.2.7 Common Fiber-Rich Food and Supplement Ingredients

Polydextrose

Three RCTs evaluated the effect of polydextrose, a common synthetic low energy, low-moderate fermentability fiber ingredient, on bowel function [48–50]. A double-blind, placebo, crossover RCT (36 healthy adults; mean age 26 years; 18 females and 18 males; 20 g polydextrose/day in muffins and cereal vs. low fiber control; 10 days with 2 weeks of washout) showed that polydextrose enriched foods significantly improved laxation activity compared with low fiber control foods (Fig. 5.4) [48]. This study shows that the addition of 20 g polydextrose in foods is well tolerated and has moderate laxative effects. Similar findings were observed for consuming 21 g/day of polydextrose in a snack bar compared to a no fiber control snack bar [49]. A triple-blind, parallel RCT (50 constipated Japanese hemodialysis patients; mean age 65 years; 60% with diabetes; 34 men and 16 women; 10 g polydextrose/day in foods vs. control; 4 weeks) demonstrated that polydextrose significantly improved stool frequency, softened the stool, and improved ease of defecation, without inducing adverse gastrointestinal effects (Fig. 5.5) [50].

Psyllium

Five RCTs support psyllium's effectiveness as a relatively low fermentable, stool bulking gel in promoting laxation and alleviating chronic constipation [52–56]. A double-blind placebo controlled RCT (60 adults with chronic constipation; 65% women; 10 g psyllium daily; 2 weeks) found that 87% of individuals receiving psyllium vs. only 30% of those in the placebo group had normal bowel movement frequency ($p < 0.001$) [52]. The other psyllium RCTs all showed similar effects in relieving chronic constipation [53–56]. These trials consistently

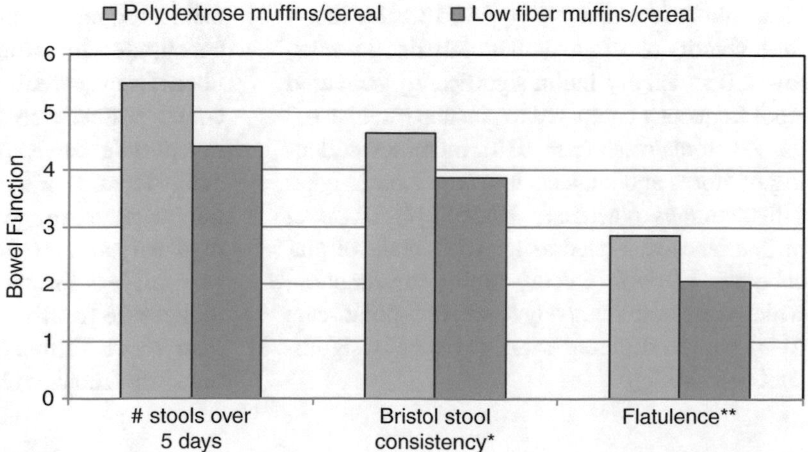

Fig. 5.4 Effect of adding 20 g/day polydextrose in the diet vs. low fiber diet ($p < .05$ for all) (adapted from [48]). * 1 (separate hard lumps) and 7 (entirely liquid) and ** 0 (none) and 10 (extreme)

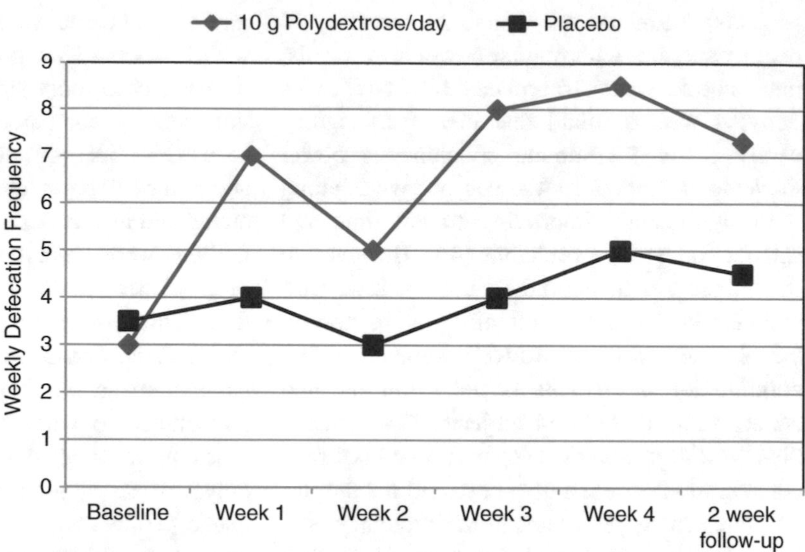

Fig. 5.5 Laxative effects of polydextrose based jelly intake on 50 constipated Japanese hemodialysis outpatients (51–79 years of age) ($p < 0.05$) (adapted from [50])

show that psyllium improved the stool frequency and softness as well as improving global symptoms including stool consistency, and reducing pain and straining on defecation in individuals with constipation. In a comparison study of psyllium and wheat bran, psyllium was shown to be more effective than wheat bran at increasing stool water (softening) and overall stool weight but wheat bran was more effective in speeding up fecal transit time verses a low fiber control [54].

Chicory Inulin

A 2017 German double blind, placebo controlled, cross-over RCT (44 healthy constipated subjects; 75% women; mean age 47 years; 12 g/day inulin from chicory or 12 g/day maltodextrin; 4 weeks) found that chicory inulin significantly increased stool frequency compared to placebo (median 4.0 vs. 3.0 stools/week ($p = .038$), increased softening of stools and subjects trended toward higher satisfaction vs. placebo ($p = .059$) [57]. The level of flatulence was rated as 1.1 with intake of placebo vs. 1.9 with chicory inulin consumption, which were both relatively low on a 5-point scale (0–4) but the difference was statistically significant ($p < 0.001$).

Conclusions

Globally constipation is a common complaint, especially among elderly adults, which affects most people at some time in their lives. The consumption of adequate fiber (>25 g/day or 14 g/1,000 kcals), recommended fluid intake, and regular physical activity, are especially beneficial in preventing and alleviating constipation. Fiber mechanisms are associated with improved laxation by increasing: stool weight and bulk (through fiber's physical volume and water holding capacity), microbiota numbers and volume, and gas volume trapped in the stool to increase bowel movement frequency and quality, especially in constipated individuals. Adequate intake of fiber from cereal, fruits, vegetables and common fiber-rich food ingredients including polydextrose, psyllium, chicory inulin and prebiotics or symbiotics have the potential to increase population-wide levels of regularity and provide constipation relief. In general, less fermentable dietary fiber tends to increase fecal weight to a greater amount than more fermentable fibers. For wheat bran, the most widely studied fiber, when baseline transit time was >48 h, each extra g/day of wheat bran significantly increased total stool weight by 3.7 g and reduced transit time by 45 min. Increased fiber intake did not change transit time in individuals with an initial time of <48 h. However, in people with an initial transit time ≥48 h, transit time was reduced by approximately 30 min per gram of cereal, fruit or vegetable fiber, regardless of fermentability. Several RCTs suggest that daily intake of prunes (dried plums) and/or kiwi fruit can help in relieving constipation symptoms similarly to psyllium.

Appendix A: Fifty High Fiber Whole or Minimally Processed Plant Foods Ranked by Amount of Fiber per Standard Food Portion Size

Food	Standard portion size	Dietary fiber (g)	Calories (kcal)	Energy density (calories/g)
High fiber bran ready-to-eat-cereal	1/3–3/4 cup (30 g)	9.1–14.3	60–80	2.0–2.6
Navy beans, cooked	1/2 cup cooked (90 g)	9.6	127	1.4
Small white beans, cooked	1/2 cup (90 g)	9.3	127	1.4
Shredded wheat ready-to-eat cereal	1–1 1/4 cup (50-60 g)	5.0–9.0	155–220	3.2–3.7
Black bean soup, canned	1/2 cup (130 g)	8.8	117	0.9
French beans, cooked	1/2 cup (90 g)	8.3	114	1.3
Split peas, cooked	1/2 cup (100 g)	8.2	114	1.1
Chickpeas (Garbanzo) beans, canned	1/2 cup (120 g)	8.1	176	1.4
Lentils, cooked	1/2 cup (100 g)	7.8	115	1.2
Pinto beans, cooked	1/2 cup (90 g)	7.7	122	1.4
Black beans, cooked	1/2 cup (90 g)	7.5	114	1.3
Artichoke, global or French, cooked	1/2 cup (84 g)	7.2	45	0.5
Lima beans, cooked	1/2 cup (90 g)	6.6	108	1.2
White beans, canned	1/2 cup (130 g)	6.3	149	1.1
Wheat bran flakes ready-to-eat cereal	3/4 cup (30 g)	4.9–5.5	90–98	3.0–3.3
Pear with skin	1 medium (180 g)	5.5	100	0.6
Pumpkin seeds. Whole, roasted	1 ounce (about 28 g)	5.3	126	4.5
Baked beans, canned, plain	1/2 cup (125 g)	5.2	120	1.0
Soybeans, cooked	1/2 cup (90 g)	5.2	150	1.7
Plain rye wafer crackers	2 wafers (22 g)	5.0	73	3.3
Avocado, Hass	1/2 fruit (68 g)	4.6	114	1.7
Apple, with skin	1 medium (180 g)	4.4	95	0.5
Green peas, cooked (fresh, frozen, canned)	1/2 cup (80 g)	3.5–4.4	59–67	0.7–0.8
Refried beans, canned	1/2 cup (120 g)	4.4	107	0.9
Mixed vegetables, cooked from frozen	1/2 cup (45 g)	4.0	59	1.3
Raspberries	1/2 cup (65 g)	3.8	32	0.5
Blackberries	1/2 cup (65 g)	3.8	31	0.4
Collards, cooked	1/2 cup (95 g)	3.8	32	0.3
Soybeans, green, cooked	1/2 cup (75 g)	3.8	127	1.4
Prunes, pitted, stewed	1/2 cup (125 g)	3.8	133	1.1
Sweet potato, baked	1 medium (114 g)	3.8	103	0.9
Multi-grain bread	2 slices regular (52 g)	3.8	140	2.7

Food	Standard portion size	Dietary fiber (g)	Calories (kcal)	Energy density (calories/g)
Figs, dried	1/4 cup (about 38 g)	3.7	93	2.5
Potato baked, with skin	1 medium (173 g)	3.6	163	0.9
Popcorn, air-popped	3 cups (24 g)	3.5	93	3.9
Almonds	1 ounce (about 28 g)	3.5	164	5.8
Whole wheat spaghetti, cooked	1/2 cup (70 g)	3.2	87	1.2
Sunflower seed kernels, dry roasted	1 ounce (about 28 g)	3.1	165	5.8
Orange	1 medium (130 g)	3.1	69	0.5
Banana	1 medium (118 g)	3.1	105	0.9
Oat bran muffin	1 small (66 g)	3.0	178	2.7
Vegetable soup	1 cup (245 g)	2.9	91	0.4
Dates	1/4 cup (about 38 g)	2.9	104	2.8
Pistachios, dry roasted	1 ounce (about 28 g)	2.8	161	5.7
Hazelnuts or filberts	1 ounce (about 28 g)	2.7	178	6.3
Peanuts, oil roasted	1 ounce (about 28 g)	2.7	170	6.0
Quinoa, cooked	1/2 cup (90 g)	2.7	92	1.0
Broccoli, cooked	1/2 cup (78 g)	2.6	27	0.3
Potato baked, without skin	1 medium (145 g)	2.3	145	1.0
Baby spinach leaves	3 ounces (90 g)	2.1	20	0.2
Blueberries	1/2 cup (74 g)	1.8	42	0.6
Carrot, raw or cooked	1 medium (60 g)	1.7	25	0.4

Dahl WJ, Stewart ML. Position of the Academy of Nutrition and Dietetics: health implications of dietary fiber. J Acad Nutr Diet. 2015;115:1861–1870.

Dietary Guidelines Advisory Committee. Scientific Report. Advisory Report to the Secretary of Health and Human Services and the Secretary of Agriculture. Part D. Chapter 1: Food and nutrient intakes, and health: current status and trends. 2015;97, 98;Table D1.8.

Slavin, J.L. Position of the American Dietetic Association: Health implications of dietary fiber. J. Am. Diet. Assoc. 2008;108:1716–1731.

U.S. Department of Agriculture and U.S. Department of Health and Human Services. Dietary Guidelines for Americans, 2010. 7th Edition, Washington, DC: U.S. Government Printing Office. 2010; Table B2.4; http://www.choosemyplate.gov/ accessed 8.22.2015.

References

1. De Giorgio R, Ruggeri E, Stanghellini V, et al. Chronic constipation in the elderly: a primer for the gastroenterologist. BMC Gastroenterol. 2015;15:130. https://doi.org/10.1186/s12876-015-0366-3.
2. Tack J, Müller-Lissner S, Stanghellini V. Diagnosis and treatment of chronic constipation–a European perspective. Neurogastroenterol Motil. 2011;23:697–710.
3. Higgins PDR, Johanson JF. Epidemiology of constipation in North America: a systematic review. Am J Gastroenterol. 2004;99(4):750–9.
4. Connell AM, Hilton C, Irvine G, et al. Variation of bowel habit in two population samples. Br Med J. 1965;5470:1095–9.
5. Bharucha AE, Dorn SD, Lembo A, Pressman A. American Gastroenterological Association medical position statement on constipation. Gastroenterology. 2013;144:211–7.
6. Bharucha AE, Pemberton JH, Locke GR III. American Gastroenterological Association technical review on constipation. Gastroenterology. 2013;144:218–38.
7. Tabbers MM, Benninga MA. Constipation in children: fibre and probiotics. BMJ Clin Evid. 2015; pii 0303. PMID:25758093.
8. Borowitz SM, Cox DJ, Tam A, et al. Precipitants of constipation during early childhood. J Am Board Fam Pract. 2003;16:213–8.
9. Wald A. Constipation. JAMA. 2016;315(2):214.
10. Wald A. Constipation: pathophysiology and management. Curr Opin Gastroenterol. 2015;31:45–9.
11. Dukas L, Willett WC, Giovannucci EL. Association between physical activity, fiber intake, and other lifestyle variables and constipation in a study of women. Am J Gastroenterol. 2003;98(8):1790–6.

12. Markland AD, Palsson O, Goode PS. Association of low dietary intake of fiber and liquids with constipation: evidence from the National Health and Nutrition Examination Survey (NHANES). Am J Gastroenterol. 2013;108(5):796–803.
13. Ford AC, Moayyedi P, Lacy BE, et al. American College of Gastroenterology Monograph on the management of irritable bowel syndrome and chronic idiopathic constipation. Am J Gastroenterol. 2014;109:S2–S26.
14. Dahl WJ, Stewart ML. Position of the Academy of Nutrition and Dietetics: health implications of dietary fiber. J Acad Nutr Diet. 2015;115:1861–70.
15. European Food Safety Authority Panel on Dietetic Products, Nutrition, and Allergies. Scientific opinion on dietary reference values for carbohydrates and dietary fibre. EFSA J. 2010;8(3):1462.
16. Committee on Nutrition, American Academy of Pediatrics. Carbohydrate and Dietary Fiber. Kleinman RE (ed). Pediatric Nutrition Handbook. 6th edition, Community on Nutrition, American Academy of Pediatrics, Illinois USA. 2009; 104.
17. Murakami K, Sasaki S, Okubo H, et al. Association between dietary fiber, water and magnesium intake and functional constipation among young Japanese women. Eur J Clin Nutr. 2007;61:616–22.
18. Wrick KL, Robertson JB, Van Soest PJ, et al. The influence of dietary fiber source on human intestinal transit and stool output. J Nutr. 1983;113:1464–79.
19. Anti M, Pignataro G, Armuzzi A, et al. Water supplementation enhances the effect of high fiber diet on stool frequency and laxative consumption in adult patients with functional constipation. Hepatogastroenterology. 1998;45(21):727–32.
20. Cummings JH. The effect of dietary fiber on fecal weight and composition. In:3rd ed. Spiller GA, ed. CRC Handbook of Dietary Fiber in Human Nutrition. 3rd ed. Boca Raton, FL: CRC Press; 2001. p. 183–241.
21. Roma E, Adamidis D, Nikolara R, et al. Diet and chronic constipation in children: role of dietary fiber. J Pediatr Gastroenterol Nutr. 1999;28(2):160–74.
22. Abdullah MM, Gules CL, Marinangeli CP, et al. Dietary fibre intake and reduction in functional constipation rates among Canadian adults: a cost-of illness analysis. Food Nutr Res. 2015;59:28646. https://doi.org/10.3402/fnr.v59.28646.
23. Schmier JK, Miller PE, Levine JA, et al. Cost savings of reduced constipation rates attributed to increased dietary fiber intake: a decision-analytical model. BMC Public Health. 2014;14:374.
24. Yang J, Wang H-P, Zhou L, Xu C-F. Effect of dietary fiber on constipation: A meta-analysis. World J Gastroenterol. 2012;18(48):7378–83.
25. Cummings JH. Constipation, dietary fibre and the control of large bowel function. Postgrad Med J. 1984;60:811–9.
26. Monro JA. Faecal bulking index: A physiological basis for dietary management of bulk in the distal colon. Asia Pacific. J Clin Nutr. 2000;9(2):74–81.
27. Jenkins DJ, Kendall CW, Vuksan V, et al. The effect of wheat bran particle size on laxation and colonic fermentation. J Am Coll Nutr. 1999;18(4):339–45.
28. Monro JA. Adequate intake values for dietary fibre based on faecal bulking indexes of 66 foods. Eur J Clin Nutr. 2004;58:32–9.
29. Tucker DM, Sandstead HH, Logan GM, et al. Dietary fiber and personality factors as determinants of stool output. Gastroenterology. 1981;81:879–83.
30. Burkitt DP, Walker AR, Painter NS. Effect of dietary fibre on stools and the transit-times, and its role in the causation of disease. Lancet. 1972;2:1408–12.
31. Yu T, Zheng YP, Tan JC, et al. Effects of prebiotics and synbiotics on functional constipation. Am J Med Sci. 2017;353(3):282–92. https://doi.org/10.1016/j.amjms.2016.09.014.
32. de Vries J, Birkett A, Hulshof T, et al. Effects of cereal, fruit and vegetable fibers on human fecal weight and transit time: a comprehensive review of intervention trials. Nutrients. 2016;8:130. https://doi.org/10.3390/nu8030130.
33. de Vries J, Miller PE, Verbeke K. Effects of cereal fiber on bowel function: A systematic review of intervention trials. World J Gastroenterol. 2015;21(29):8952–63.
34. Muller-Lissner SA. Effect of wheat bran on weight of stool and gastrointestinal transit time: a meta-analysis. BMJ. 1988;26:615–7.
35. Haack VS, Chesters JG, Vollendorf NW, et al. Increasing amounts of dietary fiber provided by foods normalizes physiologic response of the large bowel without altering calcium balance or fecal steroid excretion. Am J Clin Nutr. 1998;68:615–22.
36. Lawton CL, Walton J, Hoyland A. Short term (14 days) consumption of insoluble wheat bran fibre-containing breakfast cereals improves subjective digestive feelings, general wellbeing and bowel function in a dose dependent manner. Nutrients. 2013;5:1436–55.
37. Vuksan V, Jenkins AL, Jenkins DJA, et al. Using cereal to increase dietary fiber intake to the recommended level and the effect of fiber on bowel function in healthy persons consuming North American diets. Am J Clin Nutr. 2008;88:1256–62.
38. Hongisto S-M, Paajanen L, Saxelin M, Korpela R. A combination of fibre-rich rye bread and yoghurt containing Lactobacillus GG improves bowel function in women with self-reported constipation. Eur J Clin Nutr. 2006;60:319–24.
39. Thies F, Masson LF, Boffetta P, Kris-Etherton P. Oats and bowel disease: a systematic literature review. Br J Nutr. 2014;112:S31–43.
40. Sturtzel B, Elmadfa I. Intervention with dietary fiber to treat constipation and reduce laxative use in residents of nursing homes. Ann Nutr Metab. 2008;52(Suppl 1):54–6.
41. Wisten A, Messner T. Fruit and fibre (Pajala porridge) in the prevention of constipation. Scand J Caring Sci. 2005;19:71–6.

42. Kelsay JL, Behall KM, Prather ES. Effect of fiber from fruits and vegetables on metabolic responses of human subjects. Am J Clin Nutr. 1978;31:1149–53.
43. Lever E, Cole J, Scott SM, et al. Systematic review: the effect of prunes on gastrointestinal function. Aliment Pharmacol Ther. 2014;40:750–8.
44. Attaluri A, Donahoe R, Valestin J, et al. Randomised clinical trial: dried plums (prunes) vs. psyllium for constipation. Aliment Pharmacol Ther. 2011;33:822–8.
45. Rush EC, Patel M, Plank LD, et al. Kiwifruit promotes laxation in the elderly. Asia Pacific. J Clin Nutr. 2002;11(2):164–8.
46. Chan AO, Leung G, Tong T, Wong NYH. Increasing dietary fiber intake in terms of kiwifruit improves constipation in Chinese patients. World J Gastroenterol. 2007;13(35):4771–5.
47. Chang C-C, Lin Y-T, Lu Y-T, et al. Kiwifruit improves bowel function in patients with irritable bowel syndrome with constipation. Asia Pacific. J Clin Nutr. 2010;19(4):451–7.
48. Timm DA, Thomas W, Boileau TW, et al. Polydextrose and soluble corn fiber increase five-day fecal wet weight in healthy men and women. J Nutr. 2013;143:473–8.
49. Vester Boler BMV, Rossoni Serao MC, Bauer LL, et al. Digestive physiological outcomes related to polydextrose and soluble maize fibre consumption by healthy adult men. Br J Nutr. 2011;106:1864–71.
50. Shimada M, Nagano N, Goto S, et al. Effect of polydextrose intake on constipation in Japanese dialysis patients: a triple-blind, randomized, controlled trial. J Nutr Sci Vitaminol. 2015;61:345–53.
51. Suares NC, Ford AC. Systematic review: the effects of fibre in the management of chronic idiopathic constipation. Aliment Pharmacol Ther. 2011;33:895–901.
52. Nunes FP, Nunes CP, Levis E, et al. A double-blind trial of a celandin, Aloe vera and psyllium laxative preparation in adult patients with constipation. Rev Bras Med. 2005;62:352–7.
53. McRorie JW, Daggy BP, Morel JG, et al. Psyllium is superior to docusate sodium for treatment of chronic constipation. Aliment Pharmacol Ther. 1998;12:491–7.
54. Ashraf W, Park F, Lof J, Quigley EM. Effects of psyllium therapy on stool characteristics, colon transit and anorectal function in chronic idiopathic constipation. Aliment Pharmacol Ther. 1995;9:639–47.
55. Steven J, Van Soest PJ, Robertson JB, Levitsky DA. Comparison of the effects of psyllium and wheat bran on gastrointestinal transit time and stool characteristics. J Am Diet Assoc. 1988;88(3):323–6.
56. Fenn GC, Wilkinson PD, Lee CE, Akbar FAA. general practice study of the efficacy of regulan in functional constipation. Br J Gen Pract. 1986;40:192–7.
57. Micka A, Siepelmeyer A, Holz A, et al. Effect of consumption of chicory inulin on bowel function in healthy subjects with constipation: a randomized, double-blind, placebo-controlled trial. Int J Food Sci Nutr. 2017;68(1):82–9. https://doi.org/10.1080/09637486.2016.1212819.

Dietary Patterns, Foods and Fiber in Irritable Bowel Syndrome and Diverticular Disease

6

Keywords
Irritable bowel syndrome • Diverticular disease • Colon microbiota • Dietary fiber • Western dietary pattern • Healthy dietary pattern • Low FODMAP diets • Butyrate • Psyllium • Wheat bran • Celiac disease

Key Points

- Irritable bowel syndrome (IBS) is the most common gastrointestinal disorder occurring in people <45 years. Diverticular disease is among the most clinically and economically significant gastroenterological conditions in people ≥65 years of age. Having a history of IBS appears to increase the risk of diverticular disease in older age.
- IBS, previously called colitis, does not generally show visible structural or anatomic abnormalities, but is characterized by abdominal pain, bloating, distension, and changes in bowel habits. Celiac disease may be confounding and difficult to distinguish from IBS symptoms.
- Diverticular disease may evolve from colonic diverticulae (herniate pouches) potentially caused by high colonic intraluminal pressure which occurs in most people with aging but only approximately 20% of individuals with diverticulae develop abdominal symptoms (symptomatic uncomplicated diverticular disease). A smaller percentage of older individuals eventually develop complications such as severe bouts of diverticulitis or bleeding that may lead to sepsis and death.
- Healthy dietary patterns and low intake of fermentable oligosaccharides, disaccharides, monosaccharides and polyols (FODMAPs) may help to lower the risk and alleviate symptoms associated with IBS and diverticular disease. For IBS, psyllium is the most consistent fiber source found to help provide moderate relief of symptoms. For uncomplicated diverticular disease, fiber-rich healthy diets and low red or processed meat consumption decreases the risk, and fiber-rich diets, and foods or supplements containing wheat bran, psyllium or methylcellulose may help to alleviate diverticular disease symptoms and/or improve bowel function.
- Fiber related mechanisms that may help reduce risk or manage symptoms of IBS or uncomplicated diverticular disease are related to: (1) improved colonic health by promoting better laxation and stool bulk, and a healthier microbiota ecosystem with higher fecal ratio of probiotic to pathogenic bacteria and higher butyrate concentrations associated with lower

M.L. Dreher, *Dietary Patterns and Whole Plant Foods in Aging and Disease*, Nutrition and Health,
https://doi.org/10.1007/978-3-319-59180-3_6

colonic inflammation and improved colonocyte structure and function; and (2) reduced risk or rate of annual body weight and central abdominal fat gains (or promotion of a gradual lowering of body weight and waist circumference in overweight or obese individuals).

6.1 Introduction

Irritable bowel syndrome (IBS) and diverticular disease are both chronic and relapsing functional colonic disorders that are among the most clinically and economically significant global gastroenterological conditions [1–11]. People with IBS (and celiac disease) experience pain and disordered bowel habits that develop in childhood and young adulthood that are similar to diverticular disease symptoms which usually has onset after age 65 years. Dietary fiber (fiber) rich diets and fiber supplements have been extensively evaluated for their ability to help in both IBS and diverticular disease prevention and management. Fifty of the highest whole (minimally processed) plant food sources of fiber are summarized in Appendix A. The objective of this chapter is to review the effects of dietary patterns, low FODMAP diets and foods, especially those rich in fiber, on IBS and diverticular disease risk and symptoms.

6.1.1 Irritable Bowel Syndrome

Irritable bowel syndrome (IBS) is the most common functional gastrointestinal disorder occurring in people <45 years [1–4]. It is a chronic and relapsing functional colonic disorder that does not generally show visible structural or anatomic abnormalities, but is characterized by abdominal pain, bloating, distension, and changes in bowel habits. IBS patients often have colonic microscopic and molecular abnormalities including lowgrade inflammation and associated neuronal hyperexcitability, and microbiota dysbiosis. Previously, IBS was called colitis, mucous colitis, spastic colon, nervous colon, and spastic bowel. IBS affects 10–15% of the global population with peak prevalence in people from 20 to 39 years of age and it is twice as common in females as males [5]. Studies estimate that the IBS rate in North American children is 14% of high school students and 6% of middle school students [1, 4]. IBS accounts for as much as 12% of total visits to primary care providers with between 2.4 and 3.5 million annual physician visits for IBS in the United States alone [3]. IBS is generally diagnosed when a person has had abdominal pain or discomfort at ≥3 times a month for the previous 3 months without other disease or injury that could explain the pain [1]. The pathogenesis of IBS is multifactorial and not completely understood but potential dysfunctions that have been reported in patients with IBS include altered gastrointestinal motility, increased bloating, abnormal flatulence, colonic hypersensitivity, abdominal pain, and microbiota dysbiosis [1, 2, 5–8]. Abdominal pain is the most common symptom and often is described as a cramping sensation. Among patients about 40% of people have mild IBS, 35% moderate IBS, and 25% severe IBS [3]. IBS has four different subtypes: IBS with constipation, IBS with diarrhea, mixed IBS alternating constipation and diarrhea, and unsubtyped with a milder degree of abnormal stool consistency [1].

6.1.2 Diverticular Disease

Diverticular disease is among the most clinically and economically significant gastroenterological conditions in older people. It was virtually unknown before the expansion of low fiber diets and highly processed food in the early to mid-twentieth century [9–11]. Diverticula (diverticulosis) are colonic submucosal herniated pouches, which increase with age and occur in 5–10% in adults under 40 years, 30% by age 50 years, and 70% by the age of 85 years, but in most individuals the diverticulae remain asymptomatic showing no or few complications over one's lifetime [11–16]. Although over half of adults over 65 years old will have diverticulosis, 80% of this population remain asymptomatic or only

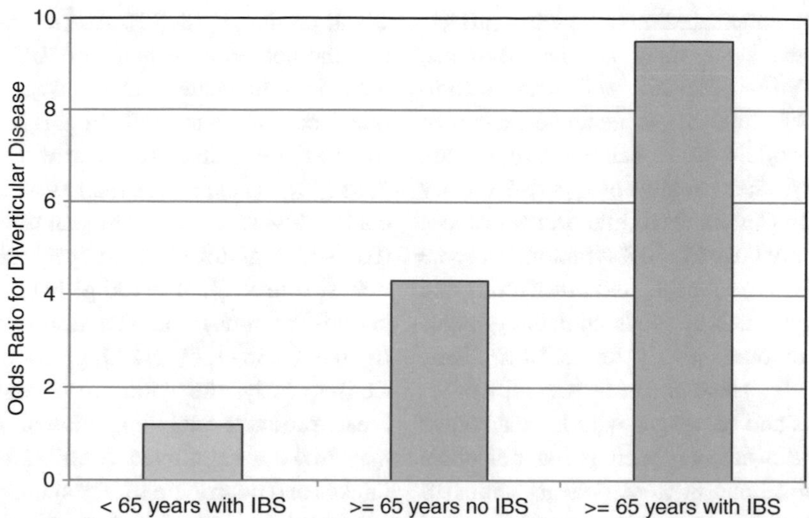

Fig. 6.1 Relation between diarrhea predominate irritable bowel syndrome (IBS) and diverticular disease risk with aging (adapted from [31])

experience infrequent, relatively minor colonic symptoms, but approximately 20% may develop abdominal symptoms (symptomatic uncomplicated diverticular disease) and, eventually, complications such as bouts of diverticulitis or bleeding [14–16]. Symptomatic uncomplicated diverticular disease is characterized by recurrent abdominal symptoms several times a year attributed to irritated diverticula, with symptoms such as abdominal pain and bloating similar to those in irritable bowel syndrome. The impact of these complaints is variable, and the severity and frequency of symptoms may range from mild and rare episodes, to a severe, chronic, recurrent disorder, impacting daily activities and the quality of life of patients. Some 15% of the patients with acute diverticulitis may have resultant complications with the development of varying levels of abscesses, perforation, fistula, peritonitis, spasms, and/or bleeding which can be associated with weakness, dizziness or light-headedness and abdominal cramping [9, 12–16]. Some of these cases may lead to emergency room visits and can be associated with sepsis or death. A meta-analysis (11 cross-sectional, 1 case-control and 1 cohort studies) found that diverticular disease can significantly increase the odds of developing colonic adenomas by 68% with a trend for increased odds of colorectal cancer by 36% [17]. In the US, complications associated with diverticular disease account for >300,000 hospital admissions, 1.5 million inpatient care days, and ≥$2.5 billion in direct costs [9–11]. The combination of an aging population, low dietary fiber (fiber) Western diets and higher intake of fermentable oligosaccharides, disaccharides, monosaccharides and polyols (FODMAPs) which are often added to processed foods, are factors that may increase the risk of diverticulosis in individuals with pre-existing colonic structural defects which potentially manifest themselves during bouts of high colonic intraluminal pressure [9, 14, 18–30]. Also, diarrhea-predominate IBS has been associated with an increased risk of developing diverticular disease, especially among people >65 years of age (Fig. 6.1) [31].

6.2 Irritable Bowel Syndrome

6.2.1 Overview of Diets and Specific Foods

Food can be a major trigger of IBS symptoms and diet management has a potentially important role in alleviating symptoms. However, there is an incomplete understanding of how food affects IBS symptoms since there are few rigorous, blinded RCTs [6–8, 32–36], so it is not uncommon for IBS individuals to generate their own theories to explain this phenomenon or seek guidance from other, usually unsupported, dietary remedies [32]. Certain foods and drinks that are: most commonly linked to IBS symptoms in some people are: beans, cabbage, and other foods that may cause gas, such as foods containing oligosaccharides or other highly fermentable fibers, foods high in fat, some higher lactose milk products, or foods and beverages with large amounts of low calorie sweeteners such as sugar alcohols [1]. Between 60 and 80% of patients with IBS report postprandial worsening symptoms and adverse reactions to one or more foods, and many patients avoid specific foods to reduce symptoms [32–35]. These symptoms tend to occur or worsen within 3 h after meal consumption in patients with IBS [33]. The relationship between fiber intake and IBS is complex and dependent on the subtype of IBS. In people with IBS-constipation, fiber can improve constipation symptoms and may help with reducing colonic pain as fiber softens stool so that it moves smoothly through the colon [1]. Fiber intake should be slowly increased with recommended levels of water to reduce the risk of increased gas and bloating and medications should be consumed at least 2 h after consuming fiber-rich meals or supplements to avoid any potential drug interactions. FODMAPs appear to increase symptoms and low FODMAP diets may improve bloating and abdominal pain or discomfort but they do not consistently improve bowel diarrhea or constipation [6, 32, 37].

6.2.2 Celiac Disease

It is difficult to clinically distinguish IBS from adult-onset celiac disease [38–40]. Both IBS and celiac disease patients can have abdominal symptoms triggered by the ingestion of wheat products. In celiac disease patients, this is due to wheat gluten intolerance, while in IBS, the effect is attributed to fructans and galactans in the wheat products [38, 39]. A meta-analysis found that the pooled prevalence of IBS symptoms in patients with treated celiac disease on a gluten free diet was up to 40%, in part because of the fructans and galactans present in gluten free diets [40]. Baked goods such as breads generally contain low to moderate in quantities of fructans (0.61–1.94 g/100 g), with rye bread being the richest source (1.94 g/100 g) [41]. Surprisingly, gluten-free bread contains similar quantities of fructan (0.36–1.79 g/100 g) to other breads. Consequently, the widespread consumption of bread products including gluten free products may make a significant contribution to fructan intakes and contribute to IBS symptoms. Despite adhering to a gluten free diet, patients with celiac disease exhibit a 5-fold higher odds of IBS symptoms compared to healthy individuals as IBS may coexist with celiac disease in some patients [33, 38–40].

6.2.3 Pathophysiology

IBS is characterized by increased susceptibility to bloating and bowel distension [42, 43]. In a study (20 patients with IBS; 20 healthy volunteers; 75% women) 90% of patients with IBS developed colonic gas retention compared to only 20% of the control subjects ($p < 0.01$). The IBS patients had excessive gas retention and impaired gas clearance from the proximal colon, as opposed to the distal colon [43]. Increased susceptibility to gas production and bloating occurs in nearly all patients with IBS, especially after the consumption of fermentable carbohydrates [42–44]. Although IBS colons generally lack visible structural or anatomic abnormalities, emerging research shows that there are colonic microscopic and molecular abnormalities from low-grade colonic inflammation and neuronal hyperexcitability, and microbiota dysbiosis. Multifactorial low grade colonic inflammation is involved in the pathogenesis of IBS with studies showing colonic microscopic and molecular abnormalities mainly characterized by an increased infiltration of mast cells [45–49]. Mast cells are innate immune cells involved in food allergies, wound healing, and protection against pathogens. Increase in the numbers of colonic mast cells in IBS patients has been related to increased colonic permeability [45]. The digestive tract contains an extensive enteric neuron network to control mucosal transport and motility and in response to persistent colonic inflammation incoming mast cells communicate with the central nervous system by release mediators such as histamine or cytokines, which can evoke neuronal hyperexcitability, a major factor for IBS pain [46–49]. Their release of various compounds, such as histamine, tryptase, and chymase can evoke neuronal hyperexcitability, a major factor for IBS pain [46–49]. Abnormalities in the colonic enteric nervous system may alter digestion, gastrointestinal motility, and cause hypersensitivity which appear to have a pivotal role in the pathogenesis of IBS in susceptible individuals [45]. Foods containing FODMAPs increase the levels of inflammatory metabolome metabolites in the urine associated with the pathophysiology of IBS [50, 51]. A single blinded, parallel RCT (40 IBS patients, 83% IBS mixed or diarrhea, 35 females, mean age 51 years; 3 weeks) found that low FODMAP diets can reduce urinary histamine 8-fold compared to high FODMAP diets [51].

Emerging research supports the link between colonic microbiota dysbiosis and the development and prolongation of IBS symptoms [52]. One of the key features of IBS is the erratic pattern of stool form, with both hard and loose stool within a time period as short as 24 h, suggesting that stool microbiota might also be unstable in IBS. It has been hypothesized that IBS may develop in predisposed individuals following an acute bout of infectious gastroenteritis, which has been linked to disturbance of the colonic microbiota with overgrowth of pathogens such as Escherichia coli, Salmonella, Shigella and Pseudomonas, 2-fold increase in the ratio of Firmicutes to Bacteroidetes and a marked reduction in diversity [52–56]. A dysbiotic colonic microbiota including increased pathogenic bacteria and decreased butyrate producing bacteria such as *F. prausnitzii* activates mucosal innate immune responses which increase colonic epithelial permeability, activate nociceptive sensory pathways and dysregulate the enteric neuromotorsensory function and brain-gut axis leading to IBS symptoms. It has been suggested that dysbiotic bowel syndrome could be another name for IBS [57].

6.2.4 Dietary Fiber

Empirical thinking suggests that increased fiber may help to promote long-term alleviation of IBS symptoms because of fiber's known ability to promote digestive health by: promoting regular bowel movements; increasing stool bulk; lowering colonic pH to protect against pathogens; supporting healthier microbiota; and controlling colonic permeability and inflammation [58, 59]. However, according to the American College of Gastroenterology monograph on IBS, the effectiveness of fiber-rich diets and supplements in relieving IBS symptoms is inconsistent as insoluble fibers such as wheat bran provide minimal relief, while some soluble fibers, especially psyllium, provide moderate relief to IBS symptoms [32]. A 2014 meta-analysis (14 RCTs; 940 subjects; 6 bran trials including 441 subjects; 7 psyllium trials including 499 subjects) found significant benefits for fiber in reducing the pooled mean IBS risk by 14% compared to a placebo, with no significant heterogeneity between studies [60]. A stratified analysis showed that bran had an insignificant effect on the treatment of IBS by lowering risk by 10%, whereas psyllium resulted in a significant 17% reduction in IBS occurance. In a 2015 systematic review and meta-analysis (22 RCTs, 1299 participants; 4–40 g fiber/day; 3–16 weeks), it was shown that fiber, especially soluble fiber, appears to have a role in improving the symptoms of IBS with a low risk of harm [41]. There was a significant improvement in global assessment of symptoms among those randomized to soluble fiber by 49% or any fiber by 27% (Fig. 6.2). Soluble fiber also reduced mean abdominal

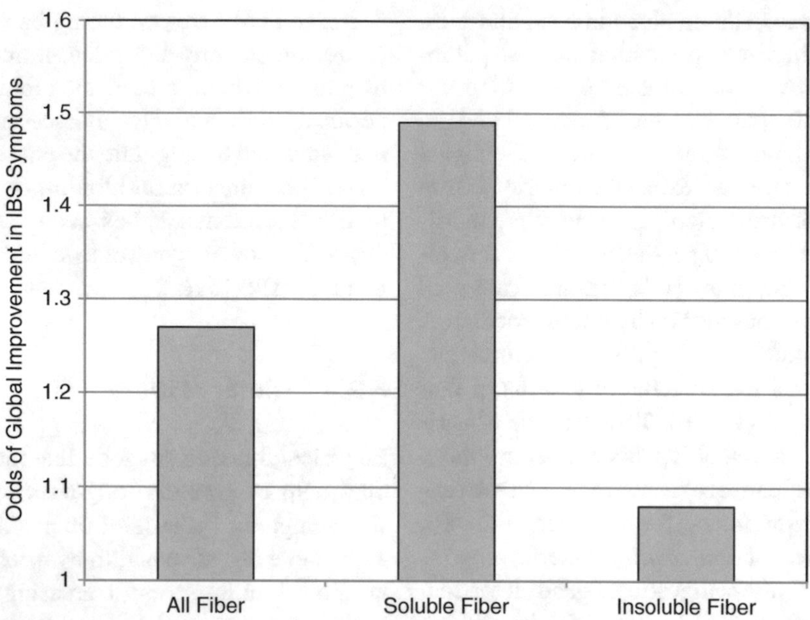

Fig. 6.2 Association between dietary fiber sub-type and management of irritable bowel syndrome (IBS) symptoms (adapted from [61])

pain scores by 1.84 units, whereas insoluble fiber did not show improvement in any outcome. The analysis concludes that soluble fiber appears to improve symptoms of IBS, whereas there is no evidence for recommending insoluble fiber for IBS. These meta-analyses identify soluble fiber, especially psyllium, if consumed with adequate water, has been shown in several RCTs to help provide varying degrees of support for alleviating IBS symptoms and promoting regularity [60, 61].

Table 6.1 provides a comprehensive summary of RCTs on the effects of fiber on IBS symptoms [62–78]. Overall, this analysis found that there is limited evidence that certain fibers have modest effectiveness in alleviating IBS symptoms without a statistically significant increase in overall adverse events compared to placebo. In a double blind RCT (275 patients in primary care; 164 completers; mean age 34 years; 78% women; 10 g psyllium or 10 g ground wheat bran added to yogurt and ingested twice daily vs. placebo yogurt with rice flour; 3 months) found that psyllium, but not wheat bran, added to yogurt was effective in the clinical management of IBS symptoms compared to the placebo (Fig. 6.3) [62]. Other soluble fibers with potential IBS protective effects similar to psyllium include partially hydrolyzed guar gum [50–52] and pectin [53]. The RCTs summarized in Table 6.1 provide evidence that psyllium is moderately effective in alleviating IBS symptoms [62–69] whereas wheat bran fiber supplementation did not improve IBS symptoms [62, 74–78]. Based on 2015 IBS global perspective guidelines and other evidence some IBS relief may be provided by the gradual introduction of a low FODMAP fiber-rich diet or with a psyllium supplement because of its soluble, stool bulking, low to moderate fermentability, along with sufficient fluids intake [79]. These dietary options have some scientific support and they are relatively inexpensive and safe, especially compared with the available drugs approved for IBS [60, 69].

6.2.5 Low FODMAPS Diets

Consumption of moderate amounts of FODMAPs by healthy individuals generally has very limited

Table 6.1 Summary of randomized controlled trials (RCTs) with specific fiber food ingredients or supplements studies and irritable bowel syndrome (IBS) symptoms

Objective	Study details	Results
Psyllium		
Bijkerk et al. (2009) To evaluate the effects of psyllium supplement for the treatment of IBS (Netherlands) [62]	**Double-blind, Parallel RCT**: 275 patients in primary care with 164 completers; mean age 34 years; 78% female; 10 g psyllium added to yogurt twice daily vs. placebo yogurt with rice flour; 12 weeks	Psyllium significantly improved relief of IBS symptoms compared to wheat bran or placebo in primary care patients (Fig. 6.3). After 3-months symptom severity was reduced with psyllium by 34% compared with 18% for the placebo (p = 0.03)
Jalihal and Kurian (1990) Assess the effects of psyllium on IBS symptoms (India) [63]	**Double-blind, Parallel RCT**: 22 patients in secondary care with 9% loss to follow-up; 20% female; 75% constipation; 30 g psyllium vs. placebo daily; 4 weeks	Psyllium significantly improved bowel satisfaction by reducing global symptoms in the majority of IBS-diarrhea subjects compared to the placebo but produced no change in abdominal pain or flatulence
Prior and Whorwell (1987) Evaluate the effects of psyllium on managing IBS symptoms (UK) [64]	**Double-blind, Parallel RCT**: 80 patients in tertiary center with 29% loss to follow-up; 90% female; 49% constipation; 3.6 g psyllium vs. placebo 3× daily; 12 weeks	Psyllium significantly improved global IBS symptoms compared to the placebo (82% vs. 53% improvement). Also, psyllium significantly improved constipation but not abdominal pain or bloating significantly
Kumar et al. (1987) Determine the optimal dose of psyllium for IBS management (India) [65]	**Dose Response, Crossover RCT**: 14 female/19 male patients; psyllium 10, 20, and 30 g/day; 14-day study; 3 days of stool collection for each dose no washout period/randomized dosing of all 3 doses for 14 days with a 1-week washout	Psyllium significantly improved 3 major IBS symptoms; constipation, abdominal pain and diarrhea. The 20 and 30 g doses were more effective than a 10-g dose but compliance was reduced with the 30-g dose. The optimum dose of psyllium in the treatment of IBS was 20 g/day
Nigam et al. (1984) Determine the effect of psyllium on alleviating IBS symptoms (India) [66]	**Double blind, Parallel RCT**: 42 patients in secondary care with no loss to follow-up; 45% female; psyllium vs. placebo; 12 weeks	Psyllium significantly reduced risk of global IBS symptoms by 38%
Arthurs and Fielding (1983) Evaluate the effects of psyllium on controlling IBS symptoms (Ireland) [67]	**Double-blind, Parallel RCT**: 80 patients in secondary care with 2.5% loss to follow-up; 78% female; 2 psyllium sachets vs. placebo; 4 weeks	Psyllium significantly reduced global IBS symptoms by 25%
Longstreth et al. (1981) Assess the effect of psyllium on IBS alleviation (US) [68]	**Double blind RCT**: 77 patients in secondary care with 60 completers; 83% female; psyllium vs. placebo; 8 weeks	Both psyllium and placebo significantly improved subjective global IBS symptoms by 70%. A strong placebo effect occurs in patients with painful IBS
Ritchie and Truelove (1979) Determine the effectiveness of psyllium on treating IBS (UK) [69]	**Double-blind, Parallel RCT**: 100 patients in tertiary care with 4% loss to follow-up; 77 women and 33 men; 2 sachets psyllium/day; 12 weeks	Psyllium significantly alleviated IBS symptoms by 42%
Partially Hydrolyzed Guar Gum (PHGG)		
Niv et al. (2016) Study the effects of PHGG on symptoms of IBS patients (Israel) [70]	**Double-blind, Parallel RCT**: 121 IBS patients with 108 completers 59% mixed, 25% diarrhea and 16% constipation IBS; 66% female; mean age 43 years; 6 g PHGG or placebo; 12 weeks; 4 weeks of follow-up	After 12 weeks, PHGG significantly lowered bloating score by 2.9 units and bloating and gas score by 3.2 units vs. placebo. The effect lasted for at least 4 weeks after the last PHGG dose. PHGG had no effect on other IBS symptoms or quality of life scores. There was a significantly higher rate of dropouts in the placebo compared with the PHGG group (49% vs. 22%)

(continued)

Table 6.1 (continued)

Objective	Study details	Results
Russo et al. (2015) Investigate the effect of PHGG on constipation -predominant IBS (Italy) [71]	**Prospective open label trial**: 86 constipated IBS subjects; mean age 37 years; mean BMI 24; 82% female; 2-week run-in baseline evaluation; 4-week intervention with 5 g PHGG consumed daily with water after breakfast	PHGG was significantly associated with improved symptom scores, stool form/ consistency, colonic transit time, and reduced use of laxatives
Parisi et al. (2002) Compare the effects of wheat bran and PHGG on IBS symptoms (Italy) [72]	**Multicenter Open RCT**: 188 patients with 59% IBS-constipation; mean age 40 years; 74% female; wheat bran diet 30 g/day vs. PHGG 5 g/day in a beverage; 12 weeks duration; after 4 weeks patients were allowed to change groups depending on symptoms	Per protocol analysis showed that both wheat bran and PHGG were effective in improving pain and bowel habits ($p > 0.05$). Intention-to-treat analysis of core IBS symptoms (abdominal pain and bowel habits) showed a significantly greater success in the PHGG group by 60% than in the wheat bran fiber group by 40%. PHGG was more effective and better tolerated than the wheat bran diet in improving core IBS symptoms
Pectin		
Xu et al. (2015) Evaluate the efficacy of pectin on diarrhea predominate IBS (China) [73]	**Parallel RCT**: 87 patients with IBS-diarrhea; 24 g pectin/day vs. placebo; 6-week intervention	In IBS-diarrhea patients, pectin significantly reduced global symptom scores, Bristol stool scale scores, and improved quality of life scores compared to placebo scores. The pectin acted as a prebiotic and no significant adverse effects were observed. Pectin appears to help alleviate symptoms of IBS- diarrhea
Wheat Bran		
Bijkerk et al. (2009) Assess the effects of wheat bran vs. psyllium supplement for the treatment of IBS (Netherlands) [62]	**Double-blind, Parallel RCT**: 275 patients in primary care with 164 completers; mean age 34 years; 78% female; 10 g ground wheat bran added to yogurt twice daily vs. psyllium and placebo yogurt with rice flour for 12 weeks	Wheat bran was less effective at relieving IBS symptoms than psyllium or placebo (Fig. 6.3). After 3 months, symptom severity was reduced for the wheat bran by 22% ($p = 0.61$) compared with 18% for the placebo. Wheat bran had insignificant benefits in IBS patients in primary care
Rees et al. (2005) Evaluate the effect of coarse wheat bran on IBS symptom management (UK) [74]	**Single-blinded, Parallel RCT**: 28 patients from tertiary center with 21% lost to follow-up; 86% female; mean age 36 years; 100% constipation predominant; 10–20 g/day of coarse wheat bran supplement added to the normal diet vs. a low fiber placebo; 8–12 weeks	Wheat bran modestly but significantly increased fecal wet weight by 28 g in 24 h compared with the placebo group. However, bran was ineffective in alleviating other bowel function measures and IBS symptoms
Lucey et al. (1987) Study the effects of wheat bran on IBS symptoms (UK) [75]	**Double-blind, Crossover RCT**: 44 patients from tertiary center with 36% lost to follow-up; 79% female; mean age 32 years; wheat bran 15.6 g fiber/day vs. placebo <0.5 g fiber/day in biscuits; 12 weeks	Wheat bran was ineffective in alleviating IBS symptoms compared to the placebo
Kruis et al. (1986) Assess the effects of wheat bran on alleviating IBS symptoms (German) [76]	**Parallel RCT**: 80 patients from tertiary center with 17.5% lost to follow-up; 62.5% female; wheat bran 15 g fiber/day vs. placebo; 16 weeks	Wheat bran significantly improved IBS symptoms vs. placebo after 12 weeks, but not after 16 weeks. The long-term effect of wheat bran vs. placebo on IBS symptoms was not confirmed

Table 6.1 (continued)

Objective	Study details	Results
Manning et al. (1977) Determine the effect of wheat bran on IBS symptoms (UK) [77]	**Parallel RCT**: 26 patients from tertiary center with 8% lost to follow-up; 46% female; 20 g wheat bran/day from bran and whole wheat bread vs. low fiber diet; 6 weeks	Wheat bran significantly improved IBS symptoms and resulted in an objective change in colonic motor activity vs. a low-fiber diet. Patients with IBS may have beneficial effects on pain symptoms with increased daily intake of wheat bran
Soltoft et al. (1977) Evaluate the effect of Miller's wheat bran on IBS symptoms (Denmark) [78]	**Double-blind, Parallel RCT**: 59 patients from tertiary center with 12% lost to follow-up; 64% women; bran 30 g/day in biscuits vs. low fiber wheat biscuits; 6 weeks	Miller's wheat bran improved subjective reported IBS symptoms by 52% compared with 65% improvement reported in the low wheat fiber control group. Miller's bran was less effective in reducing IBS symptoms than a low fiber diet

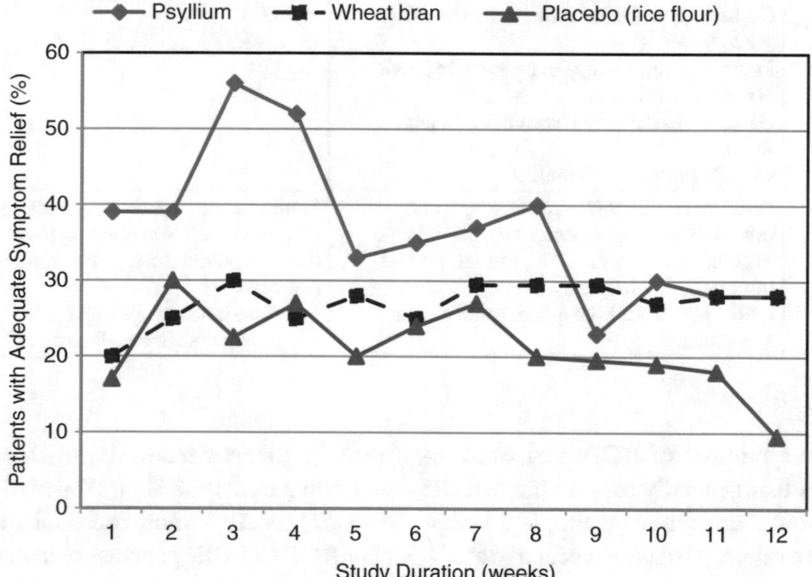

Fig. 6.3 Effect of psyllium vs. wheat bran (10 g/day each) on irritable bowel syndrome (IBS) symptom relief ($p < 0.05$) (adapted from [62])

adverse effects, but for patients with IBS they often cause IBS symptoms because they are all rapidly fermented, poorly absorbed, osmotically active and rapidly increase gas production, with additive effects contributing to IBS symptoms [6, 33]. Sources of low and high FODMAP foods are listed in Table 6.2. The validation of the effectiveness of a low FODMAP diet may involve the elimination of all known or suspected types of food with high content of FODMAPs for a period of 6–8 weeks followed by the reintroduction of individual FODMAPs to assess an individual's tolerance of each via a series of food challenges [80]. There are potential long-term challenges associated with restricting the intake of FODMAPs because it excludes a wide variety of foods from the diet, which may potentially adversely affect dietary nutrient quality and lead to colonic microbiota dysbiosis and other colonic related health concerns and require a consult with a dietitian.

Table 6.2 Potential food sources of FODMAPs (fermentable oligosaccharides, disaccharides, monosaccharides and polyols) [37, 41, 81]

Component	High FODMAP food source	Low-FODMAP food source
Fructose	**Fruit:** apple, pear, peach, mango, watermelon Other: honey or other sweeteners with fructose	**Fruit:** banana, blueberry, durian, grapefruit, grape, kiwifruit, lemon, lime, mandarin, orange, passion fruit, raspberry, and strawberry **Other:** honey substitutes (maple syrup, golden syrup)
Lactose	**Dairy:** milk (cow, goat, sheep), ice cream, soft cheeses, regular yogurt	**Dairy:** lactose free milk, hard and camembert cheese, Greek yogurt, butter **Dairy substitutes:** Ice cream Substitutes: sorbet, rice and almond milk
Polyols (e.g., sorbitol, mannitol, maltitol, xylitol, erythritol, polydextrose, and isomalt)	**Vegetable:** artichoke, asparagus, beetroot, Brussels sprout, broccoli, cabbage, cauliflower, fennel, garlic, leeks, okra, onion, peas, mushrooms, shallots **Legume:** chickpeas, lentils, red kidney beans, baked beans **Fruit**: watermelon, apple, pear, white peach, persimmon, avocado. **Cereal:** wheat and rye when eaten in large amounts **Chewing gum/hard candies**	**Vegetable:** bamboo shoots, bok choy, carrot, celery, corn, eggplant, green beans, lettuce, chives, parsnip, pumpkin, spring onion, tomato **Cereal:** gluten-free and spelt bread/cereal products
Fructans and/ or galactans	**Fruit:** nectarine, white peach, grapefruit, watermelon, longon, persimmon, cantaloupe **Vegetable:** artichoke, leeks, onions, Brussel sprouts, garlic, beet root **Grain products:** both gluten containing and gluten-free	**Fruit:** banana, blueberry, durian, grapefruit, grape, honeydew melon, kiwifruit, lemon, lime, mandarin, orange, passion fruit, raspberry **Vegetable:** most vegetables **Sweeteners:** sucrose, glucose

There are a number of RCTs and observational studies that generally support the benefits of low FODMAP diets in managing IBS symptoms but more rigorous trials are needed to establish long-term efficacy and safety. Several systematic reviews of RCTs and observational studies show that low FODMAP diets may be effective in the management IBS symptoms, especially with IBS-diarrhea [33, 81]. A 2015 systematic review of 6 RCTs on the effect of low FODMAP vs. control diets showed significantly reduced IBS symptom severity scores by 66%, abdominal pain by 81%, bloating by 75%, overall symptoms by 81% and increased quality of life by 84% [82]. The effects of seven RCTs on the effect of low FODMAP diets and IBS symptoms are summarized in Table 6.3 [44, 51, 83–87]. A single blinded, parallel RCT (40 IBS patients, 83% mixed or diarrhea predominate, 87% female, mean age 51 years; 3 weeks) showed that the IBS-symptom severity scores were significantly reduced with a low FODMAPs diet compared to a high FODMAPs diet (Fig. 6.4) [51]. A 2015 multi-center, single blind, parallel RCT (75 IBS patients, mean age 43 years; mean BMI 24; 82% female; 4 weeks) found that low FODMAPs diets had similar effectiveness to traditional IBS guidance, with regular meal pattern; avoidance of large meals; and reduced intake of fat, insoluble fibers, caffeine, and gas-producing foods, such as beans, cabbage, and onions (Fig. 6.5) [83]. A New Zealand prospective study (192 IBS patients; average age 47 years; low FODMAP diet; 84% female; 47% completers; average follow-up 15.7 months) found that IBS symptoms were significantly improved at follow-up with 72% of completers [88]. A 2017 meta-analysis (7 RCTs) found high grade evidence of an improved general symptom score in IBS patients who consumed a low FODMAP diet compared to those consuming a traditional IBS diet [89].

Table 6.3 Summary of low FODMAPs diet randomized controlled trials (RCTs) and the management of irritable bowel syndrome (IBS) symptoms

Objective	Study details	Results
McIntosh et al. (2016) Evaluate effects of low and high FODMAP diets on IBS symptoms [51]	**Single-blinded, Parallel RCT**: 40 IBS patients, 83% mixed or diarrhea predominate, with 93% completers, 87% female, mean age 51 years; low vs. high FODMAP diets; 3 weeks	Low FODMAP diet significantly reduced IBS-symptom severity scores vs. high FODMAP diet (Fig. 6.4). Low FODMAP diets significantly reduced urinary histamine levels by 8-fold but appeared to have potential adverse effects on the microbiota ecosystem in the long-term
Böhn et al. (2015) Compare the effects of a diet low in FODMAPs with traditional dietary advice in patients with IBS (Sweden) [83]	**Multi-center, Single-blind, Parallel RCT**: 75 IBS patients with 46% mixed/unsubtyped IBS; 67 completers; mean age 43 years; mean BMI 24; 82% female; low FODMAP diet vs. traditional IBS dietary guidance for 4 weeks	About 50% of patients in both the low-FODMAP and traditional IBS diet groups had reductions in IBS severity scores by ≥50 compared with baseline (p = 0.72; Fig. 6.5). Food diaries demonstrated good adherence to both diets. Low FODMAP and traditional IBS dietary advice were equally effective in reducing IBS symptoms. Combining elements from these 2 diet strategies might further reduce symptoms of IBS
Yoon et al. (2015) Examine the dose effects of FODMAP level on IBS symptoms (Korea) [84]	**Multi-center, Double-blind, Parallel RCT**: 100 IBS-diarrhea hospital patients; 84 completers; mean age 60 years; mean BMI 20; 70% male; 3 enteral diets with 1 g (low), 2.2 g (moderate), and 3.7 g (high) of FODMAPs; 14 days	Diarrhea in patients receiving low-FODMAPs was significantly improved compared with those receiving moderate- or high-FODMAPs. These results support the hypothesis that a low-FODMAP formula may reduce diarrhea leading to an improvement in nutritional status and IBS recovery
Halmos et al. (2014) Investigate the effects on IBS symptoms of a diet low in FODMAPs compared with an Australian diet (Australian) [85]	**Single-blind, Crossover RCT**: 45 out-patients with IBS with 30 completers; 43% IBS-constipation; secondary care; 70% female; median age 28 years; mean BMI 24; low <0.5 serving FODMAPs per meal diets vs. Australian diet (high in FODMAPs) and supplemented with psyllium and resistant starch; 3 weeks	IBS subjects had significantly lower overall gastrointestinal symptom scores while on a diet low in FODMAPs, compared with the usual Australian diet. Bloating, pain, and gas also were reduced while IBS patients were on the low-FODMAP diet. A diet low in FODMAPs and supplemented with psyllium and resistant starch were effective in helping to manage IBS symptoms
Pedersen et al. (2014) Investigate the effects of low FODMAP diets and probiotics on IBS symptoms (Denmark) [86]	**Unblinded, Parallel RCT**: 123 out-patients; secondary care; 108 completers; 85% IBS- diarrhea or mixed; median age 37 years; 73% female; low FODMAPs diet, probiotic Lactobacillus rhamnosus GG (LGG) supplement, and Western diet; 6 weeks	The low FODMAPs diet significantly decreased the overall IBS severity scores vs. the Western diet. LGG probiotic significantly lowered IBS symptoms but to a lesser extent than the low FODMAPs diet. Significant improvements were observed for the IBS-diarrhea and IBS-mixed subtypes only. Low FODMAPs diet and probiotic LGG are effective in controlling IBS symptoms in the IBS-diarrhea or mixed subtypes but not IBS-constipation
Biesiekierski et al. (2013) Investigate effects of gluten and a FODMAP diet on IBS symptoms (Australia) [87]	**Double-blind, Crossover RCT**: 40 IBS patients with non-celiac gluten sensitivity; primary/secondary care out- patient setting; 37 completers; 43% IBS-diarrhea, 35% IBS-constipation; median age 45 years; 84% female; low FODMAP diets, high-gluten [16 g gluten/day], low-gluten [2 g gluten/day], or control [16 g whey protein/day] diets; 1-week trial; 2 weeks of washout	IBS symptoms were significantly improved on low FODMAP diets and significantly worsened to a similar degree on regular diets including gluten or whey protein. Gluten-specific IBS effects were observed in 8% of participants. There were no specific or dose-dependent effects of gluten in patients with non-celiac gluten sensitivity placed on diets low in FODMAPs

(continued)

Table 6.3 (continued)

Objective	Study details	Results
Ong et al. (2010) Compare patterns of breath hydrogen and methane and symptoms produced in response to diets that differed only in FODMAP content (Australia) [44]	**Single-blind, Crossover RCT**: 15 IBS patients in secondary care, median age 41 years, 87% female; 15 healthy subjects, median age 23 years, 60% women; FODMAP-restricted diet (9 g/day) or a high FODMAP diet (50 g/day); 2-day trial; 7-day washout; diets were matched for total energy, starch, protein, fat and resistant starch and fiber; all food was provided to the subjects	Patients with IBS produced significantly more hydrogen gas than healthy controls while on the high FODMAP diet vs. the FODMAP-restricted diet. For IBS patients, all symptoms were significantly lower while on the FODMAP-restricted diet, including abdominal pain, bloating, passage of gas, nausea, heart burn and lethargy. The passage of gas was also significantly lower in healthy subjects while they were on the FODMAP-restricted diet. FODMAP restricted diet reduced intestinal gas and other symptoms in IBS patients compared to healthy individuals

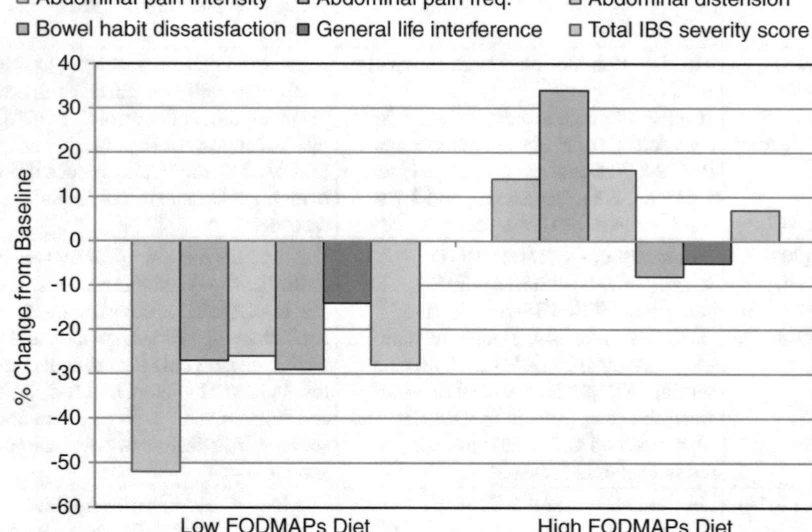

Fig. 6.4 Effect of low vs. high FODMAP diets on a range of irritable bowel syndrome (IBS) symptoms (adapted from [51])

6.3 Diverticular Disease

6.3.1 Dietary Factors

A list of specific dietary patterns and foods, and their association with diverticular disease risk are summarized in Table 6.4 [21, 90, 92].

6.3.2 Specific Foods and Beverages

Some foods and beverages historically have been linked to diverticular risk.

6.3.2.1 Nuts and Seeds

Previously there was the notion that undigested particles from nuts, seeds, and popcorn might lodge in portions of the diverticulum and hypothetically lead to diverticular disease complications, and patients were often advised in the past to avoid these foods [91, 92]. However, the Health Professionals Follow-up Study (47,228 men; mean age ranging from 51 to 60 years at baseline; mean BMI 25; 18-year follow-up; 801 incident cases of diverticulitis) observed that nuts, corn and popcorn consumption did not significantly increase the risk of

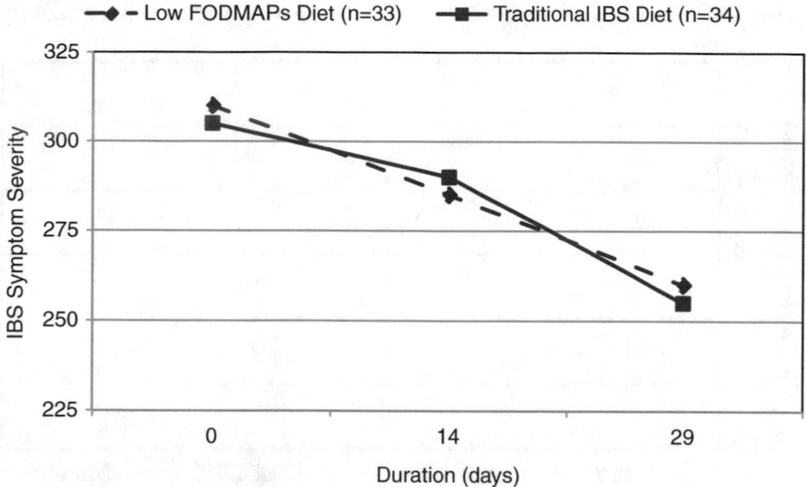

Fig. 6.5 Effect of low FODMAPs diet compared to traditional irritable bowel syndrome (IBS) dietary guidance* on IBS patient symptom severity score (p = 0.72) (adapted from [83]). *Traditional IBS dietary guidance to avoid large meals and reduce intake of fat, high lactose milk products, caffeine, and gas producing foods such as beans, cabbage and onions

Table 6.4 Examples of dietary patterns and foods associated with symptomatic diverticular disease risk [21, 30, 31]

Dietary patterns/specific foods (high intake)	Decrease risk	Increased risk
Western dietary pattern		√
Healthy dietary pattern (with adequate fiber)	√	
Beef, pork or lamb (main dish)		√
Processed meat		√
Bacon		√
Hot dogs		√
Green leafy vegetables	√	
Whole peaches, apricots, or plums	√	
Whole oranges	√	
Whole apples	√	
Blueberries	√	
Large cookie		√
Sugar sweetened beverages		√
French fried potatoes		√
White bread, cookies, donuts and so on		√

diverticulitis (Fig. 6.6) [92]. This suggests that the recommendation to avoid these foods to prevent diverticular complications should be reconsidered as these foods may actually lower risk of diverticular disease.

6.3.2.2 Coffee

Coffee consumption has not been observed to have any effect on diverticular disease [93, 94]. The Health Professionals Follow-up Study analysis (47,678 men; 40–75 years old; 4 years of follow-up) observed no association between caffeine, specific caffeinated beverages, and decaffeinated coffee and the risk of symptomatic diverticular disease [94].

6.3.2.3 Alcoholic Beverages

Among people with diverticular disease, alcoholics appear to have a 3 times greater risk of being hospitalized for diverticulitis than occasional drinkers [93]. The Health Professionals Follow-up Study analysis (47,678 men; 40–75 years old; 4 years of follow-up) observed after adjustments for age, physical activity, and energy intake of total dietary fiber and fat, that alcohol intake (comparing three standard drinks of alcohol/day to nondrinkers) was only weakly and insignificantly associated with risk of symptomatic diverticular disease [94]. When the prevalence of diverticulosis from 18 countries was analyzed against alcohol use, there was a strong correlation between diverticulosis risk and national per-capita alcohol consumption rates ($r = 0.68$; $p = 0.002$) [95]. The European Prospective Investigation into

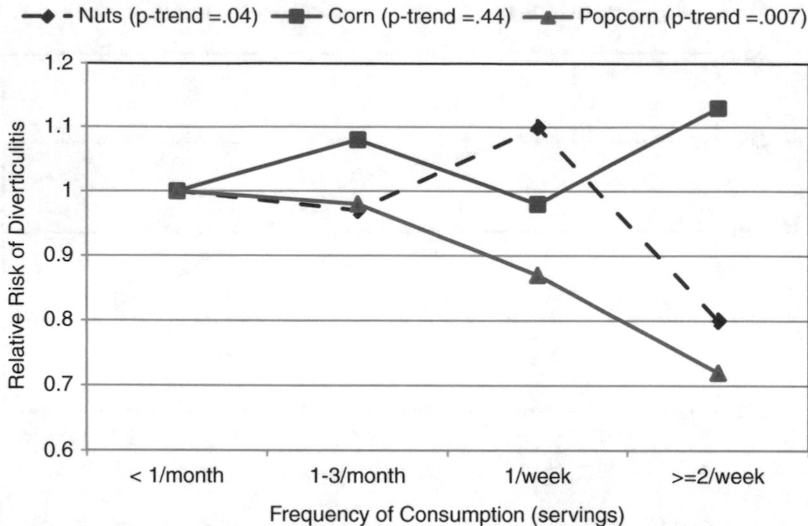

Fig. 6.6 Effect of nuts, corn and popcorn intake frequency on diverticulitis risk (adapted from [92])

Cancer and Nutrition (EPIC)-Oxford study, a cohort of mainly health conscious participants recruited from around the UK (47,033 men and women living in England or Scotland; 5459 (33%) vegetarians; mean 11.6 years of follow-up; 812 cases of diverticular disease) found that there was no significant association between the consumption of alcohol and risk of diverticular disease after adjusting for smoking [96].

6.3.3 Dietary Fiber

The National Institute of Diabetes and Digestive and Kidney Diseases (NIDDK) publication on diverticular disease indicates that the symptoms of diverticular disease may be treated with an appropriate combination of high-fiber diet or fiber supplements, medications, and possibly probiotics [97]. NIDDK suggests a (1) slow progressive increase in fiber-rich foods to minimize gas and abdominal discomfort, (2) fiber supplements methylcellulose or psyllium 1–3 times a day, along with the consumption of adequate water. A 2002 review concluded that diets high in fiber and low in total fat and red meat and a lifestyle with more physical activity might help prevent diverticular disease [98]. A 2011 review concluded that "despite the lack of high-quality supportive evidence, on the basis of low risk and theoretical benefit, a high fiber diet and/or fiber supplementation should be considered in asymptomatic diverticulosis to reduce the likelihood of disease progression and in symptomatic diverticulosis to reduce symptom episodes and prevent acute diverticulitis" [99]. FODMAPs highly fermentable fiber sources should be limited because of their risk of increasing colonic pressure due to flatulence and osmotic load, which may lead to colonic defects or diverticular disease symptoms or complications [20]. Fifty of the highest whole (minimally processed) plant food sources of dietary fiber are summarized in Appendix A.

6.3.3.1 Fiber-Rich Dietary Patterns

Observational Studies

Eight observational studies on the effect of healthy fiber-rich and lower red or processed meat diets or vegetarian diets provide insights on the risk of diverticulosis and management diverticular disease and are summarized in Table 6.5 [21, 96, 100–105].

Diverticulosis. Three observational studies assess the effects of fiber-rich dietary patterns on diverticulosis risk [100–102]. A UK case-control study (56 vegetarians for >10 years and 264 non-vegetarians; age >45 years) found that

Table 6.5 Summary of fiber-rich or healthy dietary pattern observational studies on diverticulosis and diverticular disease risk

Objective	Study details	Results
Diverticulosis		
Case-controlled study		
Gear et al. (1979) Determine the effect of fiber in vegetarian and non-vegetarian diets on diverticulosis prevalence (UK) [100]	56 vegetarians (members of the UK Vegetarian Society for ≥10 years; age > 45 years; 60% female); 264 non-vegetarians (≥ 45 years; 55% female); barium enema; food frequency questionnaire	Vegetarians had a significantly higher mean fiber intake (41.5 g/day) than non-vegetarians (21.4 g/day). Diverticulosis was significantly higher in non-vegetarians (33%) than in vegetarians (12%). Low intake of cereal fiber was associated with the presence of diverticulosis, especially for women
Cross-sectional studies		
Peery et al. (2013) Examine the link between low fiber intake and the risk of asymptomatic diverticulosis (US) [101]	539 individuals with colonic diverticula; mean age of 60 years; 1569 controls without diverticula; mean age 57 years; 60% males; mean BMI 29; mean total fiber intake 15 g/day	No association was observed between total fiber intake and diverticulosis in comparing the highest quartile to the lowest (mean intake 25 versus 8 g/day)
Peery et al. (2012) Study the association between high fiber intake and the risk of asymptomatic diverticulosis (US) [102]	878 cases of diverticulosis; mean age 59 years; 1226 controls without diverticula; mean age 54 years; mean total fiber intake 19 g/day	Higher fiber diets were not protective against asymptomatic diverticulosis
Diverticulitis/diverticular disease		
Prospective studies		
Strate et al. (2017) Examine the effect of major dietary patterns on risk of diverticulitis (Health Professionals Follow-up Study; US) [21]	46,295 men; mean baseline age 53 years; 26 years of follow-up; 1063 incident cases of diverticulitis	After adjustment for other risk factors, men in highest quintile of Western dietary pattern scores had an increased multivariate risk of diverticulitis by 55% vs. men in the lowest quintile. In contrast, men with higher prudent/healthy scores were associated with decreased risk of diverticulitis by 26–33% (Fig. 6.7). The association between dietary patterns and diverticulitis was predominantly attributable to intake of fiber (lowering risk) and red meat (raising risk)
Crowe et al. (2014) Characterize the effect of different fiber sources on diverticular disease risk (The Million Women Study, UK) [103]	690,075 women; mean age 60 years; 17,325 were admitted to hospital or died with diverticular disease; stable diet for last 5 years; mean total fiber intake 14 g/day; 6 years of follow-up	Fiber significantly reduced risk of diverticular disease related hospital admissions or death with total, cereal and fruit fiber having the strongest effects (Fig. 6.8)
Crowe et al. (2011) Assess the effect of vegetarian diets and fiber intake on risk of diverticular disease risk (European Prospective Investigation into Cancer and Nutrition [EPIC]-Oxford, UK) [96]	47,033 health conscious adults; 1/3 reported consuming a vegetarian diet; 76% female; median BMI 23; mean follow-up time of 11.6 years; 812 cases of diverticular disease	Vegetarian diets and a high intake of fiber were both associated with a reduction in diverticular disease related hospital admission or death risk. There was a significant inverse association with total fiber intake and diverticular disease risk (≥26 g/day vs. <14 g/day), after multivariate adjustments (Figs. 6.9 and 6.10)

(continued)

Table 6.5 (continued)

Objective	Study details	Results
Aldoori et al. (1998) Evaluate specific fiber types and diverticular disease risk in men (Health Professionals Follow-up Study; US) [104]	43,881 male health professionals; 40–75 years of age at baseline; 362 cases of symptomatic diverticular disease; 4 years of follow-up	Insoluble fiber was significantly associated with a decreased risk of diverticular disease by 37%, and this inverse association was particularly strong for cellulose which reduced risk by 48%
Aldoori et al. (1994) Examine the association between fiber and sources of fiber with the diagnosis of symptomatic diverticular disease in men (Health Professionals Follow-up Study; US) [105]	47,888 male health professionals; 40–75 years of age; 385 cases of symptomatic diverticular disease; 4 years of follow-up	Total fiber intake was inversely associated with the risk of diverticular disease, after adjustment for age, energy-adjusted total fat intake, and physical activity, with a significant 42% lower risk at the extremes of fiber intake; fruit and vegetable fiber were the most effective fiber sources. A high-red-meat, low-fiber diet increased risk over 2-fold compared with those on a low-red-meat, high-fiber diet

diverticulosis was significantly higher in non-vegetarians (33%) than in vegetarians (12%); vegetarians had a significantly higher mean fiber intake (41.5 g/day) than non-vegetarians (21.4 g/day) [100]. Two US cross-sectional studies (mean age of the subjects was in the mid-50s; mean fiber intake of 15–19 g/day) observed no association between total fiber intake and diverticulosis incidence [101, 102]. Scientifically, the association between diet and diverticulosis is difficult to prove because of the long latency of diverticula formation, the often lack of symptoms of diverticulosis, and the challenges of obtaining accurate dietary fiber intake.

Diverticular Disease (Diverticulitis). Five prospective studies examine the effects of dietary patterns higher in fiber and lower in red or processed meat consumption or vegetarian diets on diverticular disease risk [21, 96, 103–105]. A 2017 Health Professionals Follow-up Study (46,295 men; mean baseline age 53 years; 26 years of follow-up; 1063 incident cases of diverticulitis) found that after adjustment for other risk factors, men with highest prudent/healthy scores were associated with decreased risk of diverticulitis by 26–33% whereas men with the highest Western dietary pattern scores had an increased multivariate risk of diverticulitis by 55% (Fig. 6.7) [21]. The association between dietary patterns and diverticulitis was predominantly attributable to low intake of fiber and high red meat consumption. The UK Million Women Study (690,075 women; mean age 60 years; 17,325 were admitted to the hospital or died with diverticular disease; 6 years of follow-up) observed that fiber significantly reduced diverticular disease risk with cereal and fruit fiber having the strongest effects (Fig. 6.8) [103]. An EPIC UK/Oxford cohort (47,033 adults; 76% female; median BMI 23; 33% vegetarians; mean 11.6 years of follow-up; 812 diverticular disease hospital admissions or deaths) showed that consuming a vegetarian diet significantly lowered the multivariate adjusted risk of diverticular disease by 31% vs. meat eaters (Fig. 6.9) [96]. There was also an inverse association between fiber intake and diverticular disease with a significant 41% lower risk (≥26 g/day vs. <14 g/day) (Fig. 6.10) [96]. Two US Health Professionals Follow-up studies from the 1990s also showed similar inverse relationships between fiber intake and diverticular disease risk [104, 105].

Intervention Trials

Table 6.6 summarizes 11 intervention trials (6 RCTs and 5 open label trials) on the effects of a variety of fiber-rich dietary patterns and foods/supplement sources with adjunctive antibiotic usage on diverticular disease symptoms [106–116]. All 6 RCTs showed beneficial effects on symptoms and/or bowel function with a number of different fiber sources including fiber-rich

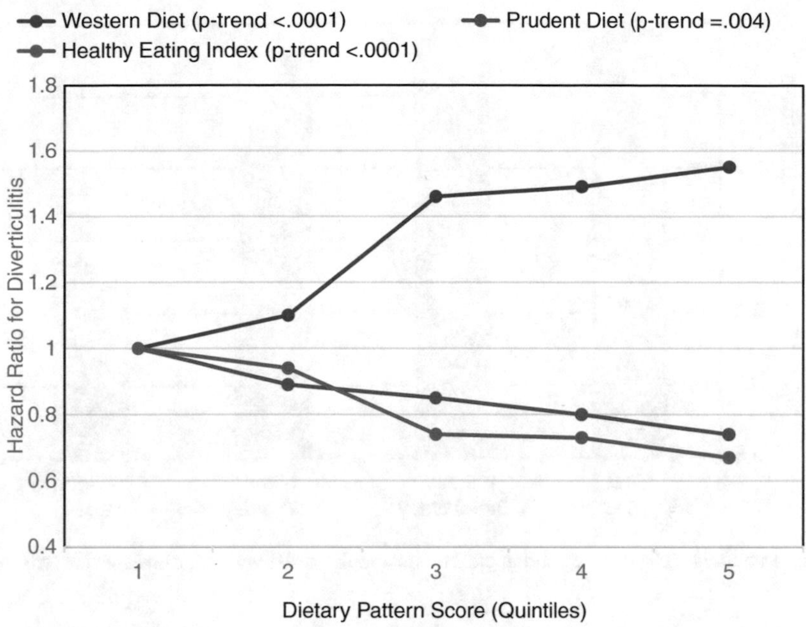

Fig. 6.7 Dietary pattern quality score and risk of diverticulitis in men (adapted from [21])

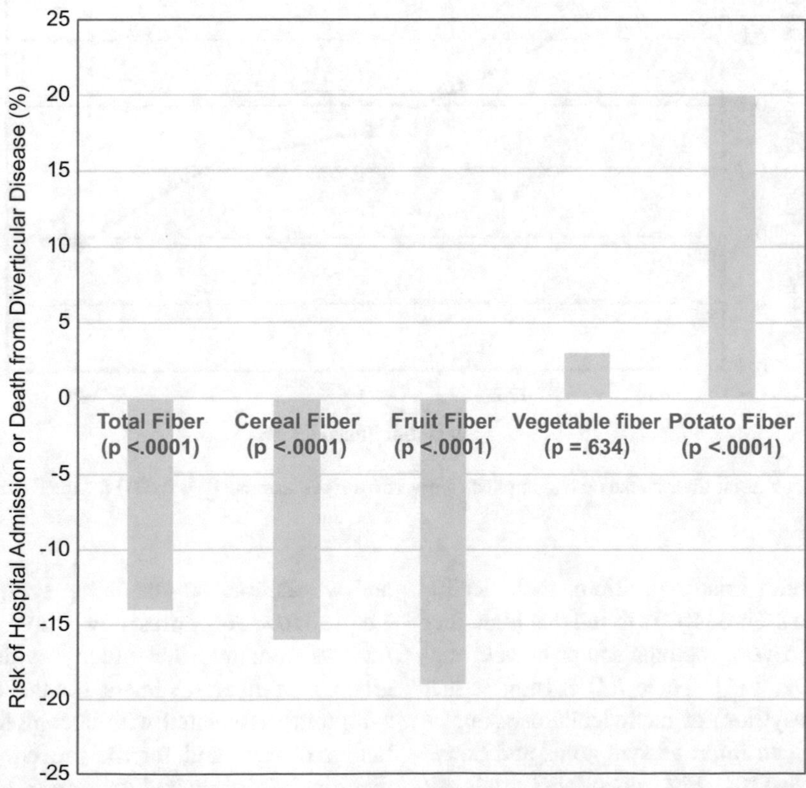

Fig. 6.8 Association between fiber intake and risk of diverticular disease related hospital admission or death risk per 5 g fiber/day intake from the UK Million Women Study (mean baseline age 60 years; 6 years of follow-up) (adapted from [103])

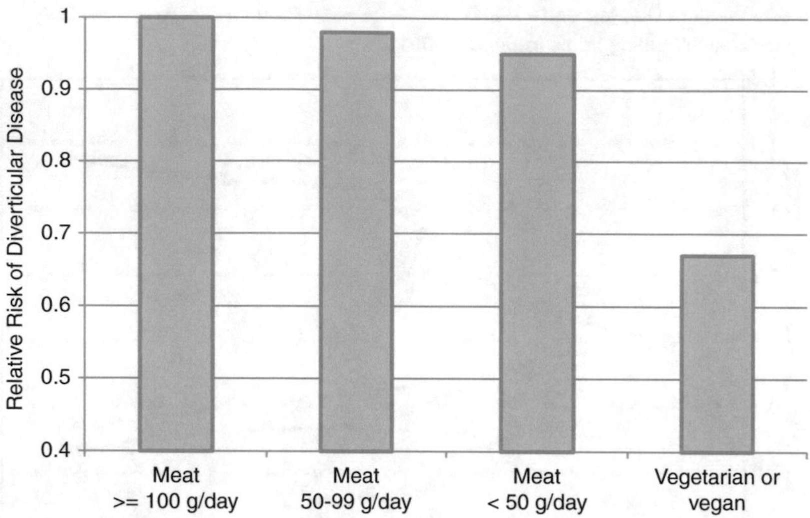

Fig. 6.9 Effect of non-vegetarian vs. vegetarian diets on uncomplicated diverticular disease risk (adapted from [96])

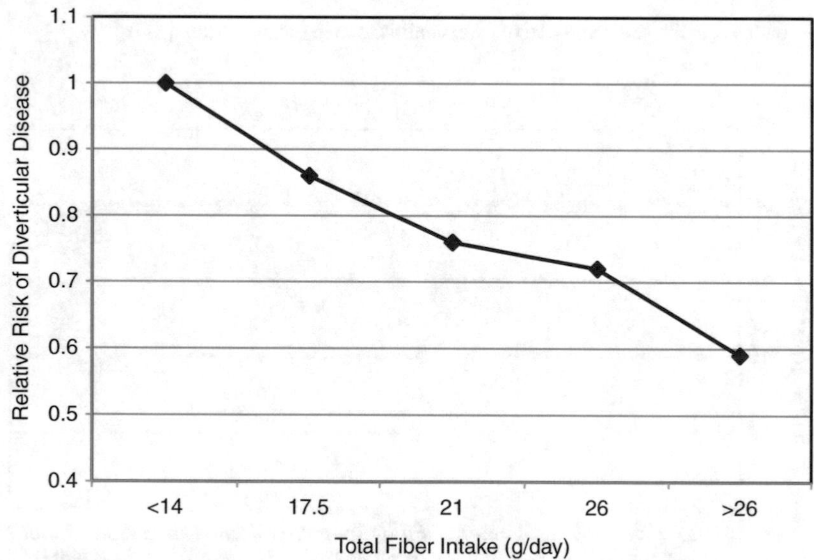

Fig. 6.10 Effect of total fiber intake on uncomplicated diverticular disease risk ($p < 0.001$) (adapted from [96])

diets, bran, bran crisps, psyllium, methylcellulose [106–111]. Three RCTs found that high fiber diets can improve symptoms and/or bowel function [106, 107, 111]. Three RCTs suggest that wheat bran, psyllium or methylcellulose supplemented diets can improve symptoms and bowel function [108–110]. Five open-label trials all support the beneficial effects of fiber-rich diets and wheat bran on alleviating symptoms [112–116]. However, presently three systematic reviews conclude that quality evidence on the efficacy of fiber treatment for the reduction of symptoms associated with uncomplicated diverticular disease and for the prevention of acute diverticulitis, is limited because of the low number of high quality RCTs [117–119].

Table 6.6 Summary of fiber-rich diet and fiber intervention trials in uncomplicated diverticular disease symptoms

Objective	Study details	Results
Randomized Controlled Trials (RCTs)		
Lahner et al. (2012) Evaluate the effects of adding a symbiotic supplement to a high fiber diet in the treatment of symptomatic diverticular disease (Italy) [106]	**Multicenter, Parallel RCT**: 45 patients; mean age 66 years; 66% female; base diet ≥30 g daily fiber plus 7 g Flortec© symbiotic formulation containing 5×10^9 CFU viable L. paracasei B12060 plus a mixture of xylo-oligosaccharides (700 mg) and arabinogalactone (1243 mg) or no supplement; ≥ 1.5 L of water/daily; 6 months	A high-fiber diet was effective in relieving abdominal symptoms. The combination of high-fiber diet and symbiotic can relieve abdominal bloating as well as abdominal pain
Smits et al. (1990) Compare the efficacy and tolerance of lactulose and a high-fiber diet in the treatment of symptomatic diverticular disease (UK) [107]	**Parallel RCT**: 43 patients; high fiber diet (30–40 g fiber daily) vs. lactulose (30 mL daily); 12 weeks	Bowel frequency and stool consistency improved similarly with both treatments. Pain on bowel movement and abdominal pain improved with both treatments in respect to frequency and severity
Ornstein et al. (1981) Compare the effects of bran and psyllium on symptomatic diverticular disease (UK) [108]	**Double-blind, Crossover RCT**: 58 patients; median age 64 years; 62% female; bran crisp bread (7 g fiber), psyllium beverage (9 g fiber) and placebo (2.3 g fiber) added to a daily habitual 15 g fiber diet; 16 weeks	The bran crisp bread and psyllium drink significantly improved symptoms of constipation when compared to the initial score. No significant differences in pain, lower bowel symptoms and total symptom scores were reported since there was only a 5–7 g difference between the test fibers and placebo
Brodribb (1977) Evaluate the effects of wheat bran on symptomatic diverticular disease [109]	**Double-blind RCT**: 18 patients; 6.7 g fiber wheat bran crisp bread daily vs. 0.6 g fiber placebo crisp bread; 3 months	Daily wheat bran crisp bread significantly decreased mean overall symptom scores vs. placebo. Although wheat bran crisp bread significantly lowered overall pain score, there were no significant differences in bowel function scores. No adverse effects were recorded
Hodgson (1977) Assess the effect of methyl cellulose on symptomatic diverticular disease (UK) [110]	**Double-blind RCT**: 30 patients; 2 tablets methylcellulose vs. 2 tablets placebo; 3 months	Patients in the methylcellulose group had significantly greater symptom decrease than those in the placebo group
Taylor and Duthie (1976) Determine the effect of bran tablets on symptomatic diverticular disease [111]	**Crossover RCT**: 20 patients; high-fiber diet, Normacol plus, and bran tablets; 1 month	Bran proved to be the most effective treatment, not only in improving the symptoms but also in returning to normal the abnormal pathophysiological changes. Bran tablets were both convenient and acceptable as well as effective
Open Label Trials		
Leahy et al. (1985) Compare the effects of higher vs. lower fiber diets on diverticular disease symptoms (UK) [112]	31 patients on high fiber diets; 25 patients; typical Western fiber diets; average follow-up 57 months	High fiber diets significantly reduced symptoms recurrence (19% vs. 44%), complications (6% vs. 20%) and required less surgery (6% vs. 32%) compared to the low fiber control group

(continued)

Table 6.6 (continued)

Objective	Study details	Results
Hyland and Taylor (1980) Evaluate the long-term effects of a high fiber diet on symptomatic diverticular disease (UK) [113]	100 patients; 75% consumed high fiber diets; 5–7 years	Of the patients consuming high fiber diets, 90% remained symptom-free
Eastwood et al. (1978) Assess the effects of different types of fiber on symptomatic diverticular disease (UK) [114]	31 patients; mean age 60 years; 20 g coarse wheat bran, 2 sachets of psyllium, and 20–40 mL/day lactulose; 4-week duration	All supplements equally alleviated symptoms
Brodribb and Humphreys (1976) Examine the effects of wheat bran on symptomatic diverticular disease (UK) [115].	40 patients; 24 g wheat bran daily; 6 months	Wheat bran decreased all symptoms by 60%, accelerated transit times in patients with >60 h, reduced intracolonic pressure. Barium enema studies showed less spasm in 8 patients and no diverticula in 3 patients after taking bran
Painter et al. (1972) Evaluate the effect of high fiber on symptomatic diverticular disease (UK) [116]	70 patients; 86% completers; high-fiber, low-sugar diet including unprocessed bran; average 22 months	89% of patients had relieved symptoms and none of the completers required surgery

6.3.3.2 Fiber Mechanisms

Fiber is known for its effects on promoting colonic health and weight control, which may contribute to reducing diverticular disease risk through a number of biological mechanisms [58, 120–125].

Colonic Health

Fiber may improve colonic health to reduce diverticular disease risk by two primary mechanisms: (1) promoting stool bulk and regular laxation and (2) maintaining a healthy colonic microbiota ecosystem [126–132]. Consistent with the original fiber hypothesis on diverticular disease, fiber promotes laxation by increasing fecal bulk and stool frequency, and reducing intestinal transit time by increasing fecal water-holding capacity, and improves the quantity and quality of microbiota for overall colonic health. Fiber sources that combine low fermentability and high water binding capacity from fiber-rich diets containing a variety of whole or minimally processed plant foods or from wheat bran, psyllium fiber, and methylcellulose containing foods or supplements are particularly effective in promoting laxation [58, 120–128]. In a 1988 RCT both wheat bran and psyllium husk fiber were shown to decrease transit time and increase daily stool regularity as well as promote healthier stool weights and structure, compared to low fiber controls [125]. Wheat bran was more effective at reducing transit time and psyllium was more effective at increasing stool water content (softer stools) and weight. A systematic review of 65 intervention studies found that wheat bran, improves bowel function by significantly increasing total wet stool weight by 3.7 g/gram intact wheat fiber and reduces transit time by 45 min/g when baseline transit time is greater than 48 h [126]. Furthermore, alterations in colonic microbiota composition related to low fiber Western diets can have an adverse effect on colonic health especially with aging, leading to increased incidence of colonic dysbiosis whereas the consumption of adequate fiber can lower the colonic lumen pH, increase the balance of healthy metabolites and inhibit the growth of pathogenic bacteria and colonic inflammation [127–132]. Bacterial fermentation of fiber to maintain an adequate colonic butyrate concentration is critical for maintaining distal colonic health. Butyrate exerts potent effects on a variety of colonic mucosal functions such as inhibition of inflammation by reinforcing various components of the colonic defense barrier and the inhibition of nuclear factor kappa B (NF-κβ) activation and histone deacetylation, and the activation of G-coupled receptors.

Body Weight Regulation

Obesity increases the risk of diverticular disease and its complications [133–136]. An increased BMI has been linked to an elevated risk for symptomatic diverticular disease and its complications with central obesity as an independent risk factor due to the release of proinflammatory cytokines from the visceral fat [133]. The Health Professionals Follow-up Study (47,228 men; baseline age range 40–75; 18 years of follow-up; 801 cases of diverticulitis) found that men with a BMI > 30 had increased risk of diverticulitis by 78% and >300% higher risk for diverticular hemorrhage compared to men with a normal BMI [135]. A Swedish prospective cohort (36,592 women; 12 years of follow-up) showed that women with an overweight or obese BMI had a higher risk of diverticular disease by 30% and a 200% higher risk of a colonic abscess or perforation compared to women with a normal BMI (20–24.9) [136]. Populations with fiber-rich diets tend to be leaner than those with low fiber diets [137–143]. In the Nurses' Health Study, women in the highest quintile of fiber intake had a significant 49% lower risk of major weight gain than women in the lowest quintile. Weight gain was inversely associated with the intake of high-fiber and whole-grain foods [139]. A systematic review of 43 prospective cohort, case-control and randomized trials found probable evidence that increased fiber intake was predictive of less weight gain and higher intake of refined grains, sweets and desserts, and high energy diets were predictive of elevated weight gain and waist size [140]. A Finnish Trial of overweight middle-aged men and women showed that lower dietary fat and higher fiber intake are significant predictors of sustained weight reduction, even after adjustment for other risk factors [141]. A long-term RCT suggests that consuming >30 g fiber/day can effectively promote weight loss similarly to that of reduced energy diet regimens [142]. After weight loss is achieved, healthy fiber rich dietary patterns, can slow weight regain to maintain a 4–10 kg weight loss after 1 year and 3–4 kg after 2 years [143].

Conclusions

Irritable bowel syndrome (IBS) is the most common gastrointestinal disorder occurring in people <45 years. Diverticular disease is among the most clinically and economically significant gastroenterological conditions in people ≥65 years of age. Having a history of IBS appears to increase the risk of diverticular disease in older age. IBS, previously called colitis, does not generally show visible structural or anatomic abnormalities, but is characterized by abdominal pain, bloating, distension, and changes in bowel habits. Celiac disease may be confounding and difficult to distinguish from IBS symptoms. Diverticular disease may evolve from colonic diverticulae (herniate pouches) potentially caused by high colonic intraluminal pressure which occurs in most people with aging but only approximately 20% of individuals with diverticulae develop abdominal symptoms (symptomatic uncomplicated diverticular disease). A smaller percentage of older individuals eventually develop complications such as severe bouts of diverticulitis or bleeding that may lead to sepsis and death. Healthy dietary patterns and low intake of FODMAPs may help to lower the risk and alleviate symptoms associated with IBS and diverticular disease. For IBS, psyllium is the fiber source most consistently found to help provide moderate relief of symptoms. For uncomplicated diverticular disease, fiber-rich healthy diets and low red or processed meat consumption decrease the risk, and fiber-rich diets, and foods or supplements containing wheat bran, psyllium or methylcellulose may help to alleviate diverticular disease symptoms and/or improve bowel function. Fiber related mechanisms that may help reduce risk or manage symptoms of IBS or uncomplicated diverticular disease are related to: (1) improved colonic health by promoting better laxation and stool bulk, and a healthier microbiota ecosystem with higher fecal ratio of probiotic to pathogenic bacteria, and higher butyrate concentration associated with lower colonic inflammation and improved colonocyte structure and function, and (2) reduced risk or rate of annual body weight and central abdominal fat gains (or promotion of a gradual lowering of body weight and waist size in overweight or obese individuals).

Appendix A: Fifty high fiber whole or minimally processed plant foods ranked by amount of fiber per standard food portion size

Food	Standard portion size	Dietary fiber (g)	Calories (kcal)	Energy density (calories/g)
High fiber bran ready-to-eat-cereal	1/3–3/4 cup (30 g)	9.1–14.3	60–80	2.0–2.6
Navy beans, cooked	1/2 cup cooked (90 g)	9.6	127	1.4
Small white beans, cooked	1/2 cup (90 g)	9.3	127	1.4
Shredded wheat ready-to-eat cereal	1–1 1/4 cup (50–60 g)	5.0–9.0	155–220	3.2–3.7
Black bean soup, canned	1/2 cup (130 g)	8.8	117	0.9
French beans, cooked	1/2 cup (90 g)	8.3	114	1.3
Split peas, cooked	1/2 cup (100 g)	8.2	114	1.1
Chickpeas (Garbanzo) beans, canned	1/2 cup (120 g)	8.1	176	1.4
Lentils, cooked	1/2 cup (100 g)	7.8	115	1.2
Pinto beans, cooked	1/2 cup (90 g)	7.7	122	1.4
Black beans, cooked	1/2 cup (90 g)	7.5	114	1.3
Artichoke, global or French, cooked	1/2 cup (84 g)	7.2	45	0.5
Lima beans, cooked	1/2 cup (90 g)	6.6	108	1.2
White beans, canned	1/2 cup (130 g)	6.3	149	1.1
Wheat bran flakes ready-to-eat cereal	3/4 cup (30 g)	4.9–5.5	90–98	3.0–3.3
Pear with skin	1 medium (180 g)	5.5	100	0.6
Pumpkin seeds. Whole, roasted	1 ounce (about 28 g)	5.3	126	4.5
Baked beans, canned, plain	1/2 cup (125 g)	5.2	120	0.9
Soybeans, cooked	1/2 cup (90 g)	5.2	150	1.7
Plain rye wafer crackers	2 wafers (22 g)	5.0	73	3.3
Avocado, Hass	1/2 fruit (68 g)	4.6	114	1.7
Apple, with skin	1 medium (180 g)	4.4	95	0.5
Green peas, cooked (fresh, frozen, canned)	1/2 cup (80 g)	3.5–4.4	59–67	0.7–0.8
Refried beans, canned	1/2 cup (120 g)	4.4	107	0.9
Mixed vegetables, cooked from frozen	1/2 cup (45 g)	4.0	59	1.3
Raspberries	1/2 cup (65 g)	3.8	32	0.5
Blackberries	1/2 cup (65 g)	3.8	31	0.4
Collards, cooked	1/2 cup (95 g)	3.8	32	0.3
Soybeans, green, cooked	1/2 cup (75 g)	3.8	127	1.4
Prunes, pitted, stewed	1/2 cup (125 g)	3.8	133	1.1
Sweet potato, baked	1 medium (114 g)	3.8	103	0.9
Multi-grain bread	2 slices regular (52 g)	3.8	140	2.7
Figs, dried	1/4 cup (about 38 g)	3.7	93	2.5
Potato baked, with skin	1 medium (173 g)	3.6	163	0.9
Popcorn, air-popped	3 cups (24 g)	3.5	93	3.9
Almonds	1 ounce (about 28 g)	3.5	164	5.8
Whole wheat spaghetti, cooked	1/2 cup (70 g)	3.2	87	1.2

Food	Standard portion size	Dietary fiber (g)	Calories (kcal)	Energy density (calories/g)
Sunflower seed kernels, dry roasted	1 ounce (about 28 g)	3.1	165	5.8
Orange	1 medium (130 g)	3.1	69	0.5
Banana	1 medium (118 g)	3.1	105	0.9
Oat bran muffin	1 small (66 g)	3.0	178	2.7
Vegetable soup	1 cup (245 g)	2.9	91	0.4
Dates	1/4 cup (about 38 g)	2.9	104	2.8
Pistachios, dry roasted	1 ounce (about 28 g)	2.8	161	5.7
Hazelnuts or filberts	1 ounce (about 28 g)	2.7	178	6.3
Peanuts, oil roasted	1 ounce (about 28 g)	2.7	170	6.0
Quinoa, cooked	1/2 cup (90 g)	2.7	92	1.0
Broccoli, cooked	1/2 cup (78 g)	2.6	27	0.3
Potato baked, without skin	1 medium (145 g)	2.3	145	1.0
Baby spinach leaves	3 ounces (90 g)	2.1	20	0.2
Blueberries	1/2 cup (74 g)	1.8	42	0.6
Carrot, raw or cooked	1 medium (60 g)	1.7	25	0.4

Dahl WJ, Stewart ML. Position of the Academy of Nutrition and Dietetics: health implications of dietary fiber. J Acad Nutr Diet. 2015;115:1861–70

Dietary Guidelines Advisory Committee. Scientific Report. Advisory Report to the Secretary of Health and Human Services and the Secretary of Agriculture. Part D. Chapter 1: Food and nutrient intakes, and health: current status and trends. 2015;97, 98; Table D1.8

Slavin JL. Position of the American Dietetic Association: health implications of dietary fiber. J Am Diet Assoc. 2008;108:1716–31

U.S. Department of Agriculture and U.S. Department of Health and Human Services. Dietary Guidelines for Americans, 2010. 7th ed. Washington, DC: U.S. Government Printing Office. 2010; Table B2.4; http://www.choosemyplate.gov/. Accessed 22 Aug 2015

References

1. National Institute of Diabetes and Digestive and Kidney Diseases. Definition and facts for irritable bowel syndrome. 2015. http://www.niddk.nih.gov/health-information/health-topics/digestive-diseases/irritable-bowel-syndrome/Pages/definition-facts.aspx www.digestive.niddk.nih.gov. Accessed 6 Jul 2016.
2. Wilkins T, Pepitone C, Alex B, Schade RR. Diagnosis and management of IBS in adults. Am Fam Physician. 2012;86(5):419–26.
3. International Foundation for Functional Gastrointestinal Disorders. Statistics. 2016. http://aboutibs.org/facts-about-ibs/statistics.html. Accessed 6 Jul 2016.
4. Lovell RM, Ford AC. Global prevalence of and risk factors for irritable bowel syndrome: a meta-analysis. Clin Gastroenterol Hepatol. 2012;10:712–21.
5. Lovell RM, Ford AC. Effect of gender on prevalence of irritable bowel syndrome in the community: systematic review and meta-analysis. Am J Gastroenterol. 2012;107:991–1000.
6. Staudacher HM, Irving PM, Lomer MCE, Whelan K. Mechanisms and efficacy of dietary FODMAP restriction in IBS. Nat Rev Gastroenterol Hepatol. 2014;1(4):256–66.
7. El-Salhy M, Ostgaardi H, Gundersen D. The role of diet in the pathogenesis and management of irritable bowel syndrome (review). Int J Mol Med. 2012;29:723–31.
8. Barbara G, Cremon C, Carini G, et al. The immune system in irritable bowel syndrome. J Neurogastroenterol Motil. 2011;17:349–59.
9. Tursi A. Diverticulosis today: unfashionable and still under-researched. Ther Adv Gastroenterol. 2016;9(2):213–28.
10. Templeton AW, Strate LL. Updates in diverticular disease. Curr Gastroenterol Rep. 2013;15(8):339–46.
11. Jacobs DO. Diverticulitis. N Engl J Med. 2007;357:2057–66.
12. Tursi A, Papagrigoriadis S. Review article: the current and evolving treatment of colonic diverticular disease. Aliment Pharmacol Ther. 2009;30:532–46.
13. Tursi A. Diverticular disease: a therapeutic overview. World J Gastrointest Pharmacol Ther. 2010;1(1):27–35.

14. Tursi A, Papa A, Danese S. Review article: the pathophysiology and medical management of diverticulosis and diverticular disease of the colon. Aliment Pharmacol Ther. 2015;42:664–84.
15. Muhammad A, Lamendola O, Daas A, et al. Association between colonic diverticulosis and prevalence of colorectal polyps. Int J Color Dis. 2014;29(8):947–51.
16. Cuomo R, Barbara G, Andreozzi P, et al. Symptom patterns can distinguish diverticular disease from irritable bowel syndrome. Eur J Clin Investig. 2013;43(11):1147–55.
17. Jaruvongvanich V, Sanguankeo A, Wijarnpreecha K, Upala S. Risk of colorectal adenomas, advanced adenomas and cancer in patients with colonic diverticular disease: Systematic review and meta-analysis. Dig Endosc. 2017;29:71–82. https://doi.org/10.1111/den12701.
18. Painter NS, Burkitt DP. Diverticular disease of the colon: a deficiency disease of western civilization. BMJ. 1971;2:450–4.
19. Reinhard T. Diverticular disease—a reexamination of the fiber hypothesis. Today's Dietitian. 2014;16(3):46.
20. Uno Y, Velkinburgh JC. Logical hypothesis: low FODMAP diet to prevent diverticulitis. World J Gastrointest Pharmacol Ther. 2016;7(4):503–12.
21. Strate LL, Keeley BR, Cao Y, et al. Western dietary pattern increases and prudent dietary pattern decreases, risk of incident diverticulitis in a prospective cohort study. Gastroenterology. 2017;152(5):1023–30. https://doi.org/10.1053/jgastro.2016.12.038.
22. Commane DM, Arasaradnam RP, Mills S, et al. Diet, ageing and genetic factors in the pathogenesis of diverticular disease. World J Gastroenterol. 2009;15(20):2479–88.
23. Wilkins T, Embey K, George R. Diagnosis and management of acute diverticulitis. Am Fam Physician. 2013;87(9):612–20.
24. Wick JY. Diverticular disease: eat your fiber? Consult Pharm. 2012;27(9):613–8.
25. Aldoori W, Ryan-Harshman M. Preventing diverticular disease. Review of recent evidence on high-fibre diets. Can Fam Physician. 2002;48:1632–7.
26. Sheth AA, Longo W, Floch MH. Diverticular disease and diverticulitis. Am J Gastroenterol. 2008;103:1550–6.
27. Tursi A, Elisei W, Picchio M, et al. Moderate to severe and prolonged left lower-abdominal pain is the best symptom characterizing symptomatic uncomplicated diverticular disease of the colon: a comparison with fecal calprotectin in clinical setting. J Clin Gastroenterol. 2015;49(3):218–21.
28. Jeyarajah S, Akbar N, Moorhead J, et al. A clinicopathological study of serotonin of the sigmoid colon mucosa in association with chronic symptoms in uncomplicated diverticulosis. Int J Color Dis. 2012;27(12):1597–605.
29. Krokowicz L, Stojcev Z, Kaczmarek FB, et al. Microencapsulated sodium butyrate administered to patients with diverticulosis decreases incidence of diverticulitis—a prospective randomized study. Int J Color Dis. 2014;29:387–93.
30. Daniels L, Budding AE, de Korte K, et al. Fecal microbiome analysis as a diagnostic test for diverticulitis. Eur J Clin Microbiol Infect Dis. 2014;33(11):1927–36.
31. Jung H-K, Choung RS, Locke GR, et al. Diarrhea-predominant irritable bowel syndrome is associated with diverticular disease: a population-based study. Am J Gastroenterol. 2010;105(3):652–61.
32. Ford AC, Moayyedi P, Lacy BE, et al. American College of Gastroenterology Monograph on the management of irritable bowel syndrome and chronic idiopathic constipation. Am J Gastroenterol. 2014;109:S2–S26.
33. Rao SSC, Yu S, Fedewa A. Systematic review: dietary fibre and FODMAP-restricted diet in the management of constipation and irritable bowel syndrome. Aliment Pharmacol Ther. 2015;41(12):1256–70.
34. Böhn L, Störsrud S, Törnblom H, et al. Self-reported food-related gastrointestinal symptoms in IBS are common and associated with more severe symptoms and reduced quality of life. Am J Gastroenterol. 2013;108:634–41.
35. Simrén M, Månsson A, Langkilde AM, et al. Food-related gastrointestinal symptoms in the irritable bowel syndrome. Digestion. 2001;63:108–15.
36. Monsbakken KW, Vandvik PO, Farup PG. Perceived food intolerance in subjects with irritable bowel syndrome-etiology, prevalence and consequences. Eur J Clin Nutr. 2006;60:667–72.
37. Cuomo R, Andreozzi P, Zito FP, et al. Irritable bowel syndrome and food interaction. World J Gastroenterol. 2014;20(27):8837–45.
38. De Giorgio R, Volta U, Gibson PR. Sensitivity to wheat, gluten and FODMAPs in IBS: facts or fiction? Gut. 2016;65:169–78.
39. El-Salhy M, Hatlebakk JG, Gilja OH, Hausken T. The relation between celiac disease, non-celiac gluten sensitivity and irritable bowel syndrome. Nutr J. 2015;14:92. https://doi.org/10.1186/s12937-015-0080-6.
40. Sainsbury A, Sanders DS, Ford AC. Prevalence of irritable bowel syndrome–type symptoms in patients with celiac disease: a meta-analysis. Clin Gastroenterol Hepatol. 2013;11:359–65.
41. Whelan K, Abrahmsohn O, David GJP, et al. Fructan content of commonly consumed wheat, rye and gluten-free breads. Int J Food Sci Nutr. 2011;62(5):498–503.
42. Lacy BE, Gabbard SL, Crowell MD. Pathophysiology, evaluation, and treatment of bloating: hope, hype, or hot air? Gastroenterol Hepatol. 2011;7(11):729–39.

43. Serra J, Azpiroz F, Malagelada JR. Impaired transit and tolerance of intestinal gas in the irritable bowel syndrome. Gut. 2001;48:14–9.
44. Ong DK, Mitchell SB, Barrett JS, et al. Manipulation of dietary short chain carbohydrates alters the pattern of gas production and genesis of symptoms in irritable bowel syndrome. J Gastroenterol Hepatol. 2010;25:1366–73.
45. Sinagra E, Pompei G, Tomasello G, et al. Inflammation in irritable bowel syndrome: myth or new treatment target? World J Gastroenterol. 2016;22(7):2242–55.
46. Zhang L, Song J, Hou X. Mast cell and irritable bowel syndrome: from the bench to the bedside. J Neurogastroenterol Motil. 2016;22(2):181–92. https://doi.org/10.5056/jnm15137.
47. Reed DE, Barajas-Lopez C, Cottrell G, et al. Mast cell tryptase and proteinase-activated receptor 2 induce hyperexcitability of guinea-pig submucosal neurons. J Physiol. 2003;547(2):531–42.
48. Barbara G, Stanghellini V, De Giorgio R, et al. Activated mast cells in proximity to colonic nerves correlate with abdominal pain in irritable bowel syndrome. Gastroenterology. 2004;126: 693–702.
49. Guilarte M, Santos J, de Torres I, et al. Diarrhoea-predominant IBS patients show mast cell activation and hyperplasia in the jejunum. Gut. 2007;56: 203–39.
50. Scalbert A, Brennan L, Manach C, et al. The food metabolome: a window over dietary exposure. Am J Clin Nutr. 2014;99:1286–308.
51. McIntosh K, Reed DE, Schneider T, et al. FODMAPs alter symptoms and the metabolome of patients with IBS: a randomised controlled trial. Gut. 2016;66(7):1241–51. https://doi.org/10.1136/gutjnl-2015-311339.
52. Distrutti E, Monaldi L, Ricci P, Fiorucci S. Gut microbiota role in irritable bowel syndrome: new therapeutic strategies. World J Gastroenterol. 2016;22(7):2219–41.
53. Simrén M, Barbara G, Flint HJ, et al. Intestinal microbiota in functional bowel disorders: a Rome foundation report. Gut. 2013;62(1):159–76.
54. Jalanka-Tuovinen J, Salojarvi J, Salonen A, et al. Faecal microbiota composition and host-microbe cross-talk following gastroenteritis and in post-infectious irritable bowel syndrome. Gut. 2014;63(11):1737–45.
55. Ponnusamy K, Choi JN, Kim J, et al. Microbial community and metabolomic comparison of irritable bowel syndrome faeces. J Med Microbiol. 2011;60(6):817–27.
56. Bonfrate L, Tack J, Grattagliano I, et al. Microbiota in health and irritable bowel syndrome: current knowledge, perspectives and therapeutic options. Scand J Gastroenterol. 2013;48:995–1009.
57. Benno P, Dahlgren A-L, Befrits R, et al. From IBS to DBS: the dysbiotic bowel syndrome. J Investig Med High Impact Case Rep. 2016;4(2):2324709616648458. https://doi.org/10.1177/2324709616648458.
58. Dahl WJ, Stewart ML. Position of the Academy of Nutrition and Dietetics: health implications of dietary fiber. J Acad Nutr Diet. 2015;115:1861–70.
59. EFSA Panel on Dietetic Products, Nutrition, and Allergies. Scientific opinion on dietary reference values for carbohydrates and dietary fibre. EFSA J. 2010;8(3):1462.
60. Moayyedi P, Quigley EMM, Lacy BE, et al. The effect of fiber supplementation on irritable bowel syndrome: a systematic review and meta-analysis. Am J Gastroenterol. 2014;109:1367–74.
61. Nagarajana N, Mordena A, Bischof D, et al. The role of fiber supplementation in the treatment of irritable bowel syndrome: a systematic review and meta-analysis. Eur J Gastroenterol Hepatol. 2015;27(9):1002–10. https://doi.org/10.1097/MEG.0000000000000425.
62. Bijkerk CJ, de Wit NJ, Muris JW, et al. Soluble or insoluble fibre in irritable bowel syndrome in primary care? Randomised placebo controlled trial. Br Med J. 2009;339:b3154. https://doi.org/10.1136/bmj.b3154.
63. Jalihal A, Kurian G. Ispaghula therapy in irritable bowel syndrome: improvement in overall well-being is related to reduction in bowel dissatisfaction. J Gastroenterol Hepatol. 1990;5:507–13.
64. Prior A, Whorwell PJ. Double blind study of ispaghula in irritable bowel syndrome. Gut. 1987;28: 1510–3.
65. Kumar A, Kumar N, Vij JC, et al. Optimum dosage of ispaghula husk in patients with irritable bowel syndrome: correlation of symptom relief with whole gut transit time and stool weight. Gut. 1987;28:150–5.
66. Nigam P, Kapoor KK, Rastog CK, et al. Different therapeutic regimens in irritable bowel syndrome. J Assoc Physicians India. 1984;32:1041–4.
67. Arthurs Y, Fielding JF. Double blind trial of ispaghula/poloxamer in the irritable bowel syndrome. Ir Med J. 1983;76:253.
68. Longstreth GF, Fox DD, Youkeles L, et al. Psyllium therapy in the irritable bowel syndrome. Ann Intern Med. 1981;95:53–6.
69. Ritchie JA, Truelove SC. Treatment of irritable bowel syndrome with lorazepam, hyoscine butylbromide, and ispaghula husk. Br Med J. 1979;1:376–8.
70. Niv E, Halak A, Tiommny E, et al. Randomized clinical study: partially hydrolyzed guar gum (PHGG) versus placebo in the treatment of patients with irritable bowel syndrome. Nutr Metab. 2016;13:10. https://doi.org/10.1186/s12986-016-0070-5.
71. Russo L, Andreozzi P, Zito FP, et al. Partially hydrolyzed guar gum in the treatment of irritable bowel syndrome with constipation: effects of gender, age and body mass index. Saudi J Gastroenterol. 2015;21(2):104–10.
72. Parisi GC, Zilli M, Miani MP, et al. High-fiber diet supplementation in patients with irritable bowel

syndrome (IBS) a multicenter, randomized, open trial comparison between wheat bran diet and partially hydrolyzed guar gum (PHGG). Dig Dis Sci. 2002;47(8):1697–704.

73. Xu L, Yu W, Jiang J, et al. Efficacy of pectin in the treatment of diarrhea predominant irritable bowel syndrome. Zhonghua Wei Chang Wai Ke Za Zhi. 2015;18(3):267–71.
74. Rees G, Davies J, Thompson R, et al. Randomised-controlled trial of a fibre supplement on the symptoms of irritable bowel syndrome. J R Soc Prom Health. 2005;125:30–4.
75. Lucey MR, Clark ML, Lowndes JO, et al. Is bran efficacious in irritable bowel syndrome? A double-blind placebo controlled crossover study. Gut. 1987;28:221–5.
76. Kruis W, Weinzierl P, Schussler P, et al. Comparison of the therapeutic effects of wheat bran and placebo in patients with the irritable bowel syndrome. Digestion. 1986;34:196–201.
77. Manning AP, Heaton KW, Harvey RF. Wheat fibre and irritable bowel syndrome. Lancet. 1977;2(8035):417–8.
78. Soltoft J, Gudmand-Hoyer E, Krag B, et al. A double-blind trial of the effect of wheat bran on symptoms of irritable bowel syndrome. Lancet. 1977;8034:270–2.
79. Quigley EMM, Fried M, Gwee K-A, et al. Irritable bowel syndrome: a global perspective. World Gastroenterol Org Guidelines 2015;19–20.
80. Gibson PR, Shepherd SJ. Evidence-based dietary management of functional gastrointestinal symptoms: The FODMAP approach. J Gastroenterol Hepatol. 2010;25:252–8.
81. Muir JG, Shepherd SJ, Rosella O, et al. Fructan and free fructose content of common Australian vegetables and fruit. J Agric Food Chem. 2007;55:6619–27.
82. Marsh A, Eslick EM, Eslick GD. Does a diet low in FODMAPs reduce symptoms associated with functional gastrointestinal disorders? A comprehensive systematic review and meta- analysis. Eur J Nutr. 2015;55(3):897–906. https://doi.org/10.1007/s00394-015-0922-1.
83. Böhn L, Störsrud S, Liljebo T, et al. Diet low in FODMAPs reduces symptoms of irritable bowel syndrome as well as traditional dietary advice: a randomized controlled trial. Gastroenterology. 2015;149:1399–407.
84. Yoon SR, Lee JH, Lee JH, et al. Low-FODMAP formula improves diarrhea and nutritional status in hospitalized patients receiving enteral nutrition: a randomized, multicenter, double-blind clinical trial. Nutr J. 2015;14:116. https://doi.org/10.1186/s12937-015-0106-0.
85. Halmos EP, Power VA, Shepherd SJ, et al. A diet low in FODMAPs reduces symptoms of irritable bowel syndrome. Gastroenterology. 2014;146:67–75.
86. Pedersen N, Andersen NN, Vegh Z, et al. Ehealth: low FODMAP diet vs lactobacillus rhamnosus GG in irritable bowel syndrome. World J Gastroenterol. 2014;20:16215–26.
87. Biesiekierski JR, Peters SL, Newnham ED, et al. No effects of gluten in patients with self-reported non-celiac gluten sensitivity after dietary reduction of fermentable, poorly absorbed, short chain carbohydrates. Gastroenterology. 2013;145:320–8.
88. de Roest RH, Dobbs BR, Chapman BA, et al. The low FODMAP diet improves gastrointestinal symptoms in patients with irritable bowel syndrome: a prospective study. Int J Clin Pract. 2013;67: 895–903.
89. Varju P, Farkas N, Hegyi P et al. Low fermentable oligosaccharides, disaccharides, monosaccharides and polyols (FODMAP) diet improves symptoms in adults suffering from irritable bowel syndrome (IBS) compared to standard IBS diet: a meta-analysis of clinical studies. PLOS ONE. 2017;12(8):e0182942.
90. Strate LL. Lifestyle factors and the course of diverticular disease. Dig Dis. 2012;30:35–45.
91. Horner JL. Natural history of diverticulosis of the colon. Am J Dig Dis. 1958;3(5):343–50.
92. Strate LL, Liu YL, Syngal S, et al. Nut, corn and popcorn consumption and the incidence of diverticular disease. JAMA. 2008;300(8):907–14.
93. Böhm SK. Risk factors for diverticulosis, diverticulitis, diverticular perforation, and bleeding: a plea for more subtle history taking. Viszeralmedizin. 2015;31:84–94.
94. Aldoori WH, Giovannucci EL, Rimm EB, et al. A prospective study of alcohol, smoking, caffeine, and the risk of symptomatic diverticular disease in men. Ann Epidemiol. 1995;5:221–8.
95. Sharara AI, El-Halabi MM, Mansour NM, et al. Alcohol consumption is a risk factor for colonic diverticulosis. J Clin Gastroenterol. 2013;47(5): 420–5.
96. Crowe FL, Appleby PN, Allen NE, Key TJ. Diet and risk of diverticular disease in Oxford cohort of European Prospective Investigation into Cancer and Nutrition (EPIC): prospective study of British vegetarians and non-vegetarians. BMJ. 2011;343:d4131. https://doi.org/10.1136/bmj. d4131.
97. The National Institute of Diabetes and Digestive and Kidney Diseases (NIDDK). Diverticular disease. 2013. NIH Publication No. 13–1163.
98. Aldoori W, Ryan-Harshman M. Preventing diverticular disease. Review of recent evidence on high-fibre diets. Can Fam Physician. 2002;48:1632–5.
99. Tarleton S, DiBaise JK. Low-residue diet in diverticular disease: putting an end to a myth. Nutr Clin Pract. 2011;26:137–42.
100. Gear JS, Ware A, Fursdon P, et al. Symptomless diverticular disease and intake of dietary fibre. Lancet. 1979;1(8115):511–4.
101. Peery AF, Sandler RS, Ahnen DJ, et al. Constipation and a low-fiber diet are not associated with diverticulosis. Clin Gastroenterol Hepatol. 2013;11(12):1622–7.
102. Peery AF, Barrett PR, Park D, et al. A high-fiber diet does not protect against asymptomatic diverticulosis. Gastroenterology. 2012;142(2):266–72.

103. Crowe FL, Balkwill A, Cairns BJ, et al. Source of dietary fibre and diverticular disease incidence: a prospective study of UK women. Gut. 2014;63:1450–6.
104. Aldoori WH, Giovannucci EL, Rockett HRH, et al. Prospective study of dietary fiber types and symptomatic diverticular disease in men. J Nutr. 1998;128:714–9.
105. Aldoori WH, Giovannucci EL, Rimm EB, et al. A prospective study of diet and the risk of symptomatic diverticular disease in men. Am J Clin Nutr. 1994;60:757–64.
106. Lahner E, Esposito G, Zullo A, et al. High fibre diet and Lactobacillus paracasei B21060 in symptomatic uncomplicated diverticular disease. World J Gastroenterol. 2012;18(41):5918–24.
107. Smits BJ, Whitehead AM, Prescott P. Lactulose in the treatment of symptomatic diverticular disease: a comparative study with high-fibre diet. Br J Clin Pract. 1990;44:314–8.
108. Ornstein MH, Littlewood ER, Baird IM, et al. Are fibre supplements really necessary in diverticular disease of the colon? A controlled clinical trial. BMJ. 1981;282:1353–6.
109. Brodribb AJ. Treatment of symptomatic diverticular disease with a high fibre diet. Lancet. 1977;1:664–6.
110. Hodgson WJ. The placebo effect. It is important in diverticular disease? Am J Gastroenterol. 1977;67:157–62.
111. Taylor I, Duthie HL. Bran tablets and diverticular disease. Br Med J. 1976;1(6016):988–90.
112. Leahy AL, Ellis RM, Quill DS, Peel ALG. High fibre diet in symptomatic diverticular disease of the colon. Ann R Coll Surg Engl. 1985;67(3):173–4.
113. Hyland JM, Taylor I. Does a high fibre diet prevent the complications of diverticular disease? Br J Surg. 1980;67:77–9.
114. Eastwood MA, Smith AN, Brydon WG, et al. Comparison of bran, ispaghula, and lactulose on colon function in diverticular disease. Gut. 1978;19:1144–7.
115. Brodribb AJ, Humphreys DM. Diverticular disease: three studies. III. Metabolic effect of bran in patients, with diverticular disease. Br Med J. 1976;1(6007):428–30.
116. Painter NS, Almeida AZ, Colebourne KW. Unprocessed bran in treatment of diverticular disease of the colon. Br Med J. 1972;2(5806):137–40.
117. Carabotti M, Annibale B, Severi C, Lahner E. Role of fiber in symptomatic uncomplicated diverticular disease: a systematic review. Forum Nutr. 2017;9:161. https://doi.org/10.3390/nu9020161.
118. Unlu C, Daniles L, Vrouenraets BC, et al. A systematic review of high-fibre dietary therapy in diverticular disease. Int J Colorectal Dis. 2012;27:419–27.
119. Maconi G, Barbara G, Bosetti C, et al. Treatment of diverticular disease of the colon and prevention of acute diverticulitis: a systematic review. Dis Colon Rectum. 2011;54(10):1326–38.
120. European Food Safety Authority (EFSA). Scientific opinion on dietary reference values for carbohydrates and dietary fibre. EFSA Panel on Dietetic Products, Nutrition, and Allergies (NDA), Parma, Italy. EFSA J. 2010;8(3):1462.
121. Slavin JL. Position of the American Dietetic Association: health implications of dietary fiber. J Am Diet Assoc. 2008;108:1716–31.
122. Slavin J. Fiber and prebiotics: mechanisms and health benefits. Forum Nutr. 2013;5:1417–35.
123. Eswaran S, Muir J, Chey WD. Fiber and functional gastrointestinal disorders. Am J Gastroenterol. 2013;108(5):718–27.
124. Cummings JH. The effect of dietary fiber on fecal weight and composition. In: Spiller GA, editor. CRC handbook of dietary fiber in human nutrition. 3rd ed. Boca Raton: CRC; 2001. p. 183–241.
125. Stevens J, VanSoest PJ, Robertson JB, Levitsky DA. Comparisons of the effects of psyllium and wheat bran on gastrointestinal transit time and stool characteristics. J Am Diet Assoc. 1988;88(3):323–6.
126. de Vries J, Miller PE, Verbeke K. Effects of cereal fiber on bowel function: a systematic review of intervention trials. World J Gastroenterol. 2015;21(29):8952–63.
127. Koh A, De Vadder F, Kovatcheva-Datchary P, Backhed F. From dietary fiber to host physiology: short-chain fatty acids as key bacterial metabolites. Cell. 2016;165:1332–45.
128. Pituch-Zdanowska A, Banaszkiewicz A, Albrecht P. The role of dietary fibre in inflammatory bowel disease. Prz Gastroenterol. 2015;10(3):135–41.
129. Conlon MA, Bird AR. The impact of diet and lifestyle on gut microbiota and human health. Forum Nutr. 2015;7:17–44.
130. Lynch DB, Jeffery IB, Cusack S, et al. Diet microbiota health interactions in older subjects: implications for healthy aging. Interdiscip Top Gerontol. 2015;40:141–54.
131. Claesson MJ, Jeffery IB, Conde S. Gut microbiota composition correlates with diet and health in the elderly. Nature. 2012;488:178–85.
132. Hamer HM, Jonkers D, Venema K, et al. Review article: the role of butyrate on colonic function. Aliment Pharmacol Ther. 2008;27:104–19.
133. Kopylov U, Ben-Horin S, Lahat A, et al. Obesity, metabolic syndrome and the risk of development of colonic diverticulosis. Digestion. 2012;86:201–5.
134. Nagata N, Sakamoto K, Arai T, et al. Visceral fat accumulation affects risk of colonic diverticular hemorrhage. Int J Color Dis. 2015;30(10):1399–406.
135. Strate LL, Liu YL, Aldoori WH, et al. Obesity increases the risks of diverticulitis and diverticular bleeding. Gastroenterology. 2009;136:115–22.
136. Hjern F, Wolk A, Hakansson N. Obesity, physical inactivity, and colonic diverticular disease requiring hospitalization in women: a prospective cohort study. Am J Gastroenterol. 2012;107:296–302.
137. Slavin JL. Dietary fiber and body weight. Nutrition. 2005;21:411–8.
138. Davis JN, Hodges VA, Gillham B. Normal-weight adults consume more fiber and fruit than their

age- and height-matched overweight/obese counterparts. J Am Diet Assoc. 2006;106:833–40.

139. Liu S, Willett WC, Manson JE, et al. Relation between changes in intakes of dietary fiber and grain products and changes in weight and development of obesity among middle-aged women. Am J Clin Nutr. 2003;78:920–7.
140. Fogelholm M, Anderssen S, Gunnarsdottir I, Lahti-Koski M. Dietary macronutrients and food consumption as determinants of long-term weight change in adult populations: a systematic literature review. Food Nutr Res. 2012:56. https://doi.org/10.3402/fnr.v56i0.19103.
141. Lindstrom J, Peltonen M, Eriksson JG, et al. High-fibre, low-fat diet predicts long-term weight loss and decreased type 2 diabetes risk: the Finnish Diabetes Prevention Study. Diabetologia. 2006;49:912–20.
142. Ma Y, Olendzki BC, Wang J, et al. Single-component versus multi-component dietary goals for the metabolic syndrome: a randomized trial. Ann Intern Med. 2015;162:248–57.
143. Dietary Guidelines Advisory Committee (DGAC). Scientific Report. Advisory report to the secretary of health and human services and the secretary of agriculture. Part D. Chapter 2: Dietary patterns, foods and nutrients and health outcomes. 2015;1–35.

Part III

Weight Management and Related Diseases

Dietary Patterns and Fiber in Body Weight and Composition Regulation

7

Keywords
Dietary patterns • Mediterranean diet • DASH diet • New Nordic diet Vegetarian diet • Western diet • Dietary fiber • Weight loss • Energy density • Obesity • Overweight • Body weight • Waist circumference Body mass index • Visceral fat

Key Points

- The human gastrointestinal and energy metabolism regulatory systems evolved with pre-agricultural high fiber diets (>50 g fiber/day).
- Prospective cohort studies and randomized controlled trials (RCTs) show that high adherence to healthy fiber-rich dietary patterns such as the Mediterranean (MedDiet), Dietary Approaches to Stop Hypertension (DASH), New Nordic, and vegetarian diets may at a minimum help to prevent weight gain and can support weight loss and lower waist circumference compared to low-fat or Western diets in overweight or obese individuals.
- Mechanisms associated with healthy fiber-rich dietary pattern effects on managing body weight and central obesity include: (1) reducing dietary energy density directly or displacing higher energy foods associated with the Western diet pattern; (2) lowering available metabolizable energy; and (3) increasing post-prandial satiety by affecting both the upper digestive tract and colonic microbiota.
- Fiber intake is inversely associated with obesity risk and populations with higher fiber diets tend to be leaner than those with low fiber diets.
- Prospective cohort studies suggest that increased total fiber intake by ≥12 g/day to a total daily fiber intake of >25 g, especially compared to refined low fiber diets, can prevent weight gain by 3.5–5.5 kg each decade.
- RCTs show that adequate fiber intake ≥28 g fiber/day from fiber-rich diets can reduce body weight and waist circumference compared to low fiber Western diets (≤20 g fiber/day). Fiber-rich diets are generally more effective at promoting weight loss than fiber supplements.

M.L. Dreher, *Dietary Patterns and Whole Plant Foods in Aging and Disease*, Nutrition and Health,
https://doi.org/10.1007/978-3-319-59180-3_7

7.1 Introduction

The worldwide overweight and obesity pandemic is among the greatest public health challenges of our time [1, 2]. Since approximately the 1980s, the global prevalence of overweight and obesity increased by more than 28% for adults and 47% for children, resulting in an increase from about 850 million overweight or obese people in 1980 to over two billion in 2013 [1]. Obesity is a complex multifactorial condition resulting from the chronic disruption between energy intake and energy expenditure, involving genetic, environmental, lifestyle, and emotional factors [3–5]. During the last several decades there has been an increased exposure to higher energy dense and lower dietary fiber (fiber) containing foods and increasingly sedentary lifestyles, which have led to net habitual positive energy balances and weight gain in western populations [1, 4–14]. A small positive energy balance of 50 kcals/day, by increased energy intake and/or reduced activity, can lead to an annual weight gain of 0.4–0.9 kg/year [5–7]. Further, a higher habitual intake of 200 kcal/day above energy balance in overweight or obese women may increase weight gain by as much as 9 kg/year [8]. Energy dense diets, common in the Western-style diet, are positively associated with higher body mass index (BMI) and risk of obesity [8–14]. Moreover, since people tend to eat approximately the same amount or volume of food on a day-to-day basis, regardless of the food energy density, the common advice of just eating less of all foods may not be the optimal approach for weight management [7]. The 2017 nationally representative Canadian Community Health Survey (11,748 adults; 18 years of age or older) found that individuals consuming diets higher in energy density (1.2 vs. 0.7 kcal/g) and lower in dietay fiber (5.9 vs. 12.2 g/1,000 kcals) significantly elevated their risk for obesity by 257% [15]. This study also found that whole fruits, dark green, orange, and non-starchy vegetables and 100% juices and yogurt were inversely associated with obesity whereas fast foods, carbonated beverages, refined grains, processed meats, sauces and dressings, and sugars and syrups were positively associated with obesity. A meta-analysis (117 trials; 4815 participants) found that hypocaloric diets were more effective for weight loss and increased exercise was more effective at reducing visceral adiposity, reducing visceral fat by a mean of 6% versus only 1% for hypocaloric diets [16]. Elevated BMI or excessive adiposity in adulthood and increasingly in childhood is a growing risk factor for major chronic diseases such as diabetes, cardiovascular disease, nonalcoholic fatty liver disease, chronic kidney disease, and a number of obesity related cancers [17–19].

For overweight or obese individuals who successfully lose weight, as many as 80% typically drift back to their original weight or more [20]. This is because after weight loss there are an array of metabolic regulatory processes at work to promote weight regain, so it is difficult to maintain weight loss [21–24]. After body fat loss, thermogenesis reduces and leads to fat loss resistance and drops in hormone levels, such as leptin and thyroid hormones, which can cause the risk of increased energy intake above energy expenditure [22, 23]. Weight loss triggers strong overeating signals sent to the brain's hypothalamus to increase appetite. Also, in this period, adipocytes face cellular stress associated with the physical forces that arise within the shrinking cells, causing them to actively promote renewed fat storage. The determinants of weight maintenance are genetics, behavior, and environment with diet behavior thought to be the most important factor that influences weight regain. A cross-sectional study of weight loss maintainers who lost >10% of their body weight and maintained that loss for ≥5 years reported that they consumed a diet with lower energy density (1.4 kcal/g) than the weight re-gain individuals (1.8 kcal/g) [21]. These weight loss maintainers consumed more fiber-rich foods such as vegetables (4.9 servings/day) and whole-grain products (2.2 servings/day) compared to less than 1 daily serving of vegetables and whole grains for the weight regainers [21]. In addition to eating a low energy dense and high fiber diet, successful long-term weight loss maintenance is associated with five additional strategies to help counteract weight regain metabolic processes: (1) engaging in physical activity; (2) eating breakfast; (3) self-monitoring weight on a regular basis; (4) limiting consumption of higher energy dense foods; and (5) catching dietary "miss-steps" before they turn into a habit [20]. Two common dietary approaches for weight loss and reducing the risk of central obesity include: (1) reducing daily energy intake by 20–35% for a negative energy balance or (2) eating lower energy dense and healthy fiber-rich dietary patterns vs. Western dietary pattern [22–25]. A 2017 meta-analysis (12 observational studies) found that highest vs. lowest adherence to healthy dietary patterns reduced central obesity risk by 19% whereas a Western dietary pattern increased risk by 16% [24]. In a randomized controlled trial (RCT) with obese adults with metabolic syndrome, it was shown that those who simply consumed a high fiber dietary pattern had similar weight loss to those on a more complex multi-component, hypocaloric diet plan after one year (Fig. 7.1) [25]. The objective of this chapter is to comprehensively review the effects of healthy dietary patterns and fiber on body weight and composition regulation.

7.2 Healthy Dietary Patterns

7.2.1 Overview

Compared with the usual Western diet, the consumption of healthy dietary patterns, including the US dietary guidelines diet, Mediterranean diet (MedDiet), Dietary Approaches to Stop Hypertension (DASH) diet, and healthy vegetarian (lacto-ovo) diets, by overweight and obese individuals can result in weight loss or at least prevent weight gain depending on the degree of adherence and fiber level [14]. Appendix A summarizes the food and nutrient composition of some major healthy dietary patterns vs. the American Western dietary pattern. The 2015 US Advisory Guidelines Advisory Committee scientific report concluded that there was strong evidence showing that overweight and obese adults, preferably as part of a comprehensive lifestyle change intervention, can achieve clinically meaningful weight loss ranging from 4 to 12 kg after 6-months through a variety of healthy dietary patterns that achieve an energy deficit [14]. Thereafter, slow weight regain is observed, with total weight loss at 1 year of 4–10 kg and at 2 years of 3–4 kg. All these healthy dietary patterns double the fiber content from about 16 g/day in the usual Western diet to >30 g/day and

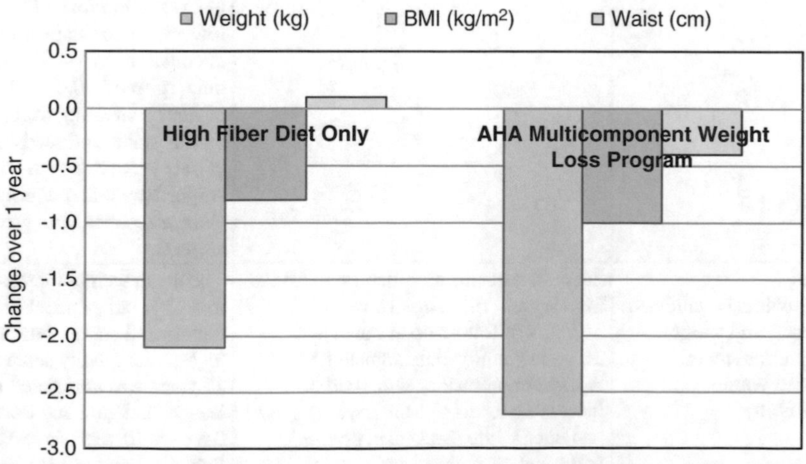

Fig. 7.1 Effect of a high fiber based weight loss diet (≥30 g fiber/day) vs. the American Heart Association (AHA) multi-component weight loss program in 240 metabolic syndrome adults after 1 year ($p > 0.05$) (adapted from [25])

decrease added sugars intake by more than half by emphasizing the increased consumption of plant-based foods, such as whole grains, fruits, vegetables, pulses, and nuts.

7.2.2 Observational Studies

The effect of dietary quality and specific healthy dietary patterns on body weight and composition regulation from observational studies are summarized studies in Table 7.1 [26–46].

7.2.2.1 Overall Diet Quality

Observational studies consistently show that habitual intake of higher overall diet quality, especially with adequate fiber intake from whole plant foods and lower intake of red meat and high energy dense processed foods and beverages, is inversely associated with weight gain and central

Table 7.1 Summary of diet quality score and specific healthy dietary pattern observational studies on body weight and composition regulation

Objective	Study details	Results
Overall dietary pattern quality		
Systematic review		
Asghari et al. (2017). Review observational studies, focusing on the association of diet quality indices with general obesity or abdominal obesity in adults [26]	34 studies (10 prospective studies and 24 cross-sectional studies)	Diet quality indices based on dietary guidelines (Healthy Eating Index) were inversely associated with parameters of weight status in most studies. Scoring on the basis of dietary diversity was directly associated with weight gain
Observational studies		
Shah et al. (2016). Investigate the relationship between dietary quality and regional adiposity in a cross-sectional analysis (Multi-Ethnic Study of Atherosclerosis [MESA]; US) [27]	5079 subjects; mean age 61 years; 47% males (multivariate adjusted)	Those with a higher diet-quality score in AHA goals and the MedDiet were generally older and female, with a lower BMI, CRP, and markers of insulin resistance. After adjustment, a higher diet-quality score (highest vs. lowest dietary score quartile) was associated with lower visceral fat: 461 cm^2/m vs. 524 cm^2/m (p-trend <0.01; Fig. 7.2), less pericardial fat (41 vs. 48 cm^3/m (p-trend <0.01), and lower hepatic steatosis (by hepatic attenuation; 59 vs. 61 Hounsfield units (p-trend <0.01). Greater intake of fiber containing fruits, vegetables, whole-grains and seeds/nuts, and yogurt was associated with decreased adiposity, while red/processed meats were associated with greater adiposity
Hu et al. (2016). Examine the previously validated diet quality score, and weight change among adolescents transitioning into young adulthood (US) [28]	2656 adolescents recruited in middle/high school; mean age 15 years; 10 years of follow-up to mean age 25 years (multivariate adjusted). A higher diet quality score had increasing levels of beans, whole grain and nuts, white meat (fish, poultry), fruits and vegetables, and low-fat dairy, while decreasing the intake of processed foods, red meat, and sweet and salty foods (eg, salty snacks, soft drinks, sweet breads, grain desserts)	The mean weight increased from 61 to 76 kg. Independent of lifestyle factors and energy intake, a 15-point higher diet quality score at age 15 years was associated with 1.5 kg less weight gain and lower BMI by 0.5 over 10 years ($p < 0.001$). Establishment of high-quality dietary patterns in adolescence may help reduce excess weight gain by young adulthood

Table 7.1 (continued)

Objective	Study details	Results
Feliciano et al. (2016). Examine whether changes in diet quality predicts changes in central adiposity among postmenopausal women (Women's Health Initiative Observational Study; US) [29]. Dietary patterns (Healthy Eating Index-2010, Alternate Healthy Eating Index-2010, Alternate MedDiet, and Dietary Approaches to Stop Hypertension (DASH)	67,175 postmenopausal women; mean baseline age was 63 years, waist size 83 cm (34.6 in.), and BMI 27; 3-year follow-up; completed FFQs, and waist size was measured; trunk fat was measured in 4254 women via dual-energy X-ray absorptiometry (DXA); 3-year changes (multivariate adjusted)	A 10% improvement in any dietary pattern quality score was associated with 0.07–0.43 cm smaller increase in waist size over 3 years (all $P < 0.05$). After adjusting for weight change, associations attenuated to 0.02–0.10 cm but remained statistically significant for all patterns except Alternate MedDiet. Results were similar for DXA trunk fat. Improvements in diet quality are modestly protective against gain in waist size, which is partially due to lesser weight gain. Achieving and maintaining a higher quality diet after menopause may help protect against gains in central adiposity
Fung et al. (2015). Evaluate the association between change of diet quality indexes and concurrent weight change over 20 years (Nurses' Health Study [NHS] I and II, and Health Professionals Follow-up Study [HPFS]; US) [30]	123,098 women and 22,973 men; mean baseline age 49 years for NHS I and 36 years for NHS II, 48 years for HPFS; mean BMIs ranged from 23–24.7; 20 years of follow-up; weight measures every 4 years (multivariate adjusted)	There was significantly less weight gain over a 4-year cycle with each standard deviation increase of diet quality score in both men and women. Improvement of diet quality was associated with less weight gain, especially in younger women and overweight individuals
Lassale et al. (2012). Assess and compare the predictive value of six different dietary scores on risk of weight gain and obesity (Supplementation en Vitamines et Mine'raux Antioxydants; France) [31]	3151 participants; 1680 men and 1471 women; mean baseline age 52 years; 13 years of follow-up (multivariate adjusted)	This study suggests that baseline diet quality, measured by different dietary scores, is a good predictor of weight gain across genders. Dietary quality score appears to be especially predictive of obesity risk in middle-aged men. These findings support the broader use of dietary scores for weight gain prevention at the population level
Wolongevicz et al. (2010). Determine how diet quality effects risk of being overweight or obese in women (Framingham Offspring and Spouse Study; US) [32]	590 normal-weight women; BMI < 25, aged 25–71 years; 16 years of follow-up (multivariate adjusted)	Women with lower diet quality were significantly 76% more likely to become overweight or obese compared with those with higher diet quality (p-trend = 0.009)
Esmaillzadeh and Azadhakht (2008). Cross-sectional evaluation of major dietary patterns and the prevalence of general obesity and central adiposity among women (Iranian) [33]	486 women, mean age 50 years; usual dietary intakes were evaluated by FFQ; with the use of factor analysis three major dietary patterns were extracted: healthy (9.5 g fiber/1000 kcal), Western (3 g fiber/1000 kcals, and Iranian 8.5 g fiber/1000 kcals) (multivariate adjusted)	Women in the upper category of the healthy pattern score were less likely to be obese by 59% and centrally obese by 52% ($p < 0.05$), whereas those in the upper quintile of the Western pattern had greater risk for general obesity by: 250% and for central obesity by 533% ($p < 0.01$). The Iranian dietary pattern was not significantly associated with general or central obesity

(continued)

Table 7.1 (continued)

Objective	Study details	Results
Schulz et al. (2005). Identify a dietary pattern predictive of subsequent annual weight change by using diet composition information (European Prospective Investigation into Cancer and Nutrition EPIC - Potsdam cohort; Germany) [34]	24,958 participants; mean baseline age 50 years, mean BMI 26; 4.4 years of follow-up (multivariate adjusted)	Mean annual weight gain gradually decreased with increasing diet quality score (p-trend <0.0001). A diet pattern characterized by low-fat, high-fiber (13.5 g fiber vs. 8.8 g fiber/1000 kcal) foods such as whole-grain bread, fruits, vegetables, and cereals was associated with body weight maintenance or prevention of excess body weight gain in non-obese subjects at baseline. This study supports the importance of adequate fiber intake for weight control
Newby et al. (2003). Assess the effect of dietary pattern on BMI and waist size (Baltimore Longitudinal Study of Aging; US) [35]	459 healthy men and women; 52% men; 95% whites; mean age for women 57 years and men 61 years; healthy diet pattern high fruit, vegetables, whole-grains, low in red meat, fast foods, and soda (27 g fiber/day) vs. white bread and meat and potato pattern (multivariate adjusted)	The mean annual gain in BMI was 0.30 units for subjects in the white bread and meat and potato pattern compared no change for those in the healthy pattern ($p < 0.01$) (Fig. 7.3). The mean annual gain in waist size was 3 times as great for subjects in the white bread and meat and potato pattern vs. those in the healthy pattern (1.3 cm vs. 0.4 cm) ($p < 0.05$)
Mediterranean diet (MedDiet)		
Li et al. (2015). Study long-term changes in anthropometric measures in a generally healthy population (Swedish women) [36]	27,544 women; mean age 40; mean BMI 22; MedDiet score 0–9; 12 years of follow-up (multivariate adjusted)	Among Swedish women, higher adherence to the MedDiet was not associated with increased body weight and waist size compared to the average median gain in body weight by 5 kg and waist size by 7.0 cm
Funtikova et al. (2014). Evaluate the association of adherence to the MedDiet and changes in waist size and 10-year incidence of abdominal obesity (Spain) [37]	3058 subjects; 51% women, mean baseline age 49 years; 10 years of follow-up (multivariate adjusted)	High adherence to the MedDiet was inversely associated with waist size by 1.5 cm ($p = 0.024$). The 10-year risk of abdominal obesity was reduced in the highest tertile score by up to 21%
May et al. (2012). Investigate the combined effect of physical activity, dietary pattern, and smoking status on prospective gain in body weight and waist size (EPIC-PANACEA) [38]	325,537 participants; 94,445 men and 231,092 women, mean age 51–58 years; mean BMI 25–27; median 5 years of follow-up (multivariate adjusted)	Men and women who reported to be physically active, never-smoking and adherent to the MedDiet gained less weight over a 5-year period for men by 537 g and women by 200 g and about 1 cm less waist size compared to participants with no or poor adherence to healthy behaviors
Beunza et al. (2010). Investigate the risk of weight gain (≥ 5 kg) or the risk of developing overweight or obesity (The Seguimiento Universidad de Navarra (SUN) Cohort; Spain) [39]	10,376 men and women; university graduates; mean age 38 years; mean 5.7 years of follow-up (multivariate adjusted)	Subjects with the lowest MedDiet adherence had an average 0.3 kg annual weight gain, whereas those with highest adherence had a loss of 0.059 kg/year and a 24% lower risk of gaining ≥5 kg over the first 4 years of follow-up

Table 7.1 (continued)

Objective	Study details	Results
Romaguera et al. (2010). Assess associations between adherence to the MedDiet, weight change, and incidence of overweight or obesity (EPIC-Physical Activity, Nutrition, Alcohol, Cessation of Smoking, Eating out of home and obesity project PANACEA; EU) [40]	325,537 participants; 94,445 men and 231,092 women, mean age 51–58 years; mean BMI 25–27; median 5 years of follow-up (multivariate adjusted)	This study found that eating a MedDiet may help to prevent weight gain and the development of overweight and obesity. High adherence to the MedDiet reduced mean weight by 0.16 kg and risk of becoming obese by 10% compared to low adherence. A similar association between adherence to the MedDiet and weight change was observed in men and women (p-interaction = 0.823). The protective effect of MedDiet against weight gain was stronger in younger people (<40 years of age), and in nonobese (BMI <30) individuals at baseline (p -interactions <0.0001)
Sanchez-Villegas et al. (2006). Evaluate the potential relation between compliance with traditional MedDiet score and subsequent weight maintenance and changes (SUN Cohort; Spain) [41]	6319 participants; mean age 34–40 years; mean BMI 23; 28-months follow-up; 7.9 g vs. 14.9 g/ fiber/1000 kcal (multivariate adjusted)	In young, normal weight adults, those in the lowest quartile of MedDiet score gained 0.73 kg compared to those in the top quartile who gained 0.45 kg. Although there was an initial inverse dose-response relationship (p-trend = 0.016), the results were not statistically significant (p-trend = 0.291)
Mendez et al. (2006). Examine whether a MedDiet pattern is associated with reduced 3-years incidence of obesity (EPIC-Spain) [42]	17,238 women, mean baseline age 47 years; 10,589 men; mean baseline age 50 years; mean of 3.3 years of follow-up (multivariate adjusted)	Higher adherence to the MedDiet was associated with a 30% lower risk of becoming obese. Associations were similar in women and men. MedDiet adherence was not associated with incidence of overweight or obesity in initially normal-weight subjects
Dietary Approaches to Stop Hypertension (DASH) diet		
Barak et al. (2014). Investigate adherence to DASH diet and general and central obesity in female nurses (cross-sectional study; Iran) [43]	293 female nurses aged >30 years; general and abdominal obesity were defined as BMI ≥25 and waist size ≥88 cm; usual dietary intakes were assessed using a validated FFQ; DASH diet score was based on foods and nutrients emphasized or minimized in the DASH diet (multivariate adjusted)	Increased adherence to the DASH diet was associated with older age ($p < 0.01$) and lower waist size ($p = 0.04$). Initially, there was no statistically significant difference in the prevalence of general obesity between extreme quartiles of the DASH diet score but after fully adjusting for dietary factors, those in the highest quartile of DASH diet score were 71% less likely to have general obesity. A marginally significant trend towards decreasing prevalence of central obesity was seen with increasing quartile of the DASH diet score with a 63% lower waist size ($p = 0.09$)

(continued)

Table 7.1 (continued)

Objective	Study details	Results
Berz et al. (2011). Study the effects of the DASH eating pattern on BMI throughout adolescence (National Growth and Health Study; US) [44]	2327 girls with ten annual visits starting at age 9 years; follow-up of 10 years (multivariate adjusted)	Adolescent girls with higher adherence to the DASH eating pattern had smaller gains in BMI. Girls in the highest vs. lowest quintile of the DASH score had significantly lower adjusted mean BMI of 24.4 vs. 26.3. The strongest individual food group predictors of BMI were total fruit with a mean BMI of 26.0 vs. 23.6 for <1 vs. ≥2 servings/day ($p < 0.001$) and low-fat dairy with a mean BMI of 25.7 vs. 23.2 for <1 vs. ≥2 servings/day ($p < 0.001$). Whole grain consumption was more weakly but beneficially associated with BMI
Vegetarian diet		
Tonstad et al. (2009). Assess the effects of different types of vegetarian diets on body weight and diabetes risk compared with non-vegetarians (The Adventist Health Study-2 cohort; US) [45]	22,434 men and 38,469 women; mean age 58 years; data from Seventh-Day Adventist church members across North America; type of vegetarian diet was categorized based on a FFQ (multivariate adjusted)	This study indicates that vegetarianism is protective against obesity and diabetes. Mean BMI was 23.6 for vegans, 25.7 for lacto-ovo vegetarians, 26.3 for pesco-vegetarians, and 27.3 for semi-vegetarians, and 28.8 for non-vegetarians. Prevalence of type 2 diabetes increased from 2.9% in vegans to 7.6% in non-vegetarians
Berkow and Barnard (2006). Review of published observational studies on the associations between vegetarian diets and reduced body weight [46]	40 studies reporting the weight status of vegetarians and non-vegetarians	29 of 40 observational studies reported that vegetarians weighed significantly less than non-vegetarians as measured by BMI or body weight. These studies found that the weight and BMI of both male and female vegetarians were 3–20% lower than those of non-vegetarians. Obesity prevalence ranges were from 0 to 6% in vegetarians and from about 5 to 45% in non-vegetarians

obesity in both men and women, especially in non-obese subjects at baseline (Table 7.1) [26–35]. A systematic review (10 cohort studies and 24 cross-sectional studies) found that high adherence to dietary quality based on the dietary guidelines (or Healthy Eating Indices) is inversely associated with obesity and other body weight parameters [26]. A cross-sectional analysis of the Multi-Ethnic Study of Atherosclerosis [MESA] (5079 adults; mean age 61 years; 47% men) demonstrated that higher intake of fiber containing fruits, vegetables, whole-grains and seeds/nuts, plus yogurt was associated with decreased adiposity, while red and processed meats were associated with greater adiposity (Fig. 7.2) [27]. A study of US adolescents (2656 middle/high school youth; mean age 15 years; 10-year follow-up to mean age 25 years) showed that a 15-point higher diet quality score (on a 100 point scale) at age 15 years was associated with 1.5 kg less weight gain and lower BMI by 0.5 kg/m^2 over 10 years ($p < 0.001$), independent of other lifestyle factors and energy intake [28]. The Women's Health Initiative Observational Study (67,175

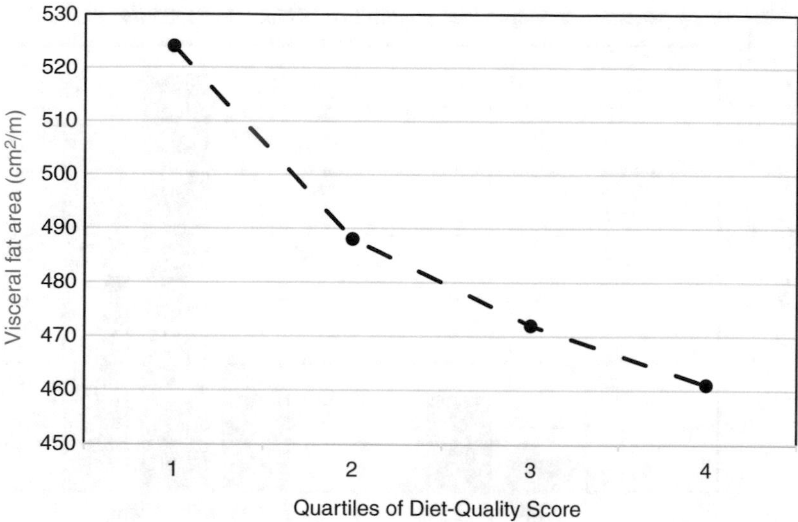

Fig. 7.2 Association between diet-quality score and visceral fat area from a cross-sectional analysis of the US Multi-Ethnic Study of Atherosclerosis ($p < 0.01$; multivariate adjusted) (adapted from [27])

postmenopausal women with waist size measurements; 3 years) found that a 10% improvement in diet quality can significantly reduce multivariate adjusted waist size by up to 0.1 cm over 3 years [29]. A pooled analysis of the large Nurses' Health Study I and II, and Health Professionals Follow-Up study (123,098 women and 22,973 men; women mean baseline age 36–48 years; men mean baseline age 58; normal BMI; 20 years of follow-up) showed that higher adherence to all types of high quality diet patterns was significantly associated with less weight gain over each 4-year weight assessment period in both men and women, especially in younger women or overweight individuals [30]. Several prospective studies report that higher dietary quality is a good predictor of lower weight gain and obesity risk in women [31, 33]. The Framingham Offspring and Spouse Study (590 normal weight women at baseline; 16-year follow-up) found that subjects with lower quality diets were associated with a 76% increased risk of becoming overweight or obese compared to subjects with high quality diets [32]. The European Prospective Investigation into Cancer and Nutrition (EPIC) - Potsdam, German cohort (24,958 participants; mean baseline age 50 years; 4.4 years of follow-up) showed that diet quality, especially low-fat, high-fiber (13.5 g fiber vs. 8.8 g fiber/1000 kcal) diets (in non-obese subjects at baseline) was inversely associated with weight gain [34]. The 2003 Baltimore Longitudinal Study of Aging (459 men and women; mean age about 60 years; healthy diet [27 g fiber/day; high in fruit, vegetables, and whole-grains, and low in red meat, fast foods, and sugary soda] vs. other types of Western diets ≤20 g/fiber/day) observed significantly less annual BMI and waist size gain for the healthy vs. Western dietary patterns (Fig. 7.3) [35].

7.2.2.2 Mediterranean Dietary Pattern (MedDiet)

Of the healthy dietary patterns, the MedDiet has been the most studied for weight control (Table 7.1) [36–42]. Higher adherence to the MedDiet has consistently been shown to be inversely associated with weight gain or risk of general or central obesity in both men and women. A prospective cohort study among Swedish women (27,544 women; mean baseline age 40; 12-years of follow-up) showed that women with higher adherence to the MedDiet were not associated with increased body weight and waist size compared to the average median gain in body

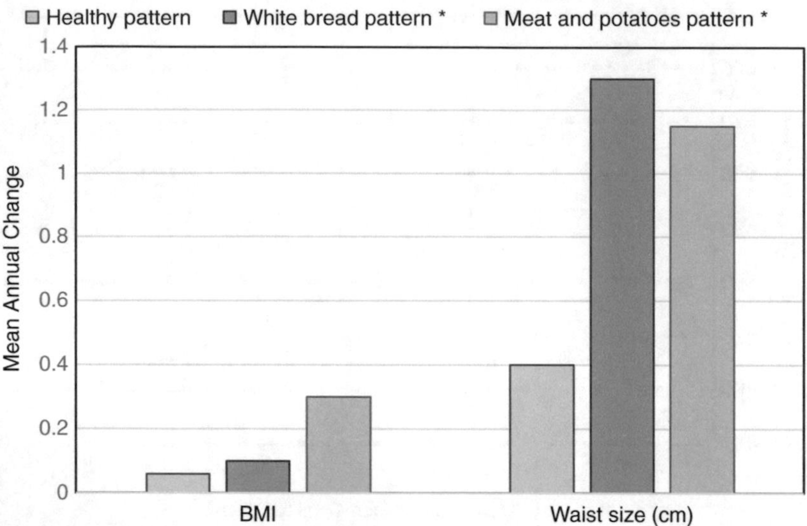

Fig. 7.3 Effect of healthy vs. Western type derived food dietary pattern on BMI and waist size in men and women from the Baltimore Longitudinal Aging Study (*$p < 0.05$) (adapted from [35]). **Healthy pattern**: contained relatively greater contributions from "healthy" foods, including fruit, high-fiber cereal, and reduced fat dairy, and relatively smaller contributions from fast food, nondiet soda, and salty snacks. **White bread pattern**: higher levels of refined carbohydrates and baked goods. **Meat and potatoes pattern**: higher levels of meats and higher energy dense vegetables such as potato products

weight by 5 kg and waist size by 7.0 cm in the overall cohort [36]. A Spanish cohort study (3058 subjects; 51% women; mean baseline age 49 years; 10 years of follow-up) found that high adherence to the MedDiet lowered waist size by 1.5 cm ($p = 0.024$; fully adjusted models) [37]. The EPIC-Spanish cohort (325,537 participants; mean baseline age 51–58 years; 5 years of follow-up) showed that non-smoking men and women with higher physical activity and high adherence to the MedDiet gained less weight and waist size compared to subjects adhering to the Western lifestyle [38]. A 2010 Spanish university study (10,376 men and women; mean baseline age 38 years; 5.7 years of follow-up) found that those subjects with the lowest MedDiet adherence had an average 0.3 kg annual weight gain, whereas those with highest MedDiet adherence lost 0.06 kg/year and had 24% lower risk of gaining ≥5 kg over the first 4 years of follow-up [39]. High adherence to the MedDiet was shown to protect against weight gain with better effects in younger people (<40 years of age) and in non-obese (BMI <30) individuals at baseline (p-interactions <0.0001) [40]. Also, several Spanish cohort studies show that higher adherence to the MedDiet significantly reduced risk of obesity by 10–30% with mean weight reductions by 0.16 kg over 3.3–5.0 years [40–42].

7.2.2.3 Dietary Approaches to Stop Hypertension (DASH) Dietary Pattern

Two studies indicate that high adherence to DASH diets helps to prevent weight gain in adolescent girls and women (Table 7.1) [43, 44]. A 2014 cross-sectional study (293 female nurses; > 30 years) showed that women with highest adherence to the DASH diet were 71% less likely to have general obesity and had a marginally significant trend towards a lower prevalence of central obesity as measured by waist size by 63% ($p = 0.09$) [43]. A 2011 US cohort study in adolescent girls (2327 girls; annual visits starting at baseline age 9 years; 10-year follow-up) found that higher adherence to the DASH eating pattern was associated with a significantly lower BMI by 1.9 units [44].

7.2.2.4 Vegetarian Dietary Pattern

Observational studies generally show that vegetarian diets protect against weight gain and may promote weight loss depending on the level of strictness or adherence [45, 46]. The Adventist Health Study-2 prospective study (60,903 subjects; mean age 58 years; 60% female; 5 years of follow-up) found that vegetarian diet strictness was inversely associated with BMI with vegans having a 5-unit lower BMI than nonvegetarians [45]. Twenty-nine of 40 observational studies reported significantly reduced BMI or body weight by 3–20% in vegetarians compared with non-vegetarians [46]. The incidence of obesity ranged from 0 to 6% in vegetarians and from about 5 to 45% in non-vegetarians.

7.2.3 Randomized Controlled Trials (RCTs)

Table 7.2 summarizes RCTs on the effects of healthy dietary patterns on body weight and composition [47–63].

7.2.3.1 Mediterranean Diet (MedDiet)

Systematic Reviews and Meta-Analyses

Four systematic reviews and meta-analyses of RCTs consistently show that *ab libitum* intake of MedDiets do not result in weight gain and high adherence to MedDiets supports weight loss and lower waist size compared to control diets such as low-fat and Western diets especially in overweight, obese or type 2 diabetic individuals, and with longer trial duration (> 6 months), or in conjunction with restricted energy intake or increased physical activity [47–50]. A meta-analysis of long-term MedDiet intake (5 RCTs; 998 subjects; comparator diets low-fat, low carbohydrate and American Diabetes Association (ADA); ≥ 12 months) showed that adherence to MedDiets resulted in greater weight loss than a low-fat diet, but produced similar weight loss to low carbohydrate or ADA diets [47]. Also, the MedDiet was more effective in lowering BMI and waist size than all the comparator diets. A meta-analysis in people with type 2 diabetes (9 RCTs; 1178 adults; age range 26–77 years; 1 month to 4 years of follow-up) found a small but significant mean loss of weight by 0.3 kg and BMI by 0.3 kg/m^2 compared to control diets along with significant improvements in glycemic control and reductions in cardiovascular disease risk factors [48]. Another meta-analysis (16 RCTs; 3436 participants; 1 month to 2 years) demonstrated that subjects on the MedDiet significantly reduced weight by 1.75 kg and BMI by 0.6 kg/m^2 compared to the control diet [49]. The effect of the MedDiet on weight loss was further improved with an energy restricted diet by 3.9 kg, with increased physical activity by 4.0 kg, or with trial durations >6 months by 2.7 kg. This analysis also showed that unrestricted intake of MedDiets does not promote weight gain, which helps to lessen weight gain concerns about the MedDiet's liberal use of olive oil and nuts. A meta-analysis of metabolic syndrome subjects (33 RCTs, and 2-cohort and 13-cross-sectional studies; 534,906 subjects) demonstrated that the MedDiet significantly reduced waist size, blood pressure, fasting blood glucose and the prevalence of metabolic syndrome, and increased HDL-C [50].

Specific RCTs

Six RCTs describe the various aspects of the effects of MedDiets, including the importance of adequate fiber intake on reducing and managing body weight and composition [51–56]. Three Spanish PREDIMED trials show impressive long-term effects of the MedDiet on maintaining and moderately lowering body weight and WC [51–53]. The PREDIMED trial (7447 subjects with type 2 diabetes or high cardiovascular risk; mean baseline age 67 years and BMI 30; MedDiet plus extra virgin olive oil or tree nuts and reduced-fat control diet; 5-year duration) showed in a long-term intervention that the unrestricted MedDiets were not associated with weight gain [51]. MedDiet plus extra virgin olive oil significantly reduced mean body weight by 0.43 kg compared to the lower fat control diet. Both MedDiets lowered waist size vs. the control diet

Table 7.2 Summary of dietary pattern randomized controlled trials (RCTs) in body weight and composition regulation

Objective	Study details	Results
Mediterranean diet (MedDiet)		
Systematic reviews and meta-analyses		
Mancini et al. (2016). Systematic review of the effect of the MedDiet on weight loss and waist size [47]	5 RCTs, 998 subjects; trials compared the MedDiet to low-fat diet, a low-carbohydrate diet, and the American Diabetes Association (ADA) diet; ≥ 12 months (12–48 months)	The MedDiet resulted in greater mean weight loss by −4.1 to −10.1 kg vs. a low-fat diet by 2.9 to −5.0 kg, but produced similar mean weight loss by −4.1 to −10.1 kg vs. low carbohydrate and ADA diets by −4.7 to −7.7 kg. Also, the MedDiet lowered mean BMI by −1.0 to −3.3 kg/m^2 vs. the other diets by 1.4 to −1.8 kg/m^2 and mean waist size vs. low-fat diets by −3.5 to −9.3 cm vs. low-fat diet by 2.6 to −3.5 cm)
Huo et al. (2014). Meta-analysis of the effects of MedDiet on glycemic control, weight loss and cardiovascular risk factors in type 2 diabetes patients [48]	9 RCTs; 1178 diabetic subjects; age range at baseline 26–77 years; 4 weeks to 4 years	In diabetic subjects, the MedDiet had greater mean reductions in BMI by 0.29 units, body weight by 0.29 kg, hemoglobin A1c by 0.30 unit, fasting plasma glucose by 0.72 mmol/L, fasting insulin by 0.55 μU/mL, total cholesterol by 0.14 mmol/L, triglycerides by 0.29 mmol/L, and both systolic and diastolic BP by 1.4 mm Hg. Also, HDL-C was increased by 0.06 mmol/L vs. control diets
Esposito et al. (2011). Evaluate the effect of MedDiets on body weight using meta-analysis [49]	16 RCTs; 3436 participants; mean age 35–69 years and BMI 26–35; 1 month to 2 years duration	MedDiet can be effective in lowering body weight, especially with energy restriction, increased physical activity, and >6 months in duration. Overall, the MedDiet significantly reduced weight by 1.75 kg and BMI by 0.57 units. In studies lasting longer than 6 months mean weight loss was 3.9 kg. Also, MedDiet accompanied with either a restricted energy diet or increased physical activity reduced weight by approximately 4 kg
Kastorini et al. (2011). Meta-analysis of the effect of a MedDiet on metabolic syndrome (MetS) and its components [50]	50 original research studies (35 RCTs, 2 prospective and 13 cross-sectional studies) through April 30, 2010; 534,906 participants	Adherence to the MedDiet was associated with significantly reduced MetS prevalence by 31%, waist size by 0.42 cm, triglycerides by 6.1 mg/dL, systolic blood pressure (BP) by 2.4 mmHg, diastolic BP by 1.6 mmHg and fasting glucose by 3.9 mg/dL and increased HDL-C by 1.2 mg/dL
Specific RCTs		
Estruch et al. (2016). Assess the long-term effects of ad libitum, high-vegetable-fat MedDiets on bodyweight and waist size in older people at risk of cardiovascular disease, most of whom were overweight or obese (PREDIMED; Spain) [51]	**Multicenter, Parallel RCT**: 7447 adults with type 2 diabetes or ≤3 CVD risk factors; mean age 67 years and BMI 30; three different *ad libitum* diets: MedDiet plus extra virgin olive oil; MedDiet plus tree nuts (total dietary fat approx. 100 g/day for both; or advice to reduced fat control diet (96 g fat/day). Advice to restrict dietary energy or promote physical activity was not advised; 5 years	This study showed that the long-term intake of plant-based, unrestricted-calorie, high-fat diets, such as the traditional MedDiet does not promote weight gain. The adjusted difference in 5-year loss in body weight in the MedDiet plus extra virgin olive oil group was 0.43 kg ($p = 0.044$) and in the plus nut group was 0.08 kg ($p = 0.730$), compared with the reduced fat control group. The adjusted difference in 5-year reduction in waist size was 0.55 cm ($p = 0.048$) in the MedDiet with extra virgin olive oil group and 0.94 cm ($p = 0.006$) in the nut group, compared with the reduced fat control group (Fig. 7.4)

Table 7.2 (continued)

Objective	Study details	Results
Alvarez-Perez et al. (2016). Assess effect of the MedDiet on anthropometric and body composition parameters (PREDIMED trial; Spain) [52]	**Parallel RCT**: 351 free-living subjects, mean age 67 years and BMI 31; 64% women; with type 2 diabetes or ≤3 CVD risk factors; ad *libitum* diets: MedDiet plus extra virgin olive oil, MedDiet plus mixed tree nuts, or a control low-fat diet guidance; study assessed changes in anthropometric measures of body weight, BMI, waist size, total body fat %; 1 year	This study found that unrestricted MedDiets that contain approximately 40% total fat can be alternative options to reduced-fat diets for weight maintenance. Significant reductions in body weight by 1 kg, BMI by 0.5 units and waist size by 1.1 cm ($p < 0.05$; all) were observed for the MedDiet plus extra virgin olive oil vs. the control group. The MedDiet plus nuts group exhibited a significant reduction in waist size by 2.3 cm ($p < 0.001$). The control group showed a significant increase in total body fat by 1% ($p = 0.02$)
Damasceno et al. (2013). Investigate effect of MedDiets on changes in adiposity and lipoprotein subfractions vs. a reduced fat control diet (PREDIMED diets; Spain) [53]	**Parallel RCT**: 169 subjects with type 2 diabetes or ≤3 CVD risk factors; mean age 67 years; 75% women; BMI 29.5; lipoprotein subclasses (particle concentrations and size) were determined by NMR spectroscopy; three different ad libitum diets: MedDiet plus extra-virgin olive oil, MedDiet plus mixed tree nuts (30 g walnuts, almonds, and hazelnuts/day), or a control reduced-fat diet; 1-year	Compared to the MedDiet plus extra virgin olive oil and reduced-fat control, participants in the tree nut-enriched MedDiet showed significantly reduced waist size by 5 cm ($p = 0.006$ for both) and increased LDL size with a net increase by 0.2 nmol/L ($p < 0.05$ for both). Also, there were increased large HDL concentrations in both the olive oil and nut supplemented MedDiets
Shai et al. (2008). Compare the effectiveness of weight-loss diets (US) [54]	**Parallel RCT**: 322 moderately obese subjects; mean age 52 years; mean BMI 31; males 86%; 3 restricted-calorie diets: low-fat, MedDiet, or low-carbohydrate; 2 years	Compared to other diet groups, the MedDiet group consumed the largest amounts of dietary fiber and the low-carbohydrate group consumed the smallest amount of carbohydrates and the largest amounts of fat, protein, and cholesterol ($P < 0.05$ for all). The mean weight loss was 4.4 kg for the MedDiet group, 4.7 kg for the low-carbohydrate group and 2.9 kg for the low-fat group ($P < 0.001$) (Fig. 7.5). MedDiet and low-carbohydrate diets appear to be effective alternatives to low-fat diets for weight loss and there are more favorable effects on glycemic control with the MedDiet and on lipids with the low-carbohydrate diet. The rate of adherence to these diets was 95% at 1 year and 85% at 2 years
Esposito et al. (2004). Assess the effect of a MedDiet on weight and cardiometabolic markers associated with metabolic syndrome (Italy) [55]	**Parallel RCT**: 180 metabolic syndrome patients (99 men and 81 women); 2 diets: MedDiet advice about how to increase daily consumption of whole grains, fruits, vegetables, nuts, and extra virgin olive oil (32 g fiber/day); control group followed a prudent diet (carbohydrates, 50–60%; proteins, 15–20%; total fat, 30%; 17 g fiber/day); 2 years	Compared to the control diet, subjects on the MedDiet had a significantly greater mean decrease in body weight by 11 kg and BMI by 4.2 units ($p < 0.001$) (Fig. 7.6). Also, compared to the control group, the MedDiet group had significantly reduced serum concentrations of hs-CRP ($p = 0.01$), lower insulin resistance ($p < 0.001$), and 50% fewer patients classified still continued to be with metabolic syndrome ($p < 0.001$)
Esposito et al. (2003). Determine the effect of an energy restricted MedDiet and physical activity on body weight, systemic inflammation, and insulin resistance (Italy) [56]	**Parallel RCT**: 120 premenopausal women; mean age 35 years and BMI 35; intervention group received detailed advice to reduce weight by ≥10% with reduced energy MedDiet and increased physical activity vs. control group given general info on healthy food choices and exercise; 2 years	The intervention group consumed 9 g fiber/day more and 310 kcals less than the usual diet control group ($p < 0.001$). Changes in body weight and BMI are shown in Fig. 7.7. The intervention was also associated with reduction in CRP by 0.8 mg/L and HOMA- insulin resistance by 0.9 units vs. control ($p = 0.008$; both)

(continued)

Table 7.2 (continued)

Objective	Study details	Results
DASH diet		
Systematic review and meta-analysis		
Soltani et al. (2016). Assess the effect of a DASH dietary pattern on body weight and composition in adults [57]	13 RCTs; 1291 participants; 10 on body weight, 6 on BMI and 2 on waist size; 8–52 weeks	Subjects on the DASH diet lost more weight by 1.42 kg in 24 weeks, reduced BMI by 0.42 units in 8–52 weeks and waist size by 1.05 cm in 24 weeks compared with controls. The effect was greater in overweight/obese participants and when compared with typical Western diet or a population's usual diets. Lower caloric DASH led to more weight reduction when compared with other low-energy diets. The DASH diet is effective for weight management, especially for weight reduction in overweight and obese participants
Healthy Nordic diets		
Nordic weight loss diet for lactating women		
Bertz et al. (2012, 2015). Assess the effect of an energy restricted diet on weight loss among overweight/obese lactating women (Lifestyle Weight Loss During Lactation Trial; Sweden) [58, 59]	**Parallel RCT with Follow-up Analysis:** 68 women; BMI 25–35; mean age 33 years and BMI 30; intervention weight loss diet based on Nordic Nutrition Recommendation: subjects were instructed to restrict energy intake by 500 kcals, limit sweets and snacks to 100 kcal/week, substitute lower fat and sugar alternatives for usual foods, cover ½ the lunch and dinner plate with vegetables, and reduce portion size vs. usual diet; 12 weeks plus 9-month follow-up	This dietary treatment was sufficient to significantly and clinically meaningfully promote weight and total fat loss, and lower BMI in lactating women, and to sustain weight loss at 9-month follow-up after the intervention ended. The intervention diet was lower in energy by approx. 400–500 kcals and increased fiber intake by 3 g/1000 kcal. Changes in body weight are shown in Fig. 7.8. BMI was reduced by ≥3 units and total weight was reduced by 5.5–6.7 kg ($p < 0.001$)
New Nordic diet		
Paulsen et al. (2014). Evaluate health effects of the New Nordic Diet, which is a food-based dietary concept recently developed in the Nordic countries in collaboration with Copenhagen's gourmet restaurant NOMA. The NND is based on regional foods in season, with a strong emphasis on palatability, healthiness, and sustainability, while aligning with regional food culture and dietary preferences (Denmark) [60]	**Parallel RCT:** 181 centrally obese men and women; 71% women; mean age of 42 years (20–66 years), mean BMI 30.2, and waist size 100 cm (39 in.); received either the New Nordic Diet (high in fruit, vegetables, dairy products whole grains, and fish, and low in sugar, cakes, pastries, and biscuits) or an average Danish diet; New Nordic Diet contained 19 g/day more total fiber and 21 kcals (87.5 kJ) less energy/100 g than average Danish diet; 26 weeks	Free-living intake of the NND reduced mean body weight by 3.2 kg (Fig. 7.9) and mean waist size by 2.9 cm ($p < 0.001$; both) compared to the average Danish diet. Also, the New Nordic Diet produced greater reductions in systolic blood pressure by 5.1 mmHg compared to the average Danish diet ($p < 0.001$). The weight loss was shown despite the fact that the diet was developed as highly palatable and offered *ad libitum*, and the study was not specifically designed as a weight-loss study

Table 7.2 (continued)

Objective	Study details	Results
Vegetarian diet		
Systematic review and meta-analysis		
Huang et al. (2016). Investigate the effects of lacto-ovo-vegetarian and vegan diets on weight reduction [61]	12 RCTs; 1151 subjects; median duration of 18 weeks	Overall, individuals assigned to the vegetarian diet groups lost significantly 2 kg more weight than those assigned to the non-vegetarian diet groups. Subgroup analysis detected significant weight reduction in subjects consuming a vegan diet by 2.5 kg and, to a lesser extent, in those given lacto-ovo-vegetarian diets by 1.5 kg. Trials on subjects consuming vegetarian diets with energy restriction revealed a significantly greater weight reduction of 2.2 kg than those without energy restriction of 1.7 kg
Barnard et al. (2015). Estimate the effect of vegetarian diets on body weight [62]	15 RCTs; 755 participants (197 ovo-lactovegetarian and 558 vegan); ≥ 4 weeks without energy intake limitations	Vegetarian diets were associated with a mean weight loss of 3.4 kg ($p < 0.001$) in an intention-to-treat analysis vs. control diet. Greater weight loss was shown in studies with higher baseline weights, smaller proportions of female participants, older participants, or longer durations, and in studies in which weight loss was a goal
Specific comparative RCT of different types of vegetarian diets		
Turner-McGrievy et al. (2015). Determine the effect of plant-based diets on weight loss (US) [63]	**Parallel RCT**: 63 overweight and obese adults; 19% non-white; 27% men; mean baseline age 48 years and BMI 35; randomized into 5 diets: a low-fat, low-glycemic index diet: vegan, vegetarian, pesco-vegetarian, semi-vegetarian, or omnivorous; 6 months	After 6 months, weight was significantly reduced in the vegan group by 7.5% and ovo-lacto vegetarian by 6.3% compared to the omnivorous, semi-vegetarian and pesco-vegetarian groups by approximately 3% ($p = 0.03$) (Fig. 7.10). Vegan diets may result in greater weight loss than more modest recommendations

after 5 years (Fig. 7.4). Two sub-cohort PREDIMED trials found that: (1) MedDiets (351 free-living subjects with type 2 diabetes or ≤3 CVD risk factors, mean age 67 years and BMI 31; 64% women) resulted in significantly lower body weight, BMI and waist size compared to the lower-fat control diet (which also significantly increased total body fat by 1%) [52]; and (2) Tree nut-enriched MedDiet (169 subjects with type 2 diabetes or ≤3 CVD risk factors; mean baseline age 67 years and BMI 29.5; 75% women; 1 year) significantly reduced waist size by 5 cm and increased LDL size by 0.2 nmol/L compared to the MedDiet plus extra virgin olive oil, and the lower-fat control diet [53]. In a US-based comparative analysis of non-energy restricted diets (322 obese subjects; 86% men; mean baseline age 52 years and BMI 31), MedDiets were as effective as low-fat or low carbohydrate diets in promoting significant weight loss over 2 years ($p < 0.001$) (Fig. 7.5) [54]. An Italian trial in 180 adults with metabolic syndrome found significant body weight, BMI and waist size lowering effects for an *ab libitum* 32 g fiber/day MedDiet (including about 500 g of whole-grains, vegetables, fruit, legumes, and nuts) compared to a 17 g fiber/day prudent diet (including about 200 g of whole-grains, vegetables, fruit, legumes, and nuts) after 2 years (Fig. 7.6) [55]. Also, an Italian weight loss trial (120 premenopausal women; mean baseline age 35 years and BMI 35; 2 years) showed significant effects of an energy restricted MedDiet compared to the usual diet along with increased physical activity on lowering body weight, BMI, CRP and insulin resistance (HOMA-IR) (Fig. 7.7) [56].

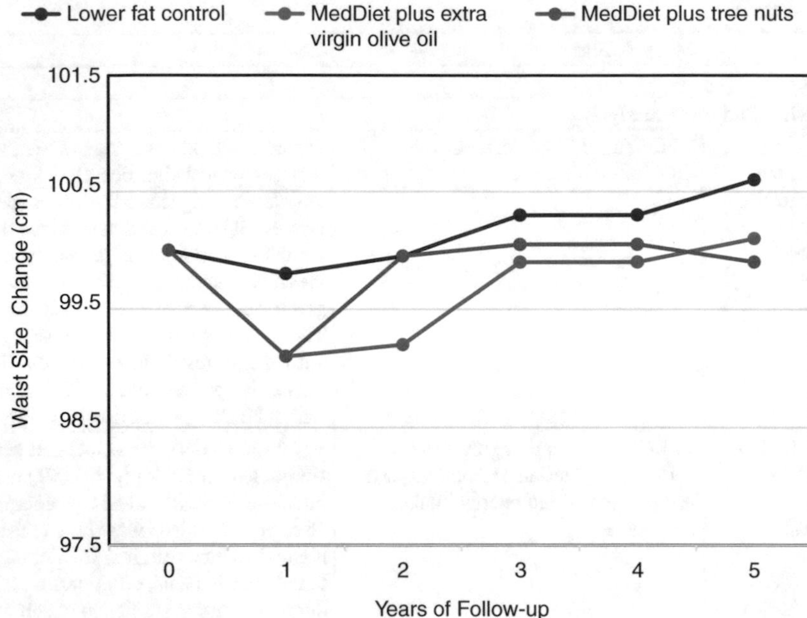

Fig. 7.4 Effect of unrestricted MedDiet and lower fat control diets on mean waist size from the PREDIMED trial over 5 years (multivariate adjusted values) (adapted from [51])

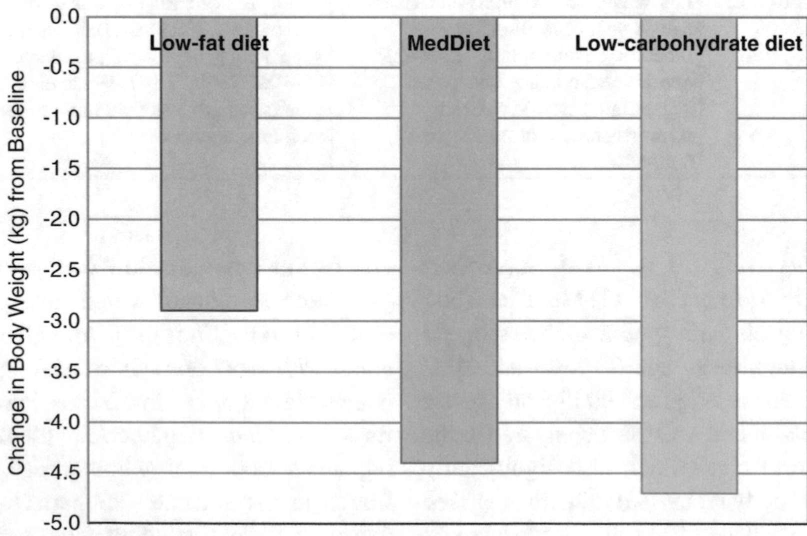

Fig. 7.5 Effect of the non-energy restricted MedDiet vs. low fat and low carbohydrate non-energy restricted diets in 322 obese adults (about 90% men) over 2 years (adapted from [54])

7.2.3.2 Other Diets

DASH Diet

A meta-analysis (13 RCTs; 1291 participants; 8–52 weeks) showed that adults on a DASH diet lost more weight by 1.42 kg and BMI by 0.42 kg m^2 in 8–24 weeks and waist size by 1 cm in 24 weeks compared with control diets [57].

Nordic Diets

Nordic Weight Loss Diet for Lactating Women. Childbearing is associated with weight gain because of gestational weight gain and

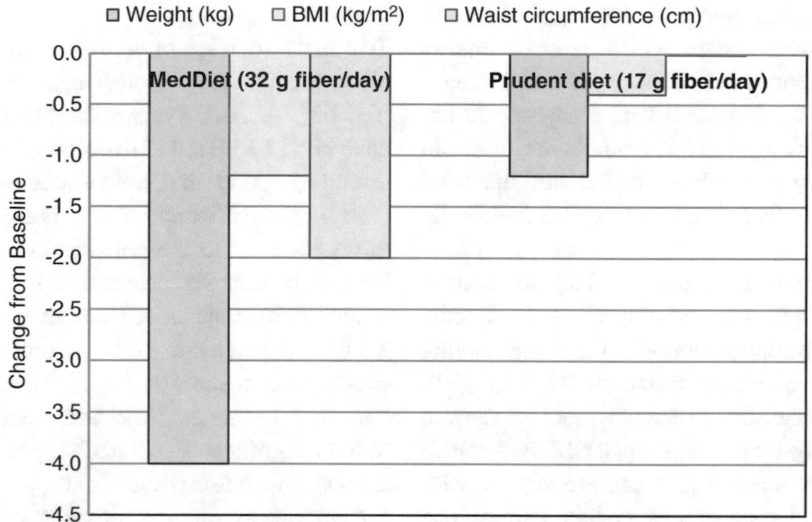

Fig. 7.6 Effect of a high fiber-rich MedDiet compared to a moderate fiber prudent diet in 180 adults with metabolic syndrome over 2 years ($p < 0.001$; all) (adapted from [55])

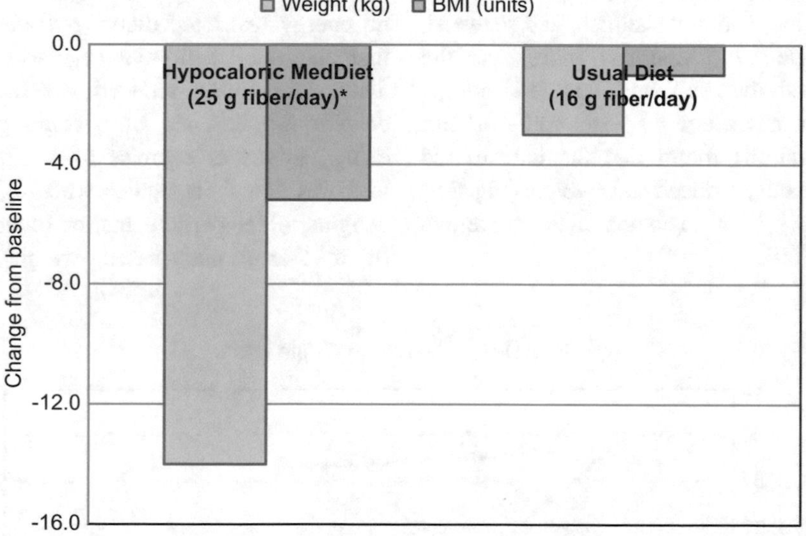

Fig. 7.7 Effect of a hypocaloric Mediterranean diet (MedDiet) plus increased physical activity vs. usual diet and exercise advice in 120 obese women over 2 years ($p < 0.001$; both) (adapted from [56])

postpartum weight retention, which can make it difficult for women to return to pre-pregnancy weight [58, 59]. The Swedish Lifestyle Weight Loss During Lactation Trial (68 women; pre-pregnancy BMI 25–35; mean age 33 years and BMI 30; intervention weight loss diet based on Nordic Nutrition Recommendation: vs. usual diet; 12 weeks duration plus 9-month follow-up) found significant and clinically meaningful promotion of weight loss, lowering of BMI, and total body fat loss in lactating women, and sustained weight loss at 9-month follow-up after the intervention ended compared to the usual diet [58, 59]. The primary guidelines for the Nordic diet was to target restricted energy intake by 500 kcals by limiting sweets and snacks to 100 kcal/week, substituting lower fat and sugar alternatives for usual foods, designating half of the lunch and dinner plate for vegetables, and reducing portion size, which reduces energy intake by approx 400–500 kcals and increase fiber intake by 3 g/1000 kcal compared to the usual diet. Changes in body weight are shown in Fig. 7.8. BMI was reduced by ≥3 units and total weight loss was reduced by 5.5–6.7 kg ($p < 0.001$).

New Nordic Diet (NND). This food-based dietary concept was developed in the Nordic countries in collaboration with the world-leading Copenhagen gourmet restaurant NOMA [60]. This diet is based on regional foods in season, with a strong emphasis on palatability, healthiness, and sustainability, which are aligned with regional food culture and dietary habits. The basic food components of the NND include: fruit and vegetables (especially berries, cabbages, root vegetables, and legumes), potatoes, fresh herbs, mushrooms, nuts, whole grain, meats from livestock and game, fish and shellfish, and seaweed, which provide 19 g fiber/day more than the average Danish diet. A Danish trial (181 adults; 71% women; mean age 42 years and BMI 30; 26-week duration) found that the unrestricted NND significantly reduced body weight (Fig. 7.9) and waist size by 2.9 cm compared to the average Danish diet [60].

Vegetarian Diets

Two meta-analyses of vegetarian diets show that all vegetarian diets protect against weight gain [61, 62]. A 2016 systematic review and meta-analysis (12 RCTs; 1151 subjects; 18-week mean duration) found that individuals on vegetarian diets lost significantly 2 kg more weight than those assigned to the non-vegetarian diets [61]. Subgroup analysis detected significant weight reduction in subjects consuming a vegan diet by 2.5 kg and, to a lesser extent, in those given lacto-ovo-vegetarian diets by 1.5 kg. Trials on subjects consuming energy restricted vegetarian diets found a significantly greater weight reduction by 2.2 kg than those without energy restriction by 1.7 kg. The weight loss for subjects with follow-up of <1 year was greater than those with follow-up of ≥1 year (−2.05 kg vs. −1.13 kg). A 2015 meta-analysis (15 RCTs; 755 adults; 197 lacto-ovo vegetarians and 558 vegans; 75% females; no energy restricted diets; ≥ 4 weeks) showed that combined lacto-ovo vegetarian and vegan diets significantly reduced weight by 3.4 kg, despite the absence of specific guidance on energy intake or exercise [62]. Greater weight loss was found in studies with higher baseline weights, older participants, or longer durations. In a 5-arm plant-based weight loss RCT

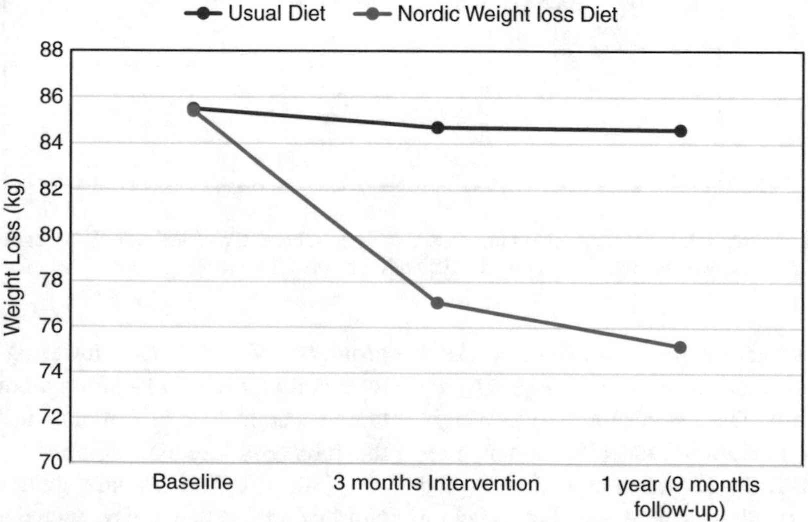

Fig. 7.8 Effects of Nordic energy restricted and higher fiber diet intervention on body weight in lactating overweight and obese women ($p < 0.001$) (adapted from [58, 59])

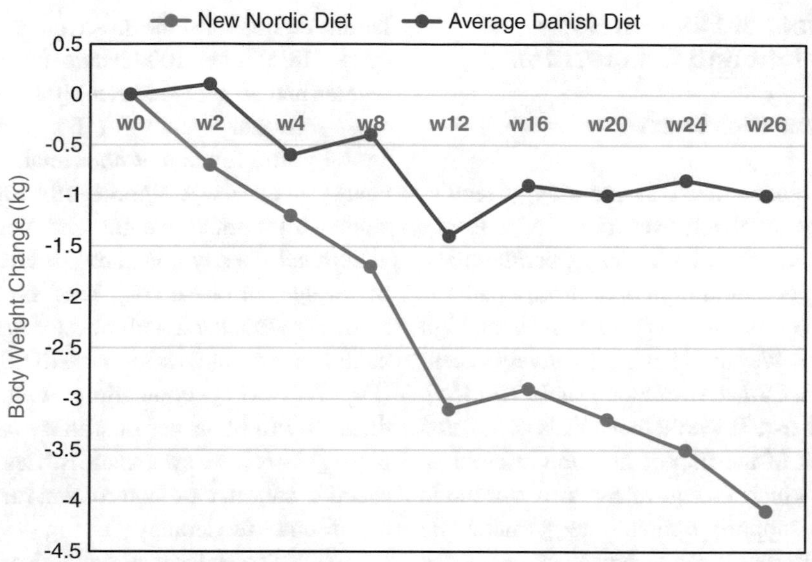

Fig. 7.9 Change in body weight (intention-to-treat) for the New Nordic Diet compared to the average Danish diet over 26 weeks ($p < 0.001$) (adapted from [60])

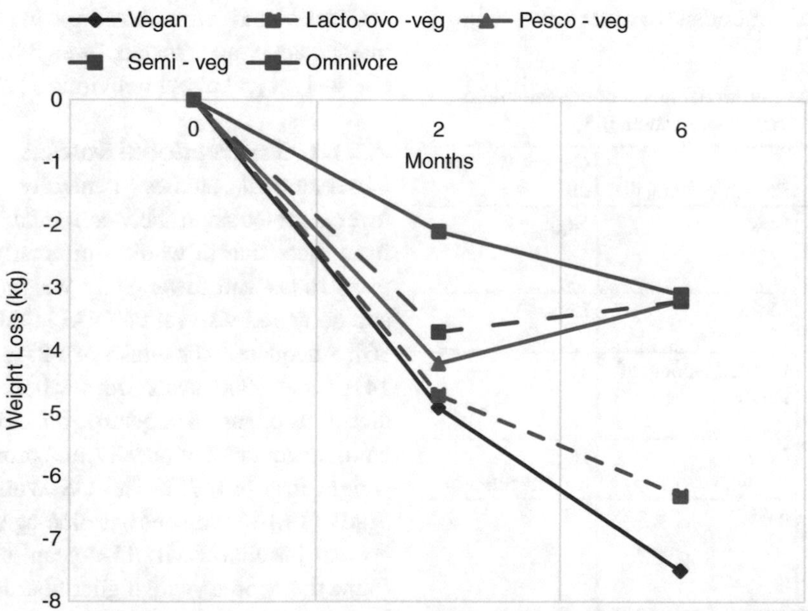

Fig. 7.10 Effect of type of vegetarian (veg) diets on weight loss in adults after 6 months (p-trend =0.01 for vegan and lacto-ovo-vegetarian diets) (adapted from [63])

(63 subjects; mean age 48 years; mean BMI 35; 73% female; vegetarian vs. omnivorous diets; 6 months) reported that vegan and lacto-ovo-vegetarian diets have similar greater effects on weight loss compared to omnivorous, semi-, and pesco-vegetarian diets (Fig. 7.10) [63].

7.3 Effect of Fiber on Body Weight and Composition

7.3.1 Fiber-Rich Diets

The human gastrointestinal and energy regulatory systems evolved over most of the last 40,000 years on diets with ≥50 g fiber/day [64]. These pre-agricultural high fiber dietary patterns are in sharp contrast to the present low fiber, high energy dense Western diets, a relatively recent occurrence in human evolution (Table 7.3) [65]. Ancestral fiber-rich whole foods diets stimulated the evolution of the important colon microbiota ecosystem, which is equivalent to a symbiotic 'organ' that supports optimal energy metabolic and cardiometabolic health processes, increased excretion of fecal metabolizable energy and fiber fermentation to short chain fatty acids (SFCAs) associated with a range of biological activities associated with better weight control [66, 67]. About 95% of Americans or other Western populations do not consume an adequate level of fiber daily (14 g fiber/1000 kcals or 25 g/day for women and 38 g/day for men) [68, 69]. A Spanish cross-sectional study (1655 adults; age 18–64 years) found that fiber intake (adjusted by energy intake) was significantly higher in subjects with normal weight and without excess abdominal obesity compared to those who were overweight or obese [70]. Total fiber intake was inversely associated with obesity risk among US adults in an analysis of NHANES 1999–2010 (Fig. 7.11) [71]. Populations with higher fiber diets tend to be leaner than those with low fiber diets [72–74]. A systematic review of 43 prospective cohort, case-control and randomized trials found moderately strong evidence that fiber-rich foods have a protective role against weight gain and increased waist size [72]. In 2010, the European Food Safety Authority (EFSA) recommended that adults should consume >25 g fiber per day (from whole-grain cereals, fruit, and vegetables) to improve weight maintenance and sustain weight reduction in overweight and obese individuals [75].

Table 7.3 Daily nutritional intake of pre-agricultural vs. present day Western dietary pattern [65]

Nutritional components	Pre-agricultural diet	Current Western diet
Diet energy density (kcal/g)	Low	High
Dietary bulk (satiating)	More	Less
Sugar and sweeteners (% energy)	Limited amount of honey	17%
Grain products	Low (all whole grain)	High (mostly refined)
Fruit, vegetables, and nuts (% energy)	65%	8%
Fiber Intake (g/day)	50–100	<15–17
Protein Intake (% energy)	37% from lean game, eggs, fish, shellfish, or nuts	15% from meat, poultry, dairy, fish, eggs, legumes, or nuts
Fat Intake (% energy)	22	32
Physical activity (kcal/day)	Active >1000 kcal/day	Sedentary (<150–490 kcal/day)

7.3.1.1 Observational Studies

Observational studies generally support an inverse association between total fiber intake from diets rich in whole (minimally processed) plant foods and lower body weight, waist size, and body and visceral fat (VAT) (Table 7.4) [76–86]. Adequate fiber intake of >25 g fiber/day or 14 g fiber/1000 kcals from whole plant-based diets is a suggested target to reduce risk of weight gain, prevent risk of obesity, and promote modest weight loss [68, 75]. The US Women's Health Study (18,146 women; baseline age ≥ 45 years; normal baseline BMI; 15.9-years of follow-up) found that women with higher fiber intake did not have significant changes in body weight or BMI [76]. A study in 252 women (mean baseline age 40 years; 20-months of follow-up) found that each 1 g/1000 kcal increase in total fiber significantly reduced body weight by 0.25 kg and body fat by 0.25%, by reducing total metabolizable energy intake [82]. Specific studies suggest that increased total fiber intake by approximately ≥12 g/day, above the typical Western diet fiber levels, especially as a replacement for refined low

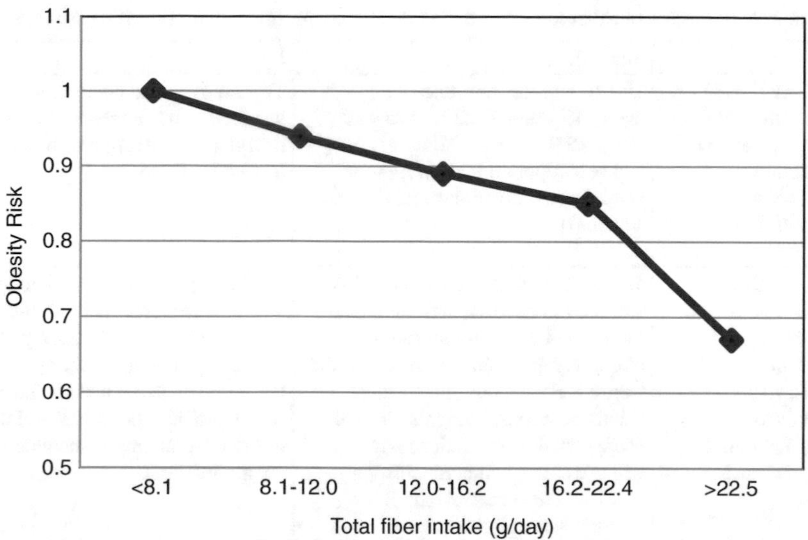

Fig. 7.11 Relationship between increasing fiber intake and adult obesity risk from the US National Health and Nutrition Examination (NHANES) Survey 1999–2010) (adapted from [71])

fiber food, can significantly prevent long-term (8–12 years) weight gain by 3.5–5.5 kg in both men and women [83, 85, 86]. For WC, studies show an inverse association with increased total fiber intake [78–80, 84]. The European Prospective Investigation into Cancer and Nutrition (EPIC) study (89,432 participants; mean baseline age 53 years; 6.5 years of follow-up) found that 10 g/day increase in total and cereal fiber reduced waist size by approximately 1 cm/year [79]. For visceral adipose tissue (VAT), several studies show an inverse association with increased fiber intake, with children appearing to be especially responsive to the effects of low fiber, energy dense diets on visceral fat gain [81].

7.3.1.2 Randomized Controlled Trials (RCT)

A systematic review of clinical studies found that increasing fiber intake by 14 g fiber/day in overweight or obese individuals, with *ad libitum* energy intake, was associated with a mean 10% decrease in energy intake and a reduction of weight by 1.9 kg after 4 months [87]. Seven RCTs found the consumption of adequate fiber intake ≥28 g fiber/day or ≥14 g fiber/1000 kcal from fiber-rich diets combined with or without a low-fat dietary pattern reduced body weight and improved body composition compared to the low fiber Western control diets (Table 7.5) [25, 88–93]. Low energy dense diets derived from higher consumption of fruits, vegetables, and fiber were shown to limit weight regain 0.3% in subjects with a history of recent weight reduction compared to an increase of 1.3% for those on the usual diet after 7 months (p = 0.002) [88]. A randomized trial (240 metabolic syndrome subjects; mean baseline age 52 years and BMI 35; 1 year) found that a high fiber diet (goal to consume >30 g fiber/day) was as effective as a reduced energy multicomponent AHA weight loss program after one year [25]. An Australian RCT (72 subjects; mean age 43 years and BMI 34; 12-week duration) demonstrated that the intake of 31 g fiber or various combinations of diets with psyllium significantly reduced body weight, BMI and % body fat compared to a 20-g fiber/day control (Fig. 7.12) [91]. The Finnish Diabetes Prevention Study (522 prediabetic subjects; 67% females; mean baseline age 55 years; 4-year duration) showed total fiber intake (>15.5 g/1000 kcal vs. <11 g/1000 kcal) significantly reduced body weight by 2.6 kg (p-trend = 0.001) and waist size by 1.3 cm (p-trend = 0.033)

Table 7.4 Summary of observational studies on fiber intake in body weight and composition regulation

Objective	Study details	Results
Rautiainen et al. (2015). Investigate the effect of fiber intake on weight change and the risk of becoming overweight or obese (Women's Health Study; US) [76]	18,146 women, baseline age ≥ 45 years; BMI 18.5 to <25; mean 15.9 years of follow-up; FFQ and self-reported body weight on annual questionnaire (multivariate adjusted)	This study found no significant association with total fiber intake and weight gain or having an overweight or obese BMI (p-trend = 0.13)
Fischer et al. (2015). Cross-sectional assessment of how usual patterns of nutrient intake are associated with visceral adipose tissue (VAT), subcutaneous, abdominal and trunk adipose tissue (German adults) [77]	583 adults; mean age 61 years; VAT volumes from MRI; nutrient intake estimated by a 112-item food-frequency questionnaire linked to the German Food Code and Nutrient Database; foods, nutrients, or total energy intake associations with adipose tissue compartments via multiple linear regression (multivariate adjusted)	VAT was positively associated with nutrients characteristic of animal products (except for dairy), (β: 0.25; p < 0.0001), but negatively with total fiber (β: −0.17; p < 0.0001), and nutrients found in milk. Subcutaneous abdominal and trunk adipose tissue were mainly associated with total energy intake
Lin et al. (2011). Assess the effect of total fiber and sources on BMI and waist size (Belgian) [78]	3083 individuals (1546 men and 1537 women); baseline age ≥ 15 years. 42% of women and 29% of men were abdominally obese. The main contributors to total fiber intake were cereals and cereal products (34%), potatoes and other tubers (18.6%), fruits (14.7%) and vegetables (14.4%) (multivariate adjusted)	Waist size was inversely related to total fiber intakes (β = −0.118, p < 0.001) and positively related to fruit-fiber intakes (β = −0.731 (p = 0.001). Intake of cereals and cereal products fiber were significantly associated with lower BMI (β = −0.045, p = 0.025), but the association was attenuated by energy intake adjustments
Du et al. (2010). Investigate the association of total dietary fiber, cereal fiber, and fruit and vegetable fiber with changes in body weight and waist size (EU EPIC) [79]	89,432 participants; mean baseline age 53 years; average 6.5 years of follow-up (multivariate adjusted)	Higher intake of total fiber, especially cereal fiber, helps to prevent body weight and waist size gain. For a 10 g/day higher total fiber intake, the mean weight loss was 39 g/year and waist size loss was 0.08 cm/year. A 10 g/day higher cereal fiber intake was associated with lower body weight/year by 77 g and lower waist size/year by 0.10 cm. Fruit and vegetable fiber were not associated with weight change but had a similar association with waist size change when compared with intake of total fiber and cereal fiber
Romaguera et al. (2010). Assess the association between dietary factors and prospective changes in waist circumference (WC) and visceral adiposity (European Prospective Investigation into Cancer and Nutrition [EPIC] Study) [80]	48,631 participants; mean baseline age 50 years; mean BMI 26; median 5.5 years of follow-up (multivariate adjusted)	In women, an increased fiber intake by 10 g fiber/day significantly reduced waist size by 0.06 cm. Waist size was also significantly increased for every 1 kcal/g higher energy density by up to 0.15 cm and for every 10 glycemic index units by up to 0.06 cm
Davis et al. (2009). Assess the relation between changes in dietary intake, and specifically sugar and fiber intakes, with changes in adiposity and risk factors for type 2 diabetes in a longitudinal analysis of overweight Latino youth (US) [81]	85 overweight Latino youth; aged 11–17 years; body composition by dual-energy X-ray absorptiometry and magnetic resonance imaging; 2 years of follow-up (multivariate adjusted)	Reduced fiber intake by 3 g/1000 kcals significantly increased visceral fat by 21% vs. an increase in fiber intake of 3 g fiber/1000 kcals, which reduced visceral fat by 4%

Table 7.4 (continued)

Objective	Study details	Results
Tucker et al. (2009). Evaluate the effects of total fiber intake on risk of gaining weight and body fat in women over time (US) [82]	252 women; mean baseline age 40 years; mean weight 65.6 kg; 20 months of follow-up; 7-day food records (multivariate adjusted)	For each 1 g/1000 kcal increase in fiber intake there was a significant decrease in body weight by 0.25 kg and fat by 0.25%. After adjustment for energy intake, there was a reduction of about 33% but the values still retained significance. Fiber's influence occurs primarily through reducing energy intake over time
Koh-Banerjee et al. (2004). Evaluate the associations between changes in cereal fiber intake and weight change (HPFS; US) [83]	27,000 men; mean baseline age 52 years; 8 years of follow-up (multivariate adjusted)	Total fiber intake was inversely related to weight gain independent of whole grains (p-trend <0.0001). The men consuming 17 g fiber/day gained 1.40 kg, whereas the men with 26 g fiber/day gained 0.39 kg. After adjusting for measurement error, there was reduced weight gain by 5.5 kg (12 lbs) for each 20-g/day increment in total fiber intake
Koh-Banerjee et al. (2003). Determine the effects of changes in diet and physical activity, on waist size among men (Health Professionals' Follow-up Study [HPFS]; US) [84]	16,587 men; mean baseline age 44–65 years; 9 years of follow-up (multivariate adjusted)	An increase of 12 g total fiber/day was associated with a 0.63 cm decrease in waist size ($p < 0.001$), whereas smoking cessation and a 20-h/week increase in television watching were associated with a 1.98 cm and 0.59 cm waist gain, respectively ($p < 0.001$). Increases of 25 metabolic equivalent hrs/week in vigorous physical activity and in weight training by ≥30 min/week were associated with 0.38-cm and 0.91-cm decreases in waist size, respectively ($p < 0.001$ for each comparison)
Liu et al. (2003). Investigate the associations between the intakes of fiber and whole- or refined-grain products and weight gain over time (Nurses' Health Study; US) [85]	74,000 female nurses; mean baseline age 50 years; 12 years of follow-up (multivariate adjusted)	Women consuming a mean total fiber intake of 20 g vs. 13 g total fiber/day gained an average of 1.52 kg (3.4 lbs) less weight (p-trend <0.0001) independent of body weight at baseline, age, and changes in covariate status; over 2–4 years women gained less weight by 0.76 kg and BMI by 0.28 units. An increase in total fiber intake by 12 g/day is estimated to reduce weight gain by 3.5 kg (8 lb) in 12 years. Women in the highest quintile of total fiber intake had a 49% lower risk of major weight gain than women in the lowest quintile (p-trend <0.0001)
Ludwig et al. (1999). Examine the role of fiber intake on weight gain, insulin status and cardiovascular disease (CVD) risk factors (The Coronary Artery Risk Development in Young Adults [CARDIA]; US) [86]	2909 healthy adults; mean baseline age 26 years; >10.5 g fiber vs. <5.9 g fiber/1000 kcal; 10 years of follow-up (multivariate adjusted)	Total fiber intake was significantly inversely associated with body weight ($p = 0.001$), waist-to-hip ratio and fasting insulin; adjusted for BMI. Increased total fiber reduced weight gain by 8 lbs., waist-hip ratio by 0.1, and fasting insulin by 0.8–1.4 μU/mL in young adults. CVD risk factor was also significantly lowered

Table 7.5 Summary of randomized controlled trials (RCTs) on fiber-rich diets in body weight and composition regulation

Objective	Study details	Results
Karimi et al. (2016). Assess effects of low energy density diet vs. a usual diet on weight maintenance, lipid profiles, and glycemic control (Iran) [88]	**Parallel RCT:** 70 subjects with recent history of weight reduction; mean age 55 years; 50% male; low energy dense diet contained 30% fat, 15% protein, and 55% carbohydrate (20 g fiber, fruit 3.7 servings and vegetables 5.5 servings) vs. usual diet including 35% fat, 15% protein, and 50% carbohydrate (14 g fiber; fruit 2.5 servings and vegetables 3.3 servings); dietary intake was assessed by using 3-day food records; 7 months	Subjects on the low energy dense diets reduced weight by 0.3% vs. subjects on the usual diet control who gained 1.3% more weight ($p = 0.002$). The results were similar for waist size with a loss of 0.4 cm on the low energy dense diet vs. a gain of 0.3 cm on the usual diet ($p = 0.004$). Also, the low energy dense diet group decreased fasting blood glucose by 9.5% vs. an increase by 0.4% on the usual diet ($p = 0.0001$). These findings support the beneficial effects of a low energy dense diet derived from higher consumption of fruits, vegetables, and fiber on attenuating weight regain
Ma et al. (2015). Evaluate the effects of a simple high fiber diet compared to a multicomponent American Heart Association (AHA) weight loss plan on body weight, waist size and BMI (US) [25]	**Parallel RCT:** 240 metabolic syndrome subjects; mean baseline age 52 years; mean BMI 35; goal ≥30 g fiber/day diet or an AHA weight loss program diet plan including caloric reduction of 500–1000 kcal/day; 1 year	At 12 months: (1) mean body weight was reduced by 2.1 kg in the high-fiber diet group vs. 2.7 kg in the AHA weight loss program (mean group difference 0.6 kg); (2) mean waist size was increased by 0.1 in. for the high fiber diet vs. a loss of 0.4 in. for the AHA weight loss program (mean group difference, 0.5 in.); and (3) mean BMI was reduced by 0.8 units for the high fiber diet and 1.0 units for the AHA weight loss program (Fig. 7.1). There were no significant differences in weight loss, BMI, or waist size between the groups. This study suggests that simply consuming a high fiber diet may be a reasonable alternative to a traditional, challenging, hypocaloric weight loss diet plan
Turner et al. (2013). Examine the effect of two high-fiber hypocaloric diets on weight loss (US) [89]	**Parallel RCT:** 20 subjects; mean age 47 years, 18 females and 2 males; mean BMI 31; high fiber, reduced energy by 300–400 kcal/day diets with either 1.5 cups beans/day or a variety of fruits, vegetables, and whole grains; 25–35 g fiber; 4 weeks	Both fiber-rich food groups increased fiber intake from about 17 g/day to about 29 g fiber/day and lowered energy density by 38% for the bean group and 29% for the variety of fiber foods group. Both diets significantly reduced body weight, with the bean diet by 1.6 kg and the variety of fiber food diet by 1.1 kg. Combined mean weight loss was 1.4 kg ($p < 0.001$)
Mecca et al. (2012). Investigate the effectiveness of a high fiber lifestyle intervention on overweight-obese adults (Brazil) [90]	**Parallel RCT:** 50 subjects; 11 males and 39 females; mean age 50 years; mean BMI 33.0; high-fiber diet group (daily 32 g fiber; 540 g fruits and vegetables) vs. control group receiving general nutrition education (17 g fiber/day); 10 weeks	Subjects on high fiber diet lost 4% more weight and BMI by 4%, and waist size by 7% vs. the lower fiber control diet ($p < 0.05$; all)
Pal et al. (2011). Assess the effects of increased fiber intake from a healthy diet, psyllium or their combinations on body weight and composition (Australia) [91]	**Parallel RCT:** 72 participants; mean age 43 years; mean BMI about 34; diets: control diet plus placebo (20 g fiber/day); control diet plus psyllium (55 g fiber/day); healthy fiber-rich food diet plus placebo (31 g fiber/day); or healthy fiber-rich food diet plus psyllium (59 g fiber/day); 12 weeks	All fiber rich diets compared to the control Western diet significantly reduced body weight, BMI, and % body fat after 12 weeks (Fig. 7.12)

Table 7.5 (continued)

Objective	Study details	Results
Ferdowsian et al. (2010). Study the effects of a high fiber, low fat vegan diet on body weight and composition in overweight subjects (US GEICO Corporate Site) [92]	**Parallel RCT:** 113 adults; BMI >25; randomized into a low-fat, vegan diet group at 29 g fiber/day vs. Western habitual diet at 15 g fiber/day; 22 weeks	The higher fiber diet group lost significantly more weight by 5.2 kg and waist size by 5.5 cm compared to the lower fiber Western diet control group ($p < 0.0001$). Weight loss of 5% of body weight was more frequently found for subjects in the high fiber group by 49% vs. control group by 11% ($p < 0.0001$)
Lindstrom et al. (2006). Investigate the effect of total dietary fiber, fat, and energy density on body weight and WC (Finnish Diabetes Prevention Study) [93]	**Parallel RCT:** 522 participants with impaired glucose tolerance; mean age 55 years; 67% female; mean BMI 31; standard lifestyle vs. high fiber, low-fat diets and exercise counseling; 15 g fiber vs. 11 g fiber/1000 kcals; 4 years	Participants consuming the low-fat, high-fiber diet lost significantly 2.4 kg more weight than those on the high-fat, low-fiber diet. The fiber density of the diet was inversely associated with weight and waist size (Figs. 7.13 and 7.14)

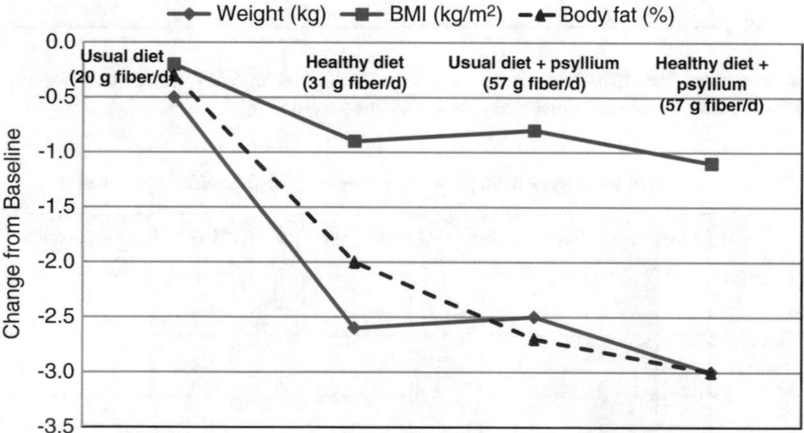

Fig. 7.12 Effect of usual diet and healthy diet with and without added psyllium (12 g 3×/day) in 72 obese adults (mean age 43 years; BMI 34) after 12 weeks ($p < 0.05$) (adapted from [91])

(Fig. 7.13) after multivariate adjustments [93]. Also, in this study, the adjusted 3-year weight reduction among those whose diets were both low in fat and high in fiber was 3.1 kg compared to 0.7 kg for subjects on the high fat and low fiber diet (Fig. 7.14). Four RCTs generally show that the consumption of 29–32 g vs. 15–20 g total fiber/day significantly reduced body weight, BMI and/or waist size over 4–22 weeks [89–92].

The daily substitution of a fiber-rich food for a lower fiber, energy dense food item at each meal and one snack is one approach to changing from a Western diet (15–17 g of daily fiber) to a healthy weight controlling diet with ≥30 g fiber/day. Examples of potential food switches to achieve ≥30 g fiber/day and lower energy density needed to prevent weight gain or to promote or maintain weight loss may include: (1) replacing a low fiber, high glycemic breakfast cereal with a fiber-rich bran breakfast cereal; (2) eating an apple instead of a cookie at lunch; (3) adding artichokes or chickpeas to a salad; and (4) snacking on nuts, sunflower seeds, or popcorn instead of potato chips. A list of 50 of the top dietary fiber containing foods are listed in Appendix B.

7.3.2 Isolated Fiber Ingredients

Three systematic reviews and 4 specific RCTs on the effects of isolated fiber ingredients on weight regulation are summarized in Table 7.6 [91, 94–99]. These RCTs showed that isolated fiber ingredients were very heterogeneous and generally less

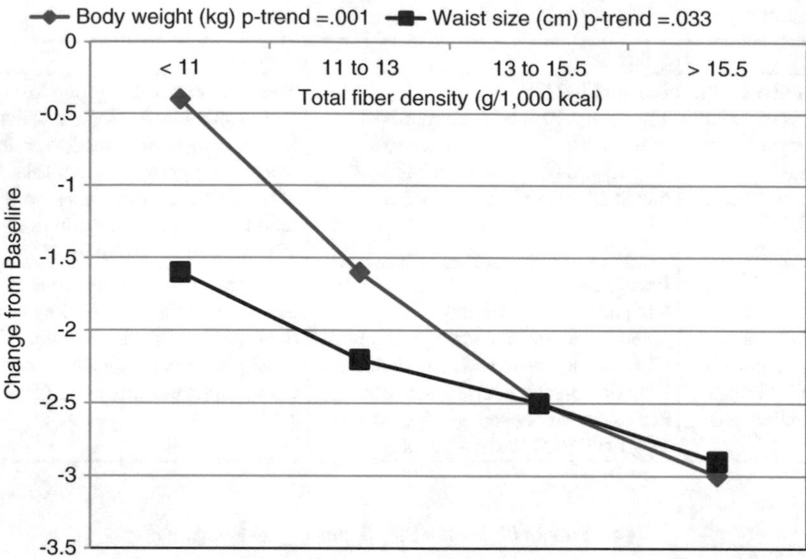

Fig. 7.13 Effect of dietary fiber density on body weight and waist size in 522 overweight/obese pre-diabetic adults over 3 years from the Finnish Diabetes Prevention Study (adapted from [93])

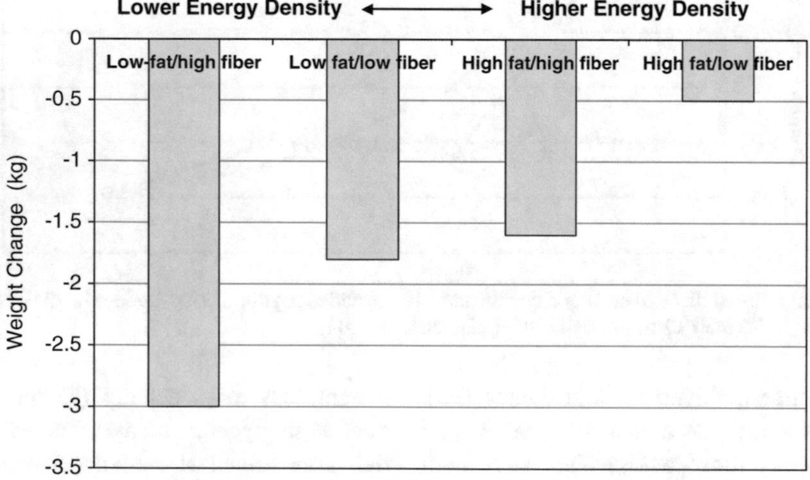

Fig. 7.14 Effect of dietary energy density on weight loss in 522 overweight/obese pre-diabetic adults over 3 years from the Finnish Diabetes Prevention Study (adapted from [93])

effective than whole foods and fiber-rich diets. In a systematic review of 66 randomized trials that examined the effects of isolated fibers, the overall weight reduction was a modest 0.1 kg per 10 g fiber after 4 weeks with a high degree of variability [95]. Two systematic reviews and clinical studies of guar gum and inulin-type fructans showed insignificant or inconsistent weight loss effects [94, 96]. Adding 12 g psyllium fiber mixed with 250 mL water, 3 times daily 5–10 min before breakfast, lunch, and dinner to a Western diet (20 g fiber/day) significantly lowered body weight, and % body fat ($p < 0.05$) with an effect similar to consuming a plant-based healthy diet with 31 g fiber/day (Fig. 7.12) [91]. During the consumption of *ad libitum* diets, the addition of 27 g/day of fermentable, soluble gel-forming/viscous fibers (pectin and β-glucan) and

Table 7.6 Summary of randomized controlled trials (RCTs) on fiber supplements and ingredients in body weight regulation

Objective	Study details	Results
Systematic reviews and meta-analysis		
Liber et al. (2013). Systematically evaluate the effects of inulin-type fructan supplementation on appetite, energy intake, and body weight (BW) in children and adults [94]	For the pediatric population; 4 RCTs; 232 children. For the adult population; 15 RCTs; 545 subjects	Very inconsistent effects on weight loss with limited data suggest that long-term use of inulin type fructans may contribute to weight reduction
Wanders et al. (2011). Systematically investigate fiber types on appetite, energy intake and body weight (systematic review) [95]	58 RCTs appetite control; 26 RCTs on acute energy intake, 38 RCTs on long-term energy intake; and 66 RCTs on body weight	Overall, effects on energy intake and body weight were relatively small, and distinct dose-response relationships were not observed. Short- and long-term effects of fiber appear to differ and have multiple mechanisms relating to their different physicochemical properties. Fibers characterized as being more viscous (e.g. pectins, β-glucans and guar gum) reduced appetite or energy intake more often than less viscous fibers
Pittler and Ernst (2001). Determine the efficacy of guar gum as a therapeutic option for reducing body weight (meta-analysis) [96]	11 RCTs; 203 subjects; 7.5–20 g guar gum/day; 4 weeks to 6 months	There was a non-significant mean body weight difference in subjects receiving guar gum compared with those receiving placebo by 0.04 kg
Specific RCTs		
Hu et al. Examine the effects of soy fiber on body weight and body composition in overweight and obese participants (China) [97]	**Parallel RCT:** 39 college students; mean age 23 years; mean BMI 26; biscuits supplemented with 27.5 g soy fiber/day for breakfast vs. control low fiber biscuits; 12 weeks	Soy fiber supplemented breakfast biscuits significantly reduced body weight by 0.7 kg and BMI 0.44 vs. a control biscuit ($p < 0.05$)
Pal et al. (2011). Compare the effects of fiber intake from a healthy diet vs. a control diet plus psyllium or a healthy diet plus psyllium on body composition (Australia) [91]	**Parallel RCT:** 72 participants; mean age 43 years; mean BMI 34; diets: control diet plus placebo (20 g fiber/day); control diet plus 12 g psyllium fiber 3 times/day; healthy fiber-rich food diet (31 g fiber/day), or healthy fiber-rich food diet plus 12 g psyllium fiber 3 times/day); 12 weeks	Adding 12 g psyllium fiber 3 times/day to a Western diet (20 g fiber/day) significantly lowers body weight, and % body fat ($p < 0.05$) with a similar effect to a 31 g fiber/day healthy diet (Fig. 7.12)
Salas-Salvado et al. (2008). Compare the effect of the administration of a mixture of fibers on body weight-loss, satiety (Spain) [98]	**Double-blind, Parallel RCT:** 200 overweight or obese subjects; mean age 48 years; mean BMI 31; 78% female; reduced calorie diet with 3 g psyllium and 1 g glucomannan either twice or three times daily vs. placebo; 16 weeks	Weight loss was higher after both doses of fiber by about 4.6 kg vs. 3.8 kg for placebo ($p = 0.43$). Also, post-prandial satiety increased in both fiber groups vs. placebo

(continued)

Table 7.6 (continued)

Objective	Study details	Results
Howarth et al. (2003). Evaluate the short-term effects of high vs. low fermentable fiber supplements on hunger, energy intake, and weight loss (US) [99]	**Crossover RCT:** 11 subjects; age 23–46 years; BMI 20–34; 27 g/day of fermentable fiber (pectin and β-glucan) and non-fermentable fiber (methylcellulose); *ad libitum* diets; 3 weeks; 4 weeks of washout; daily fiber supplements were divided into approximately three 10-g portions to be eaten 30 min before each meal with 355 mL of a non-caloric liquid, to achieve a maximum effect as a preload	This study showed a limited role for short-term use of high fermentable fiber and low fermentable fiber supplements in promoting weight loss in humans consuming an *ad libitum* diet. Over 3 weeks, fiber supplements insignificantly reduced energy intake for high fermentable fiber by 7% ($p = 0.31$) and low fermentable fiber by 9.5% ($p = 0.11$); body weight by 0.13 kg ($p > 0.05$), and % body fat for low fermentable fiber by 0.3% ($p = 0.56$); high fermentable fiber by 0.1% ($p = 0.66$)

non-fermentable fiber (methylcellulose) consumed in a non-caloric beverage 30 min before each meal was shown to insignificantly reduce body weight by 0.13 kg for both fermentable and nonfermentable fibers and reduce body fat for the fermentable fibers by 0.1% and for the non-fermentable fiber by 0.3% after 3 weeks [99]. A Chinese study (39 college students; mean age 23 years and BMI 26; 12 weeks) found that biscuits supplemented with 27.5 g isolated soy fiber significantly reduced body weight by 0.7 kg and BMI by 0.44 vs. a control biscuit ($p < 0.05$) [97]. A Spanish double-blind, placebo controlled trial with fiber supplemented hypocaloric diets (200 overweight or obese subjects; mean age 48 years and BMI 31; 78% women; 16 weeks) showed that a relatively low supplementation blend of 4 g psyllium and glucomannan 2 or 3 times/day insignificantly reduced body weight 4.6 kg compared to 3.8 kg for the placebo ($p = 0.43$), suggesting that higher levels of fiber supplementation may be required for significant additional weight loss [98]. These trials suggest that: (1) in *ab libitum* diets most fiber supplements can be effective in weight control/loss if used in high amounts when accompanied by water or noncaloric beverage prior to each meal or added to common foods as replacements for high energy dense, low fiber foods to stimulate enough physical bulking and other mechanisms to be as effective as fiber-rich whole foods [91, 97, 99]; and (2) in hypocaloric diets the addition of multiple doses of >4 g viscous soluble fiber in noncaloric beverages at each meal may boost the weight loss effects [98].

7.4 Fiber Biological Mechanisms

Postulated biological mechanisms associated with adequate fiber intake (> 25 g/day; 14 g fiber/1000 kcal) and healthy dietary patterns for the prevention of weight gain and the promotion of reduction in body weight, waist size, body and visceral fat are summarized in Fig. 7.15 [100–129].

7.4.1 Energy Density

Lower energy dense fiber-rich dietary patterns, as replacements for higher energy dense Western patterns, help to promote balanced energy intake to prevent weight gain or provide negative energy balance to help promote weight loss depending on the level of dietary fiber intake [8, 33, 42, 43, 49, 50, 98]. This is because: (1) fiber is generally considered to be 2 kcals/g or less as compared to 4 kcals/g for digestible carbohydrates such as sugar and starch as fiber is not digested in the small bowel and (2) lower energy dense fiber-rich foods displace higher density foods [100–103]. The lower fiber energy density results from most fiber sources being fermented by colonic bacteria to varying degrees into SCFA metabolites and gases (carbon dioxide, hydrogen, and methane) and/or the excretion of undigested fiber in the stool [100–105]. A 2015 longitudinal analysis (2037 obese participants; mean age 47 years; 10 years follow-up) found that the intake of energy dense and low fiber diets (1.8 kcal/g and 8 g fiber/1,000 kcal for men and 1.7 kcal/g and

Adequate Fiber Intake

Energy Density:

Lowers energy density; fiber (2 kcals/g) vs refined carbohydrates (4 kcals/g)

Post-prandial Satiety Signaling:

Increases food volume, bulk, or viscosity
Prolongs chewing time to slow eating rate
Slows gastric emptying and reduces hunger

Circulatory System:

Attenuates blood glucose, insulin and C-reactive protein
Promotes insulin sensitivity

Promotes satiety hormones such as cholecystokinin(CCK), glucagon-like peptide-1(GLP-1) and peptide YY

Colon Fermentation and Microbiotia:

Fosters healthier colonic microbiota and higher colon short chain fatty acids levels to promote satiety and leaner energy metabolism associated with a leaner phenotype.

Net Metabolizable Energy:

Higher macronutrient fecal excretion (e.g. dietary fat) for lower net metabolizable energy

Lowers Risk of Weight Gain and Obesity
Reduces Risk of Abdominal and Visceral Fat
Promotes Weight Loss

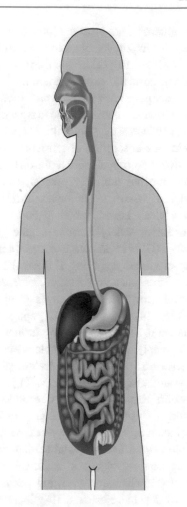

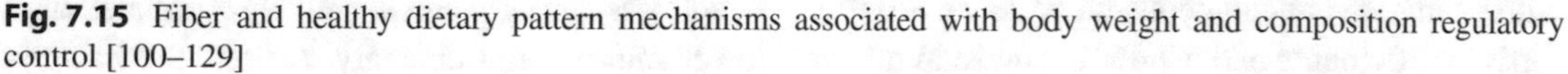

Fig. 7.15 Fiber and healthy dietary pattern mechanisms associated with body weight and composition regulatory control [100–129]

9 g fiber/1,000 kcal for women) was associated with significant increased weight gain by 1.7 kg, waist size by 1.5 cm and BMI by 0.6 kg/m^2 along with increased cardiometabolic risk factors [103].

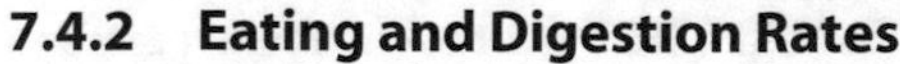

7.4.2 Eating and Digestion Rates

Fiber-rich meals tend to be more mouth filling and harder to swallow because of their higher bulk, physical density, volume, or viscosity compared with energy-matched, low-fiber meals, and more rapidly reduce hunger after ingestion [100, 105]. Fiber-rich foods or clinically proven fiber supplements, especially bulky, viscous soluble fibers, 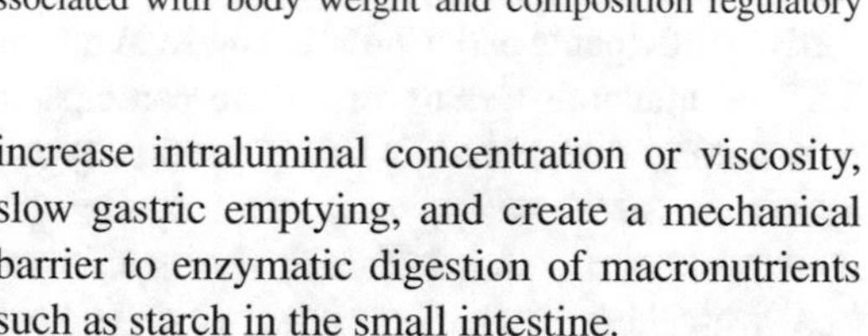 increase intraluminal concentration or viscosity, slow gastric emptying, and create a mechanical barrier to enzymatic digestion of macronutrients such as starch in the small intestine.

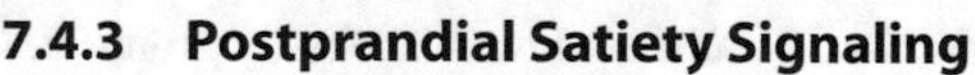

7.4.3 Postprandial Satiety Signaling

Increased fiber intake has been shown to trigger a number of hormonal satiety inducing activities [109, 110]. High fiber meals or β-glucan and psyllium supplements compared to energy matched low fiber control diets can: (1) decrease plasma ghrelin, a stomach hunger promoting hormone, and slow the rate of postprandial increases in glucose and insulin blood levels to prevent reactive hypoglycemia known to promote hunger [100, 105–110]; (2) trigger the increased secretion of the hormone cholecystokinin (CCK), a brain neuropeptide known to decrease food intake, from the proximal small intestine to slow gastric emptying and increase satiety [106, 111, 112]; and/or (3) delay the absorption of nutrients long enough to deliver a portion of them to the distal ileum, where they are not normally present, to stimulate the release of a cascade of metabolic responses called the "ileal brake" phenomenon including the release of satiety hormones glucagon-like peptide-1 (GLP-1), known to control appetite, which slows gastric emptying and small bowel transit, decreases glucagon secretion, increases pancreatic β-cell growth, and improves insulin sensitivity [113, 114] and increased peptide YY (PYY) known to reduce appetite by further slowing gastric emptying [106]. Soluble viscose fiber has been associated with an accelerated reduction in elevated visceral fat tissue (VAT) [115, 116]. The Insulin Resistance and Atherosclerosis Family Study (339 African Americans and 775 Hispanic Americans; mean age approx. 43 years; 5-year follow-up) found that soluble fiber intake and participation in vigorous activity were inversely related to change in VAT, independent of change in BMI [115]. For each 10-g increase in soluble fiber, rate of VAT accumulation decreased by 3.7% ($p = 0.01$). Soluble fiber was not associated with change in subcutaneous fat (0.2%, $p = 0.82$). Active participants had a 7.4% decrease in rate of VAT accumulation versus less active participants ($p = 0.003$). A double-blind RCT (100 subjects; age range 30-70 years; mean BMI approx 28; mean visceral fat area 125 cm^2; rice control vs. rice with high β-glucan barley (4.4 g/d) or β-glucan–free barley; 12 weeks) found that VFA was significantly reduced in both the high β-glucan barley by 10.7 cm^2 and the placebo by groups 6.8 cm^2, which was insignificantly between the groups [116]. However, a subgroup analysis of subjects with high baseline VFA (> 100 cm^2) showed a significant decrease in the β-glucan barley group VFA by 10 cm^2 more than those in the placebo group. This finding indicated that daily consumption of an amount of barley providing 4.4 g of β-glucan reduced VFA in individuals with visceral fat obesity because of increased viscosity due to high β-glucan content slowing gastric emptying, digestion, and absorption which is associated with postprandial low-glycemic index and low-insulin responses that promote favorable effects on various actions of insulin such as facilitating the induction of glycogen synthesis, fatty acid synthesis, and the esterification of fatty acids to actively reduce elevated VFA [116].

7.4.4 Colonic Effects

7.4.4.1 Microbiota

The effects of a healthy diet with adequate fiber from whole plant foods or prebiotics are increasingly being shown to have important roles in modulating the composition and metabolic function of the colonic microbial communities to help improve weight regulation and prevent obesity relative to a lower fiber, Western diet. A 2017 cross-sectional and longitudinal analysis of the Twins UK Study (1632 healthy females; mean baseline age 50 years; 9 years of follow-up) found that high colonic microbiome bacterial diversity and high-fiber intake are correlated with lower weight gain in women independently of calorie intake and other confounders [117]. Women who gained weight had a significantly lower colonic bacterial diversity and lower fiber intake as well as a higher relative concentration of Bacteroides, which was strongly and negatively correlated with lower microbiome diversity. Among the bacteria associated with lower risk of weight gain are *Clostridiales*, especially those in the *Ruminococcaceae* family. An analysis of heritability of colonic microbiome diversity estimates that 60% of the variation is dependent on lifestyle and other environmental variables and not determined by genetic make-up. A 2015 USA analysis of a double-blind RCT (21 healthy men; mean age 27.5 years; mean BMI 27; 21 g/day polydextrose or soluble corn fiber; 21 days) showed that increased fiber intake induced changes in the colonic microbiome of healthy adults [18]. A shift in the *Bacteroidetes*: *Firmicutes* ratio was observed when participants consumed soluble fiber, and changes in bacterial populations were associated with shifts in the bacterial metagenome. A 2017

Canadian double-blind RCT (42 children; mean age 10 years; mean BMI 26.5; 8 g/d oligofructose-enriched inulin vs. maltodextrin/d; 16 weeks) found that oligofructose-enriched inulin significantly decreased body weight by 3.1%, body fat by 2.4%, and trunk fat by 3.8% compared with children in the placebo group who had a slight increase in these parameters [119]. Additionally, children consuming oligofructose-enriched inulin had a significantly 35% lower interleukin (IL)-6 reduction from baseline and 16S rRNA sequencing revealed significant increases in species of the genus *Bifidobacterium* and decreases in *Bacteroides vulgatus* vs. the placebo group.

7.4.4.2 Metabolizable Energy

Compared to low fiber foods, fiber-rich foods tend to decrease the efficiency of macronutrient bioavailability, especially that of dietary fat, leading to higher fecal macronutrient excretion [117]. The consumption of >25 g fiber/day can lead to the excretion of 3–4% of macronutrient energy in the feces, which is equivalent to 80 kcals in a 2000-kcal diet [120–122].

7.4.4.3 Satiety and Energy Metabolism

SCFAs are involved in the crosstalk existing between microbes, human appetite and energy regulation [123–129]. Fiber fermentation produces SCFAs, 95% of which consist of acetate, propionate, and butyrate in a molar ratio of 60:20:20. It has been estimated that as much as 50 to 70% of the fiber from mixed diets is fermentable depending on physical properties [105, 106]. SCFAs can contribute to energy homeostasis and satiety by affecting multiple cellular metabolic pathways and receptor-mediated mechanisms [123–127]. Butyrate reduces systemic inflammation, improves insulin sensitivity, and possibly increases energy expenditure [128]. In obese subjects, propionate appears to increase the release of postprandial plasma PYY and GLP-1 from colonic cells to help reduce energy intake [129]. A 24-week study indicated that colonic generated propionate entering the circulatory system helped to reduce body weight gain and significantly reduce intra-abdominal fat accretion and intrahepatocellular lipid content in overweight adults with non-alcoholic fatty liver disease [129].

Conclusions

Weight regulation is a complex, multifactorial process involving energy intake and energy expenditure, which are affected by genetics, dietary pattern, and other lifestyle and emotional factors. The current global obesity pandemic is in large part a result of increased exposure to higher energy dense and lower fiber diets and increasingly sedentary Western lifestyles over the last several decades, which have led to net habitual positive energy balances and weight gain. Even a small daily positive energy balance of 50 kcals/day, by increased energy intake and/or reduced activity, can lead to an annual weight gain of 0.4–0.9 kg/year. The human gastrointestinal and energy metabolism regulatory systems evolved with pre-agricultural high fiber diets. Prospective cohort studies and RCTs show that high adherence to healthy fiber-rich dietary patterns such as the MedDiet, DASH, New Nordic, and vegetarian diets may at a minimum help to prevent weight gain and can support weight loss and lower waist size compared to low-fat or Western diets in overweight or obese individuals. Mechanisms associated with healthy fiber-rich dietary pattern effects on managing body weight and central obesity include: (1) reducing dietary energy density directly or displacing higher energy foods associated with the Western diet pattern; (2) lowering available metabolizable energy; and (3) increasing postprandial satiety by affecting both the upper digestive tract and colonic microbiota. Fiber intake is inversely associated with obesity risk and populations with higher fiber diets tend to be leaner than those with low fiber diets. Prospective cohort studies suggest that increased total fiber intake by ≥12 g/day to a total daily fiber intake of >25 g, compared to refined low fiber diets, can prevent weight gain by 3.5–5.5 kg each decade. RCTs show that adequate fiber intake ≥28 g fiber/day from fiber-rich diets can reduce body weight and waist circumference compared to low fiber Western diets (≤20 g fiber/day). Fiber-rich diets are generally more effective at promoting weight loss than fiber supplements.

Appendix A

Comparison of Common Dietary Patterns per 2000 kcals (Approximated Values)

Components	Western dietary pattern (US)	USDA base pattern	DASH diet pattern	Healthy Mediterranean pattern	Healthy vegetarian pattern (Lact-ovo based)	Vegan pattern
Emphasizes	Refined grains, low fiber foods, red meats, sweets and solid fats	Vegetables, fruit, whole-grain, and low-fat milk	Potassium rich vegetables, fruits, and low fat milk products	Whole grains, vegetables, fruit, dairy products, olive oil, and moderate wine	Vegetables, fruit, whole-grains, legumes, nuts, seeds, milk products, and soy foods	Plant foods: vegetables, fruits, whole grains, nuts, seeds, and soy foods
Includes	Processed meats, sugar sweetened beverages, and fast foods	Enriched grains, lean meat, fish, nuts, seeds, and vegetable oils	Whole-grain, poultry, fish, nuts, and seeds	Fish, nuts, seeds, and pulses	Eggs, non-dairy milk alternatives, and vegetable oils	Non-dairy milk alternatives
Limits	Fruits and vegetables, and whole-grains	Solid fats and added sugars	Red meats, sweets and sugar-sweetened beverages	Red meats, refined grains, and sweets	No red or white meats, or fish; limited sweets	No animal products
Estimated nutrients/components						
Carbohydrates (% Total kcal)	51	51	55	50	54	57
Protein (% Total kcal)	16	17	18	16	14	13
Total fat (% Total kcal)	33	32	27	34	32	30
Saturated fat (% Total kcal)	11	8	6	8	8	7
Unsat. fat (% Total kcal)	22	25	21	24	26	25
Fiber (g)	16	31	29+	31	35+	40+
Potassium (mg)	2800	3350	4400	3350	3300	3650
Vegetable oils (g)	19	27	25	27	19–27	18–27
Solid fats (g)	31	18	–	17	21	16
Sodium (mg)	3600	1790	1100	1690	1400	1225
Added sugar (g)	79 (20 tsp)	32 (8 tsp)	12 (3 tsp)	32 (8 tsp)	32 (8 tsp)	32 (8 tsp)
Plant food groups						
Fruit (cup)	≤1.0	2.0	2.5	2.5	2.0	2.0
Vegetables (cup)	≤1.5	2.5	2.1	2.5	2.5	2.5
Whole-grains (oz.)	0.6	3.0	4.0	3.0	3.0	3.0
Legumes (oz.)	–	1.5	0.5	1.5	3.0	3.0+
Nuts/Seeds (oz.)	0.5	0.6	1.0	0.6	1.0	2.0
Soy products (oz.)	0.0	0.5	–	–	1.1	1.5

Svetkey LP, Simons-Morton D, Vollmer WM, et al. Effects of dietary patterns on blood pressure. Arch Intern Med. 1999;159:285–93

(1) Dietary Guidelines Advisory Committee. Scientific Report of the 2010 Advisory Guidelines Advisory Report to the Secretary of Health and Human Services and the Secretary of Agriculture. Part B. Section 2: Total Diet. 2010; Table B2.4. (2) Dietary Guidelines Advisory Committee. Scientific Report of the 2015 Advisory Guidelines Advisory Report to the Secretary of Health and Human Services and the Secretary of Agriculture. Appendix E-3.7: Developing Vegetarian and Mediterranean-style Food Patterns. 2015;1–9

Appendix B

Fifty High Fiber Foods Ranked by Amount of Fiber per Standard Food Portion[a]

Food	Standard portion size	Dietary fiber (g)	Calories (kcal)	Energy density (calories/g)
High fiber bran ready-to-eat-cereal	1/3–3/4 cup (30 g)	9.1–14.3	60–80	2.0–2.6
Navy beans, cooked	1/2 cup cooked (90 g)	9.6	127	1.4
Small white beans, cooked	1/2 cup (90 g)	9.3	127	1.4
Shredded wheat ready-to-eat cereal	1–1 1/4 cup (50–60 g)	5.0–9.0	155–220	3.2–3.7
Black bean soup, canned	1/2 cup (130 g)	8.8	117	0.9
French beans, cooked	1/2 cup (90 g)	8.3	114	1.3
Split peas, cooked	1/2 cup (100 g)	8.2	114	1.1
Chickpeas (Garbanzo) beans, canned	1/2 cup (120 g)	8.1	176	1.4
Lentils, cooked	1/2 cup (100 g)	7.8	115	1.2
Pinto beans, cooked	1/2 cup (90 g)	7.7	122	1.4
Black beans, cooked	1/2 cup (90 g)	7.5	114	1.3
Artichoke, global or French, cooked	1/2 cup (84 g)	7.2	45	0.5
Lima beans, cooked	1/2 cup (90 g)	6.6	108	1.2
White beans, canned	1/2 cup (130 g)	6.3	149	1.1
Wheat bran flakes ready-to-eat cereal	3/4 cup (30 g)	4.9–5.5	90–98	3.0–3.3
Pear with skin	1 medium (180 g)	5.5	100	0.6
Pumpkin seeds. Whole, roasted	1 ounce (about 28 g)	5.3	126	4.5
Baked beans, canned, plain	1/2 cup (125 g)	5.2	120	0.9
Soybeans, cooked	1/2 cup (90 g)	5.2	150	1.7
Plain rye wafer crackers	2 wafers (22 g)	5.0	73	3.3
Avocado, Hass	1/2 fruit (68 g)	4.6	114	1.7
Apple, with skin	1 medium (180 g)	4.4	95	0.5
Green peas, cooked (fresh, frozen, canned)	1/2 cup (80 g)	3.5–4.4	59–67	0.7–0.8
Refried beans, canned	1/2 cup (120 g)	4.4	107	0.9
Mixed vegetables, cooked from frozen	1/2 cup (45 g)	4.0	59	1.3
Raspberries	1/2 cup (65 g)	3.8	32	0.5
Blackberries	1/2 cup (65 g)	3.8	31	0.4
Collards, cooked	1/2 cup (95 g)	3.8	32	0.3
Soybeans, green, cooked	1/2 cup (75 g)	3.8	127	1.4
Prunes, pitted, stewed	1/2 cup (125 g)	3.8	133	1.1
Sweet potato, baked	1 medium (114 g)	3.8	103	0.9
Multi-grain bread	2 slices regular (52 g)	3.8	140	2.7
Figs, dried	1/4 cup (about 38 g)	3.7	93	2.5
Potato baked, with skin	1 medium (173 g)	3.6	163	0.9
Popcorn, air-popped	3 cups (24 g)	3.5	93	3.9
Almonds	1 ounce (about 28 g)	3.5	164	5.8

Food	Standard portion size	Dietary fiber (g)	Calories (kcal)	Energy density (calories/g)
Whole wheat spaghetti, cooked	1/2 cup (70 g)	3.2	87	1.2
Sunflower seed kernels, dry roasted	1 ounce (about 28 g)	3.1	165	5.8
Orange	1 medium (130 g)	3.1	69	0.5
Banana	1 medium (118 g)	3.1	105	0.9
Oat bran muffin	1 small (66 g)	3.0	178	2.7
Vegetable soup	1 cup (245 g)	2.9	91	0.4
Dates	1/4 cup (about 38 g)	2.9	104	2.8
Pistachios, dry roasted	1 ounce (about 28 g)	2.8	161	5.7
Hazelnuts or filberts	1 ounce (about 28 g)	2.7	178	6.3
Peanuts, oil roasted	1 ounce (about 28 g)	2.7	170	6.0
Quinoa, cooked	1/2 cup (90 g)	2.7	92	1.0
Broccoli, cooked	1/2 cup (78 g)	2.6	27	0.3
Potato baked, without skin	1 medium (145 g)	2.3	145	1.0
Baby spinach leaves	3 ounces (90 g)	2.1	20	0.2
Blueberries	1/2 cup (74 g)	1.8	42	0.6
Carrot, raw or cooked	1 medium (60 g)	1.7	25	0.4

Dietary Guidelines Advisory Committee. Scientific Report of the 2015 Advisory Guidelines Advisory Report to the Secretary of Health and Human Services and the Secretary of Agriculture Part D. Chapter 1: Food and Nutrient Intakes, and Health: Current Status and Trends. 2015; 97, 98. Table D1.8

[a]USDA National Nutrient Database for Standard Reference, Release 27. http://www.ars.usda.gov/nutrientdata. Accessed 17 Feb 2015

References

1. World Health Organization. Obesity and overweight. Geneva. 2014. www.who.int/mediacentre/factsheets/fs311en/. Accessed 18 Jan 2015.
2. Swinburn BA, Sacks G, Hall KD, et al. The global obesity pandemic: shaped by global drivers and local environments. Lancet. 2011;378:804–14.
3. Moehlecke M, Canani LH, Lucas Oliveira L, et al. Determinants of body weight regulation in humans. Arch Endocrinol Metab. 2016;60(2):152–62.
4. Centers for Disease Control and Prevention. Overweight and obesity: causes and consequences. 2012. http://www.cdc.gov/obesity/adult/causes/index.html. Accessed 21 Feb 2015.
5. Hill JO. Can a small-changes approach help address the obesity epidemic? A report of the Joint Task Force of the American Society for Nutrition, Institute of Food Technologists, and International Food Information Council. Am J Clin Nutr. 2009;89:477–84.
6. Zhai F, Wang H, Wang Z, et al. Closing the energy gap to prevent weight gain in China. Obes Rev. 2008;9(Suppl 1):107–12.
7. Centers for Disease Control and Prevention. Low energy dense foods and weight management: cutting calories while controlling hunger. Research to Practice Series, No 5. 2015. http://www.cdc.gov/nccdphp/dnpa/nutrition/pdf/r2p_energy_density.pdf. Accessed 21 Feb.
8. Davis JN, Hodges VA, Gillham MB. Normal-weight adults consume more fiber and fruit than their age and height matched overweight/obese counterparts. J Am Diet Assoc. 2006;106:835–40.
9. Mozaffarian D, Hao T, Rimm EB, et al. Changes in diet and lifestyle and long-term weight gain in women and men. N Engl J Med. 2011;363:2392–404.
10. Rolls BJ. What is the role of portion in weight management? Int J Obes. 2014;38:S1–8.
11. Vernarelli JA, Mitchell DC, Rolls BJ, Hartman TJ. Dietary energy density is associated with obesity and other biomarkers of chronic disease in US adults. Eur J Nutr. 2015;54(1):59–65.
12. Karl JP, Roberts SB. Energy density, energy intake and body weight regulations in adults. Adv Nutr. 2014;5:835–50.
13. Raynor HA, Jeffery RW, Phelan S, et al. Amount of food group variety consumed in the diet and long-term weight loss maintenance. Obes Res. 2005;13(5):883–90.
14. Dietary Guidelines Advisory Committee. Scientific Report of the 2015 Advisory Guidelines Advisory Report to the Secretary of Health and Human Services and the Secretary of Agriculture. Part D. Chapter 2: Dietary patterns, foods and nutrients, and health outcomes. 2015;1–33.
15. Jessri M, Wolfinger RD, Lou NY, L'Abbe MR. Identification of dietary patterns associated with obesity in a nationally respresentative survey of Canadian adults: application of *a priori*, hybrid,

and simplified pattern techniques. Am J Clin Nutr. 2017;105:669–84.

16. Verheggen RJ, Maessen MF, Green DJ, et al. A systematic review and meta-analysis on the effects of exercise training versus hypocaloric diet: distinct effects on bodyweight and visceral adipose tissue. Obes Rev. 2016;17(8):664–90. https://doi.org/10.1111/obr.12406.
17. de Mutsert R, Sun Q, Willett WC, et al. Overweight in early adulthood, adult weight change, and risk of type 2 diabetes, cardiovascular diseases, and certain cancers in men: a cohort study. Am J Epidemiol. 2014;179:1353–65.
18. Wilson PW, D'Agostino RB, Sullivan L, et al. Overweight and obesity as determinants of cardiovascular risk: the Framingham experience. Arch Intern Med. 2002;162:1867–72.
19. Wang YC, McPherson K, Marsh T, et al. Health and economic burden of projected obesity trends in the USA and the UK. Lancet. 2011;378:815–25.
20. Wing RR, Phelan S. Long-term weight loss maintenance. Am J Clin Nutr. 2005;82(Suppl):222S–5S.
21. Raynor HA, Van Walleghen EL, Bachman JL. Dietary energy density and successful weight loss maintenance. Eat Behav. 2011;12(2):119–25.
22. MacLean PS, Higgins JA, Giles ED, et al. The role for adipose tissue in weight regain after weight loss. Obes Rev. 2015;16(Suppl.1):45–54.
23. Mariman ECM. An adipobiological model for weight regain after weight loss. Adipobiology. 2011; 3:7–13.
24. Rezagholizadeh F, Djafarian K, Khosravis S, Shab-Bidar S. A posteriori: healthy dietary patterns may decrease the risk of central obesity: findings froma systematic review and meta-analysis. Nutr Res. 2017;41:1-13.
25. Ma Y, Olendzki BC, Wang J, et al. Single-component versus multi-component dietary goals for the metabolic syndrome: a randomized trial. Ann Intern Med. 2015;162:248–57.
26. Asghari G, Mirmiran P, Yuzbashian E, Azizi F. A systematic review of diet quality indices in relation to obesity. Br J Nutr. 2017;117(8):1055–65. https://doi.org/10.1017/S0007114517000915.
27. Shah RV, Murthy VL, Allison JP, et al. Diet and adipose tissue distributions: The Multi-Ethnic Study of Atherosclerosis. Nutr Metab Cardiovasc Dis. 2016;26:185–93.
28. Hu T, Jacobs DR, Larson NI, et al. Higher diet quality in adolescence and dietary improvements are related to less weight gain during the transition from adolescence to adulthood. J Pediatr. 2016;178:188–93.
29. Feliciano CEM, Tinker L, Manson JE, et al. Change in dietary patterns and change in waist circumference and DXA trunk fat among postmenopausal women. Obesity. 2016;24:2176–84. https://doi.org/10.1002/oby.21589.
30. Fung TT, Pan A, Hou T, et al. Long-term change in diet quality is associated with body weight change in men and women. J Nutr. 2015;145(8):1850–6. https://doi.org/10.3945/jn.114.208785.
31. Lassale C, Fezeu L, Andreeva VA, et al. Association between dietary scores and 13-year weight change and obesity risk in a French prospective cohort. Int J Obes. 2012;36(11):1455–62.
32. Wolongevicz DM, Zhu L, Pencina MJ, et al. Diet quality and obesity in women: the Framingham Nutrition Studies. Br J Nutr. 2010;103(8):1223–9.
33. Esmaillzadeh A, Azadbakht L. Major dietary patterns in relation to general obesity and central adiposity among Iranian women. J Nutr. 2008;138:358–63.
34. Schulz M, Nothlings U, Hoffmann K, et al. Identification of a food pattern characterized by high-fiber and low-fat food choices associated with low prospective weight change in the EPIC-Potsdam cohort. J Nutr. 2005;135:1183–9.
35. Newby PK, Muller D, Hallfrisch J, et al. Dietary patterns and changes in body mass index and waist circumference in adults. Am J Clin Nutr. 2003;77:1417–25.
36. Li Y, Roswall N, Ström P, et al. Mediterranean and Nordic diet scores and long-term changes in body weight and waist circumference: results from a large cohort study. Br J Nutr. 2015;114:2093–102.
37. Funtikova AN, Benıtez-Arciniega AA, Gomez SF, et al. Mediterranean diet impact on changes in abdominal fat and 10-year incidence of abdominal obesity in a Spanish population. Br J Nutr. 2014;111:1481–7. https://doi.org/10.1017/S0007114513003966.
38. May AM, Romaguera D, Travier N, et al. Combined impact of lifestyle factors on prospective change in body weight and waist circumference in participants of the EPIC-PANACEA Study. PLoS One. 2012;7(11):e50712. https://doi.org/10.1371/journal.pone.0050712.
39. Beunza JJ, Toledo E, Hu FB, et al. Adherence to the Mediterranean diet, long-term weight change, and incident overweight or obesity: The Seguimiento Universidad de Navarra (SUN) cohort. Am J Clin Nutr. 2010;92:1484–93.
40. Romaguera D, Norat T, Vergnaud A-C, et al. Mediterranean dietary patterns and prospective weight change in participants of the EPIC-PANACEA project. Am J Clin Nutr. 2010;92:912–21.
41. Sanchez-Villegas A, Bes-Rastrollo M, Martinez-Gonzalez MA, Serra-Majem L. Adherence to a Mediterranean dietary pattern and weight gain in a follow-up study: the SUN cohort. Int J Obes. 2006;30:350–8.
42. Mendez MA, Popkin BM, Jakszyn P, et al. Adherence to a Mediterranean diet is associated with reduced 3-year incidence of obesity. J Nutr. 2006;136:2934–8.
43. Barak F, Falahi E, Keshteli AH, et al. Adherence to the Dietary Approaches to Stop Hypertension (DASH) diet in relation to obesity among Iranian female nurses. Public Health Nutr. 2014;18(4):705–12.
44. Berz JPB, Singer MR, Guo X, et al. Use of a DASH food group score to predict excess weight gain in adolescent girls in the National Growth and Health Study. Arch Pediatr Adolesc Med. 2011;165(6):540–6.

45. Tonstad S, Butler T, Yan R, Fraser GE. Type of vegetarian diet, body weight, and prevalence of type 2 diabetes. Diabetes Care. 2009;32:791–6.
46. Berkow SE, Barnard N. Vegetarian diets and weight status. Nutr Rev. 2006;64(4):175–88.
47. Mancini JG, Filion KB, Atallah R, Eisenberg MJ. Systematic review of the Mediterranean diet for long-term weight loss. Am J Med. 2016;129:407–15.
48. Huo R, Du T, Xu Y, et al. Effects of Mediterranean-style diet on glycemic control, weight loss and cardiovascular risk factors among type 2 diabetes individuals: a meta-analysis. Eur J Clin Nutr. 2014;4(11):e005497. https://doi.org/10.1136/bmjopen-2014-005497.
49. Esposito K, Kastorini CM, Panagiotakos DB, Giugliano D. Mediterranean diet and weight loss diet: meta-analysis of randomized controlled trials. Metab Syndr Relat Disord. 2011;9(1):1–12.
50. Kastorini C-M, Milionis HJ, Esposito K, et al. The effect of Mediterranean diet on metabolic syndrome and its components: a meta-analysis of 50 studies and 534,906 individuals. J Am Coll Cardiol. 2011;57(11):1299–313.
51. Estruch R, Martinez-Gonzalez MA, Corella D, et al. Effect of a high-fat Mediterranean diet on bodyweight and waist circumference: a prespecified secondary outcomes analysis of the PREDIMED randomised controlled trial. Lancet Diabetes Endocrinol. 2016;4:666–76. https://doi.org/10.1016/S2213-8587(16)30085-7.
52. Alvarez-Perez J, Sanchez-Villegas A, Diaz-Benitez EM, et al. Influence of a Mediterranean dietary pattern on body fat distribution: results of the PREDIMED–Canarias intervention randomized trial. J Am Coll Nutr. 2016;35(6):568–80. https://doi.org/10.1080/07315724.2015.1102102.
53. Damasceno NRT, Sala-Vila A, Cofán M, et al. Mediterranean diet supplemented with nuts reduces waist circumference and shifts lipoprotein subfractions to a less atherogenic pattern in subjects at high cardiovascular risk. Atherosclerosis. 2013;230:347–53.
54. Shai I, Schwarzfuchs D, Henkin Y, et al. Weight loss with a low-carbohydrate, Mediterranean, or low fat diet. N Engl J Med. 2008;359:229–41.
55. Esposito K, Marfella R, Ciotola M, et al. Effect of a Mediterranean-style diet on endothelial dysfunction and markers of vascular inflammation in the metabolic syndrome. a randomized trial. JAMA. 2004;292(12):1440–6.
56. Esposito K, Pontillo A, Di Palo C, et al. Effect of weight loss and lifestyle changes on vascular inflammatory markers in obese women: a randomized trial. JAMA. 2003;289:1799–804.
57. Soltani S, Shirani F, Chitsazi MJ, Salehi-Abargouei A. The effect of dietary approaches to stop hypertension (DASH) diet on weight and body composition in adults: a systematic review and meta-analysis of randomized controlled clinical trials. Obes Rev. 2016;17:442–54.
58. Bertz F, Winkvist A, Brekke HK. Sustainable weight loss among overweight and obese lactating women is achieved with an energy-reduced diet in line with dietary recommendations: results from the LEVA randomized controlled trial. J Acad Nutr Diet. 2015;115:78–86.
59. Bertz F, Brekke HK, Ellegard L, et al. Diet and exercise weight-loss trial in lactating overweight and obese women. Am J Clin Nutr. 2012;96:698–05.
60. Poulsen SK, Due A, Jordy AB, et al. Health effect of the New Nordic Diet in adults with increased waist circumference: a 6-mo randomized controlled trial. Am J Clin Nutr. 2014;99:35–45.
61. Huang R-Y, Huang C-C, Hu FB, Chavarro JE. Vegetarian diets and weight reduction: a meta-analysis of randomized controlled trials. J Gen Intern Med. 2016;31(1):109–16. https://doi.org/10.1007/s11606-015-3390-7.
62. Barnard ND, Levin SM, Yokoyama Y. Systematic review and meta-analysis of changes in body weight in clinical trials of vegetarian diets. J Acad Nutr Diet. 2015;115(6):954–69.
63. Turner-McGrievy GM, Davidson CR, Wingard EE, et al. Comparative effectiveness of plant-based diets for weight loss: a randomized controlled trial of five different diets. Nutrition. 2015;31:350–8.
64. Eaton SB, Konner MJ, Cordain L. Diet-dependent acid load, Paleolithic nutrition, and evolutionary health promotion. Am J Clin Nutr. 2010;91:295–7.
65. Jew S, Abumweis SS, Jones PJH. Evolution of the human diet: linking our ancestral diet to modern functional foods as a means of disease prevention. J Med Food. 2009;12(5):925–34.
66. Chambers ES, Morrison DJ, Frost G. Control of appetite and energy intake by SCFA: what are the potential underlying mechanisms? Proc Nutr Soc. 2015;74(3):328–36.
67. Deehan EC, Walter J. The fiber gap and disappearing gut microbiome: implications for human health. Trends Endocrinol Metab. 2016;27(5):239–41.
68. Dietary Guidelines Advisory Committee. Scientific Report of the 2015. Advisory Guidelines Advisory Report to the Secretary of Health and Human Services and the Secretary of Agriculture. Part D. Chapter 1: Food and nutrient intakes, and health: current status and trends. 2015; Figure D1.2:131.
69. Dahl WJ, Stewart ML. Position of the Academy of Nutrition and Dietetics: health implications of dietary fiber. J Acad Nutr Diet. 2015;115:1861–70.
70. González-Rodríguez LG, Sánchez JMP, Aranceta-Bartrina J, et al. Intake and dietary food sources of fibre in Spain: differences with regard to the prevalence of excess body weight and abdominal obesity in adults of the ANIBES Study. Forum Nutr. 2017;9:326. https://doi.org/10.3390/nu9040326.
71. Grooms KN, Ommerborn MJ, Quyen D, et al. Dietary fiber intake and cardiometabolic risk among US adults, NHANES 1999-2010. Am J Med. 2013;126(12):1059–67.
72. Lairon D. Dietary fiber and control of body weight. Nutr Metab Cardiovasc Dis. 2007;17:1–5.

73. Slavin JL. Dietary fiber and body weight. Nutrition. 2005;21:411–8.
74. Fogelholm M, Anderssen S, Gunnarsdottir I, Lahti-Koski M. Dietary macronutrients, and food consumption as determinants of long-term weight change in adult populations: a systematic literature review. Food Nutr Res. 2012;56:19103.
75. European Food Safety Authority (EFSA). EFSA Panel on Dietetic Products, Nutrition, and Allergies. Opinion on dietary reference values for carbohydrates and dietary fibre. EFSA J. 2010;8(3):1462. 27–37.
76. Rautiainen S, Wang L, Lee I-M, et al. Higher intake of fruit, but not vegetables or fiber, at baseline is associated with lower risk of becoming overweight or obese in middle-aged and older women of normal BMI at baseline. J Nutr. 2015;145:960–8.
77. Fischer K, Moewes D, Koch M, et al. MRI-determined total volumes of visceral and subcutaneous abdominal and trunk adipose tissue are differentially and sex-dependently associated with patterns of estimated usual nutrient intake in a northern German population. Am J Clin Nutr. 2015;101:794–807.
78. Lin Y, Huybrechts I, Vandevijvere S, et al. Fibre intake among the Belgian population by sex–age and sex–education groups and its association with BMI and waist circumference. Br J Nutr. 2011;105:1692–703.
79. Du H, van der AD, Boshuizen HC, et al. Dietary fiber and subsequent changes in body weight and waist circumference in European men and women. Am J Clin Nutr. 2010;91:329–36.
80. Romaguera D, Angquist L, Du H, et al. Dietary determinants of changes in waist circumference adjusted for body mass index—a proxy measure of visceral adiposity. PLoS One. 2010;5(7):e11588.
81. Davis JN, Alexander KE, Ventura EE, et al. Inverse relation between dietary fiber intake and visceral adiposity in overweight Latino youth. Am J Clin Nutr. 2009;90:1160–6.
82. Tucker LA, Thomas KS. Increasing total fiber intake reduces risk of weight and fat gains in women. J Nutr. 2009;139:576–81.
83. Koh-Banerjee P, Franz M, Sampson L, et al. Changes in whole-grain, bran, and cereal fiber consumption in relation to 8-yr weight gain among men. Am J Clin Nutr. 2004;80:1237–45.
84. Koh-Banerjee P, Chu N-F, Spiegelman DM, et al. Prospective study of the association of changes in dietary intake, physical activity, alcohol consumption, and smoking with 9-y gain in waist circumference among 16,587 US men. Am J Clin Nutr. 2003;78:719–27.
85. Liu S, Willett WC, Manson JE, et al. Relation between changes in intakes of dietary fiber and grain products and changes in weight and development of obesity among middle-aged women. Am J Clin Nutr. 2003;78:920–7.
86. Ludwig DS, Pereira MA, Kroenke CH, et al. Dietary fiber, weight gain, and cardiovascular disease risk factors in young adults. JAMA. 1999;282:1539–46.
87. Howarth NC, Saltzman E, Roberts SB. Dietary fiber and weight regulation. Nutr Rev. 2001;59(5):129–39.
88. Karimi G, Azadbakht L, Haghighatdoost F, Esmaillzadeh A. Low energy density diet, weight loss maintenance, and risk of cardiovascular disease following a recent weight reduction program: a randomized control trial. J Res Med Sci. 2016;21:32. https://doi.org/10.4103/1735-1995.181992.
89. Turner TF, Nance LM, Strickland WD, et al. Dietary adherence and satisfaction with a bean-based high-fiber weight loss diet: a pilot study. ISEN Obes. 2013;2013:5. https://doi.org/10.1155/2013/915415.
90. Mecca MS, Moreto F, Burini FHP, et al. Ten-week lifestyle changing program reduces several indicators for metabolic syndrome in overweight adults. Diabetol Metab Syndr. 2012;4:1–7.
91. Pal S, Khossousi A, Binns C, et al. The effect of a fibre supplement compared to a healthy diet on body composition, lipids, glucose, insulin and other metabolic syndrome risk factors in overweight and obese individuals. Br J Nutr. 2011;105:90–100.
92. Ferdowsian HR, Barnard ND, Hoover VJ, et al. A multi-component intervention reduces body weight and cardiovascular risk at a GEICO corporate site. Am J Health Promot. 2010;24(6):384–7.
93. Lindstrom J, Peltonen M, Eriksson JG, et al. High-fibre, low-fat diet predicts long-term weight loss and decreased type 2 diabetes risk: The Finnish Diabetes Prevention Study. Diabetologia. 2006;49:912–20.
94. Liber A, Szajewska H. Effects of inulin-type fructans on appetite, energy intake, and body weight in children and adults: systematic review of randomized controlled trials. Ann Nutr Metab. 2013; 63:42–54.
95. Wanders AJ, Van de Borne JJ, de Graaf C, et al. Effects of dietary fibre on subjective appetite, energy intake and body weight: a systematic review of randomized controlled trials. Obes Rev. 2011;12(9):724–39.
96. Pittler MH, Ernst E. Guar gum for body weight reduction meta-analysis of randomized trials. Am J Med. 2001;110:724–30.
97. Hu X, Gao J, Zhang Q, et al. Soy fiber improves weight loss and lipid profile in overweight and obese adults: a randomized controlled trial. Mol Nutr Food Res. 2013;57:2147–54.
98. Salas-Salvado J, Farres X, Luque X, et al. Effect of two doses of a mixture of soluble fibres on body weight and metabolic variables in overweight or obese patients: a randomised trial. Br J Nutr. 2008;99:1380–7.
99. Howarth NC, Saltzman E, McCrory MA, et al. Fermentable and non-fermentable fiber supplements did not alter hunger, satiety or body weight in a pilot study of men and women consuming self-selected diets. J Nutr. 2003;133:3141–4.
100. Pereira MA, Ludwig DS. Dietary fiber and body weight regulation observations and mechanism. Childhood Obes. 2001;48(4):969–79.
101. Food and Agriculture Organization of the United Nations. Food energy-methods of analysis and

conversion factors. FAO Food and Nutrition Paper. 2003;77:59.

102. Livesey G. Energy values of unavailable carbohydrate and diets: an inquiry and analysis. Am J Clin Nutr. 1990;51(4):617–37.
103. Johns DJ, Lindroos A-K, Jebb SA, et al. Dietary patterns, cardiometabolic risk factors, and the incidence of cardiovascular disease in severe obesity. Obesity. 2015;23(5):1063–70.
104. Oku T, Nakamura S. Evaluation of the relative available energy of several dietary fiber preparations using breath hydrogen evolution in healthy humans. J Nutr Sci Vitaminol. 2014;60:246–54.
105. McRorie JW. Evidence-based approach to fiber supplements and clinically meaningful health benefits, part 1. What to look for and how to recommend an effective fiber therapy. Nutr Today. 2015;50(2):82–9.
106. Sanchez D, Miguel M, Aleixandre A. Dietary fiber, gut peptides, and adipocytokines. J Med Food. 2012;15(3):223–30.
107. Holt SH, Miller JB. Particle size, satiety and the glycaemic response. Eur J Clin Nutr. 1994;48: 496–502.
108. Rebello CJ, Chu Y-F, Johnson WD, et al. The role of meal viscosity and oat β-glucan characteristics in human appetite control: a randomized crossover trial. Nutr J. 2014;13:49.
109. Vitaglione P, Lumaga RB, Stanzione A, et al. β-Glucan-enriched bread reduces energy intake and modifies plasma ghrelin and peptide YY concentrations in the short term. Appetite. 2009;53:338–44.
110. Karhunen LJ, Juvonen KR, Flander SM, et al. A psyllium fiber enriched meal strongly attenuates postprandial gastrointestinal peptide release in healthy young adults. J Nutr. 2010;140:737–44.
111. Bourdon I, Olson B, Backus R, et al. Beans, as a source of dietary fiber, increase cholecystokinin and apolipoprotein B48 response to test meals in men. J Nutr. 2001;131:1485–90.
112. Beck EJ, Tosh SM, Batterham MJ, et al. Oat beta-glucan increases postprandial cholecystokinin levels, decreases insulin response and extends subjective satiety in overweight subjects. Mol Nutr Food Res. 2009;53:1343–51.
113. Martinez-Rodriguez R, Gil A. Nutrient-mediated modulation of incretin gene expression: a systematic review. Nutr Hosp. 2012;27:46–53.
114. Hussain SS, Bloom SR. The regulation of food intake by the gut-brain axis: implications for obesity. Int J Obes (Lond). 2013;37:625–33.
115. Hairston KG, Vitolins MZ, Anderson AM, et al. Lifestyle factors and 5-year abdominal fat accumulation in a minority cohort: the IRAS family study. Obesity. 2011;20:421–27.
116. Aoe S, Ichinose Y, Kohyama N, et al. Effects of high b-glucan barley on visceral fat obesity in Japanese individuals: a randomized, doubleblind study. Nutr. 2017;42:1–6.
117. Menni C, Jackson MA, Pallister T, et al. Gut microbiome and high fibre intake are related to lower long-term weight gain. Int J Obes. 2017;41:1099–1105.
118. Holscher HD, Caporaso JG, Hooda S, et al. Fiber supplementation influences phylogenetic structure and functional capacity of the human intestinal microbiome: follow-up of a randomized controlled trial. Am J Clin Nutr. 2015;10(1):55–64.
119. Nicolucci AC, Hume MP, Martinez I, et al. Prebiotic reduce body fat and alter intestinal microbiota in children who are overweight or with obesity. Gastrenterology. 2017;153:711–22.
120. Miles CW. The metabolizable energy of diets differing in dietary fat and fiber measured in humans. J Nutr. 1992;122:306–11.
121. Miles CW, Kelsay JL, Wong NP. Effect of dietary fiber on the metabolizable energy of human diets. J Nutr. 1988;118:107–1081.
122. Baer DJ, Rumpler WV, Miles CW, Fahey GC. Dietary fiber decreases the metabolizable energy content and nutrient digestibility of mixed diets fed to humans. J Nutr. 1997;127:579–86.
123. Cani PD, Lecourt E, Dewulf EM. Gut microbiota fermentation of prebiotics increases satietogenic and incretin gut peptide production with consequences for appetite sensation and glucose response after a meal. Am J Clin Nutr. 2009;90:1236–43.
124. Everard A, Cani PD. Gut microbiota and GLP-1. Rev Endocr Metab Disord. 2014;15:189–96.
125. Kaji I, Karaki S, Kuwahara A. Short-chain fatty acid receptor and its contribution to glucagon-like peptide-1 release. Digestion. 2014;89:31–6.
126. Tarini J, Wolever TM. The fermentable fibre inulin increases postprandial serum short-chain fatty acids and reduces free-fatty acids and ghrelin in healthy subjects. Appl Physiol Nutr Metab. 2010;35(1):9–16.
127. Kasubuchi M, Hasegawa S, Hiramatsu T, et al. Dietary gut microbial metabolites, short-chain fatty acids, and host metabolic regulation. Forum Nutr. 2015;7:2839–49.
128. Conterno L, Fava F, Viola R, Tuohy KM. Obesity and the gut microbiota: does up-regulating colonic fermentation protect against obesity and metabolic disease? Genes Nutr. 2011;6:241–60.
129. Chambers ES, Viardot A, Psichas A, et al. Effects of targeted delivery of propionate to the human colon on appetite regulation, body weight maintenance and adiposity in overweight adults. Gut. 2015;64(11):1744–54.

8 Whole Plant Foods in Body Weight and Composition Regulation

Keywords
Whole plant foods • Weight maintenance • Weight loss • Body fat • Central obesity • Waist circumference • Whole grains • Fruit • Vegetables • Dietary pulses • Nuts

Key Points

- Foods commonly associated with weight gain are the high intake of French fries, sugar-sweetened beverages, and red and processed meats, and the foods that tend to be inversely associated with weight gain are non-starchy vegetables, high fiber and flavonoid rich fruits, whole grains, nuts, and plain yogurt.
- Healthy lower energy dense dietary patterns rich in whole or minimally processed plant foods (whole plant foods) tend to be associated with a lower risk of weight gain and obesity compared to the more common Western diets high in processed foods.
- Prospective cohort studies show >3 daily whole-grain servings (especially with total cereal fiber at approximately 10 g/day), can reduce body weight and waist size compared to < one half serving/day. Randomized control trials (RCTs) indicate that whole-grains are more effective in reducing body fat and waist size than body weight or BMI.
- For fruit and vegetables, cohort studies find an association with a lower risk of weight, waist size or body fat gain and obesity, especially for healthier varieties. However, higher energy dense, lower fiber fruits and vegetables may promote weight gain.
- RCTs indicate that lower energy dense, higher fiber and flavonoid rich fruits and vegetables can support lower risk of weight gain or modest weight loss and promote additional weight loss in a hypocaloric diet or help to support weight maintenance after weight loss.
- RCTs show that the daily consumption of dietary pluses and nuts do not promote weight gain, and may support modest weight loss. Nuts consumed as a snack or legumes as a meal protein source in weight loss diets do not tend to interfere with weight loss or weight maintenance after weight loss.

8.1 Introduction

Overweight and obesity status in the human population largely remained an exception until the 1970s, when increasing urbanization, sedentary

M.L. Dreher, *Dietary Patterns and Whole Plant Foods in Aging and Disease*, Nutrition and Health,
https://doi.org/10.1007/978-3-319-59180-3_8

jobs and the availability of processed foods produced a sharp rise in overweight and obesity in both children and adults [1]. The worldwide overweight and obesity pandemic is among the greatest public health challenges of our time with over two billion people now overweight or obese globally [2–4]. Obesity or excessive abdominal adiposity in adulthood and childhood is a growing risk factor for major chronic diseases [5–9]. These conditions are associated with increased health care costs and reduced workforce productivity and an estimated >300,000 premature adult deaths each year in the US [10, 11]. A small daily positive energy balance of 50 kcals/day, by increased energy intake, lower fiber diets, and/or reduced activity, can lead to an annual weight gain of 0.4–0.9 kg/year [12–16]. Further, a higher habitual intake of 200 kcal/day above energy balance in overweight or obese women may increase weight gain by as much as 9 kg/year [17]. People tend to eat similar amounts or volumes of food on a day-to-day basis regardless of the food energy density, so the common advice of just eating less of all foods may not be the optimal approach for weight management [18–22]. A systematic review found that higher energy dense, lower fiber dietary patterns may pre-dispose children to later increased risk of being overweight or obese as adults [23]. For overweight or obese individuals who successfully lose weight, as many as 80% typically drift back to their original weight or more [24]. This is because after weight loss there are an array of metabolic regulatory processes causing a cascade of dietary energy density signals designed for weight regain [25–27]. One study showed that weight loss maintainers for >5 years reported consuming a diet with a significantly lower energy density (1.4 kcal/g) than the weight regain individuals (1.8 kcal/g) [28]. The primary diet difference was that the weight maintainers consumed more fiber-rich foods such as vegetables (4.9 servings/day) and whole-grain products (2.2 servings/day) compared to less than one daily serving of vegetables and whole grains for the weight regainers. Successful long-term weight loss maintenance is associated with six key strategies to help counteract weight regain metabolic processes: (1) engaging in physical activity; (2) eating a low energy dense and high fiber diet; (3) consuming breakfast; (4) self-monitoring weight on a regular basis; (5) limiting consumption of higher energy dense foods; and (6) catching dietary miss-steps before they become a habit [15, 29–31]..A pooled prospective investigation of three cohorts from the Nurses' Health Studies and Health Professionals Follow-up (120,877 U S women and men; over 4 years) found that specific foods are independently associated with weight change (Fig. 8.1); the foods positively associated with increased weight were French fried potatoes, potato chips, sugar-sweetened beverages, red and processed meats and the foods inversely associated with weight gain were vegetables, whole grains, fruits, nuts, and yogurt ($p \leq 0.005$ for each comparison) [32]. This analysis and future research in this area have important implications for obesity prevention strategies [32]. The objective of this chapter is to review the effects of specific whole or minimally processed plant foods (whole plant foods) on weight and body composition regulation.

8.2 Whole Plant Foods

Although whole plant foods are more generally associated with lower energy density, reduced risk of weight gain or obesity than highly processed plant foods [33], whole plant foods can vary widely in nutrient composition, energy density, and physical properties (Appendix A). Thus, not all whole plant foods are equally effective in weight management. Nine intervention trials and review articles consistently show that unrestricted whole food plant-based diets are significantly more effective in lowering body weight and other anthropometric measures that the usual or Western diets [34–42]. A 2017 New Zealand based randomized controlled trial (RCT; 65 subjects; mean age 56 years; mean BMI 34; non-energy restricted whole food plant-based diet vs. usual Western type diet; regular exercise was not mandated; 6 and 12 months) showed that the whole plant food diet reduced BMI 3.9 kg/m^2 after 6 months and 4.2 kg/m^2 after 12 months compared to the usual diet [34]. A worksite 2016 US open label trial (35 subjects; mean age 43 years; 91% female; nutrient-dense, plant rich diet with

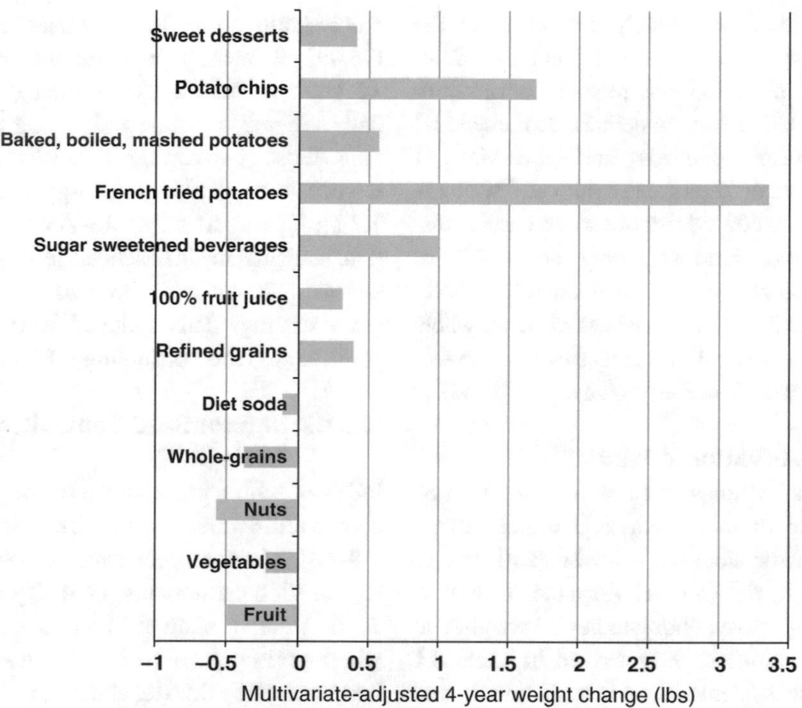

Fig. 8.1 Association between specific "whole or processed plant food" choices and 4-year weight change in US men and women from pooled Nurses' Health Studies and Health Professionals Follow-up Study data (adapted from [32])

daily greens, beans, legumes, vegetables, fresh or frozen whole fruits, nuts, seeds and whole grains and minimal intake of refined grains, vegetables oils, processed foods and meats or full-fat dairy; 6 weeks) found significant reduction in body weight, BMI, waist and hip measurements compared to baseline measurements [35]. A 2016 Australian base Mobile Health Lifestyle Program for the Prevention of Weight Gain in Young Adults RCT (250 subjects; age range 18 to 35 years; 60% women; mean BMI 27; 9 months) showed greater odds of reducing weight gain by meeting recommendations for fruit and vegetable intake by 383% and 242%, respectively, limiting intake of sugar sweetened beverages by 311%, and limiting take-out meals by 188% [36]. The 2014 Danish RCT (181 subjects; 71% women; mean age 42 years; mean BMI 30; ab libitum New Nordic Diet high in fruit, vegetables, whole-grains and fish vs. average Danish Western type diet; 26 weeks) found that the subjects on the New Nordic Diets lost 3 kg more body weight than those on the average Danish diet for the intention-to-treat analysis [42]. The New Nordic Diets also reduced systolic blood pressure by 5.1 mm Hg and diastolic blood pressure by 3.2 mm Hg compared to the average Danish diet. Ab libitum consumption of approximately 75% whole plant based diets and plus dairy products, fish and eggs with limited sweets, highly processed foods, red or processed meats is a viable option for the treatment and prevention of overweight and obesity [37–42]. The MyPlate visual educational tool was developed to encourage Americans to increase their intake of whole or minimally processed fruits, vegetables and grains to promote better health and weight control [43].

8.2.1 Whole-Grain Foods

Whole-grain products (brown rice, oatmeal, popcorn, whole wheat, or rye bread and crackers, and whole-grain/fiber-rich breakfast cereals) contain the whole intact grain kernel with natural levels of fiber, vitamins, minerals and phytochemicals [44–48]. In contrast, refined grain products (white rice and white bread, pastry, donuts and low fiber breakfast cereals) are mainly comprised of the starchy endosperm with most of the fiber, vitamins, minerals and phytonutrients removed during processing. The US dietary guidelines recommend >3 servings of whole-grains/day and <3 servings of refined grains/day to promote health and wellness associated with reduced risk of various chronic diseases [44, 49]. However, only about 1% of Americans follow the recommendation for whole-grain intake as the average intake is <1 ounce whole grains/day and 70% of Americans exceed the recommended intake for refined grains [44, 49, 50].

8.2.1.1 Observational Studies

Observational studies consistently show that higher intake of whole-grains, but not refined grains, is associated with lower BMI and/or reduced obesity risk [50, 51]. A systematic review and five prospective cohort studies on weight and body composition are summarized in Table 8.1 [52–57]. The systematic review of cohort and cross-sectional studies (15 studies; 119,829 participants) found that whole grain intake resulted in a mean reduced BMI by 0.6 units, waist size by 2.7 cm and waist- to-hip ratio by 0.023 per three servings/day compared to <0.5 serving/day [52]. This analysis also showed that the consumption of three servings of whole grains increased total fiber by 9 g/day and reduced total fat by 11 g/day in the diet. Prospective studies consistently show an inverse association between whole grain intake (rich in cereal fiber) and body weight [53–57]. In a European Prospective Investigation into Cancer and Nutrition (EPIC) Study (89,432 participants; mean baseline age 53 years; 6.5 years of follow-up) individuals with the highest intake of whole grains providing 10 g daily cereal fiber significantly reduced both weight and waist size [53]. The Physician Health Study (17,881 men; mean baseline age 53 years; follow-up at 8 and 13 years) showed an inverse association between breakfast cereal intake and weight gain with a significant 22% lower risk of >10 kg weight gain, compared with the lowest consumers [54]. The Health Professionals Follow-up Study (27,082 men; mean baseline age 52 years; 8 years of follow-up) reported that each daily 40 g increase in whole grains reduced weight gain by 0.5 kg with bran being approximately twice as effective as whole-grain [55]. In a Nurses Health Study (74,091 women; mean baseline age 50 years; 12 years of follow-up) women consuming 2.3 daily servings of whole grains weighed 0.9 kg less than those consuming 0.7 servings, whereas women with similar refined-grain intake gained 1.2 kg [56]. A Minneapolis Public School Study (240 students; mean baseline age 13 years; 2 years) showed that students who consumed >1.5 whole-grain servings daily reduced BMI by 7% compared to students consuming <0.5 servings [57].

8.2.1.2 Randomized Controlled Trials (RCTs)

RCTs of whole grain intake on weight and body composition are summarized in Table 8.2 [58–68]. A comprehensive meta-analysis (26 RCTs; 2060 participants; 18–150 g whole-grains; 2–16 weeks) showed that overall increased whole-grain intake had insignificant increased body weight by 0.06 kg and reduced waist size by 0.10 cm, and a significant reduction of body fat by 0.48% compared with control diets [58]. A subgroup analysis found that brown and black rice significantly decreased body weight by 1.1 kg and body fat by 1.2%, oats significantly decreased waist size by 1.2 cm and whole wheat cereal lowered body fat by 0.71% ($p = 0.08$) compared to control diets.

Several RCTs on increased whole-grain in ad libitum diets show mixed outcomes on weight and body composition [59–61]. A crossover RCT (33 adults, mean age 48 years; mean BMI 28; mean 168 g vs. 28 g whole grains; 6 weeks) detected a slight trend toward lower body weight for whole grains [59] whereas a parallel RCT (316 subjects; mean baseline age 46 years; mean BMI 30; <30 g, 60 g, and 120 g whole grains; 8–16 weeks) did not find a significant effect on body weight or fat (%) [61]. However, a Japanese crossover RCT (27 males; mean BMI 26; brown vs. white rice; 8 weeks for each phase) found that brown rice decreased body weight, BMI and waist size, but these weight changes returned to baseline values by the end of the white rice diet period [60]. Also, the intra-abdominal visceral fat (%) was significantly lower after 8 weeks of brown rice consumption than after a comparable period of white rice (Fig. 8.2).

Table 8.1 Summary of whole-grain prospective cohort studies on body weight and body composition regulation

Objective	Study details	Results
Systematic review		
Harland and Garton (2008). Review evidence relating to the intake of whole-grain and healthy body weight [52]	15 cohort and cross-sectional studies; 119,829 primarily European and American adults	Whole-grain significantly reduced BMI by 0.6 units, waist size by 2.7 cm, and waist: hip ratio by 0.023 in individuals consuming 3 servings/day compared to <0.5 servings/day. Higher intake of whole-grain led to increased fiber intake by 9 g/day and lowered total fat by 11 g/day and saturated fat by 3.9 g/day
Prospective cohort studies		
Du et al. (2013). Investigate the association of total fiber, cereal fiber, and fruit and vegetable fiber with changes in weight and waist size. (European Prospective Investigation into Cancer and Nutrition [EPIC]) [53]	89,432 participants, mean baseline age 53 years; average 6.5 years of follow-up (multivariate adjusted)	A 10-g/day higher cereal fiber intake was associated with annual mean weight reduction by 0.77 g and lower waist size by 0.10 cm. Fruit and vegetable fiber was not associated with weight change but had a similar association with waist size reduction as cereal fiber
Bazzano et al. (2005). Assess the association between whole-grain and refined grain breakfast cereal intakes and risk of overweight and weight gain (The Physician's Health Study; US) [54]	17,881 men; mean baseline age 53 years; mean BMI 24; >1 whole-grain servings/day vs. rarely consume; 8 and 13 years of follow-up (multivariate adjusted)	Men who consumed any type of breakfast cereal consistently weighed less than those who rarely consumed breakfast cereals (p-trend = 0.01). Those who consumed >1 serving/day of breakfast cereals were 22% less likely after 8 years and 12% less likely after 13 years to become overweight compared with men who rarely or never consumed breakfast cereals
Koh-Banerjee et al. (2004). Ascertain the associations between changes in quantitative estimates of whole-grain intake and 8-year weight gain among men (Health Professionals Follow-up Study; US) [55]	27,082 men; mean baseline age 52 years; mean BMI 25; 27 g whole-grains/day vs. 11 g WG/day; 8 years of follow-up (multivariate adjusted)	Whole-grain intake was significantly inversely associated with long-term weight gain. For every 40 g/day increased intake of whole-grain foods, a dose-response relationship was observed for a significantly reduced weight gain by 0.5 kg. Bran that was added to the diet or obtained from fortified-grain foods further reduced the risk of weight gain for every 20 g/day by 0.36 kg
Liu et al. (2003). Examine the associations between the intakes of dietary fiber and whole-grain or refined-grain products and weight gain over time (Nurses' Health Study; US) [56]	74,091 women; mean baseline age 50 years; mean BMI 25; median intake of 2.3 whole-grain servings/1000 kcals vs. 0.07 whole-grain servings/1000 kcals; 12 years of follow-up (multivariate adjusted)	Women in the highest quintile of whole-grain intake weighed 0.9 kg less than women in the lowest quintile of intake, whereas women in the highest quintile of refined-grain intake weighed 1.2 kg more than women in the lowest quintile of intake. Women in the highest quintile of fiber intake had a 49% lower risk of major weight gain than women in the lowest quintile
Steffen et al. (2003). Investigate the association between whole-grain intake and BMI in adolescents (Minneapolis Public School Students Study; US) [57]	240 students; mean baseline age 13 years; >1.5 whole-grain vs. <0.5 whole-grain servings/day; 2 years of follow-up (multivariate adjusted)	The students consuming higher whole-grain had significantly lower BMI by 1 unit compared to the students with lower whole-grain intake, after multivariate adjustments. Also, the students with higher whole-grain-intake had significantly greater insulin sensitivity

Table 8.2 Summary of whole-grain randomized controlled trials (RCTs) on body weight and composition regulation

Objective	Study details	Results
Systematic review and meta-analysis		
Pol et al. (2013). Assess the effects of whole-grain foods compared with non-whole-grain foods on changes in body weight, percentage of body fat, and waist size [58]	26 RCTs; 2060 participants; daily whole-grain dose ranged from 18 to 150 g; duration ranged from 2 to 16 weeks with the majority of studies lasting 4–6 weeks	Whole-grain intake had insignificant effects on increased body weight by 0.06 kg and decreased waist size by 0.10 cm, and a small but significant lowering effect on percentage of body fat by 0.48% compared with the non-whole-grain control. Whole wheat cereal lowered body fat more than a control by 0.71% ($p = 0.08$). A subgroup analysis for individual grains showed that only whole-grain rice decreased body weight by 1.1 kg and percentage of body fat by 1.2% compared with the white rice control. Whole-grain oats decreased waist size by 1.2 cm more than the control
RCTs		
Ad libitum energy intake		
Ampatzoglou et al. (2015). Assess the impact of increasing whole-grain intake on body weight, blood pressure, blood lipids, blood glucose, microbiota, and gastrointestinal symptoms in healthy, middle-aged adults (UK) [59]	**Crossover RCT** 33 subjects; 12 males and 21 females; mean age 48 years; mean BMI 28; mean 28 g vs. 168 g whole-grain/day; 6 weeks; 4 weeks of washout; adherence was achieved by specific dietary advice and provision of a range of cereal food products	During the whole-grain intervention, there was a significant increase in plasma alkylresorcinols and total fiber intake, without any effect on energy or other macronutrients. Although there were no effects on studied variables, there were trends toward increased 24-h fecal weight ($p = 0.08$) and reduction in body weight ($p = 0.10$) and BMI ($p = 0.08$) during the high whole-grain intervention compared with the low whole-grain period
Shimabukuro et al. (2014). Evaluate the effects of brown rice and white rice on abdominal fat distribution and metabolic parameters (BRAVO study; Japan) [60]	**Crossover RCT** 27 male subjects with metabolic syndrome; mean age 41 years; mean BMI 28; switch from brown to white rice and white to brown rice; subjects 8 weeks on each rice; no washout	In the group that ate brown rice for the first 8-weeks test period body weight, BMI and waist size were decreased but returned to baseline values by the end of the white rice diet period. In the group that are white rice in the first period body weight, BMI and waist size were comparable with the baseline values, but waist size was lower after switching to brown rice diet. Also, intra-abdominal visceral fat (%) was significantly lower after brown rice than after white rice consumption (Fig. 8.2)
Brownlee et al. (2011). Evaluate the effect of substituting whole-grain foods in the diet of habitual refined-grain consumers on markers of CVD risk and weight measures (UK) [61]	**Parallel RCT** 316 participants; mean aged 46 years; mean BMI 30; 3 diets: (1) 60 g whole-grain/day for 16 weeks; (2) 60 g whole-grains/day for 8 weeks followed by 120 g whole grains/day for 8 weeks; and (3) < 30 g whole-grain/day for 16 weeks (control)	The consumption of whole-grain from 30–120 g/day (added fiber 6–11 g/day) for 16 weeks did not significantly change weight or body fat (%)
Restricted energy intake		
Harris Jackson et al. (2014). Investigate the effect of consuming whole-grains to replace refined grains in the diets of individuals with metabolic syndrome or at risk for metabolic syndrome (US) [62]	**Parallel RCT** 50 subjects;mean age 46 years; mean BMI 33; controlled weight-loss diet containing 163–301 g whole-grain/day vs. 0 g whole-grain/day; 12 weeks	Replacing refined grains with whole-grains within a weight-loss diet did not significantly improve weight, BMI or abdominal visceral adipose tissue loss. However, the whole-grain diet significantly reduced the prevalence of prediabetes by 90% compared with 13% for the refined grain diets. Whole-grain diets were more effective at normalizing blood glucose levels and reducing the risk of individuals with prediabetes from progressing to type 2 diabetes

Table 8.2 (continued)

Objective	Study details	Results
Kristensen et al. (2012). Study the effect of replacing refined wheat with whole-grain wheat on body weight and composition (EU) [63]	**Parallel RCT** 79 postmenopausal women; mean age 68 years; mean BMI 30; energy-restricted diet (by 300 kcal/day) with 105 g whole wheat grains daily or refined wheat foods; 12 weeks	Body weight decreased significantly from baseline in refined wheat group by 2.7 kg and whole-grain wheat group by 3.6 kg with no significance between the groups ($p = 0.11$). The reduction in total body fat % was significantly greater in the whole-grain group (Fig. 8.3). Serum total and LDL cholesterol significantly increased by 5% in the refined wheat group but did not change in the whole-grain group ($p = 0.02$)
Maki et al. (2010). Investigate the effect of a whole-grain, ready to-eat (RTE) oat cereal containing viscous fiber, as part of a dietary program for weight loss (US) [64]	**Parallel RCT** 144 subjects; mean age 49 years; mean BMI 32; 78% female; 2 portions/day of whole-grain RTE oat whole grain cereal (3 g/day oat β-glucan) or energy-matched low-fiber foods (control), reduced energy diet by 500 kcal/day; 12 weeks	Both groups lost weight, in the whole-grain oat cereal group by 2.2 kg and the control by 1.7 kg ($p = 0.325$). Waist size decreased significantly more with whole-grain oat cereal by 3.3 cm compared with 1.9 cm for the control ($p = 0.012$) (Fig. 8.4)
Katcher et al. (2008). Determine whether including whole-grain foods in a hypocaloric diet (reduced by 500 kcal/day) effects weight loss and improves CVD risk factors (US) [65]	**Parallel RCT** 50 metabolic syndrome adults; 25 males and 25 females; mean age 46 years; mean BMI 36; 5 whole-grain servings/day vs. <0.25 servings in the refined grain group; all participants were given the same dietary advice in other respects for weight loss; 12 weeks	Body weight, waist size, and body fat (%) decreased significantly in both groups, but there was a significantly greater decrease in body fat (%) in the abdominal region in the whole-grain group than in the refined-grain group. C-reactive protein (CRP) decreased 38% in the whole-grain group independent of weight loss compared to no change in the refined-grain group. Total and LDL cholesterol decreased in both diet groups. Total fiber and magnesium intakes increased in the whole-grain compared to the refined-grain group
Kim et al. (2008). Assess the effect of type of rice consumed on weight control when consumed with an energy restricted diet (Korea) [66]	**Parallel RCT** 40 overweight Korean women; 20–35 years of age; energy restricted diets containing either white rice or mixture of brown rice and black rice; 6 weeks	The subjects on the brown and black rice supplemented diets showed a significantly greater reduction in weight by 1.4 kg and body fat by 1.2% compared to the white rice group
Melanson et al. (2006). Investigate the effects of exercise plus a hypocaloric whole-grain diet on weight loss (US) [67]	**Parallel RCT** 134 adults; mean age 42 years; mean BMI 31; hypocaloric diet with and without whole-grain breakfast cereals; 23 vs. 17 g fiber/day; 24 weeks	In the hypocaloric diet, consumption of whole-grain breakfast cereals insignificantly improved weight loss by 0.3 kg compared to the refined cereal diet
Saltzman et al. (2001). Evaluate the effects of oats on weight loss and body composition (US) [68]	**Parallel RCT** 43 subjects; mean BMI 26; mean age 45 years; 2 hypocaloric diets (maintenance energy minus 1000 kcals/day): (1) diet containing oats 45 g/day and (2) control diet (no added oats); 6 weeks	In the hypocaloric diets, there was no difference in weight loss by adding 45 g/day oats vs. the control diet as both groups lost about 4 kg ($p = 0.8$). The oat supplemented diet significantly lowered mean systolic blood pressure and total and LDL cholesterol

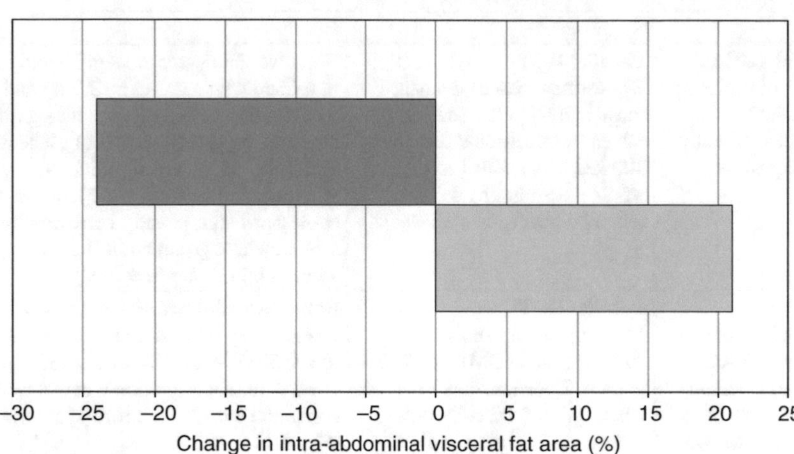

Fig. 8.2 Effect of brown vs. white rice on mean intra-abdominal visceral fat in Japanese men with metabolic syndrome after 8 weeks ($p < 0.018$) (adapted from [60])

Seven RCTs show increased whole-grain in energy restricted diets has the capacity to significantly affect abdominal or total body fat, waist circumference, CRP levels and diabetes risk if adequate whole grains are consumed [62–68]. Two RCTs suggest that whole grain from breakfast cereal or oats has no additive effect in hypocaloric diets on weight or body composition but the level of overall whole grain intake in the RCTs appears to have been relatively modest based on the fiber intake range from 13 to 23 g/day [67, 68]. Another RCT (50 subjects; mean age 46 years; mean BMI 33; controlled weight-loss diet containing 163–301 g whole-grains/day vs. 0 g whole-grains/day; 12 weeks) showed that whole grains had no effect on weight or body composition but they did significantly reduce the risk of prediabetes by 90% compared to 13% lower risk in the refined grain group [62]. A RCT in postmenopausal women (79 women; mean age 68 years; mean BMI 30; energy-restricted diet (by 300 kcal/day) with 105 g whole wheat grain daily or refined wheat foods; 12 weeks) found that body weight decreased significantly from baseline in the refined wheat group by 2.7 kg and in the whole grain wheat group by 3.6 kg with no significance between the groups ($p = 0.11$) [63]. However, the whole grain group had a significantly lower body fat (%) (Fig. 8.3). An oat breakfast cereal RCT (144 subjects; mean age 49 years; mean BMI 32; 78% female; 2 portions/day of whole-grain ready to eat (RTE) oat whole grain cereal (3 g/day oat β-glucan) or energy-matched low-fiber foods (control), as part of diet energy reduced by 500 kcal/day; 12 weeks) found that waist size decreased significantly more with oat cereal by 3.3 cm compared with 1.9 cm for the control ($p = 0.012$) (Fig. 8.4) [64]. A RCT in individuals with metabolic syndrome (50 adults; mean age 46; mean BMI 36; 5 whole grain servings vs. <0.25 servings; 12 weeks) reported a significant reduction in abdominal fat (%) and CRP levels in the whole grain vs. refined grain group [65]. In a rice based hypocaloric diet (40 Korean women; age 20–35 years; 6 weeks) consuming brown and black rice was shown to significantly reduce body weight and body fat (%) vs. white rice [66].

8.2.2 Fruits and Vegetables

8.2.2.1 Background

The Dietary Guidelines for Americans (Myplate.gov) recommends that whole or minimally processed fruits and vegetables make-up one-half of a meal's plate [43, 44]. Fruits and vegetables include a diverse group of plant foods that vary widely in their health effects due to a range of energy, fiber, glycemic index, nutrients, and phytonutrients contents, and physical properties. Adequate intake of fruits and vegetables (>400 g/day) makes important contributions to health

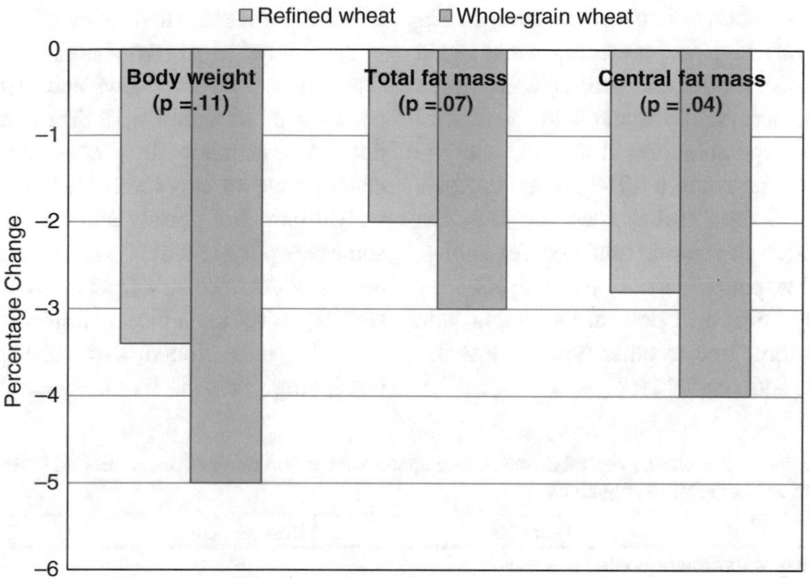

Fig. 8.3 Effect of whole-grain in an energy-restricted dietary intervention on change in body weight, total fat mass, and central fat mass in postmenopausal women after 12 weeks (adapted from [63])

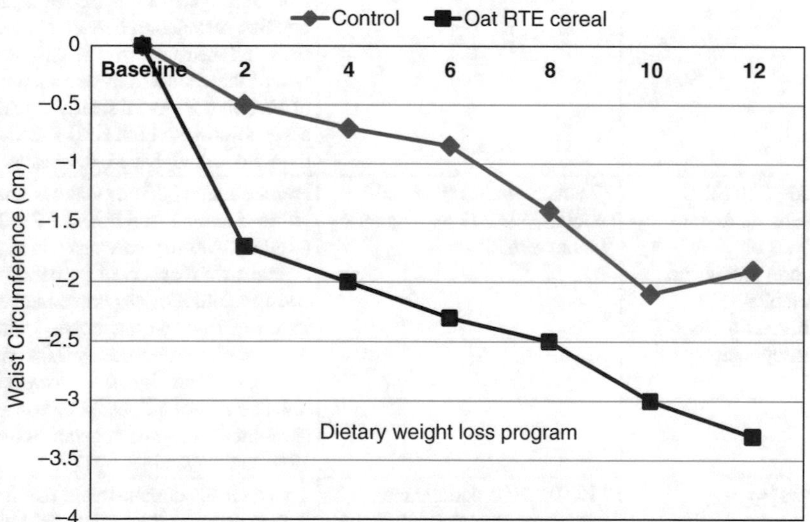

Fig. 8.4 Effect of whole-grain oat ready-to-eat (RTE) on waist size in obese adults in a dietary weight loss program with 3 g/day oat β-glucan twice daily for 12 weeks ($p = 0.012$) (adapted from [64])

because of their unique concentrations of: antioxidant vitamins and phytochemicals, especially vitamins C and A, flavonoids and carotenoids, minerals (especially electrolytes potassium and magnesium, and low sodium), and fiber [69–73]. Globally, fruits and vegetables consumption is at only a small fraction of the recommended levels [74]. Most Americans consume less than one cup of fruits and less than two cups of vegetables daily, with the primary contributors consisting of juice and processed potatoes, compared to the current recommendations of 2 cups of fruit and 2.5 cups of vegetables per day. More than 85% of the US and likely other Western population fall short of meeting the daily recommendations [43, 44]. A potential benefit of a diet rich in fruit and non-starchy vegetables is their low energy density which may help in preventing weight gain due to their water, fiber and bulk volume, which contribute to satiation compared to the typical low fruit and vegetable diets associated with the Western lifestyle. Also, a 2016 pooled analysis of 124,086 US men and women suggests that consuming high flavonoid fruits and vegetables, such as apples, pears, berries, and peppers, may be especially helpful in preventing weight gain and obesity compared to other types of low flavonoid fruits and vegetables [75].

8.2.2.2 Systematic Reviews and Meta-Analyses

Overall, systematic reviews and meta-and pooled analyses of prospective studies and RCTs show that whole or minimally processed fruits and vegetables have an important role in reducing risk of weight gain and obesity and central obesity with some exceptions (Table 8.3) [76–80]. A systematic review of potatoes on weight gain (five prospective studies; 170,413 subjects; follow-up between 2 and 20 years) found that total potato intake (excluding French fries), were inconsistently

Table 8.3 Summary of fruit and vegetable prospective cohort studies and randomized controlled trials (RCTs) studies on body weight and composition regulation

Objective	Study details	Results
Systematic review and meta-pooled analyses		
Borch et al. (2016). Evaluate the relationship between potatoes and obesity risk [76]	5 prospective studies; 170,413 subjects; follow-up between 2 and 20 years	For potatoes (excluding French fries), two studies showed a positive association with adiposity and two studies showed no association with adiposity. In the three studies that investigated French fries separately, a positive association between intake of French fries and measures of adiposity was shown. In two of these studies, it was shown that intake of French fries had a stronger positive association with both BMI and weight gain than did boiled, baked, or mashed potatoes
Schwingshackl et al. (2015). Perform a systematic review and meta-analysis of prospective cohort studies on fruits and vegetables consumption in relation to changes in anthropometric measures [77]	17 cohort studies (from 20 reports); 563,277 participants; 9 months to 20 years	Higher intake of fruits was associated with reduced annual weight by 13.7 g/100 g intake (slightly over one serving). No significant changes were observed for combined fruits and vegetables or vegetable intake. Increased intake of fruits was associated with a reduction in waist circumference by 0.04 cm/year. Comparing the highest vs. lowest intake, reduced risk of adiposity was observed for combined fruits and vegetables by 9%, fruit by 17%, and vegetables by17%
Kaiser et al. (2014). Synthesize the best available evidence on the effectiveness of the general recommendation to eat more fruits and vegetables for weight loss or the prevention of weight gain [78]	7 RCTs; 1103 participants; primary or secondary outcome of body weight; including 100% juices; >8 weeks	This analysis demonstrated that increased fruits and vegetables intake including 100% juice insignificantly increased body weight by 0.04%
Mytton et al. (2014). Quantify the relationship between changes in fruits and vegetables (excluding juices intake), energy intake and body weight [79]	8 RCTs; 1026 participants; excluding 100% juice; mean 14.7 weeks	High fruits and vegetables intake significantly reduced body weight by 0.68 kg vs. lower fruits and vegetables intake, despite no difference in daily energy intake ($p = 0.07$). Increased fruits and vegetables intake, in the absence of specific advice to decrease consumption of other foods, appears unlikely to lead to weight gain in the short-term and may subsequently have a role in weight maintenance or loss

Table 8.3 (continued)

Objective	Study details	Results
Ledoux et al. (2011). Assess the relationship between fruits and vegetables intake and adiposity [80]	12 intervention trials (11 on adults and one on children) and 11 longitudinal studies (seven on adults and four on children)	In energy restricted intervention trials, higher intake of fruits and vegetables was weakly associated with weight loss among overweight or obese adults, but not children. In longitudinal studies, high fruits and vegetables intake was associated with less or slower weight gain over lengthy time intervals among adults, but to a lesser degree among children
Prospective or longitudinal cohort studies		
Shefferly et al. (2016). Evaluate the relationship between 100% juice intake and weight status in pre-school children (Early Childhood Longitudinal Study-Birth Cohort; US) [81]	8950 children; examined at ages 2, 4 and 5 years (multivariate adjusted)	Regular 100% juice consumption between ages 2 and 4 years increased the odds of becoming overweight by 30%. However, significant increase in weight was not observed in children at age 5 years
Bertoia et al. (2015). Examine the effect of increased fruits and vegetables intake on weight change over time, including subtypes and individual fruits and vegetables (Nurses' Health Study I and II, and Health Professionals Follow-up Study; US) [82]	133,468 men and women; in women, the average baseline age was 36 and 49 years; in men, the average baseline age was 47 years; multiple 4-year weight measurement cycles over 24 years of follow-up (multivariate adjusted)	Increased intake of fruits was inversely associated with 4-year weight loss per daily serving for total fruits by 0.53 lb., berries by 1.11 lbs., and apples and pears by 1.24 lbs. (Fig. 8.5). Increased intake of several vegetables was also inversely associated with weight loss per daily serving for total vegetables by 0.25 lb., tofu/soy by 2.47 lbs. and cauliflower by 1.37 lbs. (Fig. 8.6). In contrast, increased intake of starchy vegetables, including corn, peas, and potatoes, was associated with weight gain (Fig. 8.7). Vegetables having both higher fiber and lower glycemic load were more strongly associated with weight loss compared with lower-fiber, higher-glycemic-load vegetables
Rautiainen et al. (2015). Investigate whether intake of fruits and vegetables, and total fiber is associated with weight change and the risk of becoming overweight and obese (Women's Health Study; US) [83]	18,146 women; mean baseline age 54 years; mean baseline BMI 22; mean follow-up of 15.9 years; 8125 women became overweight or obese (multivariate adjusted)	Vegetable intake was associated with greater weight gain (p-trend = 0.02) and subjects with higher fruit intake had a 13% lower risk of becoming overweight or obese (higher vs. lower intake). Overall, greater intake of fruit, but not vegetables, by middle-aged and older women with a normal BMI is associated with lower risk of becoming overweight or obese
Vergnaud et al. (2012). Assess the association between the baseline consumption of fruits and vegetables and weight change (European Prospective Investigation into Cancer and Nutrition (EPIC) study) [84]	373,803 participants; mean baseline age 52 years; mean BMI 26; country-specific validated questionnaires; per 100 g fruits and vegetables/day and weight change (g/year); mean follow-up of 5 years (multivariate adjusted)	Baseline fruits and vegetables intake was associated with weight loss in men and women who quit smoking during follow-up. There was a weak association between vegetable intake and weight loss in women who were overweight, were former smokers and weak associations between fruit intake and weight loss in women who were >50 years of age, were of normal weight, or were never smokers

(continued)

Table 8.3 (continued)

Objective	Study details	Results
Representative RCTs		
Tapsell et al. (2014). Assess the effects of higher vegetable consumption on weight loss (Australia) [85]	**Single Blind, Parallel RCT** 120 adults; mean BMI 30; mean age 49 years; two 20% energy deficit groups with healthy diet advice to consume vegetables each day. The test group was asked to consume >5 servings of low energy dense vegetables each day, but the control vegetable group consumed half the portions (0.5 vs. 1.0 cup cooked or 1 vs. 2 cups of raw, respectively); 12 months	Both groups significantly reduced intake of high energy dense vegetables and increased portions of low energy dense vegetable as instructed. The higher percentage energy from vegetables was positively associated with weight loss and sustainability (Fig. 8.8). Weight loss was sustained for 12 months by both groups, but the higher vegetable group reported significantly greater hunger satisfaction
Christensen et al. (2013). Investigate the effects of fruit intake on HbA1c, body weight, and waist size in people with type 2 diabetes (Denmark) [86]	**Parallel RCT** 63 subjects with type 2 diabetes; mean age 58 years; mean BMI 32; 78% male; diet >2 servings vs. <2 servings fruit daily, difference in fruit intake 172 g; 12 weeks	Higher fruit intake lowered mean body weight by 0.8 kg more than the lower fruit diet ($p = 0.19$; 2.5 kg vs. 1.7 kg) and mean waist size was lowered by 1.3 cm more for the higher vs. lower fruit intake ($p = 0.36$; 4.3 cm vs. 3.0 cm)
Dow et al. (2012). Evaluate the effect of red grapefruit on body weight, blood pressure and blood lipids (US) [87]	**Parallel RCT** 74 adults; mean BMI 32; 1/2 red grapefruit consumed 3 times daily vs. control diet; 6 weeks	Red grapefruit was associated with modest weight loss by 0.6 kg, significantly reduced waist size by 2.45 cm and significantly improved systolic blood pressure by 3.2 mm Hg and reduced LDL-C by 18.7 mg/dL
Peterson et al. (2011). Evaluate the effect of the consumption of dried California Mission figs (*Ficus carica* 'Mission') on serum lipid levels and body weight (US) [88]	**Crossover RCT** 102 adults; mean age 55 years; 69% females; dried California Mission Figs (120 g/day) added to their usual diet vs. their usual diet; 5 weeks	Blood lipids and lipoproteins remained unchanged with the addition of figs. Body weight insignificantly increased by 0.4 kg ($p = 0.08$)
Basu et al. (2010). Examine the effects of blueberries on metabolic syndrome parameters and body weight (US) [89]	**Parallel RCT** 48 subjects; mean age 50 years; mean BMI 38; freeze dried blueberries equivalent to 350 g blueberries/day vs. control; 8 weeks	Blueberry supplementation did not significantly affect body weight or waist size ($p > 0.05$)
Whybrow et al. (2007). Examine the effects of incorporating fruits and vegetables into diets on body weight (Scotland) [90]	**Parallel RCT** 34 males and 28 females; mean age 43 years; mean BMI 24; 300 g or 600 g fruits and vegetables daily vs. no fruits and vegetables control; isocaloric diets; 8 weeks	Increased fruits and vegetables intake reduced body weight from 0.14 to 0.29 kg compared to an increase in body weight for the no fruit and vegetable control by 0.48 kg ($p = 0.242$)
De Oliveira et al. (2003). Investigate effect of fruit intake on body weight change (Brazil) [91]	**Parallel RCT** 49 women, mean age 44 years; mean weight 79 kg; dietary supplements: apples or pears vs. oat cookies three times daily; 12 weeks	Compared to baseline, women consuming apples and pears lost 0.34 kg more body weight than women consuming oatmeal cookies ($p = 0.004$; 1.22 kg vs. 0.88 kg)

associated with increases in adiposity [76]. However, three studies that investigated French fries separately showed a positive association between intake of French fries and measures of adiposity and two of these studies indicated that intake of French fries had a stronger positive association with both BMI and weight gain than boiled, baked, or mashed potatoes. Increasing fruits and vegetables intake as a weight loss strategy has produced conflicting results mainly associated with the inclusion or exclusion of 100% fruit juice, raising the possibility that these divergent findings may be the result of the lower satiation signals when consuming fruits and vegetables as juice compared to their whole or minimally processed forms [43, 78, 79]. A meta-analysis of prospective studies (17 cohorts; 563,277 participants; follow-up from 9 months to 20 years) found that each daily 100 g fruit had a modest lowering effect on body weight by 14 g per year and that fruit intake was inversely associated with waist size and a higher intake significantly lowered the risk of adiposity by 9% [77]. Although this weight reduction is modest it represents a composite of all fruits and vegetables, and does not rule out the potential for specific healthy low energy dense, fiber and flavonoids rich fruits and vegetables to have much larger beneficial lowering effects on body weight and central obesity. A meta-analysis of whole or minimally processed fruits and vegetables, excluding 100% fruit juice, (8 RCTs; 1026 participants; mean 14.7 weeks) showed a significant reduction in body weight by 0.68 kg compared to isocaloric lower fruits and vegetables intake in diets [79]. Additionally, a systemic review of energy-restricted diets (12 intervention trials and 11 longitudinal studies) demonstrated in intervention trials that higher intake of fruits and vegetables was associated with modest weight loss in overweight and obese adults but not in children [80].

8.2.2.3 Prospective Cohort Studies

Table 8.3 provides a summary of fruits and vegetables in weight regulation [81–84]. Several prospective studies showed that specific types of fruits and vegetables vary in their effect on body weight. Pooled data from three US prospective studies including the Nurses' Health Studies and Health Professionals Follow-up Study (133,468 men and women; mean age baseline about 48 years, mean BMI approximately 25; follow-up of 4 year cycles) observed highly variable effects of specific fruits and vegetables on weight change, after adjustment for covariates [82]. Increased intake of fruits was associated with 4-year weight loss per one daily serving for total fruits by 0.53 lb, berries by 1.11 lb, and apples and pears by 1.24 lbs (Fig. 8.5). Increased intake of several vegetables was also associated with weight loss per one daily serving for total vegetables by 0.25 lb, tofu/soy by 2.47 lbs and cauliflower by1.37 lbs (Fig. 8.6). In contrast, increased intake of starchy vegetables, including corn, peas, and potatoes, was associated with weight gain (Fig. 8.7). Vegetables having higher fiber and flavonoids, and lower energy density and glycemic load were more strongly associated with weight loss compared with lower-fiber, and higher energy dense and higher-glycemic-load vegetables. The Women's Health Study (18,146 women; mean baseline age 54 years; mean 15.9 years of follow-up) found that greater intake of fruit, but not vegetables by middle-aged and older women with a normal BMI was associated with lower risk of becoming overweight or obese [83]. The EPIC Study (373,803 participants; mean baseline age 52 years; mean follow-up of 5 years) found that fruits and vegetables intake was associated with weight loss in men and in women who quit smoking during the follow-up period [84]. There was a weak association between fruit intake and weight loss in women >50 years, normal weight or never smokers. A longitudinal study in preschool children (8950 children; examined at ages 2, 4, and 5 years) reported that regular consumption of 100% juice between ages 2 and 4 years was associated with a significant 30% increased risk of being overweight but not at age 5 years [81].

8.2.2.4 Randomized Trials

Seven representative RCTs related to increased fruits and vegetables intake and change in body weight and waist circumference are summarized in Table 8.3 [85–91]. An Australian energy weight loss RCT (120 subjects; mean age 49 years; mean BMI 30; 12 months) showed that increased vegetable intake significantly lowered body weight, especially with low energy dense vegetables

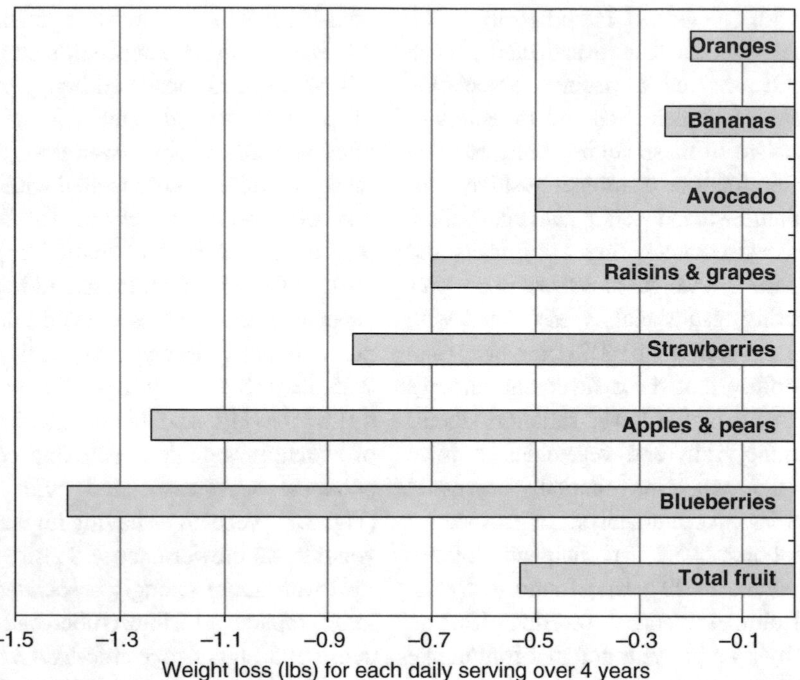

Fig. 8.5 Association between one daily serving of various fruits and weight loss in US men and women over 4 years from the Nurses' Health Studies and Health Professionals Follow-up Study (pooled data; multivariate adjusted) (adapted from [82])

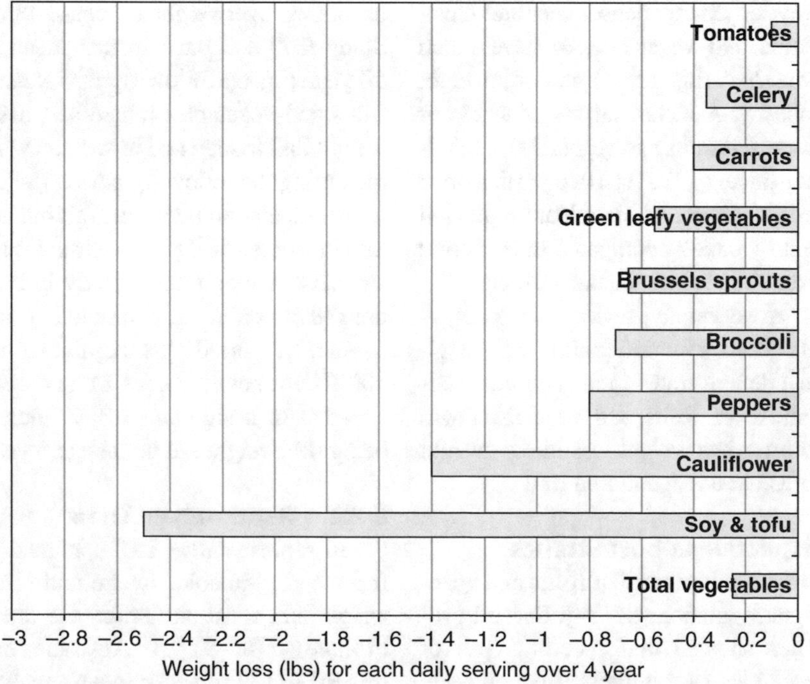

Fig. 8.6 Association between each daily serving of various vegetables and weight loss in US men and women over 4 years from the Nurses' Health Studies and Health Professionals Follow-up Study (pooled data; multivariate adjusted) (adapted from [82])

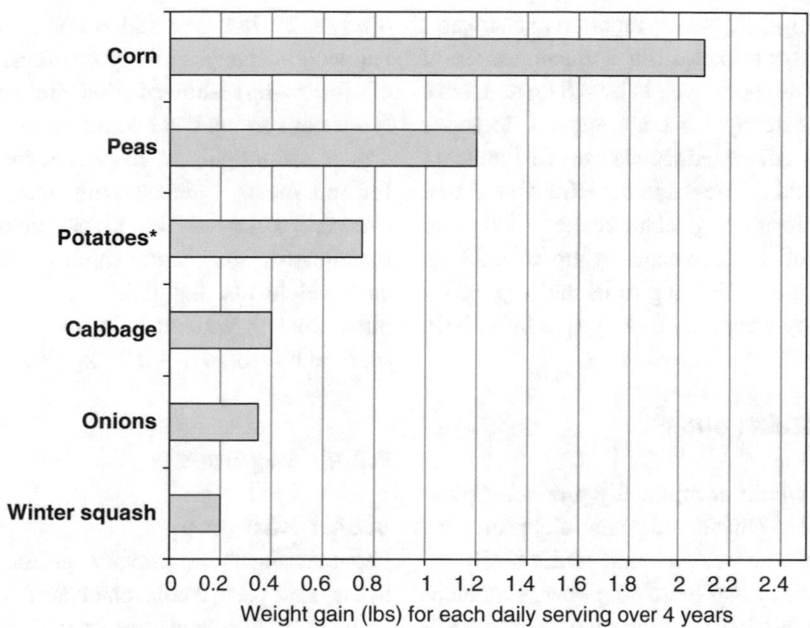

Fig. 8.7 Association between each daily serving of commonly consumed vegetables and weight gain in US men and women over 4 years from the Nurses' Health Studies and Health Professionals Follow-up Study (pooled data; multivariate adjusted) (adapted from [82]). *Includes baked, boiled, mashed white potatoes, sweet potatoes and yams and excludes French fries and potato chips

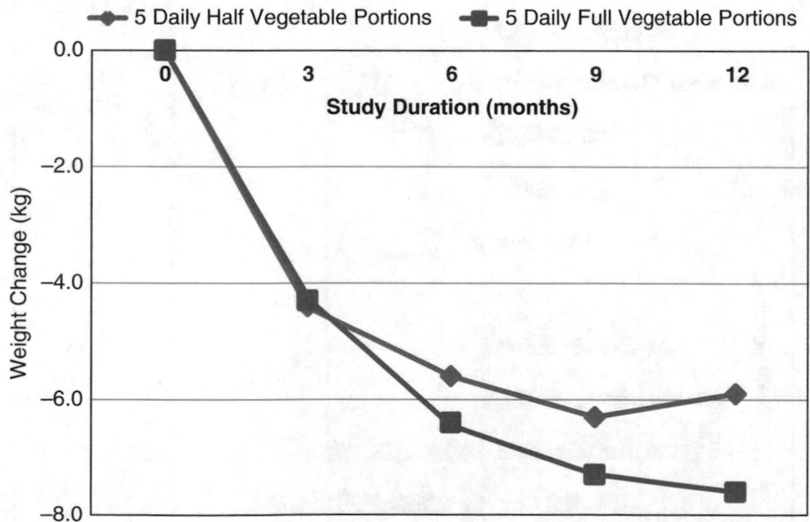

Fig. 8.8 Effect of amount of vegetables added to a diet on weight loss diet plan (20% reduced energy) in 120 obese adults over 12 months (p = 0.024) (adapted from [85])

(Fig. 8.8) [85]. A Brazilian RCT (49 women; mean age 44 years; 12 weeks) found that snacking on apples or pears significantly reduced body weight by 0.34 kg more than women snacking on oatmeal cookies [91]. Three other RCTs showed inconsistent effects of specific fruit intake on weight and waist size: (1) increased intake of a half red grapefruit three times per day modestly but significantly lowered body weight by 0.6 kg and waist size by 2.45 cm after 6 weeks [87], whereas blueberries and figs were associated with an insignificant increase in body weight [88, 89]. A Danish RCT (63 subjects with type 2 diabetes; mean age 58 years; >2 fruit servings compared to

<2 fruit servings; 12 weeks) reported that subjects with higher fruit intake (by a mean intake of 172 g) lost more body weight by 0.8 kg and had a lower waist size by 1.3 cm compared to lower fruit intake but these reductions were insignificant [86]. A Scottish dose-response RCT found that increasing fruit and vegetables intake to 300 g and 600 g reduced body weight by up to 0.29 kg whereas the diet with 0.0 g fruits and vegetables increased body weight by 0.48 kg (p = 0.24) [90].

8.2.3 Protein Foods

Protein rich whole or minimally processed plant foods have been considered potentially protective against long-term weight gain and obesity by increasing satiety and increasing energy metabolism [92]. A pooled analysis of three large US prospective cohorts including the Nurses' Health Studies and the Health Professionals Follow-up Study (120,784 men and women; protein intake and weight changes in 4 year cycles; 16–24 years of follow-up) showed that increased protein foods per serving/day had different relations with 4 year weight gain, with significant weight gain for red meats, chicken with skin, and regular cheese by 0.13–1.17 kg; no association for sugar sweetened yogurt, legumes, or eggs; and significant weight loss for plain yogurt, peanut butter, nuts, chicken without skin, low-fat cheese, and seafood by −0.14 to −0.71 kg (Fig. 8.9) [93].

8.2.4 Legumes

8.2.4.1 Background

Legumes including dietary pulses (e.g., pinto beans, split peas, lentils, chickpeas) and soybeans, are rich in fiber and protein with relatively low glycemic response properties [94]. A serving of legumes is half a cup or 90–100 g cooked legumes,

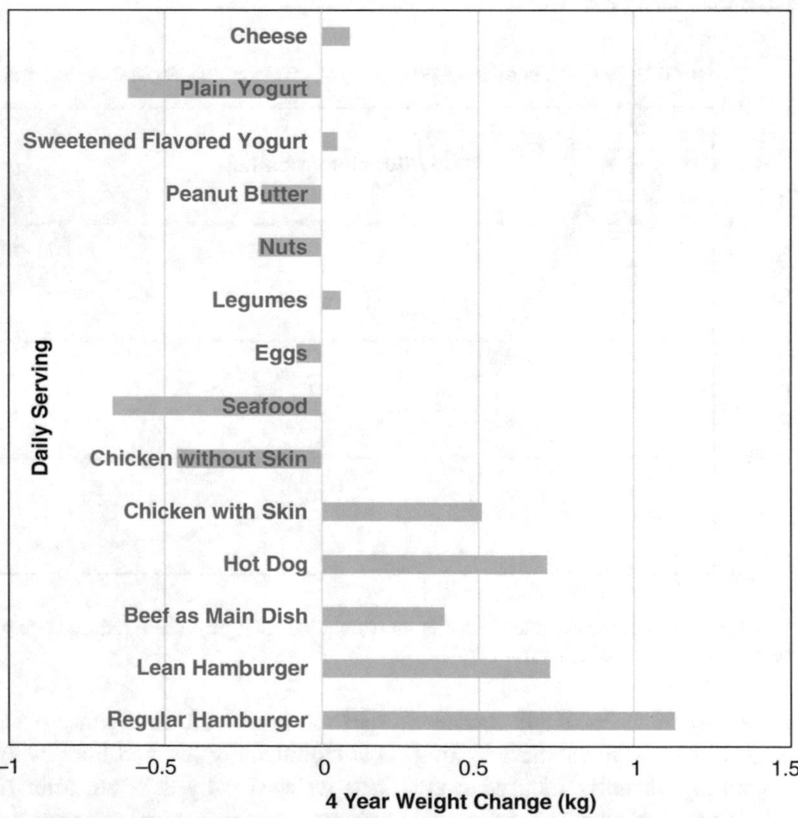

Fig. 8.9 Association between each daily serving of protein foods and weight change in US men and women over 4 years from the Nurses' Health Studies and Health Professionals Follow-up Study (pooled data; multivariate adjusted) (adapted from [93])

which contains 5–10 g of fiber, 7–8 g of protein, and <5% of energy as fat, with the exception of chickpeas and soybeans which have 15% and 47% energy from fat, respectively. Pulses promote satiety by adding bulk, and high levels of fiber (e.g., resistant starch) and protein, especially as a replacement for meat products [38]. An NHANES cross-sectional study found that bean consumers had significantly lower body weight and a 22% lower risk of being obese than non-consumers [95]. However, pulse consumption has been in decline with the global shift to Western-style diets [96]. For example, between the 1960s and 1990s, legume intake decreased by 40% in India and by 24% in Mexico. Legumes are infrequently consumed by North Americans and northern Europeans, with <8% of Americans consuming pulses daily.

8.2.4.2 Randomized Trials

Dietary pulses promote modest weight-loss even in non-energy restricted diets [97]. A meta-analysis (21 RCTs; median intake 1 serving (132 g)/day; 940 participants; median 6 weeks) showed a significant weight reduction by 0.34 kg for diets containing dietary pulses compared with control diets without them [97]. This modest weight loss with dietary pulse intake was demonstrated in both energy-restricted diets and in diets intended for weight maintenance. Six trials (509 participants) reported that dietary pulse consumption insignificantly reduced waist size by 0.37 cm. A trend was shown in six trials (340 participants) that supported lower body fat by 0.34% ($p = 0.07$) [97]. These findings are generalizable to overweight and obese populations suggesting that one daily serving of dietary pulses does not lead to weight gain and may support modest weight loss.

8.2.5 Total and Specific Nuts

8.2.5.1 Background

Nuts (e.g., almonds, pistachios, walnuts, hazelnuts, pecans, peanuts) are nutrient dense sources of fiber, protein, unsaturated fat, vitamins (e.g., B-vitamins and vitamin E), minerals (e.g., potassium and magnesium), and phytosterols, and polyphenols [35, 98]. Although nuts have a relatively high energy density (about 6 kcal/g) due primarily to a high unsaturated fat content and low water content, human studies have shown that nuts have a lower metabolizable energy than predicted from the Atwater energy tables because of the incomplete absorption of nut fat and other macronutrients [99, 100]. Human studies consistently report that the regular consumption of tree nuts, as a replacement for less healthful foods, can help prevent weight gain [101, 102]. Mechanistic studies indicate that nuts' weight control effects are largely attributable to their high satiety and low metabolizable energy (poor bioaccessibility leading to inefficient energy absorption) properties [103].

8.2.5.2 Prospective Cohort Studies

Prospective studies consistently show that increased nut consumption is protective against weight gain and obesity [104, 105]. The Spanish Seguimiento Universidad de Navarra (SUN) project (8865 men and women; mean baseline age 38 years; mean BMI 23; 28 months) indicates that people who consumed nuts >2 times/week had a 40% lower multivariate risk for weight gain compared with non-nut consumers who gained an average of 0.4 kg more over the 28 months of follow-up [104]. The Nurses' Health Study II (51,188 women in the Nurses' Health Study II; mean baseline age 36 years; mean BMI 24; 8 years of follow-up) found that women consuming nuts >2 times/week had a significant 33% lower risk of obesity and gained 0.51 kg less weight compared to non-nut consumers over 8 years of follow-up [105]. The different effects of total nuts, peanuts and tree nuts intake on obesity risk are illustrated in Fig. 8.10. A 2017 EPIC study (373,293 adults; age range 25–70 years; 5 years) showed that higher nut intake significantly reduced weight gain by 0.07 kg compared to the average weight gain of 2.1 kg for the overall population [106]. Also, this study showed that the highest nuts consumers had a significantly 5% lower risk of becoming overweight or obese.

8.2.5.3 Randomized Controlled Trials

RCTs consistently show that diets supplemented with nuts do not increase body weight, body mass index, or waist circumference compared with control diets [107–116].

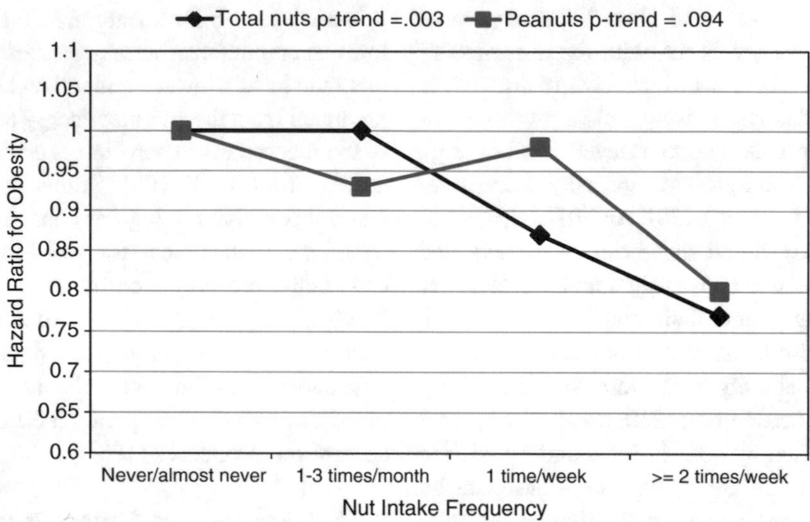

Fig. 8.10 Association between nut intake frequency and obesity risk in healthy middle-aged women over 8 years (adapted from [105])

Meta-Analysis

A systematic review and meta-analysis (33 published RCT; 75% almonds and walnuts; 1866 subjects; 2–152 weeks of duration) found that increased nut intake resulted in an insignificant decreased mean body weight by 0.47 kg, BMI by 0.40, and waist circumference by 1.25 cm [107]. Although the decreases in weight and body composition are relatively small, the results reduce any concerns that eating nuts may promote obesity in general or when eaten as a cardioprotective food. Almonds and walnuts represent 75% of the weight management research.

Almonds

Almond RCTs have consistently shown that almonds added to the habitual diet non-significantly increase body weight or when incorporated into a hypocaloric diet promote significant additional weight loss [108–113]. Two crossover RCTs demonstrate that habitual diets supplemented with two servings or 320–344 kcals of almonds daily, compared to unsupplemented control diets for 10 weeks to 6 months did not increase body weight (Fig. 8.11) [108, 109]. A parallel RCT in subjects at increased risk for type 2 diabetes (137 subjects; 48 males and 89 females; mean age approx. 30 years; almonds (43 g/day) with breakfast or lunch, alone as a morning or afternoon snack or no almonds control; 4 weeks) showed that almonds reduced hunger and did not increase the risk of weight gain [110]. A long-term weight loss RCT (123 subjects; mean baseline age 47 years; mean BMI 34; about 90% women; hypocaloric diet with 56 g almonds as snacks daily, vs. no added snack, nut free diet; 18 months) demonstrated that there was no significant 18-month weight change between the two diets with the almond group losing 3.7 kg vs. the unsupplemented group losing 5.9 kg [111]. Two shorter-term weight loss RCTs (65–108 subjects; 50–84 almonds/daily vs. nut free diets or diets rich in complex carbohydrates; 3–6 months) found significantly lower body weight and BMI with almond consumption compared to control diets [112, 113].

Walnuts

Walnuts have similar types and numbers of weight loss studies as almonds and show that adding walnuts to the habitual diet does not significantly cause weight gain. A crossover RCT (90 subjects; mean age 54 years; mean BMI 26; habitual diet plus added walnuts to 12% of energy or 28–56 g, or no added walnuts; 6 months) demonstrated that the walnut group consumed a net mean increase of 133 kcals/day compared to the control group, resulting in an insignificant weight gain of 0.4 kg vs. the 3.1 kg theoretically calculated weight gain that had been projected for that time period and intake level [114]. Another crossover RCT (46 subjects; mean age 57 years; mean BMI 33; 28 women and 18 men; 56 g

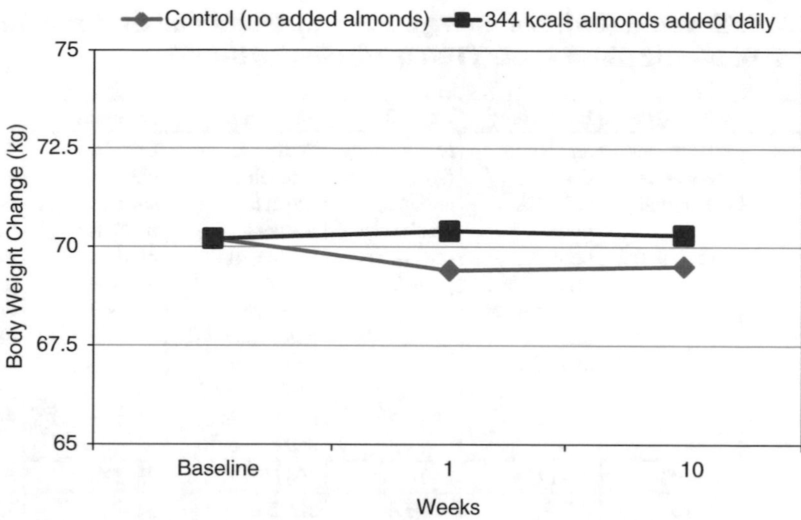

Fig. 8.11 Effect of adding two servings (344 kcals) of almonds to the habitual diet of 24 women on change in body weight over 10 weeks ($p > 0.05$) (adapted from [109])

walnuts or 350 kcals/day added to the habitual diet vs. no walnuts added to the habitual diets; 8 weeks) found that the walnut free diet resulted in small but significant mean reductions in BMI by 0.4 units and body weight by 1 kg compared to the walnut added diet. The BMI and weight increases in the walnut group were much less than expected based on the added energy intake [115]. A weight loss RCT (245 women; mean age 50 years; mean BMI 33; 42 g walnuts added; 6 months) found that women consuming walnuts (35% energy from fat), lower fat (20% energy) and low carbohydrate (45% energy from fat) weight loss diets had similar weight loss by approx 6 kg and reduction in BMI by 3 units ($p < 0.05$) but the walnut diet resulted in the most favorable changes in blood lipids [116].

Conclusions

The worldwide overweight and obesity pandemic is among the greatest public health challenges of our time with over two billion people overweight or obese globally now. Foods commonly associated with weight gain are the high intake of French fries, sugar-sweetened beverages, and red and processed meats, and the foods that tend to be inversely associated with weight gain are non-starchy vegetables, high fiber and flavonoid rich fruits, whole grains, nuts, and plain yogurt. Healthy lower energy dense dietary patterns rich in whole or minimally processed plant foods (whole plant foods) tend to be associated with a lower risk of weight gain and obesity compared to the more common Western diets high in processed foods. Prospective cohort studies show >3 daily whole-grain servings (especially with total cereal fiber at approximately10 g/day), can reduce body weight and waist size compared to < one half serving/day. RCTs indicate that whole-grains are more effective in reducing body fat and waist size than body weight or BMI. For fruits and vegetables, cohort studies find an association with a lower risk of weight, waist size or body fat gain and obesity, especially for healthier varieties. However, higher energy dense, lower fiber fruits and vegetables may promote weight gain. RCTs indicate that lower energy dense, higher fiber and flavonoid rich fruits and vegetables can support lower risk of weight gain or modest weight loss and promote additional weight loss in a hypocaloric diet or help to support weight maintenance after weight loss. RCTs show that the daily consumption of dietary pluses and nuts do not promote weight gain, and may support modest weight loss. Nuts consumed as a snack or legumes as a meal protein source in weight loss diets do not appear to interfere with weight loss or weight maintenance after weight loss.

Appendix A: Estimated range of energy, fiber, nutrients and phytochemicals composition of whole plant foods/100 g edible portion[a, b]

Components	Whole-grains	Fresh fruit	Dried fruit	Vegetables	Legumes	Nuts/seeds
Nutrients/ phytochemicals	Wheat, oats, brown rice, whole grain bread, cereal, pasta, rolls, and crackers	Apples, pears, bananas, grapes, oranges, blueberries, strawberries, and avocados	Dates, dried figs, apricots, cranberries, raisins, and prunes	Potatoes, spinach, carrots, peppers, lettuce, green beans, cabbage, onions, cucumber, cauliflower, mushrooms, and broccoli	Lentils, chickpeas, split peas, black beans, pinto beans, and soy beans	Almonds, Brazil nuts, cashews, hazelnuts, macadamias, pecans, walnuts, peanuts, sunflower seeds, and flaxseed
Energy (kcals)	110–350	30–170	240–310	10–115	85–170	520–700
Protein (g)	2.5–16	0.5–2.0	0.1–3.4	0.2–5.0	5.0–17	7.8–24
Available Carbohydrate (g)	23–77	1.0–25	64–82	0.2–25	10–27	12–33
Fiber (g)	3.5–18	2.0–7.0	5.7–10	1.2–9.5	5.0–11	3.0–27
Total fat (g)	0.9–6.5	0.0–15	0.4–1.4	0.2–1.5	0.2–9.0	46–76
SFA[a] (g)	0.2–1.0	0.0–2.1	0.0	0.0–0.1	0.1–1.3	4.0–12
MUFA[a] (g)	0.2–2.0	0.0–9.8	0.0–0.2	0.1–1.0	0.1–2.0	9.0–60
PUFA[a] (g)	0.3–2.5	0.0–1.8	0.0–0.7	0.0.0.4	0.1–5.0	1.5–47
Folate (ug)	4.0–44	<5.0–61	2–20	8.0–160	50–210	10–230
Tocopherols (mg)	0.1–3.0	0.1–1.0	0.1–4.5	0.0–1.7	0.0–1.0	1.0–35
Potassium (mg)	40–720	60–500	40–1160	100–680	200–520	360–1050
Calcium (mg)	7.0–50	3.0–25	10–160	5.0–200	20–100	20–265
Magnesium (mg)	40–160	3.0–30	5.0–70	3.0–80	40–90	120–400
Phytosterols (mg)	30–90	1.0–83	–	1.0–54	110–120	70–215
Polyphenols (mg)	70–100	50–800	–	24–1250	120–6500	130–1820
Carotenoids (ug)	–	25–6600	0.6–2160	10–20,000	50–600	0.0–1200

Ros E, Hu FB. Consumption of plant seeds and cardiovascular health epidemiological and clinical trial evidence. Circulation. 2013;128:553–65

USDA. What We Eat in America, NHANES 2011–2012, individuals 2 years and over (excluding breast-fed children). Available: www.ars.usda.gov/nea/bhnrc/fsrg

Rodriguez-Casado A. The health potential of fruits and vegetables phytochemicals: notable examples. Crit Rev Food Sci Nutr. 2016;56(7):1097–107

Rebello CJ, Greenway FL, Finley JW. A review of the nutritional value of legumes and their effects on obesity and its related co-morbidities. Obes Rev. 2014;15:392–407

Gebhardt SE, Thomas RG. Nutritive Value of Foods. 2002; U.S. Department of Agriculture, Agricultural Research Service, Home and Garden Bulletin 72

Holden JM, Eldridge AL, Beecher GR, et al. Carotenoid content of U.S. foods: an update of the database. J Food Comp An. 1999;12:169–96

Lu Q-Y, Zhang Y, Wang Y, et al. California Hass avocado: profiling of carotenoids, tocopherol, fatty acid, and fat content during maturation and from different growing areas. J Agric Food Chem. 2009;57(21):10408–13

Wu X, Beecher GR, Holden JM, et al. Lipophilic and hydrophilic antioxidant capacities of common foods in the United States. J Agric Food Chem. 2004;52:4026–37

[a]SFA (saturated fat), MUFA (monounsaturated fat) and PUFA (polyunsaturated fat)

[b]U.S. Department of Agriculture, Agriculture Research Service, Nutrient Data Laboratory. 2014. USDA National Nutrient Database for Standard Reference, Release 27. http://www.ars.usda.gov/nutrientdata. Accessed 17 Feb 2015

References

1. Haslam D. Weight management in obesity—past and present. Int J Clin Pract. 2016;70(3):206–17.
2. World Health Organization. Obesity and overweight. Geneva (Switzerland). 2014. http://who.int/mediacentre/factsheets/fs311en/. Accessed 18 Jan 2015.
3. Trust for America's Health and the Robert Wood Johnson Foundation. F as in fat: how obesity threatens America's future. 2012. http://healthyamericans.org/assets/files/TFAH2012FasInFat18.pdf. Accessed 27 Feb 2015.
4. Swinburn BA, Sacks G, Hall KD, et al. The global obesity pandemic: shaped by global drivers and local environments. Lancet. 2011;378:804–14.
5. de Mutsert R, Sun Q, Willett WC, et al. Overweight in early adulthood, adult weight change, and risk of type 2 diabetes, cardiovascular diseases, and certain cancers in men: a cohort study. Am J Epidemiol. 2014;179:1353–65.
6. Stevens J, Erber E, Truesdale KP, et al. Long- and short-term weight change and incident coronary heart disease and ischemic stroke: the Atherosclerosis Risk in Communities Study. Am J Epidemiol. 2013;178:239–48.
7. Faris MAE, Attlee A. Obesity and cancer: what's the interconnection? Adv Obes Weight Manag Control. 2015;2(4):1–6.
8. Ogden CL, Carroll MD, Kit BK, et al. Prevalence of childhood and adult obesity in the United States, 2011–2012. JAMA. 2014;311:806–14.
9. Rinella ME. Nonalcoholic fatty liver disease. A systematic review. JAMA. 2015;313(22):2263–73.
10. Flegal KM, Graubard BI, William DF, et al. Excess deaths associated with underweight, overweight and obesity. JAMA. 2005;293:1861–7.
11. Allison DB, Fontaine KR, Manson JE, et al. Annual deaths attributable to obesity in the United States. JAMA. 1999;282:1530–8.
12. Hill JO. Can a small-changes approach help address the obesity epidemic? A report of the Joint Task Force of the American Society for Nutrition, Institute of Food Technologists, and International Food Information Council. Am J Clin Nutr. 2009;89:477–84.
13. Williamson DF, Kahn HS, Remington PL, et al. The 10-year incidence of overweight and major weight gain in US adults. Arch Intern Med. 1990;150:665–72.
14. Mozaffarian D, Hao T, Rimm EB, et al. Changes in diet and lifestyle and long-term weight gain in women and men. N Engl J Med. 2011;363:2392–404.
15. Peeters A, Magliano DJ, Backholer K, et al. Changes in the rates of weight and waist circumference gain in Australian adults over time: a longitudinal cohort study. BMJ Open. 2014;4(1):e003667. https://doi.org/10.1136/bmjopen-2013-003667.
16. Heitmann BI, Garby L. Patterns of long-term weight changes in overweight developing Danish men and women aged between 30 and 60 years. Int J Obes Relat Metab Disord. 1999;23:1074–8.
17. Zhai F, Wang H, Wang Z, et al. Closing the energy gap to prevent weight gain in China. Obes Rev. 2008;9(Suppl 1):107–12.
18. Davis JN, Hodges VA, Gillham MB. Normal-weight adults consume more fiber and fruit than their age and height matched overweight/obese counterparts. J Am Diet Assoc. 2006;106:835–40.
19. Centers for Disease Control and Prevention. Low energy dense foods and weight management: cutting calories while controlling hunger. Research to Practice Series, No 5. http://www.cdc.gov/nccdphp/dnpa/nutrition/pdf/r2p_energy_density.pdf. Accessed 21 Feb 2015.
20. Rolls BJ. What is the role of portion in weight management? Int J Obes. 2014;38:S1–8.
21. Vernarelli JA, Mitchell DC, Rolls BJ, Hartman TJ. Dietary energy density is associated with obesity and other biomarkers of chronic disease in US adults. Eur J Nutr. 2015;54(1):59–65.
22. Karl JP, Roberts SB. Energy density, energy intake and body weight regulations in adults. Adv Nutr. 2014;5:835–50.
23. Ambrosini GL. Childhood dietary patterns and later obesity: a review of the evidence. Proc Nutr Soc. 2014;73:137–46.
24. Wing RR, Phelan S. Long-term weight loss maintenance. Am J Clin Nutr. 2005;82(Suppl):222S–5S.
25. Mariman ECM. An adipobiological model for weight regain after weight loss. Adipobiology. 2011;3:7–13.
26. MacLean PS, Higgins JA, Giles ED, et al. The role for adipose tissue in weight regain after weight loss. Obes Rev. 2015;16(Suppl. 1):45–54.
27. Bell ES, Roll BJ. Energy density of foods affects energy intakes across multiple levels of fat content in lean and obese women. Am J Clin Nutr. 2001;73:1010–8.
28. Raynor HA, Van Walleghen EL, Bachman JL, et al. Dietary energy and successful weight loss maintenance. Eat Behav. 2011;12(2):119–25.
29. Davey GK, Spencer EA, Appleby PN, et al. EPIC–Oxford: lifestyle characteristics and nutrient intakes in a cohort of 33,883 meat-eaters and 31,546 non meat-eaters in the UK. Public Health Nutr. 2003;6:259–68.
30. Rolls BJ, Drewnowski A, Ledikwe JH. Changing the energy density of the diet as a strategy for weight management. J Am Diet Assoc. 2005;5(Suppl 1):S98–S103.
31. Ledikwe JH, Blanck HM, Khan LK, et al. Dietary energy density is associated with energy intake and weight status in US adults. Am J Clin Nutr. 2006;83:1362–8.
32. Mozaffarian D, Hao T, Rimm EB, et al. Changes in diet and lifestyle and long-term weight gain in women and men. Engl J Med. 2011;364(25):2392–404.
33. Tuso PJ, Ismail MH, Ha BP, Bartolotto C. Nutritional update for physicians: plant-based diets. Perm J. 2013;17(2):61–6.
34. Wright N, Wilson L, Smith M, et al. The BROAD study: a randomised controlled trial using a whole plant-based diet in the community for obesity, ischemic heart disease or diabetes. Nutr Diabetes. 2017;7:e256.

35. Sutliffe JT, Fuhrman J, Carnot MJ, et al. Nutrient-dense, plant-rich dietary intervention effective at reducing cardiovascular risk factors for worksites: a pilot study. Altern Ther Health Med. 2016;2295:24–9.
36. Allman-Farinelli M, Partridge SR, McGeechan K, et al. A mobile health lifestyle program for prevention of weight gain in young adults (TxT2Bfit): nine-month outcomes of a randomized control trial. JMIR Mhealth Uhealth. 2016;4(2):e78.
37. Turner-McGrievy G, Mandes T, Crimarco A. A plant-based diet for overweight and obesity prevention and treatment. J Geriatr Cardiol. 2017;14:369–74.
38. Rebello CJ, Greenway FL, Finley JW. A review of the nutritional value of legumes and their effects on obesity and its related co-morbidities. Obes Rev. 2014;15:392–407.
39. Hever J, Cronise RJ. Plant-based nutrition for healthcare professionals: implementing diets as a primary modality in the prevention and treatment of chronic disease. J Geriatr Cardiol. 2017;14:355–68.
40. McMacken M, Shah S. A plant-based diet for the prevention and treatment of type 2 diabetes. J Geriatr Cardiol. 2017;14:342–54.
41. de Freitas Junior LM, de Almeida Jr EB. Medicinal plants for the treatment of obesity: ethnopharmacological approach and chemical and biological studies. Am J Transl Res. 2017;9(5):2050–64.
42. Poulsen SK, Due A, Jordy AB, et al. Health effects of the New Nordic diet in adults with increased waist circumference: a 6-mo randomized controlled trial. Am J Clin Nutr. 2014;99:35–45.
43. Cavallo DN, Horino M, McCarthy WJ. Adult intake of minimally processed fruits and vegetables: associations with cardiometabolic disease risk factors. J Acad Nutr Diet. 2016;116(9):1387–94. https://doi.org/10.1016/j.jand.2016.03.019.
44. Dietary Guidelines Advisory Committee. Scientific report. Advisory report to the Secretary of Health and Human Services and the Secretary of Agriculture. Part D. Chapter 1: Food and nutrient intakes, and health: current status and trends. 2015; p. 1–78.
45. Slavin J. Why whole grains are protective: biological mechanisms. Proc Nutr Soc. 2003;62:129–34.
46. Seal CJ, Brownlee IA. Whole-grain foods and chronic disease: evidence from epidemiological and intervention studies. Proc Nutr Soc. 2015;74:313–9.
47. http://wholegrainscouncil.org/whole-grains-101/What-counts-as-a-serving. Accessed 26 Dec 2015.
48. Karl JP, Saltzman E. The role of whole grains in body weight regulation. Adv Nutr. 2012;3:697–707.
49. http://health.gov/dietary guidelines/2015/guidelines/. Accessed 26 Jan 2016.
50. McGill CR, Fulgoni VL III, Devareddy L. Ten-year trends in fiber and whole grain intakes and food sources for the United States population: National Health and Nutrition Examination Survey 2001–2010. Forum Nutr. 2015;7:1119–30.
51. Giacco R, Pella-Pepo G, Luongo D, et al. Whole grain intake in relation to body weight: from epidemiological evidence to clinical trials. Nutr Metab Cardiovasc Dis. 2011;21:901–8.
52. Harland JI, Garton LE. Whole-grain intake as a marker of healthy body weight and adiposity. Public Health Nutr. 2008;11:554–63.
53. Du H, van der AD, Boshuizen HC, et al. Dietary fiber and subsequent changes in body weight and waist circumference in European men and women. Am J Clin Nutr. 2010;91:329–36.
54. Bazzano LA, Song Y, Bubes V, et al. Dietary intake of whole and refined grain breakfast cereals and weight gain in men. Obes Res. 2005;13:1952–60.
55. Koh-Banerjee P, Franz M, Sampson L, et al. Changes in whole-grain, bran, and cereal fiber consumption in relation to 8-y weight gain among men. Am J Clin Nutr. 2004;80:1237–45.
56. Liu S, Willett WC, Manson JE, et al. Relation between changes in intakes of dietary fiber and grain products and changes in weight and development of obesity among middle-aged women. Am J Clin Nutr. 2003;78:920–7.
57. Steffen LM, Jacobs DR Jr, Murtaugh MA, et al. Whole grain intake is associated with lower body mass and greater insulin sensitivity among adolescents. Am J Epidemiol. 2003;158:243–50.
58. Pol K, Christensen R, Bartels EM, et al. Whole grain and body weight changes in apparently healthy adults: a systematic review and meta-analysis of randomized controlled studies. Am J Clin Nutr. 2013;98:872–84.
59. Ampatzoglou A, Atwal KK, Maidens CM, et al. Increased whole grain consumption does not affect blood biochemistry, body composition, or gut microbiology in healthy, low-habitual whole grain consumers. J Nutr. 2015;145:215–21.
60. Shimabukuro M, Higa M, Kinjo R, et al. Effects of the brown rice diet on visceral obesity and endothelial function: the BRAVO study. Br J Nutr. 2014;111:310–20.
61. Brownlee IA, Moore C, Chatfield M, et al. Markers of cardiovascular risk are not changed by increased whole-grain intake: The WHOLEheart Study, a randomised, controlled dietary intervention. Br J Nutr. 2010;104:125–34.
62. Harris Jackson K, West SG, Heuvel JPV, et al. Effects of whole and refined grains in a weight-loss diet on markers of metabolic syndrome in individuals with increased waist circumference: a randomized controlled-feeding trial. Am J Clin Nutr. 2014;100:577–86.
63. Kristensen M, Toubro S, Jensen MG, et al. Whole grain compared with refined wheat decreases the percentage of body fat following a 12-week, energy-restricted dietary intervention in postmenopausal women. J Nutr. 2012;142:710–6.
64. Maki KC, Beiseigel JM, Jonnalagadda SS, et al. Whole-grain ready-to-eat oat cereal, as part of a

dietary program for weight loss, reduces low-density lipoprotein cholesterol in adults with overweight and obesity more than a dietary program including low-fiber control foods. J Am Diet Assoc. 2010;110:205–14.
65. Katcher HI, Legro RS, Kunselman AR, et al. The effects of a whole grain–enriched hypocaloric diet on cardiovascular disease risk factors in men and women with metabolic syndrome. Am J Clin Nutr. 2008;87:79–90.
66. Kim JY, Kim JH, Lee DH, et al. Meal replacement with mixed rice is more effective than white rice in weight control, while improving antioxidant enzyme activity in obese women. Nutr Res. 2008;28:66–71.
67. Melanson KJ, Angelopoulos TJ, Nguyen VT, et al. Consumption of whole-grain cereals during weight loss: effects on dietary quality, dietary fiber, magnesium, vitamin B-6, and obesity. J Am Diet Assoc. 2006;106:1380–8.
68. Saltzman E, Moriguti JC, Das SK, et al. Effects of a cereal rich in soluble fiber on body composition and dietary compliance during consumption of a hypocaloric diet. J Am Coll Nutr. 2001;20:50–7.
69. Slavin JL, Lloyd B. Health benefits of fruits and vegetables. Adv Nutr. 2012;3:506–16.
70. United States Department of Agriculture. 2013. Choose my plate. http://www.choosemyplate.gov/. Accessed 17 Feb 2015.
71. Boeing H, Bechthold A, Bub A, et al. Critical review: vegetables and fruit in the prevention of chronic diseases. Eur J Nutr. 2012;51:637–63.
72. WHO/FAO. Diet, nutrition and prevention of chronic disease: report of a Joint WHO/FAO Expert Consultation. Geneva, Switzerland: World Health Organization. 2003/2004. http://whqlibdoc.who.int/trs/WHO_TRS_916.pdf. Accessed 17 Feb 2015.
73. World Health Association. Global strategy on diet, physical activity and health—promoting fruit and vegetable consumption around the world. 2013. http://who.int/dietphysicalactivity/fruit/en/. Accessed 17 Feb 2015.
74. Micha R, Khatibzadeh S, Shi P, et al. Global, regional and national consumption of major food groups in 1990 and 2010: a systematic analysis including 266 country-specific nutrition surveys worldwide. BMJ Open. 2015;5(9):e008705. https://doi.org/10.1136/bmjopen-2015-008705.
75. Bertoia ML, Rimm EB, Mukamal KJ, et al. Dietary flavonoid intake and weight maintenance: three prospective cohorts of 124,086 US men and women followed for up to 24 years. BMJ. 2016;352:i17. https://doi.org/10.1136/bmj.i17.
76. Borch D, Juul-Hindsgaul N, Veller M, et al. Potatoes and risk of obesity, type 2 diabetes, and cardiovascular disease in apparently healthy adults: a systematic review of clinical intervention and observational studies. Am J Clin Nutr. 2016;104:489–98. https://doi.org/10.3945/ajcn.116.132332.
77. Schwingshackl L, Hoffmann G, Kalle-Uhlmann T, et al. Fruit and vegetable consumption and changes in anthropometric variables in adult populations: a systematic review and meta-analysis of prospective cohort studies. PLoS One. 2015;10(10):e0140846. https://doi.org/10.1371/journal.pone.0140846.
78. Kaiser KA, Brown AW, Bohan Brown MM, et al. Increased fruit and vegetable intake has no discernible effect on weight loss: a systematic review and meta-analysis. Am J Clin Nutr. 2014;100(2):567–76.
79. Mytton OT, Nnoaham K, Eyles H, et al. Systematic review and meta-analysis of the effect of increased vegetable and fruit consumption on body weight and energy intake. BMC Public Health. 2014;14:886. https://doi.org/10.1186/1471-2458-14-886.
80. Ledoux TA, Hingle MD, Baranowski T. Relationship of fruit and vegetable intake with adiposity: a systematic review. Obes Rev. 2011;12:e143–50.
81. Shefferly A, Scharf RJ, DeBoer MD. Longitudinal evaluation of 100% juice consumption on BMI status in 2–5-year-old children. Pediatr Obes. 2016;11(3):221–7.
82. Bertoia ML, Mukamal KJ, Cahill LE, et al. Changes in intake of fruits and vegetables and weight change in United States men and women followed for up to 24 years: analysis from three prospective cohort studies. PLoS Med. 2015;12(9):e1001878. https://doi.org/10.1371/journal.pmed.1001878.
83. Rautiainen S, Wang L, Lee IM, et al. Higher intake of fruit, but not vegetables or fiber, at baseline is associated with lower risk of becoming overweight or obese in middle-aged and older women of normal BMI at baseline. J Nutr. 2015;145(5):960–8. https://doi.org/10.3945/jn.114.199158.
84. Vergnaud A-C, Norat T, Romaguera D, et al. Fruit and vegetable consumption and prospective weight change in participants of the European Prospective Investigation into Cancer and Nutrition–Physical Activity, Nutrition, Alcohol, Cessation of Smoking, Eating Out of Home, and Obesity study. Am J Clin Nutr. 2012;95:184–93.
85. Tapsell LC, Batterham RL, Thorne RL, et al. Weight loss effects from vegetable intake: a 12-month randomised controlled trial. Eur J Clin Nutr. 2014;68:778–85.
86. Christensen AS, Viggers L, Hasselström K, Gregersen S. Effect of fruit restriction on glycemic control in patients with type 2 diabetes-a randomized trial. Nutr J. 2013;12:29. https://doi.org/10.1186/1475-2891-12-29.
87. Dow CA, Going SB, Chow H-H, et al. The effects of daily consumption of grapefruit on body weight, lipids, and blood pressure in healthy, overweight adults. Metabolism. 2012;61:1026–35.
88. Peterson JM, Montgomery S, Haddad E, et al. Effect of consumption of dried California mission figs on lipid concentrations. Ann Nutr Metab. 2011;58:232–8.
89. Basu A, Du M, Leyva MJ, et al. Blueberries decrease cardiovascular risk factors in obese men and women with metabolic syndrome. J Nutr. 2010;140:1582–7.

90. Whybrow S, Harrison CLS, Mayer C, Stubbs RJ. Effects of added fruits and vegetables on dietary intakes and body weight in Scottish adults. Br J Nutr. 2007;95:496–503.
91. de Oliveira MC, Sichieri R, Moura AS. Weight loss associated with a daily intake of three apples or three pears among overweight women. Nutrition. 2003;19:253–6.
92. Westerterp-Plantenga MS, Lemmens SG, Westerterp KR. Dietary protein-its role in satiety, energetics, weight loss and health. Br J Nutr. 2012;108(Suppl 2):S105–12.
93. Smith JD, Hou T, Ludwig DS, et al. Changes in intake of protein foods, carbohydrate amount and quality, and long-term weight change: results from 3 prospective cohorts. Am J Clin Nutr. 2015;101:1216–24.
94. McCrory MA, Hamaker BR, Lovejoy JC, Eichelsdoerfer PE. Pulse consumption, satiety, and weight management. Adv Nutr. 2010;1:17–30.
95. Papanikolaou Y, Fulgoni VL III. Bean consumption is associated with greater nutrient intake, reduced systolic blood pressure, lower body weight, and a smaller waist circumference in adults: results from the National Health and Nutrition Examination Survey 1999–2002. J Am Coll Nutr. 2008;27:569–76.
96. Messina V. Nutritional and health benefits of dried beans. Am J Clin Nutr. 2014;100(suppl):437S–42S.
97. Kim SJ, de Souza RJ, Choo VL, et al. Effects of dietary pulse consumption on body weight: a systematic review and meta-analysis of randomized controlled trials. Am J Clin Nutr. 2016;103:1213–23.
98. Mattes RD, Kris-Etherton PM, Foster GD. Impact of peanuts and tree nuts on body weight and healthy weight loss in adults. J Nutr. 2008;138(suppl):1741S–5S.
99. Alper CM, Mattes RD. The effects of chronic peanut consumption on energy balance and hedonics. Int J Obes. 2002;26:1129–37.
100. Novotny JA, Gebauer SK, Baer DJ. Discrepancy between the Atwater factor predicted and empirically measured energy values of almonds in human diets. Am J Clin Nutr. 2012;96:296–301.
101. Tan SY, Dhillon J, Mattes RD. Review of the effects of nuts on appetite, food intake, metabolism, and body weight. Am J Clin Nutr. 2014;100(suppl):412S–22S.
102. Jackson CL, Hu FB. Long-term associations of nut consumption with body weight and obesity. Am J Clin Nutr. 2014;100(suppl):408S–11S.
103. Mattes RD, Dreher ML. Nuts and healthy body weight maintenance mechanisms. Asia Pac J Clin Nutr. 2010;19(1):137–41.
104. Bes-Rastrollo M, Sabate J, Gomez-Gracia E, et al. Nut consumption and weight gain in a Mediterranean cohort: the SUN Study. Obesity (Silver Spring). 2007;15:107–16.
105. Bes-Rastrollo M, Wedick NM, Martinez-Gonzalez MA, et al. Prospective study of nut consumption, long-term weight change, and obesity risk in women. Am J Clin Nutr. 2009;89:1913–9.
106. Freisling H, Noh H, Slimani N, V. Nut intake and 5-year changes in body weight and obesity risk in adults: results from the EPIC-PANACEA study. Eur J Nutr. 2017; doi:10.1007/s0094-017-1513-0.
107. Flores-Mateo G, Rojas-Rueda D, Basora J, et al. Nut intake and adiposity: meta-analysis of clinical trials. Am J Clin Nutr. 2013;97:1346–55.
108. Fraser GE, Bennett HW, Jaceldo KB, Sabate J. Effect on body weight of a free 76 kilojoules (320 calorie) daily supplement of almonds for six months. J Am Coll Nutr. 2002;21(3):275–83.
109. Hollis J, Mattes R. Effect of chronic consumption of almonds on body weight in healthy humans. Br J Nutr. 2007;98:651–56.
110. Tan SY, Matter RD. Appetitive, dietary and health effects of almonds consumed with meals or as snacks: a randomized, controlled trial. Eur J Clin Nutr. 2013;67:1205–14.
111. Foster GD, Shantz KL, Veur SSV, et al. A randomized trial of the effects of an almond-enriched, hypocaloric diet in the treatment of obesity. Am J Clin Nutr. 2012;96:249–54.
112. Abazarfard Z, Salehi M, Keshavarzi S. The effect of almonds on anthropometric measurements and lipid profile in overweight and obese females in a weight reduction program. A randomized controlled clinical trial. J Res Med Sci. 2014;19(5):457–64.
113. Wien MA, Sabate JM, Ikle DN, et al, Almonds vs complex carbohydrates in a weight reduction program. Int J Obesity. 2003;27:1365–72.
114. Abazarfard Z, Eslamian G, Salehi M, Keshavarzi S. A randomized controlled trial of the effects of an almond-enriched, hypocaloric diet on liver function tests in overweight/obese women. Iran Red Crescent Med J. 2016;18(3):e23628.
115. Sabate J, MacIntyre C, Siapco G, et al. Does regular walnut consumption lead to weight gain? Br J Nutr. 2005;94:859–64.
116 Katz DL, Davidhi A, Ma Y, et al. Effects of walnuts on endothelial function in overweight adults with visceral obesity: a randomized, controlled, crossover trial. J Am Coll Nutr. 2012;31(6):415–23.

9 Dietary Patterns and Whole Plant Foods in Type 2 Diabetes Prevention and Management

Keywords
Type 2 diabetes • Dietary quality • Prediabetes • Dietary patterns Mediterranean diet • DASH diet • Vegan diet • Vegetarian diet • Nordic food index • Western diet • Whole-grains • Fruits • Vegetables • Legumes Nuts

Key Points

- A healthy lifestyle including habitual intake of a high quality dietary pattern, regular physical activity, and weight control are key components of type 2 diabetes (diabetes) prevention and management.
- Prospective cohort studies show that high quality dietary patterns including the Alternative Healthy Eating Index score have a significant inverse association with diabetes risk, and Western dietary patterns have a positive association with risk.
- Higher adherence to the Mediterranean diet (MedDiet) is associated with a 19–23% reduced risk of developing diabetes, while the results of randomized controlled trials (RCTs) show that the MedDiet can reduce risk of diabetes by 30% and can reduce glycosylated hemoglobin (HbA1c) levels by 0.30–0.47% in people with diabetes. Other healthy dietary patterns which are effective in reducing diabetes risk and in management of diabetics' health are the Dietary Approaches to Stop Hypertension (DASH), vegan and the healthy Nordic food index diets.
- Prospective cohort studies show that whole (minimally processed) plant foods including whole-grains, fruits, vegetables, dietary pulses, and nuts and flaxseed are significantly associated with lower risk of diabetes. For whole grains, 3 servings/day reduced diabetes risk by 23% and of the whole-grains oats and oat bran are the most effective in managing glycemic control in people with diabetes. For fruits and vegetables, higher intake of fruits, especially berries, and green leafy vegetables, yellow vegetables, non-starchy root and cruciferous vegetables are particularly effective in lowering diabetes risk. Three weekly servings of French fries significantly increase diabetes risk by 41% compared to only 5% for other forms of potatoes (baked, boiled or mashed). Higher intake of sugar sweetened fruit juice is significantly associated with increased diabetes risk by 28%, while higher intake of 100%

M.L. Dreher, *Dietary Patterns and Whole Plant Foods in Aging and Disease*, Nutrition and Health,
https://doi.org/10.1007/978-3-319-59180-3_9

fruit juice is not associated with diabetes risk. Higher intake of dietary pulses, peanuts, tree nuts and flaxseed are also associated with lower diabetes risk.
- Healthy dietary patterns and specific whole foods beneficially affect glycemic and cardiometabolic risk factors, which are important for preventing and managing diabetes, by helping to control body weight, visceral fat, glucose-insulin homeostasis, oxidative stress, inflammation, and endothelial health, lipoprotein concentrations, and blood pressure.

9.1 Introduction

Type 2 diabetes (diabetes) is a rapidly increasing major chronic disease (characterized by insulin dysfunction in production and utilization) and is a leading cause of premature disability and death with a global impact [1]. The prevalence of prediabetes and diabetes has increased globally in parallel with the rising levels of obesity in adults and children, a phenomenon sometimes called diabesity [1–5]. Diabesity is on track to be the largest epidemic in human history [2]. As of 2017, there are > 415 million people in the world with diabetes, which is more than the population of the USA [2]. If this global trend continues, by 2030 about one billion people are expected to be prediabetic and diabetic. Improperly managed, diabetes leads to a number of health issues, including heart diseases, stroke, blindness, nerve damage, leg and foot amputations, and death [1–5]. Adults (> 35 years of age) with newly diagnosed diabetes have a 38% higher risk of all-cause mortality compared to people without diabetes [3]. Adult-onset diabetes usually begins when a person is in his or her mid-50s, but 90% of diabetes risk can be reduced by following a healthy lifestyle, especially with healthy diets and adequate physical activity [1, 4–8]. In the US and also other Western populations it is estimated that <10% of the populations follow a diabetes preventive lifestyle [3–5, 9]. Dietary patterns, especially are a major influence on diabetes and related cardiometabolic premature mortality risk, conditions which collectively substantially increase health and economic burdens [7–10]. A 2017 meta-analysis (48 cohort studies) found that high adherence to Western dietary patterns (characterized by red and processed meats, refined grains, fried foods, high fat dairy and eggs) increased diabetes risk by 44% whereas healthy diets (characterized by fruits, vegetables, legumes, poultry and fish) reduced diabetes risk by 16% [7]. In the USA population, a nationally representative comparative risk assessment model estimated that 45% of all cardiometabolic deaths (due to heart disease, stroke, and diabetes) were associated with low intakes of fruits, vegetables, nuts and seeds, whole grains, healthy vegetable oils and seafood and excessive intake of sodium, red and processed meats and sugar sweetened beverages [10]. In USA population subgroups, suboptimal (unhealthy) diets are associated with higher mortality rates in men than in women, at younger vs older ages, among blacks and Hispanics vs whites, and among individuals with low and medium education vs higher education. Unhealthy diets and inactivity associated with increased diabetes risk may cause epigenetic changes that could lead to perpetuation of intergenerational increases in obesity and diabetes risk [2]. The objective of this chapter is to review the effects of dietary patterns and healthy whole and minimally processed plant foods (whole plant foods) in diabetes prevention and management.

9.2 Dietary Patterns

9.2.1 Overview

A lifestyle that includes a healthy dietary pattern, regular physical activity, and weight control are key components of diabetes prevention and management (along with appropriate use of pharmacotherapy) while the Western lifestyle is associated with a substantial increase in diabetes risk, especially in individuals with a high genetic predisposition [1–4, 11, 12]. Although dietary pattern varies across different populations, general guidance to increase whole plant foods (e.g., whole-grains, fruit, vegetables, legumes, nuts and seeds) and to reduce intake of refined carbohydrates, meat, processed meat, and fried foods may help reduce the growing global public health burden of diabetes. The Alternate Healthy Eating Index (AHEI), which is a measure of adherence to dietary guidelines (higher intake of vegetables, fruits, nuts and legumes, long-chain fats, and whole grains; lower intake of sugar sweetened beverages, red and processed meat, trans fat, and sodium; and moderate alcohol consumption) is strongly associated with a lower diabetes risk [13]. A review of the findings from the Nurses' Health Study on diet and diabetes is summarized in Table 9.1 [13]. For diabetes management, there are a wide range of approaches for meal planning and dietary patterns that have been shown to be clinically effective, with many including a reduced energy intake or controlling available carbohydrate intake [12]. One diet or a person with diabetes should work with their health care team on eating patterns, preferences, and metabolic goals. Multiple meal planning approaches and eating patterns can be effective for achieving metabolic goals; including carbohydrate counting, The MyPlate Method, individualized meal plans based on percentages of macronutrients, exchange lists for meal planning, glycemic index or load, and common healthy dietary patterns including the Mediterranean diet (MedDiet), Dietary Approaches to Stop Hypertension (DASH), vegetarian, vegan, low carbohydrate, and low fat diets [4, 12–14]. A summary of common healthy dietary patterns is provided in Appendix A.

Table 9.1 Summary of the findings from the Nurses' Health Studies related to diet and type 2 diabetes risk [13]

Increase type 2 diabetes risk	Decrease type 2 diabetes risk
Diets low in fiber, especially cereal fiber, and with a high glycemic index or load	Diets rich in fiber, especially from cereal products, and with a low glycemic index or load
Diets rich in animal fats	Diets rich in healthy vegetable oils
High intake of refined grains	Higher intake of whole grains; 50 g per day of cooked brown rice instead of the same amount of white rice, was associated with a 16% lower diabetes risk
High intake of french fries	Greater intake of green leafy vegetables and specific whole fruits rich in flavonoids, such as blueberries, grapes, apples, and pears
High alcohol intake	Moderate alcohol consumption Higher intake of plain yogurt Regular coffee consumption

9.2.2 Diet Nutrient Quality and Diabetes Risk

Table 9.2 summarizes systematic review and meta-analyses, individual cohort studies, and a randomized controlled trial (RCT) on diet quality related to adherence to a healthy or Western dietary pattern and diabetes risk [15–31].

9.2.2.1 Systematic Reviews and Pooled or Meta-Analyses

Eight systematic reviews and/or meta-or pooled analyses of prospective cohort studies show that diabetes risk has a significant inverse association with healthy dietary patterns with a diabetes risk reduction of 14–39% (high vs. low adherence) and Western patterns have a positive association with an increased risk by 31–300% (high vs. low adherence), after multivariate adjustments including BMI [15–22]. A 2017 systematic review and meta-analysis of the association between intake of 12 major foods and risk of diabetes (88 cohort studies) found that optimal daily consumption of risk-decreasing foods (whole grains, vegetables, fruits, and dairy) results in a 42% reduction in diabetes risk and high daily intake of risk-increasing foods (red and processed meats, sugar sweetened beverages and eggs) is associated with a threefold increased diabetes risk compared to non-consumption of these foods (Fig. 9.1) [15]. A 2016 pooled analysis of the Nurses' Health Studies and the Health Professionals Follow-up Study (124,607 men and women; >20 years of follow-up; 9361 diabetes cases) showed that diet quality, based on AHEI score assessed over

Table 9.2 Summary of prospective cohort studies on diet quality and type 2 diabetes (diabetes) and prediabetes risk

Objective	Study details	Results
Systematic reviews and meta-or pooled analyses		
Schwingshackl et al. (2017). Systematic review and meta-analysis of the relation between intake of 12 major food groups and risk of diabetes [15]	88 prospective cohort studies	Optimal daily consumption of risk-decreasing foods (2 servings whole grains; 2–3 servings vegetables; 2–3 servings fruits; 3 servings dairy) results in a 42% reduction in diabetes risk compared to non-consumption of these foods. High daily intake of risk-increasing foods of 2 servings red meat (170 g/day), 4 servings processed meat (105 g/day), 3 servings sugar sweetened beverages (750 mL/day), and one egg (55 g/day) is associated with a threefold increased diabetes risk compared to non-consumption
Ley et al. (2016). Evaluate diet quality changes during a 4-year period on diabetes incidence (Nurses' Health Studies and Health Professionals Follow-up Study; US) [16]	124,607 participants; >20 years of follow-up; 9361 cases of diabetes documented; diet quality, based on Alternate Healthy Eating Index (AHEI) score; assessed every 4 years	A >10% decrease in AHEI score over 4 years was associated with a significantly higher subsequent adjusted diabetes risk of 34%, whereas a >10% increase in AHEI score was associated with a lower risk by 16%. Greater improvement in diet quality was associated with lower diabetes risk across baseline diet quality status for low, medium, or high initial diet quality (p-trend ≤0.001) (Fig. 9.2). Changes in body weight explained 32% of the association between AHEI changes (per 10% increase) and diabetes risk
Satija et al. (2016). Examine the association of an overall plant-based diet and healthy vs. less healthy versions of a plant based diet with diabetes incidence in three cohort studies (Nurses' Health Studies and Health Professionals Follow-up Study; US) [17]	160,188 women and 40,539 men; dietary data collected every 2–4 years using a semi-quantitative food frequency questionnaire. follow-up of >20 years; 16,162 diabetes cases (multivariate adjusted including BMI). **Plant-based diet index**: (1) plant foods received positive scores, while animal foods (animal fats, dairy, eggs, fish/seafood, poultry/red meat, miscellaneous animal-based foods) received reverse scores **Healthful-plant based diet index**: (1) healthy plant foods (whole grains, fruits, vegetables, nuts, legumes, vegetable oils, tea/coffee) received positive scores, while less healthy plant foods (fruit juices, sweetened beverages, refined grains, potatoes, sweets/desserts) and animal foods received reverse scores	This analysis found an inverse association between an overall plant-based diet and diabetes incidence, which was stronger for a healthier version of the plant-based diet (Fig. 9.3). Overall plant based diet emphasizing plant foods and low in animal foods was associated with about 20% reduction in diabetes risk. Healthy plant-based diets had a larger decrease in diabetes risk by 34%. Less healthy plant foods were associated with a 16% increased diabetes risk
Maghsoudi et al. (2015). Systematically review prospective cohort studies for the association between dietary patterns and diabetes incidence, and quantify the effects using a meta-analysis [18]	Ten cohort studies; 404,528 participants; age range 27–84 years; 5–23 years of follow-up; 18,584 diabetes cases	Adherence to 'healthy' dietary patterns (vegetables, fruits and whole grains) significantly reduced the risk of diabetes by 14%, whereas 'unhealthy' dietary patterns (red and processed meats, high-fat dairy and refined grains) increased diabetes risk by 30%. Subgroup analysis showed that unhealthy dietary patterns in which foods with high phytochemical content were consumed attenuated diabetes risk to a 6% increase (Fig. 9.4)

Table 9.2 (continued)

Objective	Study details	Results
McEvoy et al. (2014). Examine the association between posteriori derived dietary patterns and risk of diabetes [19]	Nine cohort studies; 309,430 participants; 4–23 years of follow-up; 16,644 diabetes cases	Pooled results indicated a significant 15% lower diabetes risk for those in the highest category of healthy dietary pattern (greater fruit, vegetable, and complex carbohydrates) compared with those in the lowest category. Those in the highest category of the Western pattern (greater refined carbohydrates, processed meat, and fried foods) had a significant 41% increased risk of diabetes compared to those in the lowest category
Alhazmi et al. (2014). Examine the effect of dietary patterns and the risk of diabetes [20]	15 cohort studies; 378,525 participants; 4–23 years of follow-up; 23,372 diabetes cases	Healthy dietary patterns significantly reduced mean diabetes risk by 21% and unhealthy patterns increased mean risk by 44% (highest vs. lowest adherence)
Esposito et al. (2014). Assess the association between different diets and prevention of diabetes [21]	20 cohort studies; 446,213 participants; 3.2–23 years of follow-up; 21,372 diabetes cases	Leading healthy diets are equally and consistently associated with a 20% reduced risk of future diabetes. The diabetes risk did not differ by geography (USA, Europe, and Asia), the duration of follow-up (<10 and >10 years), and type of healthy diets (Mediterranean and DASH diets, Alternate Healthy Eating Index; dietary scores) with common components, including whole grains, fruit, vegetables, nuts, legumes, healthy table oils (i.e., extra virgin olive oil), protein sources such as white meat and seafood, little or moderate alcohol, and reduced intake of red and processed meats and sugar sweetened beverages
Esposito et al. (2010). Investigate the role of dietary patterns in preventing diabetes [22]	Ten cohort studies; 190,000 participants; 2–23 years of follow-up; 8932 diabetes cases	Healthy dietary patterns (high intake of fruit, vegetables, whole-grains, fish, poultry and low intake of red meat, processed foods, sugar-sweetened beverages, and starchy foods) were associated with a 39% reduction in diabetes risk compared to Western diets
Prospective cohort studies		
Doostvandi et al. (2016). Investigate the association of major dietary patterns with the risk of impaired glucose and insulin homeostasis during a 3-year follow-up (Iran; Tehran Lipid and Glucose Study) [23]	904 Iranian men and women; mean baseline age 39 years; 45% were men; measurements included: major dietary patterns were Western, traditional and healthy; fasting serum insulin, fasting serum glucose, 2-h serum glucose, impaired glucose tolerance and homeostasis model assessment of insulin resistance (HOMA-IR); 3 years of follow-up (multivariate adjusted)	There was a positive association between Western and traditional scores with change in 2 h-serum glucose levels, while the healthy pattern was negatively related to changes in fasting serum glucose, 2-h serum glucose, fasting serum insulin and HOMA-IR. Highest compared with the lowest tertile of the Western dietary pattern was accompanied by a higher risk for development of impaired glucose tolerance by 209%; a higher score on the healthy dietary pattern was associated with a significantly reduced risk of fasting serum insulin by 47%
Cespedes et al. (2016). Compare associations of four diet quality index scores with diabetes risk, by race/ethnicity, and with/without adjustment for overweight/obesity at enrollment (US; Women's Health Initiative) [24]	101,504 participants included postmenopausal women without diabetes; diets: Alternate MedDiet Index, Healthy Eating Index 2010, Alternate Healthy Eating Index 2010, and DASH diet indices; median 15 years of follow-up; 10,815 diabetes cases (multivariate adjusted)	For each diet quality index, a 1-standard-deviation higher score was associated with 10–14% lower diabetes risk ($p < 0.001$). Adjusting for overweight and obesity at baseline attenuated but did not eliminate associations to 5–10% lower risk per 1-standard-deviation higher score ($p < 0.001$). For all four dietary indices examined, higher scores were inversely associated with diabetes risk overall and across racial/ethnic groups. All the healthful diets were inversely associated with diabetes

(continued)

Table 9.2 (continued)

Objective	Study details	Results
Hong et al. (2016). Examine the associations between dietary patterns and diabetes risk (China) [25]	2900 adults; mean baseline age 51 years; mean BMI 23.5; 3 years of follow-up (multivariate adjusted)	A 1-unit increase in the 'healthy traditional' pattern score was associated with a decrease of 0.97 mg/dL in fasting plasma glucose ($p = 0.017$), while a 1-unit increase in the 'fruits, eggs and juice' pattern score was associated with an increase of 0.90 mg/dL in fasting plasma glucose ($p = 0.023$). For men, higher 'fruits, eggs and juice' pattern was associated with an 88% greater risk of hyperglycaemia vs. lower. In women, higher intake of a "healthy traditional" pattern tertile 3 was associated with a 41% lower risk compared to lower intake
Kröger et al. (2014). Assess the association between pre-defined dietary patterns and diabetes risk in European populations (EU; European Prospective Investigation into Cancer and Nutrition study (EPIC)—InterAct Study) [26]	12,403 diabetes cases and 16,154 controls; mean baseline age 53 years; mean BMI 26; 12–20 years of follow-up (multivariate adjusted)	Higher adherence to specific dietary patterns, commonly characterized by high intake of fruits or vegetables and low intake of processed meat, sugar-sweetened beverages and refined grains showed a 9–13% lower diabetes risk per standard deviation increase
Alhazmi et al. (2014). Determine the ability of two diet quality scores to predict the incidence of diabetes in women (The Australian Longitudinal Study on Women's Health) [27]	8370 women; mean baseline age 53 years; Dietary Guideline Index; 6 years of follow-up, 311 incident cases of diabetes (multivariate adjusted)	A high Dietary Guideline Index score was associated with significantly reduced diabetes risk by 49%
Gopinath et al. (2013). Assess the association between diet quality and both impaired fasting glucose and diabetes among older adults (The Blue Mountains Eye Study; Australia) [28]	2564 participants; mean age 64 years; mean BMI 26; 10-years of follow-up (multivariate adjusted)	Compared to the highest vs. lowest tertile of total diet score, there was a significant 75% decrease in risk of impaired fasting glucose in men. Also, in men, each 2-point increase in total diet score was associated with a significant 52% reduction in the 10-year incidence of impaired fasting glucose. No significant associations were observed among women or with the 10-year incidence of diabetes
de Koning et al. (2011). Evaluate the effect of diet-quality scores on diabetes risk in men (US—Health Professional Follow-up Study) [29]	41,615 men; questionnaires were mailed to participants every 2–4 years; follow-up of 20 years; 2795 cases of diabetes (multivariate adjusted)	Dietary patterns characterized by high intakes of plant-based foods such as whole grains; moderate alcohol; and low intakes of red and processed meat, sodium, sugar-sweetened beverages, and trans-fat reduce diabetes risk by 9–13% per standard deviation. High-quality diets yielded the greatest reduction in diabetes cases when followed by those with a high BMI

Table 9.2 (continued)

Objective	Study details	Results
Fung et al. (2007). Assess the association between total diet quality (Alternate Healthy Eating Index) and risk of diabetes in women (Nurses' Health Study; US) [30]	80,029 women; aged 38–63 years; follow-up of 18 years (multivariate adjusted)	Women with high total diet quality had a significant 36% lower diabetes risk. Women whose total diet improved during follow-up had a lower risk of diabetes than women whose low-quality score did not change
Randomized controlled trial (RCT)		
Kim et al. (2017). Evaluate the effect of Healthy vs. Western diets on diabetes risk factors (Australia) [31]	**Crossover RCT**: 49 subjects without diabetes; 15 men and 34 women; mean age 36 years; mean BMI 27; two 4-week weight-stable dietary interventions: Western diet—high in red and processed meat and refined grains vs. healthy diet—high in whole grains, nuts, dairy and legumes with no red meat	The Western diets reduced insulin sensitivity compared to a healthy diets in relatively insulin-resistant individuals. Dramatic improvement in diet quality increased insulin sensitivity by about 50% in only 4 weeks in people at risk of developing diabetes, whereas no effect on insulin sensitivity was seen in people with a lower risk of developing diabetes

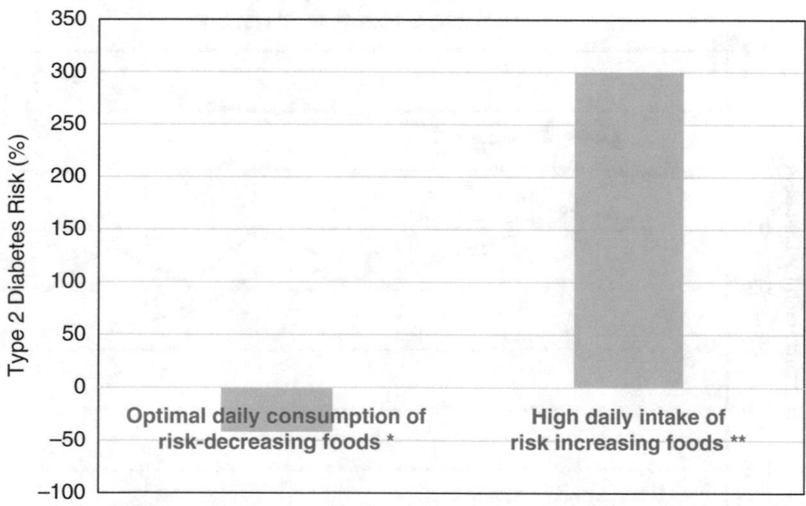

Fig. 9.1 Association between risk decreasing and risk increasing foods on type 2 diabetes risk (adapted from [15]). *Optimal daily consumption of risk-decreasing foods (2 servings whole grains; 2–3 servings vegetables; 2–3 servings fruits; 3 servings dairy) results in a 42% reduction in diabetes risk compared to non-consumption of these foods. **High daily intake of risk-increasing foods: 2 servings red meat (170 g/day), 4 servings processed meat (105 g/day), 3 servings sugar sweetened beverages (750 mL/day), and one egg (55 g/day) is associated with a threefold increased diabetes risk compared to non-consumption of these foods

4 years, showed that >10% decreased score was associated with a significantly 34% higher diabetes risk, whereas a >10% increased score was associated with a significantly 16% lower risk (Fig. 9.2) [16]. Change in AHEI score either positively or negative from baseline had a significant impact on diabetes risk. Another 2016 pooled data from the US Nurses' Health Studies and the Health Professionals Follow-up Study (160,188 women and 40,539 men; >20 years of follow-up) found that specific healthy plant-based diets emphasizing foods with higher fiber, lower glycemic index

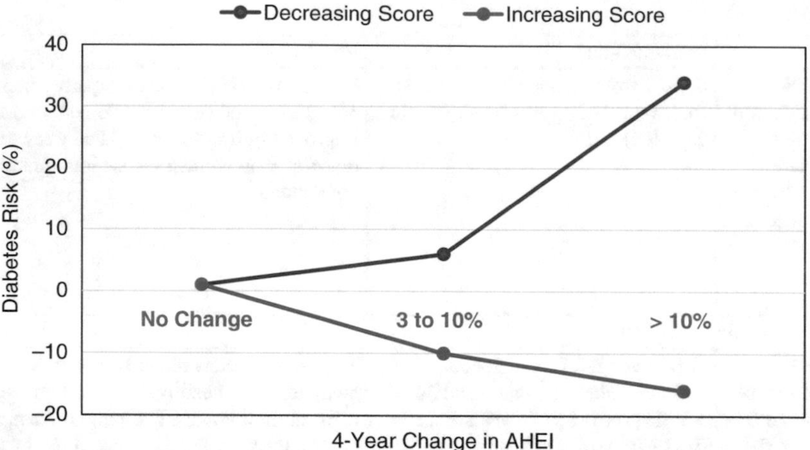

Fig. 9.2 Association between 4-year changes in Alternate Healthy Eating Index (AHEI) scores and type 2 diabetes (diabetes) risk in US men and women from pooled data from the Nurses' Health Studies and Health Professionals Follow-up Study [16]

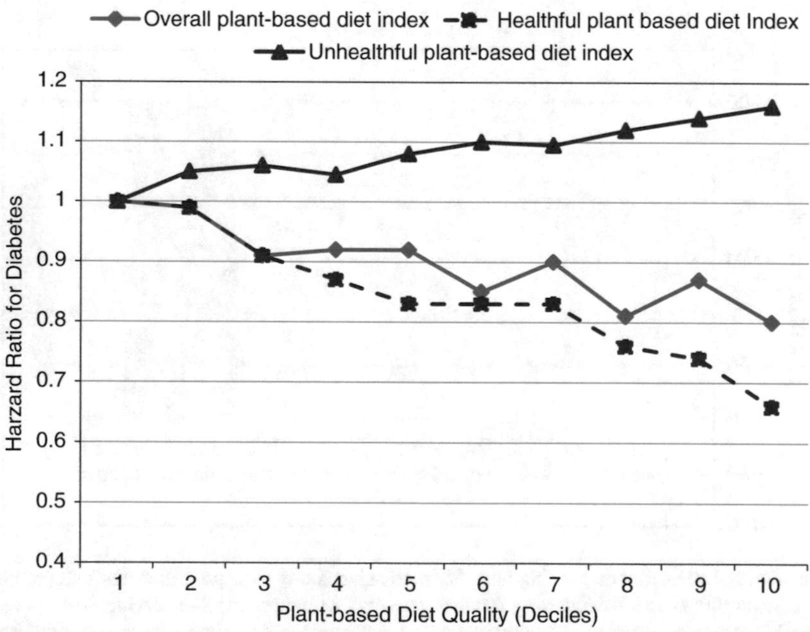

Fig. 9.3 Asssociation between type of plant-based dietary index and type 2 diabetes (diabetes) risk based on the pool analysis of men and women from the Nurses' Health Studies and Health Professionals Follow-up Study (p-trend <0.001 for all indices) (adapted from [21])

and higher amounts of phytochemicals were more effective in lowering diabetes risk than just a general recommendation to increase intake of whole plant foods (Fig. 9.3) [17]. A 2015 meta-analysis of high quality healthy vs. low quality Western diets (ten cohort studies; 404,528 participants) showed that a Western pattern significantly increased diabetes risk by 30% and a generally healthy pattern significantly reduced risk by 14%. However, in this analysis the regular inclusion of phytochemically rich fruit and vegetables, and whole-grains to the Western diet reduced risk from 30% to an insignificant 6% (Fig. 9.4) [18]. A 2014 meta-analysis of posteriori dietary patterns (nine

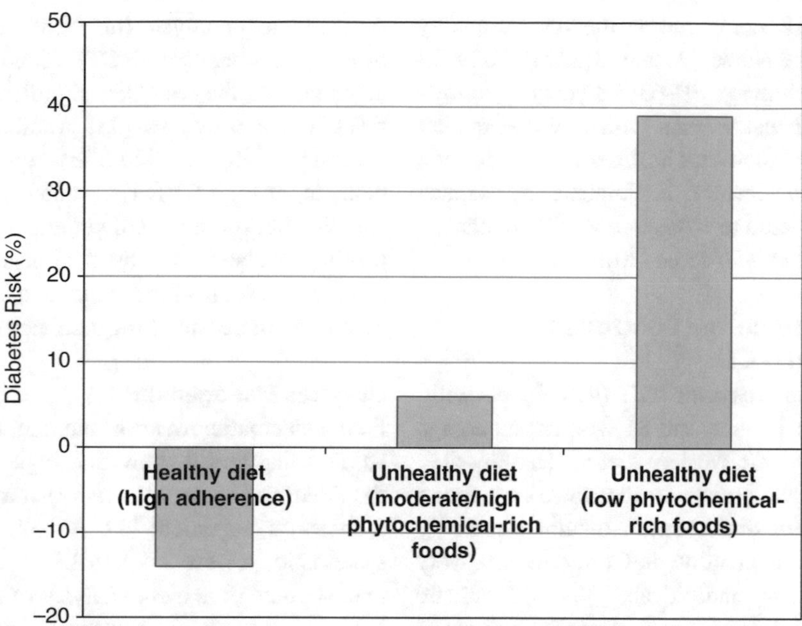

Fig. 9.4 Association between a healthy dietary pattern and two unhealthy dietary patterns with different levels of phytochemical-rich foods an d type 2 diabetes risk from a meta-analysis of ten cohort studies (adapted from [18])

cohort studies; 309,430 participants) reported that intake of fruit, vegetables and complex carbohydrates (highest vs. lowest) reduced risk by 15% and the highest intake of refined carbohydrates, processed meats, and fried foods (highest to lowest) increased risk by 41% [19]. Another 2014 meta-analysis of the adherence to a number of healthy diets including the Mediterranean (MedDiet), DASH, and Alternate Healthy Eating Index diets (20 cohort studies; 446,213 participants) found that these healthy diets are basically equally associated with a 20% lower diabetes risk and risk rate was not appreciably different in the US, Europe, or Asia [21]. Two other meta-analyses demonstrated that high adherence to healthy dietary patterns reduced diabetes risk by between 39 and 65% compared to high adherence to Western diets [20, 22].

9.2.2.2 Prospective Cohort Studies

Table 9.2 summarizes eight global cohort studies which consistently show that healthy dietary patterns protect against diabetes risk and Western patterns promote diabetes risk [23–31]. The US Women's Health Initiative (101,504 postmenopausal women; 15 years of follow-up) showed that high adherence to a range of higher quality diets, including the MedDiet, HEI 2010, AHEI, and DASH diet, all lowered diabetes risk by 5–10% with each one standard deviation increase in diet quality score [24]. Three cohort studies from Australia, China and Iran found that high adherence to a Western diet is associated with impaired glucose tolerance, high fasting glucose and insulin and impaired insulin sensitivity and higher adherence to a healthy pattern is associated with healthier glycemic control [23, 25, 28]. The European Prospective Investigation into Cancer and Nutrition study (EPIC)—InterAct Study (12,403 diabetes cases and 16,403 controls; mean baseline age 53 years; 12–20 years of follow-up) showed that a healthy dietary pattern was associated with a 9–13% lower diabetes risk per standard deviation increase [26]. The Australian Longitudinal on Women's Health (8,370 women; baseline age 45–50 years; 6 years of follow-up) found that the women with the highest diet quality score had a 49% lower diabetes risk than those with the lowest scores [27]. The Health Professionals Follow-up Study showed that high nutrient quality diets are associated with the greatest reduction in diabetes risk in men with elevated BMIs compared to the lowest quality diets [29]. The Nurses' Health Study (80,029 US women; baseline age 39–63; 18 years of follow-up) observed that women with low diet quality who improved their diet health quality even for a short time had a lower risk of diabetes by as much as 36% compared to women who did not change their low diet quality score [30].

9.2.2.3 Randomized Controlled Trial (RCT)

An Australian crossover RCT (49 subjects without diabetes; 15 men and 34 women; mean age 36 years; BMI 27; Western diet vs. Healthy diet; two 4-week weight-stable dietary trials) found that a Western diet reduced insulin sensitivity compared to a healthy diet only in relatively insulin-resistant individuals [32]. Dramatic improvement in healthy diet quality increased insulin sensitivity by about 50% in only 4 weeks in people at risk of developing diabetes.

9.2.3 Mediterranean Diet (MedDiet)

The effect of the MedDiet in preventing and managing diabetes has been the most extensively studied of the healthy dietary patterns in both prospective cohort studies and RCTs (Table 9.3) [32–42].

9.2.3.1 Meta-Analyses

Diabetes Prevention

Four meta-analyses of prospective cohort studies and RCTs consistently show that the high adherence to MedDiets significantly reduced diabetes risk [32, 34–36]. A 2015 review (seven meta-analyses) found that higher adherence to the MedDiet significantly reduced the risk of diabetes by 19–23% with a primary mechanism associated with reduced body weight [32]. Another 2015 meta-analysis (eight cohort studies and one large, long-term RCT; 122,810 subjects) showed that greater adherence to a MedDiet was associated with the primary prevention of diabetes with a higher adherence to the MedDiet significantly associated with a 19% lower risk of diabetes [34]. A 2014 meta-analysis (nine cohort studies and one large, long-term RCT) found that higher adherence to the MedDiet significantly reduced risk of diabetes by 23% [35]. Another 2014 meta-analysis (17 RCTs; 2300 overweight, obese, pre-diabetic, or high CVD risk subjects; >12 weeks) showed that higher MedDiet adherence lowered insulin resistance risk by significantly reducing hs CRP, IL-6 and intra cellular adhesion molecule 1 and increasing flow mediated dilation [37].

Diabetes Management

Four systematic reviews and meta-analyses of RCTs consistently show that high adherence to the MedDiet is an effective dietary option for diabetes management [32, 33, 37, 38]. A 2015 systematic review of MedDiets and diabetes management (five meta-analyses of RCTs including a 'de novo' meta-analyses of three RCTs with >6 months of duration) found mean HbA1c lowering by 0.3%–0.47% compared to usual care or a low-fat diet [32]. A 2015 meta-analysis (nine RCTs; 1178 diabetic patients; 4 weeks to 4 years) showed that high adherence to the MedDiet significantly lowered mean HbA1c by 0.30%, fasting blood glucose by 13 mg/dL, fasting insulin by 0.55 units, BMI by 0.29 units, weight by 0.29 kg, lowered LDL-cholesterol, triglycerides and blood pressure, and increased HDL-cholesterol [33]. This analysis demonstrates the multi-beneficial effects of the MedDiet on managing both diabetes and cardiovascular health. A 2013 meta-analysis (eight RCTs; 3–48 months) found that the MedDiet significantly improved HbA1c compared to usual care or a low-fat diet [37]. Another 2013 meta-analysis (20 RCTs, 3073 diabetic patients; >6 months) demonstrated that the MedDiet was more effective than low carbohydrate, low glycemic index, and high protein diets by significantly reducing HbA1c by 0.47% (Fig. 9.5) and promoting weight loss by 1.84 kg (Fig. 9.6) [38].

9.2.3.2 Representative Studies

Diabetes Prevention

A RCT and cohort study are representative of the MedDiet effects on diabetes risk [39, 40].

Table 9.3 Summary of Mediterranean diets (MedDiet) studies in type 2 diabetes (diabetes) risk and management

Objective	Study details	Results
Systematic reviews and meta-analyses		
Esposito et al. (2015). Assess the evidence of previous meta-analyses on efficacy of a MedDiet on the risk and management of diabetes [32]	Eight meta-analyses; diabetes patients and prediabetes subjects; five RCTs; 'de novo' meta-analysis of three long-term (> 6 months) RCTs	**(1) Diabetes Prevention**: Two meta-analyses found that higher adherence to the MedDiet significantly reduced the risk of diabetes by 19–23% and five meta-analyses showed that the MedDiet reduced body weight **(2) Diabetes Management**: A 'de novo' meta-analysis of three RCTs >6 months found in diabetic patients that the MedDiet lowered mean HbA1c levels by 0.47% compared with the usual care or a low-fat diet. Also, four meta-analyses showed that adherence to the MedDiet reduced HbA1c in diabetic patients from 0.3% to 0.47%, compared with a low-fat control diet
Huo et al. (2015). Conducted a meta-analysis of RCTs to explore the effects of MedDiet on glycemic control, weight loss and cardiovascular risk factors in diabetic patients [33]	Nine RCTs; 1178 diabetic patients; ages varied from 26 to 77 years; 4 weeks to 4 years	Compared with control diets, the MedDiet significantly reduced mean HbA1c by 0.30%; mean fasting plasma glucose by 13 mg/dL, mean fasting insulin by 0.55 μU/mL, mean BMI by 0.29 units, and mean body weight by 0.29 kg. Additionally, blood lipid and lipoprotein profiles were significantly improved with mean reductions in total cholesterol by 13 mg/dL and triglycerides by, 25.7 mg/dL and increases in HDL-C by 2.3 mg/dL; plus, a decline in systolic BP by 1.45 mm Hg and diastolic BP by 1.41 mm Hg
Schwingshackl et al. (2015). Assess the effect of MedDiet adherence on the risk of diabetes [34]	Eight cohort studies and one RCT; 122,810 subjects free of diabetes; follow-up ranged between 3.2 and 20 years	Greater adherence to a MedDiet was associated with a significant reduction in the risk of diabetes by 19% which is clinically relevant for the use of MedDiet in primary prevention of diabetes
Koloverou et al. (2014). Assess prospective studies that have evaluated the effect of a MedDiet on the development of diabetes [35]	Nine cohort studies and one RCT; 136,846 subjects; follow up ranged from 3.5 to 14 years	Higher adherence to the MedDiet was associated with 23% reduced risk of developing diabetes with no risk attenuation by region or health status
Schwingshackl et al. (2014). Assess the effects of adherence to the MedDiet on endothelial function and inflammation [36]	17 RCTs; 2300 overweight obese, prediabetic, or high cardiovascular risk subjects; >12 weeks	MedDiet significantly increased flow mediated dilation by 1.9% and adiponectin by 1.7 μg/mL, and significantly reduced hs CRP by 0.98 mg/l, interleukin (IL)-6 by 0.42 pg/mL, and intracellular adhesion molecule-1 by 23.7 ng/mL. The MedDiet improved endothelial function and reduced inflammation, which is associated with reduced risk of insulin resistance and other complications
Carter et al. (2013). Determine if the effect of the MedDiet, irrespective of weight loss, can aid in glucose control in diabetic or prediabetic persons [37]	Eight RCTs; diabetes patients and prediabetes subjects; MedDiet, low fat diet, Palaeolithic diet, or usual care; 3–48 months	The MedDiet significantly improved HbA1c levels compared to the low-fat diet and usual care but not compared to the Palaeolithic diet

(continued)

Table 9.3 (continued)

Objective	Study details	Results
Ajala et al. (2013). Assess the effect of various diets on glycemic control, lipids, and weight loss in the management of diabetic patients [38]	20 RCTs; 3073 diabetic patients; interventions that lasted >6 months that compared low carbohydrate, vegetarian, vegan, low-glycemic index (GI), high fiber, MedDiet, and high-protein diets with control diets including low-fat, high-GI, American Diabetes Association, and low-protein diets	The low carbohydrate, low-GI, MedDiet, and high-protein diets all led to significantly reduced HbA1c by 0.12%, 0.14%, 0.47%, and 0.28%, respectively, compared with their respective control diets with the MedDiet having the largest effect size (Fig. 9.5). Also, the MedDiet led to the most weight loss by 1.8 kg ($p < 0.00001$) (Fig. 9.6)
Representative studies		
Diabetes prevention		
Salas-Salvado et al. (2014). Assess the efficacy of MedDiets for the primary prevention of diabetes (Spain—Prevencion con Dieta Mediterranea trial (PREDIMED) [39]	**Multi-center Parallel RCT:** 3541 men and women without diabetes but with high cardiovascular disease risk at primary care centers; mean age 67 years; 1 of 3 diets: MedDiet plus extra-virgin olive oil, MedDiet supplemented with nuts, or a low-fat control diet; no increase in physical activity or weight loss; 4.1 years of duration	Multivariate-adjusted diabetes risk was reduced by 40% for the MedDiet supplemented with extra virgin olive oil and 18% for the MedDiet supplemented with nuts compared with the low fat control diet. There was a 30% diabetes risk reduction with both MedDiets combined when compared to the control diet
Martinez-Gonzalez et al. (2008). Assess the relation between adherence to the MedDiet and incidence of diabetes among healthy participants (Spain; Seguimiento Universidad de Navarra follow-up [SUN Project]) [40]	13,380 Spanish university graduates without diabetes; mean age 39 years; mean BMI 23; followed for a median of 4.4 years	A 2-point increase in the score was associated with a 35% relative reduction in the risk of diabetes, with a significant inverse linear trend ($p = 0.04$) in the multivariate analysis. (Fig. 9.7)
Diabetes management		
Maiorino et al. (2016). Assess the MedDiet influence on both CRP and adiponectin in newly diagnosed diabetics, and whether adherence to MedDiet affects their circulating levels (Italy RCT [41]	**Parallel RCT:** 215 men and women with newly diagnosed diabetes; MedDiet (54 males and 54 females) vs. a low-fat diet (52 males and 55 females); 1 year	The MedDiet lowered CRP by 37% and increased adiponectin by 43% compared to the low-fat diet group which remained unchanged in both outcomes. Diabetic patients with the highest MedDiet scores (6–9 points) had lower circulating CRP levels and higher circulating total adiponectin levels than the diabetic patients who scored <3 points on the scale ($p = 0.001$)
Esposito et al. (2014). Long-term effects of dietary interventions on glycemic control, need for diabetes medications, and remission of diabetes (Italy) [42]	**Parallel RCT:** 215 participants; mean age 52 years; mean BMI 29.6; 50% females; newly diagnosed diabetes; low-carbohydrate MedDiet vs. low-fat diet; 6.1–8.1 years	Lower-carbohydrate MedDiet resulted in a substantial long-term reduction of HbA1c levels, higher rate of diabetes remission, and delayed need for diabetes medication in patients with newly diagnosed diabetes vs. low fat diets (Figs. 9.8 and 9.9)

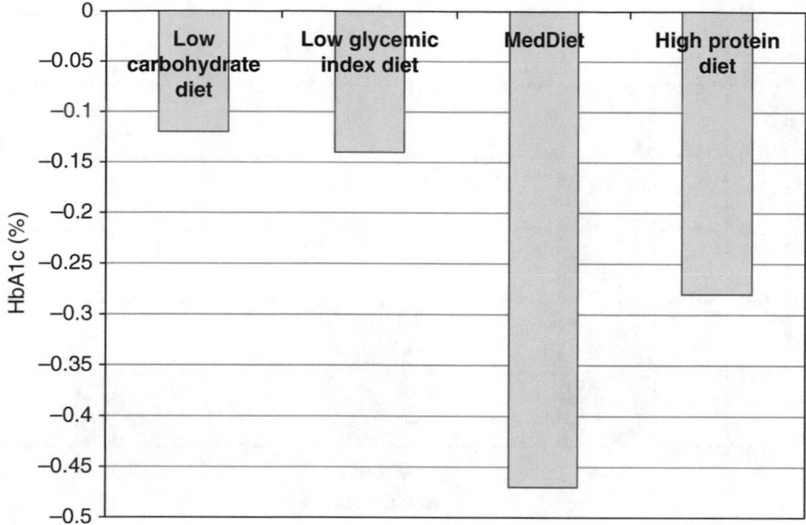

Fig. 9.5 Effect of the MedDiet vs. other dietary patterns and diabetic subject HbA1c levels from a meta-analysis of RCTs lasting >6 months (adapted from [38])

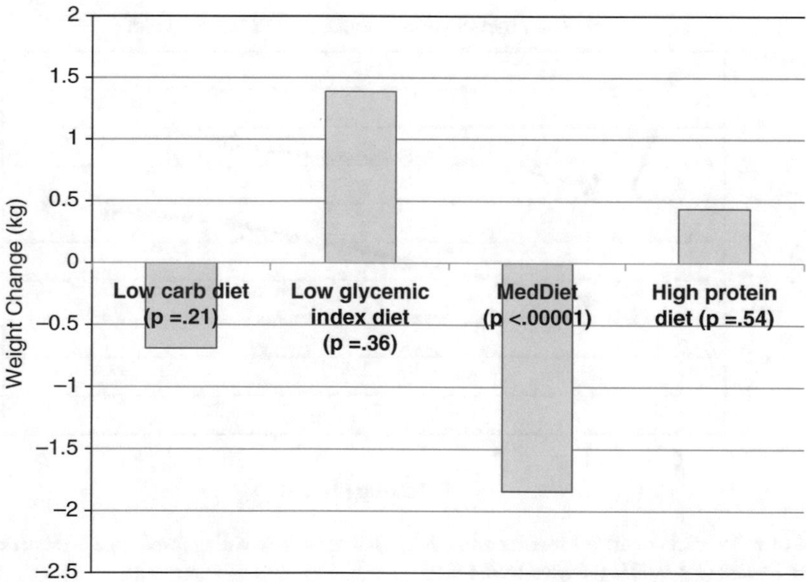

Fig. 9.6 Effect of the MedDiet vs. other dietary patterns and diabetic subject weight change from a meta-analysis of RCTs lasting >6 months (adapted from [38])

The Spanish Prevencion con Dieta Mediterranea trial [PREDIMED] (3541 men and women without diabetes but with high cardiovascular disease risk; at primary care centers; mean age 67 years; MedDiet supplemented with extra-virgin olive oil or with nuts, and a low-fat control diet; 4.1 years) found that the combined MedDiets lowered diabetes risk by 30%, when compared to the low-fat control diet [39]. The Spanish Seguimiento Universidad de Navarra (SUN) follow-up (13,380 university graduates free of diabetes; mean baseline age 39 years; median 4.4 years of follow-up) found that a 2-point increase in MedDiet score was associated with a 35% lower risk of diabetes (Fig. 9.7) [40].

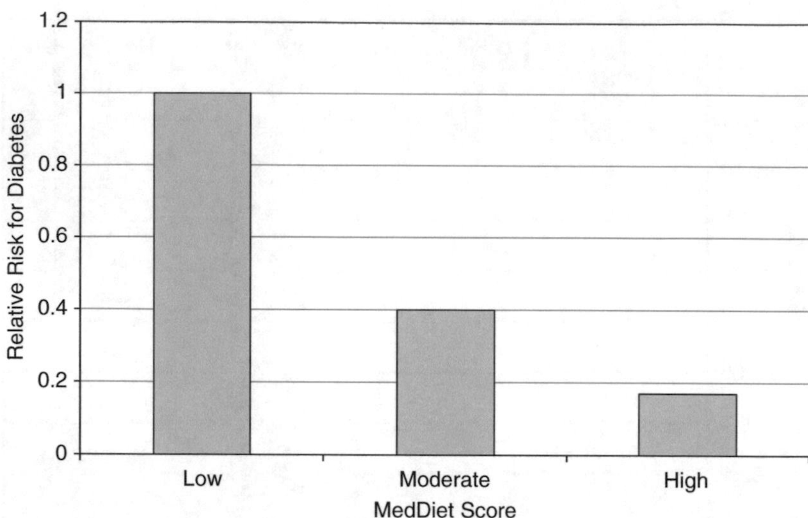

Fig. 9.7 Association between MedDiet adherence and risk for type 2 diabetes (diabetes) in 13,380 Spanish university graduates without diabetes with a median follow-up of 4.4 years ($p = 0.04$; multivariate adjusted) (adapted from [40])

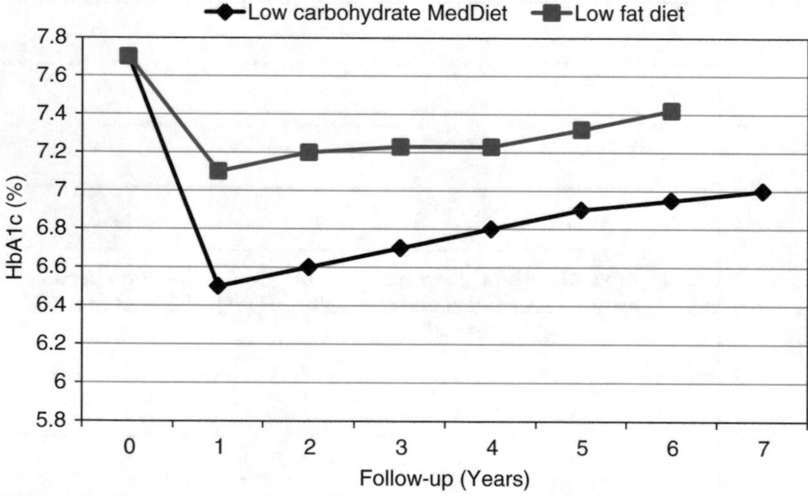

Fig. 9.8 Effect of a low carbohydrate MedDiet and HbA1c levels in newly diagnosed type 2 diabetic patients vs. a low-fat diet over 7 years ($p < 0.001$) (adapted from [42]

Diabetes Management

Two Italian RCTs are representative of MedDiet effects on diabetes management [41, 42]. The MEDITA trial (215 men and women; newly diagnosed type 2 diabetics; MedDiet vs. a low-fat diet; 1 year) found that CRP was lowered by 37% and adiponectin rose by 43% in the MedDiet group, but remained unchanged in the low-fat diet group [41]. The other RCT in newly diagnosed diabetic patients (215 participants; mean baseline age 52 years; mean BMI 29.6; 50% females; low-carbohydrate MedDiet vs. low-fat diet; 6.1–8.1 years) reported that subjects on the lower-carbohydrate MedDiet had substantial long-term reduction of HbA1c levels (Fig. 9.8), a higher rate of diabetes remission (Fig. 9.9) and delayed need for diabetes medication compared to patients on the low-fat diets [42].

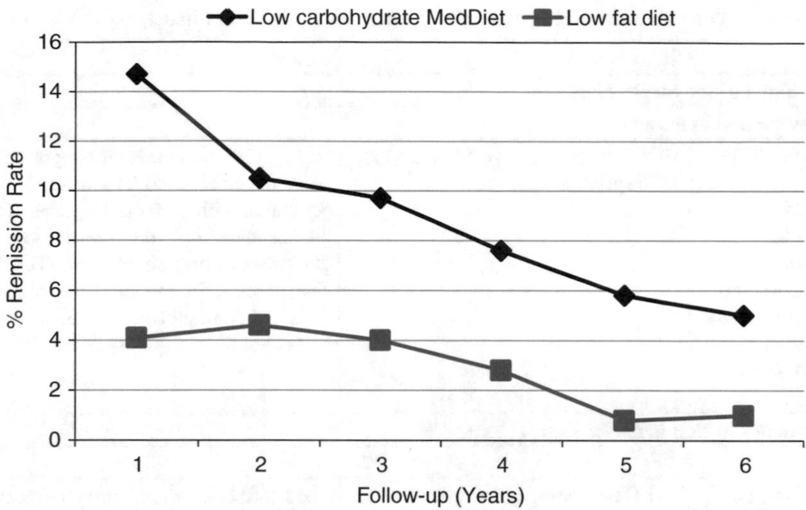

Fig. 9.9 Effect of low carbohydrate MedDiet on remission rates in newly diagnosed type 2 diabetic patients vs. low-fat diet over 6 years ($p < 0.001$) (adapted from [42])

9.2.4 Other Healthy Dietary Patterns

Prospective cohort studies and RCTs on the effect of other healthy dietary patterns in preventing and managing diabetes are summarized in Table 9.4 [43–51].

9.2.4.1 Lower Carbohydrate Diets

A 2017 meta-analysis (ten RCTs; average age 58 years; 1376 subjects) found that over 1 year, moderate carbohydrate diets (energy percentage below 45%) lowered HbA1c 0.34% compared with high carbohydrate diets and the greater the carbohydrate restriction, the better the glucose-lowering effect ($p < 0.01$) and beneficial effects on triglycerides and HDL-cholesterol levels [43].

9.2.4.2 Dietary Approaches to Stop Hypertension (DASH) Diet

A meta-analysis (20 RCTs; 2890 subjects) found that the DASH diet significantly reduced mean fasting insulin levels by 0.16 units with a modest improvement in insulin sensitivity when prescribed for more than 16 weeks [44].

9.2.4.3 Vegetarian Diets

Diabetes Management

There are a number of RCTs confirming vegetarian diets, especially low-fat vegan diets, as an effective dietary option for the management of diabetes [45–48]. A 2014 meta-analysis (six RCTs; 255 diabetic patients; 4–74 weeks) found that vegetarian diets significantly reduced HbA1c by 0.39% and directionally lowered fasting blood glucose by 7 mg/dL. This analysis showed that healthy, lower glycemic index and load vegetarian diets are an especially effective option for diabetes management [45]. A 2016 Korean RCT (93 diabetic patients; pesco-vegan diet vs. Korean Diabetes Association dietary guidance; 12 weeks) showed that the pesco-vegan diet significantly reduced HbA1C levels by 0.5% compared to the conventional diabetes diet, which lowered HbA1c levels by 0.2% after adjusting for total energy intake and waist circumference changes [46]. Two US RCTs in individuals with diabetes (99 subjects each; mean age approx 55 years; 22–74 weeks) found that low-fat vegan diets improved HbA1c more effectively than American Diabetes Association (ADA) dietary guidelines but the effect is significantly correlated with greater weight loss [47, 48].

Table 9.4 Summary of other healthy dietary patterns studies in type 2 diabetes (diabetes) risk and management

Objective	Study details	Results
Moderate vs. high carbohydrate diets		
Systematic review and meta-analysis		
Snorgaard et al. (2017). Meta-analysis comparing diets containing low to moderate amounts of carbohydrate to diets containing high amounts of carbohydrate in subjects with diabetes [43]	10 RCTs; average age 58 years; 1376 subjects	Over 1 year, moderate carbohydrate diets (energy percentage below 45%) lowered HbA1c 0.34% compared with high carbohydrate diets. The greater the carbohydrate restriction, the better the glucose-lowering effect ($R = -0.85$; $p < 0.01$). The effect of the moderate and high carbohydrate diets had similar effects on BMI, body weight, LDL cholesterol, quality of life and attrition rates
Dietary approaches to stop hypertension (DASH) diet		
Meta-analysis		
Shirani et al. (2013). Examine the effects of DASH diet consumption on the indices of glycemic control such as fasting blood glucose, serum fasting insulin level, and Homeostatic Model Assessment insulin resistance (HOMA-IR) [44]	20 RCTs; fasting blood glucose (nine RCTs; 974 subjects), fasting insulin (seven RCTs; 787 subjects), HOMA-IR (four RCTs; 677 subjects); age range 21–69 years; 3–24 weeks	The DASH diet significantly reduced mean fasting insulin levels by 0.16 units suggesting a modest improvement in insulin sensitivity when prescribed for more than 16 weeks. There were no significant beneficial effects on fasting blood glucose or HOMA-IR
Vegetarian diet		
Diabetes management		
Meta-analysis		
Yokoyama et al. (2014). Examine the association between vegetarian diets and glycemic control in diabetes [45]	Six RCTs; 255 diabetic patients; mean age 42.5 years; control diets: omnivorous, American Diabetes Association guidelines, low fat diet; BMI 26–35; 4–74 weeks	Consumption of vegetarian diets was associated with a significantly reduced HbA1c by 0.39% and a non-significantly reduced fasting blood glucose level by 7.0 mg/dL vs. control diets
Representative RCTs		
Lee et al. (2016). Compare the effects of a pesco-vegan diet and conventional diabetic diet on glycemic control (Korea) [46]	93 diabetic patients; pesco-vegan diet vs. conventional diet recommended by the Korean Diabetes Association 2011; primary endpoint change in HbA1c level; 12 weeks	The pesco-vegan diet significantly reduced HbA1c levels by 0.5% vs. the conventional diabetes diet which lowered HbA1c levels by 0.2% ($p = 0.017$). The participants with high compliance had larger reduction in HbA1c levels for pesco-vegan diet by 0.9% and control by 0.3%. The beneficial effect of pesco-vegan diets was noted even after adjusting for changes in total energy intake or waist circumference over the 12 weeks
Barnard et al. (2009). Compare the effects of a low-fat vegan diet and conventional diabetes diet recommendations on glycemia, weight, and plasma lipids (US) [47]	99 diabetic patients with medications; mean age 55 years; 61% female; low-fat vegan diet or a diet following 2003 American Diabetes Association (ADA) guidelines; primary endpoints: HbA1c and plasma lipids; 74 weeks	Weight loss was significant within each diet group but not significantly different between groups. HbA1c changes from baseline to 74 weeks was reduced for vegan diet by 0.34 units and ADA diet by 0.14 ($p = 0.43$). HbA1c reductions from baseline to last value before any medication adjustment for vegan diet was 0.40 and ADA diet 0.01 ($p = 0.03$). In analyses before alterations in lipid-lowering medications, total cholesterol decreased by 6.8 mg/dL in the vegan diet and 0.4 mg/dL in ADA diet ($p = 0.01$); LDL cholesterol decreased by 13.5 mg/dL in the vegan diet and 3.4 mg/dL in ADA diet ($p = 0.03$)

Table 9.4 (continued)

Objective	Study details	Results
Barnard et al. (2006). Evaluate the effect of a low-fat vegan diet on glycemic control in diabetic patients (US) [48]	99 diabetes patients, mean age 56 years; 40% males; low-fat vegan diet vs. the ADA dietary guidelines diet; 22 weeks	43% of the vegan group and 26% of the ADA group participants reduced diabetes medications. Including all participants, HbA1c decreased for the vegan group by 0.96 points and for the ADA group by 0.56 points ($p = 0.089$). HbA1C decreased by 1.23 points in the vegan group compared with 0.38 points in the ADA group ($p = 0.01$). Body weight decreased in the vegan group by 6.5 kg and in the ADA group by 3.1 kg ($p < 0.001$). Body weight change was significantly correlated with HbA1C change ($r = 0.51$). Among subjects not on lipid-lowering medications, vegan group LDL cholesterol was significantly lowered by 10.5% more than the ADA group
Diabetes prevention		
RCT		
Barnard et al. (2005). Investigate the effect of a low-fat, vegan diet on body weight, metabolism, and insulin sensitivity, while controlling for exercise in free-living individuals (US) [49]	64 postmenopausal women; mean age 56 years; mean BMI 33; low-fat, vegan diet or a control diet based on National Cholesterol Education Program guidelines, without energy intake limits; 14 weeks	Mean body weight decreased in vegan group by 5.8 kg, compared with 3.8 kg in the control group ($p = 0.012$). In the vegan group the mean insulin sensitivity index increased from baseline to 14 weeks by 1.1 units ($p = 0.017$), the difference between vegan and healthy control groups was 0.8 ($p = 0.19$)
Prospective study		
Tonstad et al. (2009). Assess the prevalence of diabetes in people following different types of vegetarian diets compared with that in nonvegetarians (Adventist Health Study 2; US) [50]	22,434 men and 38,469 women; mean baseline age 62.5 years; mean BMI 32; 62% female; 4 years of follow-up	Mean BMI was lowest in vegans (23.6) and incrementally higher in lacto-ovo vegetarians (25.7), pesco-vegetarians (26.3), semi-vegetarians (27.3), and nonvegetarians (28.8). Prevalence of diabetes increased from 2.9% in vegans to 7.6% in nonvegetarians; the prevalence was intermediate in participants consuming lacto-ovo (3.2%), pesco (4.8%), or semi-vegetarian (6.1%) diets. After multivariate adjustment diabetes risk increased progressively from vegans to semi-vegetarians to nonvegetarians (Fig. 9.10)
Healthy Nordic Diet		
Prospective cohort study		
Lacoppidan et al. (2015). Investigate the association between adherence to a healthy Nordic food index and the risk of diabetes (The Danish Diet, Cancer and Health Cohort Study) [51]	57,053 Danish men and women; mean baseline age 56 years; mean BMI 25; 7366 diabetes cases; median follow-up of 15.3 years	Greater adherence to the healthy Nordic food index was significantly associated with lower diabetes risk after adjusting for potential confounders. A high adherence (5–6 points) was associated with a statistically significant lower diabetes risk in women by 25% and in men by 38% compared to those with an index score of 0 points (poor adherence) (Fig. 9.11). These results suggest that regional healthy diets other than the MedDiet may also be recommended for diabetes prevention. Also, the intake of > median of specific foods such as oatmeal, root vegetables and rye bread were significantly associated with lower diabetes risk (Fig. 9.12)

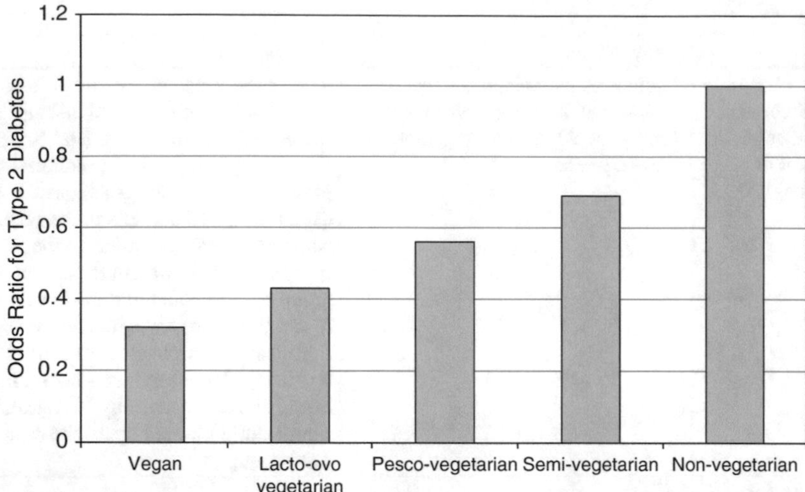

Fig. 9.10 Association between type of vegetarian diet compared to non-vegetarian diet and type 2 diabetes risk (multivariate adjusted) from the Adventist Health Study 2 (adapted from [50])

Diabetes Prevention

A representative RCT and a cohort study demonstrated the effectiveness of vegetarian diets in protecting against diabetes risk [49, 50]. A RCT in postmenopausal women (64 women; mean age 56 years; mean BMI 33; low-fat vegan diet vs. National Cholesterol Education Program guidelines; 14 weeks) demonstrated that the vegan diet was more effective than a nationally recommended cardiovascular healthy diet in lowering body weight and improving insulin sensitivity [49]. The 2009 Adventist Health Study 2 (22,434 men and 38,469 women; mean baseline age 62.5 years; mean BMI 32; 62% female; 4 years) found that all forms of vegetarian diets were more effective at lowering diabetes risk compared to non-vegetarian diets (Fig. 9.10) [50].

9.2.4.4 Healthy Nordic Food Index

The Nordic food index focuses on the intake of fish, cabbage, rye bread, oatmeal, apples and pears, and root vegetables [51]. The Danish Diet, Cancer and Health Cohort Study (57,053 Danish men and women; mean baseline age 56 years; mean BMI 25; 7366 diabetes cases; median follow-up of 15.3 years) found that greater adherence to the healthy Nordic food index was significantly associated with lower diabetes risk in women by 25% and in men by 38% (Fig. 9.11) [51]. Also, the intake of > median of specific foods such as oatmeal, root vegetables (carrots, radishes, beetroot, turnips, and other related varieties) and rye bread were significantly associated with lower diabetes risk (Fig. 9.12).

9.3 Whole Plant Foods

9.3.1 Overview

Whole plant foods collectively are an important source of healthy nutrients (e.g., vitamins, minerals), phytochemicals (e.g., polyphenols, carotenoids), fiber, and some are goods sources of protein (e.g., legumes, nuts and seeds) compared to more refined plant foods but their composition can vary widely (Appendix B). The US dietary guidelines recommend at least 3 servings/whole-grains/day and less than or equal to 3 servings of refined grains/day to promote health and wellness associated with reduced risk of diabetes and chronic diseases [52]. However, only about 1% of Americans follow the recommendation for whole-grain intake as the average American's intake is <1 ounce whole grains/day and 70% exceed the recommended intake for refined grains [52, 53]. Adequate intake of fruits and vegetables

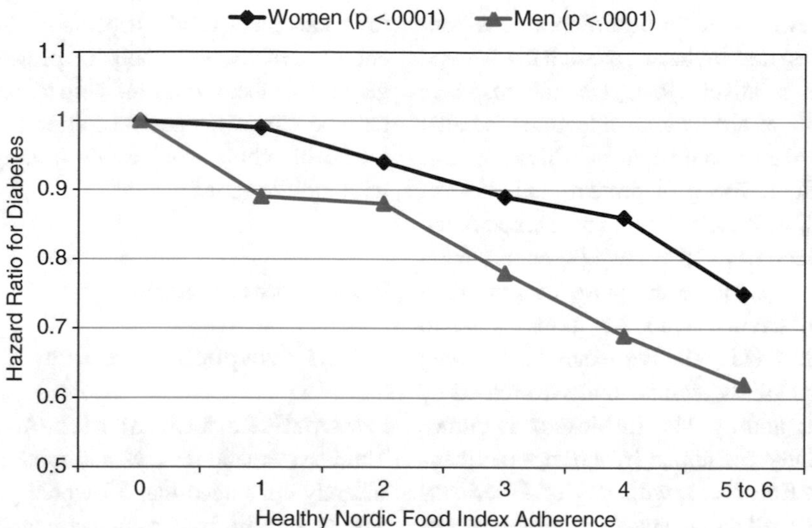

Fig. 9.11 Adherence to the Healthy Nordic Food Index and type 2 diabetes (diabetes) risk, after lifestyle adjustment (adapted from [51])

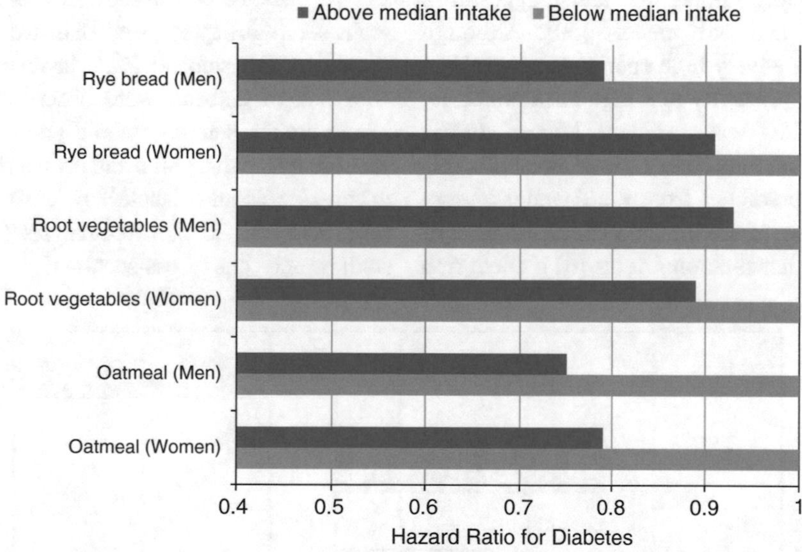

Fig. 9.12 Association between specific Healthy Nordic Food Index foods and type 2 diabetes (diabetes) risk (adapted from [51])

(> 400 g/day) makes important contributions to human health because they provide: antioxidant vitamins and phytochemicals, especially vitamins C and A, flavonoids and carotenoids, electrolytes including potassium and magnesium, with low sodium), and dietary fiber [54–56]. Globally, fruits and vegetables consumption is only a small fraction of the recommended levels [57]. More than 85% of the population fall short of meeting the daily recommendation as most Americans consume less than one cup of fruits and less than two cups of vegetables daily, with the primary contributors consisting of juice and processed potatoes, compared to the current recommendations of two cups of fruit and 2.5 cups of vegetables per day [52]. Legumes including dietary pulses (e.g., pinto beans, split peas, lentils, chickpeas) and soybeans, are rich in fiber and protein with relatively low glycemic response properties [58, 59]. A serving of legumes is half a cup or 90–100 g cooked legumes, which contains 5–10 g of fiber, 7–8 g of protein, and <5% of energy as fat, with the exception of chickpeas and soybeans which have 15% and 47% energy from fat, respectively. However, pulse consumption has been in decline with the global shift to Western-style diets [60]. For example, between the 1960s and 1990s, legume intake decreased by 40% in India and by 24% in Mexico. Legumes are infrequently consumed by North Americans and northern Europeans, with <8% of Americans consuming pulses daily. Nuts (e.g., almonds, pistachios, walnuts, hazelnuts, pecans, peanuts) are nutrient dense sources of fiber, protein, unsaturated fat, vitamins (e.g., B-vitamins and vitamin E), minerals (e.g., potassium and magnesium), phytosterols, and polyphenols [59]. Although nuts have a relatively high energy density (about 6 kcal/g) due primarily to a high unsaturated fat content and low water content, human studies have shown that nuts have a lower metabolizable energy than predicted from the Atwater energy tables because of the incomplete absorption of nut fat and other macronutrients [61]. Diets rich in whole plant foods, especially those lower in energy density, may help in preventing weight gain and diabetes risk, and help to manage longer-term health risk in people compared the minimal intake of whole plant foods in diets associated with the Western lifestyle.

9.3.2 Whole-Grains

9.3.2.1 Prospective Studies

Systematic Reviews and Meta-Analyses

Three systematic reviews and meta-analyses consistently concluded that >3 whole-grain servings/day, especially from breakfast cereals, breads, or brown rice, lowered diabetes risk by 18–40% compared to refined grains [62–64]. A 2016 meta-analysis (16 cohort studies; 643,946 participants; 29,413 diabetes cases) showed that three whole-grain servings/day reduced diabetes risk by 23% (based on ten studies) [62]. Inverse associations with risk of diabetes were observed for specific whole grains including whole grain bread, whole grain cereals, wheat bran and brown rice compared to an increased diabetes risk for white rice (Fig. 9.13). A 2015 meta-analysis (seven cohort studies and one cross-sectional study; 316,051

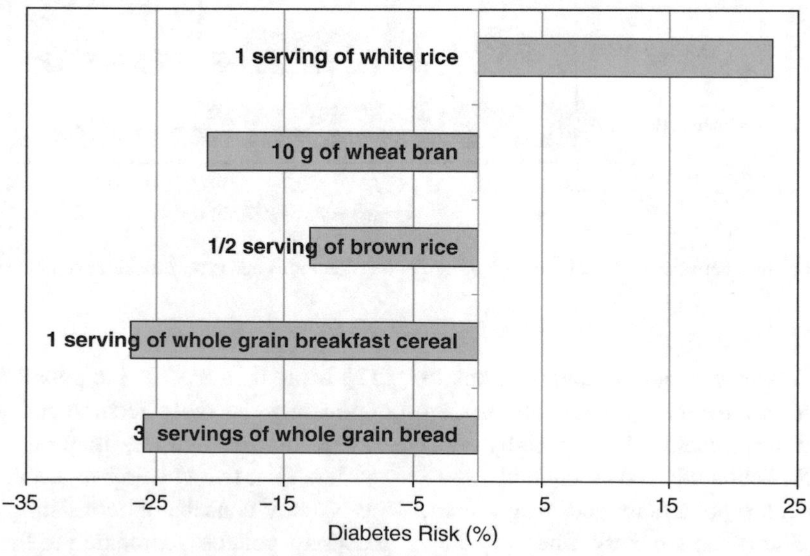

Fig. 9.13 Dose response analysis of the association of daily intake of specific grains on type 2 diabetes (diabetes) risk from a meta-analysis of 16 cohort studies (adapted from [62])

participants; follow-up ranging from 6 to 22 years; 15,573 diabetes cases) found a significant linear inverse relationship between whole grain intake and diabetes risk ($p < 0.0001$) with an overall absolute multivariate reduction of 0.3% in the diabetes risk rate for each additional 10 g of whole-grain consumed daily [63]. A 2012 systematic review and meta-analysis (45 cohort studies and 21 RCTs) showed that increased intake of whole grain and cereal fiber lowers the risk of diabetes, CVD, and weight gain when consumed at >48 g whole grains (approximately 3 servings)/day [64].

9.3.2.2 Cohort Studies

Representative prospective studies show that whole-grains are very effective at reducing diabetes risk [65–68]. The Women's Health Initiative Observational Study (72,215 postmenopausal women; mean baseline age 64 years, mean BMI 27; 7.9 years of follow-up; 3465 diabetes cases) found that women consuming >2 servings/day of whole-grains reduced multivariate diabetes risk by 37% compared to those consuming very little or no intake [65]. A Swedish prospective study (3180 women and 2297 men; mean baseline age 47 years; 8–10 years of follow-up) showed that higher intake of whole grain (59 g/day compared with 31 g/day) was associated with a 34% lower risk for deterioration in glucose tolerance from prediabetes to diabetes [66]. The Physicians' Health Study reported that men consuming whole-grain breakfast cereals had a significant 33% lower diabetes risk compared to those consuming refined breakfast cereals [67]. The pooled analysis of the Health Professionals Follow-up Study and the Nurses' Health Study (39,765 men and 157,463 women; follow-up of 14–22 years) estimated that replacing 50 g white rice/day with the same amount of brown rice was associated with a 16% lower risk of type 2 diabetes [68].

9.3.2.3 Randomized Controlled Trial (RCTs)

Diabetes Prevention

Whole-grain RCTs report inconsistent effects on insulin sensitivity, HOMA-IR scores and other diabetes risk markers [69–78]. Five RCTs found that diets rich in cereal fiber and whole-grains (approximately 28–40 g cereal fiber or >6 whole-grain servings/day) supported a significant 10–25% improvement in insulin sensitivity and/or reduced insulin resistance (HOMA-IR) scores compared to diets with <18 g fiber/day [69–73]. Five RCTs report that diets rich in cereal fiber and whole-grains (approximately 23–32 g cereal fiber or >6 whole-grain servings/day) showed insignificant effects on insulin sensitivity [74–78].

Diabetes Management

Oat and barley β-glucan are the most effective type of whole grains for improving glycemic control and glycosylated hemoglobin (HbA1c) in managing diabetes health [79–82]. A 2016 meta-analysis (four RCTs) found that compared to control, type 2 diabetes patients administrated oat β-glucan from 2.5 to 3.5 g/day for 3–8 weeks presented significantly lowered concentrations in fasting plasma glucose by 0.52 mmol/L ($p = 0.01$) and HbA1c by 0.21% ($p = 0.03$) [79]. Another 2016 meta-analysis (18 RCTs; 1024 subjects; oat products [20–136 g/day] vs. oat and barley β-glucan extract [3–10 g/day] found that higher whole oats and oat bran but not oat and barley β-glucan extracts were significantly associated with lower HbA1c, fasting glucose and fasting insulin in diabetic individuals [80].

9.3.3 Fruits and Vegetables

9.3.3.1 Systematic Reviews and Meta-Analyses

Eight systematic reviews and meta-analyses of prospective cohort studies find high variability in the effects of fruit and vegetables on diabetes risk [83–89]. A 2016 meta-analysis (23 cohort studies) found reduced diabetes risk for higher vs. lower intake of total fruit by 9%, for blueberries by 25%, for green leafy vegetables by 13%, for yellow vegetables by 28%, for cruciferous vegetables by 18% and fruit fiber lowered risk by 7% and vegetable fiber by 13% [83]. Another 2016 systematic review (six cohort studies and one nested cohort study; 326,675 subjects;

4–20 years of follow-up) showed that of potato products only French fries are consistently positively associated with diabetes risk in men and women in all three large cohort studies [84]. A 2015 meta-analysis of fruit (nine cohort studies; 403,259 participants) found a non-linear association of fruit intake and diabetes risk (p for non-linearity <0.001) with a threshold of 200 g/day total fruit intake to reduce risk of diabetes by 13% [85]. A 2012 EU InterAct meta-analysis (five cohort studies) reported that specific groups of vegetables, especially green leafy vegetables (spinach, chard, endive, lettuce, watercress) and root vegetables (carrots, radishes, beetroot, and turnips) appear to be the most beneficial in protecting against diabetes (Fig. 9.14) [87]. A meta-analysis of fruit juice (four sugar-sweetened fruit juice cohort studies, 191,686 participants; and four 100% fruit juice cohort studies, 137,663 participants) indicated that a higher intake of sugar sweetened fruit juice was significantly associated with increased diabetes risk by 28%, while higher intake of 100% fruit juice was not associated with diabetes risk (Fig. 9.15) [89]. Other meta-analyses generally report similar findings [86, 88].

9.3.3.2 Prospective Cohort Studies

Individual fruit and vegetables differ depending on fiber and caloric content, and glycemic index and load values [90–95]. A 2017 pooled analysis from the US and EU cohort studies (NIH-AARP 401,909 participants and EPIC 20,629 participants; mean baseline age approx. 64 years; mean follow-up approx. 12 years) found that the NIHAARP participants consuming higher fruit and green leafy vegetable intake were associated with a reduced diabetes risk by 5% and 13%, respectively but no significant diabetes reductions were observed in the total pooled or EPIC analyses [90]. A 2014 Finnish prospective study found that individuals in the highest quartile for intake of fruits, berries, and vegetables (with the exclusion of potatoes and fruit juices) had a significant 24% reduction in diabetes risk compared to those in the lowest quartile [91]. A pooled analysis of the Nurses' Health Studies and the Health Professionals Follow-up Study observed a high degree of heterogeneity in the effect of whole fruits on diabetes risk per three weekly servings (Fig. 9.16) [92]. For vegetables, a greater quantity (>3 servings vs. <1 serving/day) or a greater variety (11 vs. 5 varieties/week) was found to reduce

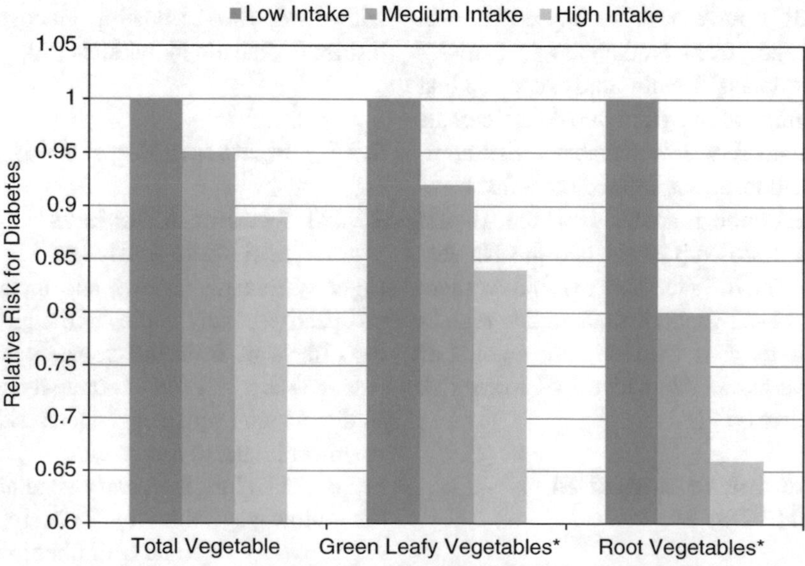

Fig. 9.14 Association between total vegetable and specific vegetable intake and type 2 diabetes (diabetes) risk from European Prospective Investigation into Cancer-InterAct study and meta-analysis (adapted from [87]). *Green leafy vegetables (spinach, chard, endive, lettuce, watercress) and root vegetables (carrots, radishes, beetroots, turnips)

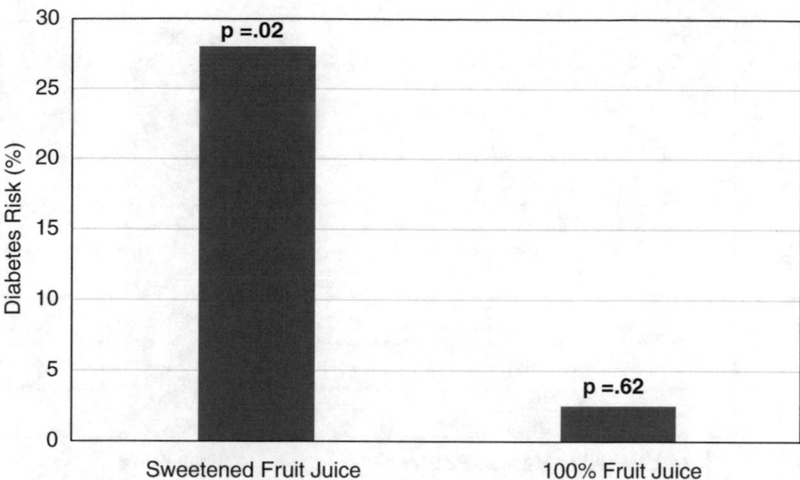

Fig. 9.15 Association between sweetened and 100% juice (highest vs. lowest intake) on type 2 diabetes (diabetes) risk from a meta-analysis of eight cohort studies (adapted from [89])

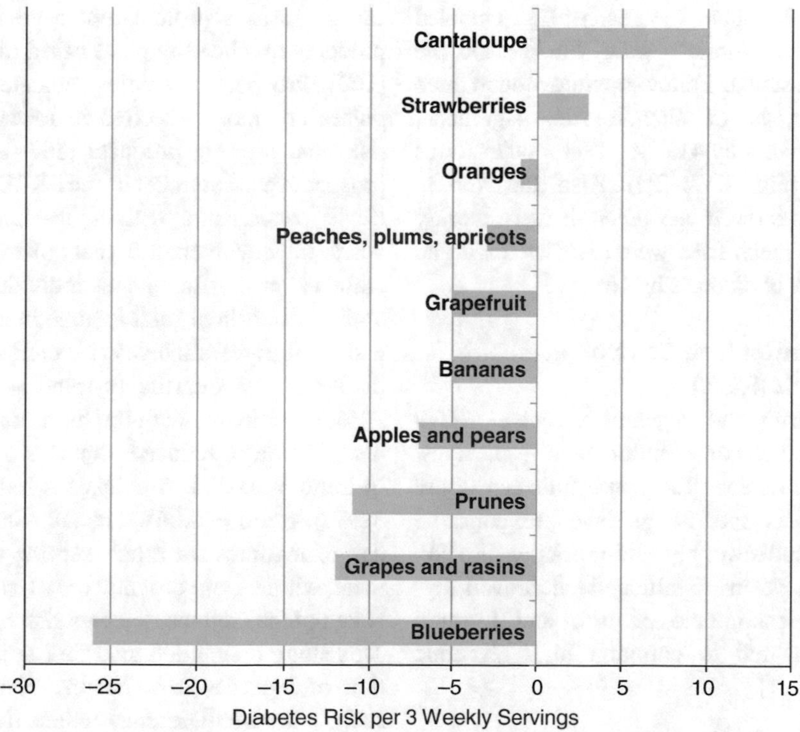

Fig. 9.16 Association between 3 servings per week of fruit varieties and type 2 diabetes (diabetes) risk from pooled data from US men and women in the Nurses' Health Studies and the Health Professionals Follow-up Study (adapted from [92])

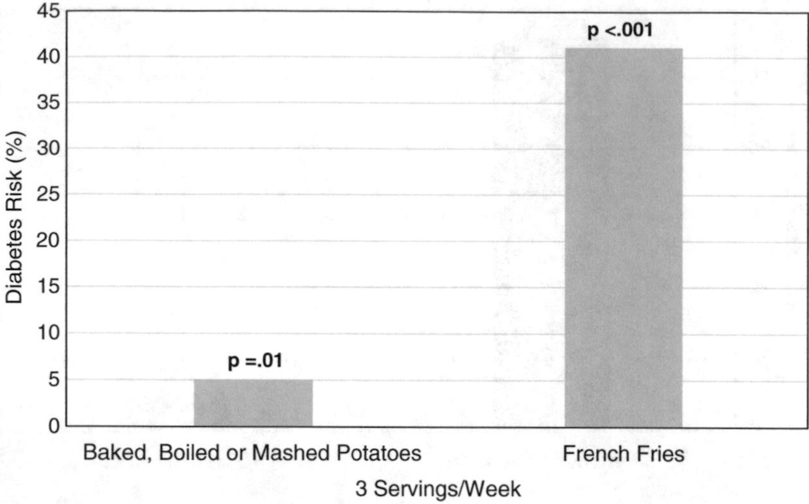

Fig. 9.17 Association between 3 servings per week of potato products and type 2 diabetes (diabetes) risk from pooled data from US men and women in the Nurses' Health Studies and the Health Professionals Follow-up Study (adapted from [94])

diabetes risk by about 24% each [93]. A pooled analysis of the Nurses' Health Studies and the Health Professionals Follow-up Study found three weekly servings of French fries significant increased diabetes by 41% vs. 5% for other forms of potatoes (Fig. 9.17) [94]. Also, the Nurses' Health Study showed in women that two weekly servings of French fries were associated with an increased risk of diabetes by 16% [95].

9.3.3.3 Randomized Controlled Trials (RCTs)

For whole fruit and vegetables, several RCTs indicate that the consumption of 5–7 portions/day has inconsistent effects on insulin sensitivity unless there is specific guidance to consume higher fiber and lower glycemic varieties [96–98]. Snacking on raisins significantly improved glycemic and insulinemic control, and lowered HbA1c compared to common high glycemic snacks [99–101].

9.3.4 Legumes

9.3.4.1 Prospective Studies

Legumes (e.g., chickpeas, lentils, beans, peas, soy and peanuts) are a good source of protein and fiber and have a low glycemic index, which can serve as a protein replacement for animal products in a healthy plant based dietary pattern [102]. Prospective studies indicate that dietary pulses are more effective in lowering diabetes risk than are soy products [102–107]. A 2017 prospective assessment of the PREDIMED study (3349 participants with a baseline age of 67 years; 62% women; 4.3 years of follow-up; 266 diabetes cases) found that individuals with the highest quartile of total legume intake (35g/day) had a 355 lower diabetes risk compared to those in the lowest quartile (p-trend = 0.04) [102]. Also, participants with the highest intake of lentils (10g/day) reduced diabetes risk by 33% (p-trend = 0.05) and chickpeas reduced risk by 32% (p-trend = 0.06). The substitution of 30g/day of legumes for a half serving of eggs, fish, meat, whole grain or white bread, rice, pasta or a baked potato reduce diabetes risk by 40 to 50%. This study concluded that the routine consumption of legumes in a healthy plant-based diet such as the MedDiet may reduce the risk of diabetes in older adults with elevated CVD risk [102]. In India's Third National Family Health Survey, non-oil seed pulses, such as lentils, were associated with a significant 30% reduced prevalence of diabetes among women but not men [103]. The Nurses' Health Study found that peanut butter was inversely associated with risk of diabetes. The consumption of >140 g (5 ounces) peanut butter/week significantly decreased diabetes risk by 21% [104]. In a study of over 43,000 Chinese Singaporeans, the consumption of tofu at least two times per week significantly reduced risk of diabetes after adjusting for BMI [105]. Pooled data from the Nurses' Health Studies and the Health Professionals Follow-up Study observed that consumption of soy foods (tofu and soy milk) was not significantly associated with a lower diabetes risk with a 7% diabetes risk reduction for >1 serving per week compared to non-consumers (p-trend = 0.14) [106]. Two representative cohort studies from Hawaii and Japan did not show significant diabetes protective benefits for soy products in either men or women [107, 108].

9.3.4.2 Randomized Controlled Trials (RCTs)

In a systematic review and meta-analysis of 41 randomized trials, non-oil-seed pulses were shown to modestly improve medium to longer term glycemic control through possible insulin-sparing mechanisms [109]. Two representative RCTs with overweight adults demonstrated that the daily consumption of 100 g cooked chickpeas or 50 g whole pea flour in muffins significantly lowered fasting insulin and insulin resistance within 4–12 weeks [110, 111].

9.3.5 Tree Nuts and Flaxseed

The effects of increased intake of tree nuts and flaxseed and diabetes risk has been evaluated in a range of prospective studies and RCTs [104, 112–120].

9.3.5.1 Prospective Cohort Studies

A 2014 systematic review and meta-analysis (five cohort studies and the PREDIMED trial) found that four weekly nut servings were significantly associated with a lower diabetes risk by 12% [112]. A 2002 Nurses' Health Study observed that the consumption of >5 nut servings/week significantly lowered diabetes risk by 27% compared to never/almost never nut consumption [104]. However, a 2013 updated Nurses' Health Study found that >2 servings/week of walnuts significantly lowered diabetes risk in women by 24% (p-trend = 0.002; after BMI adjustments) whereas the consumption of total nuts and other tree nuts was also inversely associated with diabetes risk but these associations were insignificant after adjusting for BMI (p-trend = 0.49) [113]. Further, a 2013 Nurses' Health Study and Health Professionals Follow-up Study analysis of nut intake and cause-specific mortality in men and women showed the consumption of >5 nuts servings/week lowered diabetes specific mortality by 16% [114].

9.3.5.2 Randomized Controlled Trials (RCTs)

Four representative RCTs, in adults with prediabetes or metabolic syndrome, indicate that the consumption 30 to 60 g/day of almonds, pistachios, walnuts or 30 g/day mixed nuts (50% walnuts, 25% hazelnuts and 25% almonds) significantly improved fasting insulin, insulin sensitivity, insulin resistance (HOMA-IR), and/or β-cell function after 12–16 weeks [115–118]. A 2015 walnut RCT (112 prediabetic subjects; added 56 g (366 kcals) walnuts to the habitual diet vs. no added walnuts; 6 months) showed significantly improved diet quality, endothelial function, total and LDL cholesterol, but no effects on anthropometric measures, blood glucose level, and blood pressure [115]. A 2010 almond RCT (65 prediabetic adults; hypocaloric American Diabetes Association (ADA) diet including 56 g whole almonds or a nut-free ADA control diet; 16 weeks) showed that the ADA diet supplemented with almonds significantly improved fasting insulin and HOMA-IR and β-cell function (HOMA-B) compared to the control ADA diet [117]. Also, flaxseed (13–40 g/day) has been shown to effectively improve insulin sensitivity in obese and prediabetic adults [119, 120].

9.4 Mechanisms

Healthy dietary patterns and whole plant foods influence various diabetes and cardiometabolic risk factors by improving microbiota health, body weight, visceral fat, glucose-insulin homeostasis, oxidative stress, inflammation, and endothelial health, lipoprotein concentrations, and blood pressure for lower diabetes risk and better diabetes management outcomes [4, 13, 121]. Clinical trials implicate low adiponectin, common in overweight and obese individuals with elevated visceral fat, in the pathogenesis of diabetes, coronary artery disease and hypertension [122, 123]. Healthy dietary patterns and weight loss appear to increase adiponectin concentrations, which are important for reducing diabetes risk and aiding in diabetes management by improving insulin sensitivity in the muscle and liver and through its anti-inflammatory effects. Anti-inflammatory and anti-oxidant dietary patterns are inversely related to CRP levels and positively to blood levels of carotenoids [124]. High intake of the MedDiet was associated with lower odds of diabetes by 83% (multivariate adjusted; highest compared with lowest quintile; p-trend = 0.013). High levels of antioxidant nutrients, phenolics and carotenoids in a diet abundant in fruits, berries and vegetables could potentially reduce the risk of diabetes and the associated increased risk of microvascular and macrovascular complications [124–127]. A 2017 PREDIMED substudy (1139 high CVD or diabetic risk subjects; mean baseline age 68 years; 55% women; low-fat control diet or one of two Mediterranean diets, supplemented with either extra virgin olive oil or nuts; vs lower fat diets; 1 year) found an association between increased total urinary polyphenol excretion (in spot urine samples) with decreased levels of inflammatory biomarkers and an improvement in cardiovascular risk factors such as LDL-cholesterol, HDL-cholesterol and systolic and diastolic blood pressure [126]. Also, a meta-analysis of RCTs found that the addition of >8 g of dietary fiber from food naturally rich in fiber has significant lowering effects on circulating CRP levels in overweight/obese adults [128]. A 2016 pooled analysis (124,086 US men and women) showed that consuming high flavonoid fruits and vegetables, such as apples, pears, berries, and peppers, may be especially helpful in preventing weight gain and obesity compared to other types of low flavonoid fruits and vegetables [129]. About 95% of Americans or other Western populations do not consume an adequate level of fiber daily (14 g fiber/1000 kcals or 25 g/day for women and 38 g/day for men) [130]. A 2017 analysis of the Diabetes Prevention Program (DPP) RCT data found a dietary shift toward greater intake of dietary fiber, fruits, and vegetables and lower fat diets promoted weight loss in individuals at high risk of developing diabetes, with each 5 g/day increase in fiber reducing body weight by 1.26 kg over year [131]. A 2017 Brazilian crossover RCT (19 subjects with diabetes; 53% women; mean age 66 years; isocaloric 370 kcal breakfasts; 5.4 g soluble fiber from whole fruit or guar gum supplement vs 0.8 g soluble fiber in the usual breakfast control) found that higher soluble fiber intake from a papaya and orange or guar gum at breakfast was significantly associated with similar lower postprandial glucose over 180 minutes in patients with diabetes compared to the usual low soluble fiber breakfast [132]. In contrast, polydextrose, a non-digestible prebiotic oligosaccharide used widely across most sectors of the food industry with an energy value of 1 kcal/g, was not shown in a 2017 crossover RCT to have significant effects on lowering postprandial glucose or insulin concentrations when added to beverage or low moisture bar high in carbohydrates food products because of relative low sustain intestinal viscosity or gelling properties [133]. A 2008 Canadian parallel RCT (210 participants with diabetes treated with antihyperglycemic medications; 61% men; mean age 61 years; high-cereal fiber or low-glycemic index diets; 6 months) showed that a low-glycemic index diet resulted in moderately lower HbA1c levels by 0.50% compared with a 0.18% lower HbA1c levels for high-cereal fiber diet [134]. A 2017 Japanese parallel RCT (28 participants with diabetes;

35% men; mean age 66 years; 250 kcals of brown vs white rice; 8 weeks) found that brown rice intake (which provided 5.6 g/day increase in fiber vs white rice) improved endothelial function by 20.4% vs. -5.8% for white rice ($p = 0.004$) [135]. The hs-CRP level tended to improve in the brown rice diet group compared with the white rice diet group (0.01 μg/L vs. −0.04 μg/L, $p = 0.063$). The area under the curve for postprandial glucose was modestly but consistently significantly lower in the brown rice diet group.

Conclusions

Diabetes and related obesity (diabesity) is on track to be the largest pandemic in human history, with the rate of increase in diabetes increasing at about twice as fast as predicted in 2000. Improperly managed, diabetes leads to a number of health issues, including heart diseases, stroke, kidney disease, blindness, nerve damage, leg and foot amputations, and premature death. A healthy lifestyle including habitual intake of a high quality dietary pattern, regular physical activity, and weight control are key components of diabetes prevention and management. Prospective cohort studies show that high quality dietary patterns including the Alternative Healthy Eating Index score have a significant inverse association with diabetes risk, and Western dietary patterns have a positive association with risk. Higher adherence to the MedDiet is associated with a 19–23% reduced risk of developing diabetes, while the results of RCTs show that the MedDiet can reduce risk of diabetes by 30% and can reduce HbA1c levels by 0.30–0.47% in people with diabetes. Other healthy dietary patterns which are effective in reducing diabetes risk and in management of diabetics' health are the DASH, vegan and the healthy Nordic food index diets. Prospective cohort studies show that whole (minimally processed) plant foods including whole-grains, fruits, vegetables, dietary pulses, and nuts and flaxseed are significantly associated with lower risk of diabetes. For whole grains, 3 servings/day reduced diabetes risk by 23% and of the whole-grains oats and oat bran are the most effective in managing glycemic control in people with diabetes. For fruits and vegetables, higher intake of fruits, especially berries, and green leafy vegetables, yellow vegetables, non-starchy root and cruciferous vegetables are particularly effective in lowering diabetes risk. Three weekly servings of French fries significantly increase diabetes risk by 41% compared to only 5% for other forms of potatoes (baked, boiled or mashed). Higher intake of sugar sweetened fruit juice is significantly associated with increased diabetes risk by 28%, while higher intake of 100% fruit juice is not associated with diabetes risk. Higher intake of dietary pulses, peanuts, tree nuts and flaxseed are also associated with lower diabetes risk. Healthy dietary patterns and specific whole foods beneficially affect glycemic and cardiometabolic risk factors, which are important for preventing and managing diabetes, by helping to control body weight, visceral fat, glucose-insulin homeostasis, oxidative stress, inflammation, and endothelial health, lipoprotein concentrations, and blood pressure.

Appendix A

Comparison of Western and Healthy Dietary Patterns per 2000 kcal (Approximated Values)

Components	Western dietary pattern (US)	USDA base pattern	DASH diet pattern	Healthy Mediterranean pattern	Healthy vegetarian pattern (lact-ovo based)	Vegan pattern
Emphasizes	Refined grains, low fiber foods, red meats, sweets, and solid fats	Vegetables, fruit, whole-grain, and low-fat milk	Potassium rich vegetables, fruits, and low fat milk products	Whole grains, vegetables, fruit, dairy products, olive oil, and moderate wine	Vegetables, fruit, whole-grains, legumes, nuts, seeds, milk products, and soy foods	Plant foods: vegetables, fruits, whole grains, nuts, seeds, and soy foods
Includes	Processed meats, sugar sweetened beverages, and fast foods	Enriched grains, lean meat, fish, nuts, seeds, and vegetable oils	Whole-grain, poultry, fish, nuts, and seeds	Fish, nuts, seeds, and pulses	Eggs, non-dairy milk alternatives, and vegetable oils	Non-dairy milk alternatives
Limits	Fruits and vegetables, whole-grains	Solid fats and added sugars	Red meats, sweets and sugar-sweetened beverages	Red meats, refined grains, and sweets	No red or white meats, or fish; limited sweets	No animal products allowed
Estimated nutrients/components						
Carbohydrates (% Total kcal)	49	51	55	52	55	57
Protein (% Total kcal)	16	18	18	18	14–15	13–14
Total fat (% Total kcal)	33	33	27	32	34	33
Saturated fat (% Total kcal)	11	8	6	8	8	7
Unsat. fat (% Total kcal)	22	25	21	24	26	25
Fiber (g)	16	31	29+	31	35+	40+
Potassium (mg)	2800	3350	4400	3350	3300	3650
Vegetable oils (g)	19	27	25	27	19–27	18–27
Sodium (mg)	3600	1790	1100	1690	1400	1225
Added sugar (g)	79 (20 tsp)	32 (8 tsp)	12 (3 tsp)	32 (8 tsp)	32 (8 tsp)	32 (8 tsp)
Plant food groups						
Fruit (cup)	≤1.0	2.0	2.5	2.5	2.0	2.0
Vegetables (cup)	≤1.5	2.5	2.1	2.5	2.5	2.5
Whole-grains (oz.)	0.6	3.0	4.0	3.0	3.0	3.0
Legumes (oz.)	–	1.5	0.5	1.5	3.0	3.0+
Nuts/Seeds (oz.)	0.5	0.6	1.0	0.6	1.0	2.0
Soy products (oz.)	0.0	0.5	–	–	1.1	1.5

U.S. Department of Agriculture, Agriculture Research Service, Nutrient Data Laboratory. 2014. USDA National Nutrient Database for Standard Reference, Release 27. http://www.ars.usda.gov/nutrientdata. Accessed 17 Feb 2015
Dietary Guidelines Advisory Committee. Scientific Report. Advisory Report to the Secretary of Health and Human Services and the Secretary of Agriculture. Appendix E-3.7: Developing vegetarian and Mediterranean-style food patterns. 2015;1–9
U.S. Department of Agriculture and U.S. Department of Health and Human Services. Dietary Guidelines for Americans, 2010. 7th ed. Washington, DC: U.S. Government Printing Office. 2010; Table B2.4; http://www.choosemyplate.gov/. Accessed 22 Aug 2015

Appendix B

Estimated Range of Energy, Fiber, Nutrients and Phytochemicals Composition of Whole or Minimally Processed Foods/100 g Edible Portion

Components	Whole-grains	Fresh fruit	Dried fruit	Vegetables	Legumes	Nuts/seeds
Nutrients and phytochemicals	Wheat, oats, barley, brown rice, whole grain bread, cereal, pasta, rolls and crackers	Apples, pears, bananas, grapes, oranges, blueberries, strawberries, and avocados	Dates, dried figs, apricots, cranberries, raisins, and prunes	Potatoes, spinach, carrots, peppers, lettuce, green beans, cabbage, onions, cucumber, cauliflower, mushrooms, and broccoli	Lentils, chickpeas, split peas, black beans, pinto beans, and soy beans	Almonds, Brazil nuts, cashews, hazelnuts, macadamias, pecans, walnuts, peanuts, sunflower seeds, and flaxseed
Energy (kcal)	110–350	30–170	240–310	10–115	85–170	520–700
Protein (g)	2.5–16	0.5–2.0	0.1–3.4	0.2–5.0	5.0–17	7.8–24
Available Carbohydrate (g)	23–77	1.0–25	64–82	0.2–25	10–27	12–33
Fiber (g)	3.5–18	2.0–7.0	5.7–10	1.2–9.5	5.0–11	3.0–27
Total fat (g)	0.9–6.5	0.0–15	0.4–1.4	0.2–1.5	0.2–9.0	46–76
SFA[a] (g)	0.2–1.0	0.0–2.1	0.0	0.0–0.1	0.1–1.3	4.0–12
MUFA[a] (g)	0.2–2.0	0.0–9.8	0.0–0.2	0.1–1.0	0.1–2.0	9.0–60
PUFA[a] (g)	0.3–2.5	0.0–1.8	0.0–0.7	0.0.0.4	0.1–5.0	1.5–47
Folate (ug)	4.0–44	<5.0–61	2–20	8.0–160	50–210	10–230
Tocopherols (mg)	0.1–3.0	0.1–1.0	0.1–4.5	0.0–1.7	0.0–1.0	1.0–35
Potassium (mg)	40–720	60–500	40–1160	100–680	200–520	360–1050
Calcium (mg)	7.0–50	3.0–25	10–160	5.0–200	20–100	20–265
Magnesium (mg)	40–160	3.0–30	5.0–70	3.0–80	40–90	120–400
Phytosterols (mg)	30–90	1.0–83	–	1.0–54	110–120	70–215
Polyphenols (mg)	70–100	50–800	–	24–1250	120–6500	130–1820
Carotenoids (ug)	–	25–6600	0.6–2160	10–20,000	50–600	0.0–1200

Ros E, Hu FB. Consumption of plant seeds and cardiovascular health epidemiological and clinical trial evidence. Circulation. 2013;128:553–65

USDA. What We Eat in America, NHANES 2011–2012, individuals 2 years and over (excluding breast-fed children). Available: www.ars.usda.gov/nea/bhnrc/fsrg

Rodriguez-Casado A. The health potential of fruits and vegetables phytochemicals: notable examples. Crit Rev Food Sci Nutr. 2016;56(7):1097–107

Rebello CJ, Greenway FL, Finley JW. A review of the nutritional value of legumes and their effects on obesity and its related co-morbidities. Obes Rev. 2014;15:392–407

Gebhardt SE, Thomas RG. Nutritive Value of Foods. 2002; U.S. Department of Agriculture, Agricultural Research Service, Home and Garden Bulletin 72

Holden JM, Eldridge AL, Beecher GR, et al. Carotenoid content of U.S. Foods: an update of the database. J Food Comp An. 1999;12:169–96

Lu Q-Y, Zhang Y, Wang Y, et al. California Hass avocado: profiling of carotenoids, tocopherol, fatty acid, and fat content during maturation and from different growing areas. J Agric Food Chem. 2009;57(21):10408–413

Wu X, Beecher GR, Holden JM, et al. Lipophilic and hydrophilic antioxidant capacities of common foods in the United States. J Agric Food Chem. 2004;52:4026–37

SFA saturated fat, *MUFA* monounsaturated fat, *PUFA* polyunsaturated fat

U.S. Department of Agriculture, Agriculture Research Service, Nutrient Data Laboratory. 2014. USDA National Nutrient Database for Standard Reference, Release 27. http://www.ars.usda.gov/nutrientdata. Accessed 17 Feb 2015

References

1. Asif M. The prevention and control of type-2 diabetes by changing lifestyle and dietary pattern. J Educ Health Promot. 2014;3:1. https://doi.org/10.4103/2277-9531.127541.
2. Zimmer PZ. Diabetes and its driver: the largest epidemic in human history? Clin Diabetes Endrocrinology. 2017;3:1.
3. Zucker I, Shohat T, Dankner R, Chodick G. New onset in adulthood is associated with substantial risk for mortality at all ages: a population based historical cohort study with a decade-long follow-up. Cardiovasc Diabetol. 2017;16:105.
4. Ley SH, Hamdy O, Mahan V, Hu FB. Prevention and management of type 2 diabetes: dietary components and nutritional strategies. Lancet. 2014;383:1999–2007.
5. Tabák AG, Herder C, Rathmann W, et al. Prediabetes: a high-risk state for developing diabetes. Lancet. 2012;379(9833):2279–90.
6. Salas-Salvado J, Martinez-Gonzalez MA, Bullo M, Ros E. The role of diet in the prevention of type 2 diabetes. Nutr Metab Cardiovasc Dis. 2011;21:32–48.
7. Jannasch F, Kroger J, Schulze MB. Dietary patterns and type 2 diabetes: a systematic literature review and meta-analysis of prospective studies. J Nutr. 2017;147:1174–82.
8. Tuomilehto J, Linstrom J, Eriksson JG, et al. Prevention of type 2 diabetes mellitus by changes in lifestyle among subjects with impaired glucose tolerance. N Engl J Med. 2001;344:1343–50.
9. Nield L, Summerbell CD, Hooper L, et al. Dietary advice for the prevention of type 2 diabetes mellitus in adults. Cochrane Database Syst Rev. 2008;(3). Art. No.: CD005102. https://doi.org/10.1002/14651858.CD005102.pub2.
10. Micha R, Pehalvo JL, Cudhea F, et al. Association between dietary factors and mortality from heart disease, stroke and type 2 diabetes in the United States. JAMA. 2017;317(9):912–24. https://doi.org/10.1001/jama.2017.0947.
11. Dietary Guidelines Advisory Committee (DGAC). Scientific report. Advisory report to the Secretary of Health and Human Services and the Secretary of Agriculture. Part D. Chapter 2: Dietary patterns, foods and nutrients and health outcomes. 2015;1–35.
12. Evert AB, Boucher JL, Cypress M, et al. Nutrition therapy recommendations for the management of adults with diabetes. Diabetes Care. 2014;37(suppl 1):S120–47.
13. Ley SH, Korat A, Sun Q, et al. Contribution of the Nurses' Health Studies to the uncovering risk factors for type 2 diabetes: diet, Lifestyle, biomarkers, and genetics. Am J Public Health. 2016;106(9):1624–30. https://doi.org/10.2105/AJPH.2016.303314.
14. Maghsoudi Z, Azadbakht L. How dietary patterns could have a role in prevention, progression, or management of diabetes mellitus? Review on the current evidence. J Res Med Sci. 2012;17(7):694–709.
15. Schwingshackl L, Hoffmann G, Lampousi A-M, et al. Food groups and risk of type 2 diabetes mellitus: a systematic review and meta-analysis of prospective studies. Eur J Epidemiol. 2017;32(5):363–75. https://doi.org/10.1007/s10654-0246-y.
16. Ley SH, Pan A, Li Y, et al. Changes in overall diet quality and subsequent type 2 diabetes risk: three US prospective cohorts. Diabetes Care. 2016;39:2011–8. https://doi.org/10.2337/dc16-0574.
17. Satija A, Bhupathiraju SN, Rimm EB, et al. Plant-based dietary patterns and incidence of type 2 diabetes in US men and women: results from three prospective cohort studies. PLoS Med. 2016;13(6):e1002039. https://doi.org/10.1371/journal.pmed.1002039.
18. Maghsoudi Z, Ghiasvand R, Salehi-Abargouei A. Empirically derived dietary patterns and incident type 2 diabetes mellitus: a systematic review and meta-analysis on prospective observational studies. Public Health Nutr. 2015;19(2):230–41.
19. McEvoy CT, Cardwell CR, Woodside JV, et al. Posteriori dietary patterns are related to risk of type 2 diabetes: findings from a systematic review and meta-analysis. J Acad Nutr Diet. 2014;114:1759–75.
20. Alhazmi A, Stojanovski E, McEvoy M, Garg ML. The association between dietary patterns and type 2 diabetes: a systematic review and meta-analysis of cohort studies. J Human Nutr Dietetics. 2014;27:251–60.
21. Exposito K, Chiodini P, Maiorino MI, et al. Which diet for the prevention of type 2 diabetes? A meta-analysis of prospective studies. Endocrine. 2014;47(1):107–16.
22. Esposito K, Kastorini CM, Panagiotakos DB, Giugliano D. Prevention of type 2 diabetes by dietary patterns: a systematic review of prospective studies and meta-analysis. Metab Syndr Relat Disord. 2010;8(6):471–6.
23. Doostvandi T, Bahadoran Z, Mozaffari-Khosravi H, et al. Food intake patterns are associated with the risk of impaired glucose and insulin homeostasis: a prospective approach in the Tehran Lipid and Glucose Study. Public Health Nutr. 2016;19(13):2467–74. https://doi.org/10.1017/S1368980016000616.
24. Cespedes FM, Hu FB, Tinker L, et al. Multiple healthful dietary patterns and type 2 diabetes in the Women's Health Initiative. Am J Epidemiol. 2016;183(7):622–33.
25. Hong X, Xu F, Wang Z, et al. Dietary patterns and the incidence of hyperglyacemia in China. Public Health Nutr. 2015;19(1):131–41.
26. Kröger J, Schulze MB, Romaguera D, et al. Adherence to predefined dietary patterns and incident type 2 diabetes in European populations: EPIC-InterAct Study. Diabetologia. 2014;57:321–33.
27. Alhazmi A, Stojanovski E, McEvoy M, et al. Diet quality score is a predictor of type 2 diabetes risk in women: The Australian Longitudinal Study on Women's Health. Br J Nutr. 2014; 112:945–51.
28. Gopinath B, Rochtchina E, Flood VM, Mitchell P. Diet quality is prospectively associated with

incident impaired fasting glucose in older adults. Diabet Med. 2013;30(5):557–62.
29. de Koning L, Chiuve SE, Fung TT, et al. Diet-quality scores and the risk of type 2 diabetes in men. Diabetes Care. 2011;34:1150–6.
30. Fung TT, McCullough M, van Dam RM, Hu FB. A prospective study of overall diet quality and risk of type 2 diabetes in women. Diabetes Care. 2007;30(7):1753–7.
31. Kim Y, Keogh JB, Clifton PM. Consumption of red and processed meat and refined grains for 4 weeks decreases insulin sensitivity in insulin-resistant adults: a randomized crossover study. Metabolism. 2017;68:173–83. https://doi.org/10.1016/j.metabol.2016.12.011.
32. Esposito K, Maiorino MI, Bellastella G, et al. A journey into a Mediterranean diet and type 2 diabetes: a systematic review with meta-analyses. BMJ Open. 2015;5(8):e008222. https://doi.org/10.1136/bmjopen-2015-008222.
33. Huo R, Du T, Xu Y, et al. Effects of Mediterranean-style diet on glycemic control, weight loss and cardiovascular risk factors among type 2 diabetes individuals: a meta-analysis. Eur J Clin Nutr. 2015;69:1200–8.
34. Schwingshackl L, Missbach B, König J, Hoffmann G. Adherence to a Mediterranean diet and risk of diabetes: a systematic review and meta-analysis. Public Health Nutr. 2015;18(7):1292–9.
35. Koloverou E, Esposito K, Giugliano D, Panagiotakos D. The effect of Mediterranean diet on the development of type 2 diabetes mellitus: a meta-analysis of 10 prospective studies and 136,846 participants. Metabolism. 2014;63:903–11.
36. Schwingshacki L, Hoffmann G. Mediterranean dietary pattern, inflammation and endothelial function: a systematic review and meta-analysis of intervention trials. Nutr Metab Cardiovasc Dis. 2014;24(9):923–39.
37. Carter P, Achana F, Troughton J, et al. A Mediterranean diet improves HbA1c but not fasting blood glucose compared to alternative dietary strategies: a network meta-analysis. J Hum Nutr Diet. 2014;27:280–97.
38. Ajala O, English P, Pinkney J. Systematic review and meta-analysis of different dietary approaches to the management of type 2 diabetes. Am J Clin Nutr. 2013;97:505–16.
39. Salas-Salvado J, Bullo M, Estruch R, et al. Prevention of diabetes with Mediterranean diets. Ann Inter Med. 2014;160(1):1–10.
40. Martínez-González MA, de la Fuente-Arrillaga C, Nunez-Cordoba JM, et al. Adherence to Mediterranean diet and risk of developing diabetes: prospective cohort study. BMJ. 2008;336:1348–51.
41. Maiorino ML, Bellastella G, Petrizzo M, et al. Mediterranean diet cools down the inflammatory milieu in type 2 diabetes: the MEDITA randomized controlled trial. Endocrine. 2016;54(3):634–41. https://doi.org/10.1007/s12020-016-0881-1.
42. Esposito K, Maiorino MI, Petrizzo M, et al. The effects of a Mediterranean diet on the need for diabetes drugs and remission of newly diagnosed type 2 diabetes: follow-up of a randomized trial. Diabetes Care. 2014;37:1824–30.
43. Snorgaard O, Poulsen GM, Andersen HK, et al. Systematic review and meta-analysis of dietary carbohydrate restriction in patients with type 2 diabetes. BMJ Open Diabetes Res Care. 2017;5:e000354. https://doi.org/10.1136/bmjdrc-2016-000354.
44. Shirani F, Salehi-Abargouei A, Azadbakht L. Effects of DASH diet on some risk for developing type 2 diabetes: a systematic review and meta-analysis on controlled clinical trials. Nutrition. 2013;29(7):939–47.
45. Yokoyama Y, Barnard ND, Levin SM, Watanabe M. Vegetarian diets and glycemic control in diabetes: a systematic review and meta-analysis. Cardiovasc Diagn Ther. 2014;4(5):373–82.
46. Lee Y-M, Kim S-A, Lee I-K, et al. Effect of a brown rice based vegan diet and conventional diabetic diet on glycemic control of patients with type 2 diabetes: a 12-week randomized clinical trial. PLoS One. 2016;11(6):e0155918. https://doi.org/10.1371/journal.pone.0155918.
47. Barnard ND, Cohen J, Jenkins DJA, et al. A low-fat vegan diet and a conventional diabetes diet in the treatment of type 2 diabetes: a randomized, controlled, 74-wk clinical trial. Am J Clin Nutr. 2009;89(suppl):1S–9S.
48. Barnard ND, Cohen J, Jenkins DJ, et al. A low-fat vegan diet improves glycemic control and cardiovascular risk factors in a randomized clinical trial in individuals with type 2 diabetes. Diabetes Care. 2006;29:1777–83.
49. Barnard ND, Scialli AR, Turner-McGrievy G, et al. The effects of a low-fat, plant-based dietary intervention on body weight, metabolism, and insulin sensitivity. Am J Med. 2005;118:991–7.
50. Tonstad S, Butler T, Yan R, Fraser GE. Type of vegetarian diet, body weight, and prevalence of type 2 diabetes. Diabetes Care. 2009;32:791–6.
51. Lacoppidan SA, Kyrø C, Loft S, et al. Adherence to a Healthy Nordic Food Index is associated with a lower risk of type-2 diabetes-The Danish Diet, Cancer and Health Cohort Study. Forum Nutr. 2015;7:8633–44.
52. Dietary Guidelines Advisory Committee. Scientific report. Advisory report to the Secretary of Health and Human Services and the Secretary of Agriculture. Part D. Chapter 1: Food and nutrient intakes, and health: current status and trends. 2015;1–78.
53. McGill CR, Fulgoni VL III, Devareddy L. Ten-year trends in fiber and whole grain intakes and food sources for the United States population: National Health and Nutrition Examination Survey 2001–2010. Forum Nutr. 2015;7:1119–30.
54. Slavin JL, Lloyd B. Health benefits of fruits and vegetables. Adv Nutr. 2012;3:506–16.

55. WHO/FAO. Diet, nutrition and prevention of chronic disease: report of a Joint WHO/FAO Expert Consultation. Geneva, Switzerland: World Health Organization. 2003/2004. http://whqlibdoc.who.int/trs/WHO_TRS_916.pdf. Accessed 17 Feb 2015.
56. World Health Association. Global strategy on diet, physical activity and health—promoting fruit and vegetable consumption around the world. 2013. http://who.int/dietphysical%20activity/fruit/en/. Accessed 17 Feb 2015.
57. Micha R, Khatibzadeh S, Shi P, et al. Global, regional and national consumption of major food groups in 1990 and 2010: a systematic analysis including 266 country-specific nutrition surveys worldwide. BMJ Open. 2015;5(9):e008705. https://doi.org/10.1136/bmjopen-2015-008705.
58. Rebello CJ, Greenway FL, Finley JW. A review of the nutritional value of legumes and their effects on obesity and its related co-morbidities. Obes Rev. 2014;15:392–407.
59. Ros E, Hu FB. Consumption of plant seeds and cardiovascular health epidemiological and clinical trial evidence. Circulation. 2013;128:553–65.
60. Messina V. Nutritional and health benefits of dried beans. Am J Clin Nutr. 2014;100(suppl):437S–42S.
61. Mattes RD, Kris-Etherton PM, Foster GD. Impact of peanuts and tree nuts on body weight and healthy weight loss in adults. J Nutr. 2008;138(suppl):1741S–5S.
62. Aune D, Keum N, Giovannucci E, et al. Whole grain consumption and risk of cardiovascular disease, cancer, and all cause and cause specific mortality: systematic review and dose-response meta-analysis of prospective studies. BMJ. 2016;353:i2716. https://doi.org/10.1136/bmj.i2716.
63. Chanson-Rolle A, Meynier A, Aubin F, et al. Systematic review and meta-analysis of human studies to support a quantitative recommendation for whole grain intake in relation to type 2 diabetes. PLoS One. 2015;10(6):e0131377. https://doi.org/10.1371/journal.pone.0131377.
64. Ye EQ, Chacko SA, Chou EL, et al. Greater whole-grain intake is associated with lower risk of type 2 diabetes, cardiovascular disease, and weight gain. J Nutr. 2012;142:1306–13.
65. Parker ED, Liu S, Van Horn L, et al. The association of whole grain consumption with incident type 2 diabetes: The Women's Health Initiative Observational Study. Ann Epidemiol. 2013;23(6):321–7.
66. Wirstrom T, Hilding A, Gu HF, et al. Consumption of whole grain reduces risk of deteriorating glucose tolerance, including progression to prediabetes. Am J Clin Nutr. 2013;97:179–87.
67. Kochar J, Djousse L, Gaziano JM. Breakfast cereals and risk of type 2 diabetes in the Physicians' Health Study I. Obesity. 2007;15(12):3039–44.
68. Sun Q, Spiegelman D, van Dam RM, et al. White rice, brown rice, and the risk of type 2 diabetes in US men and women. Arch Intern Med. 2010;170(11):961–9.
69. Weickert MO, Roden M, Isken F, et al. Effects of supplemented isoenergetic diets differing in cereal fiber and protein content on insulin sensitivity in overweight humans. Am J Clin Nutr. 2011;94:459–71.
70. Pereira MA, Jacobs DR, Pins JJ, et al. Effect of whole grains on insulin sensitivity in overweight hyperinsulinemic adults. Am J Clin Nutr. 2002;75:848–55.
71. Weickert MO, Mohlig M, Schofl C, et al. Cereal fiber improves whole-body insulin sensitivity in overweight and obese women. Diabetes Care. 2006;29:775–80.
72. Robertson MD, Bickerton AS, Dennis AL, et al. Insulin-sensitizing effects of dietary resistant starch and effects on skeletal muscle and adipose tissue metabolism. Am J Clin Nutr. 2005;82:559–67.
73. Landberg R, Andersson SO, Zhang JX, et al. Rye whole grain and bran intake compared with refined wheat decreases urinary C peptide, plasma insulin, and prostate specific antigen in men with prostate cancer. J Nutr. 2010;140:2180–6.
74. Giacco R, Lappi J, Costabile G, et al. Effects of rye and whole wheat versus refined cereal foods on metabolic risk factors: a randomised controlled two-centre intervention study. Clin Nutr. 2013;32:941–9.
75. Juntunen KS, Laaksonen DE, Poutanen KS, et al. High fiber rye bread and insulin secretion and sensitivity in healthy postmenopausal women. Am J Clin Nutr. 2003;77:385–91.
76. Giacco R, Clemente G, Cipriano D, et al. Effects of the regular consumption of wholemeal wheat foods on cardiovascular risk factors in healthy people. Nutr Metab Cardiovasc Dis. 2010;20:186–94.
77. Andersson A, Tengblad S, Karlström B, et al. Whole grain foods do not affect insulin sensitivity or markers of lipid peroxidation and inflammation in healthy, moderately overweight subjects. J Nutr. 2007;137:1401–7.
78. Brownlee IA, Moore C, Chatfield M, et al. Markers of cardiovascular risk are not changed by increased whole grain intake: the WHOLE heart study, a randomised, controlled dietary intervention. Br J Nutr. 2010;104:125–34.
79. Shen XL, Zhao T, Zhou Y, et al. Effect of oat β-glucan intake on glycaemic control and insulin sensitivity of diabetic patients: a meta-analysis of randomized controlled trials. Forum Nutr. 2016;8:39. https://doi.org/10.3390/nu8010039.
80. He LX, Zhao J, Huang YS, Li Y. The difference between oats and beta-glucan extract intake in the management of HbA1c, fasting glucose and insulin sensitivity: a meta-analysis of randomized controlled trials. Food Funct. 2016;7(3):1413–28. https://doi.org/10.1039/c5fo1364.
81. Thies F, Masson LF, Boffetta P, Kris-Etherton P. Oats and CVD risk markers: a systematic literature review. Br J Nutr. 2014;112:S19–30.
82. Bao L, Cai X, Xu M, Li Y. Effect of oat intake on glycaemic control and insulin sensitivity: a meta-analysis of randomised controlled trials. Br J Nutr. 2014;112:457–66.

83. Wang P-Y, Fang J-C, Gao Z-H, et al. Higher intake of fruits, vegetables or their fiber reduces the risk of type 2 diabetes: a meta-analysis. J Diabetes Investig. 2016;7:56–69.
84. Borch D, Juul-Hindsgaul N, Veller M, et al. Potatoes and risk of obesity, type 2 diabetes, and cardiovascular disease in apparently healthy adults: a systematic review of clinical intervention and observational studies. Am J Clin Nutr. 2016;104:489–98. https://doi.org/10.3945/ajcn.116.132332.
85. Li S, Miao S, Huang Y, et al. Fruit intake decreases risk of incident type 2 diabetes: an updated meta-analysis. Endocrine. 2015;48(2):454–60.
86. Li M, Fan Y, Zhang X, et al. Fruit and vegetable intake and risk of type 2 diabetes mellitus: meta-analysis of prospective cohort studies. BMJ Open. 2014;4:10. https://doi.org/10.1136/bmjopen-2014-005497.
87. Cooper AJ, Forouhi NG, Ye Z, et al. Fruit and vegetable intake and type 2 diabetes: EPIC-InterAct prospective study and meta-analysis. Eur J Clin Nutr. 2012;66(10):1082–92.
88. Carter P, Gray LJ, Troughton J, et al. Fruit and vegetable intake and incidence of type 2 diabetes mellitus: systematic review and meta-analysis. BMJ. 2010;341:c4229. https://doi.org/10.1136/bmj.c4229.
89. Xi B, Li S, Liu Z, et al. Intake of fruit juice and incidence of type 2 diabetes: a systematic review and meta-analysis. PLoS One. 9(3):e93471. https://doi.org/10.1371/journal.pone.0093471.
90. Mamluk L, O'Doherty MG, Orfanos P, et al. Fruit and vegetable intake and risk of incident of type 2 diabetes: results from the consortium on health and ageing network of cohorts in Europe and the United States (CHANCES). Eur J Clin Nutr. 2017;71(1):83–91. https://doi.org/10.1038/ejcn. 2016.143.
91. Mursu J, Virtanen JK, Tuomainen T-P, et al. Intake of fruit, berries, and vegetables and risk of type 2 diabetes in Finnish men: The Kuopio Ischaemic Heart Disease Risk Factor Study. Am J Clin Nutr. 2014;99:328–33.
92. Muraki I, Imamura F, Manson JE, et al. Fruit consumption and risk of type 2 diabetes: results from three prospective longitudinal cohort studies. BMJ. 2013;347:f5001. https://doi.org/10.1136/bmj.f5001.
93. Cooper AJ, Sharp SJ, Lentjes MAH, et al. prospective study of the association between quantity and variety of fruit and vegetable intake and incident type 2 diabetes. Diabetes Care. 2012;35:1293–300.
94. Muraki I, Rimm EB, Willett WC, et al. Potato consumption and risk of type 2 diabetes: results from three prospective cohort studies. Diabetes Care. 2016;39:376–84.
95. Halton TL, Willett WC, Liu S, et al. Potato and french fry consumption and risk of type 2 diabetes in women. Am J Clin Nutr. 2006;83:284–90.
96. Wallace IR, McEvoy CT, Hunter SJ, et al. Dose-response effect of fruit and vegetables on insulin resistance in people at high risk of cardiovascular disease. A randomized controlled trial. Diabetes Care. 2013;36(12):3888–96.
97. Taniguchi A, Yamanaka-Okumura H, Nishida Y, et al. Natto and viscous vegetables in a Japanese style meal suppress postrandial glucose and insulin responses. Asia Pac J Clin Nutr. 2008;17(4):663–8.
98. Flood A, Mai V, Pfeiffer R, et al. The effect of high-fruit and -vegetable, high-fiber, low fat dietary intervention on serum concentrations of insulin, glucose, IGF-1 and IGFBP-3. Eur J Clin Nutr. 2008;62(2):186–96.
99. Anderson JW, Waters AR. Raisin consumption by humans: effects on glycemia and insulinemia and cardiovascular risk factors. J Food Sci. 2013;78(S1):A11–7.
100. Anderson JW, Weiter KM, Christian AL, et al. Raisins compared with other snack effects on glycemia and blood pressure: a randomized, controlled trial. Postgrad Med. 2014;126(1):37–43.
101. Esfahani A, Lam J, Kendal CWC. Acute effects of raisin consumption on glucose and insulin response in healthy individuals. J Nutr Sci. 2014;3(c1). https://doi.org/10.1017/jns.2013.33.
102. Becerra-Tomas N, Diaz-Lopez A, Rosique-Esteban N, et al. Legume consumption is inversely associated wirh type 2 diabetes incidence in adults: a prospective assessment from the PREDIMED study. Clin Nutr. 2017; doi: 1016/j.clnu.2017.03.015.
103. Agrawal S, Ebrahim S. Association between legume intake and self-reported diabetes among adult men and women in India. BMC Public Health. 2013;13(1):706. https://doi.org/10.1186/1471-2458-13-706.
104. Jiang R, Manson JE, Stampfer MJ, et al. Nut and peanut butter consumption and risk of type 2 diabetes in women. JAMA. 2002;288(20):2554–60.
105. Mueller NT, Odegaard AO, Gross MD, et al. Soy intake and risk of type 2 diabetes mellitus in Chinese Singaporeans: soy intake and risk of type 2 diabetes. Eur J Nutr. 2012;51(8):1033–40.
106. Ding M, Pan A, Manson JE, et al. Consumption of soy foods and isoflavones and risk of type 2 diabetes: a pooled analysis of three US cohorts. Eur J Clin Nutr. 2016;70(12):1381. https://doi.org/10.1038/ejcn.2016. 117.
107. Nanri A, Mizoue T, Takahashi Y, et al. Soy product and isoflavone intakes are associated with a lower risk of type 2 diabetes in overweight Japanese women. J Nutr. 2010;140:580–6.
108. Morimoto Y, Steinbrecher A, Kolonel LN, et al. Soy consumption is protective against diabetes in Hawaii: The Multiethnic Cohort. Eur J Clin Nutr. 2011;65(2):279–82.
109. Sievenpiper JL, Kendall CWC, Esfahani A, et al. Effect of non-oil-seed pulses on glycaemic control: a systematic review and meta-analysis of randomised controlled experimental trials in people with and without diabetes. Diabetologia. 2009;52:1479–95.
110. Pittaway JK, Robertson IK, Ball MJ. Chickpeas may influence fatty acid and fiber intake in an ad libitum diet, leading to small improvements in serum lipid

profile and glycemic control. J Am Diet Assoc. 2008;108:1009–13.

111. Marinangeli CPF, Jones PJH. Whole and fractionated yellow pea flours reduce fasting insulin and insulin resistance in hypercholesterolaemic and overweight human subjects. Br J Nutr. 2011;105:110–7.
112. Afshin A, Micha R, Khatibzadeh S, Mozaffarian D. Consumption of nuts and legumes and risk of incident ischemic heart disease, stroke, and diabetes: a systematic review and meta-analysis. Am J Clin Nutr. 2014;100:278–88.
113. Pan A, Sun Q, Mason JE, et al. Walnut consumption is associated with lower risk of type 2 diabetes in women. J Nutr. 2013;143:512–8.
114. Bao Y, Han J, Hu FB, et al. Association of nut consumption with total and cause-specific mortality. N Engl J Med. 2013;369:2001–11.
115. Njike VY, Ayettey R, Petraro P, et al. Walnut ingestion in adults at risk for diabetes: effects on body composition, diet quality, and cardiac risk measures. BMJ Open Diabetes Res Care. 2015;3:e000115. https://doi.org/10.1136/bmjdrc-2015-000115.
116. Hernandez-Alonso P, Salas-Salvado J, Baldrich-Mora M, et al. Beneficial effects of pistachio consumption on glucose metabolism, insulin resistance, inflammation, and related metabolic risk markers: a randomized clinical trial. Diabetes Care. 2014;37(11):3098–105.
117. Wien M, Bleich D, Raghuwanshi M, et al. Almond consumption and cardiovascular risk factors in adults with prediabetes. J Am Coll Nutr. 2010;29(3):189–97.
118. Casas-Agustench P, Lopez-Uriarte P, Bullo M, et al. Effects of one serving of mixed nuts on serum lipids, insulin resistance and inflammatory markers in patients with the metabolic syndrome. Nutr Cardiovasc Dis. 2011;21(2):126–35.
119. Rhee Y, Brunt A. Flaxseed supplementation improved insulin resistance in obese glucose intolerant people: a randomized crossover design. Nutr J. 2011;10(1):44. https://doi.org/10.1186/1475-2891-10-44.
120. Hutchins AM, Brown BD, Cunnane SC, et al. Daily flaxseed consumption improves glycemic control in obese men and women with pre-diabetes: a randomized study. Nutr Res. 2013;33(5):367–75.
121. McMacken M, Shah S. A plant-based diet for the prevention and treatment of type 2 diabetes. J Geriatric Cardio. 2017;14:342–54.
122. Lopez-Jaramillo P. The role of adiponectin in cardiometabolic diseases: effects of nutritional interventions. J Nutr. 2016;146(Suppl):422S–6S.
123. Fisman EZ, Tenenbaum A. Adiponectin: a manifold therapeutic target for metabolic syndrome, diabetes, and coronary disease? Cardiovasc Diabetol. 2014;13(1):103. https://doi.org/10.1186/1475-2840-13-103.
124. McGeoghegan L, Muirhead CR, Almoosawi S. Association between an anti-inflammatory and anti-oxidant dietary pattern and diabetes in British adults: results from the national diet and nutrition survey rolling programme years 1-4. Int J Food Sci Nutr. 2015;67(5):553–61. https://doi.org/10.1080/09637486.2016.1179268.
125. Wood AD, Strachan AA, Thies F, et al. Patterns of dietary intake and serum carotenoid and tocopherol status are associated with biomarkers of chronic low-grade systemic inflammation and cardiovascular risk. Br J Nutr. 2014;112:1341–52. https://doi.org/10.1017/S0007114514001962.
126. Medina-Remón A, Rosa Casas R, Anna Tressserra-Rimbau A, et al. Polyphenol intake from a Mediterranean diet decreases inflammatory biomarkers related to atherosclerosis: a substudy of the PREDIMED trial. Br J Clin Pharmacol. 2017;83:114–28.
127. Lin D, Xiao M, Zhan J, et al. An overview of plant phenolic compounds and their importance in human nutrition and management of type 2 diabetes. Molecules. 2016;21:1374. https://doi.org/10.3390/molecules21101374.
128. Jiao J, Xu J-Y, Zhang W, et al. Effect of dietary fiber on circulating C-reactive protein in overweight and obese adults: a meta-analysis of randomized controlled trials. Int J Food Sci Nutr. 2015;66(1):114–9. https://doi.org/10.3109/09637486.2014.959898.
129. Bertoia ML, Rimm EB, Mukamal KJ, et al. Dietary flavonoid intake and weight maintenance: three prospective cohorts of 124,086 US men and women followed for up to 24 years. BMJ. 2016;352:i17. https://doi.org/10.1136/bmj.i17.
130. Dahl WJ, Stewart ML. Position of the Academy of Nutrition and Dietetics: health implications of dietary fiber. J Acad Nutr Diet. 2015;115:1861–70.
131. Sylvetsky AC, Edelstein SL, Walford G, et al. A high-carbohydrate, high-fiber, low-fat diet results in weight loss among adults at high risk of type 2 diabetes. J Nutr. 2017; doi: 10.3945/ jn.117.252395.
132. de Carvalho CM, de Paula TP, Viana LV, et al. Plasma glucose and insulin responses after consumption of breakfasts with different sources of soluble fiber in type 2 diabetes patients: a randomized crossover clinical trial. Am J Clin Nutr. 2017; doi: 10.3945/ajcn.117.157263.
133. Rahman S, Zhao A, Xiao D, et al. A randomized, controlled trial evaluating polydextrose as a fiber in a wet and dry matrix on glycemic control. J Food Sci. 2017; doi: 10.1111/1750-3841.13855.
134. Jenkins DJA, Kendall CWC, McKeown-Eyssen G, et al. Effect of a low-glycemic index or a high-cereal fiber diet on type 2 diabetes a randomized trial. JAMA. 2008;300(23):2742–53.
135. Kondo K, Morino K, Nishio Y, et al. Fiber-rich diet with brown rice improves endothelial function in type 2 diabetes mellitus: A randomized controlled trial. PLOS ONE. 2017;12(6):e0179869

10 Dietary Patterns, Foods, Nutrients and Phytochemicals in Non-Alcoholic Fatty Liver Disease

Keywords

Non-alcoholic fatty liver disease • Non-alcholic steatohepatitis • Western lifestyle • Dietary fiber • Omega-3 fatty acids • Monounsaturated fat Carotenoids • Flavonoids • Soy • Coffee • Obesity • Diet quality • Weight loss • Mediterranean diet • DASH diet • Low carbohydrate diet

Key Points

- Non-alcoholic fatty liver disease (NAFLD) is the most common cause of chronic liver disease in the world and its prevalence is increasing concurrently with the obesity pandemic.
- The high prevalence of NAFLD is generally due to unhealthy high energy dietary patterns and sedentary lifestyles leading to obesity, insulin resistance and metabolic syndrome, which are strongly associated with elevated hepatic steatosis and increased diabetes risk.
- Excessive caloric intake especially from high intake of refined carbohydrates and saturated fat promotes increased fatty liver. High intake of added sugar such as sugar sweetened beverages tends to be a stronger promoter of enzymes involved in hepatic de novo lipogenesis and NAFLD than higher-fat diets.
- Certain nutrients and phytochemicals such as omega-3 fatty acids, monounsaturated fatty acids, dietary fiber, vitamin E, carotenoids, flavonoids and caffeine, and foods and beverages including oily fish, extra virgin olive oil, oatmeal, coffee, and soy are associated with lower risk of NAFLD or its complications.
- Higher quality diets including moderate energy intake, higher intake of whole (minimally processed) plant foods, and low-fat dairy, and lower intake of red and processed meat and added sugar and salt, and adequate physical activity and sleep are associated with prevention and management NAFLD.
- The Western lifestyle is associated with higher NAFLD risk and progression to nonalcoholic steatohepatitis (NASH).
- Higher adherence to Mediterranean or Dietary Approaches to Stop Hypertension (DASH) diets, especially if energy controlled, may be effective in managing NAFLD risk and complications.

M.L. Dreher, *Dietary Patterns and Whole Plant Foods in Aging and Disease*, Nutrition and Health,
https://doi.org/10.1007/978-3-319-59180-3_10

10.1 Introduction

Nonalcoholic fatty liver disease (NAFLD) is defined by excessive fat accumulation in the liver (>5% of liver weight) and represents varying degrees of liver dysfunction and damage that is generally associated with a high adherence to the Western lifestyle, independently of excessive alcohol intake or other causes of liver disease [1–2]. The pandemic of NAFLD, which is the most common cause of chronic liver disease in the world, has emerged concurrently with the global obesity pandemic [1–5]. In the USA, over 64 million individuals are estimated to have some form of NAFLD with an annual direct medical cost of more than $100 billion [3]. Also, in four European countries (Germany, France, UK and Italy) over 52 million people have NAFLD with an annual cost of 35 billion euros. Nonalcoholic steatohepatitis (NASH) is a progression of NAFLD characterized by hepatocellular injury or hepatic steatosis and associated hepatocyte injury, inflammation, and fibrosis [1, 4]. Approximately two-thirds of obese adults have NAFLD and 20% have NASH. NASH occurs more frequently in: (1) women than in men, (2) obese Hispanics, (3) adults with morbid obesity (BMI of ≥40), and (4) older people, especially those with sarcopenia [3, 5, 6]. Higher skeletal muscle mass appears to have a beneficial effect in the prevention of NAFLD [6]. The primary clinical risk factors for NAFLD are excess body weight (e.g., abdominal fatness), insulin resistance (e.g., prediabetes or type 2 diabetes), and cardiovascular disease (e.g., elevated triglycerides or low HDL-cholesterol), which are generally associated with the Western lifestyle, including high energy dense, low fiber and nutrient dense diets and inactivity [7–13]. Two primary metabolic dysfunctions associated with the progression of NAFLD are: (1) insulin resistance has an essential role in the early stages of steatosis and (2) hepatic oxidative stress plays an important role in the progression from simple steatosis to NASH [7–9]. An overview of the pathogenesis of NAFLD is summarized in Fig. 10.1 [1, 2, 9, 10]. The primary objective of this chapter is to comprehensively review the effects of dietary patterns, specific foods, nutrients and phytochemicals on NAFLD risk and management.

10.2 Diet and Nonalcoholic Fatty Liver Disease (NAFLD) Progression

Fatty liver accumulation results from an imbalance between lipid deposition and removal, associated with excessive uptake of various blood lipids, increased de novo lipogenesis of fatty acids and triglycerides, and lower rates of very low-density lipoproteins (VLDL) release [1, 2, 4]. The progression of NAFLD to NASH involves a complex interaction of excessive hepatocellular triglyceride accumulation, reduced release of VLDL, dysfunctional mitochondrial oxidation, and epigenetic dysfunctional changes via liver specific DNA methylation. The habitual diet, especially with higher energy and added sugar intake, plays a relevant role in the pathogenesis of NAFLD, and both high risk and protective foods have been identified, but the contribution of excess calories remains critical [7–13]. The high prevalence of NAFLD is generally due to unhealthy (Western) dietary patterns and sedentary lifestyles leading to obesity and metabolic syndrome, which are strongly associated with hepatic steatosis [14]. Therefore, the first line of treatment is lifestyle modification for the prevention and management of NAFLD involving healthy dietary patterns, weight reduction and increased physical activity leading to an improvement in serum liver enzymes, reduced hepatic fatty infiltration, and, in advanced conditions, reduced degree of hepatic inflammation and fibrosis. Key dietary tips for preventing and managing NAFLD include to: (1) avoid excessive energy intake by limiting added sugar, including sugar sweetened beverages and increasing the intake of fiber-rich whole foods and (2) for heavy meat eaters, eating less red and processed meat and increasing fish intake. A 2016 Iranian case control study (159 cases and 158 controls; mean age 48 years; 57% women) found that: (1) waist size and BMI for the NAFLD participants were

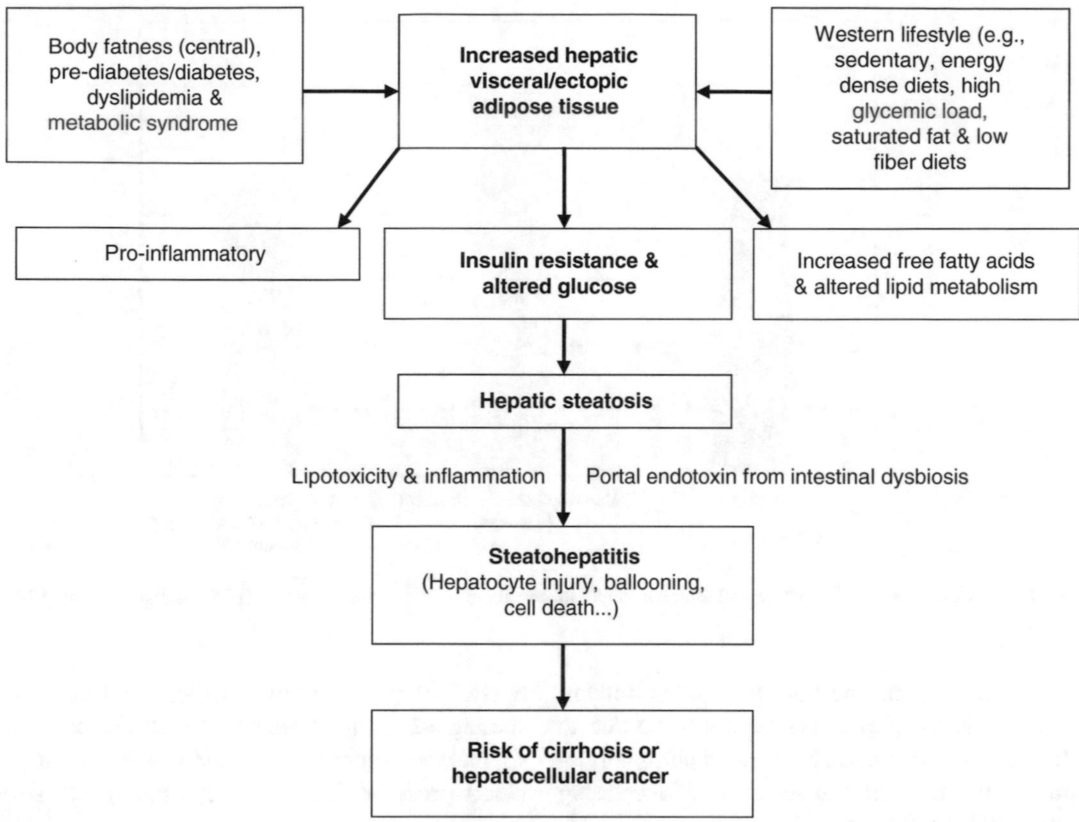

Fig. 10.1 Potential factors associated with the pathogenesis of nonalcoholic fatty liver disease (NAFLD) (adapted from [1, 2, 9, 10])

higher than the healthy participants (p < 0.05); (2) physical activity level in healthy individuals was more than in patients with NAFLD; (3) dietary intake of saturated fatty acids and sugar in patients with NAFLD was more than in healthy individuals ($p < 0.05$); and (4) intake of fiber, folic acid, vitamin D, zinc, and potassium in healthy individuals was more than in patients with NAFLD ($p < 0.05$) [15]. Weight loss is the most effective way to promote liver fat removal as 7–10% weight loss is associated with reduced liver fat, NASH remission, and reduction of fibrosis [16].

Over-consumption of processed foods and beverages high added sugar are major risk factors for development of NAFLD [17]. Hepatic lipids are derived from dietary intake, esterification of plasma free fatty acids or hepatic de novo lipogenesis. A central abnormality in NAFLD is primarily associated with increased hepatic de novo lipogenesis. Dietary fructose, especially from high added sugar intake, is a stronger promoter of enzymes involved in hepatic de novo lipogenesis than higher-fat diets. Several properties of fructose metabolism make it particularly lipogenic including its absorption via the portal vein and delivery primarily to the liver to stimulate de novo lipogenesis enzymes for its conversion into triglycerides. Also, fructose supports lipogenesis especially conjunction with insulin resistance, as fructose does not require insulin for its metabolism, and it directly stimulates sterol regulatory element-binding transcription factor 1 (SREBF1), a major transcriptional regulator of de novo lipogenesis. Also, excessive fructose intake increases liver endoplasmic reticulum stress, activates stress-related kinase caused mitochondrial dysfunction leading to increased hepatic glucose transporter type-5 (Glut5) (fructose transporter) gene expression and hepatic lipid peroxidation

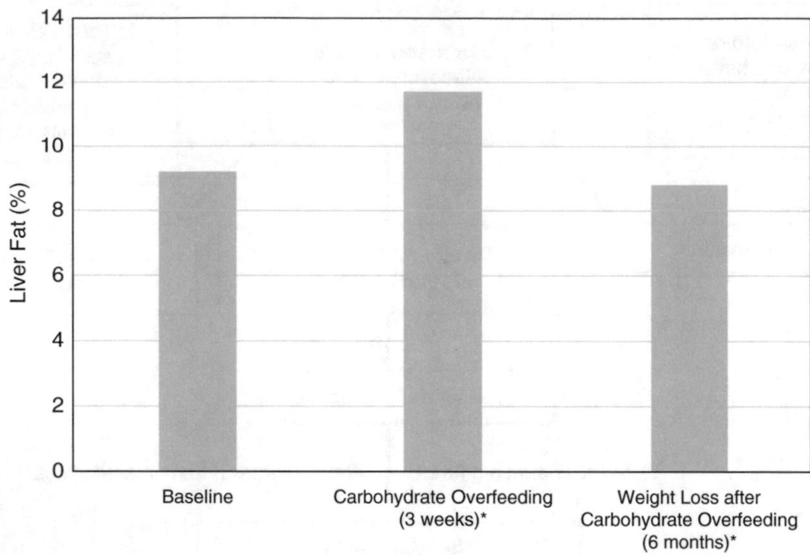

Fig. 10.2 Mean liver fat (%) before and after carbohydrate overfeeding and weight loss ($p < 0.05$*) (adapted from [18])

and inflammation. The lipogenic and proinflammatory effects of fructose appear to be due to transient ATP depletion by its rapid phosphorylation within the cell and its effect of increasing intracellular and serum uric acid levels. It is projected that population reduction of added sugar by 20% and 50% could reduce annual direct medical costs in the USA by more than 10 and 21 billion, respectively, by 2035 [12]. A clinical trial (16 obese subjects; mean BMI 31; hypercaloric diet >1000 kcal simple carbohydrates/day; 3 weeks; hypocaloric weight loss diet for 6 months) found that the overfeeding of refined carbohydrates significantly increased hepatic fat level by 27% compared to baseline levels in 3 weeks and it required 6 months on a weight loss diet to restore hepatic fat back to baseline levels (Fig. 10.2) [18]. This trial also found that the increased rate of liver fat increase was tenfold greater relative to the increase in total body weight during the high refined carbohydrate 3-week over-feeding period. Additionally, liver transaminases were significantly increased with refined carbohydrate overfeeding. An Indian cross-sectional study (242 medical students) found that the consumption of sugar sweetened soft drinks was positively correlated with increased incidence of metabolic syndrome and NAFLD (Fig. 10.3) [19]. Medical students consuming >2 sugar sweetened soft drinks/day had significantly higher BMI, waist size and diastolic blood pressure than those consuming <1 soft drink/day.

10.3 Body Weight and Central Adiposity

Obesity is associated with increased NAFLD risk [20]. A 2015 meta-analysis of the effect of adiposity on NAFLD risk (5 cohort studies; 6394 men and 4246 women; 20–88 years; 1–7 years of follow-up; diagnostic from ultrasonography and computed tomography) found a positive association with NAFLD risk for increased BMI by 19–43%, waist size by 4–115% and weight gain by 21–57% [21]. A 2016 meta-analysis (20 studies) investigating the independent relationship between central and general obesity found higher NAFLD risk for higher waist size by 34%, waist to hip ratio by 206% and BMI by 85%, which indicates that central obesity has a greater impact on NAFLD than general obesity [21]. The highest vs. lowest adiposity measures increase NAFLD for BMI by 43%, waist size by 115% and weight gain by 57%. The 2015 Copenhagen

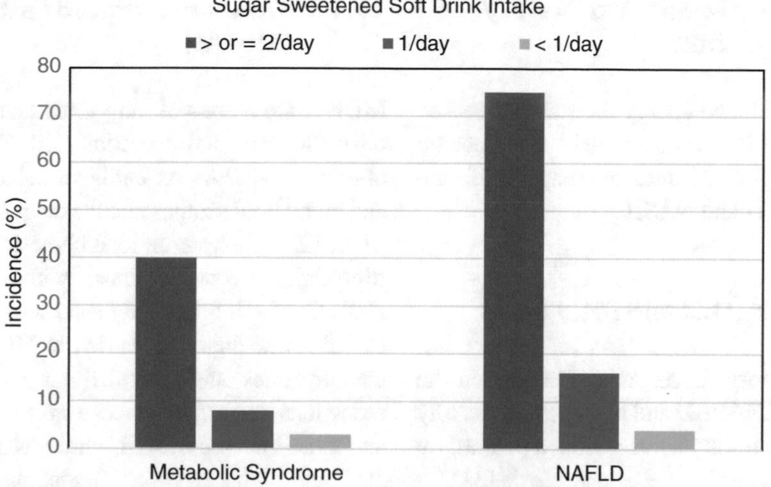

Fig. 10.3 Association between frequency of sugar sweetened soft drink intake and incidences of metabolic syndrome and nonalcohol fatty liver disease (NAFLD) in 242 Indian medical students (adapted from [19])

School Health Records Register prospective study (244,464 boys and girls, born between 1930 and 1989; heights and weights obtained from mandatory school health examinations at ages 7–13 years; NAFLD cases were observed in 1264 men and 1106 women) showed that higher BMIs between 7 and 13 years of age were positively associated with NAFLD in both sexes [22]. At age 7 years each 1 unit BMI increase was associated with a higher adult risk of NAFLD in men by 15% and women by 12%. These results suggest that BMI gain in childhood is an important indicator of the risk of development of adult NAFLD. For overweight or obese individuals, weight loss of ≥7% can help to normalize liver fat and liver enzyme levels [23]. The most effective method of treating NAFLD is the combination of weight loss and exercise [14, 24, 25]. Randomized controlled trials (RCTs) on weight loss show improved NAFLD and NASH, with the larger benefit seen with >5% weight loss [26]. A Hong Kong based RCT (154 NAFLD patients; mean baseline age 51 years; dietitian-led lifestyle modification vs. standard of care; 12 months) found that weight loss can lead to NAFLD remission (Fig. 10.4) [27]. In NAFLD patients with >10% weight loss 97% achieved NAFLD remission, compared to 13% who achieved NAFLD resolution with a weight loss of <3%. In a weight loss study of Danish children RCT (117 overweight/obese children; average age 12 years; 10-week weight-loss camp; exercised moderately for 1 h per day and restricted in their caloric intake to induce weight loss) found significant improvements in all of the parameters of liver fat, transaminases, BMI, insulin sensitivity, and parameters of the metabolic syndrome [28]. Twelve months after return to their habitual lifestyle, these improvements were maintained in only 24% of the children and 76% returned to their baseline BMI and insulin sensitivity levels. This study illustrates the need for the implementation of long-term lifestyle approaches to prevent and manage NAFLD. In a weight loss RCT of NASH patients (31 subjects; mean age 48 years; mean BMI 33; biopsy proven NASH; intensive lifestyle intervention with combination of diet, physical activity and behavior modification with a goal of 7–10% weight loss vs. limited structured education control; 48 weeks) showed that the intervention group lost an average of 9.3% of their weight vs. 0.2% in the control group ($p = 0.003$) [29]. NASH histologic activity scores improved significantly in the intervention group by 55% compared to 29% in the control group ($p = 0.05$).

10.4 Specific Foods and Dietary Components

In addition to reduced energy diets and increased physical activity to promote weight loss, specific foods or beverages and nutrients may modify the course of NAFLD and NASH [30].

10.4.1 Healthy Oils and Fatty Acids

The type of dietary fat has mixed effects on the pathogenesis of NAFLD and NASH, with healthy vegetable oils and fatty acids having a potentially protective effect against hepatic steatosis [31].

10.4.1.1 Omega 3 Fatty Acids

Omega-3 fatty acids are present in oily fish, krill oil, algae, walnuts, pine nuts, and flaxseeds. Several meta-analyses of RCTs suggest that increased intake of omega-3 PUFAs can effectively reduce NAFLD and NASH severity [32, 33]. One 2016 meta-analysis (10 RCTs; 8 trials placebo controlled; 577 NAFLD/NASH patients; median duration 12 months; median dose of omega-3 PUFAs 2.9 g/day) found omega-3 PUFAs improved liver fat, liver enzymes, triglycerides, and HDL -cholesterol in patients with NAFLD/NASH [32]. Another 2016 meta-analysis (7 RCTs with 3 double blind trials; 442 subjects [227 NAFLD or NASH patients and 215 healthy controls]; median age 49 years; duration 6–18 months; omega-3 PUFAs intake 0.83–5 g/day) showed that omega-3 PUFAs effectively lowered NAFLD and NASH severity by decreasing triglycerides, total cholesterol, alanine transaminase (ALT), and increasing HDL-cholesterol and there was a trend toward improving liver enzymes and LDL-C [33]. Omega-3 PUFAs potentially beneficial mechanisms associated with reduced NAFLD risk include: regulating gene transcription factors related to both lipid metabolism and insulin sensitivity; stimulating hepatic beta oxidation; decreasing endogenous lipid production; and down regulating the expression of pro-inflammatory molecules and of oxygen reactive species [34].

10.4.2 Monounsaturated Fatty Acids (MUFAs)

MUFAs are a class of fatty acids that are found in olive oil, nuts, and avocados [35]. The beneficial effects of MUFAs on cardiovascular disease risk and blood lipid profiles include decreasing oxidized LDL, LDL cholesterol, total cholesterol (TC), and triglycerides concentrations, without decreasing HDL-C, which is typically seen with low-fat, high carbohydrate diets. Foods rich in MUFAs displace carbohydrates and saturated fat which leads to reductions in fasting glucose and blood pressure and to an increase in HDL-cholesterol in individuals with diabetes or metabolic syndrome. Consequently, an increase in the intake of MUFAs as a replacement for high carbohydrate and saturated fat foods, may be protective against NAFLD. A RCT (37 men and 8 women with diabetes; mean age 58 years; mean BMI 30; mean HbA1c 6.6; 8 weeks) found that an isocaloric diet enriched in MUFAs significantly reduced hepatic fat content by 25% more than a high in carbohydrate diet, independent of exercise level [36]. Extra virgin olive oil is rich in both oleic acid and in phenolic compounds [37]. Several experimental studies on the biological activities of olive oil phenolic compounds suggest a potential for their regulative effect on hepatic lipid metabolism by reducing the lipogenic pathway, and thus providing protection from liver steatosis by exerting protective effects on hepatic mitochondria, a key regulator of fatty acid oxidation that counteracts excessive fat storage in hepatocytes and the pathogenesis of NAFLD.

10.4.3 Fiber-Rich Whole (Minimally Processed) Plant Foods

Increased intake of fiber-rich whole plant foods to achieve the recommended adequate fiber intake (14 g/1000 kcals) has the potential to help prevent or reduce NAFLD and NASH severity. Fiber-rich plant foods also tend to have higher antioxidant nutrients and phytochemicals (e.g., vitamin E, phenolic acids, carotenoids) density. There are several mechanisms associated with the increased intake of fiber rich diets and whole plant foods.

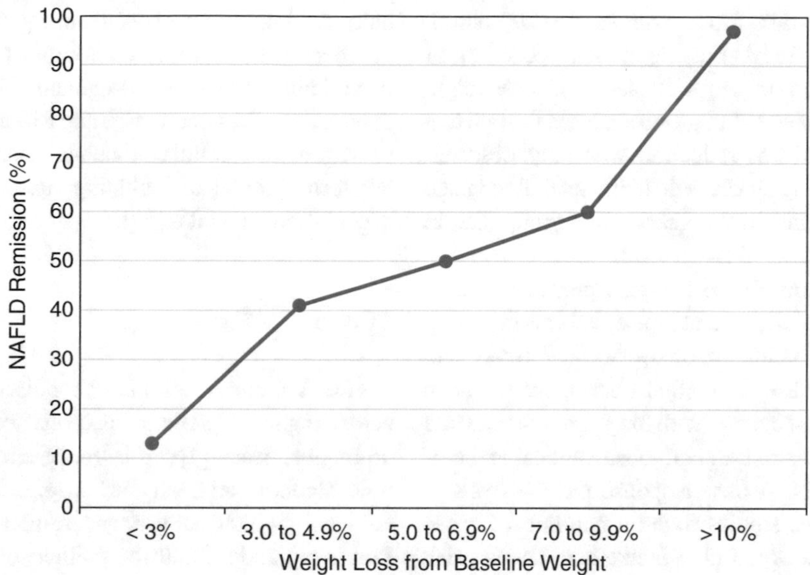

Fig. 10.4 Effect of weight loss on NAFLD remission after 12 months (p-trend p <0.001) (adapted from [27])

10.4.3.1 Body Weight and Central Obesity Control

The substitution of high-fiber, lower energy dense foods for lower fiber, higher energy dense foods typical in the Western diet has been associated with reduced weight gain and obesity risk [38–43]. Populations with higher fiber diets tend to be leaner than those with low fiber diets. A systematic review of 43 prospective and clinical studies concluded that fiber intake was inversely associated with the risk of gaining body weight and waist size [42]. Fiber-rich diets have been shown to help prevent and/or reverse visceral fat accumulation and related central body fat measures [43–45]. There are several specific RCTs that support the effects of increased fiber rich diets on preventing or attenuating NAFLD and NASH. In a double-blind RCT (40 subjects; mean age 38 years; mean BMI 29; 12 weeks), one oat cereal pack (145 kcal, with carbohydrate 25 g; protein 4.0 g; lipid 2.5 g; fiber 3.7 g and β-glucan 1.5 g) mixed with 250 mL hot water and replacing a staple food twice daily in meals was found to reduce weight and body fat, especially abdominal fat and to have liver-protective effects compared with the placebo (Fig. 10.5) [46]. In obese metabolic syndrome individuals (240 subjects; mean age 52 years; 72% women; mean BMI 35; 12 months) it was shown that a single-goal dietary recommendation to increase fiber intake (≥30 g/day) vs. a complex, multicomponent AHA dietary guidelines weight loss diet resulted in similar mean weight loss of 2.1 kg and 2.7 kg, respectively [47]. Also, there were no between-group differences in NAFLD factors including fasting plasma insulin level, HOMA-IR score, HbA1c level, total, LDL, and HDL cholesterol, triglyceride, hs-CRP, or IL-6 levels. This study suggests that a simplified approach to weight reduction emphasizing only increased fiber intake may be a reasonable alternative for persons with difficulty adhering to more complicated diet weight loss regimens to help reverse or reduce risk of NALFD or metabolic syndrome.

10.4.3.2 Systemic Inflammation and Insulin Resistance Attenuation

Elevated CRP is a biomarker of NAFLD severity or progression to NASH and increased fibrosis [48–49]. A 2017 Italian case-control study found that participants with NASH compared to healthy controls consumed significantly more liquid carbohydrates (approx 145 g vs 90 g/day) and less fiber (approx 15 g vs 28 g/day) [50]. A meta-analysis (14 RCTs) showed that intervention with dietary fiber or fiber-rich foods, compared with control, produced a slight, but significant reduction of 0.4 mg/L in circulating CRP levels in overweight and obese subjects. Subgroup analyses showed that such a significant reduction was only observed after combining studies where the total fiber intake was 8 g/d higher in the intervention group than in the control group [51].

NAFLD and NASH is highly prevalent in people with pre-diabetes and type 2 diabetes reflecting the frequent incidence of overweight/obesity and insulin resistance [52]. High fiber intake has been shown to be associated with lower pre-diabetes and type 2 diabetes risk in both observational and randomized trials. A dose-response meta-analysis of 17 prospective studies found a non-linear inverse association between fiber intake and diabetes risk [53]. In the EPIC-InterAct Study, higher total fiber and cereal fiber intake was associated with about an 18% lower risk of diabetes after adjustment for lifestyle and dietary factors [54]. The Finnish Diabetes Prevention Study (522 subjects; 31% men; mean BMI 31; mean baseline age 55 years; 4.1 years of follow-up) showed that increasing the intake of fiber-rich whole-grain cereals and fruits and vegetables, is important, not only in terms of overall health but also for sustained weight reduction and the prevention of type 2 diabetes [41].

10.4.3.3 Colonic Microbiota-Liver Axis

Adequate fiber intake is a potential important contributor to promoting colonic microbiota health and protecting against NAFLD, and reducing the adverse effects of excessive foods and beverages with added sugars [55, 56]. The health effects of dietary fiber and prebiotics against NAFLD pathology potentially include: (1) improving colonic microbiota health by increasing probiotic bacteria levels, short chain fatty acids (SCFAs) such butyrate, colonic barrier integrity and blood lipid profiles, and decreasing pathogenic bacteria levels, insulin resistance and fatty liver severity; and (2) decreased hepatic lipid content, oxidative and inflammatory stress, circulating levels of transaminases, pro-inflammatory cytokines, and endotoxaemia [55]. The SCFAs such as propionate and butyrate derived from the fermentation of fiber by the colonic microbiota bacteria have been demonstrated to up-regulate autophagy flux in hepatic cells, which may help to detoxify, repair or regenerate cellular damage associated with Western lifestyles including excessive added sugar/fructose intake [56].

10.4.4 Coffee

Coffee contains caffeine, phenols, chlorogenic acids, sugars, organic acids, polysaccharides and aromatics, triacylglycerols, tocopherols, diterphenoic alcohols and fatty acids (*e.g.*, cafestol and kahweol), which can vary according to the variety, farming practices and the method of preparation [30]. Epidemiological data suggests that coffee may have a protective effect against the development and in the management of NAFLD and NASH. A systematic review and meta-analysis (5 observational studies) found a significantly decreased risk of NAFLD among coffee drinkers by 29% and significantly decreased risk by 30% of liver fibrosis among patients with NAFLD who drank coffee on a regular basis [57]. Caffeine, the primary bioactive phytochemical in coffee, may provide a hepatoprotective effect via its strong antioxidant properties helping to reduce oxidative and inflammation stress in the liver. Also, several non-caffeine compounds, such as chlorogenic acid, are strong antioxidants that have been shown to inhibit the accumulation of lipids in hepatocytes, promote insulin sensitivity, and reduce inflammatory response.

10.4.5 Vitamin E

Vitamin E is often used in the treatment of NAFLD and NASH [58, 59]. A 2015 meta-analysis on both NAFLD and NASH (5 RCTs) found that vitamin E significantly improved liver function and histologic changes in patients with NAFLD and NASH compared to controls [58]. Specifically, vitamin E reduced steatosis in NAFLD by 0.54 U/L and in

NASH by 0.67 U/L plus lowered hepatic inflammation and enzymes and fibrosis in NASH patients. Also, another 2015 meta-analysis of NASH patients (3 RCTs) showed vitamin E supplementation had a significant and positive effect in the improvement of steatosis, ballooning degeneration, lobular inflammation and fibrosis in patients with NASH [59]. As oxidative stress plays a vital role in the progression of steatosis to NASH, vitamin E can act as a lipid-soluble antioxidant. It stabilizes free radical compounds by complexing with unpaired electrons and protecting against lipid peroxidation by acting directly with a variety of oxygen radicals [59]. Vitamin E may attenuate NASH via multiple mechanisms, including upregulating superoxide dismutase activity and inhibiting genes related to inflammation, fibrosis and hepatocellular necrosis. Almonds are a good food source of the α-tocopherol form of vitamin E.

10.4.6 Carotenoids

Carotenoids are fat-soluble pigments that give the yellow, red and orange color to fruits and vegetables with β-carotene, lycopene, α-carotene, β-cryptoxanthin, lutein and zeaxanthin among the most studied carotenoids [60]. There are multiple protective mechanisms for the effects of carotenoids in NAFLD and NASH, including antioxidant and anti-inflammatory activity. A longitudinal cohort study among middle-aged and older Japanese subjects showed that the risk of developing elevated serum liver enzymes was inversely associated with baseline serum α- and β-carotene and β-cryptoxanthin concentrations. This supports the hypothesis that antioxidant carotenoids, especially provitamin A carotenoids such as α- and β-carotene and β-cryptoxanthin might help prevent the development of NAFLD [61]. An inverse dose-response association between serum levels of carotenoids and the prevalence of NAFLD was observed in a large, community-based study of a middle-aged and elderly Chinese population [62]. Specifically, serum levels of α -carotene, β -carotene, lutein, zeaxanthin and total serum carotenoids were associated with significantly lower risk or progression of NAFLD.

10.4.7 Flavonoids and Soy

Flavonoids, commonly found in fruits, vegetables, nuts, soy, cocoa, and red wine, have been widely investigated in animal models of NAFLD in studies including soy isoflavones, green tea flavonoids, quercetin, and rutin [63]. Experimental studies have shown the protective biochemical effects of flavonoids on lipid metabolism, insulin resistance, oxidative stress, and inflammation and beneficial therapeutic effects on steatosis and liver. A RCT (45 patients with NAFLD; mean age 48 years; diets: a soy enriched low-calorie, low-carbohydrate vs. non-soy low-calorie, low-carbohydrate control; 8 weeks) found that both diets promoted similar weight loss but the soy based diet was most effective in reducing levels of aspartate aminotransferase (AST), serum fibrinogen and malondialdehyde, which suggest beneficial effects on liver function in patients with NAFLD and NASH [64]. Currently, more clinical trials are needed to confirm the efficacy of flavonoids in the treatment of NAFLD and NASH patients.

10.5 Dietary Patterns

Table 10.1 summarizes the effects of dietary quality and specific dietary patterns studies on the prevention and management of NAFLD and NASH [65–76, 78–81, 83, 84]. An overview of the food components and nutrients in specific healthy dietary patterns are summarized in Appendix A.

10.5.1 Low-Carbohydrate Diets

Low carbohydrate diets have been the focus of potential diet therapies for NAFLD in recent years but there are considerable inconsistencies among studies on these diets [65]. A 2016 systematic review and meta-analysis (10 RCTs; 230 subjects; mean age approx 47 years; 2–26 weeks) found that the consumption of low-carbohydrate diets (with <50% of calories from carbohydrates) in NAFLD patients did not significantly reduce the serum concentration of liver enzymes, but reduced the liver

Table 10.1 Summaries of dietary quality and specific dietary patterns studies on nonalcoholic fatty liver disease (NAFLD) and nonalcoholic steatohepatitis (NASH)

Objective	Study details	Results
Low-carbohydrate diets		
Haghighatdoost et al. (2016). Assess the effect of low-carbohydrate diets on managing NAFLD [65]	**Systematic review and meta-analysis:** 10 RCTs; 230 subjects; mean age approx 47 years; <50% of calories from carbohydrate, 2–26 weeks	The consumption of a low-carbohydrate diet in NAFLD patients did not reduce the serum concentration of liver enzymes, but reduced the liver fat content. Low carbohydrate diets significantly decreased mean liver fat by 11.5%
Energy-restricted diets/weight loss		
Arefhosseini et al. (2011). Examine the effects of two different compositions of low energy diets on NAFLD patients (Iran) [66]	**Double-blind RCT:** 44 ultrasonography-proven overweight NAFLD patients; mean age 41 years; approx 50% men; diets reduced energy by 500 kcal; 25 or 40% energy from fat; 6 weeks	Both energy-restricted diets decreased liver enzymes regardless of their composition, whereas the energy restricted 40% fat energy diet was more effective in reduction of weight and triglyceride levels than the diet with 25% fat energy
Rodriguez-Hernandez et al. (2011). Evaluate the effect of weight loss with a low carbohydrate diet vs. low-fat diet on aminotransferase levels in obese women with NAFLD (Mexico) [67]	**Intervention trial:** 59 women; mean age 46 years; mean BMI 38; low carbohydrate diet vs. a low-fat diet; weight loss; 6 months	After 6 months, women on both low carbohydrate and low-fat diets lost approx. 5.6% body weight along with having decreased aminotransferase levels by 22–41% (no significant difference between the diets)
Browning et al. (2011). Determine the effectiveness of dietary carbohydrate and calorie restriction in reducing hepatic triglycerides in subjects with NAFLD (US) [68]	**Intervention trial** 18 NAFLD subjects; 5 men and 13 women; mean age 45 years; BMI 35; carbohydrate-restricted to <20 g/day or calorie restricted to 1200–1500 kcal/day; 2 weeks; hepatic triglycerides were measured before and after intervention by magnetic resonance spectroscopy	Mean weight loss was similar between the groups by 4.0 kg in the calorie-restricted group and 4.6 kg in the carbohydrate-restricted group (p = 0.363). Liver triglycerides decreased significantly with weight loss but decreased more in carbohydrate-restricted subjects by 55% than in calorie-restricted subjects by 28%
Dietary quality		
Katsagoni et al. (2017). Identify dietary and lifestyle patterns effects on clinical characteristics of individuals with NAFLD (Athens, Greece) [69]	**Cross-sectional study**: 136 patients (mean age 47 years; 70% men; mean BMI 31) with ultrasound-proven NAFLD; diet and physical activity level were assessed through appropriate questionnaires. Habitual night sleep hours and duration of midday naps were recorded	A healthy dietary pattern including high consumption of low-fat dairy products, vegetables, fish, and optimal sleep duration was negatively associated with insulin resistance (p = 0.008) and liver stiffness (p = 0.05) after controlling for age, sex, BMI, energy intake, smoking habits, adiponectin, and tumor necrosis factor-α. A Western dietary pattern including high consumption of full-fat dairy products, refined cereals, potatoes, red meat, as well as high television viewing time was positively associated with insulin resistance (p = 0.005), although this association was weakened after adjusting for adiponectin and tumor necrosis factor-α

Table 10.1 (continued)

Objective	Study details	Results
Chan et al. (2017). Examine the association of diet-quality scores on NAFLD prevalence (Hong Kong) [70]	**Cross-sectional study**: 797 ethnic Chinese subjects; mean age 48 years (range 19–72 years), 42% were male; Diet Quality Index-International (DQI-I) and Mediterranean Diet Score (MDS); 28% of subjects were diagnosed with NAFLD	A 10-unit decrease in DQI-I was associated with 24% increase in the odds of having NAFLD in the age and sex adjusted model ($p = 0.009$) and the association remained significant after further adjusting for other lifestyle factors, metabolic and genetic factors ($p = 0.027$). Multivariate regression analyses showed an inverse association with the intake of vegetables and legumes, fruits and dried fruits with NAFLD prevalence ($p < 0.05$)
Katsagoni et al. (2017). Explore potential associations between dietary intake, physical activity, and sleeping habits, and the presence of NAFLD (Athens, Greece) [71]	**Case-control study**: 100 patients with ultrasound-proven NAFLD and 55 healthy controls; matched for age, sex, and BMI	NAFLD patients compared to controls consumed less vegetables and nuts, more sweets, drank less coffee and alcohol (all $p < 0.05$), and exhibited a lower level of physical activity ($p = 0.006$). High sweets consumption increased NAFLD risk by 113% ($p = 0.008$) after adjusting for multiple confounders, including body weight status. Optimal sleep duration was associated with lower NAFLD risk by 62% ($p = 0.05$)
Wehmeyer et al. (2016). Assess the association between dietary patterns on NAFLD risk and the efficacy in a real-life setting at a tertiary medical center (Germany) [72]	**Case-control study:** 55 patients diagnosed with NAFLD were compared to an age and gender-matched cohort of 88 healthy individuals. **Longitudinal sub-group analysis:** 24 NAFLD patients (16 males and 8 females); mean age 46 years; 6 months after receiving dietary advice	NAFLD patients consumed more daily calories compared with healthy controls ($p < 0.001$) and per 1000 kcals a significantly higher intake of glucose and protein but a lower intake of fiber and minerals than healthy controls. In the longitudinal analysis, patients who significantly reduced their caloric intake had lower liver enzyme alanine aminotransferase (ALT) levels after 6 months ($p < 0.001$)
Adriano et al. (2016). Assess the association of dietary patterns with NAFLD in an elderly population (Brazil) [73]	**Cross-sectional study**: 229 older adults; mean age 68 years; 103 (45%) elderly with NAFLD; diagnosis by ultrasound examination disclosed hepatic steatosis at any stage, in the absence of excess intake of alcoholic beverages; 4 dietary patterns were identified: Traditional, regional snacks, energy dense and healthy	NAFLD was inversely associated with higher adherence to a healthy dietary pattern (included fruits, vegetables/legumes, white meat, olive oil, margarine and bread/ toast, and low in red meat) with a reduced risk by 30% (p-trend = 0.037) and was directly associated with the regional snacks pattern with an increased risk of 42% (p-trend = 0.035) after adjustment for confounders. None of the other patterns were associated with NAFLD risk
Yang et al. (2015). Investigate the associations between dietary patterns and the risk of NAFLD in a middle-aged Chinese population (Hefei Nutrition and Health Study; China) [74]	**Cross-sectional study:** 999 Chinese adults; mean age 51 years; 34.5% were classified as having NAFLD; 4 major dietary patterns were identified: Traditional Chinese (coarse grains, fruits, eggs, fish and shrimp, milk, and tea), animal food (kelp/ seaweed and mushroom, pork, beef, mutton, poultry, cooked meat, eggs, fish and shrimp, beans and grease), grains-vegetables (coarse grains, tubers, vegetables, mushrooms and kelp/seaweed, beans and fish) and high-salt diets (rice, pickled vegetables, processed meat, bacon, salted duck egg, salted fish and tea)	After adjusting for potential confounders, higher intake of the animal food pattern scores had greater prevalence of NAFLD by 35% ($p < 0.05$) than those in the lowest intake and in contrast higher grains-vegetables pattern, had a lower prevalence of NAFLD by 22% ($p < 0.05$). There were no significant effects on NAFLD for the other diets

(continued)

Table 10.1 (continued)

Objective	Study details	Results
Goletzke et al. (2013). Investigate longitudinal associations between carbohydrate quality (including dietary glycaemic index (GI) and intakes of sugar, starch and fiber) and markers of liver function in an older Australian population (Blue Mountains Eye Study; Australia) [75]	**Population-based cohort study:** 866 participants not confirmed with NAFLD; median age 67 years (≥49 years); 63% women; 5 years of follow-up; multi-level mixed regression analysis was used to relate dietary GI and sugar, starch and fiber intake to the liver enzymes alanine aminotransferase (ALT), g-glutamyltransferase (GGT), and fasting trigylcerides (multivariate adjusted)	Lower fiber intake was related to significantly higher GGT and fasting triglycerides levels, with fruit fiber being the most relevant fiber source for significantly lowering GGT and TG levels
Oddy et al. (2013). Examine prospective associations between dietary patterns and NAFLD in a population-based cohort of adolescents (Western Australian Pregnancy Cohort) [76]	**Prospective cohort study:** 995 adolescents; 54.1% overweight or obese at age 14 years; follow-up at age 17 years	NAFLD was present in 15% of adolescents. A higher Western dietary pattern score at 14 years was associated with a greater risk of NAFLD at 17 years by 59% ($p < 0.005$), although those associations were no longer significant after adjusting for BMI at 14 years. A healthy dietary pattern at 14 years appeared protective against NAFLD at 17 years in centrally obese adolescents by 37% ($p = 0.033$)
Mediterranean diet (MedDiet)		
Trovato et al. (2016). Investigate the effect of Mediterranean diet (MedDiet) lifestyle on NAFLD, with ultrasound-detected fatty liver, compared to non-alcoholic healthy subjects (Italy) [78]	**Case-control study:** 532 NAFLD and 667 non-NAFLD healthy subjects, mean age 48 years (21–60 years). The adherence to MedDiet score was assessed on the basis of a 1-wk. recall computerized questionnaire which included detailed physical activity reports. The Western dietary profile score, plus a questionnaire quantifying sun exposure score and sleep habits	Poorer adherence to a MedDiet profile, sedentary habits, less sun exposure and use of Western diet foods were greater in subjects with NAFLD. Multiple linear regression analysis, weighted by years of age, BMI, and insulin resistance (HOMA-IR) were the most powerful independent predictors of fatty liver severity
Aller et al. (2015). Explore potential associations between adherence to the MedDiet and histological characteristics of patients with NAFLD (Spain) [79]	**Cross-sectional study:** 82 patients; adherence to the MedDiet pattern by 14-item assessment; 43% had a low grade of steatosis (grade 1 of classification) and 57% had a high grade of steatosis (grade 2 and 3)	One unit increase in MedDiet score was associated with a lower likehood of having steatohepatitis by 57% and steatosis by 58%. Secondly, one unit of HOMA-IR was associated with higher odds of having steatosis by 101% and liver fibrosis by 38%
Kontogianni et al. (2014). Explore the impact of adherence to the MedDiet on the presence and severity of NAFLD (Greece) [80]	**Case-control study:** 58 NAFLD patients and 58 healthy controls matched by age, sex and body mass index	MedDiet score was negatively correlated to patients' serum ALT and insulin levels, insulin resistance index and severity of steatosis and positively to serum adiponectin levels. Patients with NASH had lower adherence to the MedDiet compared to those with simple fatty liver. One unit increase in the MedDietScore was associated with 36% lower likelihood of having NASH, after adjusting for sex and abdominal fat level

Table 10.1 (continued)

Objective	Study details	Results
Ryan et al. (2013). Examine effects of the MedDiet on steatosis and insulin sensitivity (Australia) [81]	**Cross-over RCT:** 12 non-diabetic subjects; 6 females/6 males; mean age 55 years; mean BMI 32; biopsy-proven NAFLD; MedDiet and a low fat-high carbohydrate diet; 6 weeks duration on each arm; 6 weeks of wash-out	Mean weight loss was not different between the two diets (p = 0.22). There was a significant reduction in hepatic steatosis after the MedDiet by 32% compared with the control diet (p = 0.012). Insulin sensitivity improved with the MedDiet vs. no change for the control diet (p = 0.03) (Fig. 10.6)
Dietary Approaches to Stop Hypertension (DASH)		
Zade et al. (2016). Determine the effects of the Dietary Approaches to Stop Hypertension (DASH) diet on weight loss and metabolic status in overweight patients with NAFLD (Iran) [84]	**Randomized controlled trial (RCT):** 60 NAFLD patients; mean age 41 years; mean BMI 28; 50% women; randomly allocated to calorie-restricted control or DASH dietary pattern; 8 weeks; 350–700 kcal/day restricted diets consisted of 52–55% carbohydrates, 16–18% proteins and 30% total fats; however, the DASH diet was designed to be rich in fruits, vegetables, whole grains, and low-fat dairy products and low in saturated fats, cholesterol and refined grains	Adherence to the energy restricted DASH pattern, compared to the calorie restricted control diet, significantly lowered weight, BMI, alanine aminotransferase, alkaline phosphatase, insulin levels, insulin resistance (HOMA-IR) and increased insulin sensitivity check index (QUICKI). Also, compared with the control diet, the DASH diet resulted in significant reductions in serum triglycerides and total-/HDL-cholesterol ratio, hs-CRP, malondialdehyde, increased levels of nitric oxide and glutathione. Also, significantly greater percentage of patients in the DASH group had greater decrease in the severity of NAFLD than those in the usual control diet (80% vs. 43%) and greater reduction in both waist and hip circumference (Fig. 10.7)
Hekmatdoost et al. (2016). Examine the association between adherence to the DASH diet and risk of NAFLD (Iran) [85]	**Case-control study:** 102 patients with newly diagnosed NAFLD and 204 controls. Adherence to DASH-style diet was assessed using a validated food frequency questionnaire, and a DASH diet score based on food and nutrients emphasized or minimized in the DASH diet	Participants in the top quartile of a DASH diet score were 30% less likely to have NAFLD; however, after more adjustment for dyslipidemia and BMI the risk was reduced to an insignificant 8%

fat content [65]. Low carbohydrate diets significantly decreased mean liver fat by 11.5%.

10.5.2 Energy Restricted/Weight Loss Diets

Three RCTs assessed effects of energy restricted diets on the management of NAFLD [66–68]. An Iranian double blind RCT (44 ultrasonography-proven overweight NAFLD patients; mean age 41 years; approx 50% men; two diets with reduced energy by 500 kcal with 25% vs. 40% energy from fat; 6 weeks) found that both restricted energy diets decreased liver enzymes regardless of their composition, while the reduced energy diet with 40% energy from fat was more effective than the 25% fat energy diet in reduction of body weight and triglycerides levels [66]. A Mexican RCT (9 women; mean age 46 years; mean BMI 38; energy controlled diets low carbohydrate vs. a low-fat; 6 months) showed that there was no difference in weight loss and aminotransferase levels between the two diets [67]. A US RCT (18 NAFLD subjects; 5 men and 13 women; mean age 45 years; BMI 35; diets: energy and carbohydrate-restricted (<20 g/day) vs. calorie restricted; 2 weeks) found similar weight loss in both diets but liver triglycerides decreased significantly more in carbohydrate-restricted subjects by 55% than in calorie-restricted subjects by 28% [68].

10.5.3 Dietary Pattern Quality

Eight observational studies provide insights regarding the effects of dietary pattern quality on NAFLD or NASH [69–76]. A 2017 Greek cross-sectional analysis (136 NAFLD patients) observed that a healthy dietary pattern including high consumption of low-fat dairy products, vegetables, fish, and optimal sleep duration were associated with lower insulin resistance and liver stiffness whereas a Western dietary pattern including high consumption of full-fat dairy products, refined cereals, potatoes, and red meat was associated with high insulin resistance independent of BMI and energy intake [69]. Also, a 2017 Greek case-control study (100 patients with ultrasound-proven NAFLD and 55 healthy controls; matched for age, sex, and BMI) found that NAFLD patients compared to controls consumed less vegetables and nuts, more sweets, drank less coffee, ate more sweets, and had a lower level of physical activity [71]. High sweets consumption increased NAFLD risk by 113%, after adjusting for multiple confounders, including body weight status. Optimal sleep duration was associated with lower NAFLD risk by 62%. A 2017 Hong Kong cross-sectional study (797 ethnic Chinese subjects; mean age 48 years, 42% were male; 28% diagnosed with NAFLD) demonstrated that a 10-unit (100 point scale) decrease in Diet Quality Index-International was associated with 24% increase in the odds of having NAFLD whereas an inverse association with NAFLD prevalence was observed with higher intake of vegetables and legumes, fruits and dried fruits, after multivariate adjustment [70]. A 2016 German case-control study (55 patients diagnosed with NAFLD were compared to an age and gender-matched cohort of 88 healthy individuals) and Longitudinal sub-group analysis (24 NAFLD patients; 16 males and 8 females; mean age 46 years; 6 months after receiving dietary advice) found that NAFLD patients consumed more daily calories (higher glucose and lower fiber and minerals/1000 kcals) compared with healthy controls [72]. This analysis showed that NAFLD patients who significantly reduced their caloric intake had lower liver enzyme levels. A 2016 Brazilian cross-sectional study (229 older adults; mean age 68 years; 45% with confirmed NAFLD) showed that NAFLD was inversely associated with higher adherence to the healthy pattern (included fruits, vegetables/legumes, white meat, olive oil, margarine and bread/ toast, and low in red meat) with a reduced risk by 30% whereas a snacking pattern was directly associated with an increased multivariate risk of 42% [73]. A 2015 Chinese cross-sectional study (999 subjects; mean age 51 years; 34.5% confirmed NAFLD cases) found that subjects in the highest quartile of the animal food pattern scores had greater prevalence of NAFLD by 35% than those in the lowest quartile whereas high intake of a whole grains and vegetable pattern had a lower prevalence of NAFLD by 22%, after adjusting for BMI [74]. Two 2013 Australian prospective studies demonstrated the importance of a healthy diet in preventing NAFLD in both adults and children [75, 76]. A population-based cohort from the Blue Mountains Eye Study (866 participants; median age 67 years; 63% women; 5-year follow-up) found that lower fiber intake was associated with higher gamma-glutamyltransferase (GGT) and fasting triglycerides levels [75]. An evaluation of adolescents associated with the Western Australian Pregnancy Cohort (95 adolescents; 54.1% overweight or obese at age 14 years; follow-up at age 17 years) found that 15% of the adolescents had NAFLD [76]. Also, this study showed that a higher Western dietary pattern score at age 14 years was associated with a greater risk of NAFLD at 17 years by 59%, whereas a healthy dietary pattern at 14 years appeared protective against NAFLD at 17 years in centrally obese adolescents by 37%.

10.5.4 Mediterranean Diet (MedDiet)

Among several specific dietary approaches that exert positive effects in NAFLD patients, the MedDiet improves risk factors associated with NAFLD and NASH, metabolic syndrome and diabetes [77]. The main dietary features of the MedDiet include extra virgin olive oil, fish, nuts, fruits, vegetables, beans, high-fiber breads with limited meat, cheese, and sweets. The liberal use of extra virgin olive oil enhances the bioavailability of fatsoluble antioxidant vitamins and phytochemicals from the MedDiet. Specifically, MedDiet mechanisms for

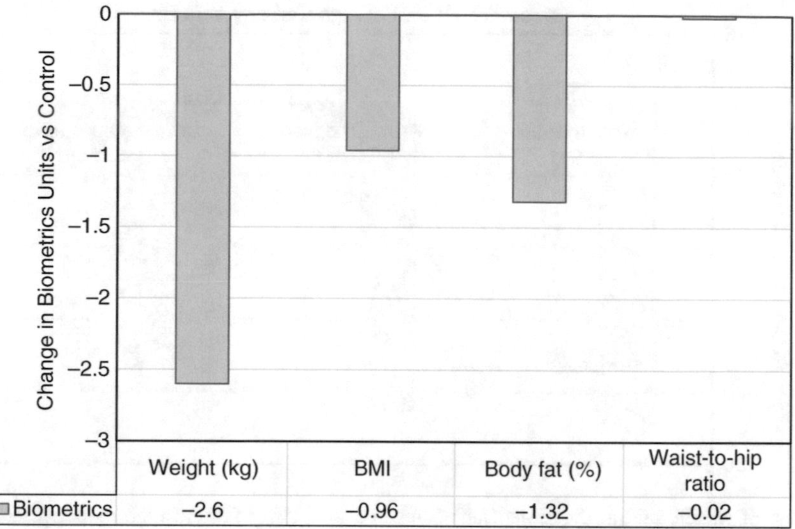

Fig. 10.5 Effect of oatmeal* as an isocaloric replacement for other foods on weight biometrics compared to control (double-blind RCT; p<.05 for all) (adapted from [46]). *Each serving of oatmeal contained 145 kcal with 3.7 g of fiber including 1.5 g of β-glucan mixed with 250 mL hot water twice daily

NAFLD protection include: fiber-rich foods which induce low glycemic response are beneficial for improved glucose and insulin metabolism; unsaturated fatty acids which are associated with better hepatic lipid metabolism; and antioxidant compounds, such as dietary polyphenols and carotenoids, which are thought to attenuate oxidation and inflammation. All these factors are thought to help to reduce NALFD risk and slow progression to NASH. Three observational [78–80] and two RCTs [81, 82] assessed the effects of the MedDiet on NAFLD or NASH risk and management. A 2016 Italian case-control study (532 NAFLD and 667 non-NAFLD healthy subjects; mean age 48 years) showed that poorer adherence to a MedDiet, sedentary habits, less sun exposure and use of "Western diet" foods were associated with greater NAFLD incidence [78]. Also, older age, higher BMI and elevated HOMA-IR were the strongest independent predictors of fatty liver severity. A 2015 Spanish cross-sectional study (82 NAFLD patients) found that a one unit increase in MedDiet score was associated with a lower likehood of having steatohepatitis by 57% and steatosis by 58% [79]. A 2014 Greek case-control study (58 NAFLD patients and 58 healthy controls matched by age, sex and body mass index) showed that the MedDiet score was negatively correlated to patients' serum alanine aminotransferase, insulin resistance index and severity of steatosis and positively to serum adiponectin levels [80]. Also, each unit increase in the MedDiet score was associated with 36% lower odds of NASH, after adjusting for sex and abdominal fat level. A 2013 Australian cross-over RCT (12 non-diabetic subjects; 6 females/6 males; mean age 55 years; mean BMI 32; with biopsy-proven NAFLD; MedDiet vs. a low fat-high carbohydrate diet; 6 weeks each, separated by a 6-week washout period) found that the mean weight loss was not different between the two diets but subjects on the MedDiet had a significant relative reduction in hepatic steatosis by 32% and increased insulin sensitivity compared with the low-fat, high carbohydrate diet (Fig. 10.6) [81]. A 2017 Italian double-blind RCT (98 adults with NAFLD; low glycemic index MedDiet vs usual (control) diet; 6 months) showed that the MedDiet significantly reduced NAFLD severity compared to the control diet [82].

10.5.5 Dietary Approaches to Stop Hypertension (DASH)

The DASH diet is rich in fruits, vegetables, whole grains, and low-fat dairy foods; includes meat, fish, poultry, nuts, and beans; and is limited

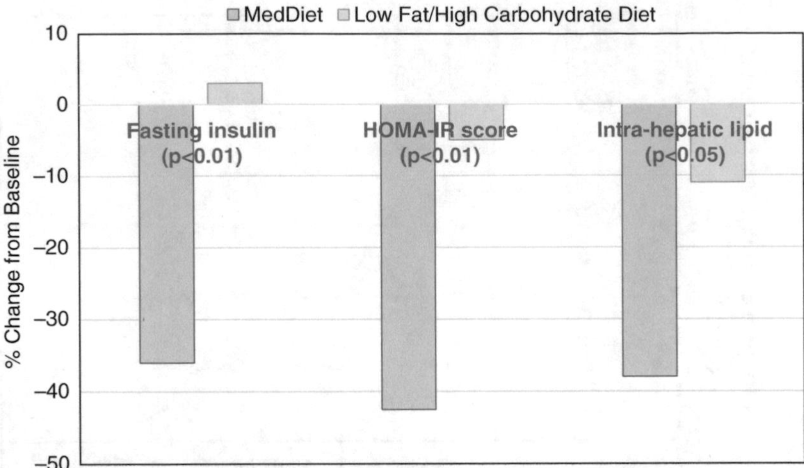

Fig. 10.6 Effect of Mediterranean diet (MedDiet) compared to a lower-fat and high carbohydrate diet from randomised, crossover 6-week trial which included 12 non-diabetic subjects (6 females/6 males) with biopsy-proven NAFLD risk factors (adapted from [81])

in sugar-sweetened foods and beverages, red meat, and added fats for a wide range of health and chronic disease risk reduction benefits [82]. A 2017 meta-analysis (7 RCTs) found that adherence to the DASH diet is effective in improving circulating serum inflammatory biomarkers in adults, compared with a usual diet; therefore, it could be an effective dietary option to suppress liver inflammation process [83]. A 2016 RCT (60 NAFLD patients; mean age 41 years; mean BMI 28; 50% women; randomly allocated to calorie-restricted DASH diet or control usual diet; 8 weeks) showed that the adherence to the energy restricted DASH pattern, compared to the energy restricted usual diet, significantly improved weight, BMI, waist size, liver enzymes, markers of insulin metabolism, serum triglycerides, hs-CRP, plasma malondialdehyde (MDA), nitric oxide (NO) and glutathione (GSH) levels [84]. Also, a significantly greater percentage of patients in the DASH group had decreased grade of NAFLD than those in the control group (80% vs. 43%) and greater reduction in both waist and hip circumference (Fig. 10.7). A 2016 case-control study (102 patients with newly diagnosed NAFLD and 204 controls) found that a higher DASH diet score was associated with 30% lower risk of NAFLD but after adjustment for dyslipidemia and BMI the risk changed to an insignificant 8% reduction [85].

Conclusions

NAFLD is the most common cause of chronic liver disease in the world and its prevalence is increasing concurrently with the obesity pandemic. The high prevalence of NAFLD is generally due to unhealthy high energy dietary patterns and sedentary lifestyles leading to obesity, insulin resistance and metabolic syndrome, which are strongly associated with elevated hepatic steatosis and increased diabetes risk. Excessive caloric intake, especially from high intake of refined carbohydrates and saturated fat, promotes increased

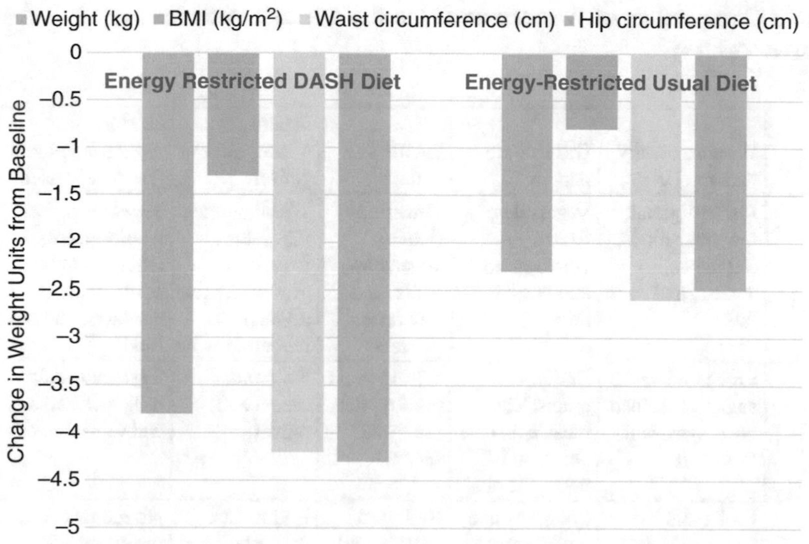

Fig. 10.7 Effect of energy restriction Dietary Approaches to Stop Hypertension (DASH) and usual diets by 350-700 kcal on body weight and composition in persons with NAFLD ($p < .01$ for all) (adapted from [84])

fatty liver. High intake of added sugar such sugar sweetened beverages tends to be a stronger promoter of enzymes involved in hepatic de novo lipogenesis and NAFLD than higher-fat diets. Certain nutrients and phytochemicals such as omega-3 fatty acids, monounsaturated fatty acids, fiber, vitamin E, carotenoids, flavonoids and caffeine, and foods and beverages including oily fish, extra virgin olive oil, oatmeal, coffee, and soy are associated with lower risk of NAFLD or its complications. Higher quality diets including moderate energy intake, higher intake of whole (minimally processed) plant foods, and low-fat dairy, and lower intake of red and processed meat and added sugar and salt, and adequate physical activity and sleep are associated with prevention and management of NAFLD. The Western lifestyle is associated with higher NAFLD risk and progression to NASH. Higher adherence to a MedDiet or DASH diets, especially if energy controlled, may be effective in managing NAFLD risk and complications.

Appendix A: Comparison of Western and Healthy Dietary Patterns per 2000 kcal (Approximated Values)

Components	Western dietary pattern (US)	USDA base pattern	DASH diet pattern	Healthy Mediterranean pattern	Healthy vegetarian pattern (Lact-ovo based)	Vegan pattern
Emphasizes	Refined grains, low fiber foods, red meats, sweets, and solid fats	Vegetables, fruit, whole-grain, and low-fat milk	Potassium rich vegetables, fruits, and low fat milk products	Whole grains, vegetables, fruit, dairy products, olive oil, and moderate wine	Vegetables, fruit, whole-grains, legumes, nuts, seeds, milk products, and soy foods	Plant foods: vegetables, fruits, whole grains, nuts, seeds, and soy foods
Includes	Processed meats, sugar sweetened beverages, and fast foods	Enriched grains, lean meat, fish, nuts, seeds, and vegetable oils	Whole-grain, poultry, fish, nuts, and seeds	Fish, nuts, seeds, and pulses	Eggs, non-dairy milk alternatives, and vegetable oils	Non-dairy milk alternatives
Limits	Fruits and vegetables, and whole-grains	Solid fats and added sugars	Red meats, sweets, and sugar-sweetened beverages	Red meats, refined grains, and sweets	No red or white meats, or fish; limited sweets	No animal products
Estimated Nutrients/Components						
Carbohydrates (% Total kcal)	51	51	55	50	54	57
Protein (% Total kcal)	16	17	18	16	14	13
Total fat (% Total kcal)	33	32	27	34	32	30
Saturated fat (% Total kcal)	11	8	6	8	8	7
Unsat. fat (% Total kcal)	22	25	21	24	26	25
Fiber (g)	16	31	29+	31	35+	40+
Potassium (mg)	2800	3350	4400	3350	3300	3650
Vegetable oils (g)	19	27	25	27	19–27	18–27
Sodium (mg)	3600	1790	1100	1690	1400	1225
Added sugar (g)	79 (20 tsp.)	32 (8 tsp.)	12 (3 tsp.)	32 (8 tsp.)	32 (8 tsp.)	32 (8 tsp.)
Plant Food Groups						
Fruit (cup)	≤1.0	2.0	2.5	2.5	2.0	2.0
Vegetables (cup)	≤1.5	2.5	2.1	2.5	2.5	2.5
Whole-grains (oz.)	0.6	3.0	4.0	3.0	3.0	3.0
Legumes (oz.)	–	1.5	0.5	1.5	3.0	3.0+
Nuts/seeds (oz.)	0.5	0.6	1.0	0.6	1.0	2.0
Soy products (oz.)	0.0	0.5	–	–	1.1	1.5

U.S. Department of Agriculture, Agriculture Research Service, Nutrient Data Laboratory. 2014. USDA National Nutrient Database for Standard Reference, Release 27. http://www.ars.usda.gov/nutrientdata. Accessed 17 Feb 2015

Dietary Guidelines Advisory Committee. Scientific Report. Advisory Report to the Secretary of Health and Human Services and the Secretary of Agriculture. Appendix E-3.7: Developing vegetarian and Mediterranean-style food patterns. 2015;1–9

U.S. Department of Agriculture and U.S. Department of Health and Human Services. Dietary Guidelines for Americans, 2010. 7th ed. Washington, DC: U.S. Government Printing Office; 2010. Table B2.4; http://www.choosemyplate.gov/. Accessed 22 Aug 2015

References

1. Rinella ME. Nonalcoholic fatty liver disease a systematic review. JAMA. 2015;313(22):2263–73.
2. Tiniakos DG, Vos MB, Brunt EM. Nonalcoholic fatty liver disease: pathology and pathogenesis. Annu Rev Pathol. 2010;5:145–71.
3. Younossi ZM, Blissert D, Blissert R, et al. The economic and clinical burden of nonalcoholic fatty liver disease in the United States and Europe. Hepatology. 2016;64:1577–86.
4. Dongiovanni P, Valenti L. A nutrigenomic approach to non-alcoholic fatty liver disease. Int J Mol Sci. 2017; 18:1534.
5. Williams CD, Stengel J, Asike MI, et al. Prevalence of nonalcoholic fatty liver disease and nonalcoholic steatohepatitis among a largely middle-aged population utilizing ultrasound and liver biopsy: a prospective study. Gastroenterology. 2011;140(1):124–31.
6. Tovo CV, Fernandes SA, Buss C, de Mattos AA. Sarcopenia and non-alcoholic fatty liver disease: is there a relationship? A systematic review. World J Hepatol. 2017;9(6):326–32. https://doi.org/10.4254/wjh.v9.i6.326.
7. Schwenger KJP, Allard JP. Clinical approaches to non-alcoholic fatty liver disease. World J Gastroenterol. 2014;20(7):1712–23.
8. Conlon BA, Beasley JM, Aebersold K, et al. Nutritional management of insulin resistance in non-alcoholic fatty liver disease (NAFLD). Forum Nutr. 2013;5:4093–114.
9. Hashiba M, Ono M, Hyogo H, et al. Glycemic variability is an independent predictive factor for development of hepatic fibrosis in nonalcoholic fatty liver disease. PLoS One. 2013;8(11):e76161.
10. Polimeni L, Ben MD, Baratta F, et al. Oxidative stress: new insights on the association of nonalcoholic fatty liver disease and atherosclerosis. World J Hepatol. 2015;7(10):1325–36.
11. Papandreou D, Andreou E. Role of diet on non-alcoholic fatty liver disease: an updated narrative review. World J Hepatol. 2015;7(3):575–82.
12. Vreman RA, Goodell AJ, Rodriquez LA, et al. Health and economic benefits of reducing sugar intake in the USA, including effects via non-alcoholic fatty liver disease: a microsimulation model. BMJ Open. 2017;7:e013543.
13. Smits MM, Ioannou GN, Boyko EJ, Utzschneider KM. Non-alcoholic fatty liver disease as an independent manifestation of the metabolic syndrome: results of a US national survey in three ethnic groups. J Gastroenterol Hepatol. 2013;28:664–70.
14. Zelber-Sagi S, Ratziu V, Oren R. Nutrition and physical activity in NAFLD: an overview of the epidemiological evidence. World J Gastroenterol. 2011;17:3377–89.
15. Zolfaghari H, Askari G, Siassi F, et al. Intake of nutrients, fiber, and sugar in patients with nonalcoholic fatty liver disease in comparison to healthy individuals. Int J Prev Med. 2016;7:98.
16. Marchesini G, Petta S, Dalle Grave R. Diet, weight loss, and liver health in nonalcoholic fatty liver disease: pathophysiology, evidence, and practice. Hepatology. 2016;63(6):2032–43. https://doi.org/10.1002/hep.28392.
17. Softic S, Cohen DE, Kahn CR. Role of dietary fructose and hepatic de novo lipogenesis in fatty liver disease. Dig Dis Sci. 2016;61(5):1282–93. https://doi.org/10.1007/s10620-016-4054-0.
18. Sevastianova K, Santos A, Kotronen A, et al. Effect of short-term carbohydrate overfeeding and long-term weight loss on liver fat in overweight humans. Am J Clin Nutr. 2012;96:727–34.
19. Siddiqi Z, Karoli R, Fatima J, et al. Soft drink consumption and the risk of nonalcoholic fatty liver disease. J Assoc Physicians India. 2017;65(5):28–32.
20. Jiménez-Cruz A, Gómez-Miranda LM, Ramírez GD, et al. Adiposity as a risk factor of nonalcoholic fat disease: a systemic review. Nutr Hosp. 2014;29(4):771–5.
21. Pang Q, Zhang JY, Song SD, et al. Central obesity and non-alcoholic fatty liver disease risk after adjusting for body mass index. World J Gastroenterol. 2015;21(5):1650–62. https://doi.org/10.3748/wjg.v21.i5.1650.
22. Zimmermann E, Gamborg M, Holst C, et al. Body mass index in school-aged children and the risk of routinely diagnosed non-alcoholic fatty liver disease in adulthood: a prospective study based on the Copenhagen School Health Records Register. BMJ Open. 2015;5:e006998.
23. Ratziu V, Bellentani S, Cortez-Pinto H, et al. A position statement on NAFLD/NASH based on the EASL 2009 special conference. J Hepatol. 2010;53:372–84.
24. Copaci I, Lupescu I, Caceaune E, et al. Noninvasive markers of improvement of liver steatosis achieved by weight reduction in patients with nonalcoholic fatty liver disease. Rom J Intern Med. 2015;53(1):54–62.
25. Montesi L, Caselli C, Centis E, et al. Physical activity support or weight loss counseling for nonalcoholic fatty liver disease. World J Gastroenterol. 2014;20(29):10128–36.
26. Hsu CC, Erik Ness E, Kowdley KV. Nutritional approaches to achieve weight loss in nonalcoholic fatty liver disease. Adv Nutr. 2017;8:253–65.
27. Wong VW, Chan RS, Wong GL, et al. Community-based lifestyle modification programme for non-alcoholic fatty liver disease: a randomized controlled trial. J Hepatol. 2013;59:536–42.
28. Grønbaek H, Lange A, Birkebaek NH, et al. Effect of a 10-week weight-loss camp on fatty liver disease and insulin sensitivity in obese Danish children. J Pediatr Gastroenterol Nutr. 2012;54(2):223–8.
29. Promrat K, Kleiner DE, Niemeier HM, et al. Randomized controlled trial testing the effects of weight loss on nonalcoholic steatohepatitis (NASH). Hepatology. 2010;51(1):121–9.
30. Gupta V, Mah XJ, Garcia MC, et al. Oily fish, coffee and walnuts: dietary treatment for nonalcoholic fatty liver disease. World J Gastroenterol. 2015;21(37):10621–35. https://doi.org/10.3748/wjg.v21.i37.10621.

31. Ferramosca A, Zara V. Modulation of hepatic steatosis by dietary fatty acids. World J Gastroenterol. 2014;20(7):1746–55. https://doi.org/10.3748/wjg.v20.i7.1746.
32. Lu W, Li S, Li J, et al. Effects of omega-3 fatty acid in nonalcoholic fatty liver disease: a meta-analysis. Gastroenterol Res Pract. 2016;1459790. https://doi.org/10.1155/2016/1459790.
33. He X-X, Wu X-L, Chen R-P, et al. Effectiveness of omega-3 polyunsaturated fatty acids in non-alcoholic fatty liver disease: a meta-analysis of randomized controlled trials. PLoS One. 2016;11(10):e0162368. https://doi.org/10.1371/journal.pone.0162368.
34. Di Minno MND, Russolillo A, Lupoli R, et al. Omega-3 fatty acids for the treatment of non-alcoholic fatty liver disease. World J Gastroenterol. 2012;18(41):5839–47. https://doi.org/10.3748/wjg.v18.i41.5839.
35. Finelli C, Tarantino G. Is there any consensus as to what diet or lifestyle approach is the right one for NAFLD patients? J Gastrointest Liver Dis. 2012;21(3):293–302.
36. Bozzetto L, Prinster A, Annuzzi G, et al. Liver fat is reduced by an isoenergetic MUFA diet in a controlled randomized study in type 2 diabetic patients. Diabetes Care. 2012;35:1429–35.
37. Priore P, Cavallo A, Gnoni A, et al. Modulation of hepatic lipid metabolism by olive oil and its phenols in nonalcoholic fatty liver disease. IUBMB Life. 2015;67(1):9–17.
38. European Food Safety Authority (EFSA). EFSA panel on dietetic products, nutrition, and allergies. Opinion on dietary reference values for carbohydrates and dietary fibre. EFSA J. 2010;8(3):1462.
39. Liu S, Willett WC, Manson JE, et al. Relation between changes in intakes of dietary fiber and grain products and changes in weight and development of obesity among middle-aged women. Am J Clin Nutr. 2003;78:920–7.
40. Slavin JL. Dietary fiber and body weight. Nutrition. 2005;21:411–8.
41. Lindstrom J, Peltonen M, Eriksson JG, et al. High-fibre, low-fat diet predicts long-term weight loss and decreased type 2 diabetes risk: the Finnish Diabetes Prevention Study. Diabetologia. 2006;49:912–20.
42. Tucker LA, Thomas KS. Increasing total fiber intake reduces risk of weight and fat gains in women. J Nutr. 2009;139:576–81.
43. Fogelholm M, Anderssen S, Gunnarsdottir I, Lahti-Koski M. Dietary macronutrients and food consumption as determinants of long-term weight change in adult populations: a systematic literature review. Food Nutr Res. 2012;56:19103.
44. Romaguera D, Angquist L, Du H, et al. Dietary determinants of changes in waist circumference adjusted for body mass index—a proxy measure of visceral adiposity. PLoS One. 2010;5(7):e11588.
45. Du H, van der AD, Boshuizen HC, et al. Dietary fiber and subsequent changes in body weight and waist circumference in European men and women. Am J Clin Nutr. 2010;91:329–36.
46. Chang H-C, Huang C-N, Yeh D-M, et al. Oat prevents obesity and abdominal fat distribution and improves liver function in humans. Plant Foods Hum Nutr. 2013;68:18–23. https://doi.org/10.1007/ s11130-013-0336-2.
47. Ma Y, Olendzki BC, Wang J, et al. Single-component versus multicomponent dietary goals for the metabolic syndrome a randomized trial. Ann Intern Med. 2015;162:248–57.
48. Yoneda M, Mawatari H, Fujita K, et al. High-sensitivity C-reactive protein is an independent clinical feature of nonalcoholic steatohepatitis (NASH) and also of the severity of fibrosis in NASH. J Gastroenterol. 2007;42(7):573–82.
49. Maleki I, Rastgar A, Hosseini V, et al. High sensitive CRP and pentraxine 3 as noninvasive biomarkers of nonalcoholic fatty liver disease. Eur Rev Med Pharmacol Sci. 2014;18(11):1583–90.
50. Federic A, Dallio M, Caprio GG, et al. Qualitative and quantitative evaluation of dietary intake in patients with non-alcoholic steatohepatitis. Nutrients. 2017; 9:1074.
51. Jiao J, Xu JY, Zhang W, et al. Effect of dietary fiber on circulating C-reactive protein in overweight and obese adults: a meta-analysis of randomized controlled trials. Int J Food Sci Nutr. 2015;66(1):114–9. https://doi.org/10.3109/09637486.2014.959898.
52. Ortiz-Lopez C, Lomonaco R, Orsak B, et al. Prevalence of prediabetes and diabetes and metabolic profile of patients with nonalcoholic fatty liver disease (NAFLD). Diabetes Care. 2012;35:873–8.
53. Yao B, Fang H, Xu W, et al. Dietary fiber intake and risk of type 2 diabetes: a dose-response analysis of prospective studies. Eur J Epidemiol. 2014;29(2):79–88.
54. The InterAct Consortium. Dietary fibre and incidence of type 2 diabetes in eight European countries: the EPIC-InterAct Study and a meta-analysis of prospective studies. Diabetologia. 2015;58(7):1394–408. https://doi.org/10.1007/s00125-015-3585-3589.
55. Mokhtari Z, Gibson DL, Hekmatdoost A. Nonalcoholic fatty liver disease, the gut microbiome, and diet. Adv Nutr. 2017;8:240–52.
56. Karkman A, Lehtimäki J, Ruokolainen L. The ecology of human microbiota: dynamics and diversity in health and disease. Ann N Y Acad Sci. 2017;1399(1):78–92. https://doi.org/10.1111/nyas.13326.
57. Wijarnpreechaa K, Thongprayoona C, Ungprasertb P. Coffee consumption and risk of nonalcoholic fatty liver disease: a systematic review and meta-analysis. Eur J Gastroenterol Hepatol. 2017;29(2):e8–e12. https://doi.org/10.1097/MEG.0000000000000776.
58. Sato K, Gosho M, Yamamoto T, et al. Vitamin E has a beneficial effect on nonalcoholic fatty acid disease: a meta-analysis of randomized controlled trials. Nutrition. 2015;31(7–8):923–30.
59. Xu R, Tao A, Zhang S. Association between vitamin E and non-alcoholic steatohepatitis: a meta-analysis. Int J Clin Exp Med. 2015;8(3):3924–34.

60. Yilmaz B, Sahin K, Bilen H, et al. Carotenoids and non-alcoholic fatty liver disease. Hepatobiliary Surg Nutr. 2015;4(3):161–71. https://doi.org/10.3978/j.issn.2304-3881.2015.01.11.
61. Sugiura M, Nakamura M, Ogawa K, et al. High serum carotenoids are associated with lower risk for developing elevated serum alanine aminotransferase among Japanese subjects: the Mikkabi cohort study. Br J Nutr. 2016;115:1462–9. https://doi.org/10.1017/S0007114516000374.
62. Cao Y, Wang C, Liu J, et al. Greater serum carotenoid levels associated with lower prevalence of nonalcoholic fatty liver disease in Chinese adults. Sci Rep. 2015;5:12951. https://doi.org/10.1038/ srep12951.
63. Van De Wier B, Koek GH, Bast A, et al. The potential of flavonoids in the treatment of non-alcoholic fatty liver disease. Crit Rev Food Sci Nutr. 2017;57(4):834–55. https://doi.org/10.1080/10408398.2014.952399.
64. Kani AH, Alavian SM, Esmaillzadeh A, et al. Effects of a novel therapeutic diet on liver enzymes and coagulating factors in patients with non-alcoholic fatty liver disease: a parallel randomized trial. Nutrition. 2014;30:814–21.
65. Haghighatdoost F, Salehi-Abargouei A, Surkan PJ, Azadbakht L. The effects of low carbohydrate diets on liver function tests in nonalcoholic fatty liver disease: a systematic review and meta-analysis of clinical trials. J Res Med Sci. 2016;21:53.
66. Arefhosseini SR, Ebrahimi-Mameghani M, Farsad Naeimi A, et al. Lifestyle modification through dietary intervention: health promotion of patients with nonalcoholic fatty liver disease. Health Promot Perspect. 2011;1:147–54.
67. Rodriguez-Hernandez H, Cervantes-Huerta M, Rodriguez-Moran M, Guerrero-Romero F. Decrease of aminotransferase levels in obese women is related to body weight reduction, irrespective of type of diet. Ann Hepatol. 2011;10:486–92.
68. Browning JD, Baker JA, Rogers T, Davis J, et al. Short-term weight loss and hepatic triglyceride reduction: evidence of a metabolic advantage with dietary carbohydrate restriction. Am J Clin Nutr. 2011;93:1048–52.
69. Katsagoni CN, Georgoulis M, Papatheodoridis GVA, et al. Associations between lifestyle characteristics and the presence of nonalcoholic fatty liver disease: a case-control study. Metab Syndr Relat Disord. 2017;15(2):72–9. https://doi.org/10.1089/met.2016.0105.
70. Chan R, Wong VW-S, Chu WC-W, et al. Diet-quality scores and prevalence of nonalcoholic fatty liver disease: a population study using proton-magnetic resonance spectroscopy. PLoS One. 2017;10(9):e0139310. https://doi.org/10.1371/journal.pone.0139310.
71. Katsagoni CN, Papatheodoridis GV, Papageorgiou MV, et al. A "healthy diet-optimal sleep" lifestyle pattern is inversely associated with liver stiffness and insulin resistance in patients with nonalcoholic fatty liver disease. Appl Physiol Nutr Metab. 2017;42(3):250–6. https://doi.org/10.1139/apnm-2016-0492.
72. Wehmeyer MH, Zyriax B-C, Jagemann B, et al. Nonalcoholic fatty liver disease is associated with excessive calorie intake rather than a distinctive dietary pattern. Medicine. 2016;95:23. https://doi.org/10.1097/MD.0000000000003887.
73. Adriano LS, de Carvalho Sampaio HA, Arruda SPM, et al. Healthy dietary pattern is inversely associated with non-alcoholic fatty liver disease in elderly. Br J Nutr. 2016;115:2189–95. https://doi.org/10.1017/S0007114516001410.
74. Yang C-Q, Shu L, Wang S, et al. Dietary patterns modulate the risk of non-alcoholic fatty liver disease in Chinese adults. Forum Nutr. 2015;7:4778–91.
75. Goletzke J, Buyken AE, Gopinath B, et al. Carbohydrate quality is not associated with liver enzyme activity and plasma TAG and HDL concentrations over 5 years in an older population. Br J Nutr. 2013;110: 918–25.
76. Oddy WH, Herbison CE, Jacoby P, et al. The western dietary pattern is prospectively associated with nonalcoholic fatty liver disease in adolescence. Am J Gastroenterol. 2013;108:778–85.
77. Godos J, Federico A, Dallio M, Scazzina F. Mediterranean diet and nonalcoholic fatty liver disease: molecular mechanisms of protection. Int J Food Sci Nutr. 2017;68(1):18–27. https://doi.org/10.1080/09637486.2016.1214239.
78. Trovato FM, Martines GF, Brischetto D, Trovato G, Catalano D. Neglected features of lifestyle: their relevance in non-alcoholic fatty liver disease. World J Hepatol. 2016;8(33):1459–65. https://doi.org/10.4254/wjh. v8. i33.1459.
79. Aller R, Izaola O, de la Fuente B, de Luis D. Mediterranean diet is associated with liver histology in patients with non-alcoholic fatty liver disease. Nutr Hosp. 2015;32(6):2518–24.
80. Kontogianni MD, Tileli N, Margariti A, et al. Adherence to the Mediterranean diet is associated with the severity of non-alcoholic fatty liver disease. Clin Nutr. 2014;33(4):678–83.
81. Ryan MC, Itsiopoulos C, Thodis T, et al. The Mediterranean diet improves hepatic steatosis and insulin sensitivity in individuals with non-alcoholic fatty liver disease. J Hepatol. 2013;59:138–43.
82. Misciagna G, Del Pilar Diaz M, Caramin DV, et al. Effect of s low glycemic index Mediterranean diet on non-clacholic fatty liver disease. A randomized controlled clinical trial. J Nutr. 2017;21(4):404–12.
83. Soltani S, Chitsazi MJ, Salehi-Abargouei A. The effect of dietary approaches to stop hypertension (DASH) on serum inflammatory markers: a systematic review and meta-analysis of randomized trials. Clin Nutr. 2017. https://doi.org/10.1016/j.clnu.2017.02.018.
84. Zade MR, Telkabadi MH, Bahmani F, et al. The effects of DASH diet on weight loss and metabolic status in adults with non-alcoholic fatty liver disease: a randomized clinical trial. Liver Int. 2016;36:563–71. https://doi.org/10.1111/liv.12990.
85. Hekmatdoost A, Shamsipour A, Melbodi M, et al. Adherence to the Dietary Approaches to Stop Hypertension (DASH) and risk of nonalcoholic fatty liver disease. Int J Food Sci Nutr. 2016;67(8):1024–9. https://doi.org/10.1080/09637486.2016.1210101.

Part IV

Cardiovascular and Cerebrovascular Diseases, and Age-Related Cognitive Function

Dietary Patterns and Coronary Heart Disease

11

Keywords

Dietary patterns • Mediterranean diet • DASH diet • Vegetarian diet • Western diet • Coronary heart disease • Carotid initima-media thickness • Lipoproteins • C-reactive protein

Key Points

- Globally coronary heart disease (CHD) is the leading cause of death and morbidity in adults. The type of dietary pattern consumed plays an important role in the risk of developing CHD.
- Healthy dietary patterns (or higher nutrient quality diets) which are associated with decreased risk of CHD include higher Healthy Eating Indices scores, Mediterranean diet (MedDiet), Dietary Approaches to Stop Hypertension (DASH) and vegetarian diets and are characterized by higher consumption of vegetables, fruits, whole-grains, low-fat dairy, and seafood, limited (or no) intake of red and processed meat, and lower intakes of refined grains, sugar-sweetened foods and beverages compared to an increased CHD risk associated with higher adherence to Western dietary patterns.
- Healthy dietary patterns have CHD protective effects because they are lower in energy density and higher in fiber, healthier fatty acid profiles, essential nutrients, antioxidants, and electrolytes, and are anti-inflammatory compared with Western diets.
- Meta-analyses estimate that healthy dietary patterns are associated with a significantly decreased CHD risk by 20–33%, while Western-type patterns are associated with an increased CHD risk by up to 45%, especially in US studies and in individuals over 50 years of age.
- A number of randomized controlled trials (RCTs) support the role for healthy dietary patterns in reducing CHD risk biomarkers including blood lipids and lipoproteins, systemic inflammatory or oxidative stress factors such as hs-CRP and oxidized LDL-C, and carotid atherosclerosis and improving endothelial health and blood pressure.
- Replacing 5% of energy intake from saturated fats with equivalent energy intake from polyunsaturated and monounsaturated fats, or carbohydrates from whole grains was associated with a significant 25%, 15%, and 9% lower risk of CHD, respectively. However, replacing saturated fat with carbohydrates from refined

M.L. Dreher, *Dietary Patterns and Whole Plant Foods in Aging and Disease*, Nutrition and Health,
https://doi.org/10.1007/978-3-319-59180-3_11

starches and/or added sugars was not significantly associated with lower CHD risk.

11.1 Introduction

Globally coronary heart disease (CHD) is the leading cause of death and morbidity in adults [1, 2]. While CHD death rates have declined over the years because of diagnostic intensity and treatment, the number of deaths remains high and this is expected to increase regardless of ethnicity with the global aging of populations [1–4]. CHD affects both men and women with prevalence increasing after the fifth decade of life in men and the sixth decade of life in women [5]. In the USA, heart disease effects someone every 43 seconds, killing over 375,000 people a year [6]. Heart disease is the leading cause of death in women, causing more deaths than all forms of cancer combined. The lifetime risk of developing heart disease after age 40 is approximately 49% for men and 32% for women. Between 2015 and 2030, annual US costs related to CHD and related atherosclerotic cardiovascular diseases are forecasted to increase from $84.8 to $202 billion.

Healthy lifestyles play an important role in preventing and managing CHD risk and include nonsmoking status, BMI <25, physical activity at goal levels, and a diet consistent with the dietary guidelines [7–11]. However, less than 1% of Americans meet all four ideal lifestyle criteria for cardiovascular health [6, 12]. Suboptimal diet quality is a leading risk factor for CHD [6] and less than 5% of the US population meet all the American Heart Association's (AHA) definition of an ideal healthy diet including consuming fruit and vegetables at ≥4.5 cups/day; whole-grains at ≥3 servings/day; fish at ≥ two 3.5 oz. servings/week; sodium at ≤2300 mg/day and sugar sweetened beverages at ≤36 oz./week) [12]. Despite the subjects consuming above the the recommended energy intake by 22% for women and 10% for men, high adherence to the AHA healthy dietary criteria has been shown to reduce the risk of BMI increase, a major risk factor for CHD (Fig. 11.1) [12]. The average US Dietary Guidelines based Healthy Eating Index score for adults is only about half the ideal healthy diet score needed to reduce CHD risk (Fig. 11.2) [13]. Thus, Americans are at heightened CHD risk levels with about 43% of American adults having total cholesterol of

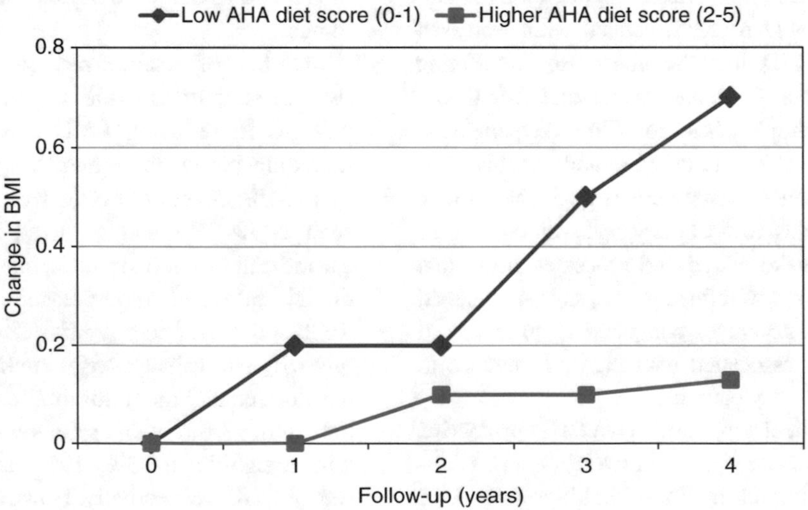

Fig. 11.1 Association between adherence to the American Heart Association's (AHA) healthy diet* and BMI over 4 years in young adults (p = 0.03) (adapted from [12]). *AHA's healthy diet: fruit and vegetables ≥4.5 cups/day; whole-grains ≥3 servings/day; fish ≥ two 3.5 oz. serving/week; sodium ≤2300 mg/day and sugar sweetened beverages ≤36 oz./week)

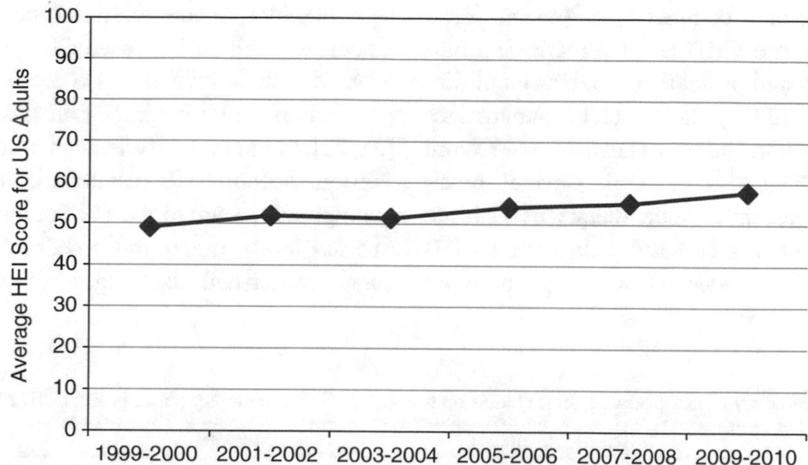

Fig. 11.2 The average US Dietary Guidelines based Healthy Eating Index (HEI) score for adults from NHANES data over 10 years (adapted from [13])

200 mg/dL or higher [6]. The French Three City Study in elderly adults (9,294 participants; 37% men; mean baseline age 74 years; median follow-up of 10.9 years) found a 67% lower risk of CHD and stroke with the highest adherence to a healthy lifestyle including a healthy diet [9]. The participants healthier lifestyles had lower BMIs, systolic blood pressure, total cholesterol, glycemia and higher HDL-cholesterol levels. Another study showed that bowel movement frequency is inversely associated with CHD mortality as a dysfunctional colon from poor quality diets may contribute to systemic oxidative and inflammatory stress [11]. The objective of this chapter is to review the effects of dietary patterns on CHD risk and its primary biomarkers.

11.2 Dietary Patterns and CHD Risk

The type of dietary pattern consumed has an important role in affecting the risk of developing CHD. Prospective cohort studies and randomized controlled trials (RCTs) have consistently demonstrated that healthy dietary patterns compared to Western dietary patterns exert clinically meaningful lowering of CHD risk and associated risk factors, including improving blood lipid profiles and maintaining normal blood pressure levels based on reduction of dietary energy density, saturated fat, cholesterol, and sodium and increased intake of fiber, potassium, and unsaturated fats [8–15]. Healthy dietary patterns have CHD protective effects because they influence a number of biological mechanisms including lowering fasting lipid profiles, circulating inflammation, abdominal and visceral fat, blood pressure; and improving insulin sensitivity and microbiota health [6–20]. The 2015 Dietary Guidelines Advisory Committee concluded that strong and consistent evidence demonstrates that healthy dietary patterns, characterized by higher consumption of vegetables, fruits, whole-grains, low-fat dairy, and seafood, and lower consumption of red and processed meat, and lower intakes of refined grains, and sugar-sweetened foods and beverages are associated with decreased CHD risk relative to high adherence to Western patterns [19]. Healthy dietary patterns based on the US Dietary Guidelines, Dietary Approaches to Stop Hypertension (DASH), Mediterranean diet (MedDiet), lacto-ovovegetarian or healthy vegan diets vs. the Western-type pattern are summarized in Appendix A.

11.2.1 Healthy vs. Western Dietary Patterns

Healthy diets reduce CHD risk by reducing known biomarker levels and slowing progression of atherosclerosis compared to Western diets known to elevate CHD risk by increasing biomarker levels and promoting progression of atherosclerosis [20]. Table 11.1 summarizes prospective cohort studies on healthy and Western diets and CHD risk [21–26]. Several meta-analyses suggest that healthy dietary patterns are associated with a significantly decreased CHD risk by 20–35% independent of age or other demographics, while Western-type patterns are associated with an increased CHD risk by up to 53% in studies involving US adults, but Asian populations had 15% increased risk (Fig. 11.3) [21, 22]. Studies on the effects of specific types of Western diets on CHD risk include the following: (1) high adherence to the US Southern diet, rich in fried foods, organ and processed meats, and sugar sweetened beverages (17,418 adults;

Table 11.1 Summary of prospective cohort studies on healthy vs. Western dietary patterns and CHD risk

Objective	Study details	Results
Systematic reviews and meta-analyses		
Zhang et al. (2015). Evaluate the effects of dietary patterns and the risk of CHD [21]	28 cohorts and 7 case-control; 983,484 participants	Healthy dietary patterns significantly decreased risk of CHD by 33% (highest vs. lowest adherence). Western-type dietary patterns increased CHD risk by 45% (highest vs. lowest adherence) (Fig. 11.3)
Hou et al. (2015). Examine potential associations between dietary patterns and CHD [22]	12 prospective studies; 409,780 participants; 6298 CHD cases	Highest adherence to a healthy dietary pattern reduced CHD risk by 20% vs. lowest adherences. In the US population, the Western dietary pattern significantly increased CHD risk by 45%
Prospective studies		
Shikany et al. (2015). Evaluate dietary pattern factors related to CHD risk (Reasons for Geographic and Racial Differences in Stroke [REGARDS]; US) [23]	17,418 adults; baseline age ≥ 45 years; 5 primary dietary patterns classified as: convenience, plant-based, sweets, southern, and alcohol and salad; median 5.8 years of follow-up; 536 acute CHD cases (multivariate adjusted)	The highest consumers of the Southern pattern (characterized by added fats, fried food, eggs, organ and processed meats, and sugar-sweetened beverages) experienced a significant 56% higher risk of CHD (comparing quartile extremes of intake). Adding BMI and medical history variables to the model attenuated the association somewhat to 37% increased risk ($p = 0.036$)
Chiuve et al. (2012). Assess the effect of a healthy diet and risk of major chronic disease (Nurses' Health Study and Health Professionals Follow-Up Studies; US) [24]	71,495 women, baseline age 30–55 years, follow-up 24 years, 4868 CVD cases; 41,029 men, ages 40–75 years; 22 years of follow-up; about 5102 cases of CVD; Alterative Healthy Eating Index (AHEI)-2010 (multivariate adjusted)	The AHEI-2010, which explicitly emphasizes high intakes of whole grains, PUFA, nuts, and fish and reductions in red and processed meats, refined grains, and sugar-sweetened beverages, was significantly associated with lower risk of CHD by 31%
Iqhal et al. (2008). Examine the association between dietary patterns and acute myocardial infarction (Canada/Global INTERHEART study) [25]	52 countries; 5761 cases of acute MI, 10,646 controls; mean baseline age 55 years;75% men; sedentary; 3 major dietary patterns including Asian (high intake of tofu and soy and other sources), Western (high in fried foods, salty snacks, eggs, and meat), and healthy diet (high in fruit and vegetables); 4 years of follow-up (multivariate adjusted)	There was an inverse association between the healthy pattern and acute myocardial infarction, with a significantly reduced risk by 30% (highest vs. lowest adherence). High adherence to the Western dietary pattern increased the adjusted acute myocardial infarction risk by 30%

Table 11.1 (continued)

Objective	Study details	Results
Hu et al. (2000). Study whether overall dietary patterns derived from a food-frequency questionnaire predict risk of CHD in men (Health Professionals Follow-up Study; US) [26]	44,875 men; aged 40–75 years; 8 years of follow-up; 2 dietary patterns: Healthy pattern, characterized by higher intake of vegetables, fruit, legumes, whole grains, fish, and poultry vs. Western pattern, characterized by higher intake of red meat, processed meat, refined grains, sweets and desserts, French fries, and high-fat dairy products (multivariate adjusted)	The healthy pattern significantly reduced CHD risk by 30% and the Western pattern significantly increased CHD risk by 64% (highest vs. lowest adherence)

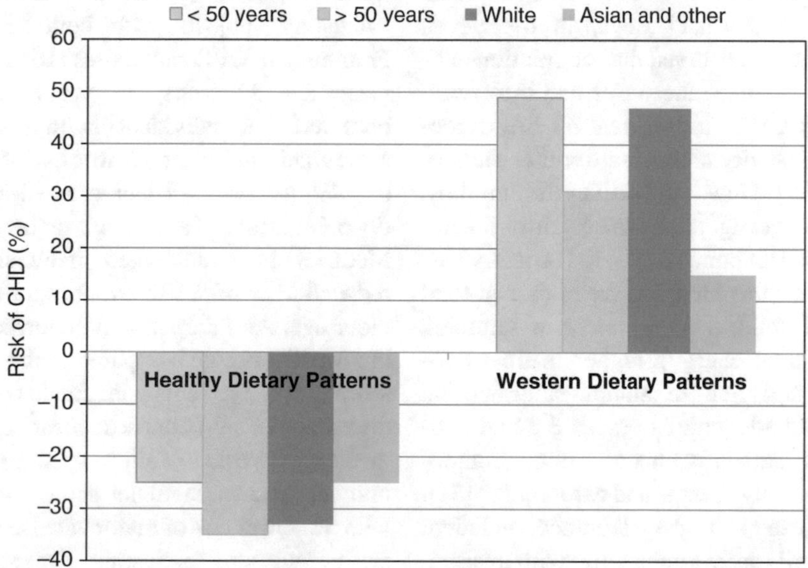

Fig. 11.3 Association between dietary patterns and coronary heart disease (CHD) risk in population sub-groups from a meta-analysis of 35 prospective studies)adapted from [21, 22])

baseline age ≥ 45 years; 5.8 years of follow-up) significantly increased CHD risk by 56% [23]; (2) diets rich in fried foods, salty snacks and meats (16,417 participants; mean baseline age 55 years; 75% men; 262 centers in 52 countries representing all geographic regions; 4 years of follow-up) significantly increased acute myocardial infarction (MI) risk by 30% [25]; and (3) higher intake of red and processed meats, refined grains, sweets, French fries and high fat dairy products (44,875 men; aged 40–75 years; 8 years of follow-up) significantly increased CHD risk by 64% [26]. These studies also show that high adherence to healthy dietary patterns significantly reduced CHD risk by about 30% [24–26]. A cross-sectional investigation from the Multi-Ethnic Study of Atherosclerosis (MESA) (2407 men and 2682 women; aged 45–84 years) observed that the inflammatory markers CRP and IL-6 were significantly increased with high adherence to Western food patterns (high in processed meats, fried potatoes, salty snacks, and desserts) and decreased with high adherence to healthy whole food patterns (rich in whole grains, fruit, nuts, and green leafy vegetables) [27]. A British RCT (165 healthy non-smoking men and women; aged 40–70 years; 12 weeks) demonstrated that high adherence to the UK Healthy

Dietary Guidelines diet reduced risk of fatal CHD by 15% and non-fatal CHD by 30% compared to the traditional British diet [28]. This RCT also showed significant reductions in systolic blood pressure by 4.2 mmHg, total/HDL-cholesterol ratio by 0.13, CRP by 36%, and weight by 1.9 kg with the UK Dietary Guidelines diet compared to the traditional British diet.

11.2.2 Mediterranean Diet (MedDiet)

Increased focus on the MedDiet first started in the 1960s when Ancel Keys, in the Seven Countries Study, observed that populations living near the Mediterranean Sea had the lowest incidence of CHD, longer healthy life expectancy and longevity compared to other parts of the world [15]. Now, the MedDiet is the most extensively investigated of the healthy dietary patterns for CHD benefits [29–31]. Dietary patterns based on the MedDiet are higher in total fat (35–40% total energy), lower in saturated fat (7–10% total energy), higher in fiber (27–37 g/day), and rich in monounsaturated fat (MUFAs) and adequate in omega-3 s and antioxidant and anti-inflammatory plant components such as polyphenols and carotenoids [31]. The criteria used to assess adherence, included: use of olive oil (or in combination with avocado oil) as the main fat; ≥2 servings/day of vegetables; ≥3 servings/day of fruits; <1 serving/day of red meat, hamburger or meat products (ham, sausage, etc.); <1 serving/day of butter, margarine, or cream; <1 serving/day of sweetened and/or carbonated beverages; ≥1 serving/day of wine; ≥3 servings/week of legumes; ≥3 servings/week of fish or shellfish; (11) <3 servings/week of commercial sweets or pastries (not homemade), such as cakes, cookies, biscuits or custard; ≥3 servings/week of nuts (including peanuts); preferential consumption of chicken or turkey meat instead of veal, pork, hamburger or sausage; and ≥2 servings/week of sofrito, a sauce made with tomato and onion, leek or garlic and simmered with olive oil or avocado oil [31]. A US study estimates that the high adherence to a MedDiet can significantly reduce CHD-related costs by up to $63 billion/year [32]. Table 11.2 summarizes the prospective studies and RCT trials on MedDiet patterns, and CHD risk and biomarkers.

11.2.2.1 Prospective Studies

Prospective studies consistently demonstrate that high adherence to the MedDiet significantly reduces CHD risk [33–39]. A meta-analysis (35 cohort studies; 4,172,412 subjects) found that each two point (18 point scale) increase in MedDiet adherence reduced risk of CVD by 10%, which is strongly associated with lower CHD risk [33]. An Italian prospective study evlauating subjects with both low and high Framingham CVD risk scores (1658 participants; mean age 52 years; 12 years of follow-up) observed that individuals with low CVD risk scores had significantly lower risk of CVD events by 21% per one unit increase in MedDiet score (9 point scale) [34]. High adherence to the MedDiet in middle-aged individuals showed reduced risk of CVD events and mortality in older age. An international cohort study assessing MedDiet score compared to the Western diet score (15,482 patients with stable coronary heart disease from 39 countries; mean age 67 years; median 3.7 years of follow-up) found that a one unit increase in MedDiet score was associated with 5% lower risk of major adverse cardiovascular events after adjusting for all covariates whereas there was no association between one unit change in Western diet score and major adverse cardiovascular events (18 point scale) [35]. This study suggests that an increased intake of healthy foods has an important role for secondary prevention of CHD. The Greek ATTICA prospective study (3042 statin using participants; age 18–89 years; 50% men; 10 years of follow-up) observed that high adherence to the MedDiet reduced CVD risk by 29% vs. a low MedDiet adherence [36]. This study also found that high adherence to MedDiets has adjunctive effects with statin use in lowering CHD risk. In the US Coronary Artery Risk Development in Young Adults (CARDIA) study (5115 subjects; aged 18–30 years; 25 years of follow-up), higher adherence to a MedDiet score was shown to reduce metabolic syndrome risk by 28%, important as metabolic syndrome is associated with

Table 11.2 Summary of Mediterranean diet (MedDiet) studies on CHD risk and biomarkers

Objective	Study details	Results
Prospective cohort studies		
Systematic review and meta-analysis		
Sofi et al. (2014). Assess the associations of MedDiet on CVD risk [33]	35 cohort studies; 4,172,412 subjects	Each 2-point increase in adherence to the MedDiet score reduced risk of CVD by 10% (18 point scale)
Prospective studies		
Bo et al. (2016). Investigate the associations of the MedDiet in a population with low CVD risk (Italy) [34]	1658 participants; low CVD risk group; mean baseline age 52 years, 58% males; high CVD, mean baseline age 58 years; 35% males; mean 12-years of follow-up; 220 CVD deaths (multivariate adjusted)	Low CVD risk individuals per unit of MedDiet score significantly reduced all-cause mortality by 17%, CVD mortality by 25%, and CVD events by 21%. High CVD risk individuals per unit MedDiet score significantly reduced CVD events by 15% while the associations with all-cause and CVD mortality were not significant (9 point scale)
Stewart et al. (2016). Determine whether MedDiet score is associated with major adverse cardiovascular events in high-risk patients with stable coronary artery disease (International) [35]	15,482 patients with stable coronary heart disease from 39 countries; mean age 67 years; MedDiet score was calculated for increasing consumption of whole grains, fruits, vegetables, legumes, fish, and alcohol, and for less meat, and a Western diet score for increasing consumption of refined grains, sweets and deserts, sugared drinks, and fried foods; median 3.7 years of follow-up (multivariate adjusted)	A one unit increase in MedDiet score was associated with 5% lower risk of major adverse cardiovascular events after adjusting for all covariates ($p = 0.002$) whereas there was no association between one unit change in the Western diet score and major adverse cardiovascular events. This study suggests that an increased intake of healthy foods may be more important for secondary prevention of CHD than avoidance of less healthy foods typical of Western diets (18 point scale)
Panagiotakos et al. (2015). Evaluate the additive protection of the MedDiet with statin therapy (ATTICA Study; Greece) [36]	3042 participants, baseline age 18–89 years; 50% men; 10-years of follow-up (multivariate adjusted)	MedDiet reduced CVD/CHD risk by 29% (highest vs. lowest adherence), independent of statin use. Patients with hyperlipidemia on a statin with low MedDiet adherence had a 75% increase in CVD/CHD risk compared to normolipidemic subjects with high adherence to MedDiet
Steffen et al. (2014). Investigate the effect of MedDiet score on metabolic syndrome risk (Coronary Artery Risk Development in Young Adults (CARDIA) study; US) [37]	5115 white and African Americans; mean baseline age 25 years; 25 years of follow-up (multivariate adjusted)	Higher MedDiet scores were associated with a significant 28% lower metabolic syndrome risk by improving risk factors including abdominal obesity, TG levels, and HDL-C levels. These findings suggest that the risk of developing the metabolic syndrome is lower when consuming diets rich in fruits, vegetables, whole grains, nuts and fish
Dilis et al. (2012). Examine the association of MedDiet adherence and CHD risk (European Prospective Investigation into Cancer and Nutrition cohort [EPIC]; Greece) [38]	23,929 adult men and women; 20–86 years; median follow-up of 10 years; 636 incident CHD cases and 240 CHD deaths were recorded (multivariate adjusted)	Each 2-point increase in the MedDiet score was associated with lower CHD mortality risk in women by 25% and in men by 19% and reduced CHD risk in women by 15% and in men by 2% (9 point scale). Among men meat intake was positively associated and in women fruit and nut intake were protective of CHD risk and mortality

(continued)

Table 11.2 (continued)

Objective	Study details	Results
Guallar-Castillon et al. (2012). Compare relationship between the Western diet and MedDiet on CHD risk (EPIC Spanish Cohort) [39]	40,757 adults; age 29–69 years; median follow-up 11 years; 606 CHD events (multivariate adjusted)	The MedDiet significantly lowered CHD risk by 27% (highest vs. lowest adherence). No association was found between the Western diet and CHD risk
Randomized controlled trials (RCTs)		
Systematic review and meta-analyses		
Liyanage et al. (2016). Evaluate the effects of the MedDiet on vascular disease and mortality [40]	6 RCTs; 10,950 subjects; 6 months to 9 years; 477 major vascular events and 315 vascular deaths; control diets include low-fat and prudent Western diets	This analysis showed that MedDiets lowered risk of major vascular events by 37%, coronary events by 35%, stroke by 35% and heart failure by 70% but did not lower CVD mortality which was insignificantly lowered by 10% compared to control diets. The MedDiet may protect against vascular disease but both the quantity and quality of the available evidence is limited and highly variable
Rees et al. (2013). Systematically review the clinical effects of the MedDiet pattern on CHD prevention (Cochrane Systematic Review) [41]	11 RCTs on the MedDiet pattern; 52,044 subjects; 5 trials with healthy individuals, 6 trials with subjects having elevated CHD risk; 3 months to 8 years	MedDiets showed modest but significant lowered TC by 6.2 mg/dL, LDL-C by 2.7 mg/dL, TG by 18.6 mg/dL, and no change in HDL-C compared to the control diets
Kastorini et al. (2011). Examine the effects of MedDiet on metabolic syndrome and its components [42]	50 studies included 35 RCTs, 2 prospective and 13 cross-sectional studies; 534,906 participants	High adherence to the MedDiet reduced metabolic syndrome risk by 31%. The MedDiet significantly reduced means for waist circumference by 0.42 cm, TG by 6 mg/dL, systolic BP by 2.4 mmHg, diastolic BP by 1.6 mmHg, and glucose by 4.0 mg/dL and increased HDL-C by 1.2 mg/dL vs. control diet
Randomized controlled trials (RCTs)		
Bedard et al. (2015). Investigate effects of the MedDiet vs. fast food on CRP in men and women (Canada) [43]	**Parallel RCT:** 35 men and 27 premenopausal women with moderate hyperlipidemia; 24–53 years; 4 weeks	Men on the MedDiet with CRP ≥2 mg/L had a significantly lowered CRP by 26.5% vs. fast food diets but in women there was no significant difference vs. fast food
Sala-Vita et al. (2014). Assess the effects of MedDiets on internal carotid intima-media thickness (ICA-IMT) and plaque height in subjects at high cardiovascular risk (Prevención con Dieta Mediterránea [PREDIMED] sub-study; Spain) [44]	**Parallel RCT:** 175 high CVD risk adults; mean age 66 years; mean BMI 30 kg/m^2; 25% male; MedDiet supplemented with extra virgin olive oil or mixed tree nuts vs. low fat control; 2.4 years	MedDiet plus nuts significantly reduced mean ICA-IMT progression by 0.084 mm vs. the low-fat control diet (Fig. 11.4). Similar results were observed for plaque height for MedDiet plus nuts. The MedDiet plus extra virgin olive oil ICA-IMT or plaque levels were not significantly different from the control diet
Estruch et al. (2013). Study the effect of the MedDiet on primary CVD/CHD prevention (PREDIMED; Spain) [45]	**Multi-center Parallel RCT:** 7447 adults with high CVD; mean age 67 years; mean BMI 30; 57% women; MedDiets with either extra virgin olive oil or mixed tree nuts vs. a low-fat diet; 4.8 years	Compared to low-fat diets, the MedDiets reduced risk of CVD/CHD with the extra virgin olive oil by 30% and with the mixed tree nuts by 28%. This primary prevention trial found that an energy-unrestricted MedDiet resulted in a substantial reduction in the risk of CVD/CHD events among high-risk persons

Table 11.2 (continued)

Objective	Study details	Results
Mitjavila et al. (2013). Investigate effects of the MedDiet on systemic lipid oxidative biomarkers in women with metabolic syndrome (Spain -PREDIMED Sub-study) [46]	**Parallel RCT:** 110 women with metabolic syndrome; mean age 69 years; mean BMI 31; MedDiet supplemented with extra virgin olive oil or mixed tree nuts vs. low fat control; 1 year	Urinary markers of levels of lipid peroxidation associated with increased atherosclerosis were reduced by high adherence to the both MedDiets vs. control diet including lower urinary F2- isoprostane and 8-oxo-7,8- dihydro-20-deoxyguanosine (DNA damage)
Murie-Fernandez et al. (2011). Study the effect of the MedDiet on carotid intima-media thickness (C-IMT) (PREDIMED-Navarra; Spain) [47]	**Parallel RCT:** 187 adults; mean age 67 years; 51% women; MedDiet supplemented with extra virgin olive oil or mixed tree nuts vs. low fat control; 1 year	Among participants with baseline C-IMT $\geq$ 0.9 mm, 1-year C-IMT changes for both MedDiets were significantly lowered compared to the low-fat control diet. No C-IMT regression was shown among participants with lower baseline IMT values <0.9 mm for any diet.
Thomazella et al. (2011). Investigate the effects of high adherence to MedDiet or low-fat therapeutic lifestyle changes diets on CHD risk (Brazil) [48]	**Parallel RCT:** 40 secondary prevention patients; mean age 55 years; MedDiet or low-fat therapeutic lifestyle changes diets including plant stanols/sterols and viscous fiber; 3 months	Both diets improved markers of redox homeostasis and metabolic effects potentially related to atheroprotection and promoted similar reduction in BMI and blood pressure. Compared to the low-fat therapeutic lifestyle changes diets, the MedDiet promoted decreases in blood leukocyte count, increases in HDL-C, and baseline brachial artery diameter. Compared to the MedDiet, the low-fat therapeutic lifestyle diets decreased LDL-C and oxidized LDL-C plasma levels, although the ratio of oxidized to total LDL-C remained unaltered
Mena et al. (2009). Examine the effects of Med-Diets vs. a low-fat diet on inflammatory biomarkers related to atherogenesis in subjects (PREDIMED sub-study; Spain) [49]	**Parallel RCT:** 112 adults with elevated CVD risk; mean age 68 years; mean BMI 28 kg/m^2; 43% women; MedDiet supplemented with extra virgin olive oil or mixed tree nuts vs. low fat control; 3 months	Both MedDiet groups had significantly reduced serum interleukin-6 (IL-6) and soluble intercellular adhesion molecule-1 vs. the low-fat diet. MedDiet plus extra virgin olive oil significantly decreased soluble vascular cellular adhesion molecule-1 and CRP vs. low-fat control diets
Fito et al. (2007). Investigate the effect of the traditional MedDiet for effects on LDL-C oxidative stress markers (PREDIMED Sub-study; Spain) [50]	**Parallel RCT:** 372 high CVD risk adults; mean age 69 years; 56% women; MedDiet supplemented with extra virgin olive oil or mixed tree nuts vs. low fat control; 3 months	Both traditional MedDiets significantly decreased mean oxidized LDL, an atherogenic risk factor, compared to the low-fat diet group
Estruch et al. (2006). Evaluate the short-term effects of MedDiets on blood lipids, glycemic control and CRP levels (PREDIMED Sub-study; Spain) [51]	**Parallel RCT:** 772 high CVD risk adults; mean age 69 years; MedDiet supplemented with extra virgin olive oil or mixed tree nuts vs. low fat control; 3 months	Both MedDiets significantly reduced plasma glucose levels by 5.4–7.0 mg/dL, systolic blood pressure by 5.9–7.1 mmHg, and TC/HDL-C ratio by 0.26–0.38 compared with the low-fat diet. The MedDiet plus nuts significantly decreased total cholesterol (TC) by 6.2 mg/dL and triglycerides (TG)13 mg/dL and the MedDiet plus extra virgin olive oil significantly reduced CRP 0.54 mg/L compared with the low-fat diet

(continued)

Table 11.2 (continued)

Objective	Study details	Results
Esposito et al. (2004). Investigate the long-term effects of a MedDiet on cardiometabolic health in subjects with metabolic syndrome (Italy) [52]	**Parallel RCT:** 180 Italian adults with metabolic syndrome; mean age 44 years; 55% men; MedDiet vs. Western type diet; 2 years	The MedDiet significantly reduced blood lipids, TC, insulin resistance, hs CRP, and body weight and reduced metabolic syndrome symptoms by 50% (Fig. 11.5)
Singh et al. (2002). Evaluate the effect of a MedDiet vs. National Cholesterol Education Program (NCEP) Step 1 diet on coronary artery disease risk [53]	**Parallel RCT:** 1000 adults with angina pectoris, MI, or surrogate risk factors for coronary artery disease; mean age 49 years; a fiber-rich MedDiet or a NCEP step I diet; 2 years	The MedDiet significantly reduced total cardiac events vs. the NCEP Step 1 diet by 49%. The MedDiet significantly lowered TC by 9%, LDL-C by 14%, and TG by 14% and increased HDL-C by 5.2% compared to the NCEP Step 1 diet
de Lorgeril et al. (1999). Investigate the effects of the MedDiet on recurrence rate after a first myocardial infarction (Lyon Diet Heart Study; France) [54]	**Parallel RCT:** 423 overweight subjects after the first MI plus CVD medications; MedDiet vs. Western type diet; 4 years; 275 events recorded	In survivors of a first infarction, the MedDiet significantly lowered myocardial infarction risk by 72% compared to those on the Western diet

significantly increased CHD risk [37]. The Greek cohort of the European Prospective Investigation into Cancer and Nutrition (EPIC) study (23,929 participants; median follow-up of 10 years) showed that a 2 point increase in MedDiet score (0–9 scale) significantly reduced CHD mortality risk by 25% in women and 19% in men and CHD incidence in women by 15% but not in men, which had an insignificant 2% reduction [38]. A Spanish EPIC study (40,757 participants; baseline age range 29–69 years; median follow-up of 11 years) found that the highest quintile of the MedDiet score reduced CHD risk by 27% compared to the lowest score [39].

11.2.2.2 Randomized Controlled Trials (RCTs)

RCTs consistently show that MedDiets significantly lower CHD risk and biomarkers compared to low fat or Western diets [40–54]. A 2016 systematic review and meta-analysis of the effect of MedDiets on vascular disease and mortality (6 RCTs; 10,950 subjects; 6 months to 9 years) showed that the MedDiet lowered risk of major vascular events by 37%, coronary events by 35%, stroke by 35% and heart failure by 70% but not CVD mortality which was insignificantly lowered by 10% compared to control diets including low fat and Western diets [40]. A Cochrane systematic review (11 RCTs; 52,044 subjects; 3 months to 8 years) concluded that MedDiets have a moderate but significant effect on lowering blood lipids and lipoproteins for beneficial effects on lowering CHD risk [41]. A meta-analysis (35 RCTs, 2 prospective and 13 cross-sectional studies; 534,906 participants) found that greater adherence to the MedDiet was associated with reduced metabolic syndrome risk by 31% including beneficial effects on all risk factors including waist circumference, TG, blood pressure, blood glucose and HDL-C [42]. A 2013 Prevención con Dieta Mediterránea (PREDIMED) RCT (7447 adults with elevated CVD risk; mean age 67 years; mean BMI 30 kg/m^2; 57% women; MedDiets with either extra virgin olive oil or mixed tree nuts vs. control low fat diets; 4.8 years) found that both MedDiets reduced CVD risk by about 30% compared to low-fat diets [45]. These findings were consistent with a 2006 PREDIMED trial (772 high CVD risk adults; mean age 69 years; MedDiet supplemented with extra virgin olive oil or mixed tree nuts vs. low fat control; 3 months) which showed that the MedDiets significantly reduced TC, TG, TC/HDL-C ratio, glucose levels, CRP, and systolic blood pressure compared with the low-fat diet [51]. A Brazilian secondary prevention RCT (40 medicated patients; mean age 55 years; MedDiet or low-fat therapeutic lifestyle changes diet including plant stanols/sterols and viscous fiber; 3 months) found that the MedDiet and therapeutic lifestyle changes diet promoted similar significant decreases in BMI and blood pressure with decreases in blood leukocyte count and increases in HDL-C and brachial artery diameter and the low-fat therapeutic lifestyle changes decreased LDL-C and oxidized LD-C plasma levels [48]. Both diets played a role in secondary prevention by improving markers of redox homeostasis and metabolic effects potentially related to atheroprotection. Several satellite PREDIMED RCTs support a potential role in promoting regression of carotid intima-media thickness and plaque with high adherence to the MedDiet supplemented with nuts, especially in individuals with elevated plaque (Fig. 11.4) [44, 47]. An Italian RCT (180 Italian adults with metabolic syndrome; mean age 44 years; 55% men; MedDiet vs. Western diet; 2 years) demonstrated that the MedDiet significantly reduced blood lipids, TC, insulin resistance, hs-CRP and body weight, and reduced metabolic syndrome risk factors by 50% compared to Western diets (Fig. 11.5) [52]. Also, a Canadian trial showed that the MedDiet was shown to reduce elevated CRP levels in men by 26.5% compared to fast food based diets [43]. Several other PREDIMED trials demonstrate that MedDiets lower systemic inflammatory markers and urinary markers of DNA damage, and lipid oxidation compared to low-fat diets [46, 49, 50]. The MedDiet protects against the development of CHD because of its beneficial role on systemic cardiovascular risk factors and its possible effect on reducing the risk of body weight gain, metabolic syndrome, and obesity [29, 55, 56].

11.2.3 Dietary Approaches to Stop Hypertension (DASH) Dietary Pattern

The DASH diet was designed for hypertension control but it also has effects on reducing several CHD risk factors, including TC, LDL-C, and inflammation [15, 19]. This pattern is rich in fruits, vegetables, and low-fat dairy products, includes whole grains, poultry, fish, and nuts, and limits saturated fat, red meat, sweets, and sugar containing beverages. Compared with the Western diet, the DASH diet provides lower total fat, saturated fat, and dietary cholesterol, and higher potassium, magnesium, calcium, fiber, and protein. Table 11.3 summarizes the DASH diet prospective studies and RCTs on the on CHD risk and biomarkers [57–67].

11.2.3.1 Prospective Cohort Studies

Prospective studies consistently show that the DASH dietary pattern helps to reduce CHD and heart failure risk [57–61]. A 2013 meta-analysis (6 studies; 260,000 adults) reports that higher

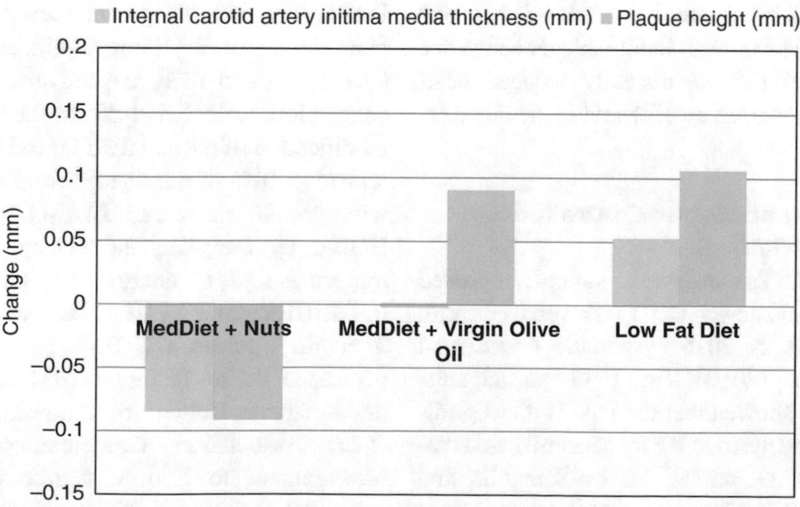

Fig. 11.4 Association between MedDiets and low-fat diets and internal carotid artery mean intima-media thickness and plaque height over 2.4 years (p = 0.047) (adapted from [44])

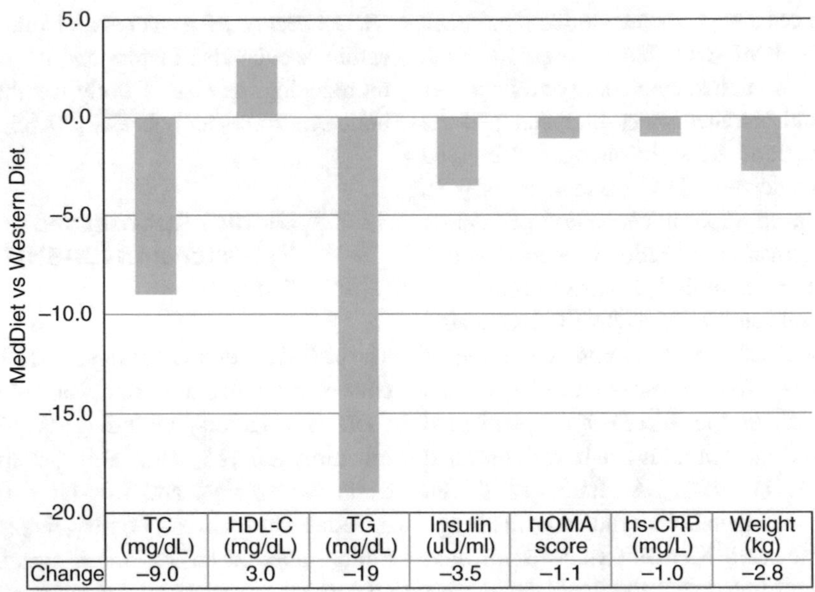

Fig. 11.5 Effect of MedDiet vs. Western diet on cardiometabolic health biomarkers in subjects with metabolic syndrome after 2 years (all p = 0.01 to <0.001) (adapted from [52]). **TC* total cholesterol, *HDL-C* high density cholesterol, *TG* triglycerides, *HOMA* measure of insulin resistance, *hs-CRP* high sensitivity C-reactive protein

adherence to the DASH diet significantly reduced risk of CHD by 21% and heart failure by 29% [57]. The EPIC Dutch cohort (33,671participants; mean age 49 years at baseline; 74% women; average follow-up of 12.2 years) observed that high adherence to the DASH diet significantly reduced CHD risk by 18% compared to low adherence [58]. The Nurses' Health Study (88,517 women; aged 34–59 years; 24 year of follow-up) found a significantly reduced total CHD risk by 24% and fatal CHD risk by 29% for high vs. low DASH diet adherence [61]. For heart failure, higher adherence to the DASH diet significantly reduced heart failure risk in women by 16% and in men by 22% [59, 60].

11.2.3.2 Randomized Controlled Trials

DASH diet RCTs consistently support improved biomarkers and lower CHD risk versus control diets [62–68]. A 2015 systematic review and meta-analysis (20 RCTs; 1917 participants; 2–24 weeks) showed that the DASH diet significantly lowered systolic BP by 25 mmHg and diastolic BP by 23 mmHg, TC by 8 mg/dL, and LDL-C by 8 mg/dL vs. control diets; these clinical changes reduced the 10-year Framingham risk score for CHD risk by 13% [62]. Four other RCTs found that higher adherence to a standard DASH diet significantly reduces the 10-year CHD risk by 12–18% [63–65, 68]. Also, the Omni Trial (164 subjects; mean age 54 years; 73% women; 6 weeks) found that the level of protein or monounsaturated fatty acids (MUFA) substituted for carbohydrate improves the 10 year CHD risk level (Fig. 11.6) [67]. For CRP, a DASH diet with 12 g added fiber from whole plant foods or psyllium significantly reduced CRP by 14 and 18%, respectively, compared to control low fiber diets [65]. In the Omni Trial a modification of the standard DASH diet made by replacing 10% of the energy from carbohydrate with protein decreased LDL-C by 3 mg/dL, HDL-C by 1 mg/dL, and TG by 16 mg/dL or replacing 10% of energy with unsaturated fat (8% MUFA and 2% PUFA) decreased LDL-C by 3 mg/dL, increased HDL-C by 1 mg/dL and decreased TG by 10 mg/dL [67]. A report from the American College of Cardiology/American Heart Association Guideline on Lifestyle Management to Reduce Cardiovascular Risk estimated that adults (TC level < 260 mg/dL,

Table 11.3 Summary of DASH diet studies on CHD risk and related biomarkers

Objective	Study details	Results
Prospective cohort studies		
Systematic review and meta-analysis		
Salehi-Abargouei et al. (2013). Investigate the effects of a DASH-style diet on the incidence of CHD [57]	6 studies; 260,000 subjects; follow-up of 7–24 years	The DASH-like diet significantly reduced risk of CVDs by 20%, CHD by 21%, and heart failure by 29%
Prospective cohort studies		
Struijk et al. (2014). Evaluate the effects of DASH diet on CHD risk (EPIC Netherlands cohort) [58]	33,671 participants; mean baseline age 49 years; 74% women; average follow-up of 12.2 years; 1630 CHD cases (multivariate adjusted)	Higher adherence to the DASH diet was associated with significantly reduced CHD risk by 9%
Levitan et al. (2013). Evaluate the effect of DASH diets on heart failure mortality in women (Women's Health Initiative; US) [59]	This study included 68,132 women. After a median follow-up of 4.6 years, 1385 women died of heart failure (multivariate adjusted)	Higher DASH diet scores were associated with significantly lower heart failure mortality in women by 16%
Levitan et al. (2009). Assess the effect of DASH diets on heart failure events in men (Sweden) [60]	38,987 men; baseline age 45 to 79 years; 9 years of follow-up; 710 were hospitalized for HF and 97 died (multivariate adjusted)	Men with the highest DASH diet adherence had a significant 22% lower heart failure event risk vs. those with the lowest adherence
Fung et al. (2008). Examine the effect of the DASH diet on CHD risk in women (Nurses' Health Study; US) [61]	88,517 women; baseline age 34 to 59 years; 24 years of follow-up; 976 CHD deaths (multivariate adjusted)	Women with the highest DASH diet adherence significantly reduced CHD risk by 24% vs. lowest adherence. Similar risk reductions were observed for nonfatal myocardial infarction and CHD deaths
Randomized controlled trials (RCTs)		
Meta-analysis		
Siervo et al. (2015). Assess the effects of the DASH diet on cardiovascular risk factors [62]	20 RCTs; 1917 participants; 2–24 weeks	The DASH diet significantly reduced systolic BP by 25 mmHg and diastolic BP by 23 mmHg, TC by 8 mg/dL and LDL-C by 8 mg/dL vs. control diets. These changes predicted a reduced 10-year Framingham risk score for CHD by 13%
Randomized controlled trials (RCTs)		
Jenkins et al. (2017). Assess the effect of dietary advice and/or food provision for the DASH diet on body weight and cardiovascular disease risk factors (Canada) [63]	**Parallel RCT:** 209 men and 710 women; mean age 45 years; mean BMI 32; 3 diets: (1) subjects encouraged to consume a DASH type diet plus increased consumption of cholesterol-lowering functional foods including soy foods, nuts, and viscous fiber sources such as oats and barley (control), (2) subjects received a weekly food basket reflecting the advice given to the first treatment group but did not receive dietary advice, and (3) subjects received both the weekly food basket and dietary advice; 6-month intervention; 12-month follow-up	Overall, at 6 months, similar reductions in all groups were found for body weight by 0.8–1.2 kg, waist size by 1.1 to 1.9 cm, and mean arterial pressure by 0.0–1.1 mmHg. After 18 months, all diets maintained the reductions in body weight, BMI and waist size that were seen at 6 months. Also, HDL-C rose between 6 and 18 months by 0.05 mmol/L ($p < 0.0001$) and the total-to-HDL-cholesterol ratio was reduced. Further, significant reductions in mean arterial pressure and Framingham CHD risk scores were seen at 18 months in all groups

(continued)

Table 11.3 (continued)

Objective	Study details	Results
Chen et al. (2010). Investigate the effects of the DASH diet on the 10-year risk of developing CHD (US) [64]	**Parallel RCT:** 459 prehypertension or stage-1 hypertension subjects not taking anti-hypertensive medication; mean age 45 years; 51% men and 60% African-American; duration 8 weeks) evaluated 3 diets: Increased fruits and vegetables (F/V), DASH diet, and low fat diet; 8 weeks	The DASH diet significantly lowered 10-year CHD risk by 18% compared to the low-fat control diet. The high F/V diet insignificantly lowered risk by 7%. Compared with F/V diet, the DASH diet significantly reduced estimated 10-year CHD risk by 11%
Maruthur et al. (2009). Examine the effects of the DASH diet on CHD risk (PREMIER Trial; US) [65]	**Parallel RCT:** 810 healthy adults with untreated pre- or stage I hypertension randomized; mean age 50 years; 61% women; active education on healthy lifestyle recommendations, or active healthy lifestyle plus DASH education vs. general advice; 6 months	Active healthy lifestyle plus DASH education significantly lowered estimated 10-year CHD risk by 14% relative to general advice
King et al. (2007). Investigate the effect of DASH diet or fiber supplemented DASH diet on CRP (US) [66]	**Crossover RCT:** 35 adults; 18 lean normotensives and 17 obese hypertensive individuals; age range 18–49 years; 80% women; evaluated 2 diets vs. baseline: High-fiber foods DASH type diet (28 g fiber/day) or psyllium fiber-supplemented DASH type diet (26 g fiber/day); mean baseline fiber intake 12 g/day; 3 weeks	Compared to baseline, CRP levels were significantly reduced in the fiber rich foods DASH diet group by 14% and in the psyllium fiber-supplemented DASH-type diet group by 18%. There were no differences in weight, TG, TC, or insulin resistance status between the two DASH diets
Apple et al. (2005). Evaluate the effects of 3 variations of the DASH diet on CHD risk (US) [67]	**Crossover RCT:** 164 adults with prehypertension or stage 1 hypertension; mean age 54 years; 73% women; 10% energy replacement of standard DASH diet carbohydrate with protein or monounsaturated fatty acids (MUFA) vs. standard DASH diet evaluate; 6 weeks	Compared with the standard DASH (carbohydrate) diet, the estimated 10-year CHD risk was reduced for the DASH diets enriched with protein by 5.8% and unsaturated fat (primarily MUFA) by 4.2% (Fig. 11.6)
Obarzanek et al. (2001). Investigate the effects of DASH diet on plasma lipids, focusing on subgroups by sex and race (US) [68]	**Parallel RCT:** 436 adults; mean age 45 years; 60% African American; baseline TC was ≤260 mg/dL; evaluated 3 diets: Control Western diet, a diet increased in fruit and vegetables, or a DASH diet, during which time subjects remained weight stable; 8 weeks	The 10-year CHD risk was significantly decreased for the DASH diet by 12.1% compared with a 0.9% increase in risk for the Western control diet

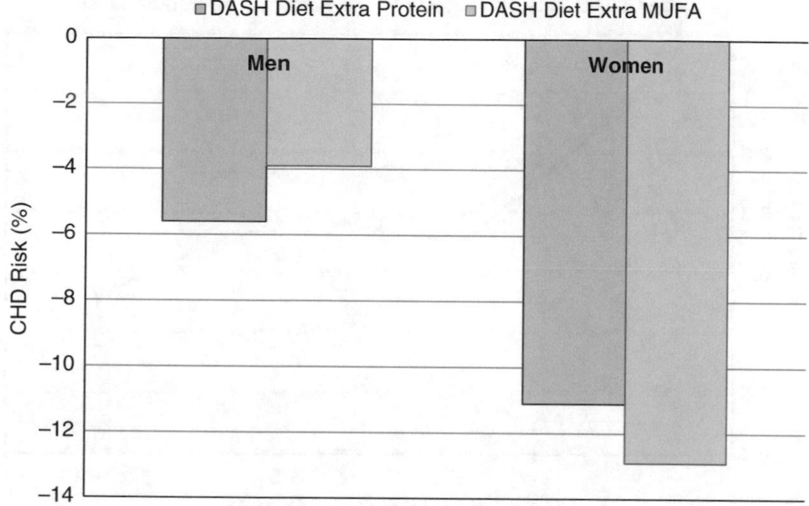

Fig. 11.6 Estimated 10-year risk of Framingham coronary heart disease (CHD) with a 10% energy replacement of standard DASH diet carbohydrate with protein or monounsaturated fatty acids (MUFA) vs. standard DASH diet (adapted from [67])

LDL-C level < 160 mg/dL and a stable body weight) with high adherence to the basic DASH diet would be projected to lower LDL-C by 11 mg/dL, reduce TC:HDL-C ratio, and have no effect on TG compared with a typical American diet of the 1990s [69]. A 2017 Canadian RCT (919 overweight men and women; mean age 45 years; mean BMI 32; 3 groups: (1) encouraged to consume a DASH type diet plus increase consumption of cholesterol-lowering functional foods including soy foods, nuts, and viscous fiber sources such as oats and barley (control), (2) weekly food basket reflecting the advice given to the first treatment group but did not receive dietary advice, and (3) both the weekly food basket plus dietary advice; 6-month intervention; 12-month follow-up) all groups showed small significant reductions in body weight by 0.8–1.2 kg, waist size by 1.1–1.9 cm, and mean arterial pressure by 0.0–1.1 mmHg at 6 months and Framingham CHD risk scores were significantly lower at 18 months regardless of food delivery or guidance approach [63].

11.2.4 Vegetarian Dietary Patterns

Vegetarian diets reduce CHD risk compared to non-vegetarian diets [69]. A meta-analysis (7 cohort studies; 124,706 adults) showed that vegetarian diets significantly reduced ischemic heart diease mortality by 29% and circulatory disease risk by 16% compared to non-vegetarian diets [70]. A meta-analysis of RCTs (11 trials; mean 24 weeks, ranging from 3 weeks to 18 months) demonstrated that vegetarian diets significantly lowered TC by 13.9 mg/dL, LDL-C by 13.1 mg/dL, and HDL-C by 3.9 mg/dL, but did not significantly affect blood TG concentrations compared to control non-vegetarian diets [71].

11.2.5 Elderly Dietary Index

The Elderly Dietary Index was constructed using ten components (ie, questions about the consumption frequency of meat, fish, fruits, vegetables, grains, legumes, olive oil, and alcohol as well as the type of bread and dairy products) according to the Modified MyPyramid for older adults and select features of the traditional Mediterranean diet [72]. Scores from 1 to 4 were assigned to each of the ten components of the index with total Elderly Dietary Index score ranging between 10 and 40. The British Regional Heart Study (3328 men; baseline mean age 68 years; 11.3 years of follow-up; 933 deaths from all causes, 327 CVD deaths, 582 CVD events, and 307 CHD events) found a that higher adherence to the Elderly Dietary Index significantly lowered risk of CVD

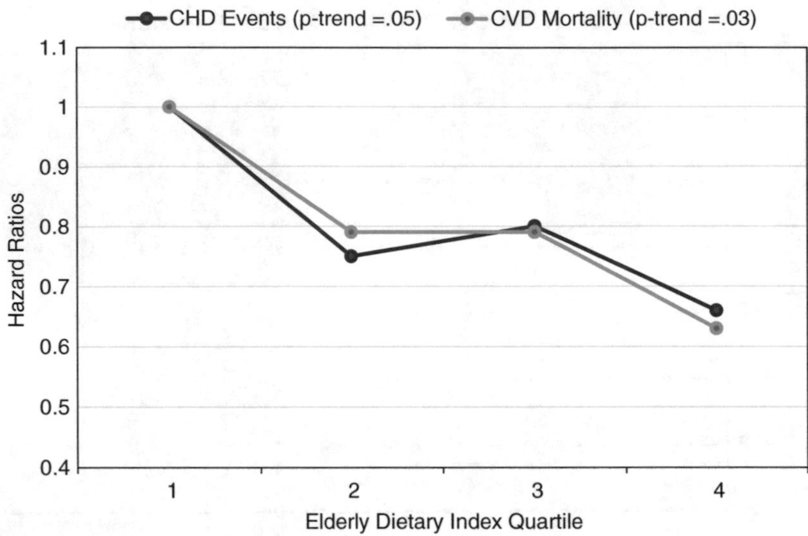

Fig. 11.7 Adherence to Elderly Dietary Index on coronary heart disease (CHD) events and cardiovascular disease (CVD) mortality in men mean baseline age 70 years over 11.3 years of follow-up from the British Regional Heart Study (multivariate adjusted) (adapted from [73])

mortality by 37% and CHD events by 33%, which was independent of sociodemographic, behavioral, and cardiovascular risk factors, compared to lower adherence (Fig. 11.7) [73].

11.3 Dietary Carbohydrates vs. Dietary Fat

There have been a number of prospective studies and RCTs on the effects of replacing dietary carbohydrate for fat intake or vice versa on CHD risk [74–78]. A meta-analysis of 8 prospective cohort studies concluded that a high dietary glycemic index and glycemic load increased the risk of CHD in women but not in men [74]. In contrast, a later cohort study found that a higher carbohydrate intake was associated with an increased CHD risk in men but not in women [75]. A pooled analysis (11 cohort studies) showed that replacing saturated fat with carbohydrates increased the risk of coronary events but not of coronary deaths [76]. Also, replacing carbohydrates with trans-fatty acids was associated with an increased CHD risk and replacing carbohydrates with PUFA or with MUFA was associated with a decreased CHD risk. The Alpha-Tocopherol, Beta-Carotene Cancer Prevention Study, double-blind RCT (21,955 men, baseline age 50–69 years; 19-years of follow-up; 4379 CHD cases) found that replacing saturated and trans-fatty acids with carbohydrates was associated with a 3% lowered CHD risk for each 2% energy intake and replacing MUFA and PUFA with carbohydrates was associated with an 8% and a 4.5% increased CHD risk for each 2% of energy intake, respectively (Fig. 11.8) [77]. A 2015 pooled analysis of the Nurses' Health Study and Health Professionals Follow-up Study (84,628 women and 42,908 men; mean baseline age 47–54 years; 24–30 years of follow-up; 7667 CHD cases) found that replacing 5% of energy intake from saturated fats with equivalent energy intake from either PUFAs, MUFAs, or carbohydrates from whole grains was associated with significant 25%, 15%, and 9% lower risks of CHD, respectively (Fig. 11.9) [78]. However, replacing saturated fat with carbohydrates from refined starches/added sugars was not significantly associated with lower CHD risk ($p > 0.10$).

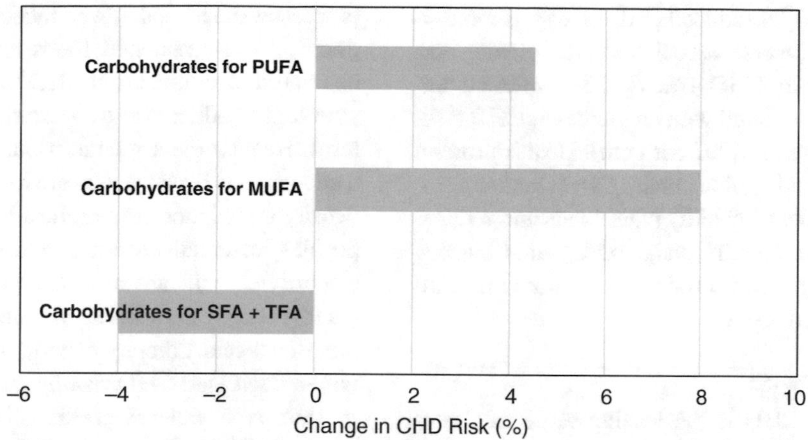

Fig. 11.8 Change in coronary heart disease (CHD) risk with the isocaloric substitution of 2% of carbohydrate energy for saturated (SFA) and trans-fat (TFA), monounsaturated fat (MUFA), or polyunsaturated fat (PUFA) in men (adapted from [77])

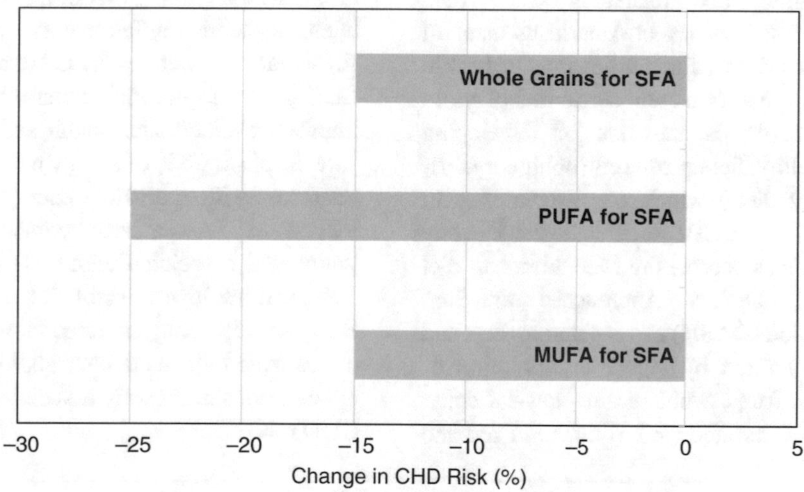

Fig. 11.9 Change in coronary heart disease (CHD) risk with the isocaloric substitution of 5% of energy from monounsaturated fat (MUFA), polyunsaturated fat (PUFA) and whole grains for saturated fat (SFA) in men and women from pooled data from the Nurses' Health Study and Health Professionals Follow-up Study; MUFA and PUFA (p = 0.02) and whole grains (p = 0.01) (adapted from [78])

11.4 Healthful vs. Unhealthful Plant Based Diets

Plant-based diets are recommended for CHD prevention and management but not all plant foods are necessarily beneficial for CHD risk reduction [79]. The association of healthy and less healthy plant based diets were examined in 73,710 women in the Nurses' Health Study (1984 to 2012), 92,329 women in Nurses' Health Study 2 (1991 to 2013), and 43,259 men in Health Professionals Follow-up Study (1986 to 2012), without CHD at baseline. An overall plant-based diet index (PDI) from repeated semiquantitative food-frequency questionnaire data, by assigning positive scores to plant foods and reverse scores to animal foods. A healthy plant-based diet index (hPDI) consisted of whole grains, fruits/vegetables, nuts/legumes, oils, tea and coffee, whereas unhealthy plant foods (uPDI) included sweetened juices/beverages, refined grains, French fries, sweets and some animal foods. Higher adherence to an overall PDI reduced CHD by 8% (p-trend = .003). This inverse association was greater for hPDI reducing CHD risk by 25% whereas an uPDI was associated with an increased CHD risk by 32% (p-trend <.001 for both). Health professionals should guide their CHD patients to increase intake of healthy plant foods and reduce intake of less healthy plant foods, sugar sweetened beverages and certain high saturated fat and energy animal foods.

Conclusions

Globally, CHD is the leading cause of death and morbidity in adults. Healthy lifestyles (e.g., BMI <25, physical activity at goal levels, a diet consistent with the dietary guidelines, and smoking avoidance) play an important role in preventing and managing CHD risk. However, less than 1% of Americans meet all four ideal criteria for cardiovascular health. The type of dietary pattern consumed plays an important role in the risk of developing CHD. Healthy dietary patterns (or higher nutrient quality diets) which are associated with decreased risk of CHD include higher Healthy Eating Indices scores, the Mediterranean diet (MedDiet), Dietary Approaches to Stop Hypertension (DASH) and vegetarian diets and are characterized by higher consumption of vegetables, fruits, whole-grains, low-fat dairy, and seafood, limited (or no) intake of red and processed meat, and lower intakes of refined grains, sugar-sweetened foods and beverages compared to an increased CHD risk associated with higher adherence to Western dietary patterns. Healthy dietary patterns have CHD protective effects because they are lower in energy density and higher in fiber, healthier fatty acid profiles, essential nutrients, antioxidants, and electrolytes, and are anti-inflammatory compared with Western diets. Meta-analyses estimate that healthy dietary patterns are associated with a decreased CHD risk by 20–33%, while Western-type patterns are associated with an increased CHD risk by up to 45%, especially in US studies and in individuals over 50 years of age. A number of RCTs support the role for healthy dietary patterns in reducing CHD risk biomarkers including blood lipids and lipoproteins, systemic inflammatory or oxidative stress factors such as hs-CRP and oxidized LDL-C, and carotid atherosclerosis and improving endothelial health and blood pressure. Replacing 5% of energy intake from saturated fats with equivalent energy intake from PUFAs, MUFAs, or carbohydrates from whole grains was associated with a significant 25%, 15%, and 9% lower risk of CHD, respectively. However, replacing saturated fat with carbohydrates from refined starches and/or added sugars was not significantly associated with lower CHD risk.

Appendix A: Comparison of Western and Healthy Dietary Patterns per 2000 kcal (Approximated Values)

Diet type	Western dietary pattern (US)	USDA base pattern	DASH diet pattern	Healthy Mediterranean pattern	Healthy vegetarian pattern (Lacto-ovo based)	Vegan pattern
Emphasizes	Refined grains, low fiber foods, red meats, sweets, solid fats	Vegetables, fruit, whole-grains, and low-fat milk	Potassium rich vegetables, fruits, and low fat milk products	Whole grains, vegetables, fruit, dairy products, olive oil, and moderate wine	Vegetables, fruit, whole-grains, legumes, nuts, seeds, milk products, and soy foods	Plant foods: Vegetables, fruits, whole grains, nuts, seeds, and soy foods
Includes	Processed meats, sugar sweetened beverages, and fast foods	Enriched grains, lean meat, fish, nuts, and seeds, vegetable oils	Whole-grains, poultry, fish, nuts, and seeds	Fish, nuts, seeds, and pulses	Eggs, non-dairy milk alternatives, and vegetable oils	Non-dairy milk alternatives

Diet type	Western dietary pattern (US)	USDA base pattern	DASH diet pattern	Healthy Mediterranean pattern	Healthy vegetarian pattern (Lacto-ovo based)	Vegan pattern
Limits	Fruits and vegetables, and whole-grains	Solid fats, and added sugars	Red meats, sweets and sugar-sweetened beverages	Red meats, refined grains, and sweets	No red or white meats, or fish; limited and sweets	No animal products
Estimated nutrients/components						
Carbohydrates (% Total kcal)	51	51	55	50	54	57
Protein (% Total kcal)	16	17	18	16	14	13
Total fat (% Total kcal)	33	32	27	34	32	30
Saturated fat (% Total kcal)	11	8	6	8	8	7
Unsat. fat (% Total kcal)	22	25	21	24	26	25
Fiber (g)	16	31	29+	31	35+	40+
Potassium (mg)	2800	3350	4400	3350	3300	3650
Vegetable oils (g)	19	27	25	27	19–27	18–27
Sodium (mg)	3600	1790	1100	1690	1400	1225
Added sugar (g)	79 (20 tsp)	32 (8 tsp)	12 (3 tsp)	32 (8 tsp)	32 (8 tsp)	32 (8 tsp)
Plant food groups						
Fruit (cup)	≤1.0	2.0	2.5	2.5	2.0	2.0
Vegetables (cup)	≤1.5	2.5	2.1	2.5	2.5	2.5
Whole-grains (oz.)	0.6	3.0	4.0	3.0	3.0	3.0
Legumes (oz.)	N/A	1.5	0.5	1.5	3.0	3.0+
Nuts/seeds (oz.)	0.5	0.6	1.0	0.6	1.0	2.0
Soy products (oz.)	0.0	0.5	–	–	1.1	1.5

U.S. Department of Agriculture, Agriculture Research Service, Nutrient Data Laboratory. 2014. USDA National Nutrient Database for Standard Reference, Release 27. http://www.ars.usda.gov/nutrientdata. Accessed 17 Feb 2015
Dietary Guidelines Advisory Committee. Scientific Report. Advisory Report to the Secretary of Health and Human Services and the Secretary of Agriculture. Appendix E-3.7: Developing vegetarian and Mediterranean-style food patterns. 2015; 1–9
U.S. Department of Agriculture and U.S. Department of Health and Human Services. Dietary Guidelines for Americans, 2010. 7th Edition, Washington, DC: U.S. Government Printing Office. 2010; Table B2.4; http://www.choosemyplate.gov/ Accessed 22 Aug 2015

References

1. Mendis S, Puska P, Norrving B. Global atlas on cardiovascular disease prevention and control. Geneva: World Health Organization; 2011.
2. Sayols-Baixeras S, Lluís-Ganella C, Lucas G, Elosua R. Pathogenesis of coronary artery disease: focus on genetic risk factors and identification of genetic variants. Appl Clin Genet. 2014;7:15–32.
3. Roger VL, Go AS, Lloyd-Jones DM, et al. Heart disease and stroke statistics-2011 update: a report from the American Heart Association. Circulation. 2011;123(4):18–209.
4. Barquera S, Pedroz-Tobias A, Medina C, et al. Global overview of the epidemiology of atherosclerosis cardiovascular disease. Arch Med Res. 2015;46(5):328–38. https://doi.org/10.1016/jarcmed.2015.06.006.
5. Lloyd-Jones DM, Larson MG, Beiser A, Levy D. Lifetime risk of developing coronary heart disease. Lancet. 1999;353:89–92.
6. Mozaffarian D, Benjamin EJ, Go AS, et al. Heart disease and stroke statistics-2015 update a report from the American Heart Association. Circulation. 2015;131:e29–322. https://doi.org/10.1161/CIR.0000000000000152.
7. Fleg JL, Forman DE, Berra K, et al. Secondary prevention of atherosclerotic cardiovascular disease in older adults a scientific statement from the American Heart Association. Circulation. 2013;128(22):2422–46.
8. Hu FB. Diet and lifestyle influences on risk of coronary heart disease. Curr Atheroscler Rep. 2009;11:257–63.
9. Gage B, Canonico M, Perier M-C, et al. Idea cardiovascular health, mortality and vascular events in elderly subjects. J Am Coll Cardiol. 2017;69:3015–26.
10. Lichtenstein AH, Appel LJ, Brands M, et al. Diet and lifestyle recommendations revision 2006: a scientific statement from the American Heart Association Nutrition Committee. Circulation. 2006;114:82–96.
11. Vermorken AJM, Andres E, Cui Y. Bowel movement frequency, oxidative stress and disease prevention (Review). Mol Clin Oncol. 2016;5:339–42. https://doi.org/10.3892/mco.2016.987.
12. Forget G, Doyon M, Lacerte G, et al. Adoption of American Heart Association 2020 Ideal Healthy Diet Recommendations prevents weight gain in young adults. J Acad Nutr Diet. 2013;113:1517–22.
13. http://health.gov/dietaryguidelines/2015/guidelines/message/. Accessed 17 Jan 2016.
14. Tuso P, Stoll SR, Li WW. A plant-based diet, atherogenesis, and coronary artery disease prevention. Perm J. 2015;19(1):62–7.
15. Bhupathiraju SN, Tucker KL. Coronary heart disease prevention: nutrients, foods, and dietary patterns. Clin Chim Acta. 2011;412:1493–514.
16. U.S. Department of Agriculture and U.S. Department of Health and Human Services. Dietary guidelines for Americans, 2010. 7th ed. Washington, DC: U.S. Government Printing Office; 2010. Table B2.4; http://www.choosemyplate.gov/. Accessed 22 Aug 2015.
17. U.S. Department of Agriculture, Agriculture Research Service, Nutrient Data Laboratory. USDA National Nutrient Database for Standard Reference, Release 27. 2014. http://www.ars.usda.gov/nutrientdata. Accessed 17 Feb 2015.
18. Dietary Guidelines Advisory Committee. Scientific Report. Advisory Report to the Secretary of Health and Human Services and the Secretary of Agriculture. Appendix E-3.7: Developing vegetarian and Mediterranean-style food patterns; 2015. p. 1–9.
19. Dietary Guidelines Advisory Committee (DGAC). Scientific Report. Advisory Report to the Secretary of Health and Human Services and the Secretary of Agriculture. Part D. Chapter 2: Dietary patterns, foods and nutrients and health outcomes; 2015. p. 1–35.
20. Mente A, de Koning L, Shannon HS, Anand SS. A systematic review of the evidence supporting a causal link between dietary factors and coronary heart disease. Arch Intern Med. 2009;169(7):659–69.
21. Zhang X-Y, Shu L, Si C-J, et al. Dietary patterns, alcohol consumption and risk of coronary heart disease in adults: a meta-analysis. Forum Nutr. 2015;7:6582–605. https://doi.org/10.3390/nu7085300.
22. Hou L, Li F, Wang Y, et al. Association between dietary patterns and coronary heart disease: a meta-analysis of prospective cohort studies. Int J Clin Exp Med. 2015;8(1):781–90.
23. Shikany JM, Safford MM, Newby PK, et al. Southern dietary pattern is associated with hazard of acute coronary heart disease in the Reasons for Geographic and Racial Differences in Stroke (REGARDS) Study. Circulation. 2015;132:804–14. https://doi.org/10.1161/CIRCULATIONAHA.115.020671.
24. Chiuve SE, Fung TT, Rimm EB, et al. Alternative dietary indices both strongly predict risk of chronic disease. J Nutr. 2012;142:1009–18.
25. Iqbal R, Anand S, Ounpuu S, et al. Dietary patterns and the risk of acute myocardial infarction in 52 countries results of the INTERHEART Study. Circulation. 2008;118:1929–37.
26. Hu FB, Rimm EB, Stampfer MJ, et al. Prospective study of major dietary patterns and risk of coronary heart disease in men. Am J Clin Nutr. 2000;72:912–21.
27. Nettleton JA, Steffen LM, Mayer-Davis EJ, et al. Dietary patterns are associated with biochemical markers of inflammation and endothelial activation in the Multi-Ethnic Study of Atherosclerosis (MESA). Am J Clin Nutr. 2006;83(6):1369–79.
28. Reidlinger DP, Darzi J, Hall WL, et al. How effective are current dietary guidelines for cardiovascular disease prevention in healthy middle-aged and older men and women? A randomized controlled trial. Am J Clin Nutr. 2015;101:922–30.
29. Ros E, Martínez-González MA, Estruch R. Mediterranean diet and cardiovascular health: teachings of the PREDIMED study. Adv Nutr. 2014;5:330S–6S.

30. de Lorgeril M. Mediterranean diet and cardiovascular disease: historical perspective and latest evidence. Curr Atheroscler Rep. 2013;15(12):370. https://doi.org/10.1007/s11883-013-0370-4.
31. Martínez-Gonzáleza MA, Salas-Salvadó J, Estruch R, et al. Benefits of the Mediterranean diet: insights from the PREDIMED study. Prog Cardiovasc Dis. 2015;58(1):50–60. https://doi.org/10.1016/ j.pcad.2015.04.003.
32. Abdullah MMH, Jones JPH, Jones PJH. Economic benefits of the Mediterranean-style diet consumption in Canada and the United States. Food Nutr Res 2015;59: 27541. https://doi.org/10.3402/fnr.v59.27541.
33. Sofi F, Macchi C, Abbate R, et al. Mediterranean diet and health status: an updated meta-analysis and a proposal for a literature-based adherence score. Public Health Nutr. 2014;17(12):2769–82.
34. Bo S, Ponzo V, Goitre I, et al. Predictive role of the Mediterranean diet on mortality in individuals at low cardiovascular risk: a 12-year follow-up population-based cohort study. J Transl Med. 2016;14:91. https://doi.org/10.1186/s12967-016-0851-7.
35. Stewart RA, Wallentin L, Benatar J, et al. Dietary patterns and the risk of major adverse cardiovascular events in a global study of high-risk patients with stable coronary heart disease. Eur Heart J. 2016;37:1993–2001. https://doi.org/10.1093/eurheartj/ehw125.
36. Panagiotakos DB, Georgousopoulou EN, Georgiopoulos GA, et al. Adherence to Mediterranean diet offers an additive protection over the use of statin therapy:results from the ATTICA study (2002-2012). Curr Vasc Pharmacol. 2015;13(6):778–87.
37. Steffen LM, Horn LV, Daviglus ML, et al. A modified Mediterranean diet score is associated with a lower risk of incident metabolic syndrome over 25 years among young adults: the CARDIA (Coronary Artery Risk Development in Young Adults) study. Br J Nutr. 2014;112:1654–61.
38. Dilis V, Katsoulis M, Lagiou P, et al. Mediterranean diet and CHD: the Greek European Prospective Investigation into Cancer and Nutrition cohort. Br J Nutr. 2012;108:699–709.
39. Guallar-Castillon P, Radriguez F, Tormo MJ, et al. Major dietary patterns and risk of coronary heart disease in middle-aged persons from a Mediterranean country: the EPIC-Spain cohort study. Nutr Metab Cardiovasc Dis. 2012;22(3):192–9.
40. Liyanage T, Ninomiya T, Wang A, et al. Effects of the Mediterranean diet on cardiovascular outcomes—a systematic review and meta-analysis. PLoS One. 2016;11(8):e0159252. https://doi.org/10.1371/journal.pone.0159252.
41. Rees K, Hartley L, Flowers N, et al. Mediterranean dietary pattern for the primary prevention of cardiovascular disease. Cochrane Database Syst Rev. 2013;8:CD009825. https://doi.org/10.1002/14651858.CD009825.pub2.
42. Kastorini C-M, Milionis HJ, Esposito K, et al. The effect of Mediterranean diet on metabolic syndrome and its components: a meta-analysis of 50 studies and 534,906 individuals. J Am Coll Cardiol. 2011;57:1299–313.
43. Bédard A, Lamarche B, Corneau L, et al. Sex differences in the impact of the Mediterranean diet on systemic inflammation. Nutr J. 2015;14:46. https://doi.org/10.1186/s12937-015-0035-y.
44. Sala-Vila A, Romero-Mamani ES, Gilabert R, et al. Changes in ultrasound-assessed carotid intima-media thickness and plaque with a Mediterranean diet. A sub-study of the PREDIMED trial. Arterioscler Thromb Vasc Biol. 2014;34:439–45.
45. Estruch R, Ros E, Salas-Salvado J, et al. Primary prevention of cardiovascular disease with a Mediterranean diet. N Engl J Med. 2013;368:1279–90.
46. Mitjavila MT, Fandos M, Salas-Salvadó J, et al. The Mediterranean diet improves the systemic lipid and DNA oxidative damage in metabolic syndrome individuals. A randomized, controlled, trial. Clin Nutr. 2013;32:172–8.
47. Murie-Fernández M, Irimia P, Toledo E, et al. Carotid intima-media thickness changes with Mediterranean diet: a randomized trial (PREDIMED-Navarra). Atherosclerosis. 2011;219:158–62.
48. Thomazella MCD, Góes MFS, Andrade CR, et al. Effects of high adherence to Mediterranean or low-fat diets in medicated secondary prevention patients. Am J Cardiol. 2011;108(11):1523–9. https://doi.org/10.1016/j.amjcard.2011.07.008.
49. Mena MP, Sacanella E, Vazquez-Agell M, et al. Inhibition of circulating immune cell activation: a molecular anti-inflammatory effect of the Mediterranean diet. Am J Clin Nutr. 2009;89:248–56.
50. Fito M, Guxens M, Corella D, et al. Effect of a traditional Mediterranean diet on lipoprotein oxidation. A randomized controlled trial. Arch Intern Med. 2007;167:1195–203.
51. Estruch R, Martinez-Gonzalez MA, Dolores Corella D, et al. Effects of a Mediterranean-style diet on cardiovascular risk factors a randomized trial. Ann Intern Med. 2006;145:1–11.
52. Esposito K, Marfella R, Ciotola M, et al. Effect of a Mediterranean-style diet on endothelial dysfunction and markers of vascular inflammation in the metabolic syndrome a randomized trial. JAMA. 2004;292:1440–6.
53. Singh RB, Dubnov G, Niaz MA, et al. Effect of an Indo-Mediterranean diet on progression of coronary artery disease in high risk patients (Indo-Mediterranean Diet Heart Study): a randomised single-blind trial. Lancet. 2002;360:1455–61.
54. de Lorgeril M, Salen P, Martin J-L, et al. Mediterranean diet, traditional risk factors, and the rate of cardiovascular complications after myocardial infarction. final report of the Lyon Diet Heart Study. Circulation. 1999;9:779–85.
55. Kastorini CM, Milionis HJ, Goudevenos JA, Panagiotakos DB. Mediterranean diet and coronary heart disease: is obesity a link? A systematic review. Nutr Metab Cardiovasc Dis. 2010;20:536–51.

56. Zidi W, Allal-Elasmi M, Zayani Y, et al. Metabolic syndrome, independent predictor for coronary artery disease. Clin Lab. 2015;61:1545–52.
57. Salehi-Abargouei A, Maghsoudi Z, Shirani F, Azadbakht L. Effects of Dietary Approaches to Stop Hypertension (DASH)-style diet on fatal or nonfatal cardiovascular disease incidence: a systematic review and meta-analysis on observational prospective studies. Nutrition. 2013;29:611–8.
58. Struijk EA, May AM, Wezenbeek NL, et al. Adherence to dietary guidelines and cardiovascular disease risk in the EPIC-NL cohort. Int J Cardiol. 2014;176(2):354–9.
59. Levitan EB, Lewis CE, Tinker LF, et al. Mediterranean and DASH diet scores and mortality in women with heart failure. The Women's Health Initiative. Circ Heart Fail. 2013;6:1116–23.
60. Levitan EB, Wolk A, Mittleman MA. Relation of consistency with the dietary approaches to stop hypertension diet and incidence of heart failure in men aged 45 to 79 years. Am J Cardiol. 2009;104(10):1416–20.
61. Fung TT, Chiuve SE, McCullough ML, et al. Adherence to a DASH-style diet and risk of coronary heart disease and stroke in women. Arch Intern Med. 2008;168(7):713–20.
62. Siervo M, Lara J, Chowdhury S, et al. Effects of the Dietary Approaches to Stop Hypertension (DASH) diet on cardiovascular risk factors: a systematic review and meta-analysis. Br J Nutr. 2015;113:1–15.
63. Jenkins DJA, Boucher BA, Ashbury FD, et al. Effect of current dietary recommendations on weight loss and cardiovascular risk factors. J Am Coll Cardiol. 2017;69:1103–12. https://doi.org/10.1016/j.jacc.2016.10.089.
64. Chen ST, Maruthur NM, Appel LJ. The effect of dietary patterns on estimated coronary heart disease risk: results from the Dietary Approaches to Stop Hypertension (DASH) Trial. Circ Cardiovasc Qual Outcomes. 2010;3(5):484–9.
65. Maruthur NM, Wang N-Y, Appel LJ. Lifestyle interventions reduce coronary heart disease risk: results from the PREMIER Trial. Circulation. 2009;119(15):2026–31.
66. King DE, Egan BM, Woolson RF, et al. Effect of a high-fiber diet vs. a fiber-supplemented diet on C-reactive protein level. Arch Intern Med. 2007;167:502–6.
67. Appel LJ, Sacks FM, Carey VJ, et al. Effects of protein, monounsaturated fat, and carbohydrate intake on blood pressure and serum lipids. Results of the OmniHeart randomized trial. JAMA. 2005;294:2455–64.
68. Obarzanek E, Sacks FM, Vollmer WM, et al. Effects on blood lipids of a blood pressure–lowering diet: The Dietary Approaches to Stop Hypertension (DASH) Trial. Am J Clin Nutr. 2001;74:80–9.
69. Eckel RH, Jakicic JM, Ard JD, et al. 2013 AHA/ACC guideline on lifestyle management to reduce cardiovascular risk: a report of the American College of Cardiology/American Heart Association Task Force on Practice Guidelines. J Am Coll Cardiol. 2014;63:2960–84.
70. Huang T, Yang B, Zheng J, et al. Cardiovascular disease mortality and cancer incidence in vegetarians: a meta-analysis and systematic review. Ann Nutr Metab. 2012;60(4):233–40.
71. Wang F, Zheng J, Yang B, et al. Effects of vegetarian diets on blood lipids: a systematic review and meta-analysis of randomized controlled trials. J Am Heart Assoc. 2015;4:e002408. https://doi.org/10.1161/JAHA.115.002408.
72. Kourlaba G, Polychronopoulos E, Zampelas A, et al. Development of a diet index for older adults and its relation to cardiovascular disease risk factors: the Elderly Dietary Index. J Am Diet Assoc. 2009;109:1022–30.
73. Atkins JL, Whincup PH, Morris RW, et al. High diet quality is associated with a lower risk of cardiovascular disease and all-cause mortality in older men. J Nutr. 2014;144:673–80. https://doi.org/10.3945/n.113.186486.
74. Dong JY, Zhang YH, Wang P, et al. Meta-analysis of dietary glycemic load and glycemic index in relation to risk of coronary heart disease. Am J Cardiol. 2012;109:1608–13.
75. Burger KN, Beulens JW, Boer JM, et al. Dietary glycemic load and glycemic index and risk of coronary heart disease and stroke in Dutch men and women: the EPICMORGEN study. PLoS One. 2011;6:e25955.
76. Jakobsen MU, O'Reilly EJ, Heitmann BL, et al. Major types of dietary fat and risk of coronary heart disease: a pooled analysis of 11 cohort studies. Am J Clin Nutr. 2009;89:1425–32.
77. Simila ME, Kontto JP, Satu Mannisto S, et al. Glycaemic index, carbohydrate substitution for fat and risk of CHD in men. Br J Nutr. 2013;110:1704–11. https://doi.org/10.1017/S0007114513000858.
78. Li Y, Hruby A, Bernstein AM, et al. Saturated fat as compared with unsaturated fats and sources of carbohydrates in relation to risk of coronary heart disease: a prospective cohort study. J Am Coll Cardiol. 2015;66(14):1538–48. https://doi.org/10.1016/j.jacc.2015.07.055.
79. Satija A, Bhupathiraju SN, Spiegelman D, et al. Healthful and unhealthful plant-based diets and the risk of coronary heart disease in US adults. J Am Coll Cardiol. 2017;70(4):411–22.

12 Whole Plant Foods and Coronary Heart Disease

Keywords
Coronary heart disease • Whole-grains • Fruit • Vegetables • Legumes Nuts • Seeds • Low density lipoprotein-cholesterol • High density lipoprotein-cholesterol • Triglycerides • C-reactive protein

Key Points

- Prospective cohort studies consistently show that diets with higher intakes of whole and minimally processed plant foods (whole plant foods) including whole-grains, fruits, vegetables, legumes, and nuts and seeds are associated with reduced coronary heart disease (CHD) risk compared to lower intake.
- Heart healthier versions of whole plant foods are higher in dietary fiber, phytosterols, healthy fatty acids (MUFAs and PUFAs), and nutrients (e.g., vitamins E and C, potassium and folate), phytochemicals (carotenoids, flavonoids and phytosterols) and lower in energy density, glycemic index and glycemic load.
- The risk of CHD incidence or mortality is significantly reduced with the intake of ≥3 servings/day of whole-grains (especially oats and barley), ≥5 servings (400 g)/day of fruits and vegetables, ≥4 weekly servings (130–150 g cooked) of legumes (both non-soy and/or soy products), and ≥5 servings/week of nuts and seeds.
- Randomized controlled trials (RCTs) generally support the beneficial effects of healthy whole plant based foods on CHD risk biomarkers including lowering serum lipids and blood pressure, improving glucose and insulin metabolism, improving endothelial function, alleviating oxidative stress and inflammation and reducing risk of weight gain compared to their refined counterparts.
- Only a small fraction of the US population meets the recommended intake levels for whole-grains, fruits, vegetables, legumes, and nuts and 70% exceed recommended refined grain intake. Approximately 45% of CHD deaths in the US are associated with suboptimal low dietary intake of fruits, vegetables, nuts and seeds, whole-grains, and seafood omega-3 PUFAs, and high intake of red and processed meats, sugar sweetened beverages, and sodium.

M.L. Dreher, *Dietary Patterns and Whole Plant Foods in Aging and Disease*, Nutrition and Health,
https://doi.org/10.1007/978-3-319-59180-3_12

12.1 Introduction

Coronary heart disease (CHD) is the leading cause of mortality worldwide, especially in countries that have acculturated to the Western lifestyle [1–6]. Although there have been some decreasing trends in overall CHD mortality rate over the last several decades because of cholesterol lowering drugs and surgical procedures, it is still a leading cause of death globally and its prevalence is expected to increase as the global population ages. The role of elevated lipids, lipoproteins and inflammation as modifiable risk factors for CHD is well established [5–9]. Healthy behaviors, including meeting the recommended intake of whole plant foods, increased physical activity, and weight control, have been shown to reduce the risk for CHD [6–9]. A recent study in the US, showed that adults with higher consumption of a plant-based diet rich in healthier plant foods (whole-grains, fruit, vegetables, legumes, nuts, seeds, vegetable oils, tea and coffee) had significantly reduced CHD risk by 25% whereas less healthy plant foods (sweetened beverages, refined grains, French fries, sweets and red and processed meats significantly increased CHD risk by 32% [10]. Whole and minimally processed plant foods (whole plant foods) are higher in fiber and nutrient density (e.g., vitamins E and C, and trace minerals such as selenium and copper), and phytochemicals (carotenoids, flavonoids and phytosterols) than refined foods (Appendix A) [11–19]. Conseqently, healthy whole plant based foods have more favorable effects on CHD risk by lowering serum lipids and blood pressure, improving glucose and insulin metabolism, improving endothelial function, alleviating oxidative stress and inflammation and reducing risk of weight gain than refined foods [7–9, 11, 13–47]. However, whole plant foods or minimally processed plant foods are consumed at low levels in the US and other Western diet consuming populations [48]. It is estimated that most of the US population falls short of meeting the recommended minimal intake levels for whole-grains by 99%, fruit by 85% and vegetables by 90%, and 70% of the US population exceeds the recommended refined grain intake.

For primary CHD prevention, the benefits achievable though diet and other lifestyle factors are likely to be similar or better than those due to drug treatment of elevated blood cholesterol or pressure because they contribute to multiple cardiometabolic health benefits [8]. Specific foods can have a positive or negative effect on CHD risk [49, 50]. A comparative analysis of the association between dietary factors and CHD risk from population dietary habits and demographic data collected by the US National Health and Nutrition Examination Surveys (NHANES; 1999–2002 and 2009–2012; 16,620 individuals) found that fruit (excluding juice), vegetables including legumes, nuts and seeds, whole grains, seafood omega-3 fat, and polyunsaturated fat reduce CHD risk and red and processed meat and sugar sweetened beverages increase CHD risk (Fig. 12.1) [49]. Similar findings were shown in a systematic review of the evidence supporting a causal link between whole plant foods and lowering of CHD risk compared to Western diets (Fig. 12.2) [50]. This is exemplified by a case study of a 60-year-old man with typical angina. After a positive stress test, he declined both drug therapy and invasive treatment and opted instead to adopt a whole food plant-based diet, which consisted primarily of vegetables, fruits, whole grains, legumes, and nuts [51]. After 4 months, his BMI fell from 26 kg/m^2 to 22 kg/m^2, his blood pressure normalized, his low-density lipoprotein- cholesterol (LDL-C) decreased from 158 mg/dL to 69 mg/dL and he was able to walk one mile without angina. The objective of this chapter is to comprehensively review the effects of whole plant foods on CHD risk and related risk factors.

12.2 Whole Plant Foods and Coronary Heart Disease Risk

The US National Center for Health Statistics reports that about 45% of cardiometabolic deaths (based on 702,308 cardiometabolic deaths in 2012) are associated with suboptimal intake of the following dietary factors including low intakes of fruits, vegetables, nuts and seeds, whole-grains, and seafood omega 3 and other polyunsaturated (PUFA) fats, and excessive intake of red and processed meats, sugar

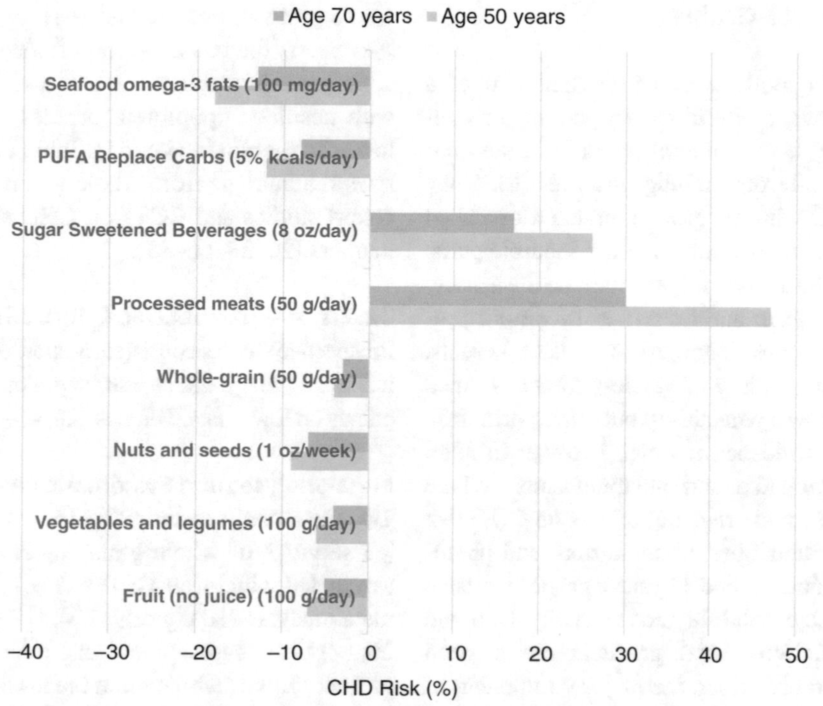

Fig. 12.1 Comparative analysis of the association between foods and beverages and coronary heart disease (CHD) risk by adult age from the US National Health and Nutrition Examination Surveys (1999–2002 and 2009–2012; 16,620 individuals) (adapted from [49])

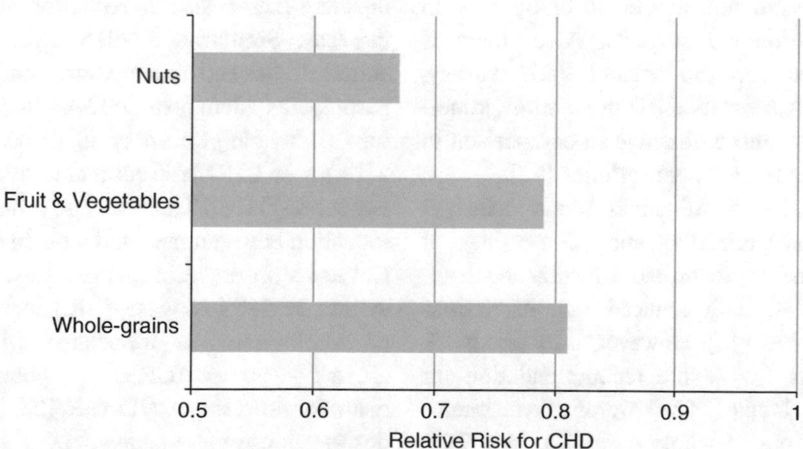

Fig. 12.2 Effect of the recommended intake of whole-grains, fruits, vegetables and nuts on a coronary heart disease (CHD) composite risk score from prospective cohort studies and RCTs (adapted from [50])

sweetened beverages, and sodium [49]. The optimal intake of these dietary factors is at least 300 g of non-juice fruit/day, 400 g vegetables including legumes/day, 5 weekly servings of nuts, 2.5–3 servings of whole-grains/day, 11% kcals from PUFA as a replacement for carbohydrates or saturated fat, and 250 mg of seafood omega-3 fat, and limiting red meat to 100 g/week and sodium to 2000 mg/day, and not or rarely consuming processed meat or sugar sweetened beverages.

12.2.1 Whole-Grains

Whole-grain foods are an important part of a healthy dietary pattern as they are major contributors of fiber, minerals, vitamins, antioxidants, phytosterols and lignans [52–56]. They consist of the intact, ground, cracked or flaked grain kernels after removal of the inedible parts, such as the husk and hull, and include the starchy endosperm, germ and bran fiber in similar proportions that are found in the intact kernels. Milling and grinding of whole-grains to refined grains improves palatability but leaves primarily the starchy endosperm, which is lower in fiber, vitamins, minerals and phytonutrients. Whole grains have a wide range of effects on CHD risk because of their fiber, micronutrient and phytochemical content, and physical properties such as particle size, solubility and viscosity. Oats and barley containing food products are a good source of soluble fiber, the major component of which is β-glucan, which is known to reduce serum LDL-C and CHD risk [56]. Daily doses of at least 3 g β-glucan may reduce plasma total and low-density lipoprotein (LDL) cholesterol levels by 5% in normocholesterolemic or by 10% in hypercholesterolemic subjects. Also, there is growing focus on the ancient grain variety, Khorasan wheat for its CHD prevention properties, which are more effective in comparison to more contemporary wheat varieties [57].

The US dietary guidelines recommend ≥3 servings/whole-grains/day and ≤3 servings of refined grains/day to promote health and wellness associated with reduced risk of various chronic diseases [48]. However, only about 1% of Americans follow the recommendation for whole-grain intake. The average American's intake is <1 ounce whole grains/day and 70% exceed the recommended intake for refined grains [48, 58]. Adequate intake of whole-grains is generally believed to have important health benefits in reducing CHD risk with recognition of health claims in the US, EU and other countries [59–63]. Large prospective cohort studies consistently associate whole-grain with improved CHD outcomes. RCTs show mixed results for CHD biomarkers due to the differing compositions and physical properties of each specific whole grain source studied [64]. In adults aged ≥45 years, the consumption of adequate whole-grain in conjunction with statins use is associated with healthier lipoprotein profiles compared to low whole-grain intake [65]. Table 12.1. summarizes the findings from whole-grains prospective cohort studies and RCTs on CHD risk and biomarkers [26, 28, 66–83].

12.2.1.1 Prospective Cohort Studies

Prospective studies consistently show that increased intake of whole-grains has significant beneficial effects on lowering CHD risk [26, 66–75].

Meta-analyses and Systematic Reviews

Two meta-analyses show that the consumption of ≥3 servings of whole grain/day is significantly associated with lower CHD risk [67, 68]. A 2016 meta-analysis (10 cohorts; 704,317 participants; 26,243 CVD cases) found that the consumption of 3 servings of whole grain breads and breakfast cereals reduced CHD risk by 19% [67]. There was a clear dose-response relationship between whole-grains and CHD risk up to 210 g/day, with a slightly steeper reduction in risk up to 3 servings/day then a slower reduction above 3 servings/day. Similarly, a 2015 meta-analysis (15 cohort studies and 3 case-control studies; 400,492 participants) demonstrated that approx. 3 servings of whole-grains/day is associated with a 21% lower CHD risk compared to a low intake (<1 serving) [68]. There was no difference in risk reduction between men and women or geographical areas observed in this analysis. Several systematic reviews suggested that increased intake of whole-grains is associated with lowering C-reactive protein (CRP) as a potential mechanism for lowering CHD risk [26, 69]. Also, a dose-response meta-analysis of whole grains (3 cohort studies; 240,532 participants; 2678 deaths from CHD) found that each serving (30 g) of whole grains/day lowered risk of CHD mortality by 8%, with significant heterogeneity [66].

Representative Cohort Studies

Six prospective cohort studies consistently show that increased whole-grain intake significantly reduced CHD risk and mortality [70–76]. A Danish cohort study (54,871 adults; mean age

Table 12.1 Summaries of whole-grain studies on CHD risk and biomarkers

Objective	Study details	Results
Prospective Cohort Studies		
Systematic Reviews and Meta-analysis		
Li et al. (2016). Investigate the effect of whole grains on the risk of CHD specific mortality according to a dose-response meta-analysis of prospective cohort studies [66]	3 cohort studies; 240,532 participants; 2678 deaths from CHD	Each 1 serving of whole grains/day lowered risk of CHD mortality by 8%, with significant heterogeneity
Aune et al. (2016). Systematically quantify the dose-response relation between consumption of whole grain and specific types of grains and the risk of cardiovascular disease (CVD) [67]	10 cohort studies; 704,317 participants; 26,243 CVD cases	There was a 19% reduction in CHD risk per 90 g/day increase in whole-grain intake (90 g is equivalent to three servings—example, two slices of bread and one bowl of cereal or one and a half pieces of pita bread made from whole-grains). A dose-response relationship between whole-grains and CHD risk was shown up to 210 g/day. There was a slightly steeper reduction in risk up to 3 servings/day then a slower reduction above 3 servings/day. The intake of whole grain bread, whole grain breakfast cereals, total breakfast cereals, and bran were inversely associated with CVD risk
Tang et al. (2015). Systematically evaluate the findings from cohort studies of the effects of whole-grain intake on CHD risk [68]	15 cohort studies and 3 case-control studies); 12 studies from the US; 400,492 participants; follow-up of 5 to 26 years; 14,427 patients with CHD	Higher intake of whole-grains (>3 servings) was significantly associated with a 21% reduced risk for CHD. In subgroup analyses, there were no differences in the overall results by geography, study duration or gender
Buyken et al. (2014). Systematically evaluate the effect of whole-grains on inflammatory markers [69]	7 observational studies; 11,295 participants; aged 27 to 62 years; BMI of 24 to 31	Five of 7 studies observed a significant association between a higher whole-grain intake and lower hs-CRP or IL-6 concentrations. One study reported only a trend for the relation between whole grain and hs-CRP. Whole-grain intake was especially effective in lowering inflammatory markers among persons with type 2 diabetes
Lefevre et al. (2012). Systematically review the effects of whole-grains on systemic inflammation [26]	13 prospective cohort studies; 35,771 participants	Each whole-grain serving significantly reduced C-reactive protein (CRP) levels by 7%. For highest vs. lowest intake, whole-grains reduced CRP by 10–29%
Prospective Cohort Studies		
Helnaes et al. (2016). Investigate the association between whole-grain intake in terms of total intake and intakes of different cereals and myocardial infarction (Denmark) [70]	54,871 adults; mean baseline age 57 years; 72% males and 28% women; mean 13.6-years of follow-up; 2329 individuals developed myocardial infarction (multivariate adjusted)	Total whole-grain intake in the highest quartile lowered risks of myocardial infarction in men by 25% and in women by 27% compared to the lowest quartile. Rye bread (in men and women) and oatmeal (in men) were associated with significantly lower risk of myocardial infarction. The effects of types of whole grain breads and oatmeal are summarized in Fig. 12.3

(continued)

Table 12.1 (continued)

Objective	Study details	Results
Johnsen et al. (2015). Investigate the effect of whole-grains on CHD mortality (Scandinavian HELGA Norwegian sub-cohort) [71]	120,000 subjects; median baseline age 51 years for women and 54 years for men; follow-up of 10–16 years; 298 women and 858 men died from CHD (multivariate adjusted)	Higher intake of breakfast cereals lowered CHD mortality for women by 9% and for men by 4%. Doubling intake of total whole-grain products lowered CHD mortality for women by 15% and for men by 8%. Among women, intake of oats and wheat was associated with a borderline statistically significant lower CHD mortality by 5%
Sonestedt et al. (2015). Examine the association between the consumption of carbohydrate-rich foods and beverages and the risk of incident ischemic CVD (The Malmö Diet and Cancer Study; Sweden) [72]	4535 subjects; mean baseline age 60 years; 62% females;14-years of follow-up (multivariate adjusted)	Higher whole grain intake significantly lowered risk for ischemic CVD by 13% (highest vs. lowest quintile). Higher intake of foods rich in added sugar (sugar and sweets, and sugar-sweetened beverages) were significantly associated with higher triglycerides and lower HDL-C concentrations
Mellen et al. (2007). Evaluate the effect of whole-grain intake on carotid intima-media thickness (C-IMT) progression (Insulin Resistance Atherosclerosis Study; US) [73]	1178 adults; mean baseline age 55 years; 56% female; follow-up of 5 years (multivariate adjusted)	Whole-grain intake was inversely associated with carotid common and internal C-IMT progression
Jensen et al. (2004). Estimate the associations of whole-grain, bran, and germ intakes with the incidence of CHD (US- The Health Professionals Follow-Up Study) [74]	42,850 men; baseline age 40–75 years; 14-years of follow-up; 1818 cases of CHD (1261 nonfatal myocardial infarctions and 557 fatal CHD) (multivariate adjusted)	CHD risk was significantly reduced by 18% between extreme quintiles of whole-grain intake. Also, CHD risk was significantly reduced by 30% with the highest intake of added bran vs. no intake of added bran (Fig. 12.4)
Liu et al. (1999). Evaluate whether high whole-grain intake affects risk of CHD in women (US -The Nurses' Health Study) [75]	75,521 women; baseline age 38–63 years; follow-up of 10 years; 761 cases of CHD (208 of fatal CHD and 553 of nonfatal myocardial infarction) (multivariate adjusted)	Whole-grain intake significantly reduced CHD risk by 25% for 2.7 servings vs. 0.13 servings. In never smokers, whole-grain CHD risk was reduced by 51%
Jacobs et al. (1998). Determine the effect of whole-grains on the risk of ischemic heart disease death (The Iowa Women's Health Study; US) [76]	34,492 postmenopausal women; baseline age 55–69 years; follow-up of 9 years (multivariate adjusted)	3.2 servings/day whole-grains was significantly inversely associated with ischemic heart disease mortality with reduced risk by 30% vs. 0.2 servings/day. Dark bread intake vs. white bread was shown to significantly lower ischemic heart disease risk (Fig. 12.5)

Table 12.1 (continued)

Objective	Study details	Results
Randomized Controlled Trials (RCTs)		
Meta-analyses and Systematic Reviews		
Hollaender et al. (2015). Systematically compare the effect of whole-grain vs. refined-grains on fasting lipids [28]	24 RCTs; 16 of the studies evaluated hypercholesterolemic subjects; 2275 participants; aged 18–75 years; the daily whole-grain dose ranged from 28 to 213 g/day; 6–8 weeks	Whole-grain intake significantly lowered mean LDL-C by 3.5 mg/dL and TC by 4.6 mg/dL compared with the refined control. Whole-grain oats was most effective in lowering TC by 6.6 mg/dL. There was no effect of whole-grain foods on HDL-C but TG was lowered by 3.5 mg/dL compared with the control (p = 0.10). A weight-loss diet improved the efficacy of whole-grains in reducing LDL-C
Zhu et al. (2015). Systematically evaluate the clinical effects of beta-glucan from oat and barley on fasting lipid levels in subjects [77]	17 RCTs; 916 hyperlipidemic subjects including 14 parallel and 3 crossover studies; 9 oat and 5 barley β-glucan studies compared to appropriate controls. The β-glucan dose ranged from 2.8 to 10.3 g/day (mean 5.5 g/day); 4–12 weeks	β-glucan significantly lowered TC by 10 mg/dL and LDL-C by 8 mg/dL with no significant differences in HDL-C, and TG vs. control diets independent of baseline TC or LDL-C, age (< or ≥50 years), duration (<or ≥8 weeks), barley-derived β-glucan, oat-derived β-glucan at > or ≤5 g day
Whitehead et al. (2015). Systematically evaluate clinical effects of oat beta-glucan/day on fasting lipid levels [78]	28 RCTs with 12 in healthy subjects, 13 in hyperlipidemic subjects, and 3 in diabetic subjects; 2700 subjects; age range 25–63 years; average β-glucan intake from food and supplements was 5.5 g/day (3–12 g/day); average 6 weeks (2–12 weeks)	Diets containing ≥3 g oat bran β glucan/day reduced serum TC and LDL-C relative to control by 9.5 and 11.5 mg/dL, respectively, with no significant effects on HDL-C or TG. LDL-C lowering was significantly greater with higher baseline LDL-C
Lefevre et al. (2012). Systematically assess the effect of whole grains on CRP [26]	7 RCTs; 742 participants; aged 46–60 years; BMI range of 27–36; 3–16 weeks	Only 1 of 7 RCTs showed significantly reduced CRP for the whole-grain high fiber group as part of a hypocaloric diet compared to the low fiber control
Representative RCTs		
Whittaker et al. (2015). Examine CHD protective effects of substituting ancient, organic khorasan wheat for modern conventional grains (Italy) [79]	**Crossover RCT:** 22 acute coronary syndrome patients; 9 females and 13 males; median age 61 years; mean BMI 26.9; assigned to consume products (bread, pasta, biscuits and crackers) made either from organic semi-whole khorasan wheat or organic semi-whole semolina control wheat; patients ingested 62 g dry weight khorasan or control/day; 8 weeks; 8-weeks washout	Ancient Khorasan wheat significantly lowered TC by 6.8%, LDL-C by 8.1%, glucose by 8% and insulin by 24.6%, independently of age, sex, traditional risk factors, medication and diet quality (Fig. 12.6). Additionally, there was a significant reduction in reactive oxygen species, lipoperoxidation of circulating monocytes and lymphocytes, and TNF-alpha vs. the contemporary semolina wheat
Vitaglione et al. (2015). To evaluate the effect of whole-wheat foods on systemic inflammation (Italy) [80]	**Parallel RCT**: 80 healthy overweight and obese subjects; mean age about 40 years; 70% female; sedentary lifestyles; diets: 70 g/day of whole-wheat foods (>4 servings; 8 g fiber/day) or refined-wheat foods (2 g fiber/day); 8 weeks	The whole-wheat group significantly reduced TNF-α and increased IL-10 (anti-inflammatory) levels compared with the refined wheat group. There was a borderline significant reduction in IL-6 compared with the refined wheat group (p = 0.06)
Giacco et al. (2013). Evaluate the effect of whole-grain vs. refined cereal foods on cardiometabolic risk factors (Italy and Finland) [81]	**Parallel RCT:** 146 metabolic syndrome subjects; aged 40–65 years; randomized into wheat and rye whole-grain (33 g fiber/day) or refined cereal products (20 g fiber/day); 12 weeks	There were no significant effects from whole- grains on TC, LDL-C, HDL-C, and TG or systemic inflammatory markers (e.g., CRP, IL-6, and TNF-α) compared to the refined grain control. No changes in anthropometric parameters were observed

(continued)

Table 12.1 (continued)

Objective	Study details	Results
Brownlee et al. (2010). Study the effect of whole-grains on CHD biomarkers in people who habitually consume refined -grains (WHOLEheart study; UK) [82]	**Parallel RCT:** 316 adult subjects; mean age 46 years; mean BMI 30; consuming <30 g whole-grains/day; randomized to 3 groups: (1) refined grain control, (2) 60 g whole-grains/day for 16 weeks and (3) 60 g whole-grains/day for 8 weeks followed by 120 g whole-grains/day for 8 weeks	Increased whole-grain intake did not significantly improve any markers of CVD risk including BMI, % body fat, waist circumference; fasting lipid profile, glucose and insulin, CRP, or endothelial function compared to refined grain
Katcher et al. (2008). To evaluate the effect of a whole-grain rich hypocaloric diet on cardiometabolic health in obese subjects [83]	**Parallel RCT:** 50 obese subjects; mean age 46 years BMI > 30; randomized into 500 kcal/day deficit groups with dietary advice to either avoid all whole-grain foods or consume only whole-grain foods; 12 weeks	There was no difference in weight loss between groups, although the whole-grain group lost a significantly greater % body fat in the abdominal region and lowered CRP levels by 38% vs. the refined grain group

57 years; 13.6 years of follow-up) observed that higher total whole-grain intake lowered myocardial infarction risk by about 25% in both men and women [70]. This was especially true for oatmeal and crispbread in men and rye bread and oatmeal in women (Fig. 12.3). The Health Professionals Follow-up Study (42,850 men; baseline aged 40–75 years; follow-up of 14 years) observed that higher whole-grain intake ≥50 g/day significantly reduced CHD risk by18% compared to about 3 g/day of whole-grains, and highest intake of added bran vs. no intake of added bran significantly reduced risk by 30%, after multivariate adjustments (Fig. 12.4) [74]. The Nurses' Health Study (75,521; 38–62 years at baseline; 10 years of follow-up) observed that about 3 daily servings vs. 0.1 servings of whole-grains significantly lowered CHD risk by 25% for all women and 51% for never smoking women [75]. The Iowa Women's Health Study (34,492 post-menopausal women; 55–69 years at baseline; 9 years of follow-up) observed an inverse association between whole grain intake and risk of death from ischemic heart disease with a 30% lower risk for about 3 servings/day of whole-grains vs. 0.2 servings, after multivariate adjustments [76]. This study also found that whole-grain dark bread significantly lowered ischemic heart disease risk compared to white bread in postmenopausal women (Fig. 12.5). The US Insulin Resistance Atherosclerosis Study (1178 adults; mean baseline age 55 years; 5 years of follow-up) observed that increased whole-grains intake was inversely associated with carotid intima-media thickness progression [73]. The Malmö Diet and Cancer Study cohort (4535 subjects; mean baseline age 60 years; 62% females; 14 years of follow-up) found that higher whole grain intake significantly lowered risk for ischemic CVD by 13% (highest vs. lowest quintile) [72]. Additionally, higher intake of foods rich in added sugar was significantly associated with higher triglycerides (TG) and lower HDL-C concentrations.

12.2.1.2 Randomized Controlled Trials (RCTs)

Intervention trials show mixed results for CHD biomarkers due to the varying compositions of whole-grains and levels of intake [26, 28, 77–83]. A 2015 meta-analysis (24 RCTs; 2275 participants) estimated that increased whole-grain intake significantly lowered mean LDL-C by 3.5 mg/dL and total cholesterol (TC) by 4.6 mg/dL compared with the refined control [28]. Oat whole-grain was twice as effective in lowering TC compared to the mean of all the other whole-grains analyzed. Whole-grains insignificantly lowered TG by 3.5 mg/dL ($p = 0.10$) and had no effect on HDL-C. The two most recent meta-analyses found that the mean intake of 5.5 g β-glucan from oat or barley whole grains significantly lowered TC and LDL-C by about

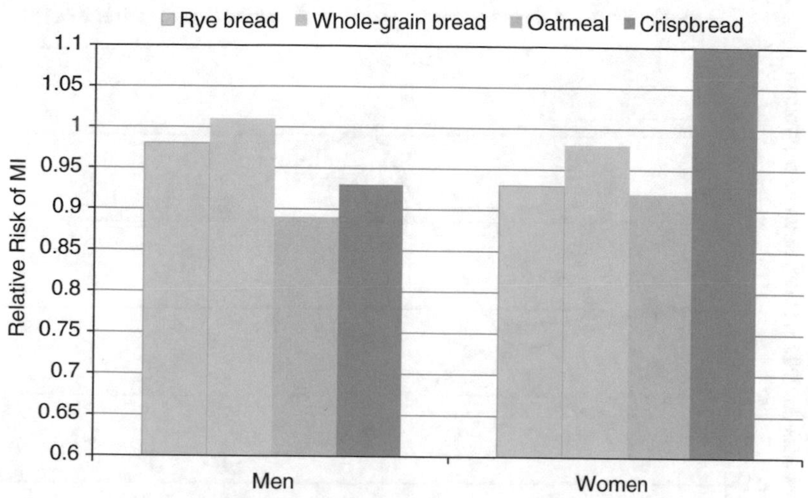

Fig. 12.3 Association between different whole-grain forms and myocardial infarction (MI) risk per 25 g intake (adapted from [70])

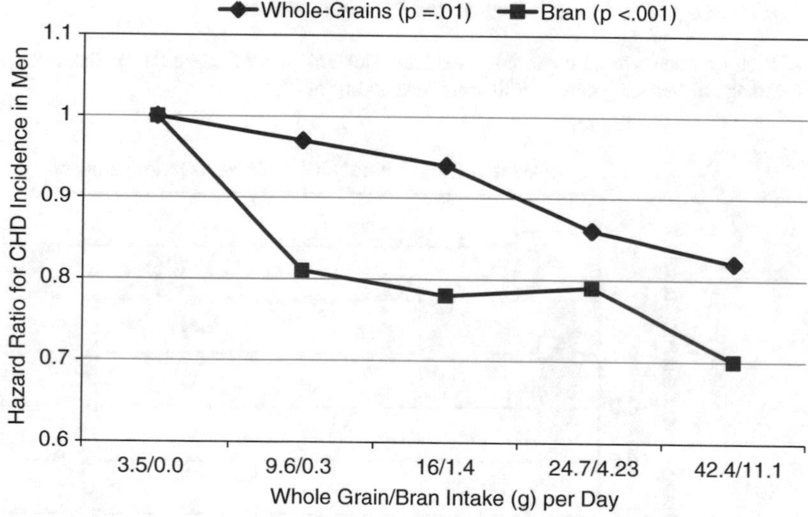

Fig. 12.4 Association between whole-grains and bran and coronary heart disease (CHD) incidence in men (adapted from [74])

10 mg/dL each [77, 78]. A review of whole-grains found that only 1 of 7 RCTs showed significantly reduced CRP compared to refined grains and that reduction was from a hypocaloric diet RCT [26]. Representative RCTs show mixed effects from whole-grain intake on CHD risk biomarkers depending on the study population, whole-grain form and overall diet [79–83]. The ancient grain khorasan wheat has been shown in several RCTs to improve lipoprotein profiles, glycemic and inflammatory biomarkers compared to modern wheat varieties but the mechanism is not completely understood (Fig. 12.6) [57, 79]. Most RCTs show that the substitution of whole grain wheat for refined wheat does not significantly reduce lipoproteins, glycemic, systemic inflammatory or endothelial markers associated with increased CHD risk but whole grain wheat may further lower circulatory inflammatory markers such as CRP in weight loss diets compared to refined grains [80–83].

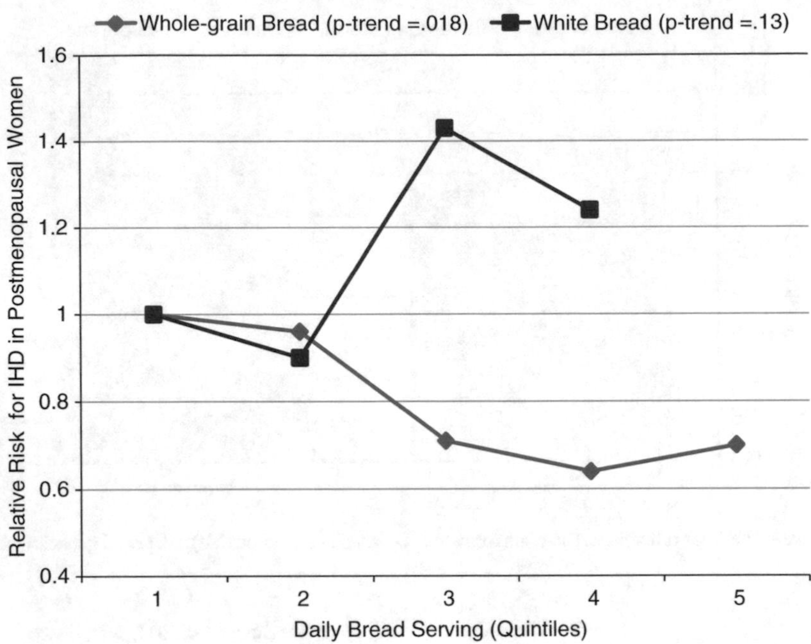

Fig. 12.5 Association between type of bread consumed and ischemic heart disease (IHD) risk in 34,492 postmenopausal women, mean age 61 years, 9 years of follow-up (adapted from [76])

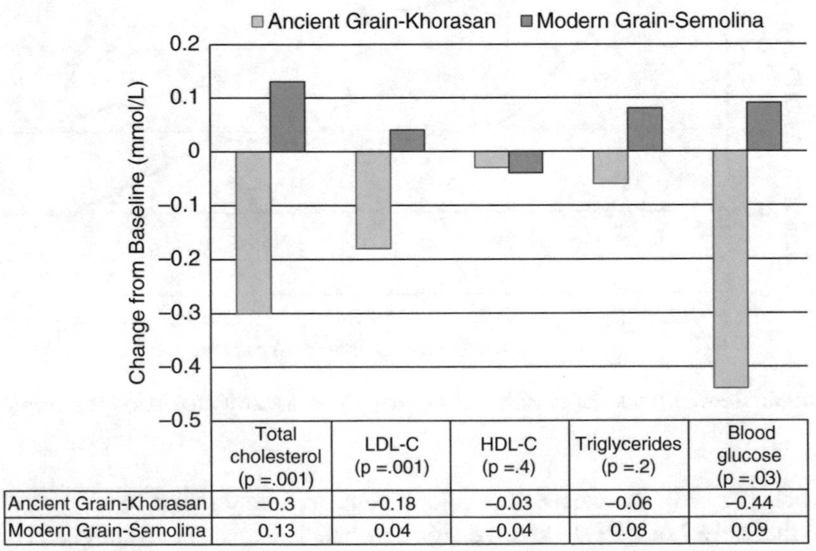

Fig. 12.6 Effect of ancient grain vs. modern grain on major coronary heart disease (CHD) risk biomarkers (adapted from [79])

12.2.2 Fruits and Vegetables

Fruit and vegetables are important parts of most global dietary guidance recommendations because of their concentrations of: antioxidant vitamins and phytochemicals, especially phenolics and carotenoids; minerals, especially electrolytes; and fiber [84]. The World Health Organization (WHO) Report recommended a minimum daily intake of 400 g of fruits and vegetables, based on evidence that higher levels are protective against CHD [85]. This led to the launch of various "eat 5 or more" fruit and vegetable campaigns in Europe, the US and Australia [86]. The USDA MyPlate educational concept, devotes one-half the plate to fruits and vegetables because they are i mportant for a healthy diet and also displace from the diet other foods of higher energy density and lower nutrient and phytochemical levels [87]. However, globally, fruit and vegetable consumption is only at a small fraction of the recommended levels [88]. In the US, >85% of the population falls short of meeting the daily fruit and vegetable intake recommendations [58]. For fruit, whole fruit comprises only about half the daily fruit intake with the remainder primarily consumed as 100% fruit juice. For vegetables, white potatoes (a good source of potassium and fiber), are the most commonly consumed single vegetable, accounting for 25% of all vegetable consumption [58]. Potatoes are consumed in a variety of forms, with about 31% being boiled (including mashed and in dishes such as potato salad, soups, and stews), 22% as chips, sticks, or puffs, 19% as French fries, 17% as baked, and 12% as home fries or hash browns. The effects of increased fruit and vegetable intake on CHD risk and related biomarkers from prospective cohort studies and RCTs is summarized in Table 12.2 [30, 31, 89–103].

12.2.2.1 Prospective Cohort Studies

Systematic Reviews and Meta-analyses

Five meta-analyses of fruit and vegetable prospective studies consistently confirm that adequate fruit and vegetable intake (e.g., 5 servings per day) is significantly associated with CHD risk reduction [89–93]. A 2017 systematic review and dose-response meta-analysis (66 CHD cohort studies, > 2 million participants; and 64 CVD cohort studies, > 600,000 participants) found that increased total and specific subtypes of fruits and vegetables significantly reduced both CHD and CVD risk [89]. CHD risk was reduced per daily 200g for fruits and vegetables by 8%, for fruits by 10% and vegetables by 16%. The intake of 800 g/day of total fruits and vegetables lowered CHD risk by 24%. For specific types of fruits and vegetables, higher intake of apples, pears, citrus fruits, 100% fruit juices, onions, green leafy vegetables, β-carotene-rich fruits and vegetables and vitamin C-rich fruits and vegetables were most effective at lowering CHD risk (Fig. 12.7). CVD risk was reduced per 200 g/day total fruits and vegetables by 8%, for fruits by 13% and vegetables by 10%. There was a 28% lower CVD risk for intakes of 800 g/day for fruits and vegetables and fruits, and 600 g/day of vegetables. Of specific types of fruits and vegetables, higher intake of apples, pears, citrus fruits, carrots, and green leafy vegetables were most effective in lowering CVD risk whereas a high intake of canned fruits increased risk (Fig. 12.8). A 2015 dose-response meta-analysis (23 cohort studies; 937,665 participants; 5–37 years of follow-up) found that the CHD risk for intakes of 500 g/day of total fruits and vegetables reduced risk by 12%, 300 g/day of fruits by 16%, and 400 g/day of vegetables by 18% [90]. In the subgroup analysis, a significant inverse association was observed in western populations, but not in Asian populations. A 2014 dose-response meta-analysis (10 cohorts; 1,147,225 participants) showed a lower risk of CVD mortality with each serving of fruit by 5% or vegetables by 4% [91]. Two other meta-analyses also found similar protective effects of increased fruit and vegetable intake on CHD risk [92, 93].

Representative Cohort Studies

Six representative cohort studies consistently support the protective benefits of fruit and vegetable consumption on CHD risk [31, 94–98]. The effects of fruit and vegetable intake were shown to be consistent across ethnic groups [94]. In the Shanghai Women's Health Study and Shanghai Men's Health Study (62,211 women, mean baseline age 54 years, 9.8 years of follow-up; 55,474 men, mean baseline age 52 years, 5.4 years of follow-up) women had a significant 6% reduction in CHD risk per 80 g fruit and vegetable intake but there was no significant lowering of CHD risk in men [31]. The pooled data from the Nurses' Health Study and Health Professionals Follow-up Study observed that

Table 12.2 Summaries of fruit and vegetable studies on CHD risk and biomarkers

Objective	Study details	Results
Prospective Cohort Studies		
Meta-Analyses		
Aune et al. (2017). Assess the dose-response relationship between fruit and vegetable intake and risk of CHD and CVD and the effects of specific types of fruits and vegetables [89]	**CHD**: 66 cohort studies; > 2 million participants **CVD**: 64 cohort studies; > 600,000 participants	**CHD**: Per 200 g/day, CHD risk was reduced for fruits and vegetables by 8%, for fruits by 10% and vegetables by 16%. There was a 24% reduction in the relative risk at an intake of 800 g/day of fruits and vegetables. There was a 21% risk reduction up to 750–800 g/day for fruits and a 30% risk reduction up to 550–600 g/day for vegetables. For specific types of fruits and vegetables: higher intake of apples, pears, citrus fruits,100% fruit juices, β-carotene- or vitamin C-rich fruits and vegetables and green leafy vegetables were among the most effective at lowering CHD risk (Fig. 12.7) **CVD**: Per 200 g/day, CVD risk was reduced for fruits and vegetables by 8%, for fruits by 13% and vegetables by 10%. There were approx. 28% risk reductions for intakes of 800 g/day for fruits and vegetables combined, and fruits, and 600 g/day of vegetables. Of specific types of fruits and vegetables, higher intake of apples and pears, citrus fruits, carrots, and green leafy vegetables were among the most effective in lowering CVD risk (Fig. 12.8)
Gan et al. (2015). Systematically evaluate the relationship of fruit and vegetable intake with CHD risk and quantify the dose-response relationship between them [90]	23 cohort studies; 937,665 participants; over 5 to 37 years of follow-up; 18,047 cases of CHD reported	In the dose-response analysis, the risk of CHD was reduced by 12% per 477 g/day in total fruits and vegetables, by 16% per 300 g/day in fruit, and by 18% per 400 g/day in vegetables
Wang et al. (2014). Systematically examine and quantify a possible dose-response relation between fruit and vegetable intake and risk of CVD [91]	Total fruits and vegetables 4 cohort studies, 469,551 participants, 6893 CVD deaths; fruits or vegetables 6 cohort studies, 677,674 participants, 9744 CVD deaths; 4.6 to 26 years of follow-up	CVD mortality was significantly reduced per daily serving of fruits and vegetables combined by 4%, for fruit consumption by 5%, and for vegetable consumption by 4%
He et al. (2007). Systematically assess the relationship of fruit and vegetable intake with CHD risk [92]	12 cohort studies; 278,459 individuals; median follow-up of 11 years; 9143 CHD events	Subjects consuming >5 daily fruit and vegetables servings significantly reduced CHD risk by 17% vs. those who ate <3 daily fruit and vegetable servings. The consumption of 3 to 5 daily servings of fruits and vegetables reduced CHD risk by 7% ($p = 0.06$)

Table 12.2 (continued)

Objective	Study details	Results
Dauchet et al. (2006). Systematically determine the strength of the association between fruit and vegetable intake and CHD risk [93]	9 studies; 91,379 men, 129,701 women; follow-up duration 5–19 years; 5007 CHD events	The risk of CHD was significantly reduced for each daily portion of fruits and vegetables by 4% and for each fruit portion by 7%
Prospective Cohort Studies		
Sharma et al. (2014). Assess the effects of fruit and vegetable intake on mortality rates from ischemic heart disease among ethnic groups (Multi- ethnic Cohort Study; US) [94]	164,617 adults; mean baseline age 66 years for males and 59 years for females; 4 years of follow-up; 1140 males and 811 females with fatal ischemic heart disease cases (multivariate adjusted)	In men, there was a significant 27% lower ischemic heart disease risk at ≥6.6 daily servings of vegetables. Inconsistent results were observed for women, where the protective association was observed only at mid-level vegetable intake levels, but not among women with the highest level of vegetable intake. There was no evidence of an association for fruit intake in men or women
Yu et al. (2014). Examine the effect of fruit and vegetable intake on CHD risk among Chinese adults (Shanghai Women's Health Study and the Shanghai Men's Health Study; China) [31]	67,211 women, mean baseline age 54 years, mean follow-up of 9.8 years; 148 CHD events; and 55,474 men, mean baseline age 52 years, mean follow-up of 5.4 years; 217 CHD events (multivariate adjusted)	Women in the highest quartile of total fruit and vegetable intake (median: 814 g/day) had a significant 38% reduced CHD risk compared with those in the lowest quartile (median: 274 g/ day). Each 80 g/day increment of total fruit and vegetable intake was associated with a 6% reduction of CHD risk among women. For men, no significant association was found for fruit and vegetable intake when analysed either in combination or individually
Bhupathiraju et al. (2013). Measure the roles of quantity and variety of fruit and vegetable intake on the incidence of CHD (US Nurses' Health Study and Health Professionals Follow-Up studies [95]	71,141 women, mean baseline age 50 years, 24-years of follow-up, 2582 cases of CHD; and 42,135 men, mean baseline age 53 years, 22-years of follow-up, 3607 CHD cases (multivariate adjusted)	The consumption of 4–5 fruit and vegetable servings/day was associated with lower CHD risk by 16%, multivariate adjusted. The intake of citrus fruit, green leafy vegetables, and β-carotene- and vitamin C-rich fruit and vegetables were more potent at lowering CHD risk vs. the general intake of fruits and vegetables (Fig. 12.9)
Griep et al. (2011). Determine the effects of fruit and vegetables of different colors (green, orange/yellow, red/purple, and white) on 10-year CHD incidence (Monitoring Project on Risk Factors and Chronic Diseases in the Netherlands Study) [96]	20,000 adults; mean baseline age 41 years; mean BMI 25; 10 years of follow-up; 245 cases of CHD (multivariate adjusted)	For each daily 25 g increase in the intake of: (1) mixed fruits and vegetables reduced CHD risk by 2% and (2) orange fruits and vegetables significantly reduced CHD risk by 24%. Specifically, carrots, were associated with a significant 32% lower risk of CHD

(continued)

Table 12.2 (continued)

Objective	Study details	Results
Griep et al. (2010). Evaluate the effects of raw vs. processed fruit and vegetable intake on CHD risk (Monitoring Project on Risk Factors and Chronic Diseases in the Netherlands Study) [97]	20,069 adults; mean baseline age 41 years; 10.5 years of follow-up; 245 CHD cases (multivariate adjusted)	Higher fruit and vegetable intake >475 g/day was associated with a 34% lower CHD risk vs. ≤241 g/day. Both raw or processed fruit and vegetables may protect against CHD risk (Fig. 12.10). A subgroup analysis indicated that increased fruit and vegetable intake was more effective in reducing CHD risk in women and subjects ≥50 years of age
Joshipura et al. (2001). Determine the dose response of specific fruits and vegetables on CHD risk (the Nurses' Health Study and the Health Professionals' Follow-Up Study; US) [98]	84,251 women, baseline 34 to 59 years of age, followed for 14 years, 1127 CHD cases; 42,148 men, 40 to 75 years; follow-up of 8 years, 1063 cases (multivariate adjusted)	Each serving/day increase in intake of fruits or vegetables was associated with a 4% lower risk for CHD. Each serving significantly reduced CHD risk for green leafy vegetables by 23% and for vitamin C-rich fruit and vegetables by 6%
Randomized Controlled Trials (RCTs)		
Systematic Review		
Hartley et al. (2013). Systematically estimate the effect of increasing fruit and vegetable intake on fasting lipids in healthy adults and those at high risk of CVD/CHD (Cochrane Systematic Review) [30]	4 RCTs; 970 participants; study duration ranged from 3 months to 1 year	The pooled data showed that increased fruit and vegetables intake insignificantly lowered LDL-C by 6.5 mg/dL, HDL-C by 0.4 mg/dL, and TG by 9.0 mg/dL compared to low fruit and vegetable control diets
Representative RCTs		
McEvoy et al. (2015). Examine the dose-response effect of fruit and vegetable intake on CHD risk factors (Northern Ireland) [99]	**Parallel RCT:** 93 overweight adults (BMI of 27–35 kg/m^2) with habitually low fruit and vegetable intake (≤160 g/day) and an elevated risk of developing CHD (estimated ≥20% over 10 years). Subjects were randomly assigned to consume 2, 4, or 7 portions fruit and vegetables (equivalent to 160 g, 320 g, or 560 g of fruits and vegetables daily); 12 weeks	There was a borderline significant dose-response effect of increasing fruit and vegetable intake on lowering LDL-C (p-trend =0.06). There were no changes in HDL-C, TG, or CRP levels with increasing fruit and vegetable intake
Wang et al. (2015). Evaluate the effect of a Hass avocado fruit on CHD biomarkers (US) [100]	**Crossover RCT:** 45 overweight/obese subjects; 3 diets: moderate-fat diets including one fresh Hass avocado; a moderate-fat (MUFA) diet avocado free; and a lower-fat diet; 5 weeks with 2 week washout	Compared with baseline, a one avocado/day diet significantly reduced LDL-C by 13.5 mg/dL and non-HDL-C by 14.6 mg/dL compared to the moderate MUFA diet reducing LDL-C by 8.3 mg/dL and non-HDL-C by 8.7 mg/dL, and lower fat diet reducing LDL-C by 7.4 mg/dL and non-HDL-C by 4.8 mg/dL. Further, only the avocado diet significantly reduced LDL, small dense LDL-C, and the ratio of LDL/HDL from baseline

Table 12.2 (continued)

Objective	Study details	Results
Rayn-Haren et al. (2013). Compare the effects of whole apples vs. apple juice on fasting lipids (Denmark) [101]	**Crossover RCT:** 23 healthy subjects evaluated the fasting lipid and CRP lowering effects of apples and apple juice over 4 weeks	Whole apples lowered LDL-C by 6.7% compared to 2.2% for apple juice. There were no significant changes in HDL-C or CRP. Fiber was identified as a primary component for whole apple cholesterol lowering effects
Choi et al. (2013). Investigate whether serum lipids are influenced by the amount of kimchi intake (Korea) [102]	**Parallel RCT:** 100 volunteers; age 23 years; BMI 21; 2 dietary groups: 15 g/day vs. 210 g/day of kimchi intake; 7 days	Triglycerides concentrations were significantly reduced with low kimchi by 6.1 mg/dL and high kimchi by 7.4 mg/dL. Total cholesterol was significantly lowered with low kimchi by 6.8 mg/dL and high kimchi by 8.9 mg/dL. Serum total antioxidant status was significantly increased dose-dependently in low kimchi by 5.2% and high kimchi by 7.5%. Fasting blood glucose was significantly decreased in the high kimchi intake
Watzl et al. (2005). Investigate the effects of low, medium, and high intakes of fruits and vegetables on markers of immune functions, including nonspecific markers of inflammation (Germany) [103]	**Parallel RCT:** 63 non-smoking men; mean age 31 years; mean BMI 24 years; run-in diet with ≤2 servings/day of fruits and vegetables for 4 weeks; diet 2, 5, or 8 fruits and vegetables servings; 4 weeks	Systemic CRP was significantly reduced in the subjects who consumed 8 servings/day of fruits and vegetables compared with those who consumed 2 servings/day

green leafy vegetables and β-carotene and vitamin C rich fruits and vegetables were among the most effective in protecting against CHD risk (Fig. 12.9) [95, 98]. A prospective Dutch study found a 24% reduction in CHD risk for a daily 25 g increase in orange fruits and vegetables compared to only 2% CHD reduction for all fruits and vegetables [96] and raw forms of fruits and vegetables were found to be more effective in lowering CHD risk than processed forms (Fig. 12.10) [97].

12.2.2.2 Randomized Controlled Trials

RCTs on the effects of fruits and vegetables on CHD biomarkers are inconsistent because of the wide variability in composition, processing, amounts consumed, subject variability, clinical designs and compliance variations [30, 99–103]. A Cochrane Systematic Review (4 RCTs; 970 subjects; duration 3–12 months) found limited evidence for the beneficial effects of fruits and vegetables on fasting lipids with mean lowering of LDL-C by 6.5 mg/dL, HDL-C by 0.4 mg/dL, and TG by 9.0 mg/dL, which were not statistically significant [30]. A dose-response RCT found a borderline significant effect of increasing self-selected fruit and vegetable intake on reducing LDL-C (p-trend = 0.06) with no change in HDL-C, TG, or CRP with increased intake [99]. A similar dose response RCT showed significant reduced CRP with increased fruit and vegetable portions [103]. RCTs showed avocados, apples and kimchi to significantly reduce blood lipids and lipoproteins to healthy levels [100–102].

12.2.3 Legumes

Legumes, including pulses (e.g., pinto beans, split peas, lentils, chickpeas) and soybeans, are rich in fiber and protein with relatively low glycemic response properties [14, 104]. A serving of legumes is 1⁄2 cup or 90–100 g cooked legumes, which contains 5–10 g of fiber and 7–8 g of protein. Most legumes contain <5% of energy as fat, with the exception of chickpeas and soybeans which have 15% and 47% energy from fat,

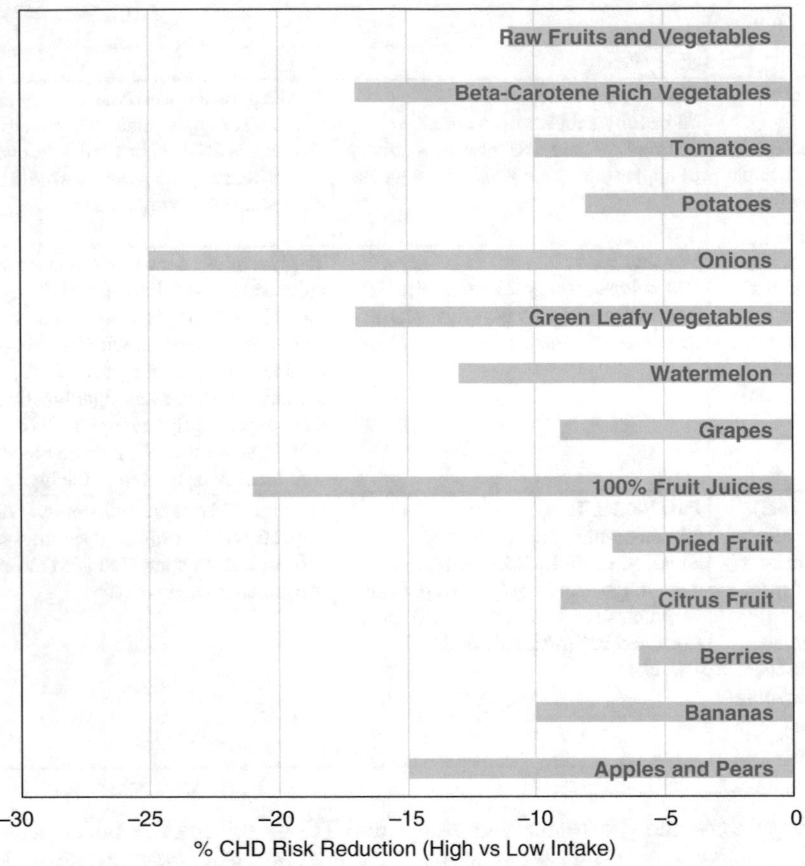

Fig. 12.7 Associations between specific fruits and vegetables and coronary heart disease (CHD) risk from 2017 meta-analysis of 66 cohort studies (adapted from [89])

respectively. Legumes contain nutritionally important amounts of the B vitamins and minerals, such as iron, calcium and potassium. They also contain bioactive phytochemicals such as phenolics, saponins and isoflavones (especially in soya foods). Legumes are often consumed as a lower energy dense, lower saturated fat, and high fiber meat or milk replacer. Legume consumption has been in decline with the global shift to Western-style diets [105]. For example, between the 1960s and 1990s, legume intake decreased by 40% in India and by 24% in Mexico. Legumes are infrequently consumed by North Americans and northern Europeans, with <8% of Americans consuming them on any given day.

12.2.3.1 Non-Soy Legumes

The prospective studies on CHD risk and RCTs on CHD related biomarkers are summarized for non-soy legumes in Table 12.3 [106–114].

Prospective Cohort Studies

A meta-analysis (5 cohort studies; 200,000 adults) and one large prospective study (9632 subjects; mean baseline age 48 years at baseline; 19 years of follow-up) support the benefits of consuming 100–130 g of non-soy legumes such as beans, peas, lentils ≥4 days per week for reducing the risk of CHD by 14–22% compared to <1 time per week, after adjusting for known CVD risk factors [106, 107].

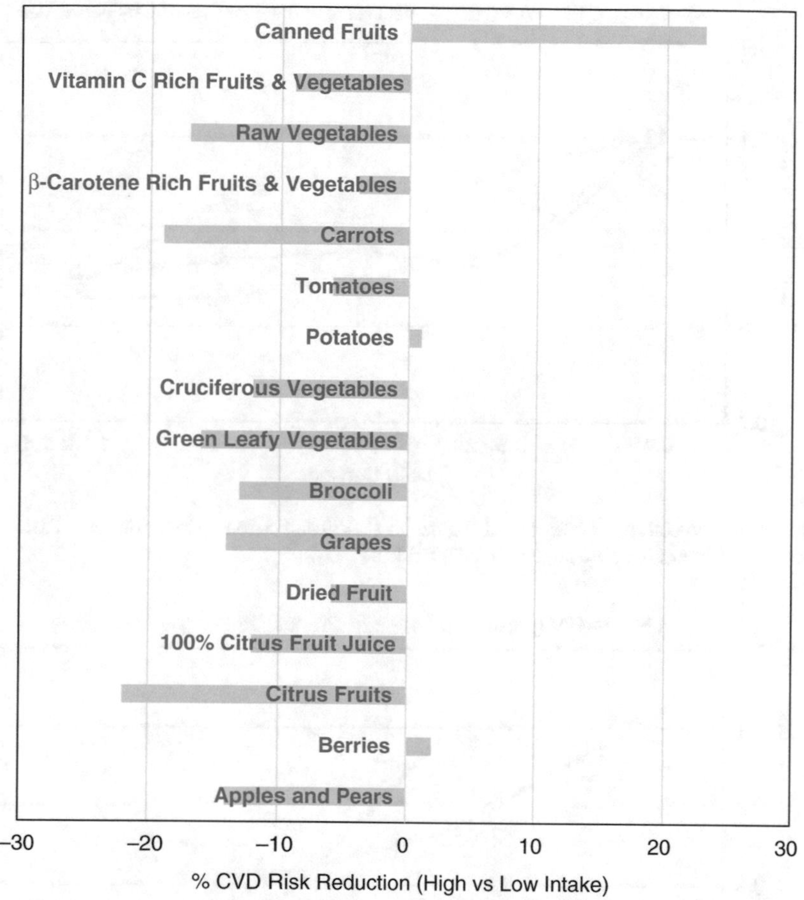

Fig. 12.8 Associations between specific fruits and vegetables and cardiovascular disease (CVD) risk from 2017 meta-analysis of 64 cohort studies (adapted from [89])

Randomized Controlled Trials

Non-soy legume RCTs find consistent beneficial effects on fasting lipid profiles and modest effects on CRP levels compared to control diets [108–114].

Fasting Lipid Profiles. A meta-analysis (26 RCTs; 1037 subjects; median age 51 years; median dose 130 g/day; duration ≥3 weeks) indicated that 130 g of pulses/day can significantly lower mean LDL-C by 6.6 mg/dL (5%) compared to control diets [109]. A systematic review showed that daily consumption of 2 servings of pulses (150 g/day) by overweight men and women with a mean age of 60 years, lowered both TC and LDL-C by about 8% after 2 months [110]. Chickpeas (100–120 g cooked/day) have been shown in several RCTs to significantly lower TC and LDL-C compared to usual or wheat-based diets [113, 114].

C-Reactive Protein. A meta-anlysis (8 RCTs; 480 subjects; duration 4–52 weeks) found that non-soy legumes lowered mean CRP by 0.21 mg/L ($p = 0.068$) [108]. In obese adults, hypocaloric legume supplemented diets significantly lowered CRP levels compared to legume free hypocaloric diets, which may be related to the 2.5% weight loss in the legume group after 8 weeks [112].

12.2.3.2 Soy Products

The prospective studies on CHD risk and RCTs on CHD related biomarkers are summarized for soy products in Table 12.4 [34, 115–124].

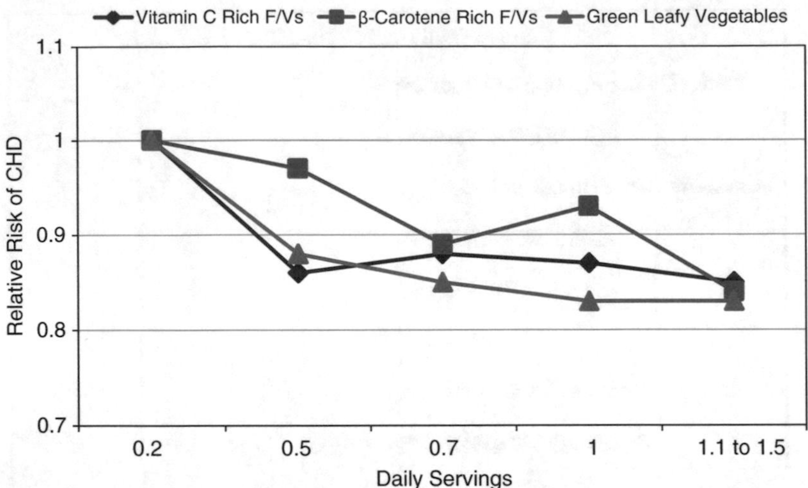

Fig. 12.9 Association between specific fruits and vegetables (F/Vs) and coronary heart disease (CHD) risk in men and women (all p < 0.003 after multivariate adjusted) (adapted from [95])

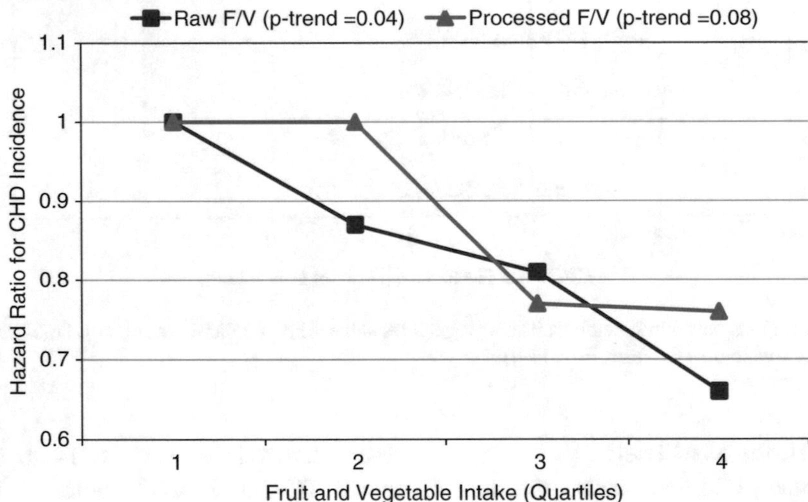

Fig. 12.10 Association between the level of raw and processed fruits and vegetables (F/V) on coronary heart disease (CHD) risk (adapted from [97])

Prospective Cohort Studies

Two prospective cohort studies show that soy product intake is associated with lower CHD risk compared to soy free diets [116, 117]. In a Japanese study, women consuming a high intake of soy foods (> 5 times/week) compared to ≤2 times/week, reduced myocardial infarction risk by 45%, but no risk reduction was observed in men [115]. In the Shanghai Women's Health Study high soy protein intake (>11 g/day) compared to low intake (<4.5 g/day) reduced CHD risk by 75% and myocardial infarction by 86% [116].

Randomized Controlled Trials

RCTs show that soy products promote improved fasting lipid profiles compared to control soy-free diets [34, 117–124].

Systematic Reviews and Meta-analyses. There are four meta-analyses and systematic reviews on soy and CHD biomarkers [34, 117–119]. A 2015 meta- analysis (35 RCTs; 2670 subjects; 82% women; 4–52 weeks; average dose 4–18 weeks) showed strong evidence that soy products resulted in significant mean reductions in serum LDL-C by 4.8 mg/dL, TG by

Table 12.3 Summaries of non-soy legumes studies on CHD risk and biomarkers

Objective	Study details	Results
Prospective Cohort Studies		
Systematic Review and Meta-analysis		
Afshin et al. (2014). Systematically estimate the effect of non-soy legume intake on ischemic heart disease risk [106]	5 prospective cohort studies; 200,000 adults; 514 ischemic heart disease cases	Four weekly 100-g servings of non-soy legumes was associated with a mean lower ischemic heart disease risk by 14%
Prospective Cohort Study		
Bazzano et al. (2001). Examine the effect of non-soy legume intake on CHD and CVD risk (National Health and Nutrition Examination Survey Epidemiological Follow-up Study; US) [107]	9632 men and women; mean baseline age 49 years; 60% women; follow-up of 19 years; 1800 CHD cases and 3680 CVD cases (multivariate adjusted)	Non-soy legume intake was significantly and inversely associated with reduced CHD and CVD risk, after adjusting for known CVD risk factors. Non-soy legume intake (≥ 4 times/week vs < 1 time/week) reduced CHD risk by 22% and CVD risk by 11%
Randomized Controlled Trials (RCTs)		
Systematic Reviews and Meta-Analyses		
Salehi-Abargouei et al. (2015). Systematically determine the effect of non-soy legume intake on systemic CRP levels [108]	8 RCTs; 480 normal, overweight and obese adults; duration 4–52 weeks	Non-soy legume intake showed a small but significant trend towards decreasing CRP by a mean of 0.2 mg/L
Ha et al. (2014). Systematically evaluate the effect of pulses (beans, chickpeas, lentils and peas) on fasting lipids [109]	26 RCTs; 1037 subjects, middle-age, normo- and hyperlipidemic adults, at moderate risk of coronary artery disease; ≥ 3 weeks	The median intake of 130 g cooked pulses/day significantly lowered mean LDL-C levels 6.6 mg/dL (5%) compared to control non-pulse diets.
Bazzano et al. (2011). Systematically evaluate the effects of non-soy legumes intake on fasting lipids [110]	10 RCTs; 268 participants; ≥ 3 weeks	Legume rich diets significantly mean lowered TC by 12 mg/dL and LDL-C by 8.0 mg/dL compared to control diets
Representative RCTs		
Abeysekara et al. (2012). Determine the effects of pulse-based diets on the fasting lipids and cardio-metabolic health of older adults (Canada) [111]	**Crossover RCT:** 108 subjects; mean age 60 years; mean weight 76 kg; randomized to consume 2 servings daily of beans, chickpeas, peas or lentils (about 150 g/day dry weight) or their regular diet (pulse-free); 2 months; 1 month washout	Compared with the regular diet, the pulse-based diet significantly decreased TC by 8.3% and LDL-C by 7.9%. Subjects consumed 36% higher fiber (69% insoluble and 31% soluble) intake while eating the pulse-based diet compared with the regular diet
Hermsdorf et al. (2011). Study the effects of hypocaloric diets with and without legumes on CRP responses (Spain) [112]	**Parallel RCT:** 30 obese subjects; mean BMI 32.5; mean age 36 years; 60% male; randomized into a calorie restricted legume free diet or calorie restricted legume based diet including 4 weekly different cooked legume servings (160–235 g chickpeas, lentils, peas and beans); 8 weeks	The legume diet significantly reduced TC, LDL-C and CRP, and promoted weight loss by 2.5% compared to the control diet

(continued)

Table 12.3 (continued)

Objective	Study details	Results
Pittaway et al. (2008). Evaluate the effects of chickpea enriched diets on *ad libitum* nutrient intake, body weight, fasting lipids, and other cardiometabolic changes (Australia) [113]	**Sequential RCT:** 45 free-living adults; 13 premenopausal women, 19 postmenopausal women, 13 men; mean age was 52 years; mean BMI 26; 120 g cooked chickpeas/day added to the habitual diet for 12 weeks, followed by 4 weeks of habitual diet without chickpeas	Chickpeas significantly lowered fasting TC by 7.7 mg/dL and LDL-C by 7.3 mg/dL, compared to the chickpea-free diet. There was also a small loss of weight by 0.45 kg ($p = 0.07$) during the chickpea phase, which was thought to be related to the increased fiber intake
Pittaway et al. (2006). Examine the effects of chickpea diets on fasting lipids (Australia) [114]	**Crossover RCT:** 47 adults; randomized to groups consuming chickpeas or wheat; 5 weeks	The chickpea group had significantly lower TC by 3.9% and LDL-C by 4.6%, compared to the wheat group

Table 12.4 Summaries of soy product studies on CHD risk and biomarkers

Objective	Study details	Results
Prospective Cohort Studies		
Kokubo et al. (2007). Assess the effect of soy and isoflavone intake on risk of cerebral and myocardial infarctions (The Japan Public Health Center–Based Prospective Study) [115]	40,462 Japanese adults; mean baseline age 50 years; BMI 23; average follow-up of 12.5 years; 587 cerebral infarctions cases, 308 myocardial infarctions cases (multivariate adjusted)	For women, there was a reduced risk of cerebral infarctions by 36% and myocardial infarctions by 45% for soy intake ≥5 times/week versus ≤2 times/week. No significant associations were observed in men
Zhang et al. (2003). Investigate the effect of soy foods on CHD risk in Chinese women (The Shanghai Women's Health Study) [116]	75,000 Chinese women; mean baseline age 51 years; mean BMI 24; mean of 2.5 years of follow-up; 62 cases of CHD (multivariate adjusted)	There was a significant reduction in adjusted CHD risk by 75% for women consuming high intake of soy protein foods (>11 g/day) vs. low intake (<4.5 g/day). Also, there was a significant 86% lower risk of nonfatal MI for the highest vs. the lowest quartile of soy intake
Randomized Controlled Trials (RCTs)		
Meta-Analyses and Reviews		
Tokede et al. (2015). Systematically estimate the clinical effect of soy products on fasting lipids [117]	35 RCTs; 2670 adults; 82% women; average dose 30 g/day (range 14–50 g/day); mean duration (4 weeks to 1 year)	Intake of soy products significantly reduced serum LDL-C by 4.8 mg/dl, TG by 4.9 mg/dl, and TC by 5.3 mg/dl and significantly increased serum HDL by 1.4 mg/dl. LDL reductions were more marked in hypercholesterolemic subjects by 7.5 mg/dl, than in healthy subjects by 3.0 mg/dl. LDL-C lowering was stronger for whole soy products (soy milk, soybeans and nuts) by 11 mg/dL vs. soy extracts by 3.2 mg/dL
Anderson et al. (2011). Systematically evaluate the clinical effects of soy foods and/or protein on fasting lipids [34]	43 RCTs (20 parallel and 23 crossover studies); median intake 30 g of soy protein daily; 4–18 weeks	Soy protein significantly lowered LDL-C by 5.5% in parallel studies and 4.2% in crossover studies vs. control diets. Also, HDL-C and TG levels were 3.2% higher and 10.7% lower, respectively, with soy vs. control diets

Table 12.4 (continued)

Objective	Study details	Results
Yang et al. (2011). Systematically review the effects of soy product intake on fasting lipid profiles and glycemic control in type 2 diabetes patients [118]	8 RCTs; soy protein (with soy isoflavones) or soy products (tofu, miso or soy nuts); 6 weeks-4 years	Soy products significantly lowered TC by 16 mg/dL, LDL-C by 12 mg/dL, and TG by 19 mg/dL along with a significantly increasing HDL-C by 2 mg/dL. There were no significant effects on fasting glucose, insulin and glycated hemoglobin
Sacks et al. (2006). Systematically review RCTs on the effect of soy protein products on fasting lipids [119]	22 RCTs; fasting lipids and other CHD risk factors; 4 weeks –1 year	The increased intake of soy products by an average of 50 g/day decreased LDL-C levels by 3%. No significant effects on HDL-C, TG, or blood pressure were reported
Representative RCTs		
Padhi et al. (2015). Determine potential dose response effects of soy protein on LDL-C in hypercholesterolemic adults (Canada) [120]	**Double-blind, Parallel RCT:** 243 hypercholesterolemic adults; mean age 55 years; mean BMI 28; randomly assigned to muffins with 25 g soy protein, 12.5 g soy protein, 12.5 g whey protein, or 25 g whey protein daily; 6 weeks while on a self-selected diet	Consuming 12.5 or 25 g protein from defatted soy flour incorporated into muffins did not reduce LDL-C or other CHD risk factors in hypercholesterolemic adults compared to similar amounts of whey protein
Azadbakht et al. (2007). Evaluate the effects of soy intake on inflammatory markers (US) [121]	**Crossover RCT**: 42 postmenopausal, metabolic syndrome women; randomly assigned to a control DASH diet, or one of 2 modified DASH diets, where a serving of red meat was replaced by soy protein, or soy nuts; 8 weeks	CRP was reduced in the soy nut diet by 8.9% and soy protein diet by1.6% compared to the control DASH diet. The soy nut diet significantly reduced IL-18 compared with the control diet by 9.2%
Jenkins et al. (2002). Assess the effects of soy foods on both lipid and nonlipid risk factors for coronary artery disease (Canada) [122]	**Parallel RCT:** 41 hyper-lipidemic men and postmenopausal women; randomized to 3 diets: a low-fat dairy food control diet; 50 g soy protein diet (73 mg isoflavones daily); or 52 g soy protein diet (10 mg isoflavones daily); 1 month	Soy diets resulted in significantly lower TC, estimated coronary artery disease risk, and LDL-C to HDL-C ratio compared to the low-fat dairy control diet. No significant differences were seen between the high and low-isoflavone soy diets. Soy diets significantly lowered coronary artery disease risk by 10% compared to low fat diary diets
Gardner et al. (2001). Determine the effect of soy protein and isoflavones on fasting lipids (US) [123]	**Double-blind, Parallel RCT:** 94 postmenopausal, moderately hypercholesterolemic women, mean age about 60 years; diets supplemented with 42 g protein/day) diets: (1) milk protein, (2) soy protein (no isoflavones), or (3) soy protein (80 mg isoflavones); 12 weeks	Soy protein with isoflavones significantly lowered LDL-C compared to soy protein without isoflavones, but neither group significantly differed from the milk group
Ashton et al. (2000). Investigate the effect on fasting lipids of replacing lean meat with tofu (Australia) [124]	**Crossover RCT:** 42 healthy men; age range 35–62 years; randomized into isocaloric and isoprotein diets with lean meat (150 g/day) vs. tofu (290 g/day); 1 month	Tofu significantly reduced TC by 9 mg/dL, TG by 13 mg/dL, and HDL-C by 3 mg/dL compared to the lean meat

4.9 mg/dL, and total cholesterol (TC) by 5.3 mg/dL. There was also a significant increase in serum HDL-C by 1.4 mg/dL [117]. Also, LDL-C reductions were more marked in hypercholesterolemic subjects by 7.5 mg/dL than in healthy subjects by 3.0 mg/dL. LDL-C reduction was stronger when whole soy products (soy milk, soybeans and nuts) were used as the intervention by 11 mg/dL, as compared to soy extracts, which lowered LDL-C by 3.2 mg/dL. Three earlier meta-analyses or systematic reviews report similar findings [34, 118, 119].

Representative RCTs. Five representative RCTs illustrate the effects of soy intake on CHD biomarkers [120–124]. Three RCTs in postmenopausal women all find beneficial effects for soy products in reducing CHD risk and associated biomarkers including CRP, TC, and LDL-C [121–123]. In a study of hypercholesterolemic men and postmenopausal women, 50 g/day of soy protein reduced coronary artery disease (CAD) risk by 10% compared to a low-fat diet without soy protein [122]. The substitution of tofu for lean meat significantly improved the fasting lipid profile [124]. In contrast, consuming 12.5 or 25 g protein from defatted soy flour incorporated into muffins did not reduce LDL-C or other any other CHD risk factors in hypercholesterolemic adults compared to matched levels of whey protein [120]. Health claims were approved by the FDA for soy products and reduced LDL-cholesterol and CHD risk in 1999 [125] but not by the European Food Safety Authority (EFSA) [126]. Equol, a bioactive metabolite of the soy isoflavone daidzein was found to be inversely associated with risk of CHD in women [127]. Although soy foods have become controversial because of concerns based primarily on animal studies that their uniquely rich phytoestrogen (isoflavone) content may be contraindicated for breast cancer patients and women at high risk of developing breast cancer, current clinical and epidemiological evidence does not support an increased breast cancer risk from soybean isoflavones intake [128, 129].

12.2.4 Nuts (Tree Nuts and Peanuts) and Seeds

Nuts and seeds are rich sources of CHD protective macronutrients, micronutrients and phytochemicals [130–132]. The consumption of a daily handful of nuts (approx. 45–60 g/day) can help to prevent or reduce weight gain, cardiometabolic dysfunction and related chronic diseases, especially if eaten as a replacement for less healthful foods [29, 133, 134]. They are compositionally low in saturated fat and sugar, rich in unsaturated fats, protein and fiber, and contain a variety of healthy vitamins, minerals and phytonutrients including carotenoids, polyphenols, and phytosterols [130, 131]. The fatty acid composition of nuts is of a healthy type since the saturated fat levels are low (range 4–16%) with 84–96% of the total fat content made up of unsaturated fat, mostly monounsaturated fatty acids (MUFAs) and polyunsaturated fatty acids (PUFAs), predominantly linoleic acid. Walnuts and flaxseed are rich sources of alpha -linolenic acid, the plant n-3 fatty acid. Nuts and seeds are good sources of protein and fiber and/or lignans per 28 g serving. Despite their relatively high Atwater metabolizable energy values of 5–6 kcal/g, they often have a 10–25% lower net metabolizable energy than the label value [135–137]. Overall, nut consumers have a significantly higher nutrient quality score than non-nut consumers, which can lead to overall better health and wellness [138]. However, in the US slightly over 60% of men and women do not consume any nuts on a given day and only14.4% of men and 11.8% of women consume ≥1.5 ounces of nuts/daily, which is similar to global nut intake [139].

Table 12.5 summarizes prospective studies and RCTs on the effects of nuts and seeds on CHD risk and CHD biomarkers [140–154]. The US FDA approved several qualified health claims for tree nuts and peanuts and CHD risk reduction with the consumption of at least 42 g (1.5 ounces)/day [132].

Table 12.5 Summaries of nut and seed studies on CHD risk and biomarkers

Objective	Study details	Results
Prospective Cohort Studies		
Systematic Reviews and Meta- and Pooled Analysis		
Mayhew et al. (2016). Systematically review the literature and quantify associations between nut intake and CHD outcomes and all-cause mortality [140]	Total CHD incidents: 3 studies; 123,971 (87,869 women); followed up of 6–26 years; 4757 CHD events. CHD mortality: 7 studies; 278,584 participants (180,734 women); follow-up of 5.4–30 years, 8454 deaths	Higher intake of nuts reduced CHD events risk by 32% and reduced the risk of CHD deaths by 30%
Ma et al. (2014). Systematically assess dose-response effects between the intake of nuts and coronary artery disease [141]	13 prospective studies; 347,477 participants; follow-up 5–30 years; 6127 coronary artery disease cases	A linear dose-response inverse relationship was reported between nuts and coronary artery disease risk, with a 5% lower risk for each nut serving/week with a significant lower risk observed for ≥2 nut servings per week. For highest vs. lowest nut intake, coronary artery disease risk was reduced by 34% (Fig. 12.11)
Luu et al. (2015). Examine the effect of peanut and tree nut intake on CVD and ischemic heart disease mortality risk (Southern Community Cohort Study, Shanghai Women's Health Study and the Shanghai Men's Health Study) [142]	3 large prospective studies; 206,029 adults; primarily peanut consumers; 5.4–12.2 years of follow-up; 14,440 deaths confirmed	A higher intake of peanuts and nuts significantly lowered ischemic heart disease mortality risk by 30–40%
Kelly and Sabate (2006). Assess the effect of nuts on CHD risk (US Adventist Health, Iowa Women's Health, Nurses' Health, and the Physicians' Health studies [143]	4 large studies; 173,000 adults; followed for 6–17 years	CHD risk was lowered by 37% for those consuming nuts ≥4 times/week compared to those who never or seldom consumed nuts
Randomized Controlled Trials (RCTs)		
Meta-analyses and Systematic Reviews		
Del Gobbo et al. (2015). Systematically assess the clinical effects of tree nuts (walnuts, pistachios, macadamia nuts, pecans, cashews, almonds, hazelnuts, and Brazil nuts) on blood lipids [144]	61 trials; 2582 subjects; 3–26 weeks	Tree nut intake (per serving/day) lowered TC by 4.7 mg/dL, LDL-C by 4.8 mg/dL, ApoB by 3.7 mg/dL, and TG by 2.2 mg/dL with no statistically significant effects on other outcomes. The dose-response between nut intake and TC and LDL-C was nonlinear with stronger effects observed for ≥60 g nuts/day. The nut dose rather than nut type is the major determinant of cholesterol lowering

(continued)

Table 12.5 (continued)

Objective	Study details	Results
Sabate et al. (2010). Systematically evaluate the effects of nut consumption on fasting lipids [145]	25 trials; 583 normo-and hypercholesterolemic adults from 7 countries (not taking lipid-lowering medications); range 3–8 weeks	A mean daily intake of 67 g (2.4 ounces) of nuts significantly reduced TC by 5.1%, LDL-C by 7.4%, and LDL-C/HDL-C by 8.3% compared to control diets. TG levels were significantly reduced by 10.2% in subjects with blood TG levels of ≥150 mg/dL but not in those with lower levels. Tree nuts (almonds, walnuts, pistachios, hazelnuts, pecans, and macadamias) had similar effects on fasting lipid levels. The lipid-lowering effects of nuts were greatest among subjects with high baseline LDL-C and among those consuming Western diets
Banel et al. (2009). Systematically assess the effect of walnuts on blood lipids and CRP [146]	13 RCTs; 365 participants; walnuts providing 10–24% of total calories; duration of 4–24 weeks	Compared with control diets, diets with walnuts significantly lowered TC by 10 mg/dL and LDL-C by 9.2 mg/dL. HDL-C and TG were not significantly affected by walnut diets more than control diets. Results for CRP were inconsistent
Phung et al. (2009). Systematically evaluate the clinical effects of almonds on fasting lipids [147]	5 RCTs; 142 subjects; almond consumption ranging from 25 to 168 g/day; 4 weeks	Almonds significantly lowered TC by 7.0 mg/dL and borderline significantly lowered LDL-C by 5.8 mg/dL vs. control diets. No significant effects on HDL-C, TG, or LDL: HDL ratio were reported
Griel et al. (2006). Systematically review the clinical evidence on tree nuts and fasting lipids [148]	22 RCTs on the effects of tree nut consumption on fasting lipids	Almonds, walnuts, pistachio nuts, hazel nuts, pecans, and macadamia nuts lowered LDL-C by11 mg/dL compared to the control diets due to healthy fatty acid profiles, fiber and phytosterol content
Representative RCTs		
Le et al. (2016). Examine the effects of walnuts on the plasma lipid profile in overweight and obese women participating in a behavioral weight loss intervention (US) [149]	**Parallel RCT (Walnuts):** 245 overweight and obese women; behavioral weight loss intervention; subjects randomly assigned to: (1) lower fat (20% energy), higher carbohydrate (65% energy) diet; (2) a lower carbohydrate (45% energy), higher fat (35% energy) diet; or (3) a walnut-rich, higher fat (35% energy), lower carbohydrate (45% energy) diet; 6 months	The walnut-rich diet resulted in the most favorable changes in lipid levels while still associated with a degree of weight loss that was comparable to the lower fat diet. TG decreased in all study arms at 6 months ($p < 0.05$). The walnut-rich diet increased HDL-C more than the lower fat or lower carbohydrate diet ($P < 0.05$). Walnuts also improved insulin sensitivity and C-reactive protein levels
Berryman et al. (2015). Evaluate the effects of fasting lipid and cardiometabolic effects of almonds in a controlled-feeding setting (US) [150]	**Crossover RCT (Almonds):** 48 subjects with moderately elevated LDL-C; randomized into a healthy diet with 42 g (1.5 oz.) of almonds/day or an identical diet with an isocaloric muffin substitution (no almonds/day); diets did not differ in saturated fat or cholesterol but the almond group had more unsaturated fat and 3 g/day more fiber vs. control group; 6 weeks	The almond diet significantly decreased non-HDL-C by 6.9 mg/dL, LDL-C by 5.3 mg/dL and HDL-C by 1.7 mg/dL compared to the control muffin diet. Also, almond consumption significantly reduced abdominal fat by 0.07 kg and leg fat by 0.12 kg, despite no differences in total body weight

Table 12.5 (continued)

Objective	Study details	Results
Edel et al. (2015). Investigate the effects of flaxseed on fasting lipids in patients with statin usage and clinically significant CVD (Canada) [151]	**Double-blind, Parallel RCT (Flaxseed):** 100 peripheral artery disease subjects; diet supplemented with 30 g of milled flaxseed or 30 g of whole-wheat; plasma lipids were measured at 0, 1, 6, and 12 months	Flaxseed ingestion resulted in an 11–15% reduction of fasting TC and LDL-C compared with placebo after 1 month into the trial (p = 0.05), which was maintained for 6 months. HDL-C and TG did not significantly change. Also, flaxseed promoted additional LDL-C lowering capabilities when used in conjunction with statins
Richmond et al. (2013). Evaluate the effects of sunflower seed or almond consumption on fasting lipids in post-menopausal women with diabetes (New Zealand) [152]	**Crossover RCT (Almonds and Sunflower seeds)**: 22 postmenopausal women with type 2 diabetes; consumed diets with the addition of 30 g sunflower kernels or almonds/day; 3 weeks; 4-week washout	TC and LDL-C decreased significantly on both sunflower seed and almond diets from baseline, with no difference between diets. Both diets showed clinically beneficial effects on reducing CVD risk
Nouran et al. (2009). Assess the effects of peanuts on lipid profiles and oxidized LDL-C in men (Iran) [153]	**Parallel RCT (Peanuts):** 54 hypercholesterolemic men; randomly assigned to: (1) peanuts (about 77 g/day) added to their habitual diet or (2) their habitual diet; 4 weeks	Compared with the habitual diet, adding peanuts to the habitual diet significantly increased HDL-C by 6.1 mg/dL and significantly reduced the LDL/HDL-C ratio by 0.7, but there was an insignificant effect on TC and LDL-C. Peanut diets reduced oxidized LDL-C by 1 mU/L (p = 0.07)
Sabate et al. (1993). Study the effects of walnuts on serum lipids (US) [154]	**Crossover RCT (Walnuts):** 18 men consuming an isocaloric NCEP Step 1 diet with and without 20% of energy from walnuts replacing common saturated fat-rich foods	The walnut enriched NCEP Step 1 diet significantly lowered TC by 12%, LDL-C by16%, HDL-C by 5%, LDL-C to HDL-C ratio by 12%, and triglycerides by 8% compared to the walnut free NCEP Step 1 diet

12.2.4.1 Prospective Cohort Studies

Four systematic reviews and meta- and pooled analyses of prospective cohort studies consistently support a CHD protective role for frequent nuts intake [140–143]. A 2016 systematic review (3 CHD incidents cohort studies, 123,971 subjects, followed up of 6–26 years; and 7 CHD mortality cohort studies; 278,584 participants, follow-up of 5.4–30 years) found that higher intake of nuts reduced CHD events risk by 32% and reduced the risk of CHD deaths by 30% [140]. A 2015 pooled prospective study (3 large prospective studies including Southern Community Cohort Study, Shanghai Women's Health Study and the Shanghai Men's Health Study; 206,029 adults; primarily peanut consumers; 5.4–12.2 years of follow-up) showed that higher nut intake (primarily from peanuts) significantly lowered ischemic heart disease mortality risk by 30–40% [142]. A 2014 dose-response meta-analysis (13 prospective studies; 347,477 participants; follow-up 5–30 years) found a linear dose-response inverse relationship between nuts and coronary artery disease risk, with a 5% lower risk for each nut serving/week with a significant lower risk observed for ≥2 nut servings per week [141]. Higher nut intake was shown to significantly reduce coronary artery disease risk by 34% (Fig. 12.11).

A 2006 pooled analysis (4 large prospective studies: US Adventist Health, Iowa Women's Health, Nurses' Health, and the Physicians' Health studies; 173,000 adults; followed for 6 to 17 years) found that CHD risk was lowered by 37% for those consuming nuts ≥4 times/week compared to those who never or seldom consumed nuts [143].

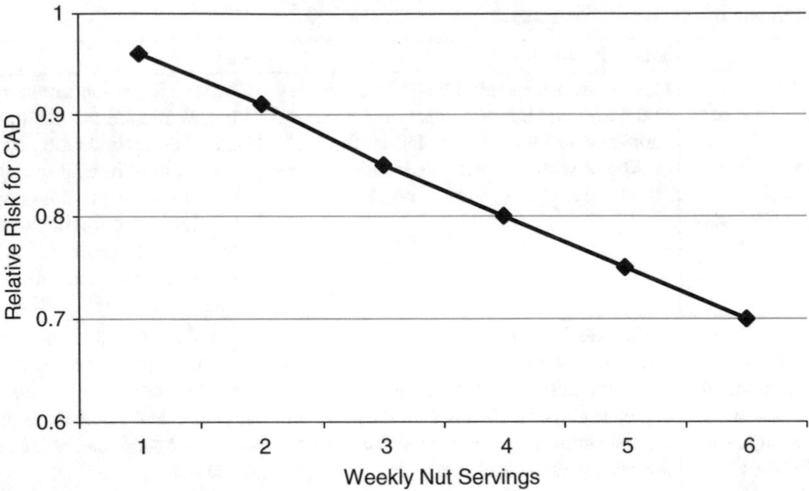

Fig. 12.11 Association between the number of weekly nut servings and coronary artery disease (CAD) risk (p-trend <0.001) (adapted from [141])

12.2.4.2 Randomized Controlled Trials

RCTs on tree nuts, seeds and peanuts consistently find similar significant effects on reducing lipids and non-HDL lipoproteins but the findings are inconsistent for lowering blood pressure and CRP [144–154]. A 2015 meta-analysis of tree nut RCTs (61 trials; 2582 subjects; duration 3–26 weeks) reported that each daily serving of nuts significantly lowered total TC by 4.7 mg/dL, LDL-C by 4.8 mg/dL, ApoB by 3.7 mg/dL, and triglycerides by 2.2 mg/dL with no statistically significant effects shown for HDL-C, blood pressure, or CRP [144]. The dose-response between nut intake and TC and LDL-C was nonlinear with stronger effects found for the consumption of ≥60 g nuts/day. There were no significant differences between nut types on lipids and lipoprotein lowering. Similar findings were reported in four previous nut meta-analyses and systematic reviews of RCTs [145–148]. RCTs on tree nuts, peanuts, flaxseed, and sunflower seeds demonstrate similar fasting lipid lowering effects [149–154]. Nuts and seeds have been shown to have adjunctive therapeutic effects on non-HDL-C lowering with statins in hypercholesterolemic individuals [151, 155].

Conclusions

Although there have been some decreasing trends in overall CHD mortality rate over the last several decades because of cholesterol lowering drugs and surgical procedures, CHD is still a leading cause of death globally and its prevalence is expected to increase as the global population ages. Healthy behaviors, including meeting the recommended intake of whole plant foods, increased physical activity, and weight control, have been shown to reduce the risk for CHD. Prospective cohort studies consistently show that diets with higher intakes of whole plant foods including whole-grains, fruits, vegetables, legumes, and nuts and seeds are associated with reduced CHD risk compared to lower intake. Heart healthier versions of whole plant foods are higher in dietary fiber, phytosterols, healthy fatty acids (MUFAs and PUFAs), and nutrients (e.g., vitamins E and C, potassium and folate), phytochemicals (carotenoids, flavonoids and phytosterols) and lower in energy density, glycemic index and glycemic load. The risk of CHD incidence or mortality is significantly reduced with the intake of ≥3 servings/day of whole-grains (especially oats and barley), ≥5 servings (400 g)/day of fruits and vegetables, ≥4 weekly servings (130–150 g cooked) of legumes (both non-soy and/or soy products), and ≥5 servings/week of nuts and seeds. RCTs generally support the beneficial effects of healthy whole plant based foods on CHD risk biomarkers including lowering serum lipids and blood pressure, improving glucose and insulin metabolism, improving endothelial function, alleviating oxidative stress and inflammation and reducing risk of weight gain compared to their refined counterparts. Only a small fraction of the US population meets the recommended intake levels for whole-grains, fruits, vegetables, legumes, and nuts and 70% exceed recommended refined grain intake. Approximately 45% of CHD deaths in the US are associated with suboptimal low dietary intake of fruits, vegetables, nuts and seeds, whole-grains, and seafood omega-3 PUFAs, and high intake of red and processed meats, sugar sweetened beverages, and sodium.

Appendix A. Estimated Range of Energy, Fiber, Nutrients and Phytochemicals Composition of Whole Plant Foods/100 g Edible Portion

Components	Whole-grains	Fresh fruit	Dried fruit	Vegetables	Legumes	Nuts/seeds
Nutrients/ Phytochemicals	Wheat, oats, brown rice, whole grain bread, cereal, pasta, rolls, and crackers	Apples, pears, bananas, grapes, oranges, blueberries, strawberries, and avocados	Dates, dried figs, apricots, cranberries, raisins, and prunes	Potatoes, spinach, carrots, peppers, lettuce, green beans, cabbage, onions, cucumber, cauliflower, mushrooms, and broccoli	Lentils, chickpeas, split peas, black beans, pinto beans, and soy beans	Almonds, Brazil nuts, cashews, hazelnuts, macadamias, pecans, walnuts, peanuts, sunflower seeds, and flaxseed
Energy (kcals)	110–350	30–170	240–310	10–115	85–170	520–700
Protein (g)	2.5–16	0.5–2.0	0.1–3.4	0.2–5.0	5.0–17	7.8–24
Available Carbohydrate (g)	23–77	1.0–25	64–82	0.2–25	10–27	12–33
Fiber (g)	3.5–18	2.0–7.0	5.7–10	1.2–9.5	5.0–11	3.0–27
Total fat (g)	0.9–6.5	0.0–15	0.4–1.4	0.2–1.5	0.2–9.0	46–76
SFA[a] (g)	0.2–1.0	0.0–2.1	0.0	0.0–0.1	0.1–1.3	4.0–12
MUFA[a] (g)	0.2–2.0	0.0–9.8	0.0–0.2	0.1–1.0	0.1–2.0	9.0–60
PUFA[a] (g)	0.3–2.5	0.0–1.8	0.0–0.7	0.0–0.4	0.1–5.0	1.5–47
Folate (μg)	4.0–44	<5.0–61	2–20	8.0–160	50–210	10–230
Tocopherols (mg)	0.1–3.0	0.1–1.0	0.1–4.5	0.0–1.7	0.0–1.0	1.0–35
Potassium (mg)	40–720	60–500	40–1160	100–680	200–520	360–1050
Calcium (mg)	7.0–50	3.0–25	10–160	5.0–200	20–100	20–265
Magnesium (mg)	40–160	3.0–30	5.0–70	3.0–80	40–90	120–400
Phytosterols (mg)	30–90	1.0–83	–	1.0–54	110–120	70–215
Polyphenols (mg)	70–100	50–800	–	24–1250	120–6500	130–1820
Carotenoids (μg)	–	25–6600	0.6–2160	10–20,000	50–600	0.0–1200

Ros E, Hu FB. Consumption of plant seeds and cardiovascular health epidemiological and clinical trial evidence. Circulation. 2013;128:553–565

USDA. What We Eat in America, NHANES 2011–2012, individuals 2 years and over (excluding breast-fed children). Available: www.ars.usda.gov/nea/bhnrc/fsrg

Rodriguez-Casado A. The health potential of fruits and vegetables phytochemicals: notable examples. Crit Rev. Food Sci Nutr. 2016;56(7):1097–1107

Rebello CJ, Greenway FL, Finley JW. A review of the nutritional value of legumes and their effects on obesity and its related co-morbidities. Obes Rev. 2014;15: 392–407
Gebhardt SE, Thomas RG. Nutritive Value of Foods. 2002; U.S. Department of Agriculture, Agricultural Research Service, Home and Garden Bulletin 72
Holden JM, Eldridge AL, Beecher GR, et al. Carotenoid content of U.S. foods: an update of the database. J Food Comp An. 1999;12:169–196
Lu Q-Y, Zhang Y, Wang Y, et al. California Hass avocado: profiling of carotenoids, tocopherol, fatty acid, and fat content during maturation and from different growing areas. J Agric Food Chem. 2009;57(21):10,408–10413
Wu X, Beecher GR, Holden JM, et al. Lipophilic and hydrophilic antioxidant capacities of common foods in the United States. J Agric Food Chem. 2004;52:4026–37
SFA (saturated fat), MUFA (monounsaturated fat) and PUFA (polyunsaturated fat)
U.S. Department of Agriculture, Agriculture Research Service, Nutrient Data Laboratory. 2014. USDA National Nutrient Database for Standard Reference, Release 27. http://www.ars.usda.gov/nutrientdata. Accessed 17 February 2015

References

1. Mendis S, Puska P, Norrving B. Global atlas on cardiovascular disease prevention and control. Geneva: World Health Organization; 2011.
2. Sayols-Baixeras S, Lluís-Ganella C, Lucas G, Elosua R. Pathogenesis of coronary artery disease: focus on genetic risk factors and identification of genetic variants. Appl Clin Genet. 2014;7:15–32.
3. Roger VL, Go AS, Lloyd-Jones DM, et al. Heart disease and stroke statistics-2011 update: a report from the American Heart Association. Circulation. 2011;123(4):18–209.
4. Enkhmaa B, Surampudi P, Anuurad E, et al. Lifestyle changes: effect of diet, exercise, functional food, and obesity treatment, on lipids and lipoproteins. [Updated 2015 Jun 8]. De Groot LJ, Beck-Peccoz P, Chrousos G, et al., editors. Endotext [Internet]. South Dartmouth (MA): MDText.com, Inc.; 2000-. PMID:26561697.
5. American Heart Association. Coronary artery disease—coronary heart disease. 2015. http://www.heart.org/HEARTORG/Conditions/More/MyHeartandStrokeNews/Coronary-Artery-Disease-Coronary-Heart-Disease_UCM_436416_Article.jsp. Accessed 14 Jul 2015.
6. Fleg JL, Forman DE, Berra K, et al. Secondary prevention of atherosclerotic cardiovascular disease in older adults a scientific statement from the American Heart Association. Circulation. 2013;128(22):2422–46.
7. Hu FB. Diet and lifestyle influences on risk of coronary heart disease. Curr Atheroscler Rep. 2009;11:257–63.
8. Hu FB, Willett WC. Optimal diets for prevention of coronary heart disease. J Am Med Assoc. 2002;288:2569–78.
9. Lichtenstein AH, Appel LJ, Brands M, et al. Diet and lifestyle recommendations revision to the 2006: a scientific statement from the American Heart Association Nutrition Committee. Circulation. 2006;114:82–96.
10. Satija A, Bhupathiraju SN, Spiegelman D, et al. Healthful and unhealthful plant-based diets and risk of coronary heart disease in US adults. J Am Coll Cardiol. 2017;70:411–22.
11. Ros E, Hu FB. Consumption of plant seeds and cardiovascular health epidemiological and clinical trial evidence. Circulation. 2013;128:553–65.
12. USDA. What We Eat in America, NHANES 2011–2012, individuals 2 years and over (excluding breast-fed children). www.ars.usda.gov/nea/bhnrc/fsrg.
13. Rodriguez-Casado A. The health potential of fruits and vegetables phytochemicals: notable examples. Crit Rev Food Sci Nutr. 2016;56(7):1097–107.
14. Rebello CJ, Greenway FL, Finley JW. A review of the nutritional value of legumes and their effects on obesity and its related co-morbidities. Obes Rev. 2014;15:392–407.
15. Gebhardt SE, Thomas RG. Nutritive value of foods, Home and Garden Bulletin 72: U.S. Department of Agriculture, Agricultural Research Service; 2002.
16. Holden JM, Eldridge AL, Beecher GR, et al. Carotenoid content of U.S. foods: an update of the database. J Food Compos Anal. 1999;12:169–96.
17. Lu Q-Y, Zhang Y, Wang Y, et al. California Hass avocado: profiling of carotenoids, tocopherol, fatty acid, and fat content during maturation and from different growing areas. J Agric Food Chem. 2009;57(21):10408–13.
18. Wu X, Beecher GR, Holden JM, et al. Lipophilic and hydrophilic antioxidant capacities of common foods in the United States. J Agric Food Chem. 2004;52:4026–37.
19. Bhupathiraju SN, Tucker KL. Coronary heart disease prevention: nutrients, foods, and dietary patterns. Clin Chim Acta. 2011;412:1493–514.
20. Appel LJ, Moore TJ, Obarzanek E, et al. A clinical trial of the effects of dietary patterns on blood pressure. N Engl J Med. 1997;336:1117–24.

21. Ornish D, Brown SE, Scherwitz LW, et al. Can lifestyle changes reverse coronary heart disease? The Lifestyle Heart Trial. Lancet. 1990;336(8708):129–33.
22. Alissa EM, Ferns GA. Dietary fruits and vegetables and cardiovascular diseases risk. Crit Rev Food Sci Nutr. 2017;57(9):1950–62. https://doi.org/10.1080/10408398.2015.1040487.
23. Bao Y, Han J, Hu FB, et al. Association of nut consumption with total and cause-specific mortality. N Engl J Med. 2013;369(21):2001–11.
24. Gupta SK, Sawhney RC, Rai L, et al. Regression of coronary atherosclerosis through healthy lifestyle in coronary artery disease patients -Mount Abu Open Heart Trial. Indian Heart J. 2011;63(5):461–9.
25. Ye EQ, Chacko SA, Chou EL, et al. Greater whole-grain intake is associated with lower risk of type 2 diabetes, cardiovascular disease, and weight gain. J Nutr. 2012;142:1304–13.
26. Lefevre M, Jonnalagadda S. Effect of whole grains on markers of subclinical inflammation. Nutr Rev. 2012;70(7):387–96.
27. Bertoia ML, Mukamal KJ, Cahill LE, et al. Changes in intake of fruits and vegetables and weight change in United States men and women followed for up to 24 years: analysis from three prospective cohort studies. PLoS Med. 2015;12(9):e1001878. https://doi.org/10.1371/journal.pmed.1001878.
28. Hollænder PLB, Alastair B, Ross AB, Kristensen M. Whole-grain and blood lipid changes in apparently healthy adults: a systematic review and meta-analysis of randomized controlled studies. Am J Clin Nutr. 2015;102(3):556–72. https://doi.org/10.3945/ajcn.115.109165.
29. Kris-Etherton PM, Hu FB, Ros E, Sabate J. The role of tree nuts and peanuts in the prevention of coronary heart disease: multiple potential mechanisms. J Nutr. 2008;138:1746S–51S.
30. Hartley L, Igbinedion E, Holmes J, et al. Increased consumption of fruit and vegetables for the primary prevention of cardiovascular diseases. Cochrane Database Syst Rev. 2013;6:CD009874. https://doi.org/10.1002/14651858.CD009874.pub2.
31. Yu D, Zhang X, Gao Y-T, et al. Fruit and vegetable intake and risk of coronary heart disease: results from prospective cohort studies of Chinese adults in Shanghai. Br J Nutr. 2014;111(2):353–62.
32. Winham DM, Hutchin AM, Johnston CS. Pinto bean consumption reduces biomarkers for heart disease risk. J Am Coll Nutr. 2007;26(3):243–9.
33. Zaheer K, Akntar MH. An updated review of dietary isoflavones: nutrition, processing, bioavailability and impacts on human health. Crit Rev Food Sci Nutr. 2017;57(6):1280–93. https://doi.org/10.1080/10408398.2014.989958.
34. Anderson JW, Bush HM. Soy protein effects on serum lipoproteins: a quality assessment and meta-analysis of randomized, controlled studies. J Am Coll Nutr. 2011;30(2):79–91.
35. Retelny VS, Neuendorf A, Roth JL. Nutrition protocols for the prevention of cardiovascular disease. Nutr Clin Pract. 2008;23:468–76.
36. National Cholesterol Education Program. Detection, evaluation, and treatment of high blood cholesterol in adults (Adult Treatment Third Report of the National Cholesterol Education Program (NCEP) expert panel III) final report. Circulation. 2002;106(25):3143–421.
37. Liu JF, Liu YH, Chen CM, et al. The effect of almonds on inflammation and oxidative stress in Chinese patients with type 2 diabetes mellitus: a randomized crossover controlled feeding trial. Eur J Nutr. 2013;52(3):927–35.
38. Kerckhoffs DAJM, Brouns F, Hornstra G, Mensink RP. Effects on the human serum lipoprotein profile of β-glucan, soy protein and isoflavones, plant sterols and stanols, garlic and tocotrienols. J Nutr. 2002;132:2494–505.
39. Wong JM, de Souza R, Kendall CW, et al. Colonic health: fermentation and short chain fatty acids. J Clin Gastroenterol. 2006;40:235–43.
40. Jiao J, Xu J-Y, Zhang W, et al. Effect of dietary fiber on circulating C-reactive protein in overweight and obese adults: a meta-analysis of randomized controlled trials. Int J Food Sci Nutr. 2015;66(1):114–9.
41. Ma Y, Olendzki BC, Wang J, et al. Single-component versus multicomponent dietary goals for the metabolic syndrome. A randomized trial. Ann Intern Med. 2015;162(4):248–57.
42. Rajaram S, Connell KM, Sabate J. Effect of almond-enriched high-monounsaturated fat diet on selected markers of inflammation: a randomised, controlled, crossover study. Br J Nutr. 2010;103:907–12.
43. McKiernan F, Lokko P, Anna Kuevi A, et al. Effects of peanut processing on body weight and fasting plasma lipids. Br J Nutr. 2010;104:418–26.
44. Esposito K, Marfella R, Ciotola M, et al. Effect of a Mediterranean-style diet on endothelial dysfunction and markers of vascular inflammation in the metabolic syndrome a randomized trial. JAMA. 2004;292:1440–6.
45. Wang Q, Ellis PR. Oat b-glucan: physico-chemical characteristics in relation to its blood-glucose and cholesterol-lowering properties. Br J Nutr. 2014;112:S4–S13.
46. Thies F, Masson LF, Boffetta P, Kris-Etherton P. Oats and CVD risk markers: a systematic literature review. Br J Nutr. 2014;112:S19–30.
47. Mozaffarian D, Kumanyika SK, Lemaitre RN, et al. Cereal, fruit, and vegetable fiber intake and the risk of cardiovascular disease in elderly individuals. JAMA. 2003;289(13):1659–66.
48. Dietary Guidelines Advisory Committee. Scientific Report. Advisory Report to the Secretary of Health and Human Services and the Secretary of Agriculture. Part D. Chapter 1: Food and nutrient intakes, and health: current status and trends. 2015; 1–78.

49. Micha R, Peñalvo JL, Cudhea F, et al. Association between dietary factors and mortality from heart disease, stroke, and type 2 diabetes in the United States. JAMA. 2017;317(9):912–24. https://doi.org/10.1001/jama.2017.0947.
50. Mente A, de Koning L, Shannon HS, Anand SS. A systematic review of the evidence supporting a causal link between dietary factors and coronary heart disease. Arch Intern Med. 2009;169(7):659–69.
51. Massera D, Zaman T, Grace E. Farren GE, et al. Case report: a whole-food plant-based diet reversed angina without medications or procedures. Case Rep Cardiol 2015; 2015:978906. doi: https://doi.org/10.1155/2015/978906.
52. U.S. Department of Agriculture and U.S. Department of Health and Human Services. Dietary Guidelines for Americans, 2010. 7th ed. Washington, DC: U.S. Government Printing Office; 2010. Table B2.4; http://www.choosemyplate.gov/. Accessed 22 Aug 2015.
53. Seal CJ, Brownlee IA. Whole-grain foods and chronic disease: evidence from epidemiological and intervention studies. Proc Nutr Soc. 2015;74:313–9.
54. Slavin J. Why whole grains are protective: biological mechanisms. Proc Nutr Soc. 2003;62:129–34.
55. Karl JP, Saltzman E. The role of whole grains in body weight regulation. Adv Nutr. 2012;3:697–707.
56. Othman RA, Moghadasian MH, Jones PJ. Cholesterol-lowering effects of oat β-glucan. Nutr Rev. 2011;69(6):299–309. https://doi.org/10.1111/j.1753-4887.2011.00401.
57. Sofi F, Whittaker A, Cesari F, et al. Characterization of Khorasan wheat (Kamut) and impact of a replacement diet on cardiovascular risk factors: cross-over dietary intervention study. Eur J Clin Nutr. 2013;67:190–5.
58. McGill CR, Fulgoni VL III, Devareddy L. Ten-year trends in fiber and whole grain intakes and food sources for the United States population: National Health and Nutrition Examination Survey 2001–2010. Forum Nutr. 2015;7:1119–30.
59. Seal CJ. Whole grains and CVD risk. Proc Nutr Soc. 2006;65:24–34.
60. Anderson JW. Whole grains protect against atherosclerotic cardiovascular disease. Proc Nutr Soc. 2003;62:135–42.
61. US Food and Drug Administration. Health claim notification for whole grain foods with moderate fat content. 2003. http://www.fda.gov/Food/LabelingNutrition/LabelClaims/FDA Modernization Act FDAMA Claims/ucm073634.htm. Accessed 18 Jul 2015.
62. EFSA Panel on Dietetic Products, Nutrition and Allergies (NDA). Scientific Opinion on the substantiation of a health claim related to whole grain (ID 831, 832, 833, 1126, 1268, 1269, 1270, 1271, 1431) pursuant to Article 13(1) of Regulation (EC) No 1924/2006. EFSA J. 2010;8(10):1766. https://doi.org/10.2903/j.efsa.2010.1766.
63. Jonnalagadda SS, Harnack L, Liu RH, et al. Putting the whole grain puzzle together: health benefits associated with whole grains-summary of American Society for Nutrition 2010 Satellite Symposium. J Nutr. 2011;141:1011S–22S.
64. Harris KA, Kris-Etherton PM. Effects of whole-grains on coronary heart disease risk. Curr Atheroscler Rep. 2010;12(6):368–76.
65. Wang H, Lichtenstein AH, Lamon-Fava S, Jacques PF. Association between statin use and serum cholesterol concentrations is modified by whole-grain consumption: NHANES 2003–2006. Am J Clin Nutr. 2014;100:1149–57.
66. Li B, Zhang G, Tan M, et al. Consumption of whole grains in relation to mortality from all causes, cardiovascular disease, and diabetes. Dose–response meta-analysis of prospective cohort studies. Medicine. 2016;95:33. https://doi.org/10.1097/MD.0000000000004229.
67. Aune D, Keum N, Giovannucci E, et al. Whole grain consumption and risk of cardiovascular disease, cancer, and all cause and cause specific mortality: systematic review and dose-response meta-analysis of prospective studies. BMJ. 2016;353:i2716. https://doi.org/10.1136/bmj.i2716.
68. Tang G, Wang D, Long J, et al. Meta-analysis of the association between whole grain intake and coronary heart disease risk. Am J Cardiol. 2015;115:625–9.
69. Buyken AE, Goletzke J, Joslowski G, et al. Association between carbohydrate quality and inflammatory markers: systematic review of observational and interventional studies. Am J Clin Nutr. 2014;99:813–33.
70. Helnæs A, Kyrø C, Andersen I, et al. Intake of whole grains is associated with lower risk of myocardial infarction: The Danish Diet, Cancer and Health Cohort. Am J Clin Nutr. 2016;103:999–1007.
71. Johnsen NF, Frederiksen K, Christensen J, et al. Whole-grain products and whole-grain types are associated with lower all-cause and cause-specific mortality in the Scandinavian HELGA cohort. Br J Nutr. 2015;114(4):608–23. https://doi.org/10.1017/S0007114515001701.
72. Sonestedt E, Hellstrand S, Schulz C-A, et al. The association between carbohydrate-rich foods and risk of cardiovascular disease is not modified by genetic susceptibility to dyslipidemia as determined by 80 validated variants. PLoS One. 2015;10(4). https://doi.org/10.1371/journal.pone.0126104.
73. Mellen PB, Liese AD, Tooze JA, et al. Whole-grain intake and carotid artery atherosclerosis in a multi-ethnic cohort: The Insulin Resistance Atherosclerosis Study. Am J Clin Nutr. 2007;85:1495–502.
74. Jensen MK, Koh-Banerjee P, Hu FB, et al. Intakes of whole grains, bran, and germ and the risk of coronary heart disease in men. Am J Clin Nutr. 2004;80:1492–9.
75. Liu S, Stampfer MJ, Hu FB, et al. Whole-grain consumption and risk of coronary heart disease: results

from the Nurses' Health Study. Am J Clin Nutr. 1999;70:412–9.
76. Jacobs DR, Meyer KA, Kushi LH, Folsom AR. Whole-grain intake may reduce the risk of ischemic heart disease death in postmenopausal women: The Iowa Women's Health Study. Am J Clin Nutr. 1998;68:248–57.
77. Zhu X, Sun X, Wang M, et al. Quantitative assessment of the effects of beta-glucan consumption on serum lipid profile and glucose level in hypercholesterolemic subjects. Nutr Metab Cardiovasc Dis. 2015;25:714–23.
78. Whitehead A, Beck EJ, Tosh S, Wolever TMS. Cholesterol-lowering effects of oat b-glucan: a meta-analysis of randomized controlled trials. Am J Clin Nutr. 2014;100:1413–21.
79. Whittaker A, Sofi F, Luisi MLE, et al. An organic Khorasan wheat-based replacement diet improves risk profile of patients with acute coronary syndrome: a randomized crossover trial. Forum Nutr. 2015;7:3401–15.
80. Vitaglione P, Mennella I, Ferracane R, et al. Whole-grain wheat consumption reduces inflammation in a randomized controlled trial on overweight and obese subjects with unhealthy dietary and lifestyle behaviors: role of polyphenols bound to cereal dietary fiber. Am J Clin Nutr. 2015;101:251–61.
81. Giacco R, Lappi J, Costabile G, et al. Effects of rye and whole wheat versus refined cereal foods on metabolic risk factors: a randomised controlled two-centre intervention study. Clin Nutr. 2013;32(6):941–9.
82. Brownlee IA, Moore C, Chatfield M, et al. Markers of cardiovascular risk are not changed by increased whole-grain intake: the WHOLE heart study, a randomised, controlled dietary intervention. Br J Nutr. 2010;104(1):125–34.
83. Katcher HI, Legro RS, Kunselman AR, et al. The effects of a whole grain-enriched hypocaloric diet on cardiovascular disease risk factors in men and women with metabolic syndrome. Am J Clin Nutr. 2008;87:79–90.
84. Slavin JL, Lloyd B. Health benefits of fruits and vegetables. Adv Nutr. 2012;3:506–16.
85. World Health Organization. Diet, nutrition, and the prevention of chronic diseases. Geneva: World Health Organization. 1990. http://www.who.int/nutrition/publications/obesity/WHO_TRS_797/en/index.html. Accessed 16 Apr 2015.
86. Rooney C, McKinley MC, Appleton KM, et al. How much is '5-a-day?' A qualitative investigation into consumer understanding of fruit and vegetable intake guidelines. J Hum Nutr Diet. 2016;30(1):105–13. https://doi.org/10.1111/jhn.12393.
87. United States Department of Agriculture. Choose my plate. 2013. http://www.choosemyplate.gov/. Accessed 17 Feb 2015.
88. Micha R, Khatibzadeh S, Shi P, et al. Global, regional and national consumption of major food groups in 1990 and 2010: a systematic analysis including 266 country-specific nutrition surveys worldwide. BMJ Open. 2015;5:e008705. https://doi.org/10.1136/bmjopen-2015-008705.
89. Aune D, Edward Giovannucci E, Boffetta P, et al. Fruit and vegetable intake and the risk of cardiovascular disease, total cancer and all-cause mortality-a systematic review and dose response meta-analysis of prospective studies. Int J Epidemiol. 2017:1–28. https://doi.org/10.1093/ije/dyw319.
90. Gan Y, Tong X, Li L. Consumption of fruit and vegetable and risk of coronary heart disease: A meta-analysis of prospective cohort studies. Int J Cardiol. 2015;183:129–37.
91. Wang X, Ouyang Y, Jun Liu J, et al. Fruit and vegetable consumption and mortality from all causes, cardiovascular disease, and cancer: systematic review and dose-response meta-analysis of prospective cohort studies. BMJ. 2014;349:g4490. https://doi.org/10.1136/bmj.g4490.
92. He FJ, Nowson CA, Lucas M, Macgregor GA. Increased consumption of fruit and vegetables is related to a reduced risk of coronary heart disease: meta-analysis of cohort studies. J Hum Hypertens. 2007;21:717–28.
93. Dauchet L, Amouyel P, Hercberg S, Dallongeville J. Fruit and vegetable consumption and risk of coronary heart disease: a meta-analysis of cohort studies. J Nutr. 2006;136:2588–93.
94. Sharma S, Vik S, Kolonel LN. Fruit and vegetable consumption, ethnicity and risk of fatal ischemic heart disease. J Nutr Health Aging. 2014;18(6):573–8.
95. Bhupathiraju SN, Wedick NM, Pan A, et al. Quantity and variety in fruit and vegetable intake and risk of coronary heart disease. Am J Clin Nutr. 2013;98:1514–23.
96. Griep LMO, Verschuren WMM, Kromhout D, et al. Colours of fruit and vegetables and 10-year incidence of CHD. Br J Nutr. 2011;106:1562–9.
97. Griep LMO, Geleijnse JM, Kromhout D, et al. Raw and processed fruit and vegetable consumption and 10-year coronary heart disease incidence in a population-based cohort study in the Netherlands. PLoS One. 2010;5(10):e13609. https://doi.org/10.1371/journal.pone.0013609.
98. Joshipura KJ, Hu FB, Manson JE, et al. The effect of fruit and vegetable intake on risk for coronary heart disease. Ann Intern Med. 2001;134:1106–14.
99. McEvoy CT, Wallace IR, Hamill L, et al. Increasing fruit and vegetable intake has no dose-response effect on conventional cardiovascular risk factors in overweight adults at high risk of developing cardiovascular disease. J Nutr. 2015;145:1464–71.
100. Wang L, Bordi PL, Fleming JA, et al. Effect of a moderate fat diet with and without avocados on lipoprotein particle number, size and subclasses in overweight and obese adults: a randomized, controlled

trial. J Am Heart Assoc. 2015;4:e001355. https://doi.org/10.1161/JAHA.114.001355.

101. Rayn-Haren G, Dragsted LO, Buch-Andersen T, et al. Intake of whole apples or clear apple juice has contrasting effects on plasma lipids in health volunteers. Eur J Nutr. 2013;52(8):1875–89.
102. Choi IH, Sook Noh JS, Han J-S, et al. Kimchi, a fermented vegetable, improves serum lipid profiles in healthy young adults: randomized clinical trial. J Med Food. 2013;16(3):223–9.
103. Watzl B, Kulling SE, Möseneder J, et al. A 4-wk intervention with high intake of carotenoid-rich vegetables and fruit reduces plasma C-reactive protein in healthy, nonsmoking men. Am J Clin Nutr. 2005;82:1052–8.
104. McCrory MA, Hamaker BR, Lovejoy JC, Eichelsdoerfer PE. Pulse consumption, satiety, and weight management. Adv Nutr. 2010;1:17–30.
105. Messina V. Nutritional and health benefits of dried beans. Am J Clin Nutr. 2014;100(suppl):437S–42S.
106. Afshin A, Micha R, Khatibzadeh S, Mozaffarian D. Consumption of nuts and legumes and risk of incident ischemic heart disease, stroke, and diabetes: a systematic review and meta-analysis. Am J Clin Nutr. 2014;100(1):278–88.
107. Bazzano LA, He J, Ogden LG, et al. Legume consumption and risk of coronary heart disease in US men and women: NHANES I epidemiologic follow-up study. Arch Intern Med. 2001;161:2573–8.
108. Salehi-Abargouei A, Saraf-Bank S, Bellissimo N, Azadbakht L. Effects of non-soy legume consumption on C-reactive protein: a systematic review and meta-analysis. Nutrition. 2015;31:631–9.
109. Ha V, Sievenpiper JL, de Souza RJ, et al. Effect of dietary pulse intake on established therapeutic lipid targets for cardiovascular risk reduction: a systematic review and meta-analysis of randomized controlled trials. CMAJ. 2014;186(8):252–62.
110. Bazzano LA, Thompson AM, Tees MT, et al. Non-soy legume consumption lowers cholesterol levels: a meta-analysis of randomized controlled trials. Nutr Metab Cardiovasc Dis. 2011;21(2):94–103.
111. Abeysekara S, Chilibeck PD, Vatanparast H, Zello GA. A pulse-based diet is effective for reducing total and LDL-cholesterol in older adults. Br J Nutr. 2012;108:S103–10.
112. Hermsdorf HH, Zulet MA, Abete I, Martinez JA. A legume-based diet reduces proinflammatory status and improves metabolic features in overweight/obese subjects. Eur J Nutr. 2011;50(1):61–9.
113. Pittaway JK, Robertson IK, Ball MJ. Chickpeas may influence fatty acid and fiber intake in an ad libitum diet, leading to small improvements in serum lipid profile and glycemic control. J Am Diet Assoc. 2008;108:1009–13.
114. Pittaway JK, Ahuja KD, Cehun M, et al. Dietary supplementation with chickpeas for at least 5 weeks results in small but significant reductions in serum total and low-density lipoprotein cholesterols in adult women and men. Ann Nutr Metab. 2006;50:512–8.
115. Kokubo Y, Iso H, Ishihara J, et al. Association of dietary intake of soy, beans, and isoflavones with risk of cerebral and myocardial infarctions in Japanese populations. The Japan Public Health Center–Based (JPHC) Study Cohort I. Circulation. 2007;116:2553–62.
116. Zhang X, Shu XO, Gao Y-T, et al. Soy food consumption is associated with lower risk of coronary heart disease in Chinese women. J Nutr. 2003;133:2874–8.
117. Tokede OA, Onabanjo TA, Yansane A, et al. Soya products and serum lipids: a meta-analysis of randomised controlled trials. Br J Nutr. 2015;114:831–43.
118. Yang B, Chen Y, Xu T, et al. Systematic review and meta-analysis of soy products consumption in patients with type 2 diabetes mellitus. Asia Pac J Clin Nutr. 2011;20(4):593–602.
119. Sacks FM, Lichtenstein A, Van Horn L, et al. Soy protein, isoflavones, and cardiovascular health: an American Heart Association Science Advisory for Professionals from the Nutrition Committee. Circulation. 2006;113:1034–44.
120. Padhi EMT, Blewett HJ, Duncan AM, et al. Whole soy flour incorporated into a muffin and consumed at 2 doses of soy protein does not lower LDL cholesterol in a randomized, double-blind controlled trial of hypercholesterolemic adults. J Nutr. 2015;145(12):2665–74. https://doi.org/10.3945/jn.115.219873.
121. Azadbakht L, Kimiagar M, Mehrabi Y, et al. Soy consumption, markers of inflammation, and endothelial function. A cross-over study in postmenopausal women with the metabolic syndrome. Diabetes Care. 2007;30:967–73.
122. Jenkins DJA, Kendall CWC, Jackson C-J, et al. Effects of high- and low-isoflavone soyfoods on blood lipids, oxidized LDL, homocysteine, and blood pressure in hyperlipidemic men and women. Am J Clin Nutr. 2002;76:365–72.
123. Gardner CD, Newell KA, Cherin R, Haskell WL. The effect of soy protein with or without isoflavones relative to milk protein on plasma lipids in hypercholesterolemic postmenopausal women. Am J Clin Nutr. 2001;73:728–35.
124. Ashton E, Ball M. Effect of soy as tofu vs. meat on lipoprotein concentrations. Eur J Clin Nutr. 2000;54(10):14–9.
125. FDA. Food labeling: health claims; soy protein and coronary heart disease. Food and Drug Administration, HHS. Final rule. Final Regist. 1999;64(206):57700–33.
126. EFSA Panel on Dietetic Products, Nutrition and Allergies (NDA). Scientific opinion on the substantiation of a health claim related to soy protein and reduction of blood cholesterol concentrations

pursuant to Article 14 of the Regulation (EC) No 1924/2006. EFSA J. 2010;8(7):1688.
127. Zhang X, Gao X-T, Yang G, et al. Urinary isoflavonoids and risk of coronary heart disease. Int J Epidemiol. 2012;41:1367–75.
128. Messina M, Messina V, Jenkins DJA. Can breast cancer patients use soya foods to help reduce risk of CHD? Br J Nutr. 2012;108:810–9.
129. Caan BJ, Natarajan L, Parker B, et al. Soy food consumption and breast cancer prognosis. Cancer Epidemiol Biomark Prev. 2011;20:854–8.
130. Ros E. Nuts and CVD. Br J Nutr. 2015;113:S111–20.
131. Prasad K. Flaxseed and cardiovascular disease. J Cardiovasc Pharmacol. 2009;54(5):369–77.
132. US Food and Drug Administration. Qualified health claims. http://www.fda.gov/Food/IngredientsPackagingLabeling/LabelingNutrition/ucm073992.htm. Accessed 11 Aug 2015.
133. Jackson CL, Hu FB. Long-term associations of nut consumption with body weight and obesity. Am J Clin Nutr. 2014;100(suppl):408S–11S.
134. Mattes RD, Kris-Etherton PM, Foster GD. Impact of peanuts and tree nuts on body weight and healthy weight loss in adults. J Nutr. 2008;138(suppl):1741S–5S.
135. Novotny JA, Gebauer SK, Baer DJ. Discrepancy between the Atwater factor predicted and empirically measured energy values of almonds in human diets. Am J Clin Nutr. 2012;96:296–301.
136. Baer DJ, Gebauer SK, Novotny JA. Walnuts consumed by healthy adults provide less available energy than predicted by the Atwater factors. J Nutr. 2016;146:9–13.
137. Traoret CJ, Lokko P, Cruz ACRF, et al. Peanut digestion and energy balance. Int J Obes. 2008;32:322–8.
138. Brown RC, Tey SL, Gray AR, et al. Nut consumption is associated with better nutrient intakes: results from the 2008/09 New Zealand Adult Nutrition Survey. Br J Nutr. 2016;115:105–12.
139. Nielsen SJ, Kit BK, Ogden CL. Nut consumption among U.S. adults, 2009–2010, NCHS data brief, no 176. Hyattsville: National Center for Health Statistics; 2014.
140. Mayhew AJ, de Souza RJ, Meyre D, et al. A systematic review and meta-analysis of nut consumption and incident risk of CVD and all-cause mortality. Br J Nutr. 2016;115:212–25.
141. Ma L, Wang F, Guo W, et al. Nut consumption and the risk of coronary artery disease: a dose-response meta-analysis of 13 prospective studies. Thromb Res. 2014;134(4):790–4.
142. Luu HN, Blot WJ, Xiang Y-B, et al. Prospective evaluation of the association of nut/peanut consumption with total and cause-specific mortality. JAMA Intern Med. 2015;175(5):755–66.
143. Kelly JH Jr, Sabate J. Nuts and coronary heart disease: an epidemiological perspective. Br J Nutr. 2006;96(2):S61–7.
144. Del Gobbo LC, Falk MC, Feldman R, et al. Effects of tree nuts on blood lipids, apolipoproteins, and blood pressure: systematic review, meta-analysis, and dose-response of 61 controlled intervention trials. Am J Clin Nutr. 2015;102:1347–56.
145. Sabate J, Oda K, Ros E. Nut consumption and blood lipid levels a pooled analysis of 25 intervention trials. Arch Intern Med. 2010;170(9):821–7.
146. Banel DK, Hu FB. Effects of walnut consumption on blood lipids and other cardiovascular risk factors: a meta-analysis and systematic review. Am J Clin Nutr. 2009;90:56–63.
147. Phung OJ, Makanji SS, White CM, Coleman CI. Almonds have a neutral effect on serum lipid profiles: a meta-analysis of randomized trials. J Am Diet Assoc. 2009;109:865–73.
148. Griel AE, Kris-Etherton PM. Tree nuts and the lipid profile: a review of clinical studies. Br J Nutr. 2006;96(2):S68–78.
149. Le T, Flatt SW, Natarajan L, et al. Effects of diet composition and insulin resistance status on plasma lipid levels in a weight loss intervention in women. J Am Heart Assoc. 2016;5:e002771. https://doi.org/10.1161/JAHA.115.002771.
150. Berryman CE, West SG, Fleming JA, et al. Effects of daily almond consumption on cardiometabolic risk and abdominal adiposity in healthy adults with elevated LDL-cholesterol: a randomized controlled trial. J Am Heart Assoc. 2015;4(1):e000993. https://doi.org/10.1161/JAHA.114.000993.
151. Edel AL, Rodriguez-Leyva D, Maddaford TG, et al. Dietary flaxseed independently lowers circulating cholesterol and lowers it beyond the effects of cholesterol-lowering medications alone in patients with peripheral artery disease. J Nutr. 2015;145:749–57.
152. Richmond K, Williams S, Mann J, et al. Markers of cardiovascular risk in postmenopausal women with type 2 diabetes are improved by the daily consumption of almonds or sunflower kernels: a feeding study. ISRN Nutr. 2013;2013:626414. https://doi.org/10.5402/2013/626414.
153. Nouran MG, Kimiagar M, Abadi A, et al. Peanut consumption and cardiovascular risk. Public Health Nutr. 2009;13(10):1581–6.
154. Sabate J, Fraser GE, Burke K, et al. Effects of walnuts on serum lipid levels and blood pressure in normal men. N Engl J Med. 1993;328:603–7.
155. Ruisinger JF, Gibson CA, Backes JM, et al. Statins and almonds to lower lipoproteins (the STALL Study). J Clin Lipidol. 2015;9:58–64.

13 Dietary Patterns and Hypertension

Keywords
Hypertension • Blood pressure • Aging • Overweight • Obesity • DASH diet • Mediterranean diet • Vegetarian diets • Dietary guidelines • Western diet

Key Points

- Elevated blood pressure (BP), including pre-hypertension and hypertension, is a common and growing public health problem. Globally, the overall prevalence of elevated BP is approaching 50% of adults age ≥ 25 years. The adult risk of cardiovascular disease (CVD) and renal disease approximately doubles for each 20/10 mm Hg incremental increase above 115/75 mm Hg.
- The major lifestyle factors associated with elevated BP and hypertension are aging, especially unhealthy aging associated with overweight and obesity, poor dietary habits, inactivity or lack of exercise, and ineffective stress management.
- There is convincing evidence that high adherence to healthy dietary patterns, including the Dietary Approaches to Stop Hypertension (DASH), the Mediterranean (MedDiet), Nordic diet, dietary guidelines-based, and vegetarian diets are effective in lowering BP, especially in older, overweight or obese hypertensive and prehypertensive adults compared to Western diets.
- Healthy dietary patterns lower sodium, excessive energy and added refined carbohydrate intake, and increase the levels of fiber, plant protein, potassium, and other essential nutrients and bioactive phytochemicals intake are associated with a lower risk of hypertension and elevated BP.
- Healthy dietary pattern mechanisms associated with reduced hypertension risk include; lowering the risk of weight gain, stimulating colon microbiota, improving vascular health by normalizing total cholesterol and LDL-C levels, reducing oxidative and inflammatory stress, improving insulin sensitivity to reduce atherosclerosis risk, and maintaining electrolyte balance.

M.L. Dreher, *Dietary Patterns and Whole Plant Foods in Aging and Disease*, Nutrition and Health,
https://doi.org/10.1007/978-3-319-59180-3_13

13.1 Introduction

Elevated blood pressure (BP), including prehypertension and hypertension, is a common and growing public health problem [1, 2]. Globally, the overall prevalence of elevated BP is approaching 50% of adults age ≥ 25 years. By 2025, because of population growth and an increasing aging population, it is projected that about 1.5 billion individuals will have hypertension [2–4]. Over nine million annual deaths worldwide are currently attributable to hypertension [1]. The World Health Organization (WHO) has identified that there is convincing evidence that obesity and poor dietary patterns are associated with increased risk of hypertension [1, 5]. Increased BP etiology is linked to the renin-angiotensin aldosterone system (RAAS), a hormonal cascade that functions in the homeostatic control of BP and extracellular fluid volume [6]. Aldosterone causes the tubules of the kidneys to increase the reabsorption of sodium and water into the blood, while at the same time causing the excretion of potassium, which increases the volume of extracellular fluid leading to elevated BP. Hypertension is a major risk factor for cardiovascular disease (CVD) stroke and renal disease [4, 7]. Also, prehypertension (120/80–139/89 mm Hg) has been associated with 1.5- to 2-fold increases in cardiovascular disease events after age 55 years and a 43% increased risk of coronary heart disease (CHD) [4].

The major factors associated with elevated BP and hypertension are aging, especially unhealthy aging associated with overweight and obesity, poor dietary habits, inactivity or lack of exercise, and ineffective stress management [1–9]. Aging is directly associated with elevated BP risk (Fig. 13.1) [4]. Excess body weight is associated with increased activity of the RAAS, insulin resistance, and reduced kidney function (especially with salt-sensitive hypertension individuals) [7–9]. Rates of hypertension are twice as likely to occur in obese vs. normal weight individuals. Dietary patterns with low dietary energy density, high fiber density and containing primarily natural sugar sources such as whole fruits tend to be associated with lower prevalence of overweight or obesity [5]. Whereas a dietary pattern with low fiber density and high in added sugars intake (primarily from chocolate and fruit drinks) was associated with increased prevalence of overweight or obesity. Dietary patterns low in fiber density and high in the ratio of sodium to potassium and high in saturated

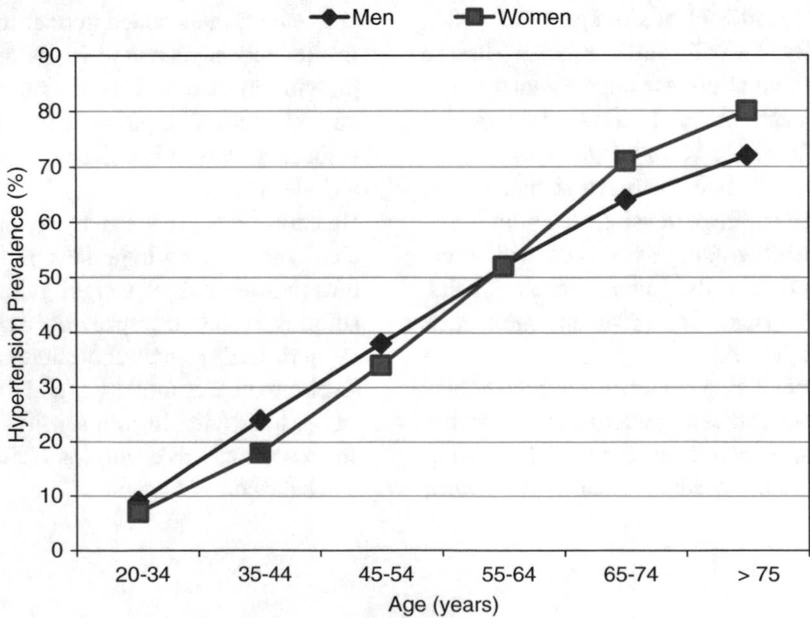

Fig. 13.1 Prevalence of hypertension in US adults ≥20 years with age (National Health and Nutrition Examination Survey [NHANES] 2007–2012) (adapted from [4])

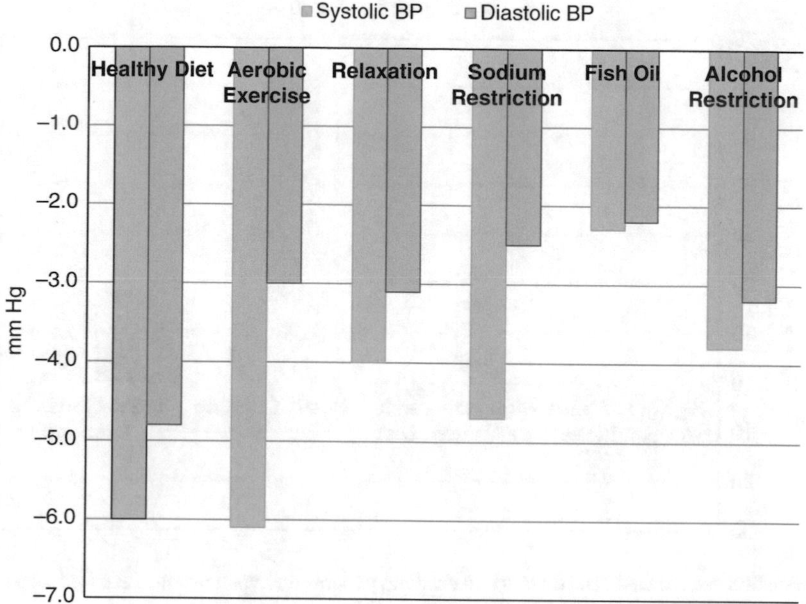

Fig. 13.2 Association between healthy lifestyle factors and blood pressure (BP) from a systematic review of RCTs (all healthy lifestyle factors $p < 0.05$) (adapted from [9, 12])

fat to polyunsaturated fat ratios are associated with increased prevalence of hypertension and prehypertension [5]. A 2017 meta-analysis of cohort studies found an inverse linear dose–response association between risk of hypertension and physical activity with a 6% lower risk of hypertension when individuals met the minimum recommended guideline levels of 150 min/week compared with inactive individuals and higher levels of physical activity reduced hypertension risk by up to 33% [8]. The Western lifestyle is associated with higher BP among both adults and adolescents [2, 9–12]. The effects of various healthy lifestyle factors associated with lower BP are summarized in Fig. 13.2 [9, 12]. Elevated BP is a major risk factor for stroke, CHD, damage to retinal blood vessels, and kidney disease/renal failure [1–9]. The adult risk of CVD and renal disease approximately doubles for each 20/10 mm Hg incremental increase above 115/75 mm Hg. Guidelines for prevention, treatment and control of elevated BP focus on lifestyle modifications including weight loss and maintenance, reduced salt intake, increased fruit and vegetables consumption, routine participation in physical activity, cessation of smoking, limiting alcohol consumption, and anxiety and stress control [1–12]. Healthy dietary patterns are more effective in reducing BP in hypertensive than normotensive individuals and they provide adjunctive BP lowering for hypertensive people already on drug therapy. The food components and compositions of several dietary patterns are summarized in Appendix A. The objective of this chapter is to comprehensively review the role of dietary patterns in hypertension prevention and management.

13.2 Dietary Patterns

High adherence to healthy diet patterns are associated with significantly lower CVD risks including hypertension and CHD compared to high adherence to the Western diet [13, 14]. Hypertension and CHD are interconnected as among individuals aged 40–90 years, each 20/10 mm Hg rise in BP doubles the risk of fatal coronary events [15, 16]. A 2016 meta-analysis (16 cohort and 11 cross-sectional studies; 295,799 participants) found that the highest adherence to a healthy dietary pattern reduced hypertension risk by 19% ($p = 0.02$) and the highest adherence to the Western diet increased hypertension risk by 4% ($p > 0.05$) compared to lowest adherence [17]. However, subgroup analysis showed that individuals >50 years were more

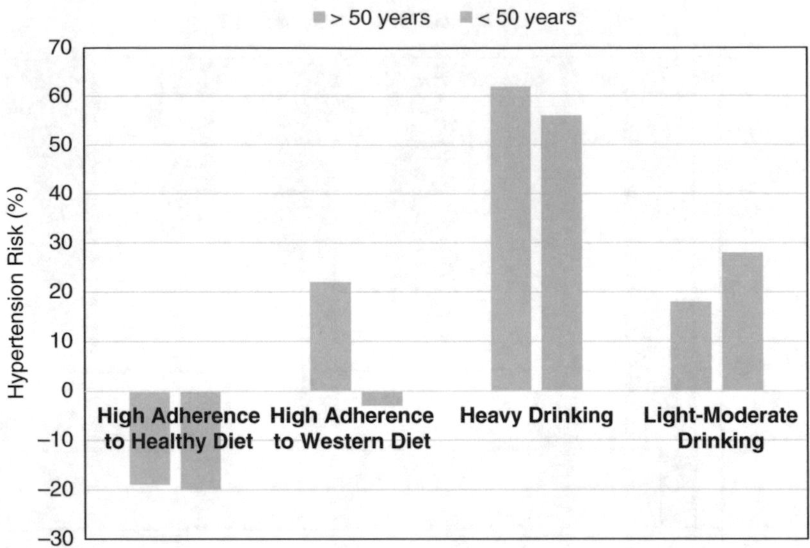

Fig. 13.3 Association between age, and dietary and drinking patterns on hypertension risk based on a meta-analysis of 27 observational studies ($p < 0.0001$, for all) (adapted from [17])

sensitive to the effects of the Western diet on hypertension risk (Fig. 13.3) [17]. Additionally, a heavy drinking pattern increased hypertension risk by 62% ($p = 0.004$), whereas light-moderate drinking patterns insignificantly increased hypertension risk by 20% ($p = 0.13$). A 2015 meta-analysis (35 cohort and case-control studies) found an inverse association between healthy dietary patterns and CHD risk with a 33% risk reduction whereas a Western diet increased CHD risk by 45% (high vs. low adherence) [18]. The high adherence to healthy dietary patterns characterized by high consumption of fruit, vegetables, whole grains, legumes, seeds, nuts, fish, and low fat dairy and low consumption of processed meat, sweets, and alcohol are generally associated with significantly lower hypertension risk [8, 19]. The US 2015 Dietary Guidelines Advisory Committee report concluded that healthy dietary patterns rich in fiber, potassium, carotenoids and other healthy components and low in saturated fat and sodium, especially the Dietary Approaches to Stop Hypertension (DASH)-style diets can lower systolic BP by 6 mm Hg and diastolic BP by 3 mm Hg compared to Western patterns [20]. A meta-analysis (17 RCTs; 4909 prehypertensive or hypertensive participants; 13 trials allowed continuation of BP-lowering medications; healthy dietary patterns such as the DASH, Nordic diet, dietary guidelines and Mediterranean diet (MedDiet); 6 weeks to 2 years) showed that healthy dietary patterns significantly lowered systolic BP by 4.3 mm Hg and diastolic BP by 2.4 mm Hg across a range of sodium intakes [21]. A cross-sectional analysis that used baseline data from the Australian HealthTrack study (328 adults; 12-month weight loss RCT) found that a dietary pattern rich in nuts, seeds, fruit, and fish with a lower sodium to potassium ratio was inversely associated with BP [22].

13.2.1 DASH Dietary Patterns

13.2.1.1 Background

The DASH diet was designed primarily for individuals with hypertension [13]. This pattern is rich in fruits and vegetables, low-fat dairy products, includes whole grains, poultry, fish, and nuts, and limits saturated fat, red meat, sweets, and sugar containing beverages. Compared with the Western diet, the DASH diet provides lower total fat, saturated fat, and dietary cholesterol, and higher potassium, magnesium, calcium, fiber, and protein. A DASH adherence score is based on the following primary food and nutrient components: increased fruits, vegetables, whole grains, nuts and legumes and low-fat dairy; and reduced red and processed meats, sweetened beverages, and sodium.

13.2.1.2 Observational Studies

A number of observational studies support the DASH diet's benefits in reducing hypertension risk factors or hypertension risk directly. In a cross-sectional analysis (2047 Irish middle-aged men and women) there was an inverse association between DASH diet score and systolic BP with significantly lower systolic BP in men by 7.5 mm Hg and in women by 5.1 mm Hg (highest vs. lowest DASH quintiles) [23]. An Iranian cross-sectional study (293 nurses) found that those in the highest vs. lowest quartile of the DASH diet scores lowered obesity risk by 71% and central obesity risk by 63%, both of which are major hypertension risk factors [24]. The Taiwanese CardioVascular Disease Risk FACtor Twotownship Study (1420 participants; mean age 45.5 years; 13-years of follow-up) found that adhering to the DASH diet was beneficial for long term BP control and reduction of stroke risk in the studied Chinese population [25]. Additionally, a 12-month WEB-based nutrition education program called 'DASH for health' longitudinal observational study (735 hypertensive or prehypertensive subjects;12 months on the program) observed a significantly lower systolic BP by 6.8 mm Hg [26]. BP and body weight were inversely associated with the number of visits to the 'DASH for health' WEB site. A 2016 Atherosclerosis Risk Communities Study (14,882 participants; age range 45-64 years; median follow-up of 23 years) found that participants with the lowest DASH diet score, which is l ike the Western dietary pattern, had a significantly increased risk of developing kidney disease by 16%, after multivariate adjustment [11].

13.2.1.3 Randomized Controlled Trials (RCTs)

RCTs have consistently demonstrated that DASH-type diets are the most effective diets for lowering elevated BP (Table 13.1) [27–37].

Meta-Analyses

Three DASH focused meta-analyses show greater BP reductions in older hypertensive individuals with elevated BMIs compared to younger, normotensive or leaner individuals [27–29]. A 2016 meta-analysis (24 RCTs; 23,858 subjects; median age 45 years; 6–48 months) found that healthy dietary patterns reduced the pooled mean systolic BP by 3 mm Hg and diastolic BP by 1.8 mm Hg [27]. The DASH diet was the most effective in BP lowering with a reduction for systolic BP by 7.6 mm Hg and diastolic BP by 4.2 mm Hg. Low-sodium; low-sodium, high-potassium; low-sodium, low-calorie; and low-calorie diets also led to significant systolic and diastolic BP reductions, whereas Mediterranean diet (MedDiet) participants experienced a significant reduction in diastolic BP but not systolic BP. A 2015 meta-analysis (20 RCTs; 1917 subjects; 2–26 weeks) showed that the DASH diet significantly decreased systolic BP by 5.2 mm Hg and diastolic BP by 2.6 mm Hg for an estimated 13% reduction in the 10-year Framingham risk score for CVD [28]. Changes in both systolic and diastolic BP were greater in participants with higher baseline BP or BMI. A 2014 meta-analysis (17 RCTs; 2561 subjects; 2–26 weeks) found that the DASH diet significantly reduced pooled mean systolic BP by 6.7 mm Hg and diastolic BP by 3.5 mm Hg; RCTs with hypertensive subjects having significantly greater decreases in BP [29].

Representative RCTs

Eight representative RCTs provide important insights on the effect of DASH diets on BP and hypertension risk [30–37]. A 2016 US crossover RCT (36 subjects; mean age 48 years and BMI 27; lower fat and higher fat DASH diets vs. Western diet; 3 weeks) showed DASH diets with full-fat or low-fat dairy food had similar effects on BP (Fig. 13.4) [30]. The low-fat dairy DASH diet significantly reduced LDL-C, HDL-C, apolipoprotein A, intermediate density lipoprotein and large LDL particles, and LDL peak diameter compared with the Western diet, but not the full-fat dairy DASH diet, which significantly reduced triglycerides levels compared with the low-fat dairy DASH diet. The OmniHeart trial (164 adults; mean age 54 years; 73% women; mean BMI 30; 80% prehypertensive; stable body weight; 6 weeks) demonstrated that replacing 10% of carbohydrate calories in the standard DASH diet with either the same

Table 13.1 Summary of Dietary Approaches to Stop Hypertension (DASH) diet RCTs in blood pressure (BP) management

Objective	Study details	Study results
Systematic reviews and meta-analyses		
Gay et al. (2016). Quantify the aggregated BP-lowering effects associated with dietary patterns and special diets interventions on BP [27]	24 RCTs; 23,858 subjects; duration ranged from 6 to 48 months of follow-up (median: 12 months); age ranged from 34 to 67 years (median: 45 years); all subjects were overweight or obese; baseline mean systolic BP 136 mm Hg and diastolic BP 86 mm Hg	Overall, all the healthy diets reduced systolic BP by 3 mm Hg and diastolic BP by 1.8 mm Hg. The DASH diet was the most effective diet with reduced systolic BP by 7.6 mm Hg and diastolic BP by 4.2 mm Hg
Siervo et al. (2015). Assess the effects of the DASH diet on BP and CVD risk factors [28]	20 RCTs; 1917 participants; male and female; age > 18 years; healthy individuals with above-optimal BP and stage 1 hypertension; 2–24 weeks	The DASH diet significantly decreased systolic BP by 5.2 mm Hg and diastolic BP by 2.6 mm Hg. Changes in both systolic and diastolic BP were greater in participants with higher baseline BP or BMI. These changes predicted a lower 10-year Framingham risk score for CVD by 13%
Saneei et al. (2014). Examine the effect of the DASH diet on BP [29]	17 RCTs; 2561 participants; 1747 participants with hypertension, 293 without hypertension, and 521 with undisclosed hypertensive status; 2–26 weeks	The DASH diet significantly reduced systolic BP by 6.7 mm Hg and diastolic BP by 3.5 mm Hg. RCTs with hypertensive subjects had significantly greater decrease in BP
Representative RCTs		
Chiu et al. (2016). Evaluate the effects of full-fat or low-fat dairy foods in the DASH diet, with a corresponding increase in fat and a reduction in sugar intake, on blood pressure and plasma lipids and lipoproteins (US) [30]	**Crossover RCT:** 36 subjects; mean age 48 years; mean BMI 27; 40% women; diets: Western diet control, a standard DASH diet, and a higher-fat, lower-carbohydrate modification of the DASH diet (HF-DASH diet); 3 weeks each, separated by 2-week washout periods	DASH diets with low-fat or full fat dairy had similar BP lowering effects compared with the Western control diet (Fig. 13.4)
Al-Solaiman et al. (2010). Evaluate the effects of the DASH diet on BP in abdominally obese hypertensive vs. lean normotensive adults (US) [31]	**Crossover RCT:** 30 adults; mean age 38 years; 80% women; 15 obese, mean BMI 35, mean baseline BP 136/89 mm Hg; 15 lean, mean BMI 23; mean BP 110/70 mm Hg; DASH diet, usual diet, or usual diet supplemented w/ potassium, magnesium and fiber to match DASH diet; 3 weeks with no washout	In obese hypertensives, the DASH diet significantly lowered systolic BP by 7.6 and diastolic BP by 5.3 mm Hg and the usual diet supplemented with potassium, magnesium and fiber lowered systolic BP by 6.2 and diastolic BP by 3.7 mm Hg compared to no BP reduction for the usual control diet. In lean normotensive subjects, BP values were not significantly different among the 3 diets
Blumenthal et al. (2010). Compare the BP lowering effects of the DASH diet alone or in combination with a weight management program (US) [32]	**Parallel RCT**: 144 overweight or obese, unmedicated outpatients; pre-hypertension or stage 1 hypertension systolic BP 130–159 mm Hg; diastolic BP 85–99 mm Hg; DASH diet alone or combined with a weight management program vs. usual diet controls; 4 months	The DASH plus weight loss significantly reduced systolic BP by 16.1 mm Hg and diastolic BP by 9.9 mm Hg vs. the DASH without weight loss which reduced systolic BP by 11.2 mm Hg and diastolic BP by 7.5 mm Hg whereas the usual diet lowered systolic BP by 3.4 mm Hg and diastolic BP by 3.8 mm Hg

Table 13.1 (continued)

Objective	Study details	Study results
Appel et al. (2005). Investigate the effects of BP on partial replacement of carbohydrates in the original DASH diet with protein and unsaturated fat (US) [33]	**3-period, crossover multi-center RCT:** 164 adults; mean age 54 years; 73% women; mean BMI 30; mean baseline BP 131/77 mm Hg; 80% prehypertensive; diets: Standard DASH diet rich in carbohydrates; DASH diet 10% energy replacement by protein, about half from plant sources; and DASH diet 10% energy replacement by unsaturated fat, primarily monounsaturated fat; 6 weeks	Compared with the DASH diet, the protein and unsaturated modified DASH diets significantly decreased systolic BP and diastolic BP among those with hypertension (Table 13.2). All DASH diets lowered estimated CHD risk by 16–21% compared with baseline
Nowson et al. (2005). Evaluate the effect of weight reduction diets: a low-fat (LF) diet and a DASH type diet on BP in men (Australia) [34]	**Parallel RCT:** 63 men; mean age 48 years; mean BMI 30; baseline BP 113/88 mm Hg; diets: Hypocaloric DASH diet or a low-fat diet. Both diet groups engaged in 0.5 h of moderate physical activity on most days of the week; 12 weeks	The hypocaloric DASH diet significantly lowered systolic BP by 7.6 mm Hg and diastolic BP by 5.4 mm Hg vs. hypocaloric low-fat diet (Fig. 13.5). Also, 5% reduction in weight decreased systolic BP by 8 mm Hg, and diastolic BP by 5 mm Hg
Appel et al. (2003). Investigate the effects of implementing several types of multi-component, lifestyle programs including the DASH diet (PREMIER study; US) [35]	**Multicenter parallel RCT:** 810 adults; mean age 50 years; mean BMI 33; 62% women; mean baseline BP 135/85 mm Hg; 5% current smokers; 38% hypertensive no BP medications; treatments: Behavioral program (e.g., weight loss, sodium reduction, increased physical activity, and limited alcohol intake); behavioral plus DASH program; or advice only as a comparison group	Compared to general advice only, the established behavioral program significantly reduced systolic BP by 3.7 mm Hg and the established behavioral program plus DASH lowered systolic BP by 4.3 mm Hg. After 6 months, the prevalence of hypertension in the advice only group, behavioral group and behavioral plus DASH diet was 26%, 17% and 12%, respectively, compared to the 38% hypertension prevalence at baseline
Miller et al. (2002). Examine the effects of a comprehensive DASH lifestyle intervention on BP and other CVD risk factors (US) [36]	**Parallel RCT:** 44 adults; mean age 54 years; 62% women; mean BMI 33; mean BP 136/84 mm Hg; all subjects on BP medications; treatments: a hypocaloric DASH diet plus moderate-intensity exercise 3 days per week vs. a control usual diet no exercise; 9 weeks	There was 4.9 kg weight loss in the DASH plus exercise group vs. control. Also, the DASH diet plus exercise group significantly lowered mean 24-hour ambulatory systolic BP by 9.5 mm Hg and diastolic BP by 5.3 mm Hg
Apple et al. (1997). Investigate the effects of a fruit and vegetable rich diet or DASH diet vs. a usual American diet on BP (US) [37]	**Multi-center parallel RCT:** 459 adults; 50% women; 60% African American; mean age 44 years; mean BMI 29; mean BP 132/85 mm Hg; diets: (1) 8–10 portions fruit and vegetable diet, (2) DASH diet with 8–10 portions of fruit and vegetables; (3) control American low fruit and vegetable diet, 8 weeks after 3-week run-in on the American diet	The DASH diet significantly reduced systolic and diastolic BP by 5.5 and 3.0 mm Hg more than the control diet (Fig. 13.6). Also, the fruit and vegetable rich diet significantly reduced systolic BP by 2.8 mm Hg and borderline significantly reduced diastolic BP by 1.1 mm Hg more than the control diet. Among the 133 hypertensive subjects, the DASH diet significantly reduced systolic and diastolic BP by 11.4 and 5.5 mm Hg more than the control diet. The DASH diet was twice as effective in lowering BP as a high fruit and vegetable diet alone

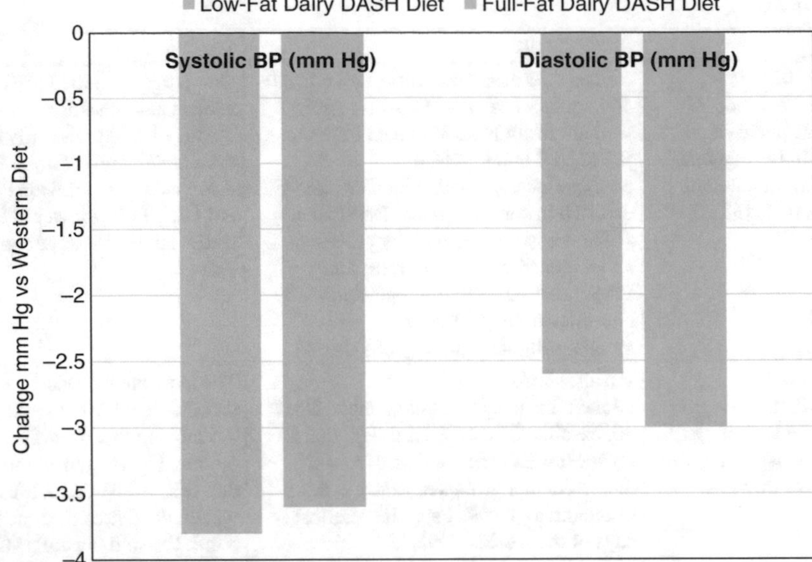

Fig. 13.4 Effects of full-fat and low-fat dairy foods in the DASH diet compared to the Western control diet on BP ($p \leq 0.017$ for all BP) [adapted from 30]

Table 13.2 Effect on blood pressure lowering of substituting 10% of carbohydrate energy in the standard DASH diet with protein or vegetable oil consisting primarily of monounsaturated fatty acids (MUFA) [33]

Blood pressure (BP)	Mean baseline BP (mm Hg)	Mean lower BP from baseline by diet		
		Carbohydrate	Protein	MUFA
Systolic BP (mm Hg)[a]				
All	131.2	8.2	9.5	9.3
Stage 1 hypertension	146.5	12.9	16.1	15.8
Prehypertension	127.5	7.0	8.0	7.7
Diastolic BP (mm Hg)[a]				
All	77.0	4.1	5.2	4.8
Stage 1 hypertension	84.2	6.3	8.6	8.2
Prehypertension	76.3	3.6	4.4	3.9

[a]All partial replacements of protein or MUFA for carbohydrate ($p < 0.02$)

calorie content of protein or monounsaturated fat significantly lowered systolic and diastolic BP as shown in Table 13.2 [33]. In a DASH weight loss RCT (63 men; mean age 48 years; hypocaloric DASH and low fat diets; mean BMI 30; BP 135/88 mm Hg; 12 weeks), the DASH diet was significantly more effective than low-fat weight loss diets in lowering BP at similar weight loss (Fig. 13.5) [34]. A 1999 DASH trial (459 adults; 50% women; 60% African American; mean age 44 years; mean BMI 29; mean BP 132/85 mm Hg; DASH diet: 8–10 portions of fruit and vegetables, increased whole-grains, low fat dairy, reduced saturated and total fat vs. American Western control diet; 8 weeks after 3-week run-in on the American Western diet) found that the DASH diet significantly reduced systolic BP by 5.5 mm Hg and diastolic BP by 3.0 mm Hg more than the Western diet control (Fig. 13.6) [37]. Among the 133 subjects with hypertension, the DASH diet more than doubled the BP lowering effects by further significantly reducing systolic BP by 11.4 mm Hg and diastolic BP by 5.5 mm Hg vs. the American Western diet. For overweight or obese individuals with elevated BP, the addition of exercise and weight loss to the DASH diet resulted in even

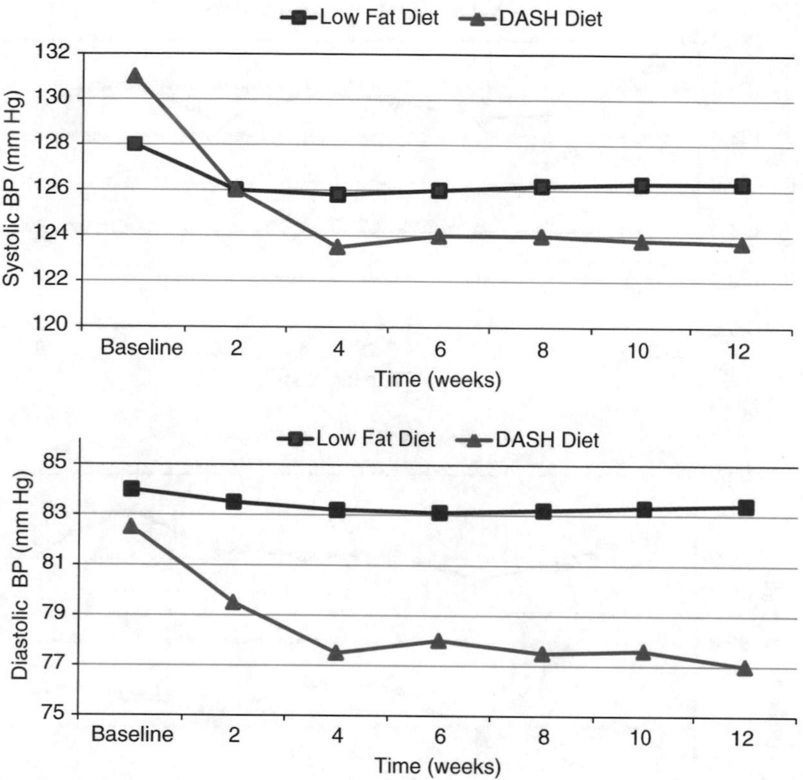

Fig. 13.5 Effect of a hypocaloric DASH-type vs. low fat weight-loss diet on blood pressure (BP) control ($p < 0.006$) [adapted from 34]

larger significant BP reductions and improvements in vascular function [31, 32, 35, 36].

13.2.2 Mediterranean Dietary Patterns (MedDiet)

The MedDiet incorporates the traditional healthy dietary habits of people from countries bordering the Mediterranean Sea, which are rich in whole plant foods such as whole-grains, fresh fruits, vegetables, beans, nuts, and seeds, along with moderate amounts of dairy foods, fish, and poultry and lower amounts of red and processed meat meat, and extra virgin olive oil as the major source of fat and moderate wine is consumed moderately with meals [2, 17, 21]. There may be some variation in food composition between regions. The BP lowering evidence for the MedDiet pattern is more limited and moderate than that for the DASH dietary pattern [7].

13.2.2.1 Observational Studies

MedDiet prospective studies generally show moderate beneficial effects on BP or hypertension risk, with higher adherence to a Mediterranean-style diet. Several studies showed a modest decrease in systolic BP by 2.4–3.1 mm Hg and diastolic by 1.3–1.9 mm Hg, which was primarily associated with olive oil, fruit and vegetable intake [38–40]. However, the SUN (Seguimiento Universidad de Navarra) prospective cohort (10,800 adults; mean age 37 years; mean BMI 23; 70% women; mean 4.6 years of follow-up) observed that higher adherence to the MedDiet did not show a significant association with lowering the incidence of hypertension, most likely because of the relative youth and normal BMI of the cohort [41]. During pregnancy, low adherence to a MedDiet pattern or high adherence to a Western dietary pattern are independently associated with higher BP [42].

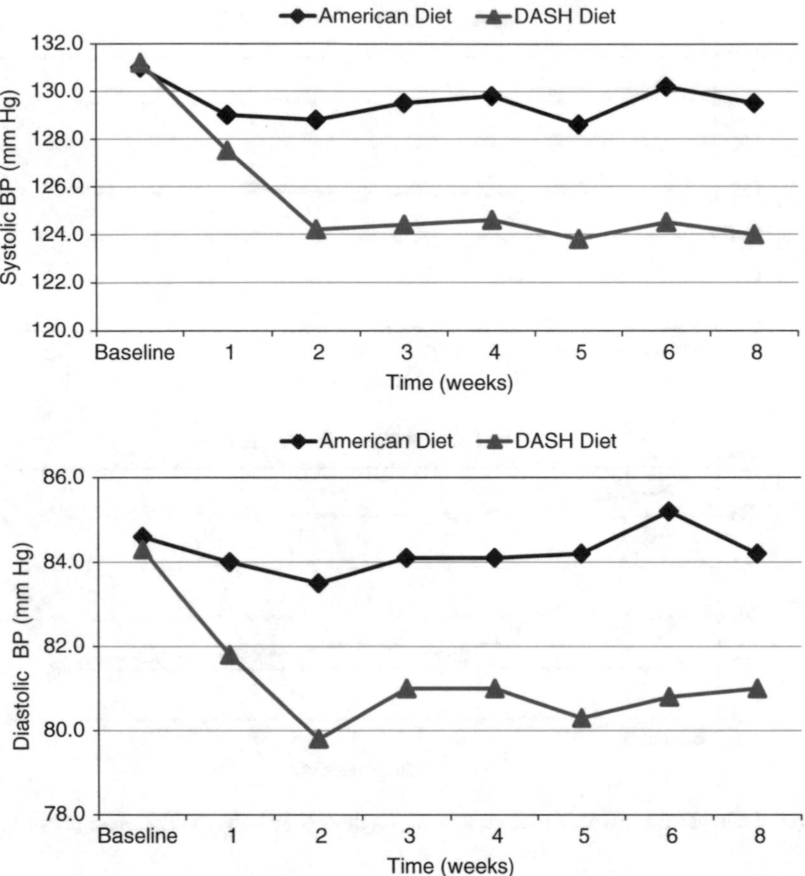

Fig. 13.6 Effect of DASH diet vs. Western-type diet on blood pressure (BP) in overweight combined normotensive and hypertensive individuals ($p < 0.001$) [adapted from 37]

13.2.2.2 Randomized Controlled Trials (RCTs)

Table 13.3 summarizes the effect of the MedDiet RCTs on BP levels in normal and hypertension subjects [43–49]. The AHA/ACC Lifestyle Guideline recommended the MedDiet over a low-fat diet for controlling BP [23].

Systematic Reviews and Meta-analyses

Three meta-analyses support a small but significant BP lowering effect for MedDiets vs. low-fat diet controls [43–45]. A 2016 meta-analysis (6 RCTs; 7000 subjects; ≥1 year) found in normal to mildly hypertensive individuals that MedDiets had a modest but significant BP lowering effect on systolic BP by 1.4 mm Hg and diastolic BP 0.7 mm Hg compared to a low-fat diet [43]. A 2015 meta-analysis (9 RCTs; 1178 type 2 diabetic subjects; 4 weeks to 4 years) showed significant mean systolic BP lowering by 1.5 mm Hg and diastolic BP by 1.4 mm Hg compared to low-fat control diets, along with greater reductions in hemoglobin A1c, fasting plasma glucose, fasting insulin, BMI, body weight, total cholesterol and triglycerides, and increased HDL-C [44]. A 2011 meta-analysis (7 RCTs; 3650 overweight or obese patients with at least one CVD risk factor or patients with established coronary artery disease; mean age 35–68 years; MedDiet vs. low fat diets; ≥6 months) found that the MedDiet significantly reduced mean systolic BP by 1.5 mm Hg and diastolic BP by 1.4 mm Hg vs. a low-fat diet; in addition the MedDiet significantly lowered body weight by 2.2 kg and BMI by 0.56 units [45].

Table 13.3 Summary of Mediterranean diets (MedDiet) RCTs in blood pressure (BP) management

Objective	Study details	Study results
Systematic reviews and meta-analyses		
Nissensohn et al. (2016). Examine MedDiet effects on BP in RCTs ≥1 year duration [43]	6 RCTs; >7000 normal and mildly hypertensive individuals; MedDiet vs. low fat diets; ≥1 year	MedDiets had modest but significant mean reductions in both systolic BP by 1.4 mm Hg and diastolic BP by 0.7 mm Hg compared to low-fat diets
Huo et al. (2015). Investigate the effects of MedDiet on cardiovascular risk factors in type 2 diabetic subjects [44]	9 RCTs; 1178 type 2 diabetic subjects; age 26–77 years; MedDiet vs. control diets; 4 weeks to 4 years	MedDiets significantly reduced mean systolic BP by 1.5 mm Hg and diastolic BP by 1.4 mm Hg vs. low-fat diets. Also, MedDiets led to greater reductions in HbA1c, fasting plasma glucose, fasting insulin, BMI, body weight, total cholesterol and triglycerides, and increased HDL-C compared to control diets
Nordmann et al. (2011). Evaluate the effects of MedDiet on BP and other CVD risk biomarkers [45]	7 RCTs; 3650 overweight/obese patients with at least one CVD risk factor or patients with established coronary artery disease; mean age 35–68 years; mean BMI ranged from 29 to 35; MedDiet vs. low fat diets; ≥ 6 months	MedDiets significantly reduced mean systolic BP by 1.7 mm Hg and diastolic BP by 1.5 mm Hg vs. low fat diets. Also, the MedDiet significantly reduced mean body weight by 2.2 kg, BMI by 0.56 kg/m^2, and total cholesterol by 7.4 mg/dL
Representative RCTs		
Storniolo et al. (2017). Evaluate the effect of MedDiets on BP and endothelial markers in hypertensive women (PREvención con DIeta MEDiterránea [PREDIMED] substudy; Spain) [46]	**Parallel RCT:** 90 high CVD risk postmenopausal women; mean age 68 years; BMI 32; mean systolic BP 155 and diastolic 84 mm Hg; diets: Traditional MedDiet supplemented with extra virgin olive oil or mixed nuts versus a control low-fat diet; 1 year	(1) for the MedDiet plus tree nuts, there was a significantly decreased diastolic BP by 5% vs. low fat control diet; significantly decreased serum endothelin-1 levels by 19% vs. baseline values. (2) For the MedDiet plus extra virgin olive oil, there was significantly increased serum stable nitric oxide metabolites by 64% vs. baseline values. (3) For the low-fat diet guidance, there were no significant changes in BP or endothelial markers
Domenech et al. (2014). Investigate the effects of MedDiets on ambulatory BP in elderly subjects at high CVD risk over 1 year (PREDIMED substudy; Spain) [47]	**Parallel RCT:** 235 high CVD risk adults; mean age 67 years; 57% women; mean BMI 30; mean systolic BP 145 mm Hg, mean diastolic BP 82 mm Hg; diets: Traditional MedDiet supplemented with extra virgin olive oil or mixed tree nuts versus a control low-fat diet; 1 year	MedDiets with both extra virgin olive oil and tree nuts significantly lowered systolic BP by 4.0 mm Hg and diastolic BP by 1.9 mm Hg vs. low fat control diets
Toledo et al. (2013). Examine the effects of the MedDiet on BP after 4 years (Primary prevention PREDIMED study; Spain) [48]	**Multi-center parallel RCT:** 7447 asymptomatic adults with high CVD risk; mean age 67 years; 57% women; mean BMI 30; mean systolic BP 143, diastolic BP 83 mm Hg; 70% subjects on anti-hypertensive medications; diets: MedDiets with either extra virgin olive oil, or mixed tree nuts vs. low-fat diet; BP measures at baseline and once yearly; 4 years	The MedDiets significantly reduced diastolic BP with extra virgin olive oil diet by 1.5 mm Hg and with tree nuts by 0.65 mm Hg vs. low fat control diet. There were no observed between-group differences in systolic BP

(continued)

Table 13.3 (continued)

Objective	Study details	Study results
Estruch et al. (2006). Evaluate the effects of the MedDiet on BP (PREDIMED sub-trial; Spain) [49]	**Parallel RCT:** 772 asymptomatic persons at high CVD risk; mean age 69 years; 59% women; 42% current smokers; mean BMI 30; all subjects on anti-hypertension medications; diets: MedDiets including nutritional education and either extra virgin olive oil, 1 L/week, or free mixed nuts, 30 g/day vs. low-fat control diet; 3 months	MedDiets significantly reduced systolic BP with extra virgin olive oil by 5.4 mm Hg and nuts by 7.1 mm Hg, and diastolic BP for extra virgin olive oil by 1.6 mm Hg and nuts by 2.7 mm Hg vs. low fat control. Significant reductions were shown for plasma glucose, cholesterol: HDL-C ratio and CRP for extra virgin olive oil MedDiet compared with the low-fat diet

Table 13.4 Potential healthy dietary pattern mechanisms associated with lower blood pressure (BP) and reduced risk of hypertension [60–77]

Target	Increase	Decrease
Food intake	Chewing Eating time	Energy density Hunger
Body weight and fat		Weight gain Abdominal fat Ectopic fat
Stomach	Satiety signals	Gastric emptying rate Lipid emulsification Lipolysis
Liver	Lipoprotein uptake Bile acid production	Lipogenesis
Small intestine	Satiety signals	Dietary fat absorption
Peripheral tissue	Insulin sensitivity	Insulin resistance
Circulatory system	Short-chain fatty acids Carotenoids (e.g., lutein) Flavonoids and metabolites Nitrate and nitric oxide Electrolyte balance	Fasting lipids (e.g, TG)[a] Fasting lipoproteins (e.g., TC, LDL-C)[a] Inflammatory markers (e.g., CRP) Oxidized LDL-C Intima-media thickness progression
Large intestine	Fermentation Short-chain fatty acids (butyrate) Microbiota health Satiety signals	Bile acid reabsorption Inflammatory activity Systemic Lipopolysaccharide (LPS)
Fecal excretion	Macronutrients (e.g., dietary fat)	Metabolizable energy

[a]*TC* total cholesterol, *LDL-C* LDL-cholesterol, *TG* triglycerides, *CRP* C-reactive protein

Representative RCTs

Four PREvención con DIeta MEDiterránea (PREDIMED) trials in older adults with high CVD risk including hypertension clearly show that MedDiets supplemented with either 1 L/week extra virgin olive oil or 30 g/day of mixed tree nuts (walnuts, almonds, and hazelnuts) significantly reduced resting BP and 24-h ambulatory BP compared with a low-fat control diet [46–49]. Two PREDIMED sub-trials (3 months - 1 year) found that the MedDiet significantly lowered systolic BP with extra virgin olive oil by 4.0–5.4 mm Hg and with tree nuts by 4.0–7.1 mm Hg, and lowered diastolic BP with extra virgin olive oil by 1.6–1.9 mm Hg and with nuts by 1.9–2.7 mm Hg compared to a low fat diet in older high CVD risk individuals [47, 49]. The large PREDIMED trial (7447 adults with high CVD risk; mean age 67 years; 57% women; mean BMI 30; elevated BP; hypertensive meds;

4 years) showed that MedDiets significantly reduced diastolic BP by 0.65–1.5 mm Hg. A 2017 mechanism focused RCT (90 high CVD risk postmenopausal women; mean age 68 years; mean BMI 32; mean BP 155/84 mm Hg; 1 year) found beneficial effects for MedDiets supplemented with extra virgin olive oil or nut polyphenols related to increased serum nitric oxide and decreased serum endothelin-1 levels, which provide potential mechanistic pathways for BP lowering [46]. A possibly related mechanism between MedDiets and BP was indicated in a crossover RCT (24 women; mean age 26 years; mean BMI 23; 10 days) which found that the MedDiet was associated with significantly elevated contentment, alertness, memory recall and calmness compared to the usual diet [50].

13.2.3 Nordic Diet

As a Northern European regional alternative to the MedDiet, the gastronomically driven, environmentally friendly, new healthy Nordic diet which focuses on fruit and vegetables (especially berries, cabbages, root vegetables, and legumes), potatoes, fresh herbs, plants and mushrooms gathered from the wild, nuts, wholegrains, meats from livestock and game, fish, shellfish, and seaweed, along with diary and eggs, has been shown to be effective in lowering BP with and without weight loss [51, 52]. One RCT (181 adults; mean age 42 years; mean BMI 30; mean baseline BP 122/81 mm Hg; 6 months) found that adherence to the new Nordic diet resulted in significant reductions in systolic BP by 5.1 mm Hg and diastolic BP by 3.2 mm Hg in addition to lowering body weight by 3.2 kg, reducing waist circumference by 2.9 cm, and improved insulin sensitivity compared to the usual Danish diet [51]. A second RCT (37 adults; mean age 55 years; 68% women; mean BMI 31; 12 weeks) found that the new healthy Nordic diet significantly lowered 24-h ambulatory diastolic BP by 4.4 mm Hg and mean arterial pressure by 4.2 mm Hg compared to the control diet, after 12 weeks, without significant changes in body weight [52].

13.2.4 Dietary Guideline Patterns

National dietary guideline based patterns, generally characterized by higher consumption of fruit, vegetables, whole grains, legumes, seeds, nuts, fish, and low fat-dairy and lower consumption of processed meat, and sweets can lower BP and hypertension risk [53, 54]. A crossover RCT (31 subjects; mean age 55 years; mean BMI 31; baseline mean BP 120/74 mm Hg; 4 weeks) found that high adherence to the 2010 US Dietary Guidelines or Healthy Eating Indices significantly reduced diastolic BP by 2.1 mm Hg, total cholesterol by 10.2 mg/dL, LDL-C by 6 mg/dL, HDL-C by 3 mg/dL, and triglycerides by 5.2 mg/dL compared to the typical Western (American) diet [53]. A RCT on UK dietary guidelines (162 adults; mean age 52 years; 60% women; 26% postmenopausal; mean BMI 25; mean BP 120/78 mm Hg; 12 weeks) showed that high adherence significantly lowered systolic BP by 3.5 mm Hg, diastolic BP by 2.1 mm Hg, CRP by 36%, LDL-C by 11.6 mg/dL, total cholesterol to HDL-C ratio by 0.13, triglycerides by 10.6 mg/dL, and waist size by 1.2 cm compared with the traditional British diet (control) [54]. Overall, high adherence to the UK dietary guidelines diet reduced the risk of CVD by one-third, in healthy middle-aged and older men and women.

13.2.5 Vegetarian Dietary Patterns

Vegetarian diets consist of increased or strict consumption of plant foods including fruits, vegetables, non-fried potatoes, whole grains, legumes, soy foods, nuts and seeds and reduction or elimination of consumption of meats, dairy products, and eggs [55]. There are a range of vegetarian diets including the vegan diet (excludes all animal products), ovo-lacto-vegetarian (excludes all meat and seafood, but contains eggs and dairy products), pesco-vegetarian (excludes meat but includes seafood), and semi-vegetarian (occasional meat allowed) [56]. A 2014 meta-analysis of RCTs (7 RCTs; 311 adults; mean age 45 years) and observational studies (32 cohorts;

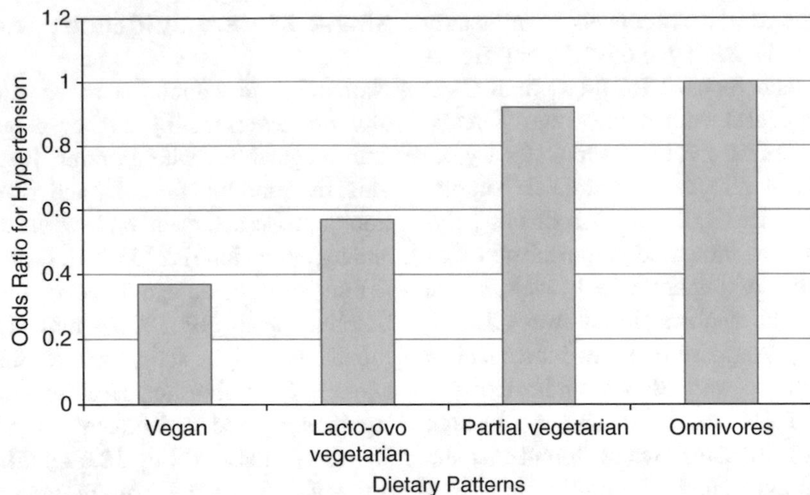

Fig. 13.7 Association between vegetarian dietary type vs. omnivore diet and hypertension risk ($p = 0.005$ for vegan; $p = 0.02$ for lacto-ovo vegetarian) [adapted from 58]

21,604 adults; mean age 47 years) suggest that vegetarian diets lower BP compared to omnivorous diets [57]. For the RCTs, vegetarian diets significantly lowered the mean systolic BP by 4.8 mm Hg and diastolic BP by 2.2 mm Hg vs. omnivorous diets. In observational studies, vegetarian diets were associated with significantly lower mean systolic BP by 6.9 mm Hg and diastolic BP by 4.7 mm Hg compared with the omnivorous diets. In the Adventist Health Study-2 cohort (500 adults; mean age 63 years; BMI 24–29) vegan and lacto-ovo vegetarians had significantly lower systolic and diastolic BP and reduced risk of hypertension compared to omnivorous Adventists (Fig. 13.7) [58]. A lifestyle comparison RCT reported that Seventh-day Adventist vegetarians had significantly less hypertension and lower BP compared with Mormon omnivores, effects which were independent of differences in BMI or sodium intake [59].

13.2.6 Potential Mechanisms

Table 13.4 summarizes potential healthy dietary patterns BP and hypertension protective mechanisms which are associated with higher dietary fiber, lower energy density and are higher in other essential nutrients and bioactive phytochemicals [60–77].

Conclusions

Prehypertension and hypertension are common and growing public health problems. Globally, the overall prevalence of elevated BP is approaching 50% of adults age ≥ 25 years. The adult risk of CVD and renal disease approximately doubles for each 20/10 mm Hg incremental increase above 115/75 mm Hg. Prehypertension is associated with 1.5- to 2-fold increases in CVD events after age 55 years and a 43% increased risk of CHD. The major factors associated with elevated BP and hypertension are aging, especially unhealthy aging associated with overweight and obesity, poor dietary habits, inactivity or lack of exercise, and ineffective stress management. High adherence to healthy dietary patterns, including the DASH, the MedDiet, Nordic Diet, dietary guidelines-based, and vegetarian diets, are effective in lowering BP, especially in older, overweight or obese hypertensive and prehypertensive adults compared to Western diets. Healthy dietary patterns reduce the intake levels of sodium, excessive energy and added refined carbohydrate intake and increase the levels of BP lowering nutrients such as fiber, plant proteins, potassium, and other essential nutrients and bioactive phytochemicals associated with a lower risk of hypertension and elevated BP. Healthy dietary pattern mechanisms associated with reduced hypertension risk include; lowering the risk of weight gain, stimulating colon microbiota, improving vascular health by normalizing total cholesterol and LDL-C levels, reducing oxidative and inflammatory stress, improving insulin sensitivity to reduce atherosclerosis risk, and maintaining electrolyte balance.

Appendix A: Comparison of Western and healthy dietary patterns per 2000 kcals (approximated values)

Components	Western dietary pattern (US)	USDA base pattern	DASH diet pattern	Healthy mediterranean pattern	Healthy vegetarian pattern (Lact-ovo based)	Vegan pattern
Emphasizes	Refined grains, low fiber foods, red meats, sweets, and solid fats	Vegetables, fruit, whole-grain, and low-fat milk	Potassium rich vegetables, fruits, and low fat milk products	Whole grains, vegetables, fruit, dairy products, olive oil, and moderate wine	Vegetables, fruit, whole-grains, legumes, nuts, seeds, milk products, and soy foods	Plant foods: Vegetables, fruits, whole grains, nuts, seeds, and soy foods
Includes	Processed meats, sugar sweetened beverages, and fast foods	Enriched grains, lean meat, fish, nuts, seeds, and vegetable oils	Whole-grain, poultry, fish, nuts, and seeds	Fish, nuts, seeds, and pulses	Eggs, non-dairy milk alternatives, and vegetable oils	Non-dairy milk alternatives
Limits	Fruits and vegetables, and whole-grains	Solid fats and added sugars	Red meats, sweets, and sugar-sweetened beverages	Red meats, refined grains, and sweets	No red or white meats, or fish; limited sweets	No animal products
Estimated nutrients/components						
Carbohydrates (% Total kcal)	51	51	55	50	54	57
Protein (% Total kcal)	16	17	18	16	14	13
Total fat (% Total kcal)	33	32	27	34	32	30
Saturated fat (% Total kcal)	11	8	6	8	8	7
Unsat. fat (% Total kcal)	22	25	21	24	26	25
Fiber (g)	16	31	29+	31	35+	40+
Potassium (mg)	2800	3350	4400	3350	3300	3650
Vegetable oils (g)	19	27	25	27	19–27	18–27
Sodium (mg)	3600	1790	1100	1690	1400	1225
Added sugar (g)	79 (20 tsp)	32 (8 tsp)	12 (3 tsp)	32 (8 tsp)	32 (8 tsp)	32 (8 tsp)

Components	Western dietary pattern (US)	USDA base pattern	DASH diet pattern	Healthy mediterranean pattern	Healthy vegetarian pattern (Lact-ovo based)	Vegan pattern
Plant food groups						
Fruit (cup)	≤ 1.0	2.0	2.5	2.5	2.0	2.0
Vegetables (cup)	≤ 1.5	2.5	2.1	2.5	2.5	2.5
Whole-grains (oz.)	0.5	3.0	4.0	3.0	3.0	3.0
Legumes (oz.)	–	1.5	0.5	1.5	3.0	3.0+
Nuts/seeds (oz.)	0.5	0.6	1.0	0.6	1.0	2.0
Soy products (oz.)	0.0	0.5	–	–	1.1	1.5

U.S. Department of Agriculture, Agriculture Research Service, Nutrient Data Laboratory. 2014. USDA National Nutrient Database for Standard Reference, Release 27. http://www.ars.usda.gov/nutrientdata. Accessed 17 Feb 2015
Dietary Guidelines Advisory Committee. Scientific Report. Advisory Report to the Secretary of Health and Human Services and the Secretary of Agriculture. Appendix E-3.7: Developing vegetarian and Mediterranean-style food patterns. 2015;1–9
U.S. Department of Agriculture and U.S. Department of Health and Human Services. Dietary Guidelines for Americans, 2010. 7th ed. Washington, DC: U.S. Government Printing Office. 2010; Table B2.4; http://www.choosemyplate.gov/. Accessed 22 Aug 2015

References

1. World Health Organization. A global brief on hypertension. Silent killer, global public health crisis. Geneva: WHO; 2013. http://www.who.int/cardiovascular_diseases/publications/global brief. hypertension/en/. Accessed April 2017.
2. Castro I, Waclawovsky G, Marcadenti A. Nutrition and physical activity on hypertension: implication of current evidence and guidelines. Curr Hypertens Rev. 2015;11(2):91–9.
3. Mendis S, Puska P, Norrving B, editors. Global atlas on cardiovascular disease prevention and control. Geneva: World Health Organization; 2011.
4. Mozaffarian D, Benjamin EJ, Go AS, et al. On behalf of the American Heart Association Statistics Committee and Stroke Statistics Subcommittee. Heart disease and stroke statistics-2016 update: a report from the American Heart Association. Circulation. 2016;133:e38–e360.
5. Livingstone KM, McNaughton SA. Dietary patterns by reduced rank regression are associated with obesity and hypertension in Australian adults. Br J Nutr. 2017;117:248–59. https://doi.org/10.1017/S0007114516004505.
6. Atlas SA. The renin-angiotensin aldosterone system: pathophysiological role and pharmacologic inhibition. J Manag Care Pharm. 2007;13(8):S9–S20.
7. Appel LJ. The effects of dietary factors on blood pressure. Cardiol Clin. 2017;35:197–212.
8. Liu X, Zhang D, Liu Y, et al. Dose-response association between physical activity and incident hypertension. A systematic review and meta-analysis of cohort studies. Hypertension. 2017;69. https://doi.org/10.1161/HypertensionAHA.116.08994.
9. Frisoli TM, Schmieder RE, Grodzicki T, Messerli FH. Beyond salt: lifestyle modifications and blood pressure. Eur Heart J. 2011;32:3081–7.
10. Steffen PR, Smith TB, Larson M, et al. Acculturation to western society as a risk factor for high blood pressure: a meta-analytic review. Psychosom Med. 2006;68:386–97.
11. Rebholz CM, Crews DC, Grams ME, et al. DASH (Dietary Approaches to Stop Hypertension) diet and risk of subsequent kidney disease. Am J Kidney Dis. 2016;68(6):853–61.
12. Dickinson HO, Mason JM, Nicolson DJ, et al. Lifestyle interventions to reduce raised blood pressure: a systematic review of randomized controlled trials. J Hypertens. 2006;24(2):215–33.
13. Bhupathiraju SN, Tucker KL. Coronary heart disease prevention: nutrients, foods, and dietary patterns. Clin Chim Acta. 2011;412:1493–514.
14. Sotos-Prieto M, Bhupathiraju SN, Mattei J, et al. Changes in diet quality and risk of cardiovascular disease among US men and women. Circulation. 2015;32(23):2212–9. https://doi.org/10.1161/circulationAHA.115.017158.
15. Wright JD, Hughes JP, Ostchega Y, et al. Mean systolic and diastolic blood pressure in adults aged 18 and over in the United States, 2001-2008. Natl Health Stat Rep. 2011;35:1–24.
16. Maraj I, Makaryus JN, Ashkar A, et al. Hypertension management in the high cardiovascular risk population. Int J Hypertens. 2013;2013:7. https://doi.org/10.1155/2013/382802.

17. Wang C-J, Shen Y-X, Liu Y. Empirically derived dietary patterns and hypertension likelihood: a meta-analysis. Kidney Blood Press Res. 2016;41:570–81. https://doi.org/10.1159/ 000443456.
18. Zhang X-Y, Shu L, Si C-J, et al. Dietary patterns, alcohol consumption and risk of coronary heart disease in adults: a meta-analysis. Forum Nutr. 2015;7:6582–605. https://doi.org/10.3390/nu7085300.
19. Eckel RH, Jakicic JM, Ard JD, et al. 2013 AHA/ACC guideline on lifestyle management to reduce cardiovascular risk: a report of the American College of Cardiology/American Heart Association Task Force on Practice Guidelines. J Am Coll Cardiol. 2014;63:2960–84.
20. Dietary Guidelines Advisory Committee. Advisory report to the Secretary of Health and Human Services and the Secretary of Agriculture. Part D. Chapter 2: Dietary patterns, foods and nutrients and health outcomes; 2015. p. 1–35.
21. Ndanuko RN, Tapsell LC, Charlton KE, et al. Dietary patterns and blood pressure in adults: a systematic review and meta-analysis of randomized controlled trials. Adv Nutr. 2016;7:76–89.
22. Ndanuko RN, Tapsell LC, Charlton KE, et al. Associations between dietary patterns and blood pressure in a clinical sample of overweight adults. J Acad Nutr Diet. 2017;117(2):228–39. https://doi.org/10.1016/j.and.2016.07.019.
23. Harrington JM, Fitzgerald AP, Kearney PM, et al. DASH diet score and distribution of blood pressure in middle-aged men and women. Am J Hypertens. 2013;26(11):1311–20.
24. Barak F, Falahi E, Keshteli AH, et al. Adherence to the Dietary Approaches to Stop Hypertension (DASH) diet in relation to obesity among Iranian female nurses. Public Health Nutr. 2014;18(4):705–12.
25. Lin P-H, Yeh W-T, Svetkey LP, et al. Dietary intakes consistent with the DASH dietary pattern reduce blood pressure increase with age and risk for stroke in a Chinese population. Asia Pac J Clin Nutr. 2013;22(3):482–91.
26. Moore TJ, Alsabeeh N, Apovian CM, et al. Weight, blood pressure, and dietary benefits after 12 months of a Web-based Nutrition Education Program (DASH for Health): longitudinal observational study. J Med Internet Res. 2008;10(4):e52. https://doi.org/10.2196/jmir.1114.
27. Gay HC, Rao SG, Vaccarino V, Ali MK. Effects of different dietary interventions on blood pressure systematic review and meta-analysis of randomized controlled trials. Hypertension. 2016;67:733–9. https://doi.org/10.1161/HypertensionAHA.115.06853.
28. Siervo M, Lara J, Chowdhury S, et al. Effects of the Dietary Approach to Stop Hypertension (DASH) diet on cardiovascular risk factors: a systematic review and meta-analysis. Br J Nutr. 2015;113:1–15.
29. Saneei P, Salehi-Abargouei A, Esmaillzadeh A, Azadbakht L. Influence of Dietary Approaches to Stop Hypertension (DASH) diet on blood pressure: a systematic review and meta-analysis on randomized controlled trials. Nutr Metab Cardiovasc Dis. 2014;24:1253–61.
30. Chiu S, Bergeron N, Williams PT, et al. Comparison of the DASH (Dietary Approaches to Stop Hypertension) diet and a higher-fat DASH diet on blood pressure and lipids and lipoproteins: a randomized controlled trial. Am J Clin Nutr. 2016;103:341–7.
31. Al-Solaiman Y, Jesri A, Mountford WK, et al. DASH lowers blood pressure in obese hypertensives beyond potassium, magnesium and fiber. J Hum Hypertens. 2010;24(4):237–46.
32. Blumenthal JA, Babyak MA, Hinderliter A, et al. Effects of the DASH diet alone and in combination with exercise and weight loss on blood pressure and cardiovascular biomarkers in men and women with high blood pressure: the ENCORE Study. Arch Intern Med. 2010;170(2):126–35.
33. Appel LJ, Sacks FM, Carey VJ, et al. Effects of protein, monounsaturated fat, and carbohydrate intake on blood pressure and serum lipids results of the OmniHeart Randomized Trial. JAMA. 2005;294:2455–64.
34. Nowson CA, Worsley A, Margerison C, et al. Blood pressure change with weight loss is affected by diet type in men. Am J Clin Nutr. 2005;81:983–9.
35. Appel LJ, Champagne CM, Harsha DW, et al. Effects of comprehensive lifestyle modification on blood pressure control: main results of the PREMIER clinical trial. JAMA. 2003;289(16):2083–93.
36. Miller ER, Erlinger TP, Young DR, et al. Results of the diet, exercise, and weight loss intervention trial (DEW-IT). Hypertension. 2002;40:612–8.
37. Appel LJ, Moore TJ, Obarzanek E, et al. A clinical trial of the effects of dietary patterns on blood pressure. N Engl J Med. 1997;336:1117–24.
38. Nunez-Cordoba JM, Valencia-Serrano F, Toledo E, et al. The Mediterranean diets and incidence of hypertension. Am J Epidemiol. 2009;169:339–46.
39. Nunez-Cordoba JM, Alonso A, Beunza JJ, et al. Role of vegetables and fruits in Mediterranean diets to prevent hypertension. Eur J Clin Nutr. 2009;63:605–12.
40. Psaltopoulou T, Naska A, Orfanos P, et al. Olive oil, the Mediterranean diet, and arterial blood pressure: the Greek European Prospective Investigation into Cancer and Nutrition (EPIC) study. Am J Clin Nutr. 2004;80:1012–8.
41. Toledo E, Carmona-Torre FD, Alonso A, et al. Hypothesis-oriented food patterns and incidence of hypertension: 6-year follow-up of the SUN (Seguimiento Universidad de Navarra) prospective cohort. Public Health Nutr. 2010;13:338–49.
42. Timmermans S, Steegers-Theunissen RPM, Vujkovic M, et al. Major dietary patterns and blood pressure patterns during pregnancy: The Generation R Study. Am J Obstet Gynecol. 2011;205:337.e1–e12. https://doi.org/10.1016/j.ajog.2011.05.013.
43. Nissensohn M, Roman-Vinas B, Sanchez-Villegas A, et al. The effect of the Mediterranean diet on hypertension: a systematic review and meta-analysis. J Nutr Educ Behav. 2016;48:42–53.

44. Huo R, Du T, Xu Y, et al. Effects of Mediterranean-style diet on glycemic control, weight loss and cardiovascular risk factors among type 2 diabetes individuals: a meta-analysis. Eur J Clin Nutr. 2015;69(11):1200–8. https://doi.org/10.1038/ejcn.2014.243.
45. Nordmann AJ, Suter-Zimmermann K, Bucher HC, et al. Meta-analysis comparing Mediterranean to low fat diets for the modification of cardiovascular risk factors. Am J Med. 2011;124(9):841–51.
46. Storniolo CE, Casillas R, Bulló M, et al. A Mediterranean diet supplemented with extra virgin olive oil or nuts improves endothelial markers involved in blood pressure control in hypertensive women. Eur J Nutr. 2017;56(1):89–97. https://doi.org/10.1007/s00394-015-1060-5.
47. Doménech M, Roman P, Lapetra J, et al. Mediterranean diet reduces 24-hour ambulatory blood pressure, blood glucose, and lipids one-year randomized, clinical trial. Hypertension. 2014;64:69–76.
48. Toledo E, Hu FB, Estruch R, et al. Effect of the Mediterranean diet on blood pressure in the PREDIMED trial: results from a randomized controlled trial. BMC Med. 2013;11:207. https://doi.org/10.1186/1741-7015-11-207.
49. Estruch R, Martínez-González MA, Corella D, et al. Effects of a Mediterranean-style diet on cardiovascular risk factors: a randomized trial. Ann Intern Med. 2006;145(1):1–11.
50. Lee J, Pase M, Pipingas A, et al. Switching to a 10-day Mediterranean-style diet improves mood and cardiovascular function in a controlled crossover study. Nutrition. 2015;31:647–52.
51. Poulsen SK, Due A, Jordy AB, et al. Health effect of the New Nordic Diet in adults with increased waist circumference: a 6-mo randomized controlled trial. Am J Clin Nutr. 2014;99:35–45.
52. Brader L, Uusitupa M, Dragsted LO, Hermansen K. Effects of an isocaloric healthy Nordic diet on ambulatory blood pressure in metabolic syndrome: a randomized SYSDIET sub-study. Eur J Clin Nutr. 2014;68:57–63.
53. Schroeder N, Park Y-H, Kang M-S, et al. A randomized trial on the effects of 2010 Dietary Guidelines for Americans and Korean Diet Patterns on cardiovascular risk factors in overweight and obese adults. J Acad Nutr Diet. 2015;115:1083–92.
54. Reidlinger DP, Darzi J, Hall WL, et al. How effective are current dietary guidelines for cardiovascular disease prevention in healthy middle-aged and older men and women? A randomized controlled trial. Am J Clin Nutr. 2015;101:922–30.
55. Orlich MJ, Jaceldo-Siegl K, Sabaté J, et al. Patterns of food consumption among vegetarians and non-vegetarians. Br J Nutr. 2014;112(10):1644–53.
56. Rizzo NS, Jaceldo-Siegl K, Sabate J, Fraser GE. Nutrient profiles of vegetarian and non-vegetarian dietary patterns. J Acad Nutr Diet. 2013;113:1610–9.
57. Yokoyama Y, Nishimura K, Barnard ND, et al. Vegetarian diets and blood pressure. A meta-analysis. JAMA Intern Med. 2014;174(4):577–87.
58. Pettersen BJ, Anousheh R, Fan J, et al. Vegetarian diets and blood pressure among white subjects: results from the Adventist Health Study-2. Public Health Nutr. 2012;15(10):1909–16.
59. Beilin LJ, Rouse IL, Armstrong BK, et al. Vegetarian diet and blood pressure levels: incidental or causal association? Am J Clin Nutr. 1988;48:806–10.
60. Sanchez-Muniz FJ. Dietary fibre and cardiovascular health. Nutr Hosp. 2012;27(1):31–45.
61. Evans CEL, Greenwood DC, Threapleton DE, et al. Effects of dietary fibre type on blood pressure: a systematic review and meta-analysis of randomized controlled trials of health individuals. J Hypertens. 2015;33(5):897–911.
62. Czernichow S, Blacher J, Hercberg S. Antioxidant vitamins and blood pressure. Curr Hypertens Rep. 2004;6(1):27–30.
63. Gammone MA, Riccioni G, D'Orazio N. Carotenoids: potential allies of cardiovascular health? Food Nutr Res. 2015;59. https://doi.org/10.3402/fnr.v59.26762.
64. Hodgson JM, Croft KD, Woodman RJ, et al. Effects of vitamin E, vitamin C and polyphenols on the rate of blood pressure variation: results of two randomised controlled trials. Br J Nutr. 2014;112(9):1551–61. https://doi.org/10.1017/S0007114514002542.
65. Koliaki C, Katsilambros N. Dietary sodium, potassium and alcohol: key players in the pathophysiology, prevention, and treatment of human hypertension. Nutr Rev. 2013;71(6):402–11.
66. Lee YP, Puddey IB, Hodgson JM. Protein, fibre, blood pressure: potential benefit of legumes. Clin Exp Pharmacol Physiol. 2008;35:473–6.
67. Rangel-Huerta OD, Pastor-Villaescusa B, Aguilera CM, Gil A. A systematic review of the efficacy of bioactive compounds in cardiovascular disease: phenolic compounds. Forum Nutr. 2015;7:5177–216.
68. Ried K, Fakler P. Protective effect of lycopene on serum cholesterol and blood pressure: meta-analyses of intervention trials. Maturitas. 2011;68:299–310.
69. Ros E, Hu FB. Consumption of plant seeds and cardiovascular health epidemiological and clinical trial evidence. Circulation. 2013;128:553–65.
70. Jayalath VH, de Souza RJ, Sievenpiper JL, et al. Effect of dietary pulses on blood pressure: a systematic review and meta-analysis of controlled feeding trials. Am J Hypertens. 2014;27(1):56–64.
71. Clark JL, Zahradka P, Taylor CG. Efficacy of flavonoids in the management of high blood pressure. Nutr Rev. 2015;73(12):799–822.
72. Hobbs DA, George TW, Lovegrove JA. The effects of dietary nitrate on blood pressure and endothelial function: a review of human intervention studies. Nutr Res Rev. 2013;26:210–22.
73. Mohammadifard N, Salehi-Abargouei A, Salas-Salvadó J, et al. The effect of tree nut, peanut, and soy nut consumption on blood pressure: a systematic review and meta-analysis of randomized controlled clinical trials. Am J Clin Nutr. 2015;101:966–82.
74. Pins JJ, Geleva D, Keenan JM. Do whole-grain oat cereals reduce the need for antihypertensive medi-

cations and improve blood pressure control? J Fam Pract. 2002;14:353–9.
75. Li B, Li F, Wang L, Zhang D. Fruit and vegetables consumption and risk of hypertension: a meta-analysis. J Clin Hypertens (Greenwich). 2016;18(5):468–76. https://doi.org/10.1111/jch.12777.
76. Yang T, Santisteban MM, Rodriguez V, et al. Gut Dysbiosis is linked to hypertension. Hypertension. 2015;65:1331–40.
77. Pluznick JL. A novel SCFA receptor, the microbiota, and blood pressure regulation. Gut Microbes. 2014;5(2):202–7.

Whole Plant Foods and Hypertension

14

Keywords

Blood pressure • Hypertension • Aging • Overweight • Obesity • Microbiota • Electrolytes • Whole grains • Fruit • Vegetables • Legumes • Soy • Nuts • Flaxseed

Key Points

- Whole (and minimally processed) plant foods usually contain some mixture of blood pressure (BP) lowering bioactive nutrients and phytochemicals such as dietary fiber, potassium, magnesium, polyphenols, unsaturated fat, and plant protein and are lower in sodium and sugar compared to highly processed plant foods.
- Whole plant foods are more effective at reducing BP in adults who are ≥45 years, hypertensive and obese than adults <45 years, normotensive, or lean.
- Prospective studies show that the consumption of healthy diets with ≥3 daily servings of whole grains, especially oats and barley rich in β-glucan, and ≥5 daily servings of fruits and vegetables, especially when including ≥4 weekly servings of broccoli, carrots, tofu or soybeans, raisins, grapes and apples, are associated with lower hypertension risk compared to Western diets.
- RCTs support the effectiveness of whole grains in lowering BP, especially at 50 g/1000 kcals or those rich in β-glucan; fruits and vegetables rich in polyphenols or nitrates and their 100% juices have been found to lower systolic BP; and two daily servings of dietary pulses or 40 g soy protein are effective in lowering BP. Flaxseeds and sesame seeds tend to be more effective than nuts in lowering BP.
- Tea and coffee have different effects on BP. Both black and green tea (> 2 cups/d) modestly lower BP in hypertensive individuals. Coffee (>3 cups/d) does not increase hypertension risk in normotensive people but hypertensive individuals may be more sensitive to acute increases in BP after coffee consumption.
- The potential mechanisms by which whole plant foods may reduce blood pressure and hypertension risk are; reducing the risk of weight gain, enhancing insulin sensitivity, improving vascular endothelial function, slowing the rate of arterial plaque build-up, maintaining electrolyte balance, and stimulating a healthier microbiota ecosystem.

M.L. Dreher, *Dietary Patterns and Whole Plant Foods in Aging and Disease*, Nutrition and Health,
https://doi.org/10.1007/978-3-319-59180-3_14

14.1 Introduction

Elevated blood pressure (BP) and hypertension are major risk factors for stroke, coronary heart disease (CHD), damage to retinal blood vessels, and kidney disease/renal failure [1–4]. The adult risk of cardiovascular disease (CVD) doubles for each 20/10 mm Hg incremental increase above 115/75 mm Hg. Elevated BP, including prehypertension (systolic BP >120–139 mm Hg or diastolic BP >80–89 mm Hg), or hypertension (systolic BP ≥140 mm Hg or diastolic BP > 90 mm Hg), is a common and growing public health problem [5, 6]. By 2025, because of population growth and an aging population, it is projected that about 1.5 billion individuals globally will have hypertension [1–4]. Aging, overweight or obesity, and lifestyle factors such as poor nutritional quality dietary patterns, excess energy intake and salt intake, sedentary lifestyles, alcohol intake, smoking, and anxiety and stress are important underlying controllable factors associated with hypertension risk, because of increased activity of the renin-angiotensin-aldosterone system, insulin resistance, and reduced kidney function [1–12]. Foods and diets with low dietary energy density, high fiber density and that contain primarily natural sugar sources such as whole fruits, tend to be associated with lower prevalence of overweight or obesity, whereas foods with low fiber density and high in added sugars intake (primarily from chocolate and fruit drinks) are associated with increased prevalence of overweight or obesity [5]. Foods low in fiber density and high in the ratio of sodium to potassium and high in saturated fat to polyunsaturated fat ratios are associated with increased prevalence of hypertension and prehypertension [5]. Guidelines for prevention, treatment and control of elevated BP/hypertension focus on lifestyle modifications including weight loss and maintenance, reduced salt intake, increased fruit and vegetable consumption, routine participation in physical activity, cessation of smoking, limiting of alcohol consumption, and anxiety and stress control [3–19]. The higher the number of risk factors (hypertension, unhealthy lipoprotein profile, and regular smoking) the faster the rate of carotid intima-media thickening or atherosclerosis progression (Fig. 14.1) [10]. Dairy products, especially lower fat products such as plain yogurt, and healthy whole plant foods have been shown to reduce the risk of elevated BP and hypertension [14]. An overview of the effects of specific foods on BP are summarized in Table 14.1 [14–30]. The primary objective of this chapter is to provide a review of the role of whole (minimally processed) plant foods in helping to prevent and manage elevated BP and hypertension.

14.2 Whole Plant Foods

Whole and minimally processed plant foods (whole plant foods) are generally higher in fiber and major dietary sources of hypertension protective nutrients (e.g., vitamins E and C, and trace minerals such as selenium and copper), and phytochemicals (carotenoids, flavonoids and phytosterols), which are often lost in the processing of highly refined foods [31–42]. Whole plant food composition is highly variable and is summarized in (Appendix A). Potential whole plant foods BP related mechanisms are: (1) reducing dietary energy density and increasing satiety and satiation, which reduce the risk of weight gain or obesity; (2) enhancing insulin sensitivity, which may improve vascular and endothelial function; (3) promoting healthier lipid and lipoprotein profiles, attenuating elevated systemic inflammation and LDL-oxidation for improved endothelial health and a slower rate of arterial plaque build-up; (4) maintaining electrolyte balance to improve RAAS homeostatic extracellular fluid volume; and (5) improving colon health via the stimulation of a healthier microbiota and increased fermentation of fiber to short chain fatty acids (SCFAs), leading to potentially improved cardiometabolic control [4, 9–11, 17, 19, 39–52]. However, whole plant foods are consumed at low levels in the typical Western diet with an estimated >90% of US adults not meeting

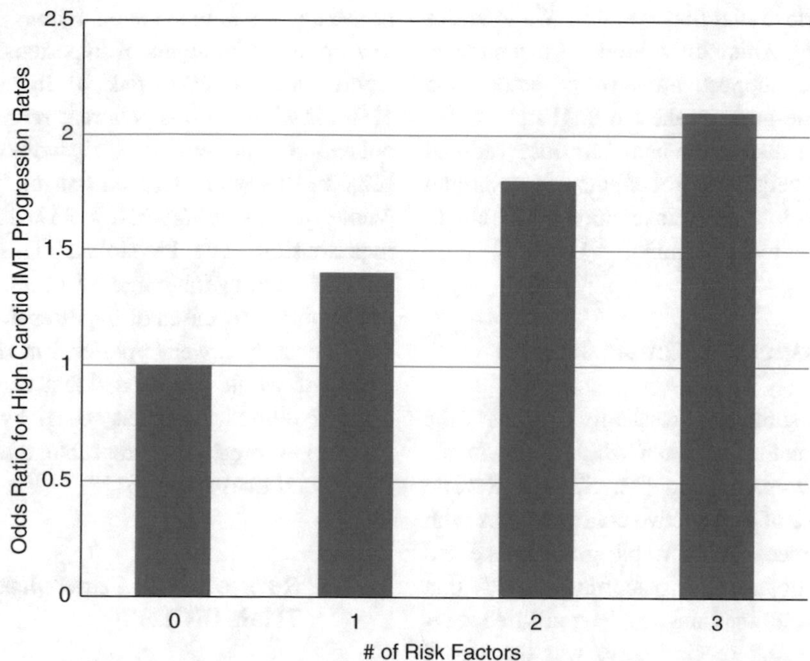

Fig. 14.1 Association between the number of risk factors (hypertension, unhealthy lipoprotein profile, and regular smoking) and carotid intima-media thickness (IMT) progression rate from The Malmo Diet and Cancer Study (adapted from [10])

Table 14.1 Effects of specific foods on risk of elevated blood pressure [14–30]

Dietary factors	Postulated effects	Strength of evidence
Low-fat dairy and milk	Decreased	+/+
High-fat dairy and cheese	Uncertain/neutral	+/–
Processed meat	Increased	+
Lean red meat	Uncertain/neutral	+/–
Whole-grains (soluble fiber, oats/psyllium)	Decreased	+
Whole-grains (insoluble fiber, wheat/rice)	Uncertain/neutral	+/–
Fruits and vegetables	Decreased	+/+
Legumes	Decreased	+
Nuts and seeds	Decreased	+

Key to evidence: +/– = limited or equivocal evidence; + = suggestive evidence from observational studies and clinical trials; +/+ = persuasive evidence, primarily from clinical trials

the recommended minimal levels of whole-grains, fruit, vegetables, legumes, or nuts/seeds to maintain optimal health and weight control outcomes [41, 53].

14.2.1 Whole-Grains

14.2.1.1 Background

Whole-grains contain basically the intact kernel with its full complement of fiber, vitamins, minerals and phytochemicals, whereas refined grain products are mainly comprised of the endosperm with most of the fiber, vitamins, minerals and phytonutrients removed during processing [54, 55]. The US dietary guidelines recommend ≥3 whole-grain servings/day and ≤3 refined grains servings/day to promote health and reduce risk of various chronic diseases [41]. However, only about 1% of Americans follow the recommendation for whole-grain intake as the average American's intake is <1 ounce whole grains/day and 70% exceed the recommended intake for refined grains [41, 53]. A 2017 RCT in healthy men and postmenopausal women found that substituting whole-grains for refined grains in the diet and increasing dietary fiber intake led to favorable effects that resulted in a 100-kcal/day energy deficit compared with the effects of a typical American diet that is low in whole grains and fiber [56]. This study provides mechanistic insights that support an inverse association between whole-grain intake and BMI and adiposity, which are also documented in observational studies. The weight control effects of consuming adequate whole-grain intake may also help to protect against hypertension [2–5].

14.2.2 Prospective Cohort Studies

Prospective studies consistently support the inverse association between whole-grain intake and risk of hypertension [22, 57–61]. Several meta-analyses of prospective cohort studies with quantitative measures of whole-grain intake and clinical cardiovascular outcomes found that greater whole grains intake (≥48 g or three servings/day vs. ≤0.2 servings/day) was associated with a 21% lower risk of cardiovascular disease (CVD) and coronary heart disease (CHD) [57–59]. The Health Professionals Follow-Up Study (31,684 men; mean age 52 years; 18 years of follow-up; 9227 cases of incident hypertension) showed that men with a median intake of about three daily whole grain servings (46 g/day) had a significantly lower risk of hypertension by19% (Fig. 14.2) [60]. The Women's Health Study (28,926 women; mean age 54 years; 10-year follow-up; 8722 incidents of hypertension) found a significantly reduced risk of hypertension by 11% for whole grains, whereas refined grain did not reduce hypertension risk in women (Fig. 14.3) [22]. In this study women consuming >4 daily whole grain servings had a 23% lower risk of hypertension. The Physicians' Health Study I (13,368 men; average age 52 years; 16 years of follow-up; 7267 cases of hypertension) observed a significantly lower hypertension risk for daily intake of whole-grain breakfast cereal by 20% and for refined breakfast cereal by 14% compared to no breakfast cereal intake in lean, overweight and obese men [61].

14.2.3 Randomized Controlled Trials (RCTs)

In general, the effects of whole-grain products on BP depends on their composition and physical properties with whole-grains rich in β-glucans (e.g., oat or barley) more effective in lowering BP than insoluble fiber (e.g., whole wheat breads and breakfast cereals) (Table 14.2) [24, 62–73]. A Swedish double blind crossover RCT (40 overweight and obese men and women; age 40 years; macronutrient composition was

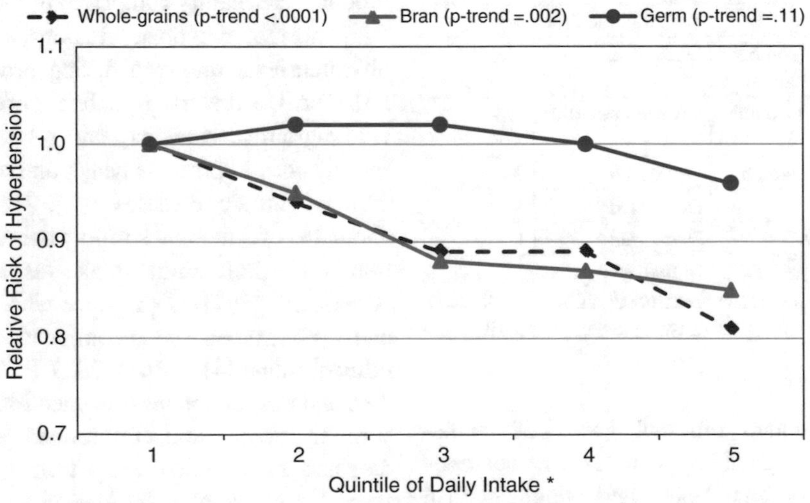

Fig. 14.2 Association between increasing whole-grains, bran and germ intake and hypertension incidence risk in men, multivariate adjusted (adapted from [59]). *Whole-grains: Q-5 (46 g); Bran: Q-5 (12 g); Germ: Q-5 (2.4 g)

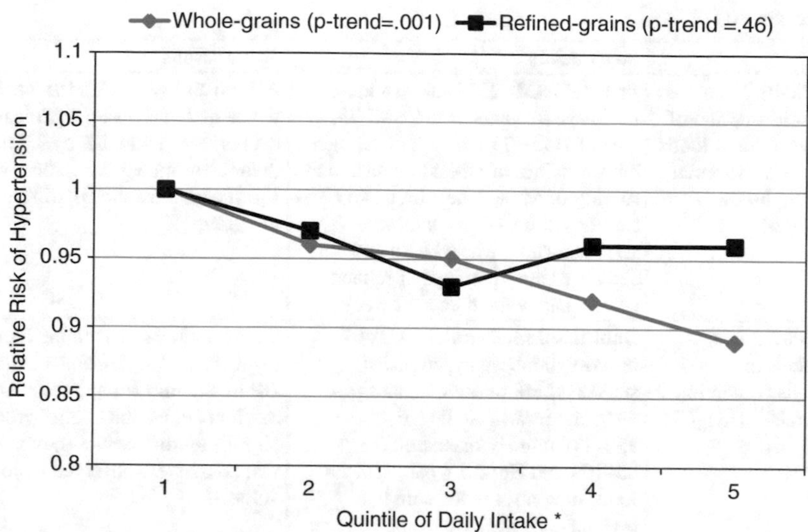

Fig. 14.3 Association between whole- and refined-grain intake and hypertension risk in women (multivariate adjusted) (adapted from [60]).*Whole-grains: Q-5 (3.1 servings); refined-grains: Q-5 (4.1 servings)

Table 14.2 Summaries of whole-grain RCTs on blood pressure (BP)

Objective	Study details	Study results
Systematic Review and Meta-analyses		
Evans et al. (2015). Assess the effects of oat and barley whole-grain foods on BP (UK) [61]	5 RCTs on oats; 400 subjects; median increase of 4 g β-glucans; ≥6 weeks	Diets rich in β-glucans with a median increase of 4 g β-glucans from whole oats or oat bran enriched foods or oat-based breakfast cereals compared with similar wheat-based test foods significantly lowered systolic BP by 2.9 mm Hg and diastolic BP by 1.5 mm Hg
Thies et al. (2014). Systematically review the literature describing long-term intervention studies that investigated the effects of oats or oat bran on CVD risk factors including BP (US) [62]	25 RCTs; primarily oat bran or breakfast cereals vs. low fiber or wheat bran cereals; β-glucan level, and design details not provided	Only three trials found oat consumption to significantly reduce BP vs. control products
Representative RCTs		
Kirwan et al. (2016). Evaluate the efficacy of whole grains compared with refined grains on body composition, hypertension, and related mediators of CVD in overweight and obese adults (Sweden) [63]	**Double-blind, Crossover RCT**: 40 overweight or obese men and women; mean age 40 years; complete whole-grain and refined-grain diets were provided for two 8-week periods, with a 10-week washout between diets. Macronutrient composition was matched, except for the inclusion of either whole grains or refined grains (50 g/1000 kcal in each diet); 33 subjects completed the trial; five participants taking antihypertensive medication were instructed to maintain medication usage throughout the study	The whole-grain diet significantly reduced diastolic BP by 5.8 mm Hg compared to a reduction of 1.6 mm Hg after the refined grain control diet (p = .01). Whole-grain intake preserved circulating total adiponectin concentrations compared with a 1.4 μg/mL decline after refined-grain intake (p = .05). Decreases in diastolic blood pressure correlated with the circulating adiponectin concentration (r = .35, p = .04) (Fig. 14.4). Substantial reductions in body weight, fat loss, systolic blood pressure, total cholesterol, and LDL cholesterol were observed during both diet periods, with no significant differences between the two diets

(continued)

Table 14.2 (continued)

Objective	Study details	Study results
Tighe et al. (2010). Examine the effects of consumption of whole-grains vs. refined foods on markers of cardiovascular disease including blood pressure (UK) [64]	**Parallel RCT**: 233 healthy adults; mean age 52 years, mean BMI 28; mean BP 131/79 mm Hg; diets: three daily servings of wheat and oats (one serving of whole wheat bread and two servings of oat cereals); three servings whole wheat bread and cereals or three servings of refined cereals and white bread; 12 weeks	After 6 and 12 weeks, the whole-grain wheat and oats group significantly decreased systolic BP by 3.7 mm Hg more than the refined group. There was no significant diastolic BP difference between the groups
Maki et al. (2007). Assess the clinical effects of consuming foods containing oat β-glucan on BP (US) [65]	**Double-blind, Parallel RCT**: 97 overweight/obese hypertensive subjects; 56% women; mean age 49 years; mean systolic BP 130–179 mm Hg/diastolic BP 85–109 mm Hg; 7.7 g oat β-glucan foods or control foods with 0 g β-glucan; 12 weeks	Obese subjects consuming foods rich in oat β-glucan had significantly lowered systolic BP by 8.3 mm Hg and diastolic BP by 3.9 mm Hg vs. the control group. No significant differences in blood pressure responses were observed in normal BMI subjects
Behall et al. (2006). Compare the effects of whole wheat and brown rice vs. barley whole-grain (β-glucan) diet on BP (US) [66]	**Crossover RCT**: 25 mildly hypercholesterolemic, overweight adults; seven men, nine premenopausal and nine post-menopausal women; mean age 47 years; mean BP 117/71 mm Hg; AHA Step 1 diet with white rice control; 20% of energy replaced with whole-grains: whole wheat/brown rice, barley, or mixture of both; 5 weeks	AHA step 1 diet with whole-grains lowered BP compared to a AHA step 1 diet with white rice; whole-grains lowered systolic BP by 1.4–6.7 mm Hg and diastolic BP 2.9–3.7 mm Hg
He et al. (2004). Investigate the effects of whole grain oats on BP (US) [67]	**Double-blind, Parallel RCT**: 110 healthy adults; age 30–65 years; stage 1 hypertension; foods containing whole-grain oats with 8 g β-glucan or control foods with 0 g β-glucan; 6 and 12 weeks	Oat β-glucan intake significantly reduced systolic BP by 2.0 mm Hg and insignificantly lowered diastolic BP by 1.0 mm Hg
Davy et al. (2002). Evaluate the clinical effect of whole-grain oat beta-glucan on BP (US) [68]	**Parallel RCT**: 36 overweight/obese men; mean age 59 years; elevated BP; addition of 14 g/day of fiber including oat cereal (5.5 g β-glucan) or wheat cereals (no β-glucan); resting and ambulatory BP; 12 weeks	Oat consumption insignificantly lowered systolic and diastolic BP by 1 mm Hg compared to wheat. Also, no significant differences in 24-h, daytime and nighttime BP observed between oat and wheat in this study. Subjects in both groups significantly increased body weight by 0.8 kg
Pins et al. (2002). Study the effects of whole-grain oat-based cereals vs. refined grain wheat-based cereals to determine their effects on BP and β blocker medications (US) [24]	**Parallel RCT:** 88 adults on antihypertensive medications; mean age 48 years; mean BP below 140/88 mm Hg; oatmeal or oat squares (3 g β-glucan) vs. wheat crisps or hot wheat cereal (0 β-glucan); 12 weeks	73% of oat β-glucan participants vs. 42% in the wheat group either stopped or reduced their β blocker medications by half. Those in the oats group who did not experience a β blocker reduction had a significant 6 mm Hg decrease in systolic BP vs. the wheat group
Keenan et al. (2002). Evaluate the anti-hypertensive effects of β-glucan-rich whole oat cereals when added to a standard American diet (US) [69]	**Parallel RCT:** 18 hypertensives and hyperinsulinemic overweight/obese adults, age 20–70 years; diets: oat cereal group (standardized to 5.5 g β-glucan/day) or a low-fiber cereal control; 6 weeks	The oat cereal group significantly lowered systolic BP by 7.5 mm Hg and diastolic BP by 5.5 mm Hg compared to the control group. In the oat cereal group, a trend toward higher insulin sensitivity suggested a possible mechanism for BP lowering

Table 14.2 (continued)

Objective	Study details	Study results
Saltzman et al. (2001). Investigate the effects of a hypo-caloric diet with and without oats on BP (US) [70]	**Parallel RCT:** 43 overweight/obese adults; mean age 45 years; mean baseline BP of 118/71 mm Hg; 8 weeks); hypocaloric diets: 45 g oats/day or no added oat control; 6-weeks	The hypocaloric oat diet significantly lowered systolic BP by 5 mm Hg and insignificantly decreased diastolic BP by 1 mm Hg vs. the control diet. There was no significant difference in weight loss between the two groups
Wheat Bran		
Kestin et al. (1990). Investigate the clinical effects of cereal brans on BP (Australia) [71]	**Double-blind, Crossover RCT**: 24 healthy men; mean BP 125/79 mm Hg; elevated blood lipids; 11.8 g fiber/day from wheat bran vs. baseline diet; 4 weeks	The baseline BP was unaltered by the addition of wheat bran
Fehily et al. (1986). To evaluate the clinical effect of wheat bran rich food on BP (UK) [72]	**Crossover RCT**: 201 healthy adults; mean age approx. 40 years; 73% men; mean baseline BP of 132/80 mm Hg; diet: 19 g cereal fiber/day (whole meal bread, whole-grain breakfast cereals with bran) vs. six cereal fiber g/day (refined white bread and breakfast cereals); 4 weeks	There was no significant difference in BP between the whole-grain wheat and refined wheat diets over 4 weeks

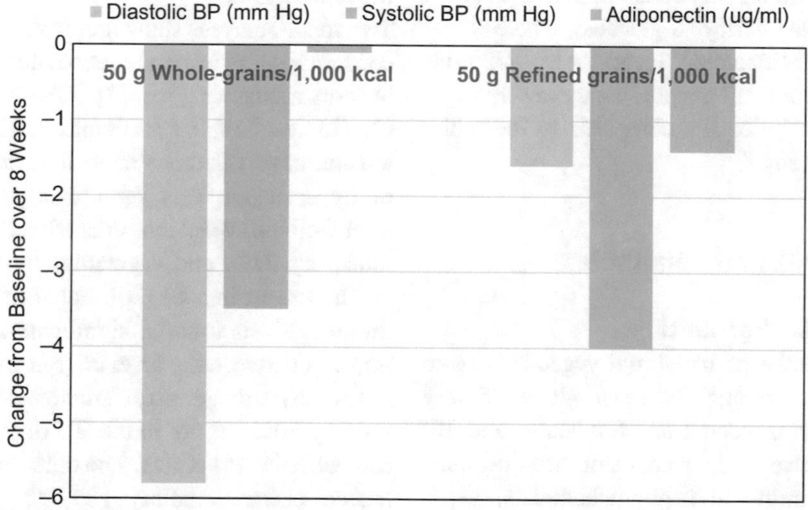

Fig. 14.4 Effect of whole vs. refined grains on blood pressure (BP) and plasma adiponectin in overweight and obese men and women (diastolic BP $p < .01$; systolic BP $p > .05$; adiponectin $p = .05$) [63]

matched, except for the inclusion of either whole grains or refined grains (50 g/1000 kcal); each diet for 8 weeks; 10-week washout) found that the whole-grain diet significantly reduced diastolic BP by 5.8 mm Hg compared to a reduction of 1.6 mm Hg after the refined grain control diet (Fig. 14.4) [63]. Whole-grain intake preserved circulating total adiponectin concentrations compared with a 1.4 μg/mL decline after refined-grain intake. Decreases in diastolic BP correlated with the circulating adiponectin concentration. In general, whole-grain rich diets, especially those containing β-glucan, are more effective at reducing BP in adults ≥45 years, hypertensive, or obese than in adults <45 years, normotensive or lean [24, 62, 63, 65–73]. A RCT

(88 adults taking β-blockers; mean age 48 years; mean BP below 140/88 mm Hg; 12 weeks) showed that the consumption of oatmeal or oat squares (3 g β-glucan) vs. wheat crisps or hot wheat cereal (0 g β-glucan) resulted in subjects either stopping or reducing β blocker by half in 73% of oat β-glucan participants vs. 42% in the wheat group [24]. Those in the oat group who did not experience a β blocker reduction had a significantly lower systolic BP by 6 mm Hg vs. the wheat group. One RCT (36 overweight and obese men; mean age 59 years; elevated BP; 5.5 g β-glucan; 12 weeks) showed whole oats to have an insignificant lowering effect on BP, which may have been confounded by a significant 0.8 kg increase in body weight during the study [68]. A USDA trial (25 mildly hypercholesterolemic, overweight adults [seven men, nine premenopausal and nine post-menopausal women; mean age 47 years; BP 117/71 mm Hg; 5 weeks) found that the consumption of an AHA step 1 diet plus barley (β-glucans), whole wheat or brown rice (insoluble fibers), or a 50/50 mixture resulted in similar significantly lowered systolic and diastolic BPs compared to the white rice control [66].

14.2.4 Fruits and Vegetables

14.2.4.1 Background

Adequate intake of fruits and vegetables is an important component of most global dietary guidance recommendations for health and BP control because of their concentrations of: antioxidant vitamins and phytochemicals, especially vitamins C and A, and carotenoids; minerals (especially electrolytes potassium and magnesium, and low sodium); and fiber [31, 34]. Fruit and vegetables include a diverse group of plant foods that vary greatly in content of energy, fiber, glycemic index value and nutrients. The World Health Organization (WHO) report recommends a minimum daily intake of 400 g of fruits and vegetables, based on evidence that higher levels are protective against cardiovascular disease (CVD) [34]. This led to the launch of various "eat 5 or more" fruit and vegetable campaigns in Europe, the US and Australia [73]. The USDA Dietary Guidelines for Americans MyPlate educational concept, devotes one-half the plate to the fruits and vegetables, partially as a displacement of other foods of higher energy density from the diet, and also as a good habit to establish for healthy aging or healthy eating at any age [74]. However, globally, fruit and vegetable consumption is at only a small fraction of the recommended levels [75]. In the US, >85% of the population fall short of meeting the daily fruit and vegetable intake recommendation [41].

14.2.4.2 Prospective Cohort Studies

The inverse association of fruit and vegetables intake and hypertension risk appears to be most strongly associated with fruit intake and weight control/loss.

Meta-analyses

Two meta-analyses show that fruit and vegetable consumption is inversely associated with hypertension incidence [76, 77]. One meta-analysis (25 studies; 334,468 participants; 41,713 hypertension cases) demonstrated that the mean risk of hypertension was significantly reduced for total fruit and vegetable intake by 19%, for fruit intake by 27%, and vegetables by 3% (highest vs. the lowest intake) [76]. For fruit intake, subgroup analysis found a significant inverse relationship between the level of fruit intake and the risk of hypertension for studies carried out in Asia by 30% but not in the EU or the US which showed a 6% lower risk. The other meta-analysis (seven cohort studies; 185,676 participants) showed that fruits or vegetables separately or total fruits and vegetables were inversely associated with hypertension risk (highest vs. lowest intake) with fruits reducing risk by 13%, vegetables by 12%, and total fruits and vegetables by 10% [77]. A dose response analysis estimated that each daily serving lowered hypertension risk for fruit by 1.9% and for total fruit and vegetables by 1.2%. Clearly, these meta-analyses support a role for increased fruit and vegetable intake in reducing the risk of developing hypertension.

Prospective Cohort and Cross-Sectional Studies

Prospective cohort studies consistently indicate that specific types of fruits and vegetables differ in their hypertension risk reduction capacity. An analysis of three large, long-term cohorts (187,453 participants from Nurses' Health Study: 62,175 women, Nurses' Health Study II: 88,475 women, and Health Professionals Follow-up Study: 36,803 men; >20 years of follow-up) found a lower mean risk of hypertension for total whole fruit by 8% and total vegetable intake by 5% (≥4 servings/day vs. ≤4 servings/week) [78]. The consumption levels of broccoli, carrots, tofu or soybeans, raisins, grapes and apples associated with significantly lower hypertension risk for ≥4 servings/week vs. <1 serving/month (Figs. 14.5 and 14.6). The Women's Health Study (29,082 US health professionals; mean age 54 years; 12.9 years of follow-up; 13,633 cases of hypertension), found that women who had a higher intake of all fruits but not all vegetables were significantly associated with reduced hypertension risk after adjustment for lifestyle and dietary factors but adding BMI to the models eliminated all significant associations [79]. This study also observed that green leafy and dark-yellow vegetables, and apples, oranges and raisins were among the most effective in lowering risk of hypertension. The Japanese Ohasama study (745 participants; mean age 56 years; mean follow-up 4 years; 222 incidents of hypertension) observed that high intake of fruit such as citrus, apples, grapes and watermelon was associated with a significant 60% lower risk of hypertension, after multivariate adjustments [80]. The Spanish Seguimiento University of Navarra (SUN) study (8594 participants; mean age 41 years; median duration 6 years) found a significant inverse association between fruit intake and BP, but not vegetable intake and hypertension risk [81]. In the population-based International Study on Macro/Micronutrients and Blood Pressure (INTERMAP) cross-sectional, cross-cultural, population-based study of middle-aged individuals (4680 participants from Japan, China, UK and US; mean age

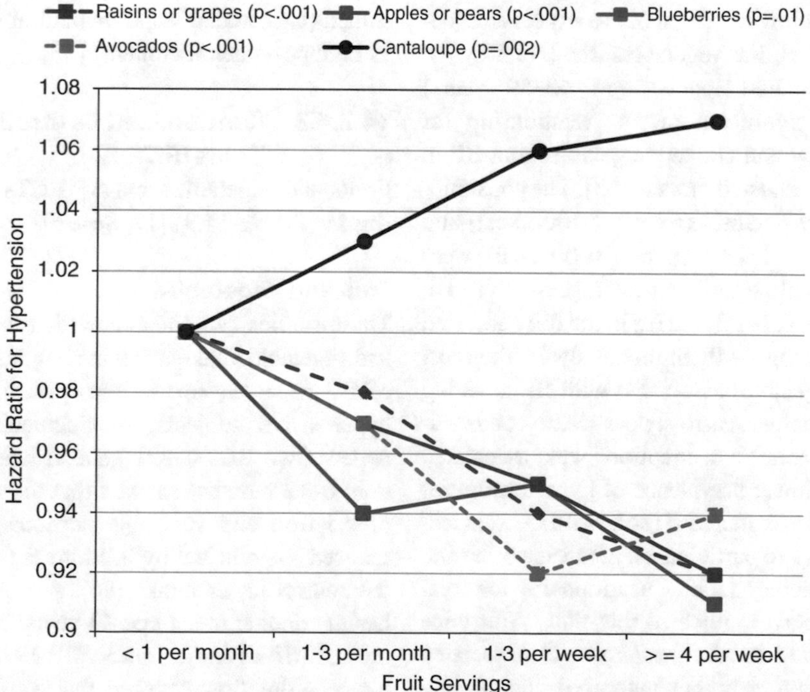

Fig. 14.5 Association between specific fruits and hypertension risk in US men and women from the Nurses' Health Studies and Health Professionals Follow-up Study (adapted from [78])

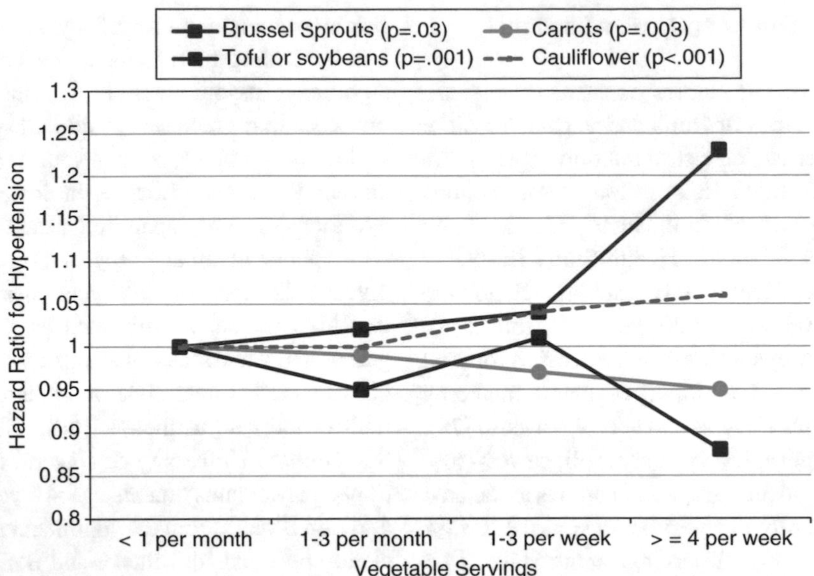

Fig. 14.6 Association between specific vegetables and hypertension risk in US men and women from the Nurses' Health Studies and Health Professionals Follow-up Study (adapted from [78])

49 years), raw fruit intake was not inversely associated with BP, but this is expected since the median fruit intake was low, 46.5 g/1000 kcals, which was below the threshold to expect a reduction in BP [82]. For vegetables, the INTERMAP study (2195 participants; age 40–59 years) observed a significant inverse relationship for both total raw and cooked vegetables and BP in multivariate-adjusted models [83]. The consumption of raw vegetables (68 g per 1000 kcal) and cooked vegetables (92 g per 1000 kcal) were associated with significant average systolic BP reductions by 0.9–1.3 mm Hg in the fully adjusted model including BMI. In this analysis, the most effective vegetables associated with BP lowering included tomatoes, carrots, peas, celery, and scallions. Gazpacho consumption was associated with a 15% lower prevalence of hypertension for each 250 g/week increase [84]. A 2015 crosssectional study (146 participants; mean age 59 years; 12 month dietary recall questionnaire for total fruit juice intake) indicated that daily fruit juice consumption (1 to >3 times/day) was associated with significantly higher increased central systolic BP, central pulse pressure, and central augmentation pressure compared to rarely (<3 times /month) or occasional juice consumption (1 to <6 times /week) but these results are expected to vary depending on the type of fruit juice consumed (e.g., added sugar vs natural sugar or low vs high polyphenol content) [85].

14.2.4.3 Randomized Controlled Trials (RCTs)

Fruits and vegetables and BP RCTs are summarized in (Table 14.3) [17, 86–96].

Fruit and Vegetables

These studies generally show that increased fruit and vegetable intake result in significant reduction of BP in older, overweight, prehypertensive or hypertensive subjects. A Cochrane systematic review (two RCTs; 891 general healthy population; 6–12 months) showed that the consumption of ≥5 fruit and vegetable portions significantly reduced systolic BP by 3.0 mm Hg compared to the control lower intake [86]. A large RCT (459 healthy adults; mean age 44 years; 50% women; mean BMI 28 kg/m^2; mean BP 132/85 mm Hg; 8-weeks duration) showed that 8–10 daily servings of fruits and vegetables significantly reduced systolic BP by 2.8 mm Hg and borderline

Table 14.3 Summaries of fruits and vegetables RCTs on blood pressure (BP)

Objective	Study details	Study results
Cochrane Systematic Review and Meta-analysis		
Hartley et al. (2013). Determine the effectiveness of increased fruits and vegetables intake for the primary prevention of CVD including BP [86]	2 RCTs; 891 generally healthy subjects; 6 months to 1 year	Advice to eat fruits and vegetables significantly reduced systolic BP by mean 3.0 mm Hg vs. low fruits and vegetables control but the reduction in diastolic BP by 0.90 mm Hg was not statistically significant
Liu et al. (2013). Quantitatively evaluate the effect of fruit juice on BP in adults (meta-analysis) [87]	8 RCTs; 197 participants; stage 1 hypertension; juices: pomegranate, concord grape juice, cranberry, orange and blueberry juice, muscadine grape juice	Fruit juice significantly reduced mean diastolic BP values by 2.1 mm Hg but insignificantly lowered systolic BP
Representative RCTs		
Jovanovski et al. (2015). Investigate the effect of spinach intake on BP (Canada) [88]	**Crossover RCT**: 27 healthy adults; mean age 25 years; mean BMI 23; 59% women; mean BP 116/69; studied high-nitrate (spinach (250 g); 845 mg nitrate/day) or low-nitrate soup (asparagus (260 g); 0.6 mg nitrate/day); BP at 3 h post-prandial; 7-day duration; 7-day washout	Spinach soup (rich in nitrates) significantly reduced mean central systolic BP by 3.4 mm Hg and diastolic BP by 2.6 mm Hg after 7-days of supplementation compared to the low-nitrate control. This highlights the potential importance of consuming specific types of components in vegetables associated with lower BP control
Tjelle et al. (2015). Assess the effects of polyphenol-rich juices on BP (Norway) [89]	**Double-blinded, Parallel RCT**: 134 healthy individuals, mean age 62 years, with high normal range BP 130/85–139/89 mm Hg; 500 mL/day of either a commercially available polyphenol-rich juice based on red grapes, cherries, chokeberries and bilberries, a similar juice enriched with polyphenol-rich extracts from blackcurrants or a placebo juice; 12 weeks	Compared with the placebo group, the polyphenol rich juices significantly reduced systolic BP in the hypertensive subjects by 2 mm Hg at 6 weeks and 2.8 mm Hg at 12 weeks. In normotensive subjects, a significant difference between placebo and polyphenolic rich juices was not observed
Novotny et al. (2015). Determine the potential of low-calorie cranberry juice on BP (US) [90]	**Double-blinded, Parallel RCT**: 56 healthy subjects; mean age 50 years; BMI 28; about 60% female; low-calorie cranberry juice vs. flavor/color/energy-matched placebo beverage; Twice daily volunteers consumed 240 mL beverage, containing 173 or 62 mg of phenolic compounds and 6.5 or 7.5 g of total sugar per 240-mL serving; 8 weeks	Low-calorie cranberry juice significantly reduced diastolic BP by 2.4 mm Hg vs. placebo
Vinson et al. (2012). Evaluate the clinical effect of purple potatoes rich in antioxidants (e.g., phenolics, anthocyanins, carotenoids) on BP in hypertensive subjects (US) [91]	**Crossover RCT**: 18 healthy adults; average age 54 years; 61% women; average BMI 29.4; 140 g of microwaved purple-pigmented potatoes twice daily vs. control biscuits; 4 weeks	Purple potatoes decreased diastolic BP by 4 mm Hg (4.3%) and systolic BP by 5 mm Hg (3.5%) vs. control. New cultivars of potatoes rich in antioxidants may help to control BP
Berry et al. (2010). Investigate the effects of increasing potassium (K) intake above usual levels by increased intakes of fruits and vegetables or supplements on BP in subjects with elevated BP (UK) [92]	**Crossover RCT**: 57 healthy adults; mean age 45 years; mean BP 137/88 mm Hg untreated; additional 20 or 40 mmol K^+/day from fruits and vegetables or 40 mmol potassium citrate capsules/day vs. low fruits and vegetables control; 6 weeks; 5-week washout	No significant differences in resting or ambulatory 24 h BP and vascular function between any of the fruit and vegetable diets. The present study provides no evidence to support dietary advice to increase K intake above usual intakes in subjects with early stages of hypertension

(continued)

Table 14.3 (continued)

Objective	Study details	Study results
McCall et al. (2009). Evaluate a potential dose-dependent effect of fruits and vegetables on BP in hypertensive subjects (UK) [93]	**Parallel RCT**: 108 adults; mean age 54 years; mean BMI 29; mean BP 143/83 mm Hg; 1, 3, or 6 daily fruit and vegetable portions added to the run-in diet. Compliance was monitored with 4-day food records and by measuring concentrations of circulating carotenoids; 4-week run-in on low fruit and vegetable diets; 8 weeks	Among hypertensive participants, there was a significant dose-response relationship between fruit and vegetable intake and vasodilation, which was correlated with serum concentrations of lutein and β- cryptoxanthin. Also, blood flow response increased by 6% after consuming just one extra daily portion of fruits and vegetables in hypertensive subjects suggesting that small increases in fruit and vegetable intake has potential benefits
John et al. (2002). Study the effect of an increase in fruit and vegetable intake on plasma antioxidant levels and BP (UK) [94]	**Parallel RCT:** 690 healthy adults; mean age 46 years; current smokers 55 + %; mean BMI 26; mean BP of 130/79 mm Hg; diets: increased daily fruit and vegetable portions by 1.4 servings vs. control diet increased by 0.1 servings; 6 months	Increased fruit and vegetable portions significantly reduced systolic BP by 4.0 mm Hg and diastolic BP by 1.5 mm Hg vs. control. At the population level, a reduction in diastolic BP by 2 mm Hg may lower the incidence of hypertension by 17%. Plasma lutein, α-carotene, β-carotene, β-cryptoxanthin, and ascorbic acid were significantly increased vs. controls
Broekmans et al. (2001) Determine the effect of fruits and vegetables and juice intake on BP (The Netherlands) [95]	**Parallel RCT:** 48 healthy adults; mean age 50 years; 50% women; mean BMI 26; mean BP of 126/80 mm Hg; two high fiber diets with 500 g fruits and vegetables/day and 200 mL fruit juice/day vs. 100 g fruits and vegetables/day and no juice; 4 weeks	Both fruit and vegetable diets significantly reduced BP for systolic BPs by 5.8–7.7 mm Hg and diastolic BP 3.9–4.4 mm Hg
Smith-Warner et al. (2000). Evaluate the effect of increased fruit and vegetable intake above recommended servings on normotensive individuals (US) [96]	**Parallel RCT:** 201 healthy adults; mean age 60 years; 71% male; BP 128/76 mm Hg; baseline diet about seven servings fruits and vegetables; intervention increased fruits and vegetables by about five servings and control decreased fruits and vegetables by about 0.5 serving; 1 year	There were no changes in BP between groups, which is not unexpected since these normotensive subjects were all consuming recommended levels of fruits and vegetables
Appel et al. (1999). Investigate the effects of fruits and vegetables rich diets, the DASH diet and the American diet on BP [17]	**Parallel RCT:** 459 healthy adults; mean age 44 years; 50% women; 60% black; mean BP 132/85 mm Hg; diet: fruit and vegetable rich diet (8–10 portions; 31 g fiber/day), DASH diet (high fruit and vegetable rich diet (8–10 portions; 31 g fiber/day) vs. control American diet (3.6 portions of fruits and vegetables; 9 g fiber/day); 3-week American diet run-in; 8 weeks	The increased fruit and vegetable diet significantly reduced systolic BP by 2.8 mm Hg and borderline significantly reduced diastolic BP by 1.1 mm Hg vs. control diet (Fig. 14.7). The DASH diet rich in fruits and vegetables, and low-fat dairy products lowered systolic BP by 5.5 mm Hg and diastolic BP by 3.0 mm Hg vs. control diet

significantly reduced diastolic BP by 1.1 mm Hg more than the control diet with 3.6 portions of fruit and vegetables/day in all subjects (non-hypertensive and hypertensive combined) (Fig. 14.7) [17]. However, when only hypertensive subjects were assessed, the BP reduction increased for systolic BP to 7.2 mm Hg ($p < .001$) and diastolic BP to 2.8 mm Hg ($p = .01$) compared to the control diet. A dose response study indicated that three and six servings of fruit and vegetables lowered systolic BP by 2.2 and 4.5 mm Hg, respectively, and each fruit and vegetable serving significantly increased forearm blood flow by 6% [93]. A longer-term RCT (690 healthy adults; mean age 46; current smokers 55%; mean BMI 26 kg/m^2; mean BP 130/79 mm Hg; 6 months) found the intake of ≥5 fruit and vegetable portions/day significantly reduced systolic BP by 4.0 mm Hg and diastolic BP by 1.5 mm Hg more than the low fruit and vegetable controls [94]. RCTs have found that spinach, rich in nitrates, reduces BP by augmenting nitric oxide status [88] and purple potatoes, rich in phenolic antioxidants, reduce BP by promoting vascular health [91].

Several trials have suggested no effects from increased intake of fruit and vegetables on BP. A crossover RCT (57 adults; mean age 45 years; BMI 28 kg/m^2; mean BP 137/88 mm Hg; 86 weeks) using both resting and ambulatory BP measurements did not see a significant change in BP in UK diets supplemented with potassium rich fruit and vegetables (20 and 40 mmol K^+/day) or potassium citrate (40 mmol K^+/day) added to the standard UK diets compared to the unsupplemented standard UK diet [92]. A parallel RCT (48 adults; mean age 50 years; mean BMI 26 kg/m^2; mean baseline BP of 126/80 mm Hg; 4-weeks duration) found that subjects adding 400 g fruits and vegetables and 200 ml fruit juice/day to a low fruit and vegetable diet (100 g/day) showed no significant differences in BP lowering effects, which was most likely due to the short study duration and normal BP levels of subjects [95]. A long-term RCT (201 healthy participants; mean age 60 years; normotensive; 1 year) observed no difference in BP with seven compared to five daily servings of fruit and vegetables [96].

Fruit Juices

Fruit juice effects on BP are heterogeneous depending on the juice composition such as the type of fruit, concentration and type of polyphenolics, as well as the BP status of the subject (normotensive vs. hypertensive) [85, 89, 90]. A meta-analysis of fruit juices (19 RCTs; 618 subjects; polyphenols contained in fruit juice ranged from 65 to 2660 mg/day (median: 927 mg/day); juices: pomegranate, concord grape, cranberry,

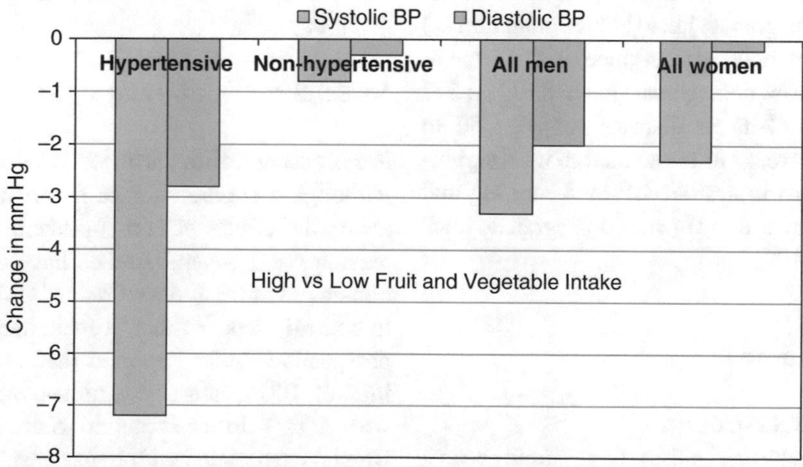

Fig. 14.7 Difference in blood pressure (BP) between a high fruit and vegetable diet and a lower fruit and vegetable control diet after 8 weeks in men and women with mean age 44 years and BMI 28 kg/m^2 ($p < .001$ for hypertensive subjects) (adapted from [17])

orange, blueberry juice, and muscadine grape juice; 2 weeks to 3 months with median: 6 weeks) found a significantly mean lower diastolic BP by 2.1 mm Hg but insignificant reductions in total cholesterol, HDL and LDL-cholesterol, and systolic BP [87]. A RCT on high polyphenol juices (134 healthy individuals, mean age 62 years, with high normal range BP 130/85–139/89 mm Hg; 12 weeks) found that 500 mL/day significantly reduced systolic BP in the hypertensive subjects by 2 mm Hg at 6 weeks and 2.8 mm Hg at 12 weeks compared to placebo but there was no difference in BP in normotensive subjects [89]. In normotensive individuals (56 healthy men and women; mean age 50 years; 8 weeks) 240 mL of low-calorie cranberry juice twice daily significantly lowered diastolic BP by 2.4 mm Hg vs. placebo [90]. A 2017 review of 100% fruit and vegetable juices concluded that although their composition is different from that of whole fruits and vegetables, they contain polyphenols, minerals such as potassium, vitamins such as vitamin C, and/or nitrates from fruits and vegetables that can lower BP [97]. The main mechanisms of action included antioxidant effects, improvement of blood flow, inhibition of platelet aggregation, and anti-inflammatory effects. This review identified three 100% fruit and vegetable juices with BP lowering effects: (1) high flavonoid (naringin and naritutin) sweetie fruit (a hybrid between grapefruit and pummelo). (2) 100% (phenolic antioxidant rich) pomegranate juice (Punica granatum L.) and (3) nitrate rich beetroot juice. A 2017 meta-analysis of 100% pomegranate juice (8 RCTs; 547 hypertensive, CVD or diabetes subjects; 50 to 500ml/day; 2 weeks to 18 months) showed significant reductions in systolic BP by 5 mm Hg and diastolic BP by 2 mm Hg after pomegranate juice consumption [98].

14.2.5 Legumes

14.2.5.1 Background

Legumes, including pulses (e.g., pinto beans, split peas, lentils, chickpeas) and soybeans, are rich in fiber and protein with relatively low glycemic response properties [35, 99]. A serving of legumes is 1⁄2 cup or 90–100 g cooked legumes, which contains 5–10 g of fiber and 7–8 g of protein. Most legumes contain <5% of energy as fat, with the exception of chickpeas and soybeans which have 15 and 47% energy from fat, respectively. Legumes, compared to cereal grains, are rich in high-quality protein [99]. The protein content of legumes ranges from 17 to 20% (dry weight) in peas and beans which is similar to meats 18–25%, and 38–40% in soybeans. This contrasts with the protein content of cereals, which is about 7–13%. A meta-analysis of 29 observational studies and RCTs of dietary protein effects on BP and hypertension concluded that the substitution of either animal or plant based protein for carbohydrate reduced the pooled systolic BP by 2.1 mm Hg for a weighted mean protein intake of 41 g/day [100]. Legumes contain nutritionally important amounts of the B vitamins and minerals, such as iron, calcium and potassium. They also contain bioactive phytochemicals such as phenolics, saponins and isoflavones (especially in soy foods). Legumes are often consumed as a lower energy dense, lower saturated fat, and high fiber meat or milk replacer. Legumes consumption has been in decline with the global shift to Western-style diets [101]. For example, between the 1960s and 1990s, legume intake decreased by 40% in India and by 24% in Mexico. Legumes are infrequently consumed by North Americans and northern Europeans, with <8% of Americans consuming them on any given day.

14.2.5.2 Non-Soy Legumes

Prospective Cohort Studies

Although there are no specific prospective studies on the effects of non-soy legumes on hypertension risk, several studies have reported that non-soy legumes reduced risk of CVD compared to control diets. Further, a meta-analysis of five prospective studies reported that 4 weekly servings of 100 g non-soy legumes was associated with a 14% lower ischemic heart disease risk, which is associated with hypertension [102].

Randomized Controlled Trials (RCTs)

A systematic review and meta-analysis 8 isocaloric dietary pulse (beans, peas, chickpeas, and lentils) RCTs; 554 mid dle aged subjects; median increase of 1 2/3 servings (160 g/day; range 81–275 g/day; median 10 weeks) found that dietary pulses significantly mean lowered systolic BP by 2.25 mm Hg and arterial BP by 0.75 mm Hg in total subjects with or without hypertension [103]. To achieve BP reductions similar to those observed in this systematic review and meta-analysis, an increase in consumption of at least two servings (1 cup)/day above current average intakes (0.1–0.3 servings/day) would need to be recommended. Dietary pulses may lower BP by increasing dietary levels of fiber, plant protein and potassium, and aid in weight control, all of which confer BP-lowering effects [104, 105].

14.2.5.3 Soy Products

Observational Studies

A limited number of observational studies suggest that soy food consumption is inversely associated with BP. The large Shanghai Women's Health Study observed that the intake of foods containing 25 g soy protein/day vs. <2.5 g/day was inversely associated with both systolic and diastolic BP, especially among women >60 years [106]. In a Japanese cross-sectional study of about 600 men, and premenopausal and postmenopausal women, there was an inverse association with soy product intake and BP in men [107].

Randomized Controlled Trials (RCTs)

Intervention trials consistently show that the consumption of soy products lowers BP. A meta-analysis (27 RCTs; soy protein varied from 18 to 66 g/day with median of 30 g/day and 100 mg isoflavones/day vs. control groups received casein or milk; 4–52 weeks with a median of 8 weeks) concluded that the consumption of soy protein products significantly lowered the pooled mean for systolic BP by 2.2 mm Hg and diastolic BP by 1.4 mm Hg compared to control diets [108]. Furthermore, the mean BP decrease was markedly greater in the hypertensive group by 8.6 mm Hg ($p = .010$) for systolic BP and 5.2 mm Hg ($p = .014$) for diastolic BP. Three double-blind RCTs suggest that partially replacing carbohydrate with soy or milk protein might help to lower elevated BP [109–111]: (1) In hypertensive adults (40 adults; mean age 48 years; 60% men; mean BP 153/100 mm Hg; 3 months) the consumption of soy milk significantly decreased BP compared to the cow's milk group (Fig. 14.8) [109]. (2) In a crossover trial (352 adults; mean age 48 years; 59% men; mean BMI 29; 33% blacks; mean BP 127/82 mm Hg; 8 weeks) 40 g/day of soy protein and milk protein significantly reduced systolic BP by 2.0 and 2.3 mm Hg, respectively, compared to the complex carbohydrate control [110]. (3) In a parallel trial (302 adults; mean age 51 years; mean BMI 27; 53% women; mean BP 135/85 mm Hg; 3 months) 40 g of isolated soy protein significantly lowered

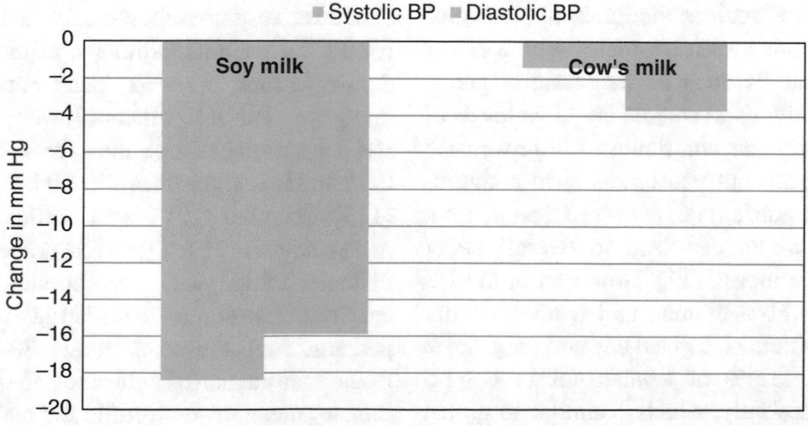

Fig. 14.8 Effect of soy milk or cow's milk-based diet (500 mL twice daily) on blood pressure (BP) in mid-age adults with essential hypertension after 3 months ($p < .0001$) (adapted from [109])

systolic BP by 4.3 mm Hg and diastolic BP by 2.8 mm Hg compared to a complex carbohydrate control; hypertensive subjects had even greater significant lowering for systolic BP by 7.9 mm Hg and for diastolic BP by 5.3 mm Hg [111].

14.2.6 Nuts and Seeds

14.2.6.1 Background

Nuts and seeds are rich sources of potentially hypertensive protective macronutrients, micronutrients and phytochemicals [32, 112, 113]. They are rich in healthy dietary fat content, with a total fat content ranging from 46% in cashews and pistachios to 76% in macadamia nuts. The fatty acid composition of nuts is of a healthy type since the saturated fat levels are low (range 4–16%) and with 84–96% of the total fat content made up of unsaturated fat, mostly monounsaturated fatty acids (MUFAs), and polyunsaturated fatty acids (PUFAs, predominantly linoleic acid). Walnuts and flaxseed are rich sources of alpha-linolenic acid, the plant n-3 fatty acid. Nuts and seeds are good sources of protein and are often rich in fiber, ranging from 1 to 7 g/28 g serving. Despite their relatively high Atwater metabolizable energy value of 5–6 kcal/g, nuts and seeds often have a 10–25% lower net metabolizable energy than the label value [114–116]. Among nut types, there are significant amounts of essential micronutrients including the B-vitamin folate, antioxidant vitamins (e.g., tocopherols), polyphenols and carotenoids such as the lutein in pistachios [112]. Also, nuts are an important source of key shortfall minerals such as magnesium, potassium and calcium and contain very low levels of sodium, which can contribute to improved BP control. Overall, nut consumers have a significantly higher nutrient quality score than non-nut consumers, which can lead to overall better health and wellness [117]. However, in the US slightly over 60% of men and women do not consume any nuts on a given day and only14.4% of men and 11.8% of women consume ≥1.5 ounces of nuts/daily, which is similar to global nut intake [118].

14.2.6.2 Prospective Cohort Studies

A number of prospective studies have reported that nuts are positively associated with CVD health and reduced risk of ischemic heart disease, compared to nut-free controls [102, 119, 120]. In Iranian adults, more frequent nut consumption (≥4 servings/week vs. no nut intake) was significantly associated with a 34% lower incidence of hypertension [121]. In US male physicians, the intake of ≥7 servings of nuts/week vs. no nut consumption was associated with a significantly lower risk of hypertension [122]. In the Atherosclerosis Risk of Communities study (9913 African-American and Caucasian adults aged 45–64 years and free of hypertension at baseline) diets rich in nuts and dairy and lower in meat were associated with a decreased risk of developing hypertension over nine years [123]. However, in a Mediterranean cohort, there was no association between nut consumption (2+ servings/week vs. never/rare nut intake) and incidence of hypertension after multivariate adjustments [124].

14.2.6.3 Randomized Controlled Trials (RCTs)

Nuts

Overall nut intake generally tends to have a modest direct clinically meaningful effect on controlling BP but the association with increased nut intake to reduce the risk of weight gain may have longer-term implication on lower hypertensive risk [23, 125]. A 2015 systematic review and dose response meta-analysis on tree nuts (61 RCTs; walnuts, almonds, pistachios, macadamia, pecans, cashews, hazel nuts and Brazil nuts) found an insignificant lower pooled mean BP per serving of tree nuts for systolic BP by 0.3 mm Hg and for diastolic BP by 0.39 mm Hg [125]. Another 2015 systematic review and meta-analysis (21 RCTs; 1652 diabetic and non-diabetic adults; walnuts, almonds, pistachios, cashews, hazelnuts, macadamia nuts, pecans, peanuts, and soy nuts; range 30–108 g/day) found that nut consumption resulted in an insignificant mean lower systolic BP by 0.9 mm Hg, but there was significant heterogeneity among studies [23]. In a subsequent revised analysis in only non-diabetic subjects, higher nut intake had modest significantly lowered systolic BP by 1.3 mm Hg. A subgroup analysis of different nut types found that pistachio nuts were the most effective, significantly reducing systolic BP by 1.8 mm Hg. Pistachios and mixed nuts significantly reduced diastolic BP by 0.8 and 1.2 mm Hg, respectively.

Seeds

Flax and sesame seeds are more effective than nuts in lowering BP [21, 126–128].

Flaxseeds

RCTs suggest that flaxseeds are effective in lowering BP because they are a rich dietary source of ω-3 fatty acids and α-linolenic acid, lignans, and fiber, with combined potential for BP lowering effects [21, 126]. A systematic review and meta-analysis (12 RCTs; 1004 health participants) showed that flaxseed consumption modestly but significantly reduced mean systolic BP by 1.8 mm Hg and mean diastolic BP by 1.6 mm Hg [21]. A double-blinded RCT (110 adults; mean age 67 years; mean BMI 28 kg/m^2; mean BP 143/78 mm Hg; 75% hypertensive; 6 months) reported that the daily consumption of a variety of foods that contained 30 g of milled flaxseed significantly lowered systolic BP by 10 mm Hg and diastolic BP by 7 mm Hg compared with a placebo (0 g flaxseed) [127]. Hypertensive subjects (systolic BP > 140 mm Hg at baseline) had a more significant lowering of systolic BP by 15 mm Hg from flaxseed intake compared to the overall study population mean. Body weight did not differ between the two groups, whereas plasma levels of ω-3 fatty acid and α-linolenic acid and enterolignans increased 2- to 50-fold in the flaxseed-fed group compared to the control group [127].

Sesame Seeds

Sesame seed consumption can reduce BP due to its high polyunsaturated fatty acids, fiber, phytosterol and lignans content [127, 128]. A 2017 systematic review and meta-analysis (8 RCTs; 843 participants) found that sesame consumption significantly reduced systolic BP by 7.8 mm Hg and diastolic BP by 5.8 mm Hg. To reduce the heterogeneity, the secondary meta-analysis was limited to four high methodology quality trials which showed a significant reduction in systolic BP by 3.2 mm Hg and a non-significant reduction in diastolic BP by 2.1 mm Hg [127]. A 2016 systematic review demonstrated that of the seven RCTs evaluated five RCTs in hypertensive individuals had a significant reduction in systolic and/or diastolic BP [128].

14.3 Tea and Coffee

Coffee and tea are among the most popular beverages in the world so the effects of how drinking them affects incident hypertension is an important public health question.

14.3.1 Tea

Tea is the second most commonly consumed beverage globally, after water, and has been traditionally associated with CVD protective properties such as antihypertensive effects in individuals with elevated BP (hypertensive or prehypertensive) [129]. Tea is rich in a class of polyphenolic compounds known as flavonoids. Tea comes from the plant Camellia sinensis and is a beverage prepared by pouring hot or boiling water over its cured leaves or leaf buds. Green and black teas have similar total flavonoid content but have different chemical structures. In green tea, flavonoids are normally found in the form of catechins, while in black tea, flavonoids are typically found as theaflavins. A 2015 meta-analysis of black and green tea combined (10 RCTs; 834 hypertensive or pre-hypertensive subjects; median duration 3 months) found that the median dosage of 456 mg of flavonoids/d (approximately 2 cups of black or green tea per day) significantly reduced systolic BP by 2.4 mm Hg and diastolic BP by 1.8 mm Hg [130]. A 2014 meta-analysis of green tea (13 RCTs; 1,367 hypertensive or pre-hypertensive subjects; 3 months) showed that median intake of 583 mg of flavonoids/d (approximately 2 ½ cups) significantly reduced both systolic and diastolic

BP by 2 mm Hg [131]. A 2014 meta-analysis of black tea (11 RCTs; 378 normotensive, hypertensive and pre-hypertensive subjects; > 1 week) found that daily consumption of 4 to 5 cups of black tea significantly reduced systolic BP by 2 mm Hg and diastolic BP by 1 mm Hg [132]. Another 2014 meta-analysis (25 RCTs; 1,476 normotensive, hypertensive and pre-hypertensive subjects) found that >12 weeks consumption of tea (green and black tea) resulted in a significant reduction of systolic BP by 2.6 mm Hg and diastolic BP by 2.2 mm Hg which was not influenced by ethnicity, caffeine intake, tea polyphenol doses, health status of participants [133]. At the population level, reductions in BP 2 to 3mm Hg are associated with lower incidence of coronary artery disease by 8% and stroke by 15% [134].

14.3.2 Coffee

Coffee is a brewed drink prepared from roasted coffee beans, which are the seeds of berries from the Coffea plant. Coffee beverages contain a mixture of several pharmacologically-bioactive compounds, including caffeine, chlorogenic acid, phenolic acids, and the diterpene alcohols, cafestol and kahweol, can also have long term effects on health [135]. A link between coffee drinking and BP was first reported nearly 75 yrs ago [136], but whether coffee intake is associated with BP or hypertension risk has mixed results. A moderate (400–600 mg/d) caffeine intake is not associated with increased risks of total cardiovascular disease, or BP among regular caffeine consumers and hypertension in baseline healthy populations [137]. Populations at risk for hypertension, or already with hypertension, may be more sensitive to some effects of caffeine. Pre- or hypertensive populations may experience acute increases in BP following caffeine intake ranging from 100 to <400 mg/d compared to normotensive people. Also, pre- or hypertensive populations may have a small increased relative risk of sustained hypertension related to high caffeine beverage consumption. Overall, studies generally suggest no association between caffeine consumption and hypertension risk in a baseline healthy population. A 2011 meta-analysis (6 cohort studies; 172,567 participants; mean follow-up 6.4 to 33 years) found that habitual coffee consumption of >3 cups/day was not associated with a significant increased hypertension risk compared with consumption of <1 cup/day, but a slightly elevated risk appeared to be associated with light-to-moderate consumption (1–3 cups/day) [138]. The Women's Health Initiative Observational Study (29,985 normotensive women; mean age 63 years; 3-year follow-up) found that the consumption of caffeinated coffee, decaffeinated coffee, and caffeine were not associated with the risk of postmenopausal incident hypertension (p-trend > 0.05 for all) [139]. In hypertensive individuals, a systematic review and meta-analysis (5 RCTs; 200–300 mg caffeine/day) showed a mean increase of 8.1 mm Hg in systolic BP and of 5.7 mm Hg in diastolic BP observed in the first hour after caffeine intake and lasting approximately 3 hrs [140]. However, after 2 weeks of coffee consumption, no increase in BP was observed after coffee was compared with a caffeine-free diet or decaffeinated coffee. There is a need to investigate directly the influence of coffee or caffeine on the degree of BP control in hypertensive individuals and its possible interaction with antihypertensive medications.

Conclusions

By 2025, because of population growth and an aging population, it is projected that about 1.5 billion individuals globally will have hypertension. Lifestyle factors such as meeting the dietary recommendation for whole plant foods is the most important action one can take to lower risk of hypertension. Whole (and minimally processed) plant foods usually contain some mixture of BP lowering bioactive nutrients and phytochemicals such as dietary fiber, potassium, magnesium, polyphenols, unsaturated fat, and plant protein and are lower in sodium and sugar compared to highly processed plant foods. Whole (and minimally processed) plant foods usually contain a number of BP lowering bioactive nutrients and phytochemicals such as fiber, potassium, magnesium, carotenoids, polyphenols, unsaturated fat, and plant protein and are lower in sodium and sugar compared to highly processed plant foods. Whole plant foods are more effective at reducing BP in adults who are ≥45 years, hypertensive and obese than adults <45 years, normotensive, or lean. Prospective studies show that the consumption of healthy diets with ≥3 daily servings of whole grains, especially grains rich in β-glucan, and ≥5 daily servings of fruits and vegetables, especially when including ≥4 weekly servings of broccoli, carrots, tofu or soybeans, raisins, grapes and apples, are associated with lower hypertension risk compared to Western diets. RCTs support the effectiveness of whole grains in lowering BP especially at 50 g/1000 kcals or those rich in β-glucan; fruits and vegetables rich in polyphenols and nitrates and their 100% juices have been shown to lower systolic BP; and 2 daily servings of dietary pulses or 40 g soy protein are effective in lowering BP. Flaxseeds and sesame seeds tend to be more effective than nuts in lowering BP. Tea and coffee have different effects on BP. Both black and green tea (>2 cups/day) modestly lower BP in hypertensive individuals. Coffee (>3 cups/day) does not increase hypertension risk in normotensive people but hypertensive individuals may be more sensitive to acute increases in BP after coffee consumption. The potential mechanisms by which whole plant foods may reduce blood pressure and hypertension risk are; reducing the risk of weight gain, enhancing insulin sensitivity, improving vascular endothelial function, slowing the rate of arterial plaque build-up, maintaining electrolyte balance, and stimulating a healthier microbiota ecosystem.

Appendix A: Estimated Range of Energy, Fiber, Nutrients and Phytochemicals Composition of Whole Plant Foods/100 g Edible Portion

Components	Whole-grains	Fresh fruit	Dried fruit	Vegetables	Legumes	Nuts/seeds
Nutrients/ phytochemicals	Wheat, oat, barley, rye, brown rice, whole grain bread, cereal, pasta, rolls and crackers	Apples, pears, bananas, grapes, oranges, blueberries, strawberries, and avocados	Dates, dried figs, apricots, cranberries, raisins and prunes	Potatoes, spinach, carrots, peppers, lettuce, green beans, cabbage, onions, cucumber, cauliflower, mushrooms, and broccoli	Lentils, chickpeas, split peas, black beans, pinto beans, and soy beans	Almonds, Brazil nuts, cashews, hazelnuts, macadamias, pecans, walnuts, peanuts, sunflower seeds, and flaxseed
Energy (kcals)	110–350	30–170	240–310	10–115	85–170	520–700
Protein (g)	2.5–16	0.5–2.0	0.1–3.4	0.2–5.0	5.0–17	7.8–24
Available carbohydrate (g)	23–77	1.0–25	64–82	0.2–25	10–27	12–33
Fiber (g)	3.5–18	2.0–7.0	5.7–10	1.2–9.5	5.0–11	3.0–27
Total fat (g)	0.9–6.5	0.0–15	0.4–1.4	0.2–1.5	0.2–9.0	46–76
SFA[a] (g)	0.2–1.0	0.0–2.1	0.0	0.0–0.1	0.1–1.3	4.0–12
MUFA[a] (g)	0.2–2.0	0.0–9.8	0.0–0.2	0.1–1.0	0.1–2.0	9.0–60
PUFA[a] (g)	0.3–2.5	0.0–1.8	0.0–0.7	0.0.0.4	0.1–5.0	1.5–47
Folate (μg)	4.0–44	<5.0–61	2–20	8.0–160	50–210	10–230
Tocopherols (mg)	0.1–3.0	0.1–1.0	0.1–4.5	0.0–1.7	0.0–1.0	1.0–35
Potassium (mg)	40–720	60–500	40–1160	100–680	200–520	360–1050
Calcium (mg)	7.0–50	3.0–25	10–160	5.0–200	20–100	20–265
Magnesium (mg)	40–160	3.0–30	5.0–70	3.0–80	40–90	120–400
Phytosterols (mg)	30–90	1.0–83	–	1.0–54	110–120	70–215

Components	Whole-grains	Fresh fruit	Dried fruit	Vegetables	Legumes	Nuts/seeds
Polyphenols (mg)	70–100	50–800	–	24–1250	120–6500	130–1820
Carotenoids (μg)	–	25–6600	1.0–2160	10–20,000	50–600	1.0–1200

SFA (saturated fat), MUFA (monounsaturated fat) and PUFA (polyunsaturated fat)

U.S. Department of Agriculture, Agriculture Research Service, Nutrient Data Laboratory. 2014. USDA National Nutrient Database for Standard Reference, Release 27. http://www.ars. usda.gov. /nutrientdata. Accessed 17 February 2015

Ros E, Hu FB. Consumption of plant seeds and cardiovascular health epidemiological and clinical trial evidence. Circulation. 2013;128:553–65

USDA. What We Eat in America, NHANES 2011–2012, individuals 2 years and over (excluding breast-fed children). Available: www.ars.usda.gov/nea/bhnrc/fsrg

Rodriguez-Casado A. The health potential of fruits and vegetables phytochemicals: notable examples. Crit Rev. Food Sci Nutr. 2016;56(7):1097–1107

Rebello CJ, Greenway FL, Finley JW. A review of the nutritional value of legumes and their effects on obesity and its related co-morbidities. Obes Rev. 2014;15:392–407

Gebhardt SE, Thomas RG. Nutritive value of foods. 2002; U.S. Department of Agriculture, Agricultural Research Service, Home and Garden Bulletin 72

Holden JM, Eldridge AL, Beecher GR, et al. Carotenoid content of U.S. foods: an update of the database. J Food Comp An. 1999;12:169–96

Lu Q-Y, Zhang Y, Wang Y, et al. California Hass avocado: profiling of carotenoids, tocopherol, fatty acid, and fat content during maturation and from different growing areas. *J* Agric Food Chem. 2009; 57(21):10408–13

Wu X, Beecher GR, Holden JM, et al. Lipophilic and hydrophilic antioxidant capacities of common foods in the United States. J Agric Food Chem. 2004;52:4026–37

References

1. WHO. In: Mendis S, Puska P, Norrving B, editors. Global atlas on cardiovascular disease prevention and control. Geneva: World Health Organization; 2011.
2. World Health Organization. A global brief on hypertension. Silent killer, global public health crisis. Geneva: WHO; 2013. http://www.who.int/cardiovascular_diseases/publications/global brief. hypertension/en/. Accessed April 2017
3. Mozaffarian D, Benjamin EJ, Go AS, on behalf of the American Heart Association Statistics Committee and Stroke Statistics Subcommittee. Heart disease and stroke statistics-2016 update: a report from the American Heart Association. Circulation. 2016;133:e38–e360.
4. Atlas SA. The renin-angiotensin aldosterone system: pathophysiological role and pharmacologic inhibition. J Manag Care Pharm. 2007;13(8):S9–S20.
5. Livingstone KM, McNaughton SA. Dietary patterns by reduced rank regression are associated with obesity and hypertension in Australian adults. Br Nutr J. 2017;117:248–59. https://doi.org/10.1017/S0007114516004505.
6. Castro I, Waclawovsky G, Marcadenti A. Nutrition and physical activity on hypertension: implication of current evidence and guidelines. Curr Hypertens Rev. 2015;11(2):91–9.
7. Savica V, Bellinghieri G, Kopple JD. Effect of nutrition on blood pressure. Ann Rev Nutr. 2010;30:365–402.
8. Dietary Guidelines Advisory Committee (DGAC). Scientific report. Advisory report to the Secretary of Health and Human Services and the Secretary of Agriculture. Part D. Chapter 2: Dietary patterns, foods and nutrients and health outcomes. 2015:1–35.
9. Frisoli TM, Schmieder RE, Grodzicki T, Messerli FH. Beyond salt: lifestyle modifications and blood pressure. Eur Heart J. 2011;32:3081–7.
10. Rosvall M, Persson M, Ostling G, et al. Risk factors for the progression of carotid intima-media thickness over a 16-year follow-up period: the Malmo Diet and Cancer Study. Atherosclerosis. 2015;239:615–21. https://doi.org/10.1016/j.atherosclerosis.2015.01.030.
11. Dickinson HO, Mason JM, Nicolson DJ, et al. Lifestyle interventions to reduce raised blood pressure: a systematic review of randomized controlled trials. J Hypertens. 2006;24(2):215–33.
12. Liu X, Zhang D, Liu Y, et al. Dose-response association between physical activity and incident hypertension. A systematic review and meta-analysis of cohort studies. Hypertension. 2017;69(5):813–20. https://doi.org/10.1161/HypertensionAHA.116.08994.
13. Briasoulis A, Agarwal V, Messerli FH. Alcohol consumption and the risk of hypertension in men and women: a systematic review and meta-analysis. J Clin Hypertens (Greenwich). 2012;14:792–8.
14. Steffen LM, Kroenke CH, Yu X, et al. Associations of plant food, dairy product, and meat intakes with 15-y incidence of elevated blood pressure in young black and white adults: the Coronary Artery Risk Development in Young Adults (CARDIA) Study. Am J Clin Nutr. 2005;82:1169–77.

15. Gay HC, Rao SG, Vaccarino V, Ali MK. Effects of different dietary interventions on blood pressure systematic review and meta-analysis of randomized controlled trials. Hypertension. 2016;67:733–9. https://doi.org/10.1161/HypertensionAHA.115.06853.
16. Alonso A, de la Fuente C, Martin-Arnau AM, et al. Fruit and vegetable consumption is inversely associated with blood pressure in a Mediterranean population with a high vegetable-fat intake: the Seguimiento Universidad de Navarra (SUN) Study. Br J Nutr. 2004;92:311–9.
17. Appel LJ, Moore TJ, Obarzanek E, et al. A clinical trial of the effects of dietary patterns on blood pressure. N Engl J Med. 1997;336:1117–24.
18. Feng J, He FJ, Li J, MacGregor GA. Effect of longer term modest salt reduction on blood pressure: Cochrane systematic review and meta-analysis of randomised trials. BMJ. 2013;346:f1325. https://doi.org/10.1136/bmj.f1325.
19. Doménech M, Roman P, Lapetra J, et al. Mediterranean diet reduces 24-hour ambulatory blood pressure, blood glucose, and lipids one-year randomized, clinical trial. Hypertension. 2014;64:69–76.
20. Jayalath VH, de Souza RJ, Sievenpiper JL, et al. Effect of dietary pulses on blood pressure: a systematic review and meta-analysis of controlled feeding trials. Am J Hypertens. 2014;27(1):56–64.
21. Khalesi S, Irwin C, Schubert M. Flaxseed consumption may reduce blood pressure: a systematic review and meta-analysis of controlled trials. J Nutr. 2015;145(4):758–65. https://doi.org/10.3945/jn.114.205302.
22. Kochar J, Gaziano M, Djoussé L. Breakfast cereals and risk of hypertension in the physicians' health study. Clin Nutr. 2012;31(1):89–92.
23. Mohammadifard N, Salehi-Abargouei A, Salas-Salvadó J, et al. The effect of tree nut, peanut, and soy nut consumption on blood pressure: a systematic review and meta-analysis of randomized controlled clinical trials. Am J Clin Nutr. 2015;101:966–82.
24. Pins JJ, Geleva D, Keenan JM. Do whole-grain oat cereals reduce the need for antihypertensive medications and improve blood pressure control? J Fam Pract. 2002;14:353–9.
25. Ahhmed AM, Muguruma M. A review of meat protein hydrolysates and hypertension. Meat Sci. 2010;86(1):110–8.
26. Appleby PN, Davey GK, Key TJ. Hypertension and blood pressure among meat eaters, fish eaters, vegetarians and vegans in EPIC–Oxford. Public Health Nutr. 2002;5(5):645–54.
27. Mattei J, Noel S, Tucker KL. A meat, processed meat, and French fries dietary pattern is associated with high allostatic load in Puerto Rican older adults. J Am Diet Assoc. 2011;111(10):1498–506.
28. Lajous M, Bijon A, Fagherazzi G, et al. Processed and unprocessed red meat consumption and hypertension in women. Am J Clin Nutr. 2014;100:948–52.
29. Soedamah-Muthu SS, Verberne LDM, Ding EL, et al. Dairy consumption and incidence of hypertension a dose-response meta-analysis of prospective cohort studies. Hypertension. 2012;60:1131–7.
30. Ballard KD, Bruno RS. Protective role of dairy and its constituents on vascular function independent of blood pressure-lowering activities. Nutr Rev. 2014;3(1):36–50.
31. U.S. Department of Agriculture, Agriculture Research Service, Nutrient Data Laboratory. 2014. USDA National Nutrient Database for Standard Reference, Release 27. http://www.ars. usda.gov./nutrientdata. Accessed 17 Feb 2015.
32. Ros E, Hu FB. Consumption of plant seeds and cardiovascular health epidemiological and clinical trial evidence. Circulation. 2013;128:553–65.
33. USDA. What we eat in America, NHANES 2011-2012, individuals 2 years and over (excluding breast-fed children). Available: www.ars.usda.gov/nea/bhnrc/fsrg.
34. Slavin JL, Lloyd B. Health benefits of fruits and vegetables. Adv Nutr. 2012;3:506–16.
35. Rebello CJ, Greenway FL, Finley JW. A review of the nutritional value of legumes and their effects on obesity and its related co-morbidities. Obes Rev. 2014;15:392–407.
36. Gebhardt SE, Thomas RG. Nutritive value of foods. Washington, DC: U.S. Department of Agriculture, Agricultural Research Service, Home and Garden Bulletin 72; 2002.
37. Holden JM, Eldridge AL, Beecher GR, et al. Carotenoid content of U.S. foods: an update of the database. J Food Comp An. 1999;12:169–96.
38. Lu Q-Y, Zhang Y, Wang Y, et al. California Hass avocado: profiling of carotenoids, tocopherol, fatty acid, and fat content during maturation and from different growing areas. J Agric Food Chem. 2009;57(21):10408–13.
39. Wu X, Beecher GR, Holden JM, et al. Lipophilic and hydrophilic antioxidant capacities of common foods in the United States. J Agric Food Chem. 2004;52:4026–37.
40. Bhupathiraju SN, Tucker KL. Coronary heart disease prevention: nutrients, foods, and dietary patterns. Clin Chim Acta. 2011;412:1493–514.
41. Dietary Guidelines Advisory Committee. Scientific Report. Advisory Report to the Secretary of Health and Human Services and the Secretary of Agriculture. Part D. Chapter 1: Food and nutrient intakes, and health: current status and trends 2015;1–78. http://health.gov/ dietary guidelines/2015/guidelines/. Accessed 26 Jan 2016.
42. Sanchez-Muniz FJ. Dietary fibre and cardiovascular health. Nutr Hosp. 2012;27(1):31–45.
43. Yang T, Santisteban MM, Rodriguez V, et al. Gut dysbiosis is linked to hypertension. Hypertension. 2015;65:1331–40.
44. Pluznick JL. A novel SCFA receptor, the microbiota, and blood pressure regulation. Gut Microbes. 2014;5(2):202–7.

45. Leermakers ETM, Darweesh SKL, Baena CP, et al. The effects of lutein on cardiometabolic health across the life course: a systematic review and meta-analysis. Am J Clin Nutr. 2016;103:481–94.
46. Lillioja S, Neal AL, Tapsell L, et al. Whole grains, type 2 diabetes, coronary heart disease, and hypertension: links to the aleurone preferred over indigestible fiber. Biofactors. 2013;39(3):242–58.
47. Karl JP, Saltzman E. The role of whole grains in body weight regulation. Adv Nutr. 2012;3:697–707.
48. Seal CJ. Whole grains and CVD risk. Proc Nutr Soc. 2006;65:24–34.
49. Medina-Remón A, Tresserra-Rimbau A, Pons A, et al. Effects of total dietary polyphenols on plasma nitric oxide and blood pressure in a high cardiovascular risk cohort. The PREDIMED randomized trial. Nutr Metab Cardiovasc Dis. 2015;25(1):60–7. https://doi.org/10.1016/j.numecd. 2014.09.001.
50. Clark JL, Zahradka P, Taylor CG. Efficacy of flavonoids in the management of high blood pressure. Nutr Rev. 2015;73(12):799–822.
51. Hobbs DA, George TW, Lovegrove JA. The effects of dietary nitrate on blood pressure and endothelial function: a review of human intervention studies. Nutr Res Rev. 2013;26:210–22.
52. Micha R, Peñalvo JL, Cudhea F, et al. Association between dietary factors and mortality from heart disease, stroke, and type 2 diabetes in the United States. JAMA. 2017;317(9):912–24. https://doi.org/10.1001/jama.2017.0947.
53. http://wholegrainscouncil.org/whole-grains-101/what-counts-as-a-serving. Accessed 26 Dec 2015.
54. Seal CJ, Brownlee IA. Whole-grain foods and chronic disease: evidence from epidemiological and intervention studies. Proc Nutr Soc. 2015;74:313–9.
55. Karl JP, Meydani M, Barnett JB, et al. Substituting whole grains for refined grains in a 6-wk randomized trial favorably affects energy-balance metrics in healthy men and postmenopausal women. Am J Clin Nutr. 2017;105:589–99.
56. Mellen PB, Walsh TF, Herrington DM. Whole grain intake and cardiovascular disease: a meta-analysis. Nutr Metab Cardiovasc Dis. 2008;18(4):283–90.
57. Tang G, Wang D, Long J, et al. Meta-analysis of the association between whole grain intake and coronary heart disease risk. Am J Cardiol. 2015;115(5):625–9.
58. Ye EQ, Chacko SA, Chou EL, et al. Greater whole-grain intake is associated with lower risk of type 2 diabetes, cardiovascular disease, and weight gain. J Nutr. 2012;142:1304–13.
59. Flint AJ, FB H, Glynn RJ, et al. Whole grains and incident hypertension in men. Am J Clin Nutr. 2009;90:493–8.
60. Wang L, Gaziano JM, Liu S, et al. Whole- and refined-grain intakes and the risk of hypertension in women. Am J Clin Nutr. 2007;86:472–9.
61. Evans CEL, Greenwood DC, Threapleton DE, et al. Effects of dietary fibre type on blood pressure: a systematic review and meta-analysis of randomized controlled trials of health individuals. J Hypertension. 2015;33(5):897–911.
62. Thies F, Masson LF, Boffetta P, Kris-Etherton P. Oats and CVD risk markers: a systematic literature review. Br J Nutr. 2014;112:S19–30.
63. Kirwan JP, Malin SK, Scelsi AR, et al. Whole-grain diet reduces cardiovascular risk factors in overweight and obese adults: a randomized controlled trial. J Nutr. 2016;146:2244–51.
64. Tighe P, Duthie G, Vaughan N, et al. Effect of increased consumption of whole-grain foods on blood pressure and other cardiovascular risk markers in healthy middle-aged persons: a randomized controlled trial. Am J Clin Nutr. 2010;92:733–40.
65. Maki KC, Galant R, Samuel P, et al. Effects of consuming foods containing oat beta-glucan on blood pressure, carbohydrate metabolism and biomarkers of oxidative stress in men and women with elevated blood pressure. Eur J Clin Nutr. 2007;61:786–95.
66. Behall KM, Scholfield DJ, Hallfrisch J. Whole-grain diets reduce blood pressure in mildly hypercholesterolemic men and women. J Am Diet Assoc. 2006;106:1445–9.
67. He J, Streiffer RH, Muntner P, et al. Effect of dietary fiber intake on blood pressure: a randomized, double-blind, placebo-controlled trial. J Hypertens. 2004;22:73–80.
68. Davy BM, Melby CL, Beske SD, et al. Oat consumption does not affect resting casual and ambulatory 24-h arterial blood pressure in men with high-normal blood pressure to stage I hypertension. J Nutr. 2002;132:394–8.
69. Keenan JM, Joel J, Pins JJ, et al. Oat ingestion reduces systolic and diastolic blood pressure in patients with mild or borderline hypertension: a pilot trial. J Fam Pract. 2002;51:369–75.
70. Saltzman E, Das SK, Lichtenstein AH, et al. An oat-containing hypocaloric diet reduces systolic blood pressure and improves lipid profile beyond effects of weight loss in men and women. J Nutr. 2001;131:1465–70.
71. Kestin M, Moss R, Clifton PM, Nestel PJ. Comparative effects of three cereal brans on plasma lipids, blood pressure, and glucose metabolism in mildly hypercholesterolemic men. Am J Clin Nutr. 1990;52:661–6.
72. Fehily AM, Burr ML, Butland BK, Eastham RD. A randomised controlled trial to investigate the effect of a high fibre diet on blood pressure and plasma fibrinogen. J Epid Commun Health. 1986;40:334–7.
73. Rooney C, McKinley MC, Appleton KM, et al. How much is '5-a-day'? A qualitative investigation into consumer understanding of fruit and vegetable intake guidelines. J Hum Nutr Diet. 2017;30(1):105–13. https://doi.org/10.1111/jhn.12393.
74. United States Department of Agriculture. 2013. Choose my plate. http://www choosemyplategov/. Accessed 17 Feb 2015.
75. Micha R, Khatibzadeh S, Shi P, et al. Global, regional and national consumption of major food groups in

1990 and 2010: a systematic analysis including 266 country-specific nutrition surveys worldwide. BMJ Open. 2015;5(9):e008705. https://doi.org/10.1136/bmjopen-2015-008705.

76. Li B, Li F, Wang L, Zhang D. Fruit and vegetables consumption and risk of hypertension: a meta-analysis. J Clin Hypertens (Greenwich). 2016;18(5):468–76. https://doi.org/10.1111/jch.12777.
77. Wu L, Sun D, He Y. Fruit and vegetable consumption and incident hypertension: dose response meta-analysis of prospective cohort studies. J Hum Hypertens. 2016;30(10):573–80. https://doi.org/10.1038/jhh.2016.44.
78. Borgi L, Muraki I, Satija A, et al. Fruit and vegetable consumption and the incidence of hypertension in three prospective cohort studies. Hypertension. 2016;67:288–93.
79. Wang L, Manson JE, Gaziano JM, et al. Fruit and vegetable intake and the risk of hypertension in middle-aged and older women. Am J Hypertens. 2012;25(2):180–9.
80. Tsubota-Utsugi M, Ohkubo T, Kikuya M. High fruit intake is associated with a lower risk of future hypertension determined by home blood pressure measurement: the OHASAMA study. J Hum Hypertens. 2011;25(3):164–71.
81. Nunez-Cordoba JM, Alonso A, Beunza JJ, et al. Role of vegetables and fruits in Mediterranean diets to prevent hypertension. Eur J Clin Nutr. 2009;63:605–12.
82. Griep LMO, Stamler J, Chan Q, et al. Association of raw fruit and fruit juice consumption with blood pressure: the INTERMAP study. Am J Clin Nutr. 2013;97:1083–91.
83. Chan Q, Stamler J, Brown IJ, et al. Relation of raw and cooked vegetable consumption to blood pressure: the INTERMAP study. J Hum Hypertens. 2014;28:353–9.
84. Medina-Remon A, Vallverdu-Queralt A, Arranz S, et al. Gazpacho consumption is associated with lower blood pressure and reduced hypertension in a high cardiovascular risk cohort. Cross-sectional study of the PREDIMED trial. Nutr Metab Cardiov Dis. 2013;23(10):944–52.
85. Pase MP, Grima N, Cockerell R, Pipingas A. Habitual intake of fruit juice predicts central blood pressure. Appetite. 2015;84:68–72.
86. Hartley L, Igbinedion E, Holmes J, et al. Increased consumption of fruit and vegetables for the primary prevention of cardiovascular diseases. Cochrane Database of Systematic Rev. 2013;6:CD009874. https://doi.org/10.1002/14651858.CD009874.pub2.
87. Liu K, Xing A, Chen K. Effect of fruit juice on cholesterol and blood pressure in adults: a meta-analysis of 19 randomized controlled trials. PLoS One. 2013;8(4). https://doi.org/10.1371/journal. pone. 0061420.
88. Jovanovski E, Bosco L, Khan K, et al. Effect of spinach, a high dietary nitrate source, on arterial stiffness and related hemodynamic measures: a randomized, controlled trial in healthy adults. Clin Nutr Res. 2015;4:160–7.
89. Tjelle TE, Holtung L, Bøhn SK, et al. Polyphenol-rich juices reduce blood pressure measures in a randomised controlled trial in high normal and hypertensive volunteers. Br J Nutr. 2015;114:1054–63.
90. Novotny JA, Baer DJ, Khoo C, et al. Cranberry juice consumption lowers markers of cardiometabolic risk, including blood pressure and circulating C-reactive protein, triglyceride, and glucose concentrations in adults. J Nutr. 2015;145:1185–93.
91. Vinson JA, Demkosky CA, Navarre DA, Smyda MA. High-antioxidant potatoes: acute in vivo antioxidant source and hypotensive agent in humans after supplementation to hypertensive subjects. J Agric Food Chem. 2012;60:6749–54.
92. Berry SE, Mulla UZ, Chowienczyk PJ, et al. Increased potassium intake from fruit and vegetables or supplements does not lower blood pressure or improve vascular function in UK men and women with early hypertension: a randomised controlled trial. Br J Nutr. 2010;104:1839–47.
93. McCall DO, McGartland CP, McKinley MC, et al. Dietary intake of fruits and vegetables improves microvascular function in hypertensive subjects in a dose-dependent manner. Circulation. 2009;119:2153–60.
94. John JH, Ziebland S, Yudkin P, et al. Effects of fruit and vegetable consumption on plasma antioxidant concentrations and blood pressure: a randomized controlled trial. Lancet. 2002;359:1969–74.
95. Broekmans WMR, Klopping-Ketelaars WAA, Kluft C, et al. Fruit and vegetables and cardiovascular FV intake and risk of CVD risk profile: a diet controlled intervention study. Eur J Clin Nutr. 2001;55:636–42.
96. Smith-Warner SA, Elmer PJ, Tharp TM, et al. Increasing vegetable and fruit intake: randomized intervention and monitoring in an at-risk population. Cancer Epidemiol Biomarkers Prev. 2000;9(3):307–17.
97. Zheng J, Zhou Y, Li S, et al. Effects and mechanisms of fruit and vegetable juices on cardiovascular diseases. Int J Mol Sci. 2017;18:555. https://doi.org/10.3390/ijms18030555.
98. Sahebkar A, Ferri C, Giorgini P, et al. Effects of pomegranate juice on blood pressure: a systematic review and meta-analysis of randomized controlled trials. Pharmacological Res. 2017;115:149–61.
99. Bouchenak M, Lamri-Senhadji M. Nutritional quality of legumes, and their role in cardiometabolic risk prevention: a review. J Med Food. 2013;16(3):185–98.
100. Tielemans SMAJ, Altorf-van der Kuil W, Engberink MF, et al. Intake of total protein, plant protein and animal protein in relation to blood pressure: a meta-analysis of observational and intervention studies. J Human Hypertension. 2013;27:564–71.
101. Messina V. Nutritional and health benefits of dried beans. Am J Clin Nutr. 2014;100(suppl 1):437S–42S.
102. Afshin A, Micha R, Khatibzadeh S, Mozaffarian D. Consumption of nuts and legumes and risk of incident ischemic heart disease, stroke, and diabetes: a systematic review and meta-analysis. Am J Clin Nutr. 2014;100(1):278–88.

103. Jayalath VH, de Souza RJ, Sievenpiper JL, et al. Effect of dietary pulses on blood pressure: a systematic review and meta-analysis of controlled feeding trials. Am J Hypertension. 2014;27(1):56–64.
104. Lee YP, Puddey IB, Hodgson JM. Protein, fibre and blood pressure: potential benefit of legumes. Clin Exp Pharm Physiol. 2008;35:473–6.
105. Appel LJ, Sacks FM, Carey VJ, et al. Effects of protein, monounsaturated fat, and carbohydrate intake on blood pressure and serum lipids results of the OmniHeart Randomized Trial. JAMA. 2005;294:2455–64.
106. Yang G, Shu XO, Jin F, et al. Longitudinal study of soy food intake and blood pressure among middle-aged and elderly Chinese women. Am J Clin Nutr. 2005;81:1012–7.
107. Nagata C, Shimizu H, Takami R, et al. Association of blood pressure with intake of soy products and other food groups in Japanese men and women. Prev Med. 2003;36:692–7.
108. Dong J-Y, Tong X, Z-W W, et al. Meta-analysis: effect of soya protein on blood pressure: a meta-analysis of randomised controlled trials. Br J Nutr. 2011;106:317–26.
109. Rivas M, Garay RP, Escanero JF, et al. Soy milk lowers blood pressure in men and women with mild to moderate essential hypertension. J Nutr. 2002;132:1900–2.
110. He J, Wofford MR, Reynolds K, et al. Effect of dietary protein supplementation on blood pressure: a randomized controlled trial. Circulation. 2011;124(5):589–95.
111. He J, Gu D, Xigui W, et al. Effect of soybean protein on blood pressure: a randomized, controlled trial. Ann Intern Med. 2005;143(1):1–9.
112. Ros E. Nuts and CVD. Br J Nutr. 2015;113:S111–20.
113. Prasad K. Flaxseed and cardiovascular disease. J Cardiovasc Pharmacol. 2009;54(5):369–77.
114. Novotny JA, Gebauer SK, Baer DJ. Discrepancy between the Atwater factor predicted and empirically measured energy values of almonds in human diets. Am J Clin Nutr. 2012;96:296–301.
115. Mattes RD, Kris-Etherton PM, Foster GD. Impact of peanuts and tree nuts on body weight and healthy weight loss in adults. J Nutr. 2008;138(suppl):1741S–5S.
116. Traoret CJ, Lokko P, Cruz ACRF, et al. Peanut digestion and energy balance. Int J Obes. 2008;32:322–8.
117. Brown RC, Tey SL, Gray AR, et al. Nut consumption is associated with better nutrient intakes: results from the 2008/09 New Zealand Adult Nutrition Survey. Br J Nutr. 2016;115:105–12.
118. Nielsen SJ, Kit BK, Ogden CL. Nut consumption among U.S. adults, 2009-2010. NCHS data brief, no 176. Hyattsville, MD: National Center for Health Statistics 2014.
119. Luu HN, Blot WJ, Xiang Y-B, et al. Prospective evaluation of the association of nut/peanut consumption with total and cause-specific mortality. JAMA Intern Med. 2015;175(5):755–66.
120. Ma L, Wang F, Guo W, et al. Nut consumption and the risk of coronary artery disease: a dose-response meta-analysis of 13 prospective studies. Thromb Res. 2014;134(4):790–4.
121. Yazdekhasti N, Mohammadifard N, Sarrafzadegan N, et al. The relationship between nut consumption and blood pressure in an Iranian adult population: Isfahan Healthy Heart. Program. 2013;23(10):929–36.
122. Djoussé L, Rudich T, Gaziano JM. Nut consumption and risk of hypertension in US male physicians. Clin Nutr. 2009;28(1):10–4.
123. Weng L-C, Steffen LM, Szklo M, et al. Diet pattern with more dairy and nuts, but less meat is related to lower risk of developing hypertension in middle-aged adults: the Atherosclerosis Risk in Communities (ARIC) study. Forum Nutr. 2013;5: 1719–33.
124. Martınez-Lapiscina EH, Pimenta AM, Beunza JJ, et al. Nut consumption and incidence of hypertension: the SUN prospective cohort. Nutr Metab Cardiov Dis. 2010;20(5):359–65.
125. Del Gobbo LC, Falk MC, Feldman R, et al. Effects of tree nuts on blood lipids, apolipoproteins, and blood pressure: systematic review, meta-analysis, and dose-response of 61 controlled intervention trials. Am J Clin Nutr. 2015;102(6):1347–56. https://doi.org/10.3945/ajcn. 115.110965.
126. Rodriguez-Leyva D, Weighell W, Edel AL, et al. Potent antihypertensive action of dietary flaxseed in hypertensive patients. Hypertension. 2013;62: 1081–89.
127. Khosravi-Boroujeni H, Nikbakht E, Natanelov E, Khalesi S. Can sesame consumption improve blood pressure? A systematic review and meta-analysis of controlled trials. J Sci Food Agric. 2017; doi: https://doi.org/10.1002/jsfa.8361.
128. Cardoso CA, de Oliveira GM, Gouveia LA, et al. The effect of dietary intake of sesame (Sesamumindicum L.) derivatives related to the lipid profile and blood pressure: a systematic review. Crit Rev Food Sci Nutr. 2016; doi: https://doi.org/10.1080/10408398.2015.1137858.
129. Yarmolinsky J, Gon G, Edwards P. Effect of tea on blood pressure for secondary prevention of cardiovascular disease: a systematic review and meta-analysis of randomized controlled trials. Nutr Rev. 2015;73(4):236–46.
130. Peng X, Zhou R, Wang B, et al. Effect of green tea consumption on blood pressure: a meta-analysis of 13 randomized controlled trials. Sci Rep. 2014;4:6251.
131. Greyling A, Ras RT, Zock PL et al. The effect of black tea on blood pressure: a systematic rReview with meta-analysis of randomized controlled trials. PLoS ONE. 2014;9(7):e103247.
132. Liu G, Mi X-N, Zheng X-X, et al. Effects of tea intake on blood pressure: a meta-analysis of randomised controlled trials. Br J Nutr. 2014;112(7): 1043–54.

133. Cook NR. Implications of small reductions in diastolic blood pressure for primary prevention. Arch Intern Med. 1995;155(7):701–9.
134. Miranda A, Steluti J, Fisberg R, Marchioni D. Association between coffee consumption and its polyphenols with cardiovascular risk factors: a population-based study. Nutrients. 2017;9(3):276.
135. Loader TB, Taylor cG, Zahradka P, Jones PJH. Chlorogenic acid from coffee beans: evaluating the evidence for a blood pressure – regulating health claim. Nutr Rev. 2017;75(2):114–33.
136. Horst K, Robinson WD, Jenkins WL, Bao DL. The effect of caffeine, coffee and decaffeinated coffee upon blood pressure, pulse rate and certain motor reactions of normal young men. J Pharmacol Exp. 1934;52:307–21.
137. Turnbull D, Rodricks JV, Mariano GF, Chowdhury F. Caffeine and cardiovascular health. Regul Toxicol Pharmacol. 2017;89:165–85.
138. Zhang Z, Hu G, Caballero B, et al. Habitual coffee consumption and risk of hypertension: a systematic review and meta-analysis of prospective observational studies. Am JClin Nutr. 2011;93(6):1212–19.
139. Rhee JJ, Qin F, Hedlin HK, et al. Coffee and caffeine consumption and the risk of hypertension in postmenopausal women. Am J Clin Nutr. 2016;103(1):210–17.
140. Mesas AE, Leon-Munoz LM, Rodriguez-Artalejo F, Lopez-Garcia E. The effect of coffee on blood pressure and cardiovascular disease in hypertensive individuals: a systematic review and meta-analysis. Am J Clin Nutr. 2011;94(4):1113–26.

Dietary Patterns, Foods and Beverages in Chronic Kidney Disease

15

Keywords
Chronic kidney disease • Dietary fiber • Dietary patterns • Hypertension • Inflammation • Microalbuminuria • Obesity • Glomercular filtration rate • Whole foods

Key Points

- The prevalence of chronic kidney disease (CKD) is high (estimated 200 million people worldwide) and steadily increasing, especially in older populations, and it is associated with increased risk of renal cancer, cardiovascular disease, and bone disorders and fractures.
- The Western diet is associated with increased renal dysfunction, CKD risk and progression to end stage renal disease (ESRD).
- A healthy diet for CKD patients should help to slow the rate of progression of kidney failure, reduce uremic toxicity, decrease proteinuria, and lower the risk of secondary complications including cardiovascular disease, bone disease, and hypertension.
- Lower dietary energy density and higher fiber healthy dietary patterns can play a role in lowering the risk of CKD. Protein sources vary in their effect on CKD risk with red and processed meat consumption significantly increasing risk whereas higher intake of nuts, legumes, and low-fat dairy products may lower risk.
- Increased fiber intake triggers a number of physiologic processes in both the colon microbiota and systemically that support the detoxification of the kidneys, via influences on the gut barrier, gastrointestinal immune and endocrine responses, nitrogen cycling, and microbial metabolism which alter the physiology and biochemistry of the kidneys to help re-establish homeostasis.
- Healthy dietary patterns including fiber-rich whole-grains, fruits and vegetables may improve renal function, and decrease metabolic acidosis compared to poor quality diets low in fruits and vegetables and high in processed foods and animal products. High adherence to healthy dietary patterns such as the Dietary Approaches to Stop Hypertension (DASH), especially a modified version of the DASH diet for people with CKD, and the Mediterranean diet (MedDiet) may help to reduce CKD risk, progression to later stages and mortality.

M.L. Dreher, *Dietary Patterns and Whole Plant Foods in Aging and Disease*, Nutrition and Health,
https://doi.org/10.1007/978-3-319-59180-3_15

15.1 Introduction

The kidney is a highly-vascularized organ, which plays a major role regulating electrolyte concentrations, blood pressure, energy metabolic hormones, and excretion of waste metabolites. The prevalence of chronic kidney disease (CKD) is high (estimated 200 million people worldwide) and steadily increasing, especially in older populations, and it is associated with increased risk of renal cancer, cardiovascular disease, and bone disorders and fractures [1–9]. In the US, the estimates of CKD in the general population is 14% with approximately 500,000 individuals on dialysis and 200,000 living with kidney transplants [7]. The prevalence of CKD in individuals over age 60 is estimated to be up to 25% [3–5]. African Americans have a four-fold higher risk of CKD compared to Caucasians. CKD patients experience an increased rate of mortality by 59% compared with healthy individuals as more people die from CKD each year than from breast or prostate cancer. CKD usually develops over many years and leads to end-stage kidney (or renal) disease (ESRD) [7]. There are 5 stages of CKD: (1) normal kidney function (estimated glomerular filtration rate (eGFR) ≥90 mL/min per 1.73 m^2) with persistent proteinuria (≥3 months); (2) kidney damage with mild loss of kidney function (eGFR 60–89 mL/min per 1.73 m^2) and persistent proteinuria (≥3 months); (3) mild-to-severe loss of kidney function (eGFR 30–59 mL/min per 1.73 m^2); (4) severe loss of kidney function (eGFR 15–29 mL/min per 1.73 m^2); and (5) kidney failure or ESRD (eGFR <15 mL/min per 1.73 m^2) requiring dialysis or transplant for survival [7].

Western dietary patterns, diabetes and obesity are important risk factors associated with the increased risk of CKD [10, 11]. Western dietary patterns, rich in refined carbohydrates, salt, fat and protein from red meat, and low in fiber-rich foods, are generally associated with increased risk of CKD. A systematic review and meta-analysis (39 cohort studies; 630,677 participants; mean 6.8 years of follow-up) found that obesity in the general population increased risk of low eGFR by 28% and albuminuria by 51% [12]. A high BMI predicts onset of albuminuria without kidney failure (CKD stages 1–2) as well as CKD stages 3 and higher. Abdominal obesity is considered a major risk factor for CKD development and progression (Fig. 15.1) [13–16]. An analysis

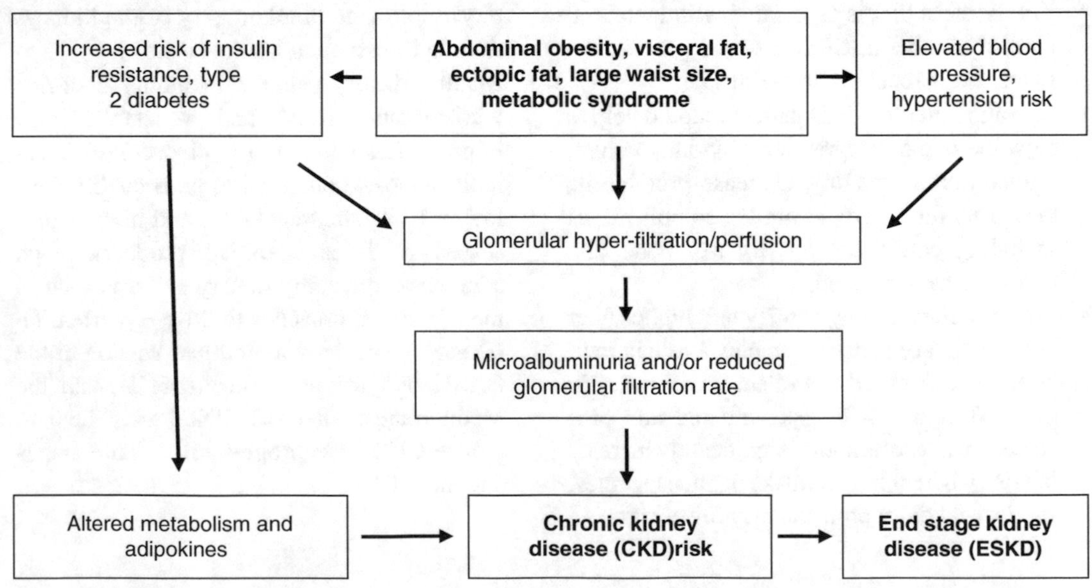

Fig. 15.1 Effect of abdominal obesity related conditions and chronic kidney disease (CDK) risk (adapted from [13–16])

of data from the US NHANES 1999–2010 (6918 young adults; ages 20–40 years) found that abdominal obesity in young adults, especially in Mexican-Americans, was independently associated with 3.5-fold higher odds of the CKD risk factor albuminuria even with normal blood pressures, normoglycemia and normal insulin levels [17]. Initially, ectopic fat causes renal vasodilation and glomerular hyper-filtration, which act as compensatory mechanisms to maintain sodium balance but the increased arterial pressure and metabolic abnormalities, may ultimately lead to glomerular injury [18]. Specifically, increased ectopic fat in the kidney can cause physical compression of the kidney's renal vein and artery that pass through the renal sinus increasing renal interstitial pressure, decreasing sodium excretion and stimulating inflammation, oxidative stress, and lipotoxicity factors that may also contribute to renal dysfunction associated with hypertension and CKD.

Healthy diets are important for patients with CKD as proper nutrition helps to prevent infection and prevent kidney disease from worsening. Nutrition requirements differ depending on the level of kidney function and the presence of co-morbid conditions, including hypertension, diabetes, and cardiovascular disease. The CKD patients' diet should help to slow the rate of progression of kidney failure, reduce uremic toxicity, decrease proteinuria, and lower the risk of secondary complications including cardiovascular disease, bone disease, and hypertension. The objective of this chapter is to comprehensively review the effects of dietary patterns, foods, nutrients and beverages on CKD risk and management.

15.2 Lifestyle and Chronic Kidney Disease (CKD)

The American Heart Association (AHA) Life's Simple 7, which includes: (1) non-smoking or quit >1 year ago; (2) BMI < 25; (3) blood pressure (BP) <120/80 mm Hg; (4) ≥ 150 min/week of physical activity; (5) a healthy dietary pattern (high in fruits and vegetables, fish, fiber-rich whole grains, (6) low intake of sodium, and (7) limiting or avoiding sugar-sweetened beverages, has been shown to reduce CKD risk [19]. The Atherosclerosis Risk in Communities (ARIC) cohort study (14,832 participants; mean age 54 years; 55% female; 26% blacks; BMI range 23–31; median 22-year follow-up; 2743 CKD cases) showed a significant inverse association between the adherence to Life's Simple **7** goals and incident CKD (Fig. 15.2) [19]. Individual factors significantly associated with lower CKD risk were non-cigarette smoking, BMI < 25, increased physical activity, and lower BP and fasting blood glucose but not healthy diet score or total cholesterol. The Chronic Renal Insufficiency Cohort (CRIC) Study (3006 persons with mild-to-moderate CKD; mean age 58 years; 48% female; 47% non-Hispanic white, 45% diabetes; median follow-up of 4 years; 726 CKD progression events, 353 atherosclerotic events, and 437 deaths) found that greater adherence to all components of a healthy lifestyle were associated with 68% reduced risk for adverse outcomes, including progression of CKD, atherosclerotic events and all-cause mortality [20].

15.3 Protein and Dietary Fiber

15.3.1 Protein

Dietary proteins are digested to amino acids, including acidic amino acids such as aspartic and glutamic and basic amino acids with an amine functional such as lysine, arginine, and histidine [21]. Proteins from meat products (from a typical Western diet) generate predominantly acidic products including hydrogen chloride, sulfuric acid, and phosphoric acids. These acids are non-volatile and rely on the kidneys for their excretion (primarily in the form of ammonium salts and phosphoric salts). A healthy individual generates net acids, approximately 1 mEq/kg/day (mmol/kg/day), which is rapidly buffered by sodium bicarbonate to form sodium salts. During this process, bicarbonate is consumed, which needs to be regenerated, a task accomplished by the kidneys. In patients with reduced kidney function, nonvolatile acids can accumulate

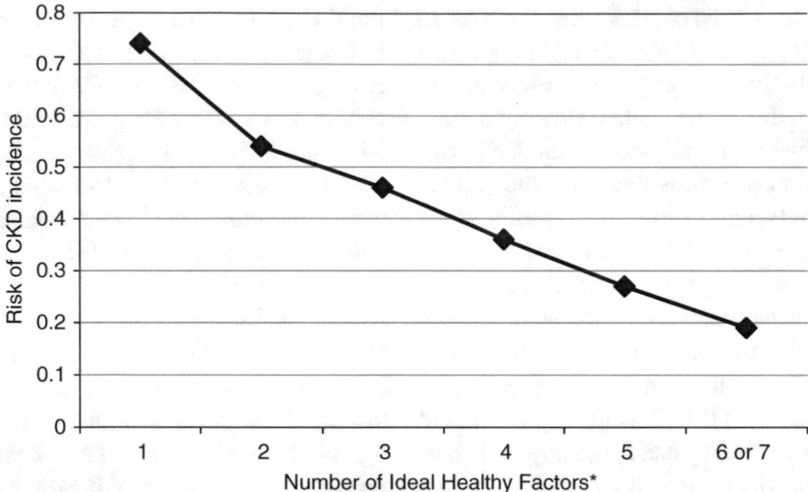

Fig. 15.2 Dose-response relationship between number of ideal Life's Simple 7 health factors and chronic kidney disease (CKD) incidence (p-trend <0.001; multivariate adjusted) (adapted from [19]). * (1) non-smoking or quit >1 year ago; (2) BMI < 25; (3) blood pressure (BP) <120/80 mm Hg; (4) ≥ 150 min/week of physical activity; (5) healthy dietary pattern (high in fruits and vegetables, fish, fiber-rich whole grains; (6) low intake of sodium; and (7) low intake or avoidance of sugar-sweetened beverages

causing metabolic acidosis and leading to progressive kidney damage associated with defects in acid excretion, systemic inflammation, end-organ hormone resistance and uremic toxin accumulation. Consequently, dietary protein restriction is recommended for patients with moderate to severe renal insufficiency with plant and low-fat dairy protein sources more effective than red and processed meat sources in reducing the risk and progression of CKD [22]. In the 2017 US Atherosclerosis Risk in Communities study (11,952 adults; aged 44–66 years; estimated baseline glomerular filtration rate (eGFR) ≥ 60 mL/min/1.73 m^2; 23 years of follow-up; 2.632 CKD cases) found that red and processed meat consumption was associated with significantly increased CKD risk by 23% whereas higher intake of nuts, legumes, and low-fat dairy products was associated with a significantly lower CKD risk by 12 to 17% (Fig. 15.3) [22]. The Netherlands Doetinchem Cohort study (3798 participants, mean baseline age 45 years; 52% women; examined 3 times 5 years apart) found that the daily consumption of ≥2 servings milk and milk products or low-fat dairy was associated with less annual decline in the eGFR in the subgroup of participants with mildly decreased eGFR [23]. Intakes of total and plant protein, and dairy products are generally not associated with eGFR changes.

15.3.2 Dietary Fiber

Lower dietary energy density and higher fiber intake from fruits , vegetables, whole grains, legumes and nuts are associated with better overall health and lower risk of CKD risk and progression [24–26]. However, fruits and vegetables, important fiber sources but rich in potassium, are often restricted in advanced CKD to prevent or correct hyperkalemia [26]. Examples, of fiber-rich lower potassium fruit and vegetables include apples, blueberries, cabbage, red bell peppers, cauliflower and onions. Adequate fiber intake is particularly important for promoting kidney health and protecting against advanced stage CKD by triggering a number of physiologic processes in both the colon microbiota and systemically that lead to the detoxification of kidneys, via its influences on the gut barrier, gastrointestinal immune and endocrine responses, nitrogen cycling and microbial metabolism which alter the physiology and

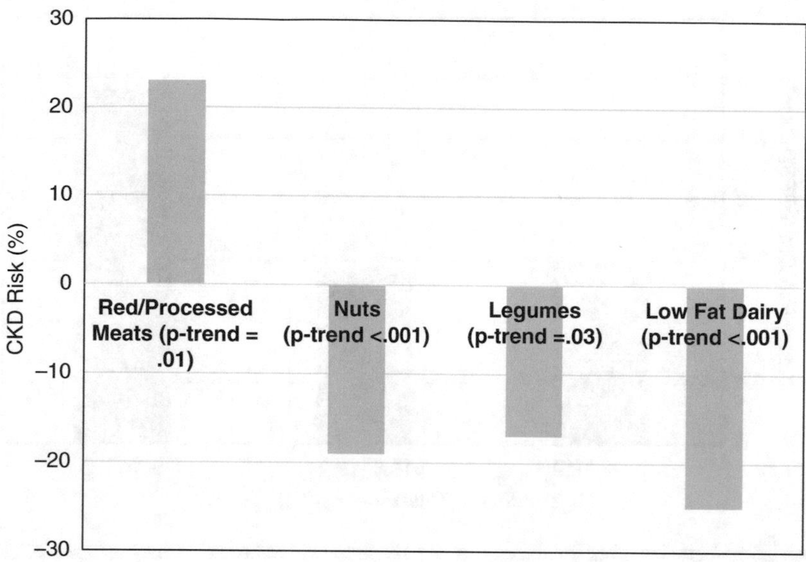

Fig. 15.3 Association between protein source and chronic kidney disease (CKD) risk (adapted from [22])

biochemistry of the kidneys to help re-establish homeostasis [27]. Further, higher fiber intake increases microbial sequestration of nitrogen in the colon, resulting in increased fecal nitrogen excretion and reduced concentrations of nitrogenous metabolites in the blood, which reduces nitrogenous burden on the kidneys helping reduce risk of CKD development or progression. A systematic review and meta-analysis (14 RCTs;143 CKD patients; median age 52 years; fiber supplemented/high fiber diets vs. non-supplemented/ low-fiber diets; median fiber 27 g/day; median protein 60 g/day; median follow-up 4.5 weeks) found that fiber supplementation significantly reduced serum urea by 1.8 mmol/L and serum creatinine by 22.8 mmol/L [28]. Several observational studies demonstrated that increased fiber intake may be especially effective at reducing systemic inflammation in CKD patients and mortality risk [29, 30]. The Third National Health and Nutrition Examination Survey (NHANES III) (14,533 adults; mean age 45 years; 48% males; prevalence of CKD 5.8%) found that for each 10 g/day increase in total fiber intake, the odds of elevated serum C-reactive protein levels were decreased in individuals without CKD by 11% and with CKD by 38% [29]. Also, total fiber intake was not significantly associated with overall mortality in those without CKD but was inversely related to mortality in those with kidney disease. Each 10 g/day increase in intake was associated with reduced overall mortality risk for total fiber by 17%, for insoluble fiber by 23% and soluble fiber by 33%. This study suggests that increased fiber intake in CKD individuals may lower systemic inflammation and mortality risk. The Uppsala Longitudinal Study of Adult Men (1110 community-dwelling elderly men from Sweden; mean age 71 years; mean BMI 26; median 10 years of follow-up; 300 deaths, 138 cardiovascular disease, 111cancer, 19 infections, 33 other causes) showed that high fiber intake was associated with significantly better kidney function (Fig. 15.4), lower odds of having C-reactive protein (CRP) >3 mg/L and reduced risk of mortality [30]. Total fiber was independently and directly associated with significantly improved eGFR (adjusted difference, 2.6 mL/min per 1.73m^2) per 10 g/day higher intake. Meta-analysis (14 RCTs) showed that increased fiber intake by 8 g/day from supplements or fiber-rich foods compared with control significantly reduced CRP levels by about 0.5 mg/L and for those individuals with elevated CRP the reduction was 0.72 mg/dL (p = 0.06) [31]. Lowering CRP has been associated with reduced incidence and complication of CKD as

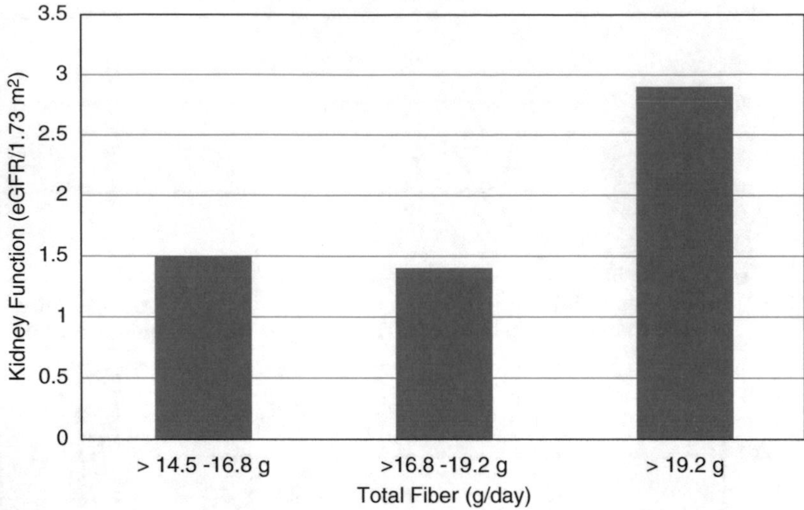

Fig. 15.4 Association between fiber intake/day in elderly men with chronic kidney disease (CKD) and kidney glomerular filtration rate (eGFR) ($p = 0.02$) (adapted from [30])

elevated CRP has been associated with impaired eGFR in hypertensive adults with a mean age of 60 years [32]. There is increasing clinical evidence that individuals at risk or patients with CKD have distinctly dysbiotic colonic microbiota, which can activate a cascade of metabolic abnormalities, including uremic toxin production, inflammation, and immunosuppression, that may lead to CKD or ultimately promotes progressive kidney failure [33, 34]. Several human studies show that increased fiber intake can lower circulating p-cresol and indoxyl sulfate [34, 35]. A single-blind RCT (6 males and 7 females; mean age 65 years; eGFR <50 mL/min/1.73m^2) showed that increasing fiber intake from 17 g to 27 g/day significantly reduced circulating p-cresol by 20% [35]. In a cross-sectional analysis (40 CKD patients; mean age 69; 60% male; 45% diabetic; mean estimated eGFR of 24 mL/min/1.73 m^2), it was demonstrated that total fiber intake was significantly associated with lower free and total serum p-cresol sulfate but not indoxyl sulfate [36]. This kidney-colonic axis may provide new nutritional CKD therapeutic opportunities involving the microbiota and fiber, prebiotics, probiotics, and symbiotics. Appendix A provides a list of 50 top fiber-rich plant foods.

15.4 Whole Plant Foods

15.4.1 Whole-grains

Organizations such as the National Kidney Foundation, the American Kidney Fund, the National Institute of Diabetes and Digestive and Kidney Diseases, and the US Department of Health and Human Services have previously recommended not including whole grains as part of the renal diet because of the potential risk of excessive phosphorus intake [37]. However, the phosphorus content in whole-grains is covalently bound to organic molecules (primarily phytate) and requires the enzyme phytase to be released to become available for absorption. While some phytase is contained in some raw whole grains (corn, oats, and millet have little to no phytase activity), the enzyme is decreased in milling, food preparation and over time. Also, since the enzyme required for the release of phosphorus from phytate is not present in the human intestinal lumen, when ingesting cooked food, the bioavailability of phosphorus from whole grains is low. The Australian Blue Mountains Eye Study (2600 participants; aged ≥50 years; 19.4% had moderate CKD and 80.6% did not have CKD; 5 years of follow-up) found

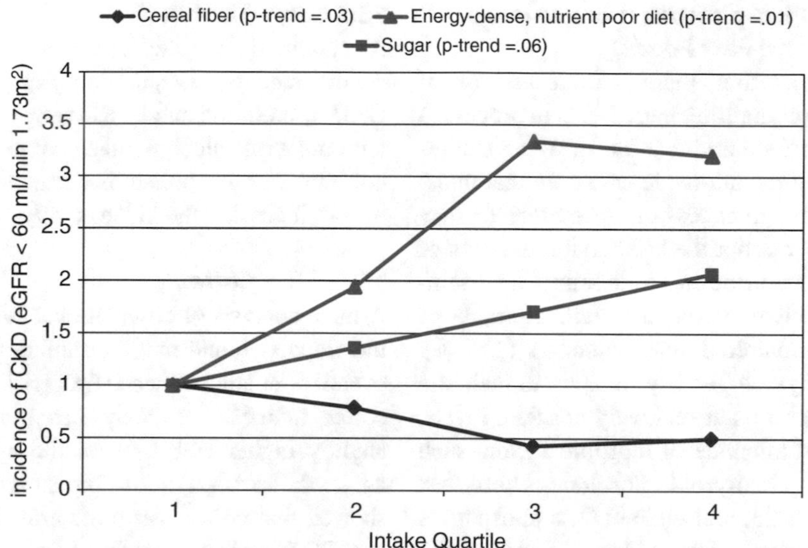

Fig. 15.5 Dietary factors associated with 5-year incidence of chronic kidney disease (CKD) from a cross-sectional analysis of 2600 Australian adults (≥50 years) in the Blue Mountains Eye Study (adapted from [38])

that fiber from cereal (predominantly from rolled oats and wholemeal/wholegrain breads) significantly lowered adjusted incidence of CKD by 50% and energy dense, nutrient poor foods significantly increased risk by 220% (Fig. 15.5) [38]. Consequently, it has been proposed that modest consumption of whole-grains by CKD patients may provide benefits to help protect against CKD and other chronic diseases. A parallel RCT (52 CKD patients; control diet vs. control plus 50 g oats/day) found that the added oats beneficially lowered serum albumin and serum potassium [39], This is consistent with the fiber -colon microbiota-kidney detoxification axis described previously [28].

15.4.2 Fruits and Vegetables

A highly adhered to Western-type diet is deficient in fruits and vegetables and contains excessive red and processed meat products which can promote metabolic acidosis, which increases progressively with aging due to the physiological decline in kidney function [40]. Two RCTs in stage 3 or 4 CKD patients suggest that increased fruit and vegetable intake or oral bicarbonate are equally effective in reducing urinary acidosis and in preserving glomerular filtration rate [41, 42]. An Australian prospective cohort study (145 adults with stage 3 or 4 CKD; 3 years of follow-up) found that increased fruits and vegetables lowered risk of CKD progression by 39% and improved survival by 65% [43].

15.5 Food Ingredients and Beverages

15.5.1 Minerals

15.5.1.1 Sodium (Salt)

High salt intake is associated with both increased blood pressure (BP) and worsening of kidney function. A 2015 Cochrane Systematic Review (8 RCTs; 258 subjects with CKD; 1 to 26 weeks) found that salt reduction in people with CKD reduced BP, 24-hour sodium excretion and proteinuria, which are predictive of long-term improvement of kidney function, slower progression to ESRD and reduced mortality risk [44]. However, longer-term RCTs with CKD patients on restricted salt diets are needed to confirm the benefits suggested by the current short-term RCTs.

15.5.1.2 Phosphorous (Convenience and Fast Foods)

In the Western diet, there is increased use of phosphorus-containing ingredients in processed convenience food and fast foods. Acute studies in healthy young adults demonstrate that phosphorus intakes in excess of nutrient needs may significantly disrupt the hormonal regulation of phosphorus contributing to dysfunctional mineral metabolism, vascular calcification, bone loss, and impaired kidney function [45, 46]. Although physiological systems try to maintain serum phosphorus at relatively constant levels, through the influence of multiple factors-such as aging, parathyroid hormone, fibroblast growth factor 23, and vitamin D, a phosphorus imbalance can affect kidney, bone health (osteoporosis), and the digestive system. Excessive dietary phosphate intake can elevate serum phosphate even in individuals with normal kidney function and higher serum phosphorus has been associated with increased adverse events and cardiovascular-related mortality both in people with CKD and in those with no evidence of disease.

15.5.1.3 Magnesium

The Healthy Aging in Neighborhoods of Diversity Across the Life Span Study (177 participants; mean age 47 years; 5-year follow-up) found that low magnesium intake was significantly associated with a doubling of the odds for rapid eGFR decline, after multivariate adjustments [47]. Good sources of magnesium include: green leafy vegetables, such as spinach, legumes, nuts, seeds, and whole grains.

15.5.2 Beverages

15.5.2.1 Sugar Sweetened Beverages

A systemic review and meta-analysis (5 sugar and 4 artificially sweetened cohorts) found that high intake of sugar sweetened beverages was associated with a 25% higher risk CKD progression than artificially sweetened sodas [48].

15.5.2.2 Alcohol

A systematic review and meta-analysis (20 cohort studies; 292,431 subjects) found that CKD, proteinuria and ESRD were not associated with moderate alcohol intake but excessive alcohol intake or alcoholism is detrimental to health overall including the kidneys [49].

15.5.2.3 Coffee

A meta-analysis (4 observational studies; 14,898 individuals) found that consuming coffee in the overall population reduced CKD risk by 29%, and coffee intake >1 cup/day was associated with slightly higher eGFR in middle age and older adults (> 46 years) [50]. The subgroup analysis showed that coffee was more effective in reducing CKD risk in women than in men. Overall, this study concludes that coffee consumption should not be a concern for CKD risk in the general population. The various components of coffee that may preserve the glomerular endothelial cells from oxidative stress include caffeine, hydroxychloroquine, quinides, niacin and chlorogenic acid.

15.6 Dietary Patterns

Western diets have resulted in increased intake of animal protein, refined carbohydrates, phosphate- and sodium-based preservatives, and led to higher risk of abdominal obesity, and systemic inflammation associated with CKD risk and progression to end stage renal disease (ESRD) [10, 11, 41]. Healthy dietary patterns consisting of mostly whole plant foods and lower in processed foods and meats have been shown to improve renal function, reduce CKD risk and delay progression and mortality risk in older adults at increased risk of CKD. While healthy dietary patterns, such as the DASH or Mediterranean diets (MedDiets), may help prevent CKD progression in early stage, specific renal diets with lower protein, sodium and phosphorus may be required in advance stages of renal insufficiency. Table 15.1 provides a summary of 2 meta-analyses, 9 prospective cohort studies and 2 intervention trials including one DASH diet and one MedDiet [51–63].

Table 15.1 Summary of dietary quality and dietary pattern studies on the risk and progression of chronic kidney disease (CKD) and mortality

Objective	Study details	Results
Meta-analyses		
Kelly et al. (2017) Assess the effect of healthy dietary patterns on CKD risk of end stage renal disease (ESRD) and mortality [51]	7 cohort studies; 15,285 participants with CKD; 3983 events; healthy dietary patterns generally consisted of higher fruits and vegetables, fish, legumes, cereals, whole grains and fiber and lower in red meats, salt and added sugar	Six studies showed that healthy dietary patterns were consistently associated with 27% lower mortality risk. One study found no significant association with a healthy diet and ESRD risk
Prospective cohort studies		
Lui et al. (2017) Explore the association between a DASH diet and CKD end points ([Healthy Aging in Neighborhoods of Diversity Across the Life Span study; US) [52]	1534 participants; mean age 48 years; 59% African-American; baseline estimated globular filtration rate (eGFR) > 60 mL/min/1.73 m^2; 5 years of follow-up (multivariate adjusted)	High energy intake and low DASH diet intake in participants with hypertension had a 68% increased risk of rapid decline of eGFR but not among participants without hypertension
Rebholz et al. (2016) Assess the effect of the DASH diet on risk of CKD (Atherosclerosis Risk in Communities (ARIC) Study; US) [53]	3720 participants with baseline eGFR >60 mL/min/1.73 m^2; 23 years of follow-up (multivariate adjusted)	A low DASH diet score was associated with 16% higher risk of CKD (p-trend <0.001; multivariate adjusted)
Smyth et al. (2016) Investigate the effect of diet quality on renal outcomes (NIH-AARP Diet and Health Study; US) [54]	544,635 participants; age 51–70 years; diets: Alternate Healthy Eating Index (AHEI), Healthy Eating Index (HEI), Mediterranean diet (MedDiet) score, Dietary Approach to Stop Hypertension (DASH) scores; 14.3 years of follow-up (multivariate adjusted)	All the healthy dietary patterns were associated with significantly improved renal function by 18–29%. Greater than 3.6 g sodium/day was associated with a 17% increased risk of renal dysfunction and adequate potassium was associated with a 17% reduced risk of renal dysfunction
Banerjee et al. (2015) Examine the association between dietary acid load and progression to ESRD (US National Health and Nutrition Examination Survey III; US) [55]	1486 adults with CKD; median 14.2 years of follow-up; 311 (20.9%) participants developed ESRD (multivariate adjusted)	Higher levels of dietary acid load typical of the Western diet were associated with a doubling of the risk of ESRD; for the highest tertile and 81% for the middle tertile compared with the lowest tertile in the fully adjusted model
Foster et al. (2015) Determine the association of lifestyle characteristics with estimated glomerular filtration rate (eGFR) <60 mL/min/1.73 m^2 and rapid eGFR decline in older adults (Framingham Offspring Study; US) [56]	1802 participants; mean age 59 years, 54.8% women; measures of diet quality, physical activity, alcohol intake, current smoking status; 6.6 years of follow-up; 9.5% of participants developed incident eGFR <60 (multivariate adjusted)	Higher diet quality was associated with a significant 37% reduced odds of renal dysfunction in fully adjusted models. Higher diet quality was associated with 31% lower risk of rapid eGFR decline. No associations were observed with physical activity, smoking status, or alcohol intake with incident eGFR <60 or rapid eGFR decline

(continued)

Table 15.1 (continued)

Objective	Study details	Results
Gutierrez et al. (2014) Assess relationships between dietary patterns and health outcomes in persons with CKD. (Reasons for Geographic and Racial Differences in Stroke (REGARDS) study; US) [57]	3972 participants with CKD; mean age 69 years; 5 empirically derived dietary patterns identified via factor analysis: convenience (Chinese and Mexican foods, pizza, other mixed dishes), plant-based (fruits, vegetables); sweets/fats (sugary foods); Southern (fried foods, organ meats, sweetened beverages); and alcohol/salads (alcohol, green-leafy vegetables, salad dressing); 6 years of follow-up; 816 deaths and 141 ESRD events (multivariate adjusted)	Higher plant-based pattern scores were associated with lower risk of mortality by 23% whereas higher Southern pattern scores were associated with greater risk of mortality by 51% (highest vs. lowest quartiles) (Fig. 15.6). There were no associations of dietary patterns with incident ESRD in multivariable-adjusted models
Chang et al. (2013) Investigate the effect of the DASH diet on risk of coronary heart disease and CKD (Coronary Artery Risk Development in Young Adults [CARDIA] Study; US) [58]	2354 African-American and white participants; mean age 35 years; 47% male; DASH vs. Western diets; 15-year follow-up; 3.3% developed incident Microalbuminuria (multivariate adjusted)	Poor diet quality and obesity were significantly associated with about a 100% increased risk of microalbuminuria after multivariate adjustments. Also, compared to individuals with no unhealthy lifestyle-related factors (poor diet quality, current smoking and obesity), those with 1, 2 and 3 unhealthy lifestyle factors had increased risk of microalbuminuria by 31%, 173%, and 534%, respectively
Huang et al. (2013) Test the hypothesis that adherence to the MedDiet may better preserved kidney function (Uppsala Longitudinal Study of Adult Men cohort; Sweden) [59]	1110 men; mean age 70 years; MedDiet Score; follow-up of 9.9 years; 168 deaths (multivariate adjusted)	Adherence to the MedDiet was associated with lower odds of CKD or mortality in elderly men. Compared with low adherence, medium and high MedDiet adherences were significantly associated with lower risk of CKD by 23% and 42%, respectively (Fig. 15.7). Also, moderate and high adherence had lower mortality risk by 25% and 23%, respectively. Phosphate intake and net endogenous acid production were progressively lower across increasingly adherent groups
Lin et al. (2011) Evaluate the effect of healthier eating patterns vs. the Western dietary pattern (Nurses' Health Study; US) [60]	3121 women, mean age 67 years; 54% hypertensive and 23% diabetic subjects; microalbuminuria or eGFR decline; 11 years of follow-up (multivariate adjusted)	The Western pattern score was directly associated with microalbuminuria by 117% and rapid eGFR decline of ≥3 mL/min/1.73 m^2 per year by 77% (high vs. low quartile; multivariate adjusted). The DASH score decreased risk for rapid eGFR decline by 45%, but had no association with microalbuminuria (high vs. low quartile; multivariate adjusted; Fig. 15.8). The general healthy dietary pattern was not associated with microalbuminuria or eGFR decline
Intervention trials		
Meta-analysis		
Oyabu et al. (2016) Determine the effect of a low-carbohydrate diet (LCD) on renal function in overweight and obese individuals without CKD [61]	9 RCTs, 1687 participants; 46% male; 4 studies in diabetic patients; 861 were fed LCD and 826 were fed the control diet; carbohydrate consumption was 4–45% of total energy intake; 6–24 months	The mean eGFR in the low carbohydrate diet group was improved compared to the higher carbohydrate control diet by 0.13 mL/min/1.73m^2

Table 15.1 (continued)

Objective	Study details	Results
Representative trials		
Tyson et al. (2016) Test the effects of the DASH diet on serum electrolytes and blood pressure (BP) in adults with moderate CVD [62]	11 adults with an estimated glomerular filtration rate of 30–59 mL/min/1.73 m^2 and medication-treated hypertension; reduced-sodium, run-in diet for 1 week followed by a reduced sodium, DASH diet for 2 weeks	The DASH diet had no significant effect on potassium and serum bicarbonate was significantly reduced by 2.5 mg/dL at 2 weeks, compared to baseline values. Neither incident hyperkalemia nor new onset metabolic acidosis was observed. Clinic BP and mean 24-h ambulatory BP was unchanged. DASH significantly reduced mean nighttime BP by 5.3 mm Hg
Díaz-López et al. (2012) Investigate the effects of Med Diets on kidney function (Spain) [63]	**Prevención con Dieta Mediterránea (PREDIMED) sub-RCT:** 785 participants; 55% women; mean age 67 years; diets: a MedDiet supplemented with extra virgin olive oil or mixed nuts, or a control low-fat diet; 1-year	The 3 dietary approaches were associated with improved kidney function, with similar average increases in eGFR, but no changes in urinary albumin-creatinine ratio after full adjustment. Both the MedDiet and low-fat diet are equally beneficial in elderly individuals at high cardiovascular risk

15.6.1 Prospective Cohort Studies

15.6.1.1 Meta-analysis

A meta-analysis (7 cohort studies; 15,285 subjects with CKD) found that CKD patients with a healthy dietary pattern, generally higher in fruit and vegetables, fish, legumes, cereals, whole grains, and fiber, and lower in red meat, and added salt and sugar, had a 27% lower risk of mortality compared consuming Western diets [51].

15.6.1.2 Prospective Studies

Nine prospective studies provide strong evidence that healthy dietary patterns reduce and Western diets increase CKD risk, progression and mortality [52–60]. All variations of higher quality or healthy dietary patterns based on minimizing meat, salt, added sugar, and heavily processed foods while emphasizing phytochemical-rich whole plant foods have generally similar significant effects on improving renal function [54, 56, 57, 59, 60]. In contrast, Western dietary patterns are associated with increased CKD risk and poor renal function [52, 53, 55, 57, 58, 60]. Two studies show that low Dietary Approaches to Stop Hypertension (DASH) scores increase risk of CKD by 16% [52] or increase rapid decline in eGFR by 68% in individuals with hypertension [53]. Dietary patterns with greater than 3.6 g sodium/day were associated with a 17% increased risk of renal dysfunction and adequate potassium was associated with a 17% reduced risk of renal dysfunction [54]. This study also showed that higher Alternate Healthy Eating Index (AHEI), Healthy Eating Index (HEI), MedDiet score, and DASH diet scores improved renal function by 18–29% compared to lower adherence [54]. The US National Health and Nutrition Examination Survey III (1486 CKD patients; 14.2 years of follow-up) found that a high dietary acid load typical of the Western dietary pattern doubled the risk of end stage renal disease for the highest tertile [55]. The Framingham Offspring Study (1802 participants; mean age 59 years; 6.6 years of follow-up) showed that higher diet quality was associated with a significant 37% reduced odds of renal dysfunction in fully adjusted models [56]. Higher diet quality was associated with 31% lower risk of rapid eGFR decline. A US study in patients with CKD consuming higher intake of plant based diets found reduced mortality by 23% whereas Western diets increased mortality risk by 51% [57]. The US Coronary Artery Risk Development in Young Adults (CARDIA) (2354 African American and Caucasian participants; mean baseline age of 35 years; 15 years of follow-up) demonstrated that that poor diet quality and obesity was associated with a significant 100% increased risk of microalbuminuria, a risk factor for CKD [58]. The Swedish, Uppsala Longitudinal Study of Adult Men (1110 men; mean baseline age 70 years; 9.9 years of follow-up) found in older men that the higher adherence to a MedDiet lowered the risk of CDK by 23% and risk of mortality by 42% [59]. The Nurses' Health Study (3121 women; mean baseline age 67 years; 11 years of follow-up) showed that those with high adherence to the Western diet had a 117% increased risk of microalbuminuria whereas those who followed healthy diets, especially the DASH diet, had no association with microalbuminuria after an 11-year follow-up (Fig. 15.6) [60]. Also, women with high Western diet scores had a significantly increased risk of rapid eGFR decline of ≥3 mL/min/1.73 m^2 per year by 77% compared to a significant risk reduction by 45% in women with the highest DASH scores, or no eGFR decline with a generally healthy diet.

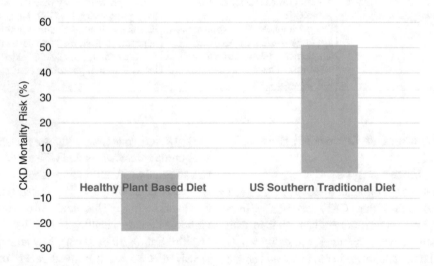

Fig. 15.6 Association between higher dietary pattern and chronic kidney disease (CKD) mortality risk in older US adults (baseline age 69 years; 6 years of follow-up) (adapted from [57])

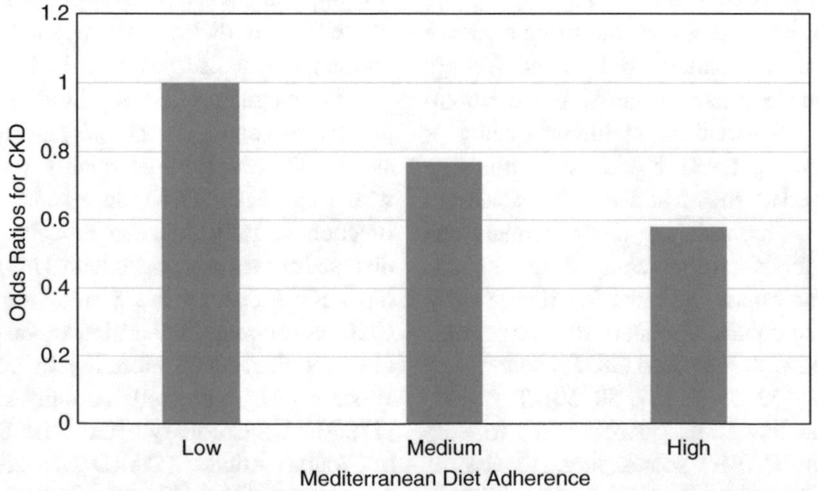

Fig. 15.7 Association between adherence to the Mediterranean diet (MedDiet) and chronic kidney disease (CKD) risk in older Swedish adults (mean baseline age 70 years; 9.9-years follow-up (p-trend = 0.04) (adapted from [59])

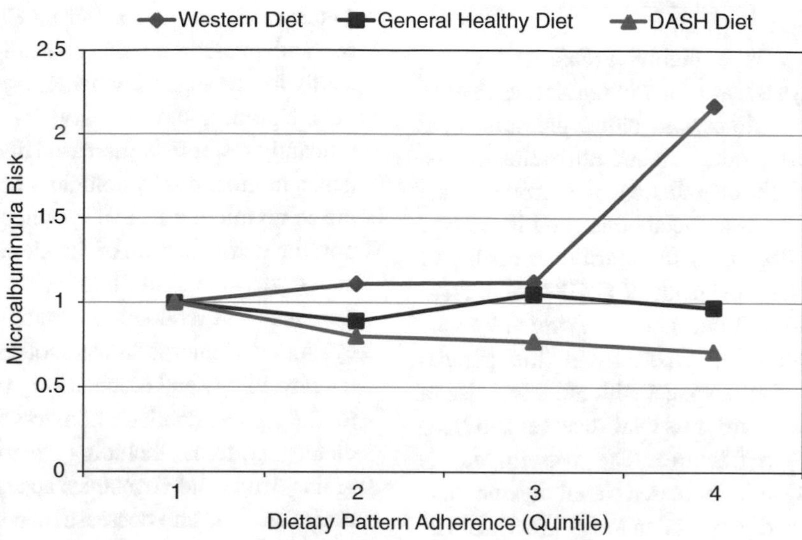

Fig. 15.8 Association between dietary pattern adherence and microalbuminuria risk in older women (mean baseline age 67 years; after 11 years; p-trend = 0.01) (adapted from [60])

15.6.2 Randomized Controlled Trials

A meta-analysis (9 RCTs; 1687 overweight or obese non-CKD subjects) showed that low-carbohydrate dietary patterns improved renal glomerular function vs. typical or higher carbohydrate dietary patterns [61]. A 2016 pilot intervention trial (11 adults with moderate CKD and medication-treated hypertension; reduced-sodium, run-in diet for 1 week followed by a reduced sodium, DASH diet for 2 weeks) found that the DASH diet had no significant effect on potassium and that serum bicarbonate was significantly reduced by 2.5 mg/dL at 2 weeks, compared with baseline [62]. Also, no incident hyperkalemia, new onset metabolic acidosis or change in blood pressure (BP) and mean 24-h ambulatory BP were observed. A 2012 Prevención con Dieta Mediterránea (PREDIMED) RCT (785 participants with high CVD risk; 55% women; mean age 67 years; diets: a MedDiet supplemented with extra virgin olive oil or mixed nuts, or a control low-fat diet; 1-year) found that MedDiets and low-fat diets were equally effective for improving kidney function, with similar average increases in eGFR, but no changes in urinary albumin-creatinine ratio was noted at full adjustment after 1 year [63]. A 2017 Cochrane Systematic Review (17 RCTs; 1,639 subjects with CKD; median 12 months) found that healthier dietary patterns improved CKD patient quality of life, and lowered BP and total cholesterol compared to usual diet controls [64].

15.6.3 Nutritional Guidelines

A modified version of the DASH diet is available for people with CKD with a protein intake of 0.6–0.8 g/kg of body weight/day, as well as lower phosphorus (0.8–1.0 g/day) and potassium (2–4 g/day) intake [10, 65]. Protein intake may be restricted to 0.6 g/kg body weight per day when eGFR decreases to <60 mL/min/1.73 m^2. High-protein diets should be avoided in persons with established later CKD stages who are not receiving dialysis. Adequate fiber intake should be encouraged for CKD patients. No specific levels of fiber intake are suggested, but the adequate intake level of 14 g/1000 kcal should be a good target intake level, which is typical of most healthy diets, including increased fruit and vegetable intake which may help to reduce risk of metabolic acidosis and reduce urine albumin and slow loss of renal function.

Conclusions

The kidney is a highly-vascularized organ, which plays a major role in regulating electrolyte concentrations and blood pressure, lipid metabolism, production and utilization of systemic glucose, degradation of hormones, and excretion of waste metabolites, and is affected to a large degree by the nutritional quality of the diet. The prevalence of CKD is high (estimated 200 million people worldwide) and steadily increasing, especially in older populations, and it is associated with increased risk of renal cancer, cardiovascular disease, and bone disorders and fractures. The Western diet is associated with increased renal dysfunction, CKD risk and progression to ESRD. The CKD patients' diet should help to slow the rate of progression of kidney failure, reduce uremic toxicity, decrease proteinuria, and lower the risk of secondary complications including cardiovascular disease, bone disease, and hypertension. Healthy lower dietary energy density and higher fiber healthy dietary patterns lower risk of CKD and its progression. Protein sources vary in their effect on CKD risk with red and processed meat consumption significantly increasing risk whereas higher intake of nuts, legumes, and low-fat dairy products significantly lower risk. Increased fiber intake triggers a number of physiologic processes in both the colon microbiota and systemically that support the detoxification of the kidneys, via influences on the gut barrier, gastrointestinal immune and endocrine responses, nitrogen cycling, and microbial metabolism which alter the physiology and biochemistry of the kidneys to help re-establish homeostasis. Healthy dietary patterns including fiber-rich wholegrains, fruits and vegetables appear to improve renal function, and decrease metabolic acidosis compared to poor quality diets low in fruits and vegetables and high in processed foods and animal products. High adherence to healthy dietary patterns such as the DASH diet, especially a modified version of the DASH diet for people with CKD, and the Mediterranean diet (MedDiet) may help to reduce CKD risk, progression to later stages and mortality.

Appendix A: Fifty high fiber whole or minimally processed plant foods ranked by amount of fiber per standard food portion size

Food	Standard portion size	Dietary fiber (g)	Calories (kcal)	Energy density (calories/g)
High fiber bran ready-to-eat-cereal	1/3–3/4 cup (30 g)	9.1–14.3	60–80	2.0–2.6
Navy beans, cooked	1/2 cup cooked (90 g)	9.6	127	1.4
Small white beans, cooked	1/2 cup (90 g)	9.3	127	1.4
Shredded wheat ready-to-eat cereal	1–1 1/4 cup (50-60 g)	5.0–9.0	155–220	3.2–3.7
Black bean soup, canned	1/2 cup (130 g)	8.8	117	0.9
French beans, cooked	1/2 cup (90 g)	8.3	114	1.3
Split peas, cooked	1/2 cup (100 g)	8.2	114	1.1
Chickpeas (Garbanzo) beans, canned	1/2 cup (120 g)	8.1	176	1.4
Lentils, cooked	1/2 cup (100 g)	7.8	115	1.2
Pinto beans, cooked	1/2 cup (90 g)	7.7	122	1.4
Black beans, cooked	1/2 cup (90 g)	7.5	114	1.3
Artichoke, global or French, cooked	1/2 cup (84 g)	7.2	45	0.5
Lima beans, cooked	1/2 cup (90 g)	6.6	108	1.2
White beans, canned	1/2 cup (130 g)	6.3	149	1.1
Wheat bran flakes ready-to-eat cereal	3/4 cup (30 g)	4.9–5.5	90–98	3.0–3.3

Food	Standard portion size	Dietary fiber (g)	Calories (kcal)	Energy density (calories/g)
Pear with skin	1 medium (180 g)	5.5	100	0.6
Pumpkin seeds. whole, roasted	1 ounce (about 28 g)	5.3	126	4.5
Baked beans, canned, plain	1/2 cup (125 g)	5.2	120	0.9
Soybeans, cooked	1/2 cup (90 g)	5.2	150	1.7
Plain rye wafer crackers	2 wafers (22 g)	5.0	73	3.3
Avocado, Hass	1/2 fruit (68 g)	4.6	114	1.7
Apple, with skin	1 medium (180 g)	4.4	95	0.5
Green peas, cooked (fresh, frozen, canned)	1/2 cup (80 g)	3.5–4.4	59–67	0.7–0.8
Refried beans, canned	1/2 cup (120 g)	4.4	107	0.9
Mixed vegetables, cooked from frozen	1/2 cup (45 g)	4.0	59	0.7
Raspberries	1/2 cup (65 g)	3.8	32	0.5
Blackberries	1/2 cup (65 g)	3.8	31	0.4
Collards, cooked	1/2 cup (95 g)	3.8	32	0.3
Soybeans, green, cooked	1/2 cup (75 g)	3.8	127	1.4
Prunes, pitted, stewed	1/2 cup (125 g)	3.8	133	1.1
Sweet potato, baked	1 medium (114 g)	3.8	103	0.9
Multi-grain bread	2 slices regular (52 g)	3.8	140	2.7
Figs, dried	1/4 cup (about 38 g)	3.7	93	2.5
Potato baked, with skin	1 medium (173 g)	3.6	163	0.9
Popcorn, air-popped	3 cups (24 g)	3.5	93	3.9
Almonds	1 ounce (about 28 g)	3.5	164	5.8
Whole wheat spaghetti, cooked	1/2 cup (70 g)	3.2	87	1.2
Sunflower seed kernels, dry roasted	1 ounce (about 28 g)	3.1	165	5.8
Orange	1 medium (130 g)	3.1	69	0.5
Banana	1 medium (118 g)	3.1	105	0.9
Oat bran muffin	1 small (66 g)	3.0	178	2.7
Vegetable soup	1 cup (245 g)	2.9	91	0.4
Dates	1/4 cup (about 38 g)	2.9	104	2.8
Pistachios, dry roasted	1 ounce (about 28 g)	2.8	161	5.7
Hazelnuts or filberts	1 ounce (about 28 g)	2.7	178	6.3
Peanuts, oil roasted	1 ounce (about 28 g)	2.7	170	6.0
Quinoa, cooked	1/2 cup (90 g)	2.7	92	1.0
Broccoli, cooked	1/2 cup (78 g)	2.6	27	0.3
Potato baked, without skin	1 medium (145 g)	2.3	145	1.0
Baby spinach leaves	3 ounces (90 g)	2.1	20	0.2
Blueberries	1/2 cup (74 g)	1.8	42	0.6
Carrot, raw or cooked	1 medium (60 g)	1.7	25	0.4

Dahl WJ, Stewart ML. Position of the Academy of Nutrition and Dietetics: health implications of dietary fiber. J Acad Nutr Diet. 2015;115:1861–70

Dietary Guidelines Advisory Committee. Scientific Report. Advisory Report to the Secretary of Health and Human Services and the Secretary of Agriculture. Part D. Chapter 1: Food and nutrient intakes, and health: current status and trends. 2015;97–98; Table D1.8

Slavin JL. Position of the American Dietetic Association: Health implications of dietary fiber. J Am Diet Assoc 2008;108:1716–31

U.S. Department of Agriculture and U.S. Department of Health and Human Services. Dietary Guidelines for Americans, 2010. 7th ed. Washington, DC: U.S. Government Printing Office. 2010; Table B2.4; http://www.choosemyplate.gov/. accessed 22 Aug 2015

References

1. Jha V, Garcia-Garcia G, Iseki K, et al. Chronic kidney disease: global dimension and perspectives. Lancet. 2013;382:260–72.
2. Lozano R, Naghavi M, Foreman K, et al. Global and regional mortality from 235 causes of death for 20 age groups in 1990 and 2010: a systematic analysis for the Global Burden of Disease Study 2010. Lancet. 2013;380:2095–128.
3. Ojo A. Addressing the global burden of chronic kidney disease through clinical and translational research. Trans Am Clin Climatol Assoc. 2014;125:229–46.
4. Sharma K. Obesity, oxidative stress, and fibrosis in chronic kidney disease. Kidney Int Suppl. 2014;4:113–7.
5. Hall ME, de Carmo JM, da Silva AA, et al. Obesity, hypertension, and chronic kidney disease. Int J Nephrol Renovasc Dis. 2014;7:75–88.
6. McCullough K, Sharma P, Ali T, et al. Measuring the population burden of chronic kidney disease: a systematic literature review of the estimated prevalence of impaired kidney function. Nephrol Dial Transplant. 2012;27(5):1812–21.
7. National Institutes for Diabetes and Digestive and Kidney Diseases. Kidney disease. Kidney disease statistics for the United States. https://www.niddk.nih.gov/health-information/health-statistics/Pages/kidney-disease-statistics-united-states.aspx. Accessed April 2017.
8. American Kidney Fund. End stage renal disease. 2015. http://www.kidneyfund.org/kidney-disease/kidney-failure/end-stage-renal-disease/. Accessed 31 May 2015.
9. Said S, Hernandez GT. The link between chronic kidney disease and cardiovascular disease. J Nephropathol. 2014;3(3):99–104.
10. Hariharan D, Vellanki K, Kramer H. The Western diet and chronic kidney disease. Curr Hypertens Rep. 2015;17:16. https://doi.org/10.1007/s11906-014-0529-6.
11. Odermatt A. The Western-style diet: a major risk factor for impaired kidney function and chronic kidney disease. Am J Physiol Renal Physiol. 2011;301:919–31.
12. Garofalo C, Borrelli S, Minutolo R, et al. A systematic review and meta-analysis suggest obesity predicts onset of chronic kidney disease in the general population. Kidney Int. 2017;91(5):1224–35. https://doi.org/10.1016/k.kint.2016.12.013.
13. Garland JS. Elevated body mass index as a risk factor for chronic kidney disease: current perspectives. Diabetes Metab Syndr Obes. 2014;7:347–55.
14. Navarroa G, Ardiles L. Association between obesity and chronic renal disease. Rev Med Chil. 2015;143:77–84.
15. Foster MC, Hwang S-J, Porter SA, et al. Fatty kidney, hypertension, and chronic kidney disease: The Framingham Heart Study. Hypertension. 2011;58(5):784–90.
16. Kang SH, Cho KH, Park JW, et al. Association of visceral fat area with chronic kidney disease and metabolic syndrome risk in the general population: analysis using multi-frequency bioimpedance. Kidney Blood Press Res. 2015;40:223–30.
17. Sarathy H, Henriquez G, Abramowitz MK, et al. Abdominal obesity, race and chronic kidney disease in young adults: results from NHANES 1999-2010. PLoS One. 2016;11(5). https://doi.org/10.1371/journal.pone.0153588.
18. de Vries AP, Ruggenenti P, Ruan XZ, et al. Fatty kidney: emerging role of ectopic lipid in obesity-related renal disease. Lancet Diabetes Endocrinol. 2014;2(5):417–26.
19. Rebholz CM, Anderson CAM, Grams ME, et al. Relationship of the American Heart Association's impact goals (Life's Simple 7) with risk of chronic kidney disease: results from the Atherosclerosis Risk in Communities (ARIC) Cohort Study. J Am Heart Assoc. 2016;5:e003192. https://doi.org/10.1161/JAHA.116.003192.
20. Ricardo AC, Anderson CA, Yang W, et al. Healthy lifestyle and risk of kidney disease progression, atherosclerotic events, and death in CKD: findings from the chronic renal insufficiency cohort (CRIC) study. Am J Kidney Dis. 2015;65(3):412–24.
21. Zha Y, Qian Q. Protein nutrition and malnutrition in CKD and ESRD. Forum Nutr. 2017;9:208. https://doi.org/10.3390/nu9030208.
22. Haring B, Selvin E, Liang M, et al. Dietary protein sources and risk for incident chronic kidney disease: results from the Atherosclerosis Risk in Communities (ARIC) Study. J Ren Nutr. 2017;27(4):233–42. https://doi.org/10.1053/j.jrn.2016.11.004.
23. Herber-Gast G-CM, Biesbroek S, Verschuren WMM, et al. Association of dietary protein and dairy intakes and change in renal function: results from the population-based longitudinal Doetinchem cohort study. Am J Clin Nutr. 2016;104:1712–9.
24. Rouhani MH, Najafabadi MM, Esmaillzadeh A, et al. Dietary energy density, renal function, and progression of chronic kidney disease. Adv Med. 2016;2675345. https://doi.org/10.1155/2016/2675345.
25. Díaz-López A, Bulló M, Basora J, et al. Cross-sectional associations between macronutrient intake and chronic kidney disease in a population at high cardiovascular risk. Clin Nutr. 2013;32:606e612. https://doi.org/10.1016/j.clnu.2012.10.013.
26. Evenepoel P, Meijers BK. Dietary fiber and protein: nutritional therapy in chronic kidney disease and beyond. Kidney Int. 2012;81:227–9.
27. Kieffer DA, Martin RJ, Adams SH. Impact of dietary fibers on nutrient management and detoxification organs: gut, liver, and kidneys. Adv Nutr. 2016;7:1111–21. https://doi.org/10.3945/an.116.013219.
28. Chiavaroli L, Mirrahimi A, Sievenpiper JL, et al. Dietary fiber effects in chronic kidney disease: a systematic review and meta-analysis of controlled feeding trials. Eur J Clin Nutr. 2014. https://doi.org/10.1038/ejcn.2014.237.
29. Krishnamurthy VMR, Wei G, Baird BC, et al. High dietary fiber intake is associated with decreased

inflammation and all-cause mortality in patients with chronic kidney disease. Kidney Int. 2012;81:300–6.

30. Xu H, Huang X, Riserus U, et al. Dietary fiber, kidney function, inflammation, and mortality risk. Clin J Am Soc Nephrol. 2014;9(12):2104–10.
31. Jiao J, Xu J, Zhang W, et al. Effect of dietary fiber on circulating C-reactive protein in over-weight and obese adults: a meta-analysis of randomized controlled trials. Int J Food Sci Nutr. 2015;66(1):114–9.
32. Shu H-S, Tai Y-Y, Chang K-T, et al. Plasma high-sensitivity C-reactive protein level is associated with impaired estimated glomerular filtration rate in hypertensives. Acta Cardiol Sin. 2015;31:91–7.
33. Rossi M, Johnson DW, Campbell KL. The kidney-gut axis: implications for nutrition care. J Ren Nutr. 2015;25(5):399–403.
34. Ramezani A, Raj DS. The gut microbiome, kidney disease, and targeted interventions. J Am Soc Nephrol. 2014;25:657–70.
35. Salmean YA, Segal MS, Palil SP, Dahl WJ. Fiber supplementation lowers plasma p-cresol in chronic kidney disease patients. J Ren Nutr. 2015;25(3):316–20.
36. Rossi M, Johnson DW, Xu H, et al. Dietary protein-fiber ratio with circulating levels of indoxyl sulfate and p-cresyl sulfate in chronic kidney disease patients. Nutr Metab Cardiovasc Dis. 2015;25(9):860–5.
37. Williams C, Ronco C, Kotanko P. Whole grains in the renal diet - is it time to reevaluate their role? Blood Purif. 2013;36:210–4.
38. Gopinath B, Harris DC, Flood VM, et al. Carbohydrate nutrition is associated with the 5-year incidence of chronic kidney disease. J Nutr. 2011;141:433–9.
39. Rouhani MH, Mortazavi Najafabadi M· et al. The impact of oat (Avena sativa) consumption on biomarkers of renal function in patients with chronic kidney disease: A parallel randomized clinical trial. Clin Nutr. 2016. https://doi.org/10.1016/j.clnu.2016.11.022.
40. Adeva MM, Souto G. Diet-induced metabolic acidosis. Clin Nutr. 2011;30:416–21.
41. Goraya N, Simoni J, Jo C-H, Wesson DE. A comparison of treating metabolic acidosis in CKD stage 4 hypertensive kidney disease with fruits and vegetables or sodium bicarbonate. Clin J Am Soc Nephrol. 2013;8:371–81.
42. Goraya N, Simoni J, Jo C-H, Wesson DE. Treatment of metabolic acidosis in patients with stage 3 chronic kidney disease with fruits and vegetables or oral bicarbonate reduces urine angiotensinogen and preserves glomerular filtration rate. Kidney Int. 2014;86(5):1031–8.
43. Wai SN, Kelly JT, Johnson DW, Campbell KL. Dietary patterns and clinical outcomes in chronic kidney disease; The CKD.QLD Nutrition Study. J Ren Nutr. 2016;27(3):175–82. https://doi.org/10.1053/j.jrn.2016.10.005.
44. McMahon EJ, Campbell KL, Bauer JD, Mudge DW. Altered dietary salt intake for people with chronic kidney disease. Cochrane Database of Systematic Rev. 2015;(2). https://doi.org/10.1002/14651858.CD010070.pub2.
45. Uribarri J, Calvo MS. Dietary phosphorus excess: a risk factor in chronic bone, kidney, and cardiovascular disease? Adv Nutr. 2013;4:542–4. https://doi.org/10.3945/an.113.004234.
46. Suki WN, Moore LW. Phosphorus regulation in chronic kidney disease. Methodist Debakey Cardiovasc J. 2016;12(4 Suppl):6–9. 10.14797/mdcj-12-4s1-6.
47. Rebholz CM, Tin A, Liu Y, et al. Dietary magnesium and kidney function decline: the healthy aging in neighborhoods of diversity across the life span study. Am J Nephrol. 2016;44(5):381–7. https://doi.org/10.1159/000450861.
48. Cheungpasitporn W, Thongprayoon C, O'Corragain OA, et al. Associations of sugar-sweetened and artificially sweetened soda with chronic kidney disease: a systematic review and meta-analysis. Nephrology. 2014;19(12):791–7. https://doi.org/10.1111/nep.12343.
49. Cheungpasitporn W, Thongprayoon C, Kittanamongkolchai W, et al. High alcohol consumption and the risk of renal damage: a systematic review and meta-analysis. Q J Med. 2015;108:539–48. https://doi.org/10.1093/qjmed/hcu247.
50. Wijampreecha K, Thongprayoon C, Thamcharoen N, et al. Association of coffee consumption and chronic kidney disease: a meta-analysis. Int J Clin Pract. 2017;71:e12919. https://doi.org/10.1111/ijcp.12919.
51. Kelly JT, Palmer SC, Wai SN, et al. Healthy dietary patterns and risk of mortality and ESRD in CKD: a meta-analysis of cohort studies. Clin J Am Soc Nephrol. 2017;12(2):272–9. https://doi.org/10.2215/CJN.06190616.
52. Liu Y, Kuczmarski MF, Miller ER 3rd, et al. Dietary habits and risk of kidney function decline in urban population. J Ren Nutr. 2017;27(1):16–25. https://doi.org/10.1053/j.jrn.2016.08.007.
53. Rebholz CM, Crews DC, Grams ME, et al. DASH (Dietary Approaches to Stop Hypertension) diet and risk of subsequent kidney disease. Am J Kidney Dis. 2016;68(6):853–61. https://doi.org/10.1053/j.ajkd.2016.05.019.
54. Smyth A, Griffin M, Yusuf S, et al. Diet and major renal outcomes: a prospective cohort study. The NIH-AARP Diet and Health Study. J Ren Nutr. 2016;26(5):288–98. https://doi.org/10.1053/ j.jrn.2016.01.016.
55. Banerjee T, Crews DC, Wesson DE, et al. High dietary acid load predicts ESRD among adults with CKD. J Am Soc Nephrol. 2015;26:1693–700.
56. Foster MC, Hwang SJ, Massaro JM, et al. Lifestyle factors and indices of kidney function in the Framingham heart study. Am J Nephrol. 2015;41:267–74.
57. Gutierrez OM, Muntner P, Rizk DV, et al. Dietary patterns and risk of death and progression to ESRD in individuals with CKD: a cohort study. Am J Kidney Dis. 2014;64(2):204–13.
58. Chang A, Van Horn L, Jacobs DR, et al. Lifestyle-related factors, obesity, and incident

microalbuminuria: the CARDIA (Coronary Artery Risk Development in Young Adults) study. Am J Kidney Dis. 2013;62(2):267–75.
59. Huang X, Jimenez-Moleon JJ, Lindholm B, et al. Mediterranean diet, kidney function, and mortality in men with CKD. Clin J Am Soc Nephrol. 2013;8:1548–55.
60. Lin J, Fung TT, Hu FB, Curhan GC. Association of dietary patterns with albuminuria and kidney function decline in older white women: a subgroup analysis from the Nurses' Health Study. Am J Kidney Dis. 2011;57(2):245–54.
61. Oyabu C, Hashimoto Y, Fukuda T. Impact of low-carbohydrate diet on renal function: a meta-analysis of over 1000 individuals from nine randomised controlled trials. Br J Nutr. 2016;116(4):632–8. https://doi.org/10.1017/S00071145516002178.
62. Tyson CC, Lin P-H, Corsino L, et al. Short-term effects of the DASH diet in adults with moderate chronic kidney disease: a pilot feeding study. Clin Kidney J. 2016;9(4):592–8. https://doi.org/10.1093/ckj/sfw046.
63. Díaz-López A, Bulló M, Martínez-González MA, et al. Effects of Mediterranean diets on kidney function: a report from the PREDIMED trial. Am J Kidney Dis. 2012;60(3):380–9.
64. Palmer SC, Maggo JK, Campbell KL, et al. Dietary interventions for adults with chronic kidney disease. Cochrane Database of Systematic Rev. 2017; Issue 4. Art No.CD011998.
65. Kidney Disease Outcomes Quality Initiative (K/DOQI). K/DOQI clinical practice guidelines on hypertension and antihypertensive agents in chronic kidney disease. Am J Kidney Dis. 2004;43(5 Suppl 1):1–290. PMID:15114537.

16 Dietary Patterns and Stroke Risk

Keywords
Ischemic stroke risk • Life's Simple 7 • Healthy dietary patterns • Western diet • DASH diet • Mediterranean diet • Healthy Nordic diet • Obesity • Inactivity

Key Points

- Approximately 75% of stroke risk is attributable to smoking, poor diet quality, low physical activity, and excessive body weight, which are associated with sub-optimal cardiometabolic health.
- Cohort studies show that healthy dietary patterns are significantly protective against stroke risk by 11–23% whereas the Western dietary pattern increases stroke risk by 5–6%.
- A large Spanish PREDIMED trial found that the Mediterranean diet (MedDiet) significantly reduced stroke risk by 39% in older adults with high cardiovascular disease risk over 4.8 years.
- Prospective studies show that high adherence to MedDiets, Dietary Approaches to Stop Hypertension (DASH) and the Healthy Nordic Diet Index significantly reduces total or ischemic stroke risk.
- Potential healthy dietary pattern mechanisms for lowering stroke risk are through aiding in weight and glycemic control; improving vascular function, and blood lipids and lipoprotein profiles; and contributing to a healthier colonic microbiota ecosystem and lower systemic inflammation and oxidative stress.

16.1 Introduction

Stroke is the brain equivalent of a heart attack and the leading cause of neurological functional impairment by a vascular cause and includes blockage (ischemic stroke) or rupture of a blood vessel (hemorrhagic stroke). Stroke is a major cause of disability and death worldwide, and changes the lives not only of the stroke victims but also of their families as many stroke victims become dependent in their activities of daily living due to significant stroke related cognitive and physical disabilities [1–5]. Stroke is the second most common cause of death worldwide, accounting for 6.2 million deaths or about 11% of total deaths [1–3]. Forecast projections estimate that there will be a 20% increase in stroke prevalence by 2030 compared to 2012 rates, because of the increase in aging populations.

M.L. Dreher, *Dietary Patterns and Whole Plant Foods in Aging and Disease*, Nutrition and Health,
https://doi.org/10.1007/978-3-319-59180-3_16

The objective of this chapter is to comprehensively assess the effects of dietary patterns on stroke events and mortality risk.

16.2 Modifiable Behavior Risk Factors

Over 90% of stroke risk is attributable to modifiable risk factors, including 74% due to behavioral factors such as smoking, poor diet, and low physical activity [5]. The American Heart Association developed the "Life's Simple 7" plan for ideal cardiovascular health and lower stroke risk which includes the following criteria: (1) non-smoking or quit >1 year ago; (2) BMI < 25; (3) blood pressure (BP) <120/80 mmHg; (4) ≥ 150 min/week of physical activity; (5) healthy dietary pattern (high in fruits and vegetables, fish, fiber-rich whole grains, (6) low intake of sodium, and (7) limiting or avoiding sugar-sweetened beverages [6]. Less than 2% of the US population meets all the criteria for cardiovascular health with adherence to a healthy dietary pattern the most difficult to achieve and maintain [7, 8].

Adherence to "Life's Simple 7" or similar healthy lifestyle criteria has been shown to reduce stroke and mortality risk [6, 8, 9]. A National Health and Nutrition Examination Survey prospective study (420 US adults with previous stroke experience; mean baseline age ≥65 years; median 9 years of follow-up) found an inverse dose-dependent relationship between the number of "Life's Simple 7" metrics met and 10-year mortality after a stroke (Fig. 16.1) [6]. The Reasons for Geographic and Racial Differences in Stroke Study (22,914 participants; with data on "Life's Simple 7" and no previous CVD; mean age 65 years, 42% were black, 58% women; 432 incident strokes; mean 4.9 years of follow-up) found that a 1-point higher "Life's Simple 7" score was associated with an 8% lower risk of stroke (Fig. 16.2) [8]. Those who met ≥4 health metrics had significantly lower all-cause mortality by 49% than those who met 0 to 1. Specifically adhering to "Life's Simple 7" goals might be the most effective approach for reducing stroke risk and extending survival after stroke. Also, the Women's Health Study (37,634 US women without stroke at baseline; 17.2 years of follow-up, 867 total stroke cases) found that higher healthy lifestyle index measures including non-smoking, regular physical activity, healthier BMI, limited alcohol consumption, and a healthy diet were significantly associated with reduced stroke risk [9].

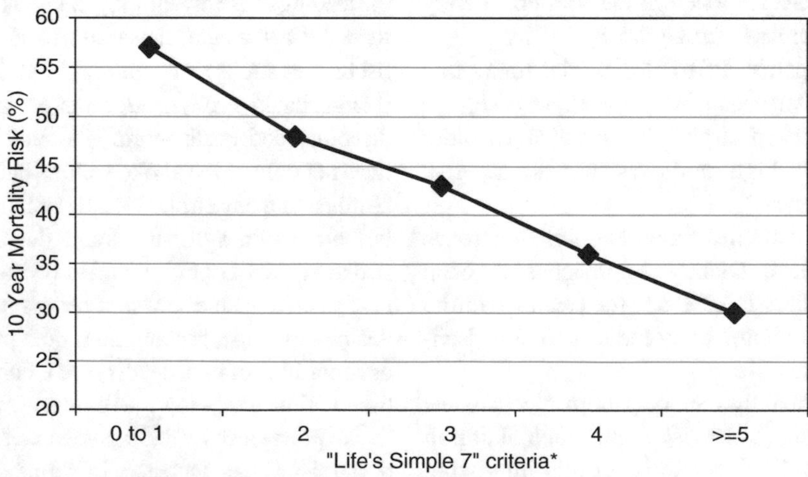

Fig. 16.1 Association between the number of "Life's Simple 7" criteria adopted and long-term mortality risk after stroke (p-trend = 0.022; multivariate adjusted) (adapted from [6]). *Non-smoking, regular physical activity, healthy diet, maintaining normal weight, and controlling cholesterol, blood pressure, and blood glucose levels

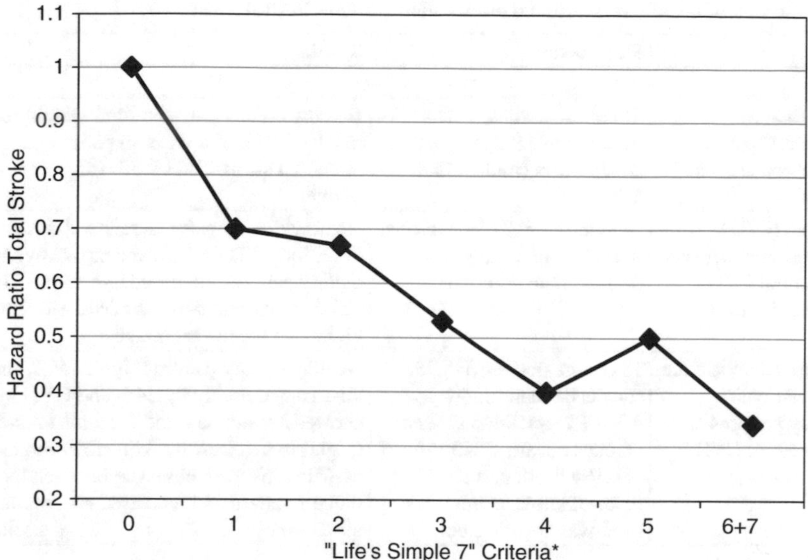

Fig. 16.2 Association between the number of "Life's Simple 7" criteria met and total stroke risk in 22,914 healthy subjects (mean age 65 years; 58% women; 4.9 years of follow-up) (adapted from [8]). *Not smoking, regular physical activity, healthy diet, maintaining normal weight, and controlling cholesterol, blood pressure, and blood glucose levels

Those women in the highest healthy lifestyle adherence category had reduced total stroke risk by up to 57% compared to women in the lowest adherence group. Even women in the modest healthy lifestyle index group had significant decreases in total and ischemic stroke risk.

16.3 Dietary Patterns

16.3.1 Background

The type of dietary pattern adhered to has a major effect on body weight, central obesity, blood lipids, blood pressure, and glycemic and insulinemic control, which are important factors associated with stroke risk [2–23]. An overview of characteristics and composition of common dietary patterns including the Western diet, dietary guideline based diets, Dietary Approaches to Stop Hypertension (DASH), the Mediterranean diet (MedDiet), lacto-ovo-vegetarian, and healthy vegan dietary patterns are summarized in Appendix A. Whole (minimally processed) plant foods rich in stroke protective nutrients and phytochemicals such as fiber, vitamins E and C, trace minerals, carotenoids, flavonoids and phytosterols are characterizing components of healthy dietary patterns [22–28]. Potential mechanisms for healthy dietary patterns to lower stroke risk are: (1) reduce dietary energy density and increase satiety and satiation, which reduces the risk of weight gain or obesity; (2) enhance insulin sensitivity, which may improve vascular and endothelial function, (3) promote healthier LDL-C, HDL-C and triglyceride profiles for improved endothelial health and a slower rate of arterial plaque build-up, (4) attenuate elevated systemic inflammation and LDL-oxidation, and (5) stimulate healthier colonic microbiota which is associated with increased fiber fermentation to short chain fatty acids for colon and cardiometabolic health [29–49].

16.3.2 Healthy vs. Western Dietary Patterns

Studies on the effects of healthy vs. Western diets on stroke risk are summarized in Table 16.1 [50–55].

Table 16.1 Summary of healthy vs. western dietary patterns studies in stroke risk

Objective	Study details	Results
Meta-analyses		
Zhang et al. (20105). Investigate the association between dietary patterns and stroke risk [50]	21 cohort studies; 1,023,131 subjects; age range 20–79 years (multivariate adjusted)	Healthy dietary patterns significantly reduced stroke risk by 23% and a Western pattern insignificantly increased stroke risk by 5% (highest to the lowest intake)
Rodriguez et al. (2015). Assess the association between dietary patterns and CVD, CHD and stroke risk [51]	19 cohorts; 610,691 subjects; follow-up of 1–18 years (multivariate adjusted)	Healthy dietary patterns reduced risk for CVD by 31%, for CHD by 17% and stroke by14%. Western dietary patterns increased risk for CVD by 14%, CHD by 3% and stroke by 5%. All comparisons were highest to the lowest intake
Li et al. (2015). Elucidate the potential associations between dietary patterns and the risk of all-cause, CVD and stroke mortality [52]	13 cohort studies; 338,787 subjects; mean follow-up of 5.7–18 years; 9465 cases of all-cause death, 5543 cases of CVD death and 1918 cases of stroke death (multivariate adjusted)	Healthy dietary patterns significantly reduced risk of all-cause mortality by 24% and CVD by 19%, and showed an inverse trend for stroke mortality by 11% (highest vs. lowest intake). However, no significant associations were observed between the Western dietary pattern and increased risk of mortality from all-cause by 7%, CVD by 1% and stroke by 6%
Prospective cohort studies		
Stricker et al. (2013). Evaluate different dietary patterns and CHD and stroke risk (Dutch cohorts of the European Prospective Investigation into Cancer (EPIC) Study) [53]	40,011 men and women; 13 years of follow-up; 588 stroke cases (multivariate adjusted)	The high adherence to healthy dietary patterns (high intake of fish, high fiber foods, raw vegetables and moderate wine intake) reduced stroke risk by 21% compared to the Western dietary pattern (high intake of French fries, fast food, low-fiber products, soft drinks with sugar, and alcoholic drinks)
Judd et al. (2013). Assess the effect of US dietary patterns on stroke risk (REasons for Geographic and Racial Differences in Stroke (REGARDS) cohort study) [54]	30,239 American adults; aged ≥45 years; median 5.7 years of follow-up; 490 stroke cases (multivariate adjusted)	Higher adherence to the healthy (plant-based pattern) was significantly associated with lower stroke risk by 29%. This association was attenuated to 15–25% after addition of income, education, total energy intake, smoking, and sedentary behavior. Participants with a higher adherence to the Southern pattern had a significant 39% increased risk of stroke
Fung et al. (2004). Investigate the effect of dietary patterns on stroke risk in women (The Nurses' Health Study) [55]	71,768 women; 38–63 years; 29% hypertension; 23% smokers; 14 years of follow-up; 791 stroke cases (multivariate adjusted)	The Western diet significantly increased risk for total stroke by 58% and for ischemic stroke by 56%. The healthy patterns reduced risk for total stroke by 22% and ischemic stroke by 26% ($p = 0.13$ for both) (Fig. 16.3). Healthy dietary patterns were characterized by higher intakes of fruits, vegetables, legumes, fish, and whole-grains, whereas the Western pattern by higher intakes of red and processed meats, refined grains, and sweets and desserts. All comparisons highest vs. lowest adherence

16.3.2.1 Prospective Cohort Studies

Systematic Reviews and Meta-analyses

Three meta-analyses support the protective effects of consuming health dietary patterns and the adverse effects of a Western dietary pattern on stroke risk or mortality [50–52]. A 2015 meta-analysis (21 cohort studies; 1,023,131 subjects; age range 20–79 years) found that higher adherence to healthy dietary patterns significantly reduced stroke risk by 23% and higher adherence to a Western pattern insignificantly increased stroke risk by 5% [50]. A second 2015 meta-analysis (19 cohorts; 610,691 subjects; follow-up of 1–18 years) showed that higher adherence to

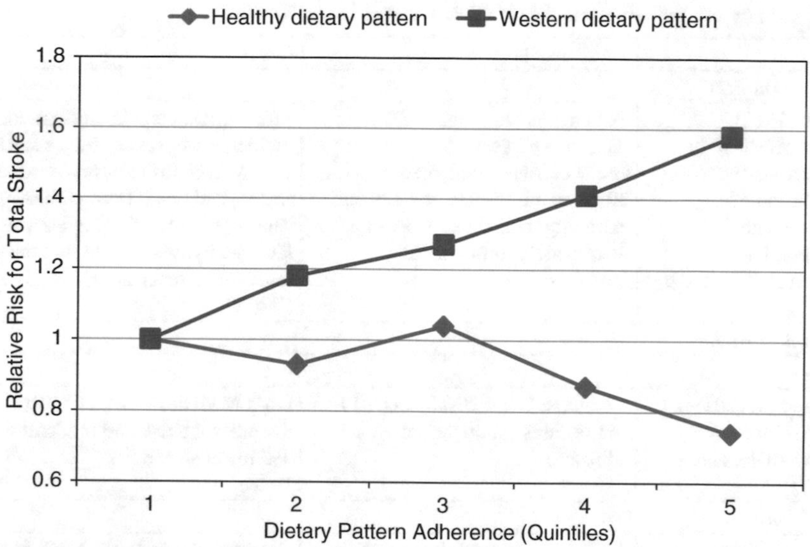

Fig. 16.3 Association between level of dietary pattern adherence and total stroke risk in US women (age ranging from 38 to 63 years; 14 years of follow-up) (adapted from [55])

healthy dietary patterns reduced risk for CVD by 31%, for CHD by 17% and stroke by14% whereas higher adherence to Western dietary patterns increased risk for CVD by 14%, CHD by 3% and stroke by 5% [51]. A third 2015 meta-analysis (13 cohort studies; 338,787 subjects; mean follow-up of 6–18 years) indicated that higher adherence to healthy dietary patterns lowered stroke mortality by 11% whereas higher adherence to a Western dietary pattern increased risk of mortality from stroke by 6% [52].

Specific Studies

Three prospective studies provide insights on dietary patterns and stroke risk [53–55]. A 2013 Dutch European Prospective Investigation into Cancer [EPIC] Study (40,011 men and women; 13 years of follow-up) observed that high adherence to healthy dietary patterns (high intake of fish, high fiber foods, raw vegetables and moderate wine intake) significantly reduced stroke risk by 21% compared to the Western diet pattern (high intake of French fries, fast food, low-fiber products, soft drinks with sugar, and alcoholic drinks) [53]. A 2013 Southern US REasons for Geographic and Racial Differences in Stroke (REGARDS) study (30,239 Americans; aged ≥45 years; median 5.7 years of follow-up) observed that greater adherence to a healthy (plant-based pattern) significantly lowered stroke risk by 29% whereas higher adherence to the Southern pattern had a significantly increased risk of stroke by 39% [54]. A 2004 Nurses' Health Study (71,768 women; baseline age 38–63 years; 14 years of follow-up) observed that high adherence to the Western diet significantly increased risk for total stroke by 58% and for ischemic stroke by 56% whereas high adherence to healthy patterns reduced risk for total stroke by 22% and ischemic stroke by 26% (Fig. 16.3) [55].

16.3.3 Mediterranean Diet (MedDiet)

A primary prevention trial and cohort studies on the MedDiet and stroke risk are summarized in Table 16.2 [56–63]. Notable beneficial nutrients that are abundant in the MedDiet are monounsaturated fatty acids, a balanced ratio of omega-6/omega-3 essential fatty acids, high amounts of fiber, and antioxidants such as vitamins E and C, and polyphenols.

Table 16.2 Summary of Mediterranean diet (MedDiet) studies in stroke risk

Objective	Study details	Results
Primary prevention RCT		
Estruch et al. (2013). Investigate the effect of the MedDiet pattern on the primary prevention of cardiovascular events ([Prevención con Diet Mediterránea [PREDIMED]; Spain) [56]	7447 adults with high CVD risk; mean age 67 years; 57% women; two MedDiets supplemented with 30 g/day mixed nuts or 1 L/week extra virgin olive oil vs. low fat diet; median follow-up of 4.8 years	The MedDiet significantly reduced the incidence of primary major cardiovascular events (composite of myocardial infarction, stroke, and death from cardiovascular causes) by 30%. Stroke risk was significantly lowered by39%, which was the only specific outcome to reach statistical significance (Fig. 16.4)
Prospective cohort studies		
Meta-analysis		
Psaltopoulou et al. (2013). Evaluate the association between the MedDiet and stroke risk [57]	9 cohorts; 162,092 subjects, 3176 stroke cases (multivariate adjusted)	High MedDiet adherence resulted in a 16% lower stroke risk and moderate adherence in 4% lower stroke risk
Specific cohort studies		
Tsivgoulis et al. (2015). Evaluate the effect of adherence to MedDiet on stroke risk (REasons for Geographic and Racial Differences in Stroke (REGARDS) study; US) [58]	30,239 US adults; mean baseline age of 65 years; 44% male; 56% from the stroke-belt region; MedDiet score 0–9; 6.5 years of follow-up; 565 stroke cases (multivariate adjusted)	High adherence to the MedDiet (5–9 on MedDiet scale) was associated with lower risk of incident ischemic stroke by 21% ($p = 0.016$) after adjustment for demographics, vascular risk factors, blood pressure levels, and antihypertensive medications. When the MedDiet was evaluated as a continuous variable, a 1-point increase in MedDiet score was independently associated with a 5% reduction in the risk of incident ischemic stroke
Hoevenaar-Blom (2012). Evaluate the effect of MedDiet score on incidence of total and specific CVD and stroke risk (Dutch EPIC Study) [59]	40,011 participants; MedDiet score 0–9; mean 11.8 years of follow-up; 4881 CVD events (multivariate adjusted)	There was an inverse association between the MedDiet and stroke incidence by 30% (highest compared to lowest adherence) and a 2-point increase in MedDiet score reduced stroke risk by 12%
Misirli et al. (2012). Investigate the effect of the traditional MedDiet on cerebrovascular disease risk in a Mediterranean population (Greek segment of the EPIC Study) [60]	23,601 participants; age 42% > 55 years; 76% ≥ 25 BMI; 59% women; MedDiet score 0–9; median 10.6 years of follow-up; 395 stroke incident cases and 196 stroke deaths (multivariate adjusted)	Compared to a low MedDiet score of 0–3 points, a high score of 6–9 significantly lowered ischemic stroke risk by 46%. MedDiets appear to be more effective in lowering stroke risk in women than men (Fig. 16.5)
Agnoli et al. (2011). Assess the association between the Italian MedDiet Index and stroke risk (EPIC Italy) [61]	47,021 Italians adults; mean baseline age 50 years; 68% women; 37% with hypertension; 25% smokers; mean 7.9 years of follow-up; 178 stroke cases were diagnosed (multivariate adjusted)	Higher adherence to the Italian MedDiet Index reduced risk for total stroke by 53% ischemic stroke by 63% and hemorrhagic stroke by 49%
Gardner et al. (2011). Examine the MedDiet effects on vascular events (Northern Manhattan Study; US) [62]	2568 adults; mean age 69 years; 64% women; mean 9 years of follow-up; 171 ischemic stroke cases, 133 myocardial infarctions, 314 vascular deaths (multivariate adjusted)	The MedDiet score was inversely associated with risk of the composite outcome of ischemic stroke and myocardial infarction (p-trend = 0.04) and with vascular related death (p-trend = 0.02). Moderate and high MedDiet scores were marginally associated with decreased risk of MI. There was no significant association between MedDiet scores and risk of ischemic stroke

Table 16.2 (continued)

Objective	Study details	Results
Fung et al. (2009). Evaluate the effects of the MedDiet on CHD and stroke incidence and mortality in women (Nurses' Health Study; US) [63]	74,886 women; age range 38–63 years; 20 years of follow-up; 2391 incident cases of CHD, 1763 incident cases of stroke, and 1077 cardiovascular disease deaths (multivariate adjusted)	Women in the top Alternate MedDiet Score quintile were at significantly lower risk for CHD by 29% and stroke by 13% vs. lowest score; CVD mortality by 39% vs. the lowest quintile

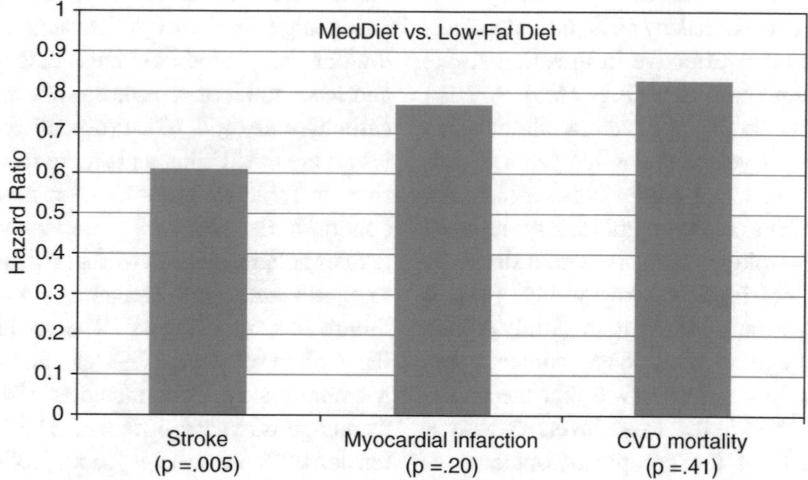

Fig. 16.4 Association between high adherence to a Mediterranean diet (MedDiet) vs. low-fat diet and stroke, myocardial infarction, and cardiovascular disease (CVD) mortality from the PREDIMED Primary Prevention Trial, multivariate adjusted (adapted from [56])

16.3.3.1 Randomized Controlled Trial (RCT)

A multicenter Spanish PREDIMED (Prevención con Dieta Mediterránea) trial (7500 adults with high CVD risk; mean age 67 years; 57% women; diets: a MedDiet supplemented with extra-virgin olive oil, a MedDiet supplemented with mixed nuts, or a control low fat diet; 4.8 years) found that an energy-unrestricted MedDiets significantly reduced stroke risk by 39% (Fig. 16.4) [56].

16.3.3.2 Prospective Cohort Studies

Meta-analysis

A meta-analysis (nine cohorts; 162,092 subjects) found that high adherence to the MedDiet pattern was associated with reduced risk for stroke by 16% whereas moderate adherence only reduced risk by 4% [57].

Specific Studies

Six prospective cohort studies consistently show that the MedDiet is protective against stroke risk [58–63]. A 2015 US Southern regional REGARDS study (30,239 US adults; mean baseline age of 65 years; 6.5 years of follow-up) observed that high adherence to the MedDiet (5–9 on MedDiet scale) was associated with significantly lower ischemic stroke risk by 21% [58]. When the MedDiet was evaluated as a continuous variable, a 1-point increase in MedDiet score was independently associated with a 5% reduction in ischemic stroke risk. A 2012 Dutch EPIC Study (40,011 adults; mean 11.8 years of follow-up) found that higher adherence to the MedDiet significantly reduced stroke incidence by 30% and a 2-point increase in MedDiet score reduced stroke risk by 12% [59]. Another 2012 EPIC study in Greece (23,601 adults; median 10.6 years of follow-up) showed that higher MedDiet adherence scores significantly lowered ischemic stroke risk by 46% [60]. MedDiets appear to be more effective in lowering stroke risk in women than men (Fig. 16.5). A 2011 Italian EPIC study (47,021 Italians adults; mean baseline age 50 years; mean 7.9 years of follow-up) observed that higher adherence to the Italian MedDiet Index significantly reduced risk for total stroke by 53%, ischemic stroke by 63% and hemorrhagic stroke by 49% [61]. A 2011 US Northern Manhattan Study (2568 adults; mean age 69 years; 64% women; mean 9 years of follow-up) observed that the higher adherence to the MedDiet was inversely associated with risk of the composite outcome of ischemic stroke and myocardial infarction and with vascular related death [62]. A 2009 US Nurses' Health Study (74,886 women; age range 38–63 years; 20 years of follow-up) observed that women with high adherence to the Alternate MedDiet Score had significantly lower stroke risk by 13% and lower CVD mortality by 39% [63].

16.3.4 DASH Diet

The DASH diet was designed and clinically validated to prevent and treat hypertension by emphasizing high intake of fruits, vegetables, grains, low-fat dairy products, nuts, chicken, and fish and low intake of red meat, sweets, and refined carbohydrates [64–67]. Prospective cohort studies on the DASH diet and stroke risk are summarized in Table 16.3 [68–73]. A meta-analysis (six cohort studies; 150,000 participants) found that greater adherence to DASH-like diets was shown to significantly protect against stroke, and heart failure risk by 19% [68]. The pooled data from the Cohort of Swedish Men and the Swedish Mammography Cohort studies (74,404 adults; mean age 60 years; 50% had BMI ≥ 25; hypertension 20%; mean 11.9 years of follow-up; 3896 ischemic strokes) observed that the modified DASH score was significantly inversely associated with ischemic stroke risk with a reduction of 14% (highest vs. lowest score quartile) (Fig. 16.6)

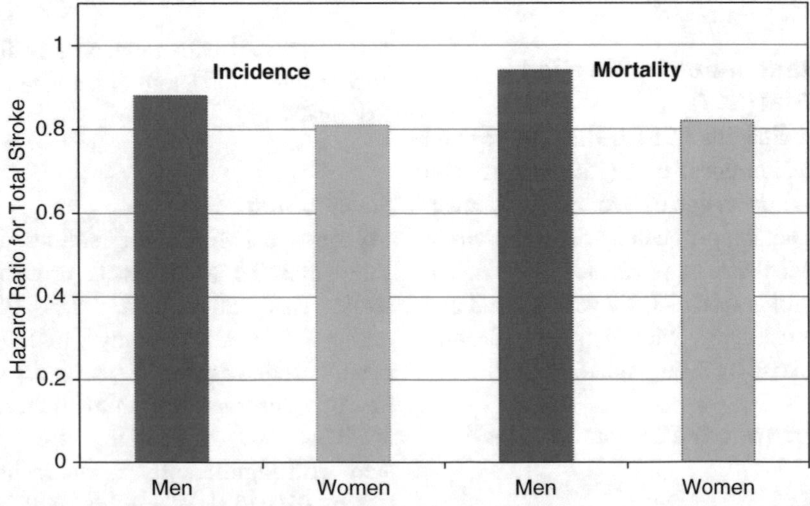

Fig. 16.5 Effect per 2-point increase in adherence to Mediterranean diet on total stroke incidence and mortality (multivariate adjusted) (adapted from [60])

Table 16.3 Summary of DASH diet cohort studies in stroke risk

Objective	Study details	Results
Systematic review and meta-analysis		
Salehi-Abargouei (2013). Evaluate and quantify the effects of the DASH diet on stroke risk [68]	3 cohort studies for stroke; 150,191 adults; 8–24 years of follow-up (multivariate adjusted)	The DASH-style diets significantly decreased stroke risk by 19%
Specific prospective cohort studies		
Larsson et al. (2016). Assess the effect of adherence to the DASH diet and stroke risk (Cohort of Swedish Men and the Swedish Mammography Cohort studies) [69]	74,404 adults; mean age 60 years; mean 11.9 years of follow-up; 3896 ischemic strokes, 560 intracerebral hemorrhages, and 176 subarachnoid hemorrhages (multivariate adjusted)	High adherence to the DASH diet was significantly associated with a reduced risk of ischemic stroke in generally healthy adults (p-trend = 0.002), with a multivariable relative risk reduction by 14% (highest vs. lowest quartile) (Fig. 16.6)
Struijk et al. (2014). Investigate the effects of dietary patterns such as the DASH diet and risk of CVD, CHD or stroke (Dutch EPIC study cohort) [70].	33,671 Dutch adults; mean age 49 years; 74% women; 30% smokers; 21% hypertension; average 12.2 years of follow-up; 2752 CVD cases including 1630 CHD and 527 stroke cases (multivariate adjusted)	Higher adherence to the DASH diet significantly lowered risk of CVD by 14%, CHD by 18% and stroke by13% (highest vs. lowest tertile; or per standard deviation)
Chan et al. (2013). Examine the effect of the MedDiet and DASH diet scores on stroke risk in older Chinese adults [71].	2735 Chinese adults; age ≥ 65 years; 51% women; mean follow-up of 5.7 years; 156 stroke cases (multivariate adjusted)	The DASH diet score was borderline significantly (p = 0.068) associated with lower stroke risk of 38% (≥4.5 vs. ≤4 score) in men but not in women
Fung et al. (2008). Evaluate the association between the DASH diet score and CHD and stroke risk (The Nurses' Health Study; US) [72]	88,517 women; age 34–59 years; 24 years of follow-up; 2317 cases of CHD and 1682 cases of stroke, of which 1242 were ischemic and 440 hemorrhagic (multivariate adjusted)	The DASH score was significantly inversely associated with CHD risk by 24% and stroke risk by 18% for extremes of adherence (Fig. 16.7). Cross-sectional analysis showed that the DASH score was significantly associated with lower plasma levels of C-reactive protein and interleukin 6
Folsom et al. (2007). Evaluate the effect of DASH diet and risk of CVD mortality (Iowa Women's Health Study; US) [73]	20,993 women; mean baseline age 61 years; mean 16 years of follow-up; 236 stroke death cases (multivariate adjusted)	Risk of stroke death was insignificantly reduced by 18%

[69]. In an older Chinese cohort (2735 Chinese adults; age baseline age ≥65 years; 51% women; mean follow-up of 5.7 years) it was observed that a higher DASH diet score (≥4.5 vs.≤4 score) was associated with a 38% lower stroke risk in men, but not in women [71]. The Nurses' Health Study (88,517 women; age 34–59 years; 24 years of follow-up) found that higher adherence to the DASH-style diet was inversely associated with a lower risk of CHD and stroke among middle aged women (Fig. 16.7) [72]. A sub-group analysis of women suggests that the DASH score was significantly associated with lower plasma levels of C-reactive protein (CRP) and interleukin 6 (IL-6).

16.3.5 Healthy Nordic Dietary Pattern

The Healthy Nordic diet is based on healthy foods traditionally eaten in the Nordic countries and contains high intakes of fish, apples and pears, cabbages, root vegetables, whole grains from oats,

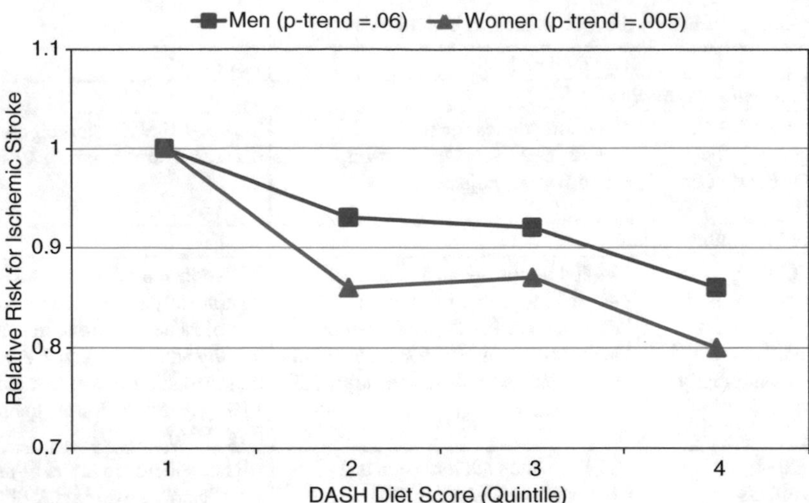

Fig. 16.6 Association between DASH diet adherence and ischemic stroke risk in men and women (mean baseline age 60 years; mean follow-up of 11.9 years) from the Cohort of Swedish Men and the Swedish Mammography Cohort (multivariate adjusted) (adapted from [69])

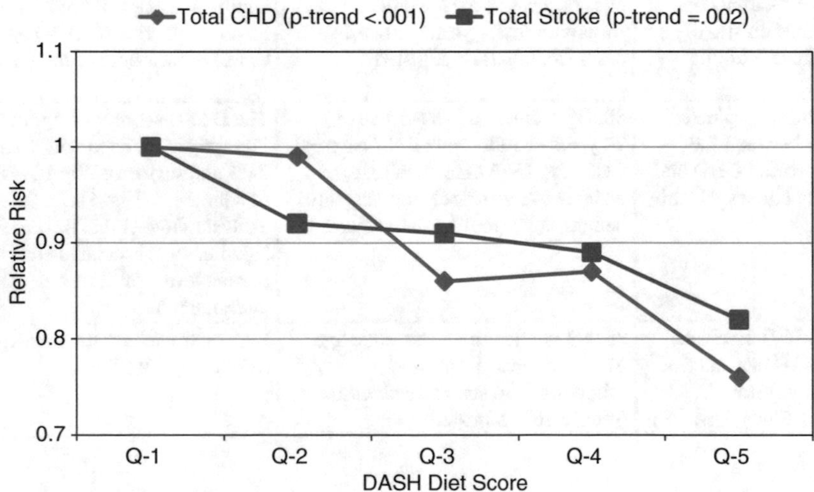

Fig. 16.7 Association between DASH score on total coronary heart disease (CHD) and stroke risk in mid-life women followed for 24 years from the Nurses' Health Study (adapted from [72])

barley and rye, and berries [74]. The vegetable oil used is rapeseed oil (Canola oil), which has been shown in several RCTs of high-risk populations (obese, hypercholesterolemic, or hyperlipidemic subjects) to have beneficial effects on cardiovascular risk markers, such as blood pressure, cholesterol, and adiposity [75]. The 2017 Danish Diet, Cancer and Health cohort (55,338 men and

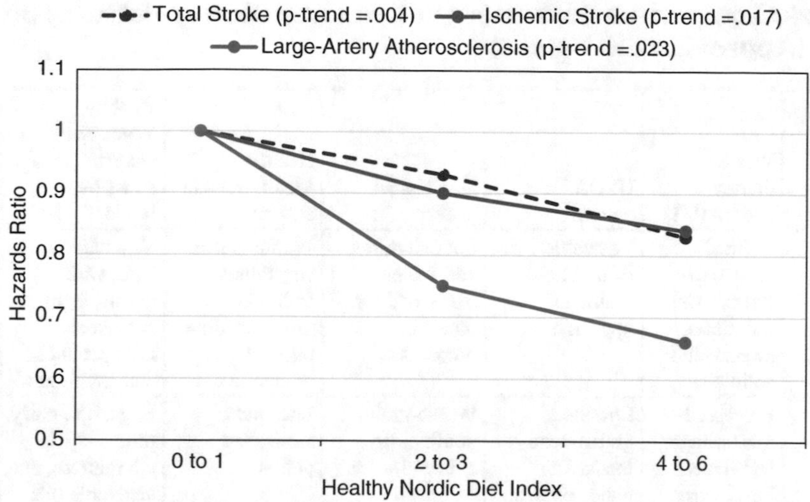

Fig. 16.8 Association between the Healthy Nordic Food Index score and stroke risk (adapted from [74])

women; baseline age 56 years; 52% women; median 13.5 years of follow-up) found that a higher healthy Nordic diet index score was associated with a lower risk of stroke and large-artery atherosclerosis (Fig. 16.8) [74].

Conclusions

Stroke is the second most common cause of death worldwide and forecast projections estimate that there will be a 20% increase in stroke prevalence by 2030 compared to 2012 rates, because of the increase in aging populations. Approximately 75% of stroke risk is attributable to smoking, poor diet quality, low physical activity, and excessive body weight, which are associated with sub-optimal cardiometabolic health. Cohort studies show that healthy dietary patterns are significantly protective against stroke risk by 11–23% whereas the Western dietary pattern increases stroke risk by 5–6%. A large Spanish PREDIMED trial found that the MedDiet significantly reduced stroke risk by 39% in older adults with high cardiovascular disease risk over 4.8 years. Prospective studies show that high adherence to MedDiets, DASH diets and the Healthy Nordic Diet Index significantly reduces total or ischemic stroke risk. MedDiets and DASH diets tend to be more effective at lowering stroke risk in women than men. Potential healthy dietary pattern mechanisms for lowering stroke risk are through aiding in weight and glycemic control; improving vascular function, and blood lipids and lipoprotein profiles; and contributing to a healthier colonic microbiota ecosystem and lower systemic inflammation and oxidative stress.

Appendix A: Comparison of Western and Healthy Dietary Patterns per 2000 kcal (Approximated Values)

Components	Western dietary pattern (US)	USDA Base pattern	DASH Diet pattern	Healthy Mediterranean pattern	Healthy Vegetarian pattern (Lact-ovo based)	Vegan pattern
Emphasizes	Refined grains, low fiber foods, red meats, sweets, and solid fats	Vegetables, fruit, whole-grain, and low-fat milk	Potassium rich vegetables, fruits, and low fat milk products	Whole grains, vegetables, fruit, dairy products, olive oil, and moderate wine	Vegetables, fruit, whole-grains, legumes, nuts, seeds, milk products, and soy foods	Plant foods: vegetables, fruits, whole grains, nuts, seeds, and soy foods
Includes	Processed meats, sugar sweetened beverages, and fast foods	Enriched grains, lean meat, fish, nuts, seeds, and vegetable oils	Whole-grain, poultry, fish, nuts and seeds	Fish, nuts, seeds, and pulses	Eggs, non-dairy milk alternatives, and vegetable oils	Non-dairy milk alternatives
Limits	Fruits and vegetables, and whole-grains	Solid fats and added sugars	Red meats, sweets, and sugar-sweetened beverages	Red meats, refined grains, and sweets	No red or white meats, or fish; limited sweets	No animal products
Estimated nutrients/components						
Carbohydrates (% total kcal)	51	51	55	50	54	57
Protein (% total kcal)	16	17	18	16	14	13
Total fat (% total kcal)	33	32	27	34	32	30
Saturated fat (% total kcal)	11	8	6	8	8	7
Unsat. fat (% total kcal)	22	25	21	24	26	25
Fiber (g)	16	31	29+	31	35+	40+
Potassium (mg)	2800	3350	4400	3350	3300	3650
Vegetable oils (g)	19	27	25	27	19–27	18–27
Sodium (mg)	3600	1790	1100	1690	1400	1225
Added sugar (g)	79 (20 tsp)	32 (8 tsp)	12 (3 tsp)	32 (8 tsp)	32 (8 tsp)	32 (8 tsp)

Components	Western dietary pattern (US)	USDA Base pattern	DASH Diet pattern	Healthy Mediterranean pattern	Healthy Vegetarian pattern (Lact-ovo based)	Vegan pattern
Plant food groups						
Fruit (cup)	≤1.0	2.0	2.5	2.5	2.0	2.0
Vegetables (cup)	≤1.5	2.5	2.1	2.5	2.5	2.5
Whole-grains (oz.)	0.5	3.0	4.0	3.0	3.0	3.0
Legumes (oz.)	–	1.5	0.5	1.5	3.0	3.0+
Nuts/seeds (oz.)	0.5	0.6	1.0	0.6	1.0	2.0
Soy products (oz.)	0.0	0.5	–	–	1.1	1.5

U.S. Department of Agriculture and U.S. Department of Health and Human Services. Dietary Guidelines for Americans, 2010. 7th Edition, Washington, DC: U.S. Government Printing Office. 2010; Table B2.4; http://www.choosemyplate.gov/accessed 8.22.2015

U.S. Department of Agriculture, Agriculture Research Service, Nutrient Data Laboratory. 2014. USDA National Nutrient Database for Standard Reference, Release 27. https://www.ars.usda.gov/nutrientdata. Accessed 17 February 2015

Dietary Guidelines Advisory Committee. Scientific Report. Advisory Report to the Secretary of Health and Human Services and the Secretary of Agriculture. Appendix E-3.7: Developing vegetarian and Mediterranean-style food patterns. 2015; 1–9

References

1. Mendis S, Puska P, Norrving B (editors). Global atlas on cardiovascular disease prevention and control. The underlying pathology of heart attacks and strokes. Geneva: World Health Organization. 2011. ISBN 978-92-4-156437-3.
2. Mozaffarian D, Benjamin EJ, Go AS, et al. Heart disease and stroke statistics-2015 update: a report from the American Heart Association. Circulation. 2015;131:29–322.
3. Meschia JF, Bushnell C, Boden-Albala B, et al. Guidelines for the primary prevention of stroke. a statement for healthcare professionals from the American Heart Association/American Stroke Association. Stroke. 2014;45:3754–832.
4. Goldstein LB, Bushnell CD, Adams RJ, et al. Guidelines for the primary prevention of stroke. a guideline for healthcare professionals from the American Heart Association/American Stroke Association. Stroke. 2011;42:517–84.
5. Feigin VL, Roth GA, Naghavi M, et al. Global burden of stroke and risk factors in 188 countries, during 1990-2013: a systematic analysis for the global burden of disease study 2013. Lancet Neurol. 2016;15(9):913–24. https://doi.org/10.1016/S1474-4422(16)30073-4.
6. Lin MP, Ovbiagele B, Markovic D, Towfighi A. "Life's Simple 7" and long-term mortality after stroke. J Am Heart Assoc. 2015;4(11). https://doi.org/10.1161/JAHA.114.001470.
7. Younus A, Aneni EC, Spatz ES, et al. A systematic review of the prevalence and outcomes of ideal cardiovascular health in US and non-US populations. Mayo Clin Proc. 2016;91(5):649–70.
8. Kulshreshtha A, Vaccarino V, Judd SE, et al. Life's Simple 7 and risk of incident stroke the reasons for geographic and racial differences in Stroke study. Stroke. 2013;44:1909–14.
9. Rist PM, Buring JE, Kase CS, Kurth T. Healthy lifestyle and functional outcomes from stroke in women. Am J Med. 2016;129(7):715–724.e2. https://doi.org/10.1016/j.amjmed.2016.02.002.
10. Sipahi I, Swaminathan A, Natesan V, et al. Effect of antihypertensive therapy on incident stroke in cohorts with prehypertensive blood pressure levels: a meta-analysis of randomized controlled trials. Stroke. 2012;43:432–40.
11. Lackland DT, Roccella EJ, Deutsch A, et al. Factors influencing the decline in stroke mortality: a statement from the American Heart Association/American Stroke Association. Circulation. 2014;45:315–53.
12. Chen X, Zhou L, Zhang Y, et al. Risk factors of stroke in Western and Asian countries: a systematic review and meta-analysis of prospective cohort studies. BMC Public Health. 2014;14(776.) http://www.biomedcentral.com/1471-2458/14/776
13. Strazzullo P, D'Elia L, Cairella G, et al. Excess body weight and incidence of stroke: meta-analysis of prospective studies with 2 million participants. Stroke. 2010;41:418–26.

14. Neter JE, Stam BE, Kok FJ, et al. Influence of weight reduction on blood pressure: a meta-analysis of randomized controlled trials. Hypertension. 2003;42:878–84.
15. Lee CD, Folsom AR, Blair SN. Physical activity and stroke risk: a meta-analysis. Stroke. 2003;34:2475–81.
16. Wendel-Vos GC, Schuit AJ, Feskens EJ, et al. Physical activity and stroke: a meta-analysis of observational data. Int J Epidemiol. 2004;33:787–98.
17. Hopper I, Billah B, Skiba M, Krum H. Prevention of diabetes and reduction in major cardiovascular events in studies of subjects with prediabetes: meta-analysis of randomised controlled clinical trials. Eur J Cardiovasc Prev Rehabil. 2011;18:813–23.
18. Zhang Y, Tuomilehto J, Jousilahti P, et al. Total and high-density lipoprotein cholesterol and stroke risk. Stroke. 2012;43:1768–74.
19. Varbo A, Nordestgaard BG, Tybjaeg-Hansen A, et al. Nonfasting triglycerides, cholesterol, and ischemic stroke in the general population. Ann Neurol. 2011;69(4):628–34.
20. Lu Y, Hajifathalian K, Ezzati M, et al. Metabolic mediators of the effects of body-mass index, overweight, and obesity on coronary heart disease and stroke: a pooled analysis of 97 prospective cohorts with 1.8 million participants. Lancet. 2014;383(9921):970–83.
21. Peters SA, Huxley RR, Woodward M. Smoking as a risk factor for stroke in women compared with men: a systematic review and meta-analysis of 81 cohorts, including 3,980,359 individuals and 42,401 strokes. Stroke. 2013;44(10):2821–8.
22. Kontogianni MD, Panagiotakos DB. Dietary patterns and stroke: A systematic review and re-meta-analysis. Maturitas. 2014;79:41–7.
23. Sherzai A, Heim LT, Boothby C, Sherzai AD. Stroke, food groups, and dietary patterns: a systematic review. Nutr Rev. 2012;70(8):423–35.
24. Dietary Guidelines Advisory Committee. Scientific Report. Advisory Report to the Secretary of Health and Human Services and the Secretary of Agriculture. Part D. Chapter 1: Food and nutrient intakes, and health: current status and trends 2015; 1–78.
25. Dietary Guidelines Advisory Committee. Scientific Report. Advisory Report to the Secretary of Health and Human Services and the Secretary of Agriculture. Appendix E-37: Developing vegetarian and Mediterranean-style food patterns 2015; 1–9.
26. USDA. What We Eat in America, NHANES 2011–2012, individuals 2 years and over (excluding breast-fed children). Available: www.ars.usda.gov/nea/bhnrc/fsrg.
27. U.S. Department of Agriculture, Agriculture Research Service, Nutrient Data Laboratory. 2014. USDA National Nutrient Database for Standard Reference, Release 27. http://www.ars. usda.gov/nutrientdata. Accessed 17 Feb 2015.
28. U.S. Department of Agriculture and U.S. Department of Health and Human Services. Dietary Guidelines for Americans, 2010. 7th edition, Washington, DC: U.S. Government Printing Office. 2010; Table B2.4; http://www.choosemyplate.gov/accessed 8.22.2015.
29. Ascherio A, Rimm EB, Hernan MA, et al. Intake of potassium, magnesium, calcium, and fiber and risk of stroke among US men. Circulation. 1998;98:1198–204.
30. Crump C, Sundquist J, Winkleby MA, Sundquist K. Interactive effects of physical fitness and body mass index on risk of stroke: a national cohort study. Int J Stroke. 2016;11(6):683–94. pii: 1747493016641961
31. Evans CEL, Greenwood DC, Threapleton DE, et al. Effects of dietary fibre type on blood pressure: a systematic review and meta-analysis of randomized controlled trials of healthy individuals. J Hypertens. 2015;33(5):897–911.
32. Davis JN, Hodges VA, Gillham MB. Normal-weight adults consume more fiber and fruit than their age- and height-matched overweight/obese counterparts. J Am Diet Assoc. 2006;106:833–40.
33. Slavin JL. Dietary fiber and body weight. Nutrition. 2005;21:411–8.
34. Fogelholm M, Anderssen S, Gunnarsdottir I, Lahti-Koski M. Dietary macronutrients and food consumption as determinants of long-term weight change in adult populations: a systematic literature review. Food Nutr Res. 2012;56. https://doi.org/10.3402/fnr.v56i0.19103.
35. Genser B, Silbernage G, De Backer G, et al. Plant sterols and cardiovascular disease: a systematic review and meta-analysis. Eur Heart J. 2012;33:444–51.
36. Lau C, Faerch K, Glumer C, et al. Dietary glycemic index, glycemic load, fiber, simple sugars, and insulin resistance: the Inter99 study. Diabetes Care. 2005;28:1397–403.
37. Tosh SM. Review of human studies investigating the post-prandial blood-glucose lowering ability of oat and barley food products. Eur J Clin Nutr. 2013;67:310–7.
38. Silva FM, Kramer CK, de Almeida JC, et al. Fiber intake and glycemic control in patients with type 2 diabetes mellitus: a systematic review with meta-analysis of randomized controlled trials. Nutr Rev. 2013;71(12):790–801.
39. Sen A, Marsche G, Freudenberger P, et al. Association between higher plasma lutein, zeaxanthin, and vitamin C concentrations and longer telomere length: results of the Austrian Stroke Prevention Study. J Am Geriatr Soc. 2014;62:222–9.
40. Winek K, Meisel A, Dirnagl U. Gut microbiota impact on stroke outcome: fad or fact? J Cereb Blood Flow Metab. 2016;36(5):891–8. https://doi.org/10.1177/0271678X16636890.
41. Whitehead A, Beck EJ, Tosh S, Wolever TMS. Cholesterol-lowering effects of oat β-glucan: a meta-analysis of randomized controlled trials. Am J Clin Nutr. 2014;100:1413–21.
42. Leermaker ET, Darweesh SK, Baena CP, et al. The effects of lutein on cardiometabolic health across the life course: a systematic review and meta-analysis. Am J Clin Nutr. 2016;103(2):481–94.
43. Berni Canani R, Di Costanzo M, Leone L, et al. Potential beneficial effects of butyrate in intestinal and extraintestinal diseases. World J Gastroenterol. 2011;17(12):1519–28.
44. Zhou Y, Han W, Gong D, Fan Y. Hs-CRP in stroke: a meta-analysis. Clin Chim Acta. 2016;435:21–7.

45. McCall DO, McGartland CP, McKinley MC, et al. Dietary intake of fruits and vegetables improves microvascular function in hypertensive subjects in a dose-dependent manner. Circulation. 2009;119: 2153–60.
46. Noad RL, Rooney C, McCall D, et al. Beneficial effect of a polyphenol-rich diet on cardiovascular risk: a randomised control trial. Heart. 2016;102(17):1371–9. https://doi.org/10.1136/heartjnl-2015-309218.
47. Jiao J, JY X, Zhang W, et al. Effect of dietary fiber on circulating C-reactive protein in overweight and obese adults: a meta-analysis of randomized controlled trials. Int J Food Sci Nutr. 2015;66(1):114–9.
48. North CJ, Venter CS, Jerling JC. The effects of dietary fibre on C reactive protein, an inflammation marker predicting cardiovascular disease. Eur J Clin Nutr. 2009;63:921–33.
49. Maukonen J, Saarela M. Human gut microbiota: does diet matter? Proc Nutr Soc. 2015;74:23–36.
50. Zhang X, Shu L, Si C, et al. Dietary patterns and risk of stroke in adults: a systematic review and meta-analysis of prospective cohort studies. J Stroke Cerebrovascular Dis. 2015;24(10):2173–82.
51. Rodríguez-Monforte M, Flores-Mateo G, Sánchez E. Dietary patterns and CVD: a systematic review and meta-analysis of observational studies. Br J Nutr. 2015;114:1341–59.
52. Li F, Hou L, Chen W, et al. Associations of dietary patterns with the risk of all-cause, CVD and stroke mortality: a meta-analysis of prospective cohort studies. Br J Nutr. 2015;13:16–24.
53. Stricker MD, Onland-Moret NC, Boer JM, et al. Dietary patterns derived from principal component and k-means cluster analysis: long-term association with coronary heart disease and stroke. Nutr Metab Cardiovasc Dis. 2013;23(3):250–6.
54. Judd SE, Gutiérrez OM, Newby PK, et al. Dietary patterns are associated with incident stroke and contribute to excess risk of stroke in black Americans. Stroke. 2013;44:3305–11.
55. Fung TT, Stampfer MJ, Manson JE, et al. Prospective study of major dietary patterns and stroke risk in women. Stroke. 2004;35:2014–9.
56. Estruch R, Ros E, Salas-Salvado J, for the PREDIMED Study Investigators, et al. Primary prevention of cardiovascular disease with a Mediterranean diet. N Engl J Med. 2013;368:1279–90.
57. Psaltopoulou T, Sergentanis TN, Panagiotakos DB, et al. Mediterranean diet, stroke, cognitive impairment, and depression: a meta-analysis. Ann Neurol. 2013;74:580–91.
58. Tsivgoulis G, Psaltopoulou T, Wadley VG, et al. Adherence to a Mediterranean diet and prediction of incident stroke. Stroke. 2015;46:780–5.
59. Hoevenaar-Blom MP, Nooyens ACJ, Kromhout D, et al. Mediterranean style diet and 12-year incidence of cardiovascular diseases: the EPIC-NL cohort study. PLoS One. 2012;7(9). https://doi.org/10.1371/journal.pone.0045458.
60. Misirli G, Benetou V, Lagiou P, et al. Relation of the traditional Mediterranean diet to cerebrovascular disease in a Mediterranean population. Am J Epidemiol. 2012;176(12):1185–92.
61. Agnoli C, Krogh V, Grioni S, et al. A priori-defined dietary patterns are associated with reduced risk of stroke in a large Italian cohort. J Nutr. 2011;141: 1552–8.
62. Gardener H, et al. Mediterranean-style diet and risk of ischemic stroke, myocardial infarction, and vascular death: the Northern Manhattan Study. Am J Clin Nutr. 2011;94(6):1458–64.
63. Fung TT, Rexrode KM, Mantzoros CS, et al. Mediterranean diet and incidence of and mortality from coronary heart disease and stroke in women. Circulation. 2009;119:1093–100.
64. Appel LJ, Moore TJ, Obarzanek E, et al. A clinical trial of the effects of dietary patterns on blood pressure. N Engl J Med. 1997;336:1117–24.
65. Appel LJ. ASH position paper: dietary approaches to lower blood pressure. J Clin Hypertension. 2009;11(7):358–68.
66. Moore TJ, Conlin PR, Ard J, Svetkey LP. DASH (Dietary Approaches to Stop Hypertension) diet is effective treatment for stage 1 isolated systolic hypertension. Hypertension. 2001;38:155–8.
67. Sacks FM, Obarzanek E, Windhauser MM, et al. Rationale and design of the Dietary Approaches to Stop Hypertension (DASH) trial. A multicenter controlled-feeding study of dietary patterns to lower blood pressure. Ann Epidemiol. 1995;5:108–18.
68. Salehi-Abargouei A, Maghsoudi Z, Shirani F, Azadbakht L. Effects of Dietary Approaches to Stop Hypertension (DASH)-style diet on fatal or nonfatal cardiovascular diseases-incidence: a systematic review and meta-analysis on observational prospective studies. Nutrition. 2013;29:611–8.
69. Larsson SC, Wallin A, Wolk A. Dietary Approaches to Stop Hypertension diet and incidence of stroke results from 2 prospective cohorts. Stroke. 2016;47(4):986–90. https://doi.org/10.1161/STROKEAHA. 116.012675.
70. Struijk EA, May AM, Wezenbeek N, et al. Adherence to dietary guidelines and cardiovascular disease risk in the EPIC-NL cohort. Int J Cardiol. 2014;176(2):354–9.
71. Chan R, Chan D, Woo J. The association of *a priori* and *posterior* dietary patterns with the risk of incident stroke in Chinese older people in Hong Kong. J Nutr Health Aging. 2013;17:866–74.
72. Fung TT, Chiuve SE, McCullough ML, et al. Adherence to a DASH-style diet and risk of coronary heart disease and stroke in women. Arch Intern Med. 2008;168(7):713–20.
73. Folsom AR, Parker ED, Harnack LJ. Degree of concordance with DASH diet guidelines and incidence of hypertension and fatal cardiovascular disease. Am J Hypertens. 2007;20:225–32.
74. Hansen CP, Overvad K, Kyrø C, et al. Adherence to a healthy Nordic diet and risk of stroke a Danish cohort study. Stroke. 2017;48:259–64. https://doi.org/10.1161/STROKEAHA.116.015019.
75. Lin L, Allemekinders H, Dansby A, et al. Evidence of health benefits of canola oil. Nutr Rev. 2013;71(6):370–85. https://doi.org/10.1111/nure.12033.

Whole Plant Foods and Stroke Risk 17

Keywords
Stroke • Ischemic stroke • Hemorrhagic stroke • Whole plant foods Whole-grains • Fruits • Vegetables • Green leafy vegetables • Apples Legumes • Nuts • Peanuts • Tea • Coffee

Key Points

- Stroke and related cerebrovascular diseases make-up the second most common cause of death worldwide, accounting for 6.2 million deaths (11% of total deaths). Regular consumption of specific foods and beverages may have significant effects on stroke risk with potential stroke protective foods including low fat dairy, whole grains, fruits, vegetables, nuts, tea and coffee whereas high intake of red meat, sugar-sweetened beverages and alcohol may increase stroke risk.
- The consumption of ≥3 daily servings of whole grains is associated with lower total stroke risk by 8–14% and ischemic stroke by 25% compared to never or rare intake.
- Increased consumption by 200 g (or 2 1/2 servings)/day reduces total stroke for total fruits and vegetables by 16%, fruits by 18% and vegetables by 13%. Raw fruits and vegetables are more effective than processed forms; examples of effective specific varieties for reducing ischemic stroke risk are green leafy vegetables, white fruits and vegetables (e.g., apples, cauliflower, mushrooms) and vitamin C rich fruits and vegetables (e.g., citrus, bell peppers, broccoli).
- Plant protein sources such as legumes and nuts have mixed effects on stroke risk. Dietary pulses or total legumes are not associated with stroke risk but nuts and soy foods are associated with lower stroke risk.
- Whole plant foods containing a variety of nutrients and phytochemicals such as fiber, antioxidant vitamins, potassium, magnesium, carotenoids, flavonoids and phytosterols may provide potential stroke protection by mechanisms associated with promoting vascular health by attenuating elevated blood pressure, lowering LDL-cholesterol levels and systemic inflammation associated with atherosclerosis, and promoting better insulin sensitivity, blood glucose control, weight control, and microbiota health compared to less healthy or highly processed plant foods.

M.L. Dreher, *Dietary Patterns and Whole Plant Foods in Aging and Disease*, Nutrition and Health,
https://doi.org/10.1007/978-3-319-59180-3_17

17.1 Introduction

Strokes are caused by a disruption of the blood supply to the brain due to either blockage (ischemic stroke) or rupture of a blood vessel (hemorrhagic stroke) [1]. Of all strokes, 87% are ischemic [2]. Stroke and related cerebrovascular diseases make-up the second most common cause of death worldwide, accounting for 6.2 million deaths (11% of total deaths) [2]. Over 90% of stroke risk can be attributed to modifiable risk factors, including 74% due to behavioral factors (smoking, poor diet, and low physical activity) and their association with metabolic factors including high systolic blood pressure (BP), high BMI, high fasting plasma glucose, high total cholesterol, and low glomerular filtration rate [2–12]. Stroke is a major cause of disability and death worldwide, and changes the lives not only of the stroke victims but also of their families as many become dependent in their activities of daily living due to significant stroke related cognitive and physical deficits [1–5]. Forecasts suggest a >20% increase in stroke prevalence by 2030 compared to 2012 rates, because of the increase in aging populations [2–4]. Stroke carries a high risk of death and survivors can experience loss of vision and/or speech, paralysis, and confusion. Intervention trials and observation studies suggest that lifestyle habits are the primary factors associated with stroke risk. The type and amount of foods and beverages consumed can have an important effect on stroke risk and prevention. An overview of commonly consumed foods and beverages that may have potential effects on stroke risk are summarized in Table 17.1 [13–37]. The primary objective of this chapter is to comprehensively review the effects of whole and minimally processed plant foods (whole plant foods) on stroke risk and prevention.

17.2 Whole Plant Foods

Whole plant foods contain a variety of nutrients and phytochemicals that may be associated with lower stroke risk, such as fiber, vitamins E and C, trace minerals, carotenoids, flavonoids and phytosterols (Appendix A) [38–46]. Potential mechanisms by which whole plant foods amplify support for reduced stroke risk in contrast to the effects of highly processed refined foods by: (1) reducing dietary energy density and increasing satiety and satiation, which reduces the risk of weight gain or obesity; (2) enhancing insulin sensitivity, which may improve vascular and endothelial functions, (3) promoting healthier LDL-C, HDL-C and triglyceride profiles for improved endothelial health and a slower rate of arterial plaque build-up, (4) attenuating elevated systemic inflammation and LDL-oxidation, and (5) stimulating healthier microbiota and increased fermentation to short chain fatty acids (SCFAs) such as butyrate for colon and cardiometabolic health and body weight control [47–69]. However, whole plant foods are consumed at low levels in the typical Western diet with an estimated >90% of US adults not meeting the recommended minimal levels of whole-grains, fruits, vegetables, legumes, or nuts and seeds to maintain optimal health and weight control outcomes [47–49].

Table 17.1 Overview of foods and beverages with potential effects on stroke risk

Increase stroke risk	Little or No effect on risk	Decrease stroke risk
Total red meat >50 g/day and fresh red meat >70 g/day [26–28] Sugar sweetened beverages ≥2 servings/day [35–37] Heavy alcohol intake [13, 14]	Moderate whole-fat dairy, butter or cream [20, 21] Refined grains (≤ 3 servings/day) [29, 30] Lean, fatty or total fish [33, 34] Moderate alcohol intake [13, 14]	Total dairy, low fat diary and cheese ≥2 servings daily [22, 23] Extra virgin olive oil 1 L/week [19] Dark chocolate >50 g/week [18, 19]. Fruits and vegetables ≥200 g/day [31, 32] Whole-grains ≥3 servings [29, 30] Nuts ≥5 days of the week [24, 25] Tea ≥3 cups/day; green or black [17] Coffee 3–5 cups/day [15, 16] Low alcohol intake ≤1 drink (10 g ethanol)/day [13, 14]

17.2.1 Whole-Grains

17.2.1.1 Background

Whole-grain products (brown rice, oatmeal, whole oats, popcorn, whole rye, and graham and whole wheat flour) consist of the starchy endosperm, germ and bran found in similar proportions to that of the whole intact kernel with fiber, vitamins, minerals and phytochemicals [70, 71]. In contrast, refined grain products (white rice and flour, and white bread, pastry, and low fiber breakfast cereals) are mainly comprised of the starchy endosperm with most of the fiber, vitamins, minerals and phytonutrients removed during processing. The US dietary guidelines recommend ≥3 servings/whole-grains/day and ≤3 servings of refined grains/day to promote health and wellness associated with reduced risk of various chronic diseases [48, 49]. However, only about 1% of Americans follow the recommendation for whole-grain intake as the average American's intake is <1 ounce whole grains/day and 70% exceed the recommended intake for refined grains [48, 72].

17.2.1.2 Prospective Cohort Studies

A summary of prospective cohort studies examining the effects of whole-grain and refined grains on stroke risk is provided in Table 17.2 [30, 73–80].

Systematic Reviews and Meta-analyses

Four meta-analyses provide insights on the effects of increased intake of whole-grains and stroke risk [30, 73–75]. Three analyses conclude that the consumption of ≥3 daily servings of whole grains is associated with lower total stroke risk by 8–14% and ischemic stroke by 25% vs. infrequent intake [30, 73, 74]. The effects of whole-grain intake on stroke risk was non-linear with no additional reduction in risk above 120–150 g/day (4–5 servings) [73]. The increased intake of refined grains was not significantly associated with stroke risk [75].

Specific Prospective Cohort Studies

Five prospective cohort studies provide specific insights into the effect of increased whole-grain intake on stroke risk [76–80]. Two Iowa Women's Health Studies in post-menopausal women (approx. 30,000 women; mean baseline age 61 years; 9–17 years of follow-up) observed that ≥2.7 servings/day of whole-grains had a trend for reduced stroke mortality risk by 13–15% and similar increased intake of refined grain intake showed an increased trend for stroke mortality risk by 30–33% [76, 80]. A 2005 Nurses' Health Study (78,770 women;18 years of follow-up) showed that whole-grain cereal fiber was inversely associated with stroke risk outcomes [77]. A 2000 Nurses' Health Study (75,521 US women; mean baseline age 50 years;12 years of follow-up) observed that increased intake of whole-grains was inversely associated with ischemic stroke risk in women and increased refined grain intake positively associated with increased risk (Fig. 17.1) [29]. The Atherosclerosis Risk in Communities cohort (15,792 adults; mean baseline age 53 years; 11 years of follow-up) showed that ≥3 servings/day of whole-grains reduced ischemic stroke risk by 25%, whereas 3–5 servings of refined-grains did not significantly increase ischemic stroke risk [78].

17.2.2 Fruits and Vegetables

17.2.2.1 Background

Adequate intake of fruits and vegetables is an important component of most global dietary guidance recommendations for health and BP control because of their concentrations of: antioxidant vitamins and phytochemicals, especially vitamins C and A, and carotenoids; minerals (especially electrolytes, high potassium and magnesium, and low sodium); and dietary fiber and lower energy density; but their composition is highly variable leading to diverse BP and hypertension effects [38, 41]. The World Health Organization (WHO) report recommended a minimum daily intake of 400 g of fruit and vegetables in 1990s, based on emerging evidence that higher levels are protective against cardiovascular disease (CVD) [81]. This led to the launch of various "eat 5 or more" fruit and vegetable campaigns in Europe, the US and Australia

Table 17.2 Summary of prospective cohort studies on whole- and refined-grain intake in stroke risk

Objective	Study details	Results
Systematic reviews and meta-analyses		
Aune et al. (2016). Quantify the dose-response relation between intake of whole grain and stroke risk [73].	6 cohort studies; 245,012 participants; 2337 stroke cases.	For high vs. low intake of whole grains, there was a 13% lower stroke risk; and a 12% lower risk per three servings (90 g/day). There was evidence of non-linearity between whole grain and risk of stroke ($p < 0.001$) with no further reduction in risk above 120–150 g/day
Chen et al. (2016). Investigate the association of whole and refined grain and stroke risk [30].	7 cohort studies; 446,451 participants; 5892 stroke events).	Total stroke risk was reduced for total grains by 5%, for whole grain by 8%, and for refined grains by 1% (highest vs. lowest intake). Whole grains were inversely associated with ischemic stroke risk by 25%. Refined grain was not associated with total stroke risk.
Fang et al. (2015). Examine the evidence for the effects of whole-grains on stroke risk [74].	6 cohort studies; 247,487 subjects; mean age range 38–74 years; 1635 stroke cases, mean follow-up of 5.5–24 years; 5 studies from US and 1 study from Finland.	Whole-grains were significantly associated with reduced risk of stroke by 14% (≥2.7 servings vs. rare intake).
Wu et al. (2015). Evaluate the association between refined-grains and stroke risk [75].	8 cohort studies; 410,821 participants; 8284 stroke events.	Diets higher in refined-grains had insignificantly increased stroke risk by 2% in men and women.
Prospective cohort studies		
Jacobs et al. (2007). Assess the association between whole-grain intake and inflammatory disease and stroke mortality risk (US Iowa Women's Health Study) [76].	27,312 healthy postmenopausal women; mean baseline age 61 years, mean BMI 27; 17 years of follow-up; 1071 deaths from inflammatory causes (multivariate adjusted).	Compared with women who rarely or never ate whole-grain foods, women consuming ≥2.7 servings/day whole-grains had a trend for lower stroke mortality risk by15% and similar intakes of refined grains showed a trend toward increased stroke mortality risk by 30%.
Oh et al. (2005). Assess the association between high carbohydrate intake, a high glycemic index diet, and a high glycemic load diet and stroke risk (Nurses' Health Study; US) [77].	78,779 women; mean baseline age 46 years;18-years of follow-up; 1020 stroke cases (multivariate adjusted).	Carbohydrate intake and glycemic load were significantly associated with elevated risk of hemorrhagic stroke for extreme quintiles but not with ischemic stroke, especially among women with a BMI of ≥25. Cereal fiber intake was inversely associated with total stroke by 34% and hemorrhagic stroke risk by 49% at highest vs. lowest intake.
Steffen et al. (2003). Evaluate the association between whole grain intake on risk of total mortality and the incidence of coronary artery disease (CAD) and ischemic stroke (Atherosclerosis Risk in Communities cohort; US) [78].	15,792 adults; mean baseline age 53 years; mean BMI 27; 11 years of follow-up; 214 ischemic strokes (multivariate adjusted).	Whole-grain intake was inversely associated with ischemic stroke incidence. Subjects consuming ≥3 whole-grain foods servings / day had significantly reduced ischemic stroke risk by 25% (p-trend =0.15) Compared to rare or never intake. Refined grain was not associated with ischemic stroke incidence.

Table 17.2 (continued)

Objective	Study details	Results
Liu et al. (2003). Evaluate the association between whole- and refined-grain breakfast cereal intakes and mortality in men (The Physicians' Health Study; US) [80].	86,190 men; mean baseline age 56 years; mean follow-up of 5.5 years; 146 stroke deaths (multivariate adjusted).	The consumption of ≥1 serving/day of total, whole-grain or refined grain breakfast cereal vs. rarely or never consuming breakfast cereal was insignificantly associated with stroke mortality risk.
Liu et al. (2000). Investigate the relationship between whole-grain intake and ischemic stroke risk (The Nurses' Health Study) [29].	75,521 US women; mean baseline age 50 years; 12 years of follow-up; 352 ischemic stroke incident cases (multivariate adjusted).	Whole-grain intake was inversely associated with ischemic stroke risk (median intake: 2.7 servings/day vs. 0.13 servings/day) with risk reductions by 31% (p-trend = 0.08) whereas refined grain insignificantly reduced stroke risk by 3% (Fig. 17.1).
Jacobs et al. (1999). Investigate the association between whole-grains and mortality risk (The Iowa Women's Health Study; US) [80].	34,333 healthy postmenopausal women; mean baseline age 61.5 years; 9 years of follow-up (multivariate adjusted).	Women in the highest category of whole-grain cereal intake (≥3 servings/day) had trend for lower stroke mortality risk by 13% and similar refined grains intake showed an increased trend for stroke mortality risk by 33%.

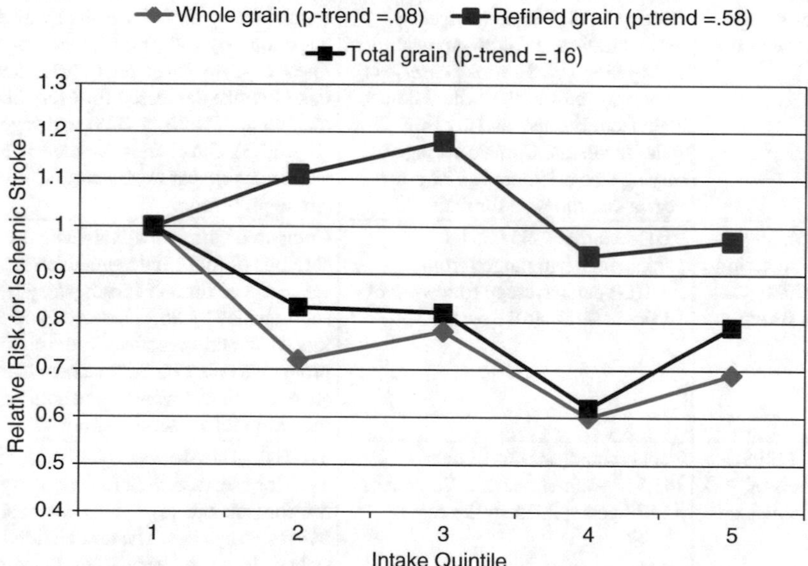

Fig. 17.1 Association between whole, refined and total grain intake and ischemic stroke risk in women from the Nurses' Health Study after 12 years (adapted from [29])

[82]. The USDA MyPlate educational concept, which devotes one-half the plate to fruits and vegetables, as a displacement of other foods of higher energy density from the diet, is a good habit to establish for healthy aging or healthy eating at any age [83]. However, globally, fruit and vegetable consumption is only a small fraction of the recommended levels [84]. In the US, >85% of the population fall short of meeting the daily fruit and vegetable intake recommendation [48].

17.2.2.2 Prospective Studies

Fruit and vegetable intake is consistently shown to be inversely related to stroke risk with certain specific fruits and vegetables being uniquely more effective than others (Table 17.3) [31, 32, 78, 85–93].

Systemic Reviews and Meta-analyses

Four meta-analyses all show that fruits and vegetables are inversely associated with stroke risk [31, 85–87]. A 2017 dose-response meta-analysis (43 cohort studies) found that 200 g/day reduced total stroke risk for fruits and vegetables by 16%,

Table 17.3 Summary of fruit and vegetable intake studies in stroke risk

Objective	Study details	Results
Systematic reviews and meta-analyses		
Aune et al. (2017). Conduct a systematic review and meta-analysis to clarify the effects of fruit and vegetable intake on stroke risk [85].	43 cohort studies; >2 million participants.	Per 200 g fruits and vegetables/day the total stroke risk was reduced by 16%; fruits by 18% and vegetables by 13%. There was evidence of a non-linear association for total stroke, risk was reduced for 800 g/day of fruits and vegetables combined by 33% and for 200–350 g/day by 20% whereas 500 g/day of vegetables reduced risk by 28%. For ischemic stroke, risk was reduced per 200 g/day for fruits by 12% and for vegetables by 14%. For hemorrhagic stroke, risk was reduced per 200 g/day for fruits by 34% and vegetables by 24%. The effects of individual fruits and vegetables on stroke risk are summarized in Fig. 17.2.
Hu et al. (2014). Investigate the effect of fruits and vegetables on stroke risk [31].	20 cohort studies published up to January 2014; 760,629 subjects; mean duration of follow-up was 3–37 years; 16,981 stroke cases; six studies were from the United States, eight from Europe, and six from Asia (Japan and China); average serving was calculated as 77 g for vegetables and 80 g for fruits.	Stroke risk was reduced for total fruits and vegetables by 21%, for fruits by 23% and for vegetables by 14% (highest vs. lowest intake). The linear dose–response relationship showed that the risk of stroke decreased for every 200 g/day increment of fruits by 32% and vegetables by 11% (Fig. 17.3). Citrus fruits, apples, pears, and leafy vegetables appear to be uniquely effective for stroke protection.
He et al. (2006). Evaluate the association between fruits and vegetables and stroke risk [86].	9 cohort studies; 257,551 participants; age ranged from 25–103 years; average follow-up of 13 years; 4917 stroke cases.	Compared with individuals who consumed ≤3 servings of fruits and vegetables/day, stroke risk was reduced for 3–5 servings/day by 11% and >5 servings/day by 26%. Subgroup analyses showed that fruits and vegetables had a significant protective effect on both ischemic and hemorrhagic stroke. Men and women had similar stroke risk reduction for >5 servings/day.
Dauchet et al. (2005). Assess the effects of fruits and vegetables on stroke risk [87].	7 cohort studies; 90,513 men, 141,536 women; mean follow-up of 3 to 20 years; 2955 stroke cases.	The risk of stroke was significantly decreased by 11% for each additional serving/day of fruits, by 5% for fruit and vegetables, and insignificantly by 3% for vegetables. The association between fruits only or fruits and vegetables and stroke was linear, suggesting a dose-response relationship.
Prospective cohort studies		
Larsson et al. (2013). Examine the relationship between intake of specific fruit and vegetable subgroups and stroke risk in a cohort of Swedish women and men (Swedish Mammography Cohort and the Cohort of Swedish Men) [32].	74,961 adults; mean baseline age 60 years; 46% women; 50% overweight; 25% current smokers; 20% with hypertension; 10.2 years of follow-up; 4089 stroke cases (multivariate adjusted).	Total stroke risk for fruit and vegetable intake was significantly reduced by13% (> 6 servings/day vs. <2.3 servings/day). Sub-group analysis showed that the risk for normotensive individuals was significantly reduced by 19%. The reduced total stroke risk per serving for apples and pears was 11% and for green leafy vegetables was 8% (Fig. 17.4).

Table 17.3 (continued)

Objective	Study details	Results
Oude Grieo et al. (2011). Investigate the effect of fruit and vegetable color groups and stroke risk (Dutch cohorts of the European Prospective Investigation into Cancer [EPIC] Study) [88].	20,069 adults; mean baseline age 41 years, 45% men; mean BMI 25; 37% smokers; 10 years of follow-up; 233 stroke cases (multivariate adjusted).	Higher intake of white fruits and vegetables was inversely associated with stroke risk by 52% (>171 g/day vs. ≤78 g/day). Each 25-g/d increase in white fruits and vegetables consumption was associated with a 9% lower risk of stroke. Apples and pears were the most commonly consumed of the white fruit and vegetables (55%) (Fig. 17.5).
Oude Grieo et al. (2011). Evaluate effect of raw or processed fruits and vegetables and stroke risk (Dutch cohorts of the EPIC study) [89].	20,069 adults; mean baseline age 41 years, 45% men; mean BMI 25; 37% smokers; 10 years of follow-up; 233 stroke cases (multivariate adjusted).	High intake of raw fruits and vegetables may protect against stroke (median intake: 337 g/day vs. 56 g/day) whereas no significant inverse association was observed between processed fruit and vegetable consumption and stroke risk (median intake: 301/day vs. 86 g/day) (Fig. 17.6).
Mizrahi et al. (2009). Study the effect of whole plant foods on cerebrovascular disease incidence (Finnish Mobile Clinic Health Examination Survey Follow-up Study) [90].	3932 adults; mean baseline age 54 years; 53% men; mean BMI 27; 30% current smokers; 24% with hypertension; 24 years of follow-up; 625 cases of cerebrovascular incidence or death (multivariate adjusted).	The intake of fruits, especially citrus, and cruciferous vegetables may protect against cerebrovascular diseases. An inverse association was found between fruit consumption and the incidence of cerebrovascular diseases by 25%, ischemic stroke by 27% and intracerebral hemorrhage by 53%, which was primarily due to the consumption of citrus fruits. The consumption of cruciferous vegetables, reduced risk of ischemic stroke by 33% and intracerebral hemorrhage by 51%.
Sauvaget et al. (2003). Investigate effects of a diet rich in fruits and vegetables on total stroke mortality (Hiroshima/Nagasaki Life Span Study) [91].	40,349 Japanese adults; mean baseline age 56 years; 38% men; 73% from Hiroshima city; mean radiation dose115mSv; 18 years of follow-up; 1926 stroke deaths (multivariate adjusted).	Daily consumption of green-yellow vegetables and fruits was associated with a lower risk of total stroke, ischemic and stroke mortality. A daily serving of green-yellow vegetables was associated with a significant 26% reduction in the risk of death from total stroke in men and women compared with an intake of ≤1 serving/week. A daily fruit serving was associated with a significant 35% reduction in risk of total stroke death in men and a 25% reduction in women vs. ≤1 serving/week.
Steffen et al. (2003). Evaluate the effect of fruit and vegetable intakes on the risk of total mortality and the incidence of coronary artery disease (CAD) and ischemic stroke (Atherosclerosis Risk in Communities cohort; US) [78].	15,792 adults; mean baseline age 53 years; 11 years of follow-up; 270 fatal or nonfatal incident stroke, with 21 ischemic strokes (multivariate adjusted).	Compared with a mean intake of 1.5 servings of fruits and vegetables/day, those with a mean intake of 7.5 servings/day had a 22% lower risk of total mortality. There was no association between the intake of fruit and vegetables and the risk of incident ischemic stroke.
Bazzano et al. (2002). Investigate the effect of fruit and vegetable intake and CVD and stroke risk (National Health and Nutrition Examination Survey Epidemiologic Follow-up Study; US) [92].	9608 adults; mean baseline age 50 years; 40% men; mean BMI 25; mean BP 134/84 mm Hg; 19 years of follow-up; 888 stroke cases (multivariate adjusted).	Consuming fruits and vegetables ≥3 times/day compared with < once/day was associated with a significant 27% lower stroke incidence and a significant 42% lower stroke mortality.

(continued)

Table 17.3 (continued)

Objective	Study details	Results
Joshipura et al. (1999). Examine the effect of fruit and vegetable intake on ischemic stroke risk (Nurses' Health Study and Health Professionals' Follow-up Study; US) [93].	75,596 women; mean baseline age 46 years; 14 years of follow-up; 366 stroke cases; and 38,683 men, mean baseline age 54 years; 8 years of follow-up; 204 stroke cases (multivariate adjusted).	Pooled data from men and women showed that each daily serving of fruit and vegetables was associated with lower ischemic stroke risk by 6%. Risk reductions per serving of specific fruit and vegetable subtypes are shown in Fig. 17.7.

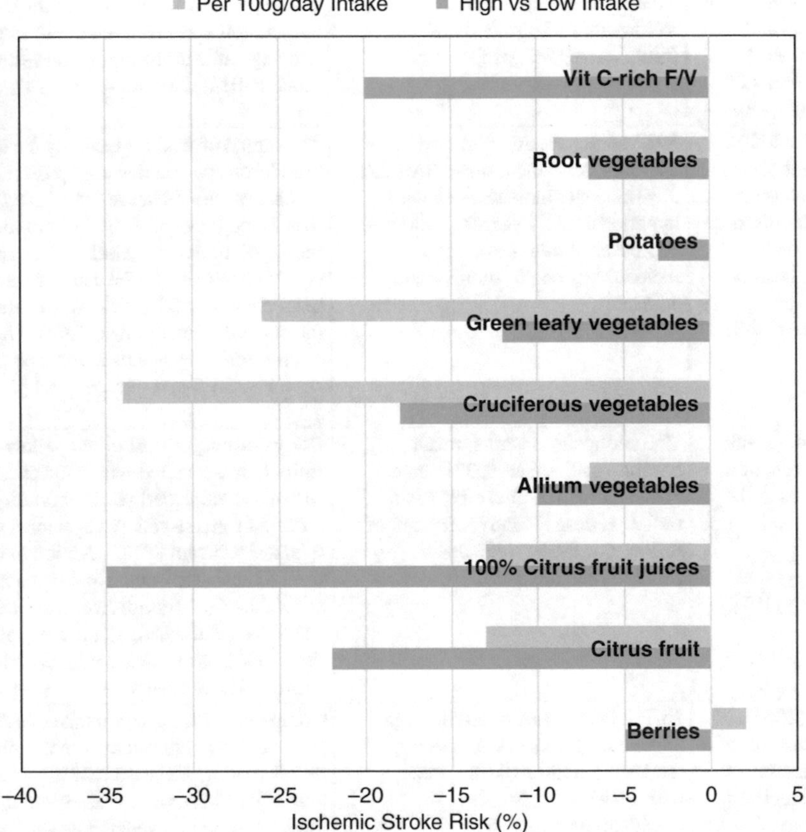

Fig. 17.2 Association between fruit and vegetable (F/V) subtypes and ischemic stroke risk from a 2017 meta-analysis of 43 cohort studies (adapted from [85])

for fruits by 18% and vegetables by 13% [85]. There was evidence of a nonlinear association between total fruits and vegetables, fruit, and vegetables, and lower total stroke risk. Total risk was reduced for 800 g/day of fruits and vegetables by 33%, for 500 g/day of vegetables by 28% and for 200–350 g/day of fruits and vegetables by 20%. Per 200 g/day, ischemic stroke risk was reduced for fruit and vegetables combined by 8%, for fruits by 12% and for vegetables by 14%. The effects of individual fruits and vegetable subtypes on stroke risk are summarized in Fig. 17.2. A 2014 meta-analysis (20 cohort studies; 760,629 adults; mean follow-up of 3–37 years) found that total stroke risk was reduced for higher total fruits and vegetables consumption by 21%, for fruits by

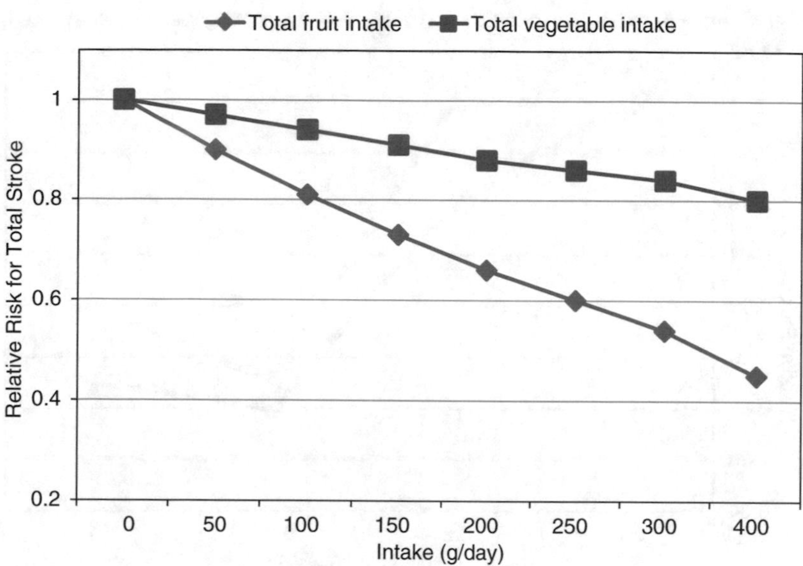

Fig. 17.3 The dose-response analysis between fruit and vegetable consumption and stroke risk from a meta-analysis of 20 prospective cohort studies (760,629 participants) (adapted from [31])

23% and for vegetables by 14% vs. the lowest intake [31]. The linear dose-response relationship showed that every daily 200 g (2 1/2 servings) of fruits reduced total stroke risk by 32% and vegetables reduced risk by 11% (Fig. 17.3). Data suggests that citrus fruits, apples, pears, and green leafy vegetables might be uniquely effective for stroke protection. Two other meta-analyses report similar findings on the effects of fruits and vegetables on stroke risk [86, 87].

Specific Prospective Cohort Studies

Eight cohort studies provide important insights regarding increased intake of total and specific fruits and vegetables on stroke risk [32, 78, 88–93]. A 2013 Swedish Mammography Cohort and the Cohort of Swedish Men studies (74,961 adults; mean baseline age 60 years; 46% women; 50% overweight; 10.2 years of follow-up) identified apples, pears and green leafy vegetables most effective at lowering total stroke risk (Fig. 17.4) [32]. The Dutch cohorts of the European Prospective Investigation into Cancer (EPIC) Study (20,069 adults; mean baseline age 41 years; 45% men; 10 years of follow-up) identified white fruits (e.g., apples, pears, bananas) and vegetables (e.g., cauliflower, cucumber, and mushrooms, garlic, leeks and onions) as the most effective at reducing stroke risk by 52% (>171 g/day vs. ≤78 g/day) (Fig. 17.5) [88]. Each 25 g/day increased intake of apples and pears was associated with a 7% lower stroke risk. There was also an inverse association with stroke for raw fruits and vegetables, with a significantly reduced stroke risk by 31% compared to an 11% increased risk trend for processed fruits and vegetables (Fig. 17.6) [89]. The Hiroshima/Nagasaki Life Span Study (40,349 adults; mean baseline age 56 years; 38% men; 18 years of follow-up) found that daily fruit intake was associated with a reduction in total stroke mortality risk in men by 35% and in women by 25% [91]. For vegetables, green-yellow vegetables were the most effective for stroke protection, reducing mortality risk by 26% (daily intake vs. ≤1/week). A 1999 pooled analysis of Nurses' Health Study and Health Professionals' Follow-up Study (75,596 women; mean baseline age 46 years;14 years of follow-up, 366 stroke cases; 38,683 men, mean baseline age 54 years, mean BMI 26, 8 years of follow-up) found that in US men and women each serving of fruits and vegetables was associated with a 6% lower risk of ischemic stroke [93]. Risk reductions per serving of specific fruits and vegetables are shown in Fig. 17.7.

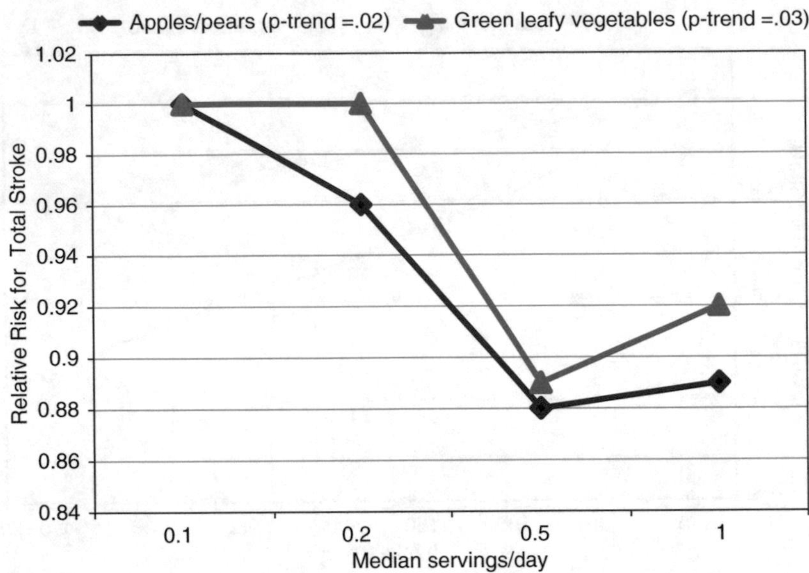

Fig. 17.4 Association between apples and pears, and green leafy vegetables and total stroke risk among men and women (adapted from [32])

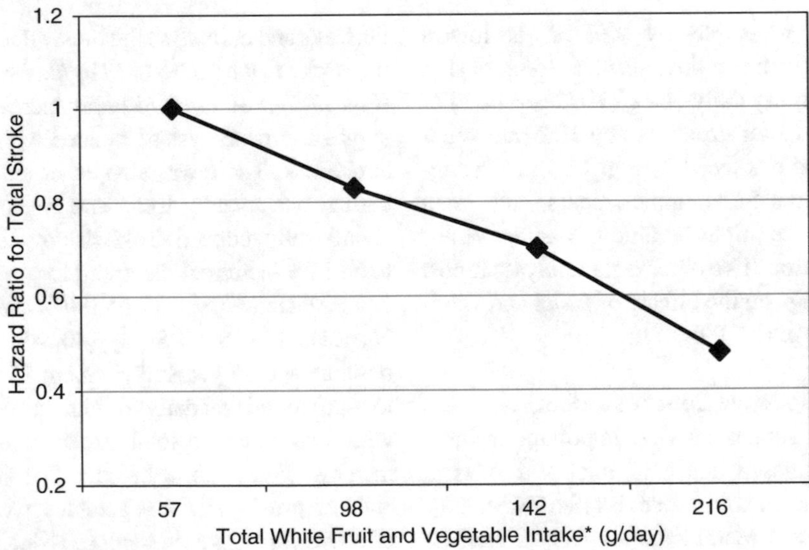

Fig. 17.5 Association between total white fruits and vegetables intake and total stroke risk (p-trend = 0.002) (adapted from [88]). *55% apples, pears, apple sauce, and cloudy apple juice; 35% bananas, cauliflower, cucumber, and mushrooms; 10% garlic, leek and onion

17.2.3 Dietary Protein Sources

Dietary protein sources have variable effects on stroke risk [94]. The pooled data from the Nurse's Health Study and Health Professionals Follow-up Study (84,010 women aged 30–55 years at baseline and 43,150 men aged 40–75 years at baseline; during 26 and 22 years of follow-up) found that the intake of red meat and potentially legumes increased total stroke risk whereas intake of poul-

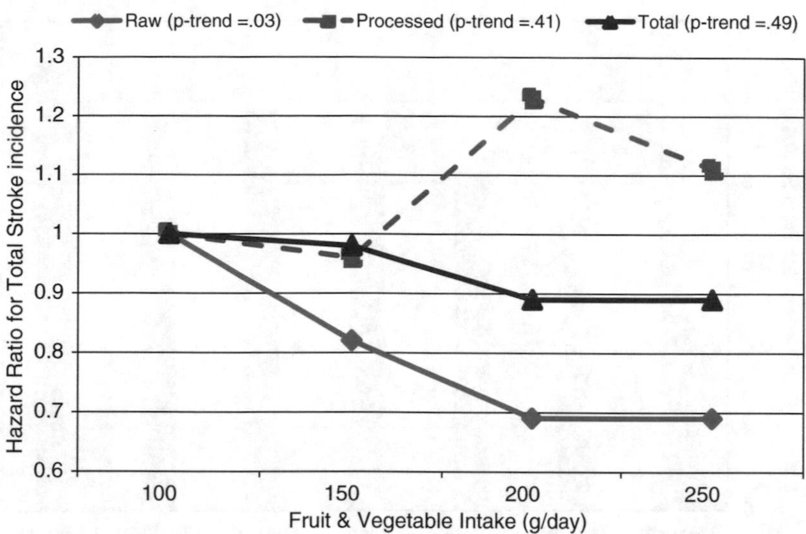

Fig. 17.6 Association between raw and processed fruits and vegetables and total stroke risk (multivariate adjusted) (adapted from [89])

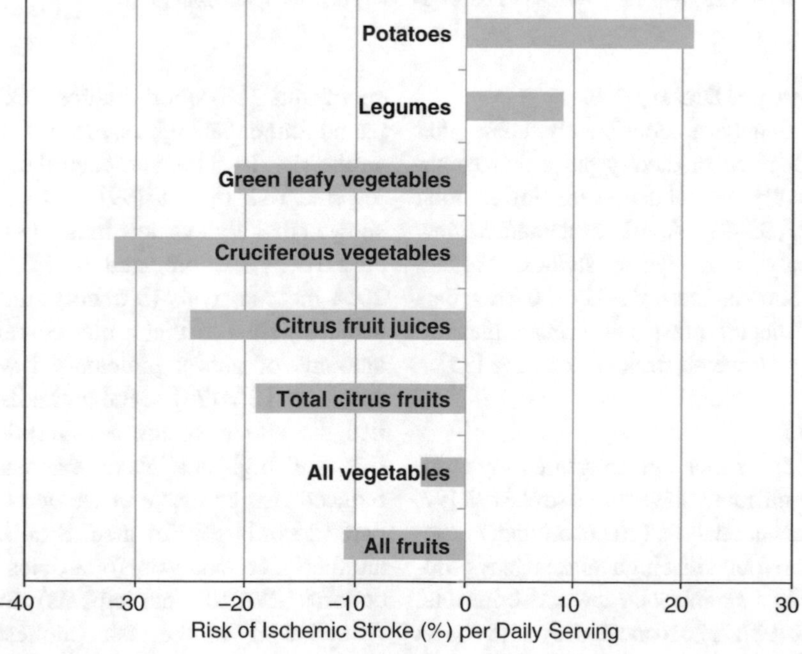

Fig. 17.7 Association between specific fruits and vegetables per serving and ischemic stroke risk in women and men (adapted from [93])

try, nuts, fish, and both whole-fat and low-fat dairy lowered risk (Fig. 17.8) [94]. These associations were independent of other major stroke risk factors. The two-primary plant based protein sources, legumes and nuts, will be reviewed in more detail.

17.2.3.1 Legumes

Total legumes or dietary pulses show variable effects but they are generally not associated with total stroke risk whereas soy products have been shown to lower total stroke risk [25, 95–98].

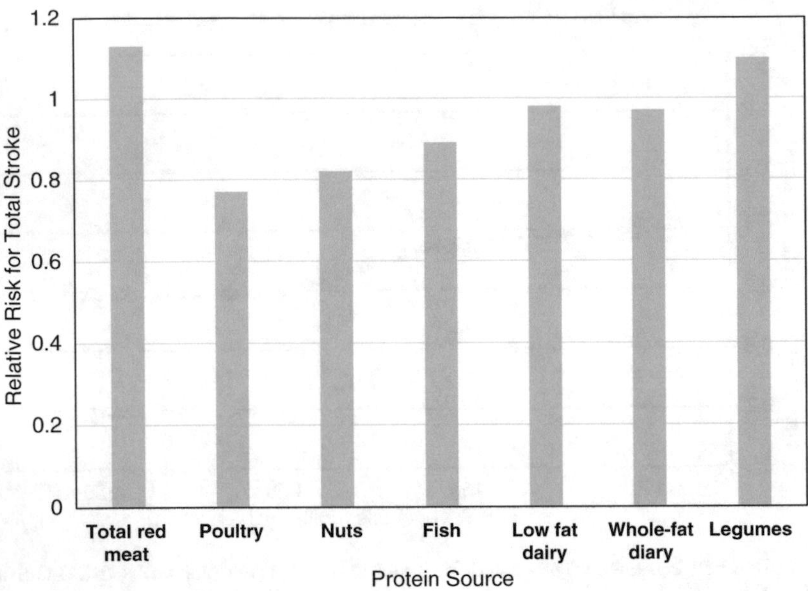

Fig. 17.8 Association between protein source (per serving) and total stroke risk in men and women from the pooled Nurses' Health Study and Health Professionals Follow-up Study data (adapted from [94])

Total Legume and Dietary Pulses

Several meta-analyses consistently show that higher total legume or dietary pulse intakes are not significantly associated with lower total stroke risk [25, 95–97]. A 2017 systematic review and meta-analysis (6 legume studies; 254,628 participants) showed that 4 weekly 100 g servings of legumes (dietary pulses) was insignificantly associated with lowered stroke risk by 2% [95].

Soy Products

Two meta-analyses found that increased soy products intake significantly lowers total stroke risk [97, 98]. A 2017 meta-analysis (10 cohort and 7 case-control studies) found that high intake of soy products resulted in a significantly lower risk for total stroke by 18% [98]. A 2016 meta-analysis (5 cohort studies and 6 case-control studies) showed a significant inverse association between soy intake and total stroke risk but there was not an association between soy isoflavones intake and stroke risk [97].

17.2.3.2 Tree Nuts and Peanuts

Meta-analyses

Meta-analyses of tree nuts and peanuts consistently show a stroke risk protective effect [24, 25, 96, 99]. A 2016 dose-response meta-analysis of nuts (11 cohort studies; 396,768 participants) found that high vs. low nut intake lowered stroke risk by 11% and each daily nut serving lowered risk by 7% [99]. Sub-group analysis showed that high vs. low intake of tree nuts lowered risk by 7% compared to 17% for peanuts. A 2014 meta-analysis (8 cohort studies; 468,887 subjects) showed that a diet containing greater amounts of nuts significantly lowered risk of stroke by 10% [25]. Gender significantly modified the effects of nut consumption on stroke risk, and high nut intake was associated with reduced risk of stroke in women by 15% compared to only 5% for men. Similar findings in another meta-analysis (6 articles including 9 cohorts; 476,181 participants) found a 10% reduction in stroke risk (highest vs. lowest intake), which was significant for females only [24]. Another 2014 meta-analysis (3 cohort studies and one RCT; 155,685 participants) showed a trend that 4 weekly servings of nuts lowered total stroke risk by 11% [96]. A systematic review and meta-analysis (32 cohort studies; 841,211 participants) found that higher intake of monounsaturated fat (MUFA), oleic acid, and higher MUFA: SFA ratio reduced stroke risk by 17%, which is characteristic of most nuts [100].

Prospective Cohort Studies
Several cohort studies provide insights on the effects of nuts on stroke risk [101, 102]. Three large cohorts (71,764 US participants in the Southern Community Cohort Study in the southeastern United States, and the other 2 cohorts included 134,265 participants in the Shanghai Women's Health Study and the Shanghai Men's Health Study in Shanghai, China; 5.4–12.2 years of follow-up) found that peanuts significantly lowered ischemic stroke and hemorrhagic stroke by 23% in Asians [101]. The US Physicians' Health Study (21,078 men; mean baseline age 55 years; 21 years of follow up) found that the consumption of ≥7 weekly nut servings showed a trend toward reduced ischemic stroke risk by 7% [102].

17.3 Tea and Coffee on Stroke Risk

Tea and coffee are the most frequently consumed beverages worldwide and also important sources of polyphenols, which have potential beneficial effects on cardiovascular health [17]. The polyphenols in these beverages may reduce the risk of stroke through multiple beneficial mechanisms, including antihypertensive, hypo-cholesterolemic, antioxidative and anti-inflammatory, vascular endothelial function and insulin sensitivity effects.

17.3.1 Prospective Cohort Studies

17.3.1.1 Tea

There is a large body of scientific evidence that tea is associated with reduced hypertension risk and other major risk factors associated with stroke [17]. A 2012 meta-analysis (14 cohort studies; 513,804 participants; median 11.5 years of follow-up) showed that 3 cups of green and black tea were associated with a reduction in total stroke risk for green tea by 17% ($p < 0.01$) and black tea by 9% ($p = 0.17$) [103]. Three cups of overall tea consumption were associated with a significant 13% lower risk of total stroke and a 24% lower ischemic stroke risk. The Finnish Alpha-Tocopherol, Beta-Carotene Cancer Prevention Study (26,556 male smokers; mean age 58 years at baseline; 13.6 years of follow-up) showed that those drinking > 2 cups tea/day significantly reduced ischemic stroke by 21% compared to non-tea drinkers [104].

17.3.1.2 Coffee

Coffee is a complex mixture of biologically active substances with both potential beneficial and adverse effects on cardiovascular or cerebrovascular health [15, 17]. The phenolic compounds in coffee, such as caffeic, ferulic, and chlorogenic ac ids, have a strong antioxidant activity and may reduce the oxidation of low density lipoprotein cholesterol and systemic inflammatory markers, and increase insulin sensitivity with inconsistent effects on BP depending on whether the subjects are normotensive or hypertensive and new or habitual coffee drinkers. A 2011 meta-analysis (11 cohort studies; 479,689 participants; 2-24 years of follow-up) found that the consumption of 1 to 6 cups of coffee/d was significantly inversely associated with risk of total stroke, with the strongest association (17% lower risk) being observed for 3 to 4 cups/day [15]. Heavy coffee consumption >7 cups/day was not significantly associated with total stroke risk. The associations were similar for ischemic stroke and hemorrhagic stroke, but only results for ischemic stroke was significant. The Finnish Alpha-Tocopherol, Beta-Carotene Cancer Prevention Study (26,556 male smokers; mean age 58 years at baseline; 13.6 years of follow-up) showed that drinking > 8 cups coffee/d significantly reduced ischemic stroke by 23% compared to those drinking < 2 cups/day [104].

Conclusions

Stroke and related cerebrovascular diseases make-up the second most common cause of death worldwide, accounting for 6.2 million deaths (11% of total deaths). Over 90% of stroke risk is attributable to modifiable risk factors such as smoking, poor diet, and low physical activity. Stroke is a major cause of disability and death worldwide, which changes the lives not only of the stroke victims but also of their families as many become dependent in their activities of daily living due to significant stroke related cognitive and other physical deficits. Forecasts suggest a >20% increase in stroke prevalence by 2030 compared to 2012 rates, because of the increase in aging populations. Regular consumption of specific foods and beverages may have significant effects on stroke risk with potential stroke protective foods including low fat dairy, whole grains, fruits, vegetables, nuts, tea and coffee whereas high intake of red meat, sugar-sweetened beverages and alcohol may increase stroke risk. The consumption of ≥3 daily servings of whole grains is associated with lower total stroke risk by 8–14% and ischemic stroke by 25% compared to never or rare intake. Increased consumption by 200 g (or 2 1/2 servings)/day reduces total stroke for fruits and vegetables by 16%, fruits by 18% and vegetables by 13%. Raw fruits and vegetables are more effective than processed forms; examples of effective specific varieties for reducing ischemic stroke risk are green leafy vegetables, white fruits and vegetables (e.g., apples, cauliflower, mushrooms) and vitamin C rich fruits and vegetables (e.g., citrus, bell peppers, broccoli). Plant protein sources such as legumes and nuts have mixed effects on stroke risk. Dietary pulses or total legumes are not associated with stroke risk but nuts and soy foods are associated with lower stroke risk. Whole plant foods containing a variety of nutrients and phytochemicals such as fiber, antioxidant vitamins, potassium, magnesium, carotenoids, flavonoids and phytosterols may provide potential stroke protection by mechanisms associated with promoting vascular health by attenuating elevated blood pressure, lowering LDL-cholesterol levels and systemic inflammation associated with atherosclerosis, and promoting better insulin sensitivity, blood glucose control, weight control, and microbiota health compared to less healthy or refined plant foods.

Appendix A: Estimated Range of Energy, Fiber, Nutrients and Phytochemicals Composition of Whole Plant Foods/100 g Edible Portion

Components	Whole-Grains	Fresh Fruit	Dried Fruit	Vegetables	Legumes	Nuts/Seeds
Nutrients/ Phytochemicals	Wheat, oat, barley, rye, brown rice, whole grain bread, cereal, pasta, rolls, and crackers	Apples, pears, bananas, grapes, oranges, blueberries, strawberries, and avocados	Dates, dried figs, apricots, cranberries, raisins, and prunes	Potatoes, spinach, carrots, peppers, lettuce, green beans, cabbage, onions, cucumber, cauliflower, mushrooms, and broccoli	Lentils, chickpeas, split peas, black beans, pinto beans, and soy beans	Almonds, Brazil nuts, cashews, hazelnuts, macadamias, pecans, walnuts, peanuts, sunflower seeds, and flaxseed
Energy (kcals)	110–350	30–170	240–310	10–115	85–170	520–700
Protein (g)	2.5–16	0.5–2.0	0.1–3.4	0.2–5.0	5.0–17	7.8–24
Available carbohydrate (g)	23–77	1.0–25	64–82	0.2–25	10–27	12–33
Fiber (g)	3.5–18	2.0–7.0	5.7–10	1.2–9.5	5.0–11	3.0–27
Total fat (g)	0.9–6.5	0.0–15	0.4–1.4	0.2–1.5	0.2–9.0	46–76
SFA (g)	0.2–1.0	0.0–2.1	0.0	0.0–0.1	0.1–1.3	4.0–12
MUFA (g)	0.2–2.0	0.0–9.8	0.0–0.2	0.1–1.0	0.1–2.0	9.0–60
PUFA (g)	0.3–2.5	0.0–1.8	0.0–0.7	0.0.0.4	0.1–5.0	1.5–47
Folate (ug)	4.0–44	<5.0–61	2–20	8.0–160	50–210	10–230
Tocopherols (mg)	0.1–3.0	0.1–1.0	0.1–4.5	0.0–1.7	0.0–1.0	1.0–35
Potassium (mg)	40–720	60–500	40–1160	100–680	200–520	360–1050
Calcium (mg)	7.0–50	3.0–25	10–160	5.0–200	20–100	20–265
Magnesium (mg)	40–160	3.0–30	5.0–70	3.0–80	40–90	120–400
Phytosterols (mg)	30–90	1.0–83	—	1.0–54	110–120	70–215
Polyphenols (mg)	70–100	50–800	—	24–1250	120–6500	130–1820
Carotenoids (ug)	—	25–6600	1.0–2160	10–20,000	50–600	1.0–1200

Ros E, Hu FB. Consumption of plant seeds and cardiovascular health epidemiological and clinical trial evidence. Circulation. 2013;128: 553–565

USDA. What We Eat in America, NHANES 2011–2012, individuals 2 years and over (excluding breast-fed children). Available: www.ars.usda.gov/nea/bhnrc/fsrg

Rodriguez-Casado A. The health potential of fruits and vegetables phytochemicals: notable examples. Crit Rev. Food Sci Nutr. 2016; 56(7):1097–1107

Rebello CJ, Greenway FL, Finley JW. A review of the nutritional value of legumes and their effects on obesity and its related co-morbidities. Obes Rev. 2014;15: 392–407

Gebhardt SE, Thomas RG. Nutritive Value of Foods. 2002; U.S. Department of Agriculture, Agricultural Research Service, Home and Garden Bulletin 72.

Holden JM, Eldridge AL, Beecher GR, et al. Carotenoid content of U.S. foods: an update of the database. J Food Comp An. 1999; 12:169–196

Lu Q-Y, Zhang Y, Wang Y, et al. California Hass avocado: profiling of carotenoids, tocopherol, fatty acid, and fat content during maturation and from different growing areas. *J* Agric Food Chem. 2009; 57(21):10408–10413

Wu X, Beecher GR, Holden JM, et al. Lipophilic and hydrophilic antioxidant capacities of common foods in the United States. J Agric Food Chem. 2004; 52: 4026–4037

SFA (saturated fat), MUFA (monounsaturated fat) and PUFA (polyunsaturated fat)

U.S. Department of Agriculture, Agriculture Research Service, Nutrient Data Laboratory. 2014. USDA National Nutrient Database for Standard Reference, Release 27. http://www.ars.usda.gov/nutrientdata. Accessed 17 Feb 2015

References

1. Mendis S, Puska P, Norrving B, editors. Global atlas on cardiovascular disease prevention and control. The underlying pathology of heart attacks and strokes. Geneva: World Health Organization; 2011.
2. Mozaffarian D, Benjamin EJ, Go AS, et al. Heart disease and stroke statistics-2015 update: a report from the American Heart Association. Circulation. 2015;131:29–322.
3. Feigin VL, Roth GA, Naghavi M, et al. Global burden of stroke and risk factors in 188 countries, during 1990-2013: a systematic analysis for the Global Burden of Disease Study. Lancet Neurol. 2016;15(9):913–24. https://doi.org/10.1016/S1474-4422(16)30073-4.
4. Meschia JF, Bushnell C, Boden-Albala B, et al. Guidelines for the primary prevention of stroke. A statement for healthcare professionals from the American Heart Association/American Stroke Association. Stroke. 2014;45(12):3754–832. https://doi.org/10.1161/STR.0000000000000046.
5. Goldstein LB, Bushnell CD, Adams RJ, et al. Guidelines for the primary prevention of stroke. A guideline for healthcare professionals from the American Heart Association/American Stroke Association. Stroke. 2011;42(2):517–84. https://doi.org/10.1161/STR.0b013e3181fcb238.
6. Niewadaa M, Michel P. Lifestyle modification for stroke prevention: facts and fiction. Curr Opin Neurol. 2016;29:9–13.
7. Kontogianni MD, Panagiotakos DB. Dietary patterns and stroke: a systematic review and re-meta-analysis. Maturitas. 2014;79:41–7.
8. Neter JE, Stam BE, Kok FJ, et al. Influence of weight reduction on blood pressure: a meta-analysis of randomized controlled trials. Hypertension. 2003;42:878–84.
9. Strazzullo P, D'Elia L, Cairella G, et al. Excess body weight and incidence of stroke: meta-analysis of prospective studies with 2 million participants. Stroke. 2010;41:e418–26.
10. Lee CD, Folsom AR, Blair SN. Physical activity and stroke risk: a meta-analysis. Stroke. 2003;34: 2475–81.
11. Wendel-Vos GC, Schuit AJ, Feskens EJ, et al. Physical activity and stroke: a meta-analysis of observational data. Int J Epidemiol. 2004;33: 787–98.
12. Masson P, Webster AX, Hong M, et al. Chronic kidney disease and the risk of stroke: a systematic review and meta-analysis. Nephrol Dial Transplant. 2015;30(7):1162–9.
13. Reynolds K, Lewis B, Nolen JD, et al. Alcohol consumption and risk of stroke: a meta-analysis. JAMA. 2003;289:579–88.
14. Zhang C, Qin YY, Chen Q, et al. Alcohol intake and risk of stroke: a dose-response meta-analysis of prospective studies. Int J Cardiol. 2014;174(3):669–77.
15. Larsson SC, Orsini N. Coffee consumption and risk of stroke: a dose-response meta-analysis of prospective studies. Am J Epidemiol. 2011;174:993–1001.
16. Kim B, Nam Y, Kim J, et al. Coffee consumption and stroke risk: a meta-analysis of epidemiologic studies. Korean J Fam Med. 2012;33:356–65.
17. Larsson SC. Coffee, tea, and cocoa and risk of stroke. Stroke. 2014;45:309–14.
18. Larsson SC, Virtamo J, Wolk A. Chocolate consumption and risk of stroke: a prospective cohort of men and women. Neurology. 2012;79(12):1223–9.
19. Martınez-Gonzalez MA, Dominguez LJ, Delgado-Rodriguez M. Olive oil consumption and risk of CHD and/or stroke: a meta-analysis of case–control, cohort and intervention studies. Br J Nutr. 2014;112:248–59.
20. Yakoob MY, Shi P, Hu FB, et al. Circulating biomarkers of dairy fat and risk of incident stroke in U.S. men and women in 2 large prospective cohorts. Am J Clin Nutr. 2014;100(6):1437–47.
21. Pimpin L, Wu JHY, Haskelberg H, et al. Is butter back? A systematic review and meta-analysis of butter consumption and risk of cardiovascular disease, diabetes, and total mortality. PLoS One. 2016;11(6):e0158118. https://doi.org/10.1371/ journal. pone. 0158118.
22. Hu D, Huang J, Wang Y, et al. Dairy foods and risk of stroke: a meta-analysis of prospective cohort studies. Nutr Metab Cardiovasc Dis. 2014;24(5):460–9.
23. de Goede J, Soedamah-Muthu SS, Pan A, et al. Dairy consumption and risk of stroke: a systematic review and updated dose–response meta-analysis of prospective cohort studies. J Am Heart Assoc. 2016;5(5). https://doi.org/10.1161/JAHA.115.002787.
24. Zhang Z, Xu G, Wei Y, et al. Nut consumption and risk of stroke. Eur J Epidemiol. 2015;30(3):189–96.
25. Shi ZQ, Tang JJ, Wu H, et al. Consumption of nuts and legumes and risk of stroke: a meta-analysis of prospective cohort studies. Nutr Metab Cardiovasc Dis. 2014;24(12):1262–71.
26. Kaluza J, Wolk A, Larsson SC. Red meat consumption and risk of stroke a meta-analysis of prospective studies. Stroke. 2012;43:2556–60.
27. Yang C, Pan L, Sun C, et al. Red meat consumption and the risk of stroke: a dose-response meta-analysis of prospective cohort studies. J Stroke Cerebrovasc Dis. 2016;25(5):1177–86.
28. Chen GC, Lv DB, Pang Z, Liu QF. Red and processed meat consumption and risk of stroke: a meta-analysis of prospective cohort studies. Eur J Clin Nutr. 2013;91(1):91–5.
29. Liu S, Manson JE, Stampfer MJ, et al. Whole grain consumption and risk of ischemic stroke in women a prospective study. JAMA. 2000;284:1534–40.
30. Chen J, Huang Q, Shi W, et al. Meta-analysis of the association between whole and refined grain consumption and stroke risk based on prospective cohort studies. Asia Pac J Public Health. 2016;28(7):563–75. https://doi.org/10.1177/1010539516650722.

31. Hu D, Huang J, Wang Y, et al. Fruits and vegetables consumption and risk of stroke a meta-analysis of prospective cohort studies. Stroke. 2014;45:1613–9.
32. Larsson SC, Virtamo J, Wolk A. Total and specific fruit and vegetable consumption and risk of stroke: a prospective study. Atherosclerosis. 2013;227:147–52.
33. Chowdhury R, Stevens S, Gorman D, et al. Association between fish consumption, long chain omega 3 fatty acids, and risk of cerebrovascular disease: systematic review and meta-analysis. BMJ. 2012;345:e6698. https://doi.org/10.1136/bmj.e6698.
34. Amiano P, Chamosa S, Etxezarreta N, et al. No association between fish consumption and risk of stroke in the Spanish cohort of the European Prospective Investigation into Cancer and Nutrition (EPIC-Spain): a 13.8-year follow-up study. Public Health Nutr. 2015;19(4):674–81.
35. Larsson SC, Akesson A, Wolk A. Sweetened beverage consumption is associated with increased risk of stroke in women and men. J Nutr. 2014;144:856–60.
36. Bernstein AM, de Koning L, Flint AJ, et al. Soda consumption and the risk of stroke in men and women. Am J Clin Nutr. 2012;95:1190–9.
37. Jayalath VH, de Souza RJ, Ha V, et al. Sugar-sweetened beverage consumption and incident hypertension: a systematic review and meta-analysis of prospective cohorts. Am J Clin Nutr. 2015;102:914–21.
38. U.S. Department of Agriculture, Agriculture Research Service, Nutrient Data Laboratory. USDA National Nutrient Database for Standard Reference, Release 27; 2014. http://www.ars.usda.gov/nutrientdata. Accessed 17 Feb 2015.
39. Ros E, Hu FB. Consumption of plant seeds and cardiovascular health epidemiological and clinical trial evidence. Circulation. 2013;128(5):553–65. https://doi.org/10.1161/CIRCULATIONAHA.112.001119.
40. USDA. What We Eat in America, NHANES 2011–2012, individuals 2 years and over (excluding breast-fed children). www.ars.usda.gov/nea/bhnrc/fsrg.
41. Slavin JL, Lloyd B. Health benefits of fruits and vegetables. Adv Nutr. 2012;3:506–16.
42. Rebello CJ, Greenway FL, Finley JW. A review of the nutritional value of legumes and their effects on obesity and its related co-morbidities. Obes Rev. 2014;15:392–407.
43. Gebhardt SE, Thomas RG. Nutritive value of foods. U.S. Department of Agriculture, Agricultural Research Service, Home and Garden Bulletin 72; 2002.
44. Holden JM, Eldridge AL, Beecher GR, et al. Carotenoid content of U.S. foods: an update of the database. J Food Comp Anal. 1999;12:169–96.
45. Lu Q-Y, Zhang Y, Wang Y, et al. California Hass avocado: profiling of carotenoids, tocopherol, fatty acid, and fat content during maturation and from different growing areas. J Agric Food Chem. 2009;57(21):10408–13.
46. Wu X, Beecher GR, Holden JM, et al. Lipophilic and hydrophilic antioxidant capacities of common foods in the United States. J Agric Food Chem. 2004;52:4026–37.
47. Bhupathiraju SN, Tucker KL. Coronary heart disease prevention: nutrients, foods, and dietary patterns. Clin Chim Acta. 2011;412:1493–514.
48. Dietary Guidelines Advisory Committee. Scientific Report. Advisory Report to the Secretary of Health and Human Services and the Secretary of Agriculture. Part D. Chapter 1: Food and nutrient intakes, and health: current status and trends; 2015. p. 1–78.
49. http://health.gov/dietary guidelines/2015/guidelines/. Accessed 26 Jan 2016.
50. Ascherio A, Rimm EB, Hernan MA, et al. Intake of potassium, magnesium, calcium, and fiber and risk of stroke among US men. Circulation. 1998;98:1198–204.
51. Lackland DT, Roccella EJ, Deutsch A, et al. Factors influencing the decline in stroke mortality: a statement from the American Heart Association/American Stroke Association. Circulation. 2014;45:315–53.
52. Evans CEL, Greenwood DC, Threapleton DE, et al. Effects of dietary fibre type on blood pressure: a systematic review and meta-analysis of randomized controlled trials of healthy individuals. J Hypertens. 2015;33(5):897–911.
53. Davis JN, Hodges VA, Gillham MB. Normal-weight adults consume more fiber and fruit than their age- and height-matched overweight/obese counterparts. J Am Diet Assoc. 2006;106:833–40.
54. Slavin JL. Dietary fiber and body weight. Nutrition. 2005;21:411–8.
55. Fogelholm M, Anderssen S, Gunnarsdottir I, Lahti-Koski M. Dietary macronutrients and food consumption as determinants of long-term weight change in adult populations: a systematic literature review. Food Nutr Res. 2012;56. https://doi.org/10.3402/fnr.v56i0.19103.
56. Genser B, Silbernage G, De Backer G, et al. Plant sterols and cardiovascular disease: a systematic review and meta-analysis. Eur Heart J. 2012;33:444–51.
57. Lau C, Faerch K, Glumer C, et al. Dietary glycemic index, glycemic load, fiber, simple sugars, and insulin resistance: the Inter99 study. Diabetes Care. 2005;28:1397–403.
58. Tosh SM. Review of human studies investigating the post-prandial blood-glucose lowering ability of oat and barley food products. Eur J Clin Nutr. 2013;67:310–7.
59. Silva FM, Kramer CK, de Almeida JC, et al. Fiber intake and glycemic control in patients with type 2 diabetes mellitus: a systematic review with meta-analysis of randomized controlled trials. Nutr Rev. 2013;71(12):790–801.
60. Sen A, Marsche G, Freudenberger P, et al. Association between higher plasma lutein, zeaxanthin, and vitamin C concentrations and longer telomere length: results of the Austrian Stroke Prevention Study. J Am Geriatr Soc. 2014;62:222–9.

61. Varbo A, Nordestgaard BG, Tybjaeg-Hansen A, et al. Nonfasting triglycerides, cholesterol, and ischemic stroke in the general population. Ann Neurol. 2011;69(4):628–34.
62. Whitehead A, Beck EJ, Tosh S, Wolever TMS. Cholesterol-lowering effects of oat β-glucan: a meta-analysis of randomized controlled trials. Am J Clin Nutr. 2014;100:1413–21.
63. Leermaker ET, Darweesh SK, Baena CP, et al. The effects of lutein on cardiometabolic health across the life course: a systematic review and meta-analysis. Am J Clin Nutr. 2016;103(2):481–94.
64. Berni Canani R, Di Costanzo M, Leone L, et al. Potential beneficial effects of butyrate in intestinal and extraintestinal diseases. World J Gastroenterol. 2011;17(12):1519–28.
65. Zhou Y, Han W, Gong D, Fan Y. Hs-CRP in stroke: a meta-analysis. Clin Chim Acta. 2016;435:21–7.
66. McCall DO, McGartland CP, McKinley MC, et al. Dietary intake of fruits and vegetables improves microvascular function in hypertensive subjects in a dose-dependent manner. Circulation. 2009;119:2153–60.
67. Noad RL, Rooney C, McCall D, et al. Beneficial effect of a polyphenol-rich diet on cardiovascular risk: a randomised control trial. Heart. 2016;102(17):1371–9. https://doi.org/10.1136/heartjnl-2015-309218.
68. Jiao J, Xu JY, Zhang W, et al. Effect of dietary fiber on circulating C-reactive protein in overweight and obese adults: a meta-analysis of randomized controlled trials. Int J Food Sci Nutr. 2015;66(1):114–9.
69. Maukonen J, Saarela M. Human gut microbiota: does diet matter? Proc Nutr Soc. 2015;74:23–36.
70. http://wholegrainscouncil.org/whole-grains-101/what-counts-as-a-serving. Accessed 26 Dec 2015.
71. Seal CJ, Brownlee IA. Whole-grain foods and chronic disease: evidence from epidemiological and intervention studies. Proc Nutr Soc. 2015;74:313–9.
72. McGill CR, Fulgoni VL III, Devareddy L. Ten-year trends in fiber and whole grain intakes and food sources for the United States population: National Health and Nutrition Examination Survey 2001–2010. Forum Nutr. 2015;7:1119–30.
73. Aune D, Keum NN, Giovannucci E, et al. Whole grain consumption and risk of cardiovascular disease, cancer, and all cause and cause specific mortality: systematic review and dose-response meta-analysis of prospective studies. BMJ. 2016;353:i2716. https://doi.org/10.1136/bmj.i2716.
74. Fang L, Li W, Zhang W, et al. Association between whole grain intake and stroke risk: evidence from a meta-analysis. Int J Clin Exp Med. 2015;8(9):16978–83.
75. Wu D, Guan Y, Lv S, et al. No evidence of increased risk of stroke with consumption of refined grains: a meta-analysis of prospective cohort studies. J Stroke Cerebrovasc Dis. 2015;24(12):2738–46. https://doi.org/10.1016/j.jstrokecerebrovasdis.2015.08.004.
76. Jacobs DR Jr, Andersen LF, Blomhoff R. Whole-grain consumption is associated with a reduced risk of non-cardiovascular, non-cancer death attributed to inflammatory diseases in the Iowa Women's Health Study. Am J Clin Nutr. 2007;85:1606–14.
77. Oh K, Hu FB, Cho E, et al. Carbohydrate intake, glycemic index, glycemic load, and dietary fiber in relation to risk of stroke in women. Am J Epidemiol. 2005;161(2):161–9.
78. Steffen LM, Jacobs DR Jr, Stevens J, et al. Associations of whole-grain, refined-grain, and fruit and vegetable consumption with risks of all-cause mortality and incident coronary artery disease and ischemic stroke: The Atherosclerosis Risk in Communities (ARIC) Study. Am J Clin Nutr. 2003;78:383–90.
79. Liu S, Sesso HD, Manson JE, et al. Is intake of breakfast cereals related to total and cause-specific mortality in men? Am J Clin Nutr. 2003;77:594–9.
80. Jacobs DR, Meyer KA, Kushi LH, Folsom AR. Is whole grain intake associated with reduced total and cause-specific death rates in older women? The Iowa Women's Health Study. Am J Public Health. 1999;89:322–9.
81. World Health Organization. Diet, nutrition, and the prevention of chronic diseases. Geneva: World Health Organization; 1990. http://www.who.int/nutrition/publications/obesity/WHO_TRS_797/en/index.html. Accessed 16 April 2015.
82. Rooney C, McKinley MC, Appleton KM, et al. How much is '5-a-day'? A qualitative investigation into consumer understanding of fruit and vegetable intake guidelines. J Hum Nutr Diet. 2017;30(1):105–13. https://doi.org/10.1111/jhn.12393.
83. United States Department of Agriculture. Choose my plate. 2013. http://www.choosemyplate.gov/. Accessed 17 Feb 2015.
84. Micha R, Khatibzadeh S, Shi P, et al. Global, regional and national consumption of major food groups in 1990 and 2010: a systematic analysis including 266 country-specific nutrition surveys worldwide. BMJ Open. 2015;5. https://doi.org/10.1136/bmjopen-2015-008705.
85. Aune D, Giovannucci E, Boffetta P, et al. Fruit and vegetable intake and the risk of cardiovascular disease, total cancer and all-cause mortality-a systematic review and dose response meta-analysis of prospective studies. Int J Epidemiol. 2017:1–28. https://doi.org/10.1093/ije/dyw319.
86. He FJ, Nowson CA, MacGregor GA. Fruit and vegetable consumption and stroke: meta-analysis of cohort studies. Lancet. 2006;367:320–6.
87. Dauchet L, Amouyel P, Dallongeville J. Fruit and vegetable consumption and risk of stroke: a meta-analysis of cohort studies. Neurology. 2005;65(8):1193–7.
88. Oude Griep LM, Verschuren WM, Kromhout D, et al. Colors of fruit and vegetables and 10-year incidence of stroke. Stroke. 2011;42:3190–5.
89. Oude Griep LM, Verschuren WM, Kromhout D, et al. Raw and processed fruit and vegetable consumption and 10-year stroke incidence in a population-based cohort study in the Netherlands. Eur J Clin Nutr. 2011;5:791–9.

90. Mizrahi A, Knekt P, Montonen J, et al. Plant foods and the risk of cerebrovascular diseases: a potential protection of fruit consumption. Br J Nutr. 2009;102:1075–83.
91. Sauvaget C, Nagano J, Allen N, Kodama K. Vegetable and fruit intake and stroke mortality in the Hiroshima/Nagasaki Life Span Study. Stroke. 2003;34:2355–60.
92. Bazzano LA, He J, Ogden LG, et al. Fruit and vegetable intake and risk of cardiovascular disease in US adults: the first National Health and Nutrition Examination Survey Epidemiologic Follow-up Study. Am J Clin Nutr. 2002;76:93–9.
93. Joshipura KJ, Ascherio A, Manson JE, et al. Fruit and vegetable intake in relation to risk of ischemic stroke. JAMA. 1999;282:1233–9.
94. Bernstein AM, Pan A, Rexrode KM, et al. Dietary protein sources and the risk of stroke in men and women. Stroke. 2012;43:637–44. https://doi.org/10.1161/STROKEAHA.111.633404.
95. Marventano S, Pulido MI, Sánchez-González C, et al. Legume consumption and CVD risk: a systematic review and meta-analysis. Public Health Nutr. 2017;20(2):245–54. https://doi.org/10.1017/S1368980016002299.
96. Afshin A, Micha R, Khatibzadeh S, Mozaffarian D. Consumption of nuts and legumes and risk of incident ischemic heart disease, stroke, and diabetes: a systematic review and meta-analysis. Am J Clin Nutr. 2014;100(1):278–88.
97. Lou D, Li Y, Yao G, et al. Soy consumption with risk of coronary heart disease and stroke: a meta-analysis of observational studies. Neuroepidemiology. 2016;46(4):242–52.
98. Yan Z, Zhang X, Li C, et al. Association between consumption of soy and risk of cardiovascular disease: a meta-analysis of observational studies. Eur J Prev Cardiol. 2017;24(7):735–47. https://doi.org/10.1177/2047487316686441.
99. Aune D, Keum NN, Giovannucci E, et al. Nut consumption and risk of cardiovascular disease, total cancer, all-cause and causespecific mortality: a systematic review and dose-response meta-analysis of prospective studies. BMC Med. 2016;14:207. https://doi.org/10.1186/s12916-016-0730-3.
100. Schwingshackl L, Hoffmann G. Monounsaturated fatty acids, olive oil and health status: a systematic review and meta-analysis of cohort studies. Lipids Health Dis. 2014;13:154. https://doi.org/10.1186/1476-511X-13-154.
101. Luu HN, Blot WJ, Xiang YB, et al. Prospective evaluation of the association of nut/peanut consumption with total and cause-specific mortality. JAMA Intern Med. 2015;175(5):755–66. https://doi.org/10.1001/jamainternmed.2014.8347.
102. Djoussé L, Gaziano JM, Kase C, Kurth T. Nut consumption and risk of stroke in US male physicians. Clin Nutr. 2010;29(5):605–9.
103. Shen L, Song L-G, Hong MA, et al. Tea consumption and risk of stroke: a dose-response meta-analysis of prospective studies. Biomed Biotech. 2012;13(8):652–62.
104. Larsson SC, Mannisto S, Virtanen MJ, et al. Coffee and tea consumption and risk of stroke subtypes in male smokers. Stroke. 2008;39(6):1681–87

18 Dietary Patterns, Foods and Beverages in Age-Related Cognitive Performance and Dementia

Keywords

Western diet • Diet quality • Healthy diet • Mediterranean diet • DASH diet • MIND diet • Fruits • Vegetables • Soy • Nuts • Dairy • 100% fruit juice • Coffee • Tea • Cocoa • Alcohol • Polyphenols • Flavanols • Anthocyanins • Lutein • Macular pigment density

Key Points

- All measures of cognitive performance decline with age, with executive functioning (e.g., working memory, reasoning, task flexibility, problem solving and planning) showing the largest rate of decline with every successive decade of age. There is a considerable degree of heterogeneity in cognitive performance across populations, which can be significantly affected by dietary pattern and specific foods and beverages.
- In general, following dietary advice for lowering the risk of cardiovascular and metabolic disorders, such as consuming high levels of healthy fats from fish or vegetable oils, non-starchy vegetables, low glycemic index fruits and a diet low in foods with added sugars should be encouraged for cognitive health. There is significant evidence from human studies that low quality diets reduce and high-quality diets enhance global cognitive performance with aging.
- The Mediterranean diet (MedDiet), DASH diet, and MIND diet (a hybrid of both the MedDiet and DASH diet with an emphasis on specific brain protective foods) are effective in protecting cognitive performance with aging.
- A number of randomized controlled trials (RCTs) and prospective cohort studies support the benefits of high polyphenolic fruits and vegetables, dairy (especially yogurt), 100% juices (polyphenol rich), coffee, tea, flavanol-rich cocoa beverages, and low-moderate wine consumption on improving age-related cognitive performance and reducing risk of dementia, but excessive alcohol consumption can have negative effects on cognitive performance and lead to higher risk of dementia.
- Lutein has been shown to preferentially accumulate in the human brain and its content in neural tissue as reflected in macular pigment density has been positively correlated with cognitive performance and reduced risk of dementia.

M.L. Dreher, *Dietary Patterns and Whole Plant Foods in Aging and Disease*, Nutrition and Health,
https://doi.org/10.1007/978-3-319-59180-3_18

18.1 Introduction

All measures of cognitive performance decline with age, with the most rapid loss rate for information processing speed [1]. Executive functioning (e.g., working memory, reasoning, task flexibility, problem solving and planning) shows the largest rate of decline with every further decade of age. There is a considerable degree of heterogeneity in cognitive performance across populations. In the Mini–Mental State Examination (MMSE), a 30-point questionnaire that is used extensively in clinical and research settings to measure cognitive impairment and to estimate the severity and progression of cognitive impairment, males declined at a slightly slower rate than females, and every additional year of education was associated with a slightly slower rate of MMSE decline. Although apolipoprotein E (Apo-E) is a major cholesterol carrier that supports lipid transport and injury repair in the brain, individuals that are *APOE* ε4 allele carriers tend to have a slightly more rapid decline in most cognitive measures than those who are non-*APOE* ε4 allele carriers due to increased risk of cerebral amyloid angiopathy and age-related cognitive impairment, especially in processing speed [1]. The World Health Organization (WHO) reports that 50 million people are affected by dementia worldwide and the number of cases is expected to triple by 2050 [2]. Dementia is a syndrome, typically chronic or progressive in development, in which there is deterioration in cognitive function beyond what might be expected from normal aging and which progressively interferes with a person's ability to function at work or in other everyday activities [2]. It affects memory, thinking, orientation, comprehension, calculation, learning capacity, language, and judgement. Pathological mechanisms for age related dementia are complex including; (1) reduced vascular function related to chronic systemic inflammation, hyperinsulinemia or elevated systolic blood pressure; (2) neuroinflammation, microglial dysfunction and brain cellular senescence are associated with overweight and obesity related colonic microbiota dysfunction; and (3) brain injuries such as Alzheimer's disease (cerebral accumulation of amyloid-β peptides) or stroke [2–8]. With aging populations, there are eight million new dementia cases each year and the burden of illness it creates approaches pandemic proportions. Dementia affects each person in a different way, depending upon the impact of the disease and the person's personality. There are typically three stages: (1) The early stage of dementia is often gradual and often overlooked; common symptoms include: forgetfulness, losing track of the time and becoming lost in familiar places; (2) As dementia progresses to the middle stage, the signs and symptoms become clearer and more restricting; common symptoms include: becoming forgetful of recent events and people's names, becoming lost at home, and having increasing difficulty with communication such as repeating questions and personal care; and (3) Late stage of dementia is one of near total dependence and inactivity; common symptoms include: becoming unaware of the time and place, having difficulty recognizing relatives and friends, having an increasing need for assisted self-care, having difficulty walking and experiencing behavior changes such as increased aggression. Alzheimer's disease is the most common form of dementia and may contribute to 60–70% of late stage cases. Lifestyle factors such as diet quality, levels of physical activity and smoking play important roles in determining the risk of age-related cognitive impairment [2, 6–8]. Figure 18.1 provides an overview of the biological process. Poor quality Western diets adversely influence cognitive health and are a major factor in cognitive decline and dementia and the opposite is associated with high quality healthy diets [7, 8]. In general, following dietary advice including the consumption of healthy fats from fish or vegetable oils, non-starchy vegetables, low glycemic index fruits and a diet low in foods with added sugars should be encouraged for lowering the risk of cardiovascular and metabolic disorders to help support cognitive health and reduce the risk of dementia [6]. The objective of this chapter is to comprehensively review the effects of dietary pattern quality, foods, beverages, and individual dietary components on age-related cognitive function and dementia.

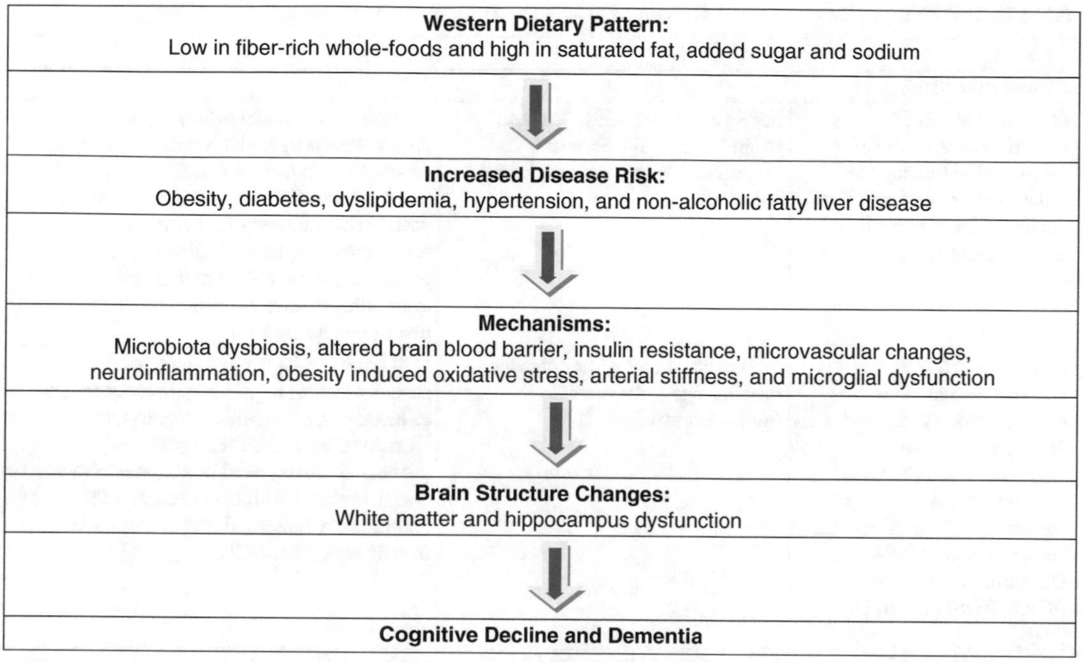

Western Dietary Pattern: Low in fiber-rich whole-foods and high in saturated fat, added sugar and sodium
⇓
Increased Disease Risk: Obesity, diabetes, dyslipidemia, hypertension, and non-alcoholic fatty liver disease
⇓
Mechanisms: Microbiota dysbiosis, altered brain blood barrier, insulin resistance, microvascular changes, neuroinflammation, obesity induced oxidative stress, arterial stiffness, and microglial dysfunction
⇓
Brain Structure Changes: White matter and hippocampus dysfunction
⇓
Cognitive Decline and Dementia

Fig. 18.1 Mechanisms associated with the Western diet and cognitive decline and dementia (adapted from [7, 8])

18.2 Diet Quality

Table 18.1 summarizes the findings from 10 prospective cohort studies and two randomized controlled trials (RCTs) on the protective effects of higher quality diets on cognitive function and dementia [9–20]. A 2017 UK Whitehall II Study (5083 participants; mean baseline age 56 years; 29% women; 10 years of follow-up) found that a major inflammatory diet consisted of higher red and processed meats, peas, fried foods and lower whole grains, which was associated with higher systemic inflammation and accelerated cognitive decline [9]. The US Reasons for Geographic and Racial Differences in Stroke (REGARDS) study in the Southeast (18,080 subjects; baseline age $\geq$ 49 years; cross-sectional analysis) found that diets rich in plant-based foods were associated with higher cognitive scores and reduced risk of cognitive impairment whereas diets high in fried food and processed meat were associated with lower cognitive scores and significantly increased risk of cognitive impairment (Fig. 18.2) [10]. The UK Newcastle 85+ Study (302 men and 489 women; 85 years +; global cognition measured at 3–5 years) showed that diets high in red/processed meat, gravy, and potatoes/potato dishes or butter may predispose very old adults to cognitive impairment [11]. The Australian Personality and Total Health Through Life project longitudinal investigation of older adults (255 subjects; aged 63 years at baseline; 4 years of follow-up) showed that those participants with a high adherence to unhealthy diets or moderate adherence to healthy diets had significantly smaller left hippocampal volumes compared to those with high adherence to healthy diets (Fig. 18.3) [12]. The Swedish National Study on Aging and Care (2223 healthy participants; mean baseline age 71 years; 39% men; 6-years follow-up) demonstrated that higher adherence to the Western diet was associated with faster cognitive decline whereas higher adherence to higher quality healthy diets was inversely associated with cognitive decline [13]. The Taiwan Longitudinal Study of Aging (1926 Chinese men and 1744 Chinese women; baseline age > 65 years; 8-years follow-up) showed that Western diets or high meat and low fish, beans/legumes, vegetables and fruits diets were positively associated with up to an eightfold increase

Table 18.1 Summaries of studies on diet quality and age-related cognitive performance

Objective	Study details	Results
Prospective Studies		
Ozawa et al. (2017). Investigate the association between diet quality and inflammation and cognitive decline (The Whitehall II Study; UK) [9]	5083 participants; 29% women; mean baseline age 56 years; 10 years of follow-up (multivariate adjusted)	A major inflammatory dietary pattern characterized by higher intake of red meat, processed meat, peas, and fried food, and lower intake of whole grains was associated with high circulating IL-6 levels and accelerated cognitive decline (significant reductions in reasoning and global cognition after adjustment for demographics and health related factors)
Pearson et al. (2016). Evaluate associations between empirically derived dietary patterns and cognitive function in the Southeast USA known as the stroke belt. (Reasons for Geographic and Racial Differences in Stroke (REGARDS) cohort; US) [10]	18,080 black and white subjects; baseline age ≥ 49 years (multivariate adjusted)	Diets rich in plant-based foods were associated with higher cognitive scores and reduced risk of cognitive impairment whereas diets rich in fried food and processed meat typical of a Southern diet was associated with lower scores and significantly increased risk of cognitive impairment (Fig. 18.2)
Granic et al. (2016). Investigate the association between diet quality and global and attention-specific cognition (Newcastle 85+ Study; UK) [11]	302 men and 489 women; 85 years +; global cognition [measured by the Standardized Mini-Mental State Examination (SMMSE)] over 5 y and attention assessed by the cognitive drug research attention battery over 3 years (multivariate adjusted)	Diets high in red/processed meat, gravy, and potatoes/potato dishes or butter may predisposed older adults to cognitive impairment
Jacka et al. (2015). Examine the association between diet quality and hippocampal volume in humans (Personality and Total Health Through Life project; Australian) [12]	255 healthy adults; mean baseline age 63 years; follow-up 4 years (multivariate adjusted)	Increased adherence to a healthy quality diet was associated with a larger left hippocampal volume, while higher adherence to an unhealthy Western diet was (independently) associated with a smaller left hippocampal volume (Fig. 18.3)
Shakersaina et al. (2015). Evaluate the effect of diet quality on cognitive changes with aging (Swedish National study on Aging and Care) [13]	2223 healthy participants; mean baseline age 71 years; 39% men; 6-years follow-up; mini-mental state examination	Higher adherence to the Western diet vs. lower adherence was associated with cognitive decline whereas higher adherence to a healthy diet was inversely associated with cognitive decline
Tsai (2015). Examine the effect of diet quality on cognitive decline in older Taiwanese (Taiwan Longitudinal Study of Aging [14]	1926 Chinese men and 1744 Chinese women; baseline age > 65 years; 8-years of follow-up (multivariate adjusted)	A Western diet was positively associated with an eightfold increased risk of cognitive decline over 8 years (adjusted) whereas traditional and healthy diets were not. Diets rich in meats and infrequent consumption of fish, beans/legumes, vegetables and fruits may adversely affect cognitive function in older Taiwanese

Table 18.1 (continued)

Objective	Study details	Results
Gardener (2015). Investigate the associations of diet quality and change in cognitive performance (Australian Imaging, Biomarkers and Lifestyle study of Ageing) [15]	527 subjects; mean baseline age 69 years; 40% male; 3 years of follow-up; 3 diets: Australian MedDiet, prudent, and Western diets (multivariate adjusted)	The primary findings from this study is that higher baseline adherence to a 'healthy' diet is associated with less decline in the executive function composite score in apolipoprotein E (APO-E) ε4 allele carriers. By contrast, higher baseline adherence to the 'unhealthy' Western diet score is associated with increased cognitive decline in the visuospatial functioning composite in APO-E ε4 allele non-carriers
Zhu et al. (2015). Evaluate the associations between diet quality and cognitive function in middle age years (The Coronary Artery Risk Development in Young Adults (CARDIA) Study; US) [16]	2435 participants; 18–30 years at baseline; 5 and 25 years of follow-up (multivariate adjusted)	Those participants with higher quality diet at age 18–30 maintained or improved cognitive performance 5 and 25 years later; with especially better word memory recall
Ozawa et al. (2013). Investigate the associations of diet quality and risk of dementia in older Japanese (Hisayama Study) [17]	1006 healthy community-dwelling Japanese subjects; baseline age 60–79 years; median follow-up 15 years;144 Alzheimer disease cases, 88 vascular dementia cases (multivariate adjusted)	High quality diets, high intakes of soybeans and soybean products, vegetables, seaweed, milk and dairy products and a low intake of rice was associated with 35% lower risk of Alzheimer's disease and a 55% lower risk of vascular dementia
Wengreen et al. (2009). Examine associations between diet quality and cognitive performance among elderly men and women (Cache County Study on Memory and Aging in Utah) [18]	3634 resident men and women; mean baseline age 75 years; recommended food score (RFS) and non-RFS; cognition assessed by the modified mini-mental state examination (3MS) at baseline and 3 subsequent interviews over 11 years (multivariate adjusted)	Participants in the highest quartile of RFS scored 1.8 points higher on the baseline cognitive function test than those in the lowest quartile of RFS ($p < .001$). This effect was strengthened over 11 years of follow-up. Those with the highest RFS declined by 3.4 points over 11 years compared with the 5.2-point decline experienced by those with the lowest RFS ($p = .0013$). Consuming a healthy diet with a variety of recommended foods may help to attenuate age-related cognitive decline among the elderly
RCTs		
Attuquayefio et al. (2017). Investigate the impacts of high saturated fat and added sugar from the Western diet on hippocampal related functioning (Australia) [19]	**Parallel RCT**: 102 participants completed the trial; mean age 20 years; mean BMI 20; breakfasts high in saturated fat and added sugar (experimental group) vs. similar breakfast food types but significantly lower in saturated fat and added sugar (control group); 4 days	The experimental group showed a marked increase in blood glucose and triglyceride response to their breakfast compared to controls. Larger changes in blood glucose were associated with greater reductions in hippocampal-dependent learning and memory, similar to findings from animal studies (Fig. 18.4)

(continued)

Table 18.1 (continued)

Objective	Study details	Results
Smyth et al. (2015). Determine the association of dietary factors and risk of cognitive decline in a population at high risk of cardiovascular disease (CVD) (2 international parallel trials of the ONTARGET (Ongoing Telmisartan Alone and in Combination with Ramipril Global Endpoint Trial) and TRANSCEND (Telmisartan Randomised Assessment Study in ACE Intolerant Subjects with CVD) [20]	**2 Large parallel RCTs**: 27,860 men and women; 26% women; 56 months of follow-up, 4699 cases of cognitive decline; Alternative Healthy Eating Index	Those in the highest healthy eating quintile had significantly lower risk of cognitive decline by 24% compared with the lowest quintile. The healthy diet was primarily associated with an improvement in attention and calculation ability. Lower risk of cognitive decline was consistent regardless of baseline cognitive level. The interaction with diet quality and activity is summarized in Fig. 18.5

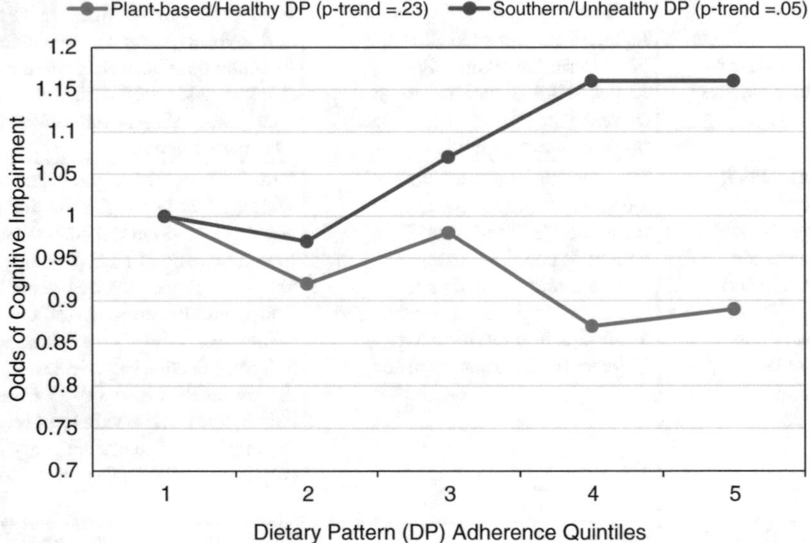

Fig. 18.2 Risk of cognitive impairment and type of dietary pattern (DP) from the Reasons for Geographic and Racial Differences in Stroke (REGARDS) cohort (adapted from [10])

in the rate of cognitive decline over 8 years compared to healthy or traditional diets [14]. The Australian Imaging, Biomarkers and Lifestyle Study of Ageing (527 subjects; mean baseline age 69 years; 40% male; 3-years follow-up) found that higher adherence to a healthy diet is important to reduce risk for cognitive decline, whereas the Western diet was associated with faster decline, especially related to executive function and visuospatial functioning [15]. The US Coronary Artery Risk Development in Young Adults (CARDIA) Study (2435 participants; 18–30 years at baseline; 5 and 25 years of follow-up) showed that those participants with a higher quality diet at age 18–30 maintained or improved cognitive performance 5 and 25 years later and were especially better in word memory recall [16]. The Japanese Hisayama Study (1006 healthy community-dwelling Japanese subjects; baseline age 60–79 years; median follow-up 15 years)

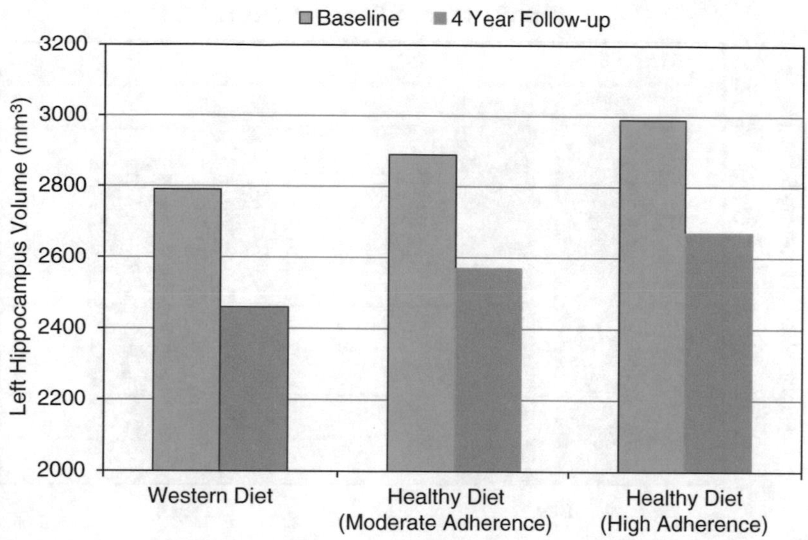

Fig. 18.3 Association between dietary pattern and left hippocampus volume in adults aged 60–64 years at baseline and at 4 years of follow-up (p = .008 high healthy diet adherence vs. other diets) (adapted from [12])

demonstrated that a healthy diet with high intake of soybeans and soybean products, vegetables, seaweed, milk and dairy products and a low intake of rice, was associated with 35% lower risk of Alzheimer's disease and a 55% lower risk of vascular dementia [17]. The Cache County Study on Memory and Aging in Utah (3634 resident men and women; mean baseline age 75 years; recommended food score (RFS) and non-RFS; 11 years of follow-up) found that participants in the highest quartile of RFS had significantly slower cognitive declined by 34% compared with those with the lowest RFS (p = .0013) [18]. A 2017 RCT (102 participants; mean age 20 years; breakfasts high in saturated fat and added sugar (experimental group) vs. a similar breakfast food type but significantly lower in saturated fat and added sugar (control group); 4 days) demonstrated that the experimental group showed a marked increase in blood glucose and triglyceride responses to their breakfast, which was associated with greater reductions in hippocampal-dependent learning and memory compared to the controls (Fig. 18.4) [19]. The pooled data from two large international trials with populations at high risk of cardiovascular disease (27,860 men and women; 26% women; 56 months of follow-up, 4699 cases of cognitive decline) found that those subjects in the healthiest dietary quintile of the modified Alternative Healthy Eating Index had significantly lower risk of cognitive decline by 24% compared with those in the lowest quintile. The healthy diet was primarily associated with an improvement in attention and calculation [20]. The interaction of diet quality and activity is summarized in Fig. 18.5. Studies on higher quality diets generally show they help to attenuate age-related cognitive decline and protect against dementia (among the elderly).

18.3 Healthy Dietary Patterns

Numerous prospective cohort studies and several RCTs support the beneficial effects of high adherence to the Mediterranean diet, (MedDiet) Dietary Approaches to Stopping Hypertension (DASH) diet, MIND diet (a hybrid of MedDiet and DASH) and/or the Nordic diet in protecting against age-related cognitive decline and dementia which are summarized in Table 18.2 [15, 21–42]. The composition of the Western diet vs common healthy dietary patterns is summarized in Appendix A.

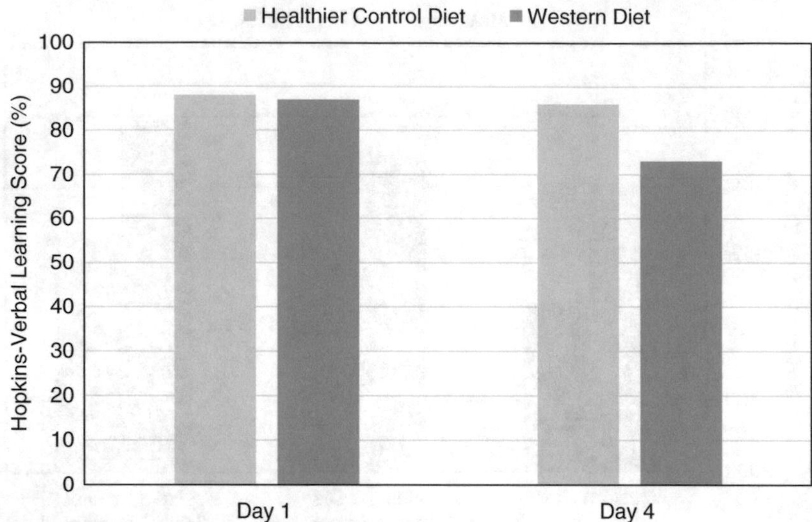

Fig. 18.4 Effect of four days on a high saturated fat and added sugar Western diet on hippocampal dependent learning in young adults ($p < .001$) (adapted from [19])

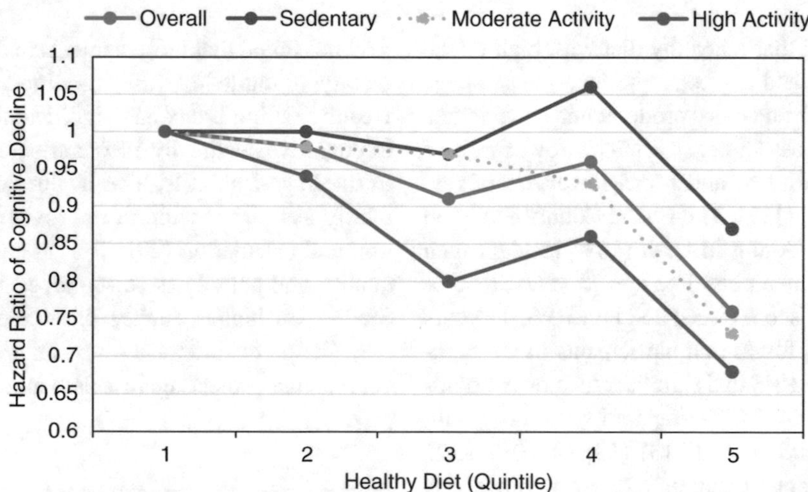

Fig. 18.5 Interaction between adherence to a healthy diet and level of physical activity in 27,860 older adults (mean baseline age 66 years) over 56 months (adapted from [20])

18.3.1 Mediterranean Diet (MedDiet)

18.3.1.1 Systematic Reviews and Meta-Analyses

Seven systematic reviews and meta-analyses consistently show that MedDiets are associated with lower risk for age-related cognitive decline and the development of Alzheimer disease [21–27]. A 2017 analysis of the effect of (1) the MedDiet and (2) omega-3 fatty acids on cognitive outcomes in a cognitively healthy older population (24 studies including 16 cohort studies, 3 cross-sectional studies, and 5 RCTs) found that higher adherence to the MedDiet was associated with better cognitive outcomes in 75% of the studies. Highly consumed foods in the MedDiet, such as fish, nuts and vegetables, had protective effects against cognitive decline across the studies [21]. Also, increased dietary and circulating blood omega-3 fatty acids were shown to improve cognition in

Table 18.2 Summary of specific dietary patterns studies in age-related cognitive performance

Objective	Study details	Results
Mediterranean (MedDiet)		
Systematic Reviews and Meta-Analyses		
Masana et al. (2017). Evaluate the effect of (1) the MedDiet and (2) omega-3 fatty acids on cognitive outcomes in a cognitively healthy aged population [21]	24 studies including 16 cohort studies (8.5 months to 11 years), 3 cross-sectional studies, 5 RCTs (12 weeks to 6.5 years); 45–16,058 participants	(1) Adherence to the MedDiet was associated with better cognitive outcomes in 75% of the studies, while 25% found no association. Also, there was some evidence that certain food groups that are highly consumed in the MedDiet, such as fish, nuts and vegetables, had a protective effect on cognitive decline across included studies. (2) Increased dietary and circulating blood omega-3 fatty acids were shown to improve cognition in 62.5% of the studies and 37.5% of the studies found no association
Wu and Sun (2017). Evaluate the association and dose-response of the MedDiet and cognitive function [22]	9 cohort studies; 34,168 participants; baseline age ≥ 45 years (45–98 years); 2–12 years of follow-up	Compared with the lowest category, the pooled analysis showed that the highest MedDiet scores were inversely associated with developing cognitive disorders by 21%. Subgroup analysis showed that the MedDiet was inversely associated with mild cognitive impairment by 17% and Alzheimer's disease by 40% (Fig. 18.6)
Hardman et al. (2016). Evaluate the effect of the MedDiet on cognitive processes and Alzheimer's disease (AD) over time [23]	18 longitudinal and prospective studies	Of the 18 studies, 13 showed that higher adherence to a MedDiet was related to slowing the rate of cognitive decline, minimizing the conversion to AD, or improving the cognitive function. Five of the 18 studies did not demonstrate that MedDiet adherence had a protective effect against cognitive decline or show improved cognition. The specific cognitive domains that benefit from higher MedDiet score were memory (delayed recognition, long-term, and working memory), executive function, and visual constructs
Petersson et al. (2016). Provide an update on the effects of the MedDiet on cognitive function, cognitive impairment, AD, and all-type dementia [24]	32 studies (5 RCTs and 27 observational studies)	A majority of studies found that the MedDiet was associated with improved cognitive function, a decreased risk of cognitive impairment, dementia, or AD. Five studies found no association between the MedDiet and cognitive function; 3studies found no correlation between the MedDiet and AD, and another 3 studies found no association between the MedDiet and cognitive impairment. Although there was large heterogeneity and differences in study quality, the authors concluded that higher adherence to the MedDiet is associated with better cognitive performance
Singh et al. (2014). Determine whether there is an association between the Mediterranean diet (MedDiet) and risk of cognitive impairment [25]	6 cohorts; 8019 subjects, mean baseline age mid-70s; cognitively normal; follow-up of 4–8 years	Subjects in the highest MedDiet tertile had significantly lower adjusted risk of cognitive impairment by 33% as compared to the lowest tertile. Among cognitively normal individuals, higher adherence to the MedDiet was associated with significantly reduced risk of mild cognitive impairment by 27% and Alzheimer's disease by 36%

(continued)

Table 18.2 (continued)

Objective	Study details	Results
Lourida et al. (2013). Evaluate the association between MedDiet adherence and cognitive function or dementia [26]	13 studies [7 cohort, 1 longitudinal, 1 nested case-control, 3 cross-sectional studies and 1 single blind RCT]; 25–3790 subjects; mean follow-up ranged from 10 days to 8 years	Higher adherence to the MedDiet was associated with better cognitive function, lower rates of cognitive decline, and reduced Alzheimer disease risk in 10 out of 13 studies, whereas results for mild cognitive impairment were inconsistent
Sofi et al. (2010). Assess the effect of adherence to the MedDiet on neurodegenerative diseases [27]	18 cohorts; 2,190,627 subjects; follow-up of 4–20 years.	A 2-point increase in adherence to the MedDiet was associated with a significant reduction in neurodegenerative diseases by 13%
Prospective Studies		
Gardener et al. (2015). Investigate the association of three well-recognised dietary patterns with cognitive change (Australian Imaging, Biomarkers and Lifestyle study of Ageing) [15]	527 subjects; mean baseline age 69 years; 40% male; 3-years of follow-up (multivariate adjusted)	Of the diets, higher adherence to the MedDiet was significantly associated after 36 months with better performance in the executive function in apolipoprotein E (APOE) ε4 allele carriers compared to higher Western diet adherence, which was significantly associated with greater cognitive decline
Galbete et al. (2015). Evaluate the association between adherence to the MedDiet and cognitive function (SUN Project; Spain) [28]	823 participants; mean baseline age 62 years; 10-point (0–9) MedDiet Score was used to categorize adherence to MedDiet; telephone interview of cognitive status-modified range 0–54 points; 2-year change (multivariate adjusted)	Higher cognitive decline was observed among participants with low or moderate baseline adherence to the MedDiet than among those with better adherence. A higher adherence to the MedDiet might be associated with better cognitive function but the differences were of small magnitude
Tangney et al. (2014). Estimate the effects of DASH and MedDiet on age-related cognitive function (Memory and Aging Project; US) [29]	826 participants; mean baseline age 81.5 years; 26% men; 4.1 years of follow-up; (multivariate adjusted)	A 1-unit increase in DASH score was associated with a slower rate of global cognitive decline by 0.007 standardized units ($p = .03$). Similarly, a 1-unit-higher MedDiet score was associated with a slower rate of global cognitive decline by 0.002 standardized units ($p = .01$)
Samieri et al. (2013). Assess the long-term effect of the MedDiet on cognitive function and decline (Nurses' Health Study; US) [30]	16,058 women; mean baseline age 74 years; 6 years of follow-up (multivariate adjusted)	Each higher quintile of MedDiet score was linearly positively associated with an increase in mean cognitive global cognition and verbal memory, a loss in these cognitive functions are strong early predictors of Alzheimer disease at older age (Fig. 18.7). These associations were similar to those observed in women 1–1.5 years of younger age

Table 18.2 (continued)

Objective	Study details	Results
Wengreen et al. (2013). Examine associations between DASH and MedDiet dietary patterns and age-related cognitive change in a prospective, population-based study (Cache County Study on Memory, Health and Aging; US) [31]	3831 men and women; Mean baseline age 74 years and BMI 26; cognitive function was assessed by using the Modified Mini-Mental State Exam; 4 times over 11 years (multivariate adjusted)	Higher DASH and MedDiet scores were associated with higher average cognitive function. People in quintile 5 of DASH averaged 0.97 point higher than those in quintile 1 ($p = .001$). The corresponding difference for MedDiet quintiles was 0.94 ($p = .001$). Higher intakes of whole grains, nuts, and legumes were also associated with higher average cognitive function scores by approx. 20% each
Samieri et al. (2013). Examine the effect of adherence to the alternate MedDiet on cognitive function and decline (Women's Health Study; US) [32]	6174 women; baseline age 72 years; 5 years of follow-up. Alternate MedDiet (aMedDiet) adherence is based on intakes of: vegetables, fruits, legumes, whole grains, nuts, fish and lower intake of red and processed meats, moderate alcohol, and the healthy ratio of monounsaturated-to-saturated fats (multivariate adjusted)	The aMedDiet score was not associated with trajectories of repeated cognitive scores (p-trend across quintiles = .26 and .40 for global cognition and verbal memory, respectively). Overall global cognition and verbal memory at older ages were assessed by averaging the three cognitive measures (p-trend =.63 and .44, respectively). Among alternate MedDiet components, higher monounsaturated-to-saturated fats ratio (or higher olive oil) was associated with more favorable cognitive trajectories (p-trend = .03 and 0.05 for global cognition and verbal memory, respectively). Greater whole-grain intake was associated with better average global cognition (p-trend = .02)
Randomized Controlled Trials (RCTs)		
Valls-Pedret et al. (2015). Investigate the effect of adherence to the MedDiet on cognitive function in older adults (PREDIMED trial; Spain) [33]	**Parallel RCT**: 447 cognitively healthy volunteers with high cardiovascular disease (CVD) risk; mean baseline age 67 years; 51% women; randomly assigned to a MedDiet plus extra-virgin olive oil (1 L/week) or mixed tree nuts (30 g/day) vs. a control diet (advice to reduce dietary fat); median of 4.1 years (multivariate adjusted)	The MedDiet supplemented with olive oil or mixed nuts was associated with significantly improved cognitive function. Compared with the low-fat control diets, MedDiet plus tree nuts significantly improved memory and MedDiet plus extra virgin olive oil improved frontal and global cognition
Martinez-Lapiscina et al. (2013). Assess effects of MedDiets on cognitive function (PREDIMED-NAVARRA; Spain) [34]	**Parallel RCT**: 522 participants at high CVD risk; mean baseline age 75 years; 45% men; randomly assigned to a MedDiet plus extra virgin olive oil or mixed tree nuts vs. advice to reduce dietary fat; 6.5 years of follow-up (multivariate adjusted)	The MedDiet supplemented with extra virgin olive oil or mixed nuts significantly enhanced cognitive function as measured by the Mini-Mental State Exam and clock draw test vs. a low-fat diet
Martinez-Lapiscina et al. (2013). Assess the effect of MedDiets on cognition in a controlled intervention (PREDIMED-NAVARRA; Spain) [35]	**Parallel RCT**: 285 high CVD risk participants; 45% men; mean baseline age 74 years; 3 diets: MedDiets plus extra-virgin olive oil; MedDiets plus mixed tree nuts; a low-fat control diet; 6.5 years (multivariate adjusted)	Better post-trial cognitive performance versus control in all cognitive domains and significantly better performance across fluency and memory tasks were observed for participants allocated to the MedDiet extra virgin olive oil vs. control; mild cognitive impairment was significantly reduced by 66% compared with control group (Fig. 18.8). Participants assigned to MedDiet plus tree nuts group did not differ from controls

(continued)

Table 18.2 (continued)

Objective	Study details	Results
Valls-Pedret et al. (2012). Assess whether consumption of antioxidant-rich foods in the MedDiet relates to cognitive function in the elderly (PREDIMED trial; Spain) [36]	**Cross-sectional assessment of Parallel RCT**: 447 cognitively healthy volunteers with high CVD risk; mean baseline age 67 years; 52% women; MedDiet (multivariate adjusted)	MedDiet adherence as measured by increasing consumption of polyphenol rich foods and beverages was associated with better cognitive performance. Higher intakes of extra virgin olive oil, coffee, walnuts, and wine known to be rich in polyphenols were associated with better memory function and global cognition. Increased urinary polyphenol excretion directly reflected cognitive/memory improvements as summarized in Figs. 18.9 and 18.10
Dietary Approaches to Stop Hypertension (DASH) Diet		
Prospective Cohort Studies		
Berendsen et al. (2017). Examine the association between long-term adherence to the Dietary Approaches to Stop Hypertension (DASH) diet and cognitive function and decline in older American women (The Nurses' Health Study; US) [37]	16,144 women; mean baseline age 74 years; 6 years of follow-up (multivariate adjusted)	Greater DASH diet score adherence was associated with better average cognitive function, irrespective of apolipoprotein E 4 allele status. High DASH diet adherence was not associated with a decline in cognitive function over 6 years and the data suggests an improved cognitive function of 1 year younger in age
Haring et al. (2016). Determine the effect of dietary patterns on cognitive function in older women (Women's Health Initiative Memory Study; Germany) [38]	6425 postmenopausal women; baseline age 65–79 years; DASH diet score and other healthy dietary patterns; median follow-up of 9.1 years; 499 cases of mild cognitive impairment and 390 probable dementia cases (multivariate adjusted)	The DASH diet was insignificantly associated with cognitive decline in older women especially those women with hypertension
Mediterranean-DASH Diet Intervention for Neurodegenerative Delay [MIND] Diet		
Cross-over Study		
McEvoy et al. (2017). evaluate the association between the Mediterranean diet (MedDiet) and the Mediterranean-DASH diet Intervention for Neurodegeneration Delay (MIND diet) and cognition in a nationally representative population of older adults (Health and Retirement Study; US) [39]	5907 community-dwelling older adults; mean age 68 years (multivariate adjusted) The MIND diets emphasizes brain healthy foods (green leafy vegetables, other vegetables, nuts, berries, beans, whole grains, seafood, poultry, olive oil and wine) and restricts unhealthy foods (red meats, stick margarine, pastries and sweets, and fried/fast food)	In this large nationally representative US population of older adults, greater adherence to the MedDiet and MIND diet was associated with improved cognitive performance and lower risk of cognitive impairment by 35% (p-trend <.001)

Table 18.2 (continued)

Objective	Study details	Results
Prospective Cohort Studies		
Morris et al. (2015). Assess the effects of combining key effects of the MedDiet and DASH diet on slowing cognitive decline with the MIND diet; Memory and Aging Project [MAP]; US) [40]	960 participants; average baseline 81 years of age; 75% women; 4.7 years of follow-up (multivariate adjusted)	The MIND score was positively associated with slower decline in global cognitive score ($p < .0001$) (Fig. 18.11). The difference in decline rates for being in the top tertile of MIND diet scores vs. the lowest was equivalent to being 7.5 years younger in cognitive age
Morris et al. (2015). Assess combining key effects of the MedDiet and DASH diet on Alzheimers' disease incidence with the MIND diet; MAP; US) [41]	923 participants; average baseline age 81 years; 75% women; 4.5 years of follow-up; 144 cases of Alzheimers' disease (multivariate adjusted)	Participants in the top and middle tertile of MIND diet scores had significant 53 and 35% reductions in the rate of developing Alzheimers' disease compared with participants in the lowest tertile (Fig. 18.12). These data suggest that even modest adherence to the MIND diet score may help substantially in the prevention of Alzheimers' disease. By contrast, only the highest adherence to the DASH and MedDiet diets were associated with Alzheimers' disease prevention
Nordic Diet – Prospective Cohort Study		
Mannikko et al. (2015). Estimate the cross-sectional and longitudinal associations of the Nordic diet with cognitive function (Sweden and Finland) [42]	1140 women and men; mean baseline age 66 years and BMI 27; 4 years of follow-up (multivariate adjusted) The Nordic diet is characterized by a wide selection of berries, root vegetables, whole-grain products (primarily rye, oat and barley being eaten in bread and porridge) with higher fiber contents; rapeseed (canola) oil with oleic acid and essential fatty acids linoleic acid and α-linolenic acid at 2- and 20-fold higher amounts, respectively, compared with olive oil used in the MedDiet	A higher Nordic diet score was positively associated with verbal fluency ($p = .039$) and word list learning ($p = .022$) but better global cognitive performance and lower Alzheimer's disease related cognitive indicators were only significant, after excluding individuals with impaired cognition at baseline

62.5% of the studies. A 2017 dose-response analysis of the MedDiet on cognitive function (9 cohort studies; 34,168 participants; baseline age ≥ 45 years; 2–12 years of follow-up) showed that the highest MedDiet scores were inversely associated with the developing of cognitive disorders by 21% compared to low scores; subgroup analysis showed that the MedDiet was inversely associated with mild cognitive impairment by 17% and Alzheimer's disease by 40% (Fig. 18.6) [22]. A 2016 analysis of the effects of the MedDiet on cognitive processes and Alzheimer's disease (18 longitudinal and prospective studies) found that 13 of these studies showed that higher adherence to a MedDiet either slowed the rate of cognitive decline, minimized the conversion to Alzheimer's disease or improved the cognitive function [23]. The specific cognitive domains benefiting from higher MedDiet score were memory (delayed recognition, long-term, and working memory), executive function, and visual constructs. Another 2016 analysis (32 studies (5 RCTs and 27 observational studies) showed that 21 of the 32 studies found that the MedDiet was associated with improved cognitive function, a decreased risk of cognitive impairment or

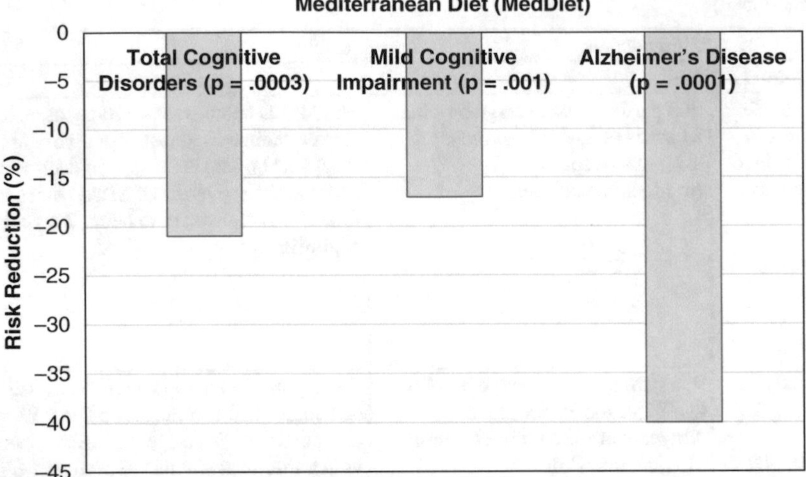

Fig. 18.6 Association between high adherence to the MedDiet and risk of age-related cognitive decline and dementia in adults (≥ 45 years; highest vs. lowest adherence) from a metaanalysis of 9 cohort studies (adapted from [22])

decreased risk of dementia or Alzheimer's disease [24]. Although there was large heterogeneity and differences in study quality, the authors concluded that higher adherence to the MedDiet is associated with better cognitive performance. A 2014 analysis (6 cohorts; 8019 subjects, mean baseline age mid-70s; cognitively normal; follow-up 4–8 years) found that the highest MedDiet tertile had significantly lower adjusted risk of cognitive impairment by 33% as compared to the lowest tertile [25]. Among cognitively normal individuals, higher adherence to the MedDiet was associated with significantly reduced risk of mild cognitive impairment by 27% and Alzheimer's disease by 36%. A 2013 analysis (12 studies: 7 cohort, 1 longitudinal, 1 nested case-control, 3 cross-sectional studies and 1 single blind RCT; 25–3790 subjects; mean follow-up ranged from 10 days to 8 years) showed that higher adherence to the MedDiet was associated with better cognitive function, lower rates of cognitive decline, and reduced Alzheimer disease risk in 9 out of 12 studies, whereas results for mild cognitive impairment were inconsistent [26]. A 2010 analysis (18 cohorts; 2,190,627 participants; follow-up for 4–20 years) demonstrated a 2-point increase in adherence to the MedDiet was associated with a significant reduction in neurodegenerative diseases by 13% [27].

18.3.1.2 Prospective Cohort Studies

Six prospective studies summarize the range of effects of the MedDiet on age related cognitive performance [15, 28–32]. The Australian Imaging, Biomarkers and Lifestyle Study of Ageing (527 subjects; mean baseline age 69 years; 40% male; 3-years follow-up; 3 diets: MedDiet, prudent and Western diets) showed that higher baseline adherence to the MedDiet was associated with less decline in the executive function composite score in apolipoprotein E (APO-E) ε4 allele carriers. By contrast, higher baseline adherence to the Western diet score was associated with increased cognitive decline in the visuospatial functioning composite in APO-E ε4 allele non-carriers [15]. Overall, this study shows that adherence to the MedDiet is important to reduce risk for cognitive decline, especially in executive function and visuospatial functioning. A 2015 Spanish study (823 participants; mean baseline age 62 years; 2 year changes; telephone interviews of cognitive status-modified cognition assessment) found a faster rate of cognitive decline with lower to moderate adherence to the MedDiet than for those with high adherence [28]. The 2014 US Memory and Aging Project (826 participants; mean baseline age 82.5 years; 74% women; 4.2 years of follow-up) found that each 1-unit-higher MedDiet score was associated with a significantly slower rate of global cognitive decline by 0.002 standardized units [29]. A 2013 Nurses' Health Study (16,058 women; mean baseline age 74 years; 6 years of follow-up) showed that each higher quintile of MedDiet score was linearly associated with better mean global cognition and verbal memory (multivariable-adjusted), declines in which are strong early predictors of Alzheimer disease at older age (Fig. 18.7) [30]. The 2013 US Cache County Study on Memory, Health and Aging (3831 men and women; mean baseline age 74 years and BMI 26; 11 years of follow-up; cognitive function was assessed by using the modified mini-mental state examination) found that higher MedDiet scores were associated with higher average cognitive function by 0.94 units ($p = .001$) [31]. Also, higher intakes of whole grains, nuts, and legumes were also associated with higher average cognitive function scores by approximately 20%. A 2013 Women's Health Study (6174 women; baseline age 72 years; 5 years of follow-up) showed that higher adherence to the alternative MedDiet, a simplified guidance based on the intake of vegetables, fruits, legumes, whole-grains, nuts, fish, red meat, moderate alcohol and higher ratio of monounsaturated (MUFA)-to-saturated fats was not significantly associated with better global cognition or verbal memory scores [32]. However, specifically higher MUFA to saturated fat ratio significantly improved global cognitive performance and verbal memory scores and greater whole-grain intake was associated with significantly improved global cognitive performance [32].

18.3.1.3 Randomized Controlled Trials

Three Spanish RCTs demonstrated consistent protective effects of the MedDiet on age related cognitive performance in older subjects with high CVD risk [33–36]. A 2015 PREDIMED trial (447 cognitively healthy volunteers with high CVD risk; mean baseline age 67 years; 51% women; randomly assigned to a MedDiet supplemented with extra virgin olive oil or (one L/week) or mixed nuts (30 g/day) vs. a control diet (advice to reduce dietary fat); median of 4.1 years) found that both MedDiets were associated with significantly improved cognitive function compared to the lower-fat control [33]. Also, a 2013 PREDIMED trial from Navarra, Spain (522 participants at high vascular risk; mean baseline age 75 years; 45% men; 6.5 years of follow-up) showed that MedDiets supplemented with extra virgin olive oil or mixed nuts significantly enhanced cognitive function as measured by the Mini-Mental State Exam and clock draw test vs. a low-fat diet [34]. However, another 2013 PREDIMED-Navarra analysis (285

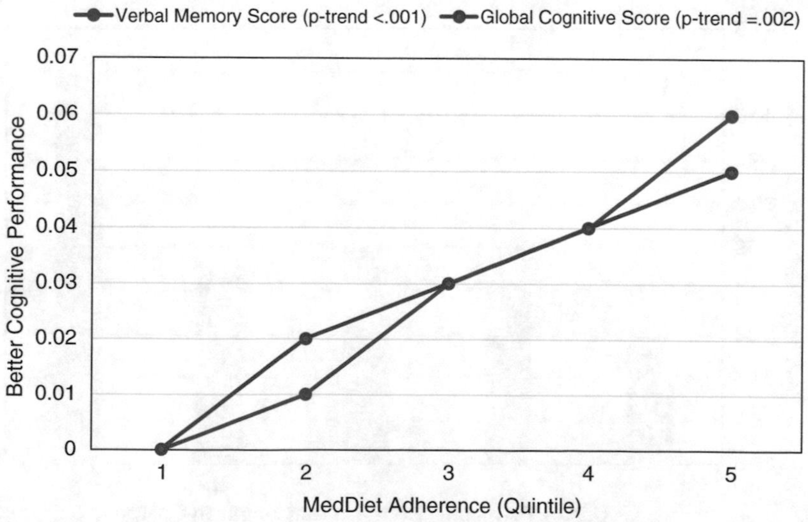

Fig. 18.7 Association between cognitive performance and Mediterranean diet (MedDiet) adherence in women from the Nurses' Health Study (mean baseline age 74 years; 6 years of follow-up) (adapted from [30])

high vascular risk participants; 45% men; mean baseline age 74 years: 6.5 years) found that only the MedDiet plus extra virgin olive oil group significantly reduced mild cognitive impairment by 66% compared to the lower fat control diet (Fig. 18.8) [35]. Results from the participants assigned to MedDiet plus nuts group did not differ from the control group. A cross-sectional analysis of a PREDIMED trial (447 cognitively healthy volunteers with high CVD risk; mean baseline age 67 years; 52% women) found that MedDiet adherence with increasing consumption of polyphenol rich foods and beverages was associated with better cognitive performance [36]. Higher intakes of extra virgin olive oil, coffee, walnuts, and wine were associated with better memory function and global cognition. The relationship between increasing urinary polyphenols excretion and cognitive performance are summarized in Figs. 18.9 and 18.10.

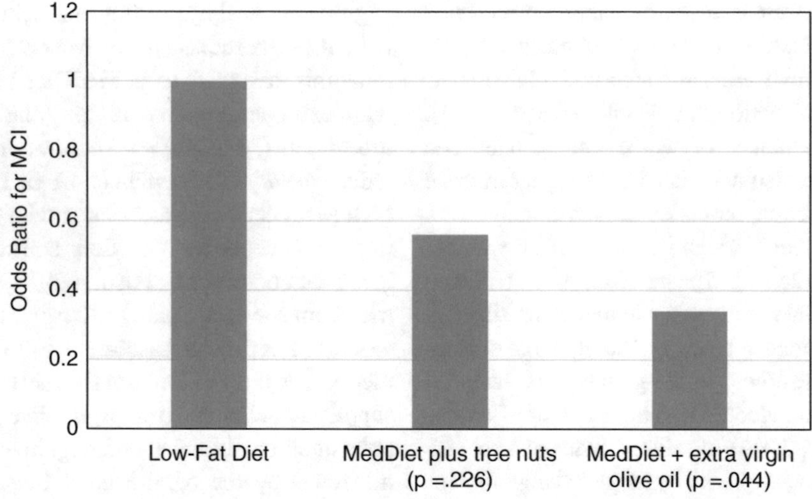

Fig. 18.8 Risk of mild cognitive impairment (MCI) after 6.5 years of two MedDiets (supplemented with 30 g mixed tree nuts/day or 1 liter extra virgin olive oil/week) vs. guidance for a low-fat diet (PREDIMED-Navarra RCT) (adapted from [35])

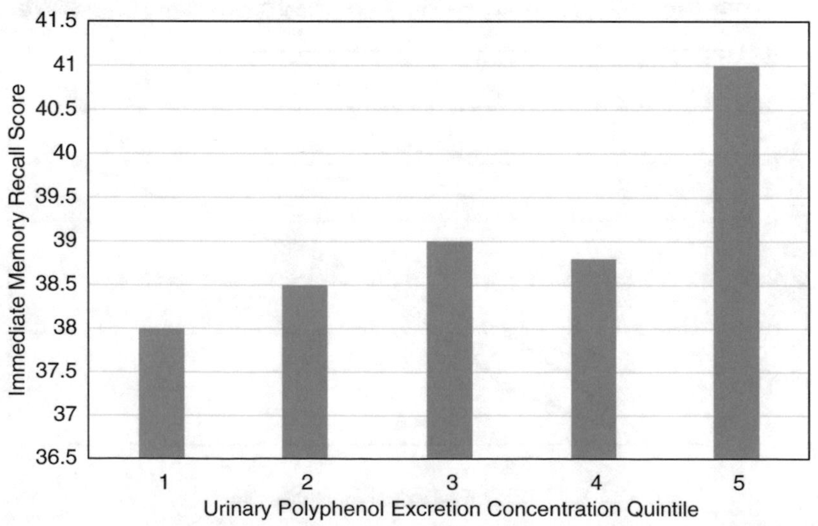

Fig. 18.9 Association between Mediterranean diet (MedDiet) adherence as measured by urinary polyphenol excretion and immediate memory recall score (p-trend = .018) (adapted from [36])

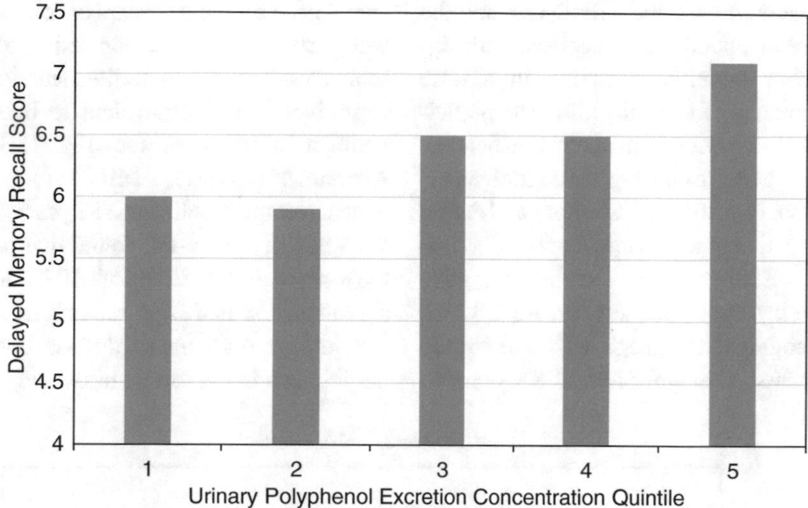

Fig. 18.10 Association between Mediterranean diet (MedDiet) adherence as measured by urinary polyphenol excretion and delayed memory recall score (p-trend = .003) (adapted from [36])

18.3.2 Dietary Approaches to Stop Hypertension (DASH) Diets

Several prospective cohort studies generally show that higher adherence to the DASH diet improves cognitive function in older adults [29, 31, 37, 38]. A 2017 The Nurses' Health Study (16,144 women; mean baseline age 74 years; 6 years of follow-up) found that high adherence to the DASH diet was not associated with a decline in cognitive function over 6 years and suggested the equivalent to being 1 year younger in age [37]. Also, greater adherence to the DASH diet was associated with better cognitive function irrespective of apolipoprotein E ε4 allele status. The 2014 US Memory and Aging Project (826 participants; mean baseline age 81.5 years; 26% men; 4.1 years of follow-up) found that a 1-unit increase in DASH score was associated with a slower rate of global cognitive decline by 0.007 standardized units (p = .03) [29]. The US Cache County Study on Memory, Health and Aging (3831 men and women; mean baseline age 74 years and BMI 26; 11 years of follow-up; cognitive function by modified mini-mental state examination) showed that those participants with the highest DASH diet averaged 0.97 points higher in cognitive function than those in the lowest DASH diet quintile (p = .001) [31]. Higher intakes of whole grains, nuts, and legumes were also associated with higher average cognitive function scores by approximately 20%. However, a 2016 German study (6425 postmenopausal women; baseline age 65–79; 9.1 years of follow-up) found that higher adherence to the DASH diet was not significantly associated with less cognitive decline especially in women with hypertension [38].

18.3.3 Mediterranean-DASH Diet Intervention for Neurodegenerative Delay (MIND)

The MIND diet score combines the cognitive promoting dietary components from both the MedDiet and DASH diet, with emphasizes on brain healthy foods including green leafy vegetables, other vegetables, nuts, berries, beans, whole grains, seafood, poultry, extra virgin olive oil and red wine or high polyphenolic 100% juices (in moderation) and the restriction of unhealthy foods (red meats, stick margarine, pastries and sweets, and fried/fast foods) [20]. Several studies support the MIND diet as being one of the most effective dietary patterns for promoting better age related cognitive performance and reducing the risk of dementia such a Alzheimer's disease [39–41]. The Health and Retirement Study, a large US population-based cross-sectional study (5907 participants; mean age 68 years) showed that high adherence scores to both the MIND diet and the MedDiet were independently associated with significantly better cognitive function in a dose response manner (p < .001, all) [39]. The participants in this study with high dietary adherence were 35% less likely to have poor cognitive performance. Also, two 2015 US Memory and Aging Project prospective studies support the effectiveness of the MIND diet on slowing cognitive decline and delaying Alzheimers disease [39, 40]. For slowing cognitive decline, a MIND diet study (960 participants; average baseline 81 years of age; 75% women; 4.7 years of follow-up) showed that participants in the top tertile of MIND diet scores vs. the lowest tertile had slower rates of cognitive decline equivalent to being 7.5 years younger in cognitive age (Fig. 18.11) [40]. For Alzheimer's disease, a MIND study (923 participants; average baseline age 81 years; 75% women; 4.5 years of follow-up) found that participants in the top and middle tertile of MIND diet scores had significant 53 and 35% reductions in the rate of developing Alzheimers disease compared with participants in the lowest tertile (Fig. 18.12) [41].

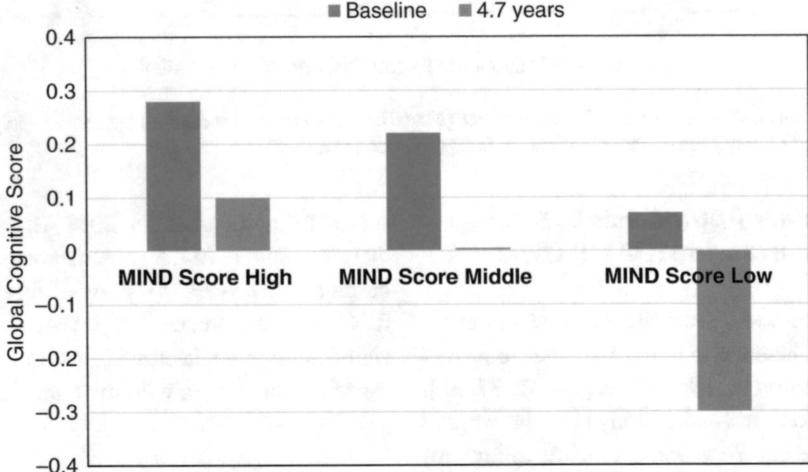

Fig. 18.11 Change in global cognitive score as a function of MIND diet score over 4.7 years with an average baseline age of 81 years (p = .01) (adapted from [40])

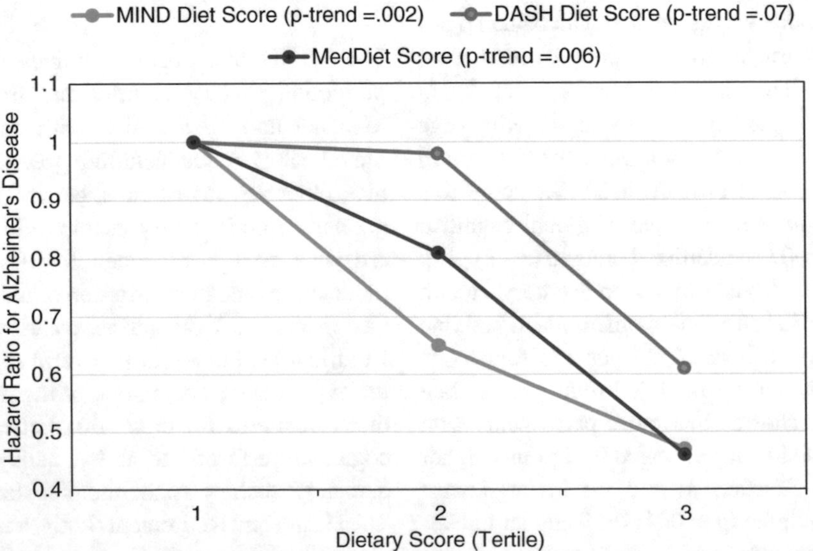

Fig. 18.12 Risk of Alzheimer's disease as a function of dietary pattern over 4.5 years w ith an average baseline age of 81 years (adapted from [41])

18.3.4 Nordic Diets

The Nordic diet is characterized by a wide selection of berries, root vegetables, and whole-grain products (primarily rye, oat and barley) being eaten in bread and porridge (i.e. products that have high fiber contents). The vegetable oil used is rapeseed (canola), which is high in unsaturated fatty acids including oleic acid and essential fatty acids linoleic acid and α-linolenic acid which are 2- and 20 times higher, respectively, compared with olive oil used in the MedDiet [42]. A longitudinal assessment of the Nordic diet (1140 women and men from Sweden and Finland; mean baseline age 66 years; 4 years of follow-up) showed that a higher Nordic diet score was positively associated with verbal fluency ($p = .039$) and word list learning ($p = .022$) but only better global cognitive performance and lower Alzheimer's disease related cognitive indicators were significant, after excluding individuals with impaired cognition at baseline [42].

18.4 Foods and Beverages

18.4.1 Whole Plant Foods and Dairy Products

Aging brain protective foods include higher intake of vegetables, fruit, whole grains, fish, low fat dairy products and nuts, and lower intake of sweets, fried potatoes, processed meat, high-fat dairies and butter [43]. A Western Norway cross-sectional study (2031 older subjects; aged 70–74 years; 55% women; extensive cognitive testing; completed a comprehensive validated and self-reported food frequency questionnaire) found that participants with higher intakes of fruits, vegetables, whole grain products and mushrooms performed significantly better in cognitive tests than those with very low or no intake [44]. The associations were strongest between cognition and the combined intake of fruits and vegetables, with a marked dose-dependent relationship up to about 500 g/day. The dose-related increase of intakes of whole grain products and potatoes reached a plateau at about 100–150 g/day, levelling off or decreasing thereafter, whereas the associations were linear for mushrooms. Individual plant foods, carrots, cruciferous vegetables, citrus fruits and high-fiber bread were most effective at improving cognitive performance whereas high intake of white bread was negatively associated with cognitive function. Tables 18.3 and 18.4 provide summaries of the effects of whole (minimally processed) plant foods, and soy and dairy products on cognitive performance. The composition of whole plant foods is summarized in Appendix B.

18.4.1.1 Fruits and Vegetables

Two systematic reviews, 5 prospective cohort studies, and 2 RCTs summarize the range of positive effects of increased fruit and vegetable intake on age-related cognitive performance (Table 18.3) [45–53]. Fruit and vegetable sources with higher levels of nutrient and phytochemical antioxidants tend to be more effective in attenuating brain oxidative or inflammatory stress or elevating serum levels of brain-derived neurotrophic factor.

Systematic Reviews

Two systematic reviews support the protective effect of fruit and vegetable intake on improving age related cognitive performance [45, 46]. A 2014 systematic review found statistically significant benefits of fruits, vegetables, or 100% juice consumption for improved cognitive function in older adults reported in 17 of 19 observational studies and 3 of 6 intervention trials [45]. However, there was a high degree of variability in cognitive effects depending on the type of fruit, vegetable or juice consumed. A 2012 systematic review (6 cohort studies; ≥ 6 months of follow-up) showed in 5 of 6 studies that higher consumption of vegetables, but not fruit, was associated with a decreased risk of cognitive decline or dementia [46]. In these studies, the vegetables most associated with slower cognitive decline included cruciferous vegetables, legumes, and green leafy vegetables, particularly cabbage, zucchini, squash, broccoli, and lettuce, at a daily intake of 3 servings (200 g). The effect of vegetables may be associated with the fact that people frequently consume vegetables with added healthy oils, which aid in absorption of fat soluble antioxidants such as vitamins A and E, and carotenoids.

Table 18.3 Summaries of fruit, vegetable, whole-grain and nut studies in age-related cognitive performance

Objective	Study details	Results
Fruits and Vegetables		
Systematic Reviews		
Lamport et al. al. (2014). Summarize the association between polyphenol intake from fruit, vegetable, and juice consumption and cognition [45]	19 observational studies and 6 intervention studies	17 observational studies and 3 intervention studies reported significant benefits of fruit, vegetable, or juice consumption for cognitive performance. The data suggest that chronic intake of fruits, vegetables, and juices are beneficial for cognition in healthy older adults. However, there was a high degree of variability in cognitive effects depending on the type of fruit, vegetable or juice consumed
Loef and Walach (2012). Summarize the effects of fruit and vegetable intake on age related cognitive function [46]	6 cohort studies on fruits and vegetables with a follow-up of 6 months or longer	Five of the 6 studies that analyzed fruit and vegetable consumption separately found that higher consumption of vegetables, but not fruit, was associated with a decreased risk of cognitive decline or dementia. In these studies, the vegetables most associated with slower cognitive decline included cruciferous vegetables, legumes, and green leafy vegetables, particularly cabbage, zucchini, squash, broccoli, and lettuce, at a daily intake of 3 servings (200 g) a day. The authors suggest that these beneficial effects might be due to higher intake of flavonoids or antioxidants in both fruits and vegetables, or increased vitamin E in vegetables, compared to fruits, which have more vitamin C. Furthermore, people frequently consume vegetables with added fats (e.g., oils) which may aid in absorption of nutrients/phytochemicals
Prospective Cohort Studies		
Devore et al. (2012). Evaluate the effect of berries and flavonoids on cognitive decline (The Nurses' Health Study; US) [47]	16,010 participants, mean baseline age 74 years; follow-up assessments were conducted twice, at two-year intervals for 4 years of follow-up (multivariate adjusted)	Greater intakes of blueberries and strawberries were associated with slower rates of cognitive decline. For blueberries, high intake improved mean global score (averaging six cognitive tests) by 0.04 units (p-trend = .014 (Fig. 18.13). For strawberries, high intake improved mean global cognitive score by 0.03 units (p-trend = .022). Berries delayed cognitive aging by 1.5–2.5 years of age. Greater intakes of anthocyanidins and total flavonoids were associated with slower rates of cognitive decline (p-trends = .015 and .053)
Chen et al. (2012). Investigate the association between dietary habits and declines in cognitive function among Chinese illiterate elderly (Chinese Longitudinal Health Longevity Study) [48]	6911 illiterate participants; baseline age ≥ 65; 3 years of follow-up (multivariate adjusted)	Lower intakes of vegetables and legumes were associated with cognitive decline among illiterate elderly Chinese. Intake of vegetables and legumes were inversely associated with cognitive decline with significantly lower risk of cognitive decline for high intake of vegetables by 34% and legumes by 22%

Table 18.3 (continued)

Objective	Study details	Results
Nooyens et al. (2011). Evaluate the effect of habitual fruit and vegetable intake during mid-age on cognitive function (Doetinchem Cohort Study; The Netherlands) [49]	2613 men and women; baseline age 43–70 years (mean 55 years); examined for cognitive function twice over a 5-year follow-up (multivariate adjusted)	Higher vegetable intake was associated with smaller decline in information processing speed ($p < .01$) and global cognitive function ($p = .02$) over 5 years. High intakes of some subgroups of vegetables (i.e. cabbage and root vegetables such as carrots, red beets, mushrooms) were associated with a smaller decline in cognitive function. Total intakes of fruits, legumes and juices were not associated with change in cognitive function
Peneau et al. (2011). Examine the association between fruit and vegetable intake and cognitive performance in a sample of adults (Supplementation with Antioxidant Vitamins and Minerals 2; France) [50]	2533 subjects; baseline age 45–60 years; mean age at evaluation 66 years; 13 years of follow-up (multivariate adjusted)	Higher intakes of fruit and vitamin C–rich fruits and vegetables were associated with better verbal memory. In contrast, higher intakes of vegetables, and β-carotene-rich fruits and vegetables were associated with poorer executive function. Further research is required to better understand the complex associations between different groups of fruits and vegetables on specific elements of age related cognitive function
Kang et al. (2005). Examine the effect of fruit and vegetable intake on cognitive function and decline in older women (The Nurses' Health Study; US) [51]	13,388 women; mean baseline age 67 years; 6 years of follow-up (multivariate adjusted)	Specific vegetable intake was significantly associated with a lower rate of cognitive decline. For the highest quintile of cruciferous vegetables, the decline was slower by 0.04 units (p-trend = .01) compared to the lowest intake. Women consuming the highest intake of green leafy vegetables had a slower decline by 0.05 units (p-trend <.001). The cognitive improvement was equal to 1–2 years of younger cognitive age
RCTs		
Lee et al. (2016). Assess effects of polyphenol rich grapes on regional cerebral metabolism in older adults (US) [52]	**Double-blinded, Parallel RCT:** 10 subjects with mild decline in cognition; mean age 72 years; 50% women; high polyphenol grape formulation vs. placebo grape formulation free of polyphenols; 6 months; cognitive performance was measured through neuropsychological assessments. Changes in brain metabolism occurring with each therapy regimen were assessed by brain PET scans with the radiotracer	Polyphenol rich grapes increased metabolic activity in the right superior parietal cortex and left inferior anterior temporal cortex which was correlated with improvements in attention/working memory, as measured with WAIS-III Digital Span ($r = -0.69$, $p = .04$). The placebo low polyphenol grapes lowered metabolic activity in brain area of cognitive function especially the right posterior cingulate cortex ($p = .01$), and left superior posterolateral temporal cortex metabolic activity ($p = 0.04$). The placebo group also showed significant declines in the left prefrontal, cingulate, and left superior posterolateral temporal cortex ($p < .01$). Although there was no significant difference in behavior cognitive performance, this study suggests a protective effect of polyphenol rich grapes against early brain pathologic metabolic decline

(continued)

Table 18.3 (continued)

Objective	Study details	Results
Neshatdousta et al. (2016). Investigate effect of fruit and vegetable flavonoid levels on serum brain-derived neurotrophic factor (BDNF) and cognitive performance (UK) [53]	**Parallel RCT**: 154 men and women; aged 26–70 years; intervention diet averaged 3 portions of fruit and vegetables per day to deliver high-or low-levels of flavonoids; intake was increased by 2 portions every 6 weeks; 2, 4 and 6 portions were 49, 121 and 198 mg flavonoids/day, respectively vs < 6 mg flavonoids/day (habitual diet); 18-weeks	High-flavonoid intake from fruits and vegetables induced significant improvements in cognitive performance and increases in serum brain-derived neurotrophic factor (BDNF) levels (p = <.001) compared to low flavonoid fruits and vegetables habitual diets (Figs. 18.14 and 18.15) Flavonoid rich fruits and vegetables include: apples, pears, berries, oranges, peppers, broccoli, onions, cabbage
Whole-grains		
Prospective Cohort Studies		
Samieri et al. (2013). Examine the effect of adherence to the alternate MedDiet on cognitive function and decline (Women's Health Study; US) [35]	6174 women; baseline age 72 years; 5 years of follow-up	Greater whole-grain intake was associated with better average global cognition (p-trend = .02)
Wengreen et al. (2013). Evaluate associations between DASH and MedDiet dietary patterns and age-related cognitive changes in a prospective, population-based study (Cache County Study on Memory, Health and Aging; US) [37]	3831 men and women; Mean baseline age 74 years and BMI 26; cognitive function was assessed by using the Modified Mini-Mental State Examination 4 times over 11 years	Higher intakes of whole grains were associated with higher average cognitive function scores by approx. 20%
Nuts		
Prospective Cohort Studies		
O'Brien et al. (2014). Examine the effects of long-term nuts intake on cognition in older women (The Nurses' Health Study; US) [54]	16,010 women; mean baseline age 74 years; 6 years of follow-up (multivariate adjusted)	Women consuming ≥5 servings of nuts/week had higher cognitive scores than non-consumers with a mean improvement by 0.08 standard units (p-trend = .003). This mean difference of 0.08 is equivalent to a mean 2-year improved cognitive age

Table 18.3 (continued)

Objective	Study details	Results
RCT		
Cardoso et al. (2016). Evaluate whether Brazil nuts, rich in selenium, preserve cognitive function in older adults via enhancement of selenoprotein antioxidant systems (Brazil) [55]	**Parallel RCT:** 31 older adults with mild cognitive impairment (MCI); mean age 78 years; 70% women; randomly assigned to ingestion of Brazil nuts (290 μg selenium/day) or to the low selenium control; blood selenium concentrations, erythrocyte glutathione peroxidase (GPx) activity, oxygen radical absorbance capacity; 6 months	Selenium levels were increased with Brazil nuts whereas the control group had no change. Among the parameters related to the antioxidant system, only erythrocyte GPx activity change was significantly different between the groups ($p = .006$). Improvements in verbal fluency ($p = .007$) and constructional praxis (the ability to build, assemble, or draw objects) ($p = .031$) were significantly greater in the Brazil nuts group when compared with the control group. These findings suggest that the intake of Brazil nuts helps to correct selenium deficiency and provides preliminary evidence that Brazil nut consumption can have positive effects on some cognitive functions of older adults with MCI
Valls-Pedret et al. (2015). Examine the effect of MedDiets supplemented with nuts or olive oil vs. lower fat diets on age-related cognitive decline (PREDIMED; Spain) [33]	**Parallel RCT**: 447 cognitively healthy adults at high CVD risk; mean baseline age 67 years; 3 dietary interventions: control (low-fat) diet, MedDiet supplemented with virgin olive oil, or MedDiet supplemented with nuts; median follow-up 4.1 years	Multivariate analysis found that the MedDiet plus nuts improved performance above the baseline in memory test ($p = .04$) whereas the subjects on MedDiet plus extra virgin olive oil performed better in tests of frontal ($p < .003$) and global cognition ($p < .005$). All cognitive tests on the lower fat control diets were significantly decreased ($p < .05$)
Sanchez-Villegas et al. (2011). Assess the role of a MedDiet on plasma brain-derived neurotrophic factor (BDNF) levels (PREDIMED; Spain) [56]	**Parallel RCT**: 243 cognitively healthy adults at high CVD risk; mean baseline age 67 years; 3 dietary interventions: control (low-fat) diet, MedDiet plus extra virgin olive oil, or MedDiet plus nuts. Plasma BDNF levels were measured after 3 years of intervention	Participants assigned to MedDiet + nuts showed a significantly lower risk by 78% of low plasma BDNF values (<13 μg/mL) as compared to the low-fat control group. Among participants with depression at baseline, significantly higher BDNF levels were found for those assigned to the MedDiet plus nuts

Prospective Cohort Studies

Four representative prospective studies illustrate the effects of increased fruit and vegetable intake on age-related cognitive function [47–51]. A 2012 Nurses' Health Study (16,010 participants, mean baseline age 74 years; 4 years of follow-up) found that higher intake of berries was associated with slower rates of cognitive decline [47]. For blueberries, high intake significantly improved mean global score (averaging six cognitive tests) (Fig. 18.13) and slightly less similar findings were observed for strawberries. Greater intakes of anthocyanidins and total flavonoids were associated with significantly slower rates of cognitive decline. A 2005 Nurses' Health Study (13,388 women; mean baseline age 67 years; 6 years of follow-up) showed that specific vegetables were significantly associated with a lower rate of cognitive decline [51]. For cruciferous and green leafy vegetables, the highest quintile of intake significantly reduced cognitive decline by 0.04 and 0.05 units, respectively, compared to the lowest intake. The Chinese Longitudinal Health Longevity Study (6911 illiterate participants; baseline age ≥ 65; 3 years of follow-up) found that the intake of vegetables and legumes was inversely associated with cognitive decline with significant lower risk of cognitive decline for high

Table 18.4 Summary of soy food/supplements and dairy foods studies in age related cognitive performance

Objective	Study details	Results
Soy Products		
Meta-Analysis		
Cheng et al. (2015). Quantify the effects of soy isoflavone intake on improving cognitive function in post-menopausal women [57]	10 placebo-controlled RCTs; 1024 participants; 6 weeks to 30 months	Overall global cognitive function was significantly improved by 0.08 units (p = .014). Visual memory was significantly improved by 0.10 units (p = .016). In subgroup analyses, statistically significant improvements were observed in non-US countries and with a mean age younger than 60 years
RCT		
St John et al. (2014). Determine effects of change in urine excretion of isoflavonoids on cognitive change (Women's Isoflavone Soy Health Clinical Trial; US) [58]	**Placebo-controlled, double-blind RCT:** 350 healthy postmenopausal women; mean age 61 years; 25 g of isoflavone-rich soy protein (91 mg of aglycone weight isoflavones) or milk protein-matched placebo, provided daily; mean 2.5 years	Mean increased urine excretion of isoflavonoids from baseline was not significantly associated with change in a composite score of global cognition. Secondary analyses indicated that change in urine excretion of isoflavonoids was inversely associated with general intelligence, but not with factor scores representing verbal or visual episodic memory. Postmenopausal women considering long-term soy protein supplementation should consider consuming less than 25 g soy protein or 91 mg of isoflavones per day
Henderson et al. (2012). Determine the cognitive effects of long-term dietary soy isoflavones in a daily dose comparable to that of traditional Asian diets (Women's Isoflavone Soy Health Clinical Trial; US) [59]	**Placebo-controlled, double-blind RCT:** 350 healthy postmenopausal women; mean age 61 years; 25 g of isoflavone-rich soy protein (91 mg of aglycone weight isoflavones) or milk protein-matched placebo, provided daily; mean 2.5 years	Women consuming soy protein or milk protein placebo showed improved global cognitive composite scores. Soy protein improved global cognition from baseline by 58% whereas milk protein improved score by 69% but there was no significant difference between the two groups. Secondary analyses indicated that soy protein improved visual memory by 67% but there were no significant between-group differences on other cognitive factors or individual test scores
Fournier et al. (2007). Investigate the effect of soy isoflavones (soy milk and supplement) on cognitive functioning in healthy, postmenopausal women (US) [60]	**Double-blind, placebo-controlled RCT:** 79 postmenopausal women; mean age 56 years; diets: cow's milk (control); soy milk, (72 mg isoflavones/day); isoflavone supplement (70 mg isoflavones/day); placebo supplement; 16 weeks	Soy milk or soy isoflavone supplements over a 16-week period did not improve or appreciably affect cognitive functioning in healthy, postmenopausal women compared to cow's milk. Soy milk and supplements did not improve selective attention (Stroop task), visual long-term memory (pattern recognition), short-term visuospatial memory (Benton Visual Retention Test), or visuo-spatial working memory (color match task). Also, the soy milk group showed a decline in verbal working memory (Digit Ordering Task) compared to cow's milk groups
Dairy Products		
Systematic Review		
Crichton et al. (2010). Systematic review to assess evidence for an association between dairy intake and cognitive functioning [61]	3 cross-sectional and 5 prospective studies; 449–4809 subjects; subjects >60 years in prospective studies	Poorer cognitive performance and an increased risk for vascular dementia were found to be associated with a lower consumption of milk or dairy products. However, the consumption of whole-fat dairy products may be associated with cognitive decline in the elderly. No significant associations were found between milk and yogurt, or cheese consumption and cognitive decline

Table 18.4 (continued)

Objective	Study details	Results
Prospective Cohort Studies and RCTs		
Kesse-Guyot et al. (2016). Examine the associations of total and specific dairy product intake with cognitive performance in aging adults (Supplémentation en Vitamines et Minéraux Antioxydants (SU. VI. MAX) RCT and the SU.VI.MAX 2 observational follow-up study; France) [62]	3076 participants from the general population; mean age 66 years; cognitive assessment; 13 years of follow-up; dairy product consumption was estimated using 10 × 24 h recalls	Higher yogurt consumption was significantly associated with better verbal memory performance
Crichton et al. (2012). Determine the effect of reduced fat dairy on cognitive performance (Australia) [63]	**Crossover RCT:** 38 participants with habitually low dairy intakes (<2 servings/day); 60% women; mean age 52 years; mean BMI 31.5; randomized to 4 vs. one servings/day of reduced fat dairy foods; 6 months	Spatial working memory performance was improved by 8% (p = .046) following the high dairy diet compared with the low dairy diet. Spatial working memory requires simultaneous storing and manipulating visual-spatial information mediated by the prefrontal cortex

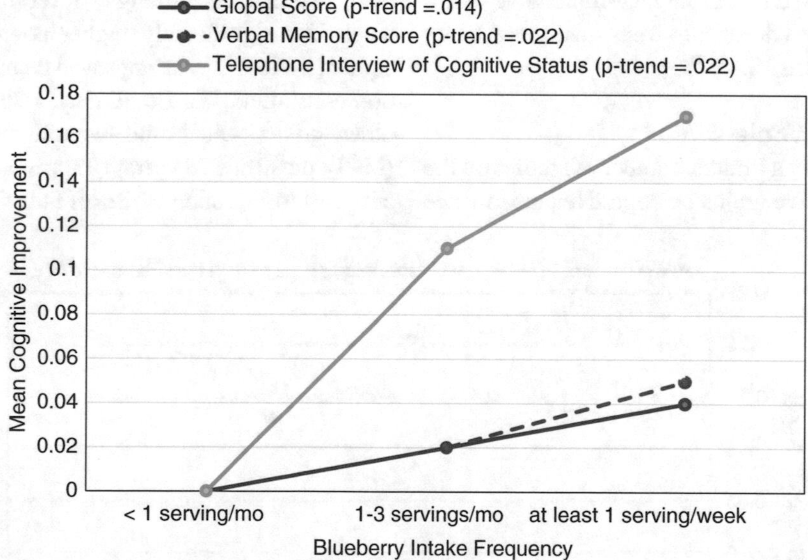

Fig. 18.13 Association between blueberry intake frequency and cognitive function in older women (baseline age 74 years) over 4 years from the Nurses' Health Study (adapted from [47])

intake of vegetables by 34% and legumes by 22% [48]. The Dutch Doetinchem Cohort Study (2613 adults; mean age 55 years; 5 years of follow-up) reported that higher vegetable intake, especially from root vegetables, such as carrots, red beets and mushrooms, significantly slowed the decline in information processing speed and global cognitive function [49]. A French cohort study (2533 subjects; mean age at evaluation 66 years; 13 years of follow-up) found that higher intake of fruit and vitamin C rich fruits and vegetables was associated with better verbal memory [50].

Randomized Controlled Trials (RCTs)

Two RCTs show the effects of flavonoid-rich fruits and vegetables on age related cognitive performance with aging [52, 53]. A 2017 RCT (10 subjects with mild decline in cognition; mean age 72 years; 50% women; polyphenol-rich grapes vs. placebo low polyphenol grapes; 6 months; brain PET scans with the radiotracer) found that the polyphenol rich grapes increased metabolic activity in the right superior parietal cortex and left inferior anterior temporal cortex which was correlated with improvements in attention/working memory whereas subjects consuming the low polyphenol grape placebo had significant metabolic decline in brain areas of cognitive interest [52]. This study suggests a protective effect of grapes against early pathologic brain metabolic decline. A 2016 RCT (154 adults; aged 20–70 years; 18 weeks) found that high flavonoid fruits and vegetables such as berries, oranges, apples, pears, peppers, or broccoli significantly improved cognitive performance and serum brain-derived neurotrophic factor compared to a usual low fruit and vegetable diet or low flavonoid fruits and vegetables (Figs. 18.14 and 18.15) [53].

18.4.1.2 Whole-Grains

There are only a limited number of studies on the effects of whole grains on cognitive performance (Table 18.3) [35, 37]. The Women's Health Study (6174 women; baseline age 72 years; 5 years of follow-up) showed that greater whole-grain intake was associated with better average global cognition (p-trend = 0.02) [35]. The Cache County Study on Memory, Health and Aging (3831 men and women; mean baseline age 74 years and BMI 26; cognitive function assessed over 11 years) found that higher intakes of whole grains were associated with higher average cognitive function scores by approx. 20% [37].

18.4.1.3 Nuts

One prospective cohort study and three RCTs show the effects of increased nut intake on improving age related cognitive performance (Table 18.3) [33, 54–56]. A 2014 Nurses' Health Study (15,467 women; mean age 74 years; 15–21 years of follow-up) found that higher total nut intake was associated with better average cognitive status for all cognitive attributes measured [54]. Women consuming ≥5 servings of nuts/week had significantly higher cognitive scores equivalent to a 2-year improved cognitive age vs. non-consumers. For Brazil nuts, a 2016 RCT (31 older adults with mild cognitive impairment (MCI); mean age 78 years; 70% women; randomly assigned to ingestion of Brazil nuts (290 µg sele-

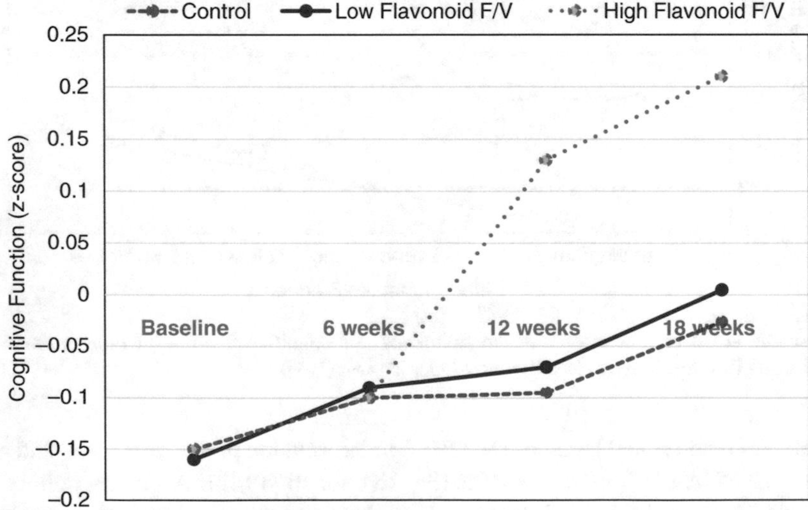

Fig. 18.14 Effect of fruits and vegetables (F/V) flavonoid level on cognitive function after 18 weeks from a RCT with 154 adults ($p < 0.001$ for high flavonoid F/V at 12 and 18 weeks) (adapted from [53])

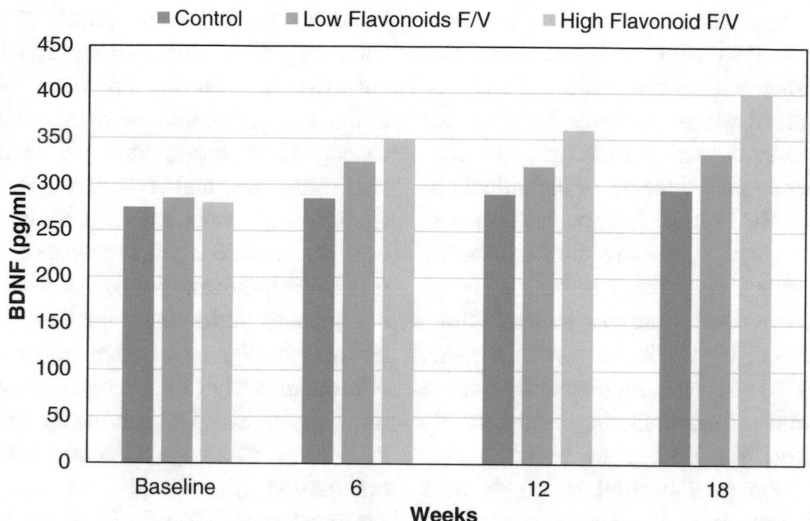

Fig. 18.15 Effect of fruits and vegetables (F/V) flavonoid level on serum brain-derived neurotrophic factor (BDNF) concentration over 18 weeks from a randomized controlled trial with 154 adults ($p < .001$ for high flavonoid F/V after 18 weeks) (adapted from [53])

nium/day) or to the low selenium control; 6 months) found that Brazil nuts significantly improved verbal fluency and constructional praxis (the ability to build, assemble, or draw objects) compared with the control group [55]. These findings support a possible role for Brazil nuts in correcting selenium deficiency and preserving cognitive function in older adults via its enhancement of selenoprotein antioxidant systems. Two Spanish PREDIMED RCTs (243 and 447 cognitive healthy adults at high risk of CVD; mean baseline age 67 years; 30 g mixed nuts/day; 3–4.1 years) found that the MedDiet plus nuts significantly improved memory and increased levels of plasma brain derived neurotrophic factor, known to improve brain function compared to lower fat control diets [33, 56].

18.4.1.4 Soy vs. Milk Protein

Table 18.4 summarizes a meta-analysis, systematic review and key studies on the effects of soy and milk protein or foods on cognitive performance [57–63].

Isolated Soy Protein

Isoflavone-rich isolated soy protein (soy protein) intake is often considered for improving quality of life and cognitive performance in postmenopausal women [57–60]. A 2015 meta-analysis (10 placebo-controlled RCTs; 1024 participants; 6 weeks to 30 months) found that soy protein significantly improved global cognitive performance by 0.08 units and visual memory by 0.10 units. In subgroup analyses, the statistically significant improvements were observed for non-US countries and mean age younger than 60 years [57]. The 2014 Women's Isoflavone Soy Health Clinical Trial (350 healthy postmenopausal women; mean baseline age 61 years; 25 g of soy protein or milk protein-matched placebo, provided daily; 2.5 years) found that women with increased urine excretion of isoflavonoids from baseline showed an insignificant trend for better composite score of global cognition [58]. However, a secondary analysis suggests that higher urinary excretion of isoflavonoids was associated with lower general intelligence, which needs to be confirmed. A 2012 Women's Isoflavone Soy Health Clinical Trial found that both soy protein and the milk protein placebo were associated with similarly improved global cognitive composite scores from baseline levels [59]. Specifically, soy protein improved global cognition from baseline by 58% whereas milk protein improved scores by 69% but there was no significant difference between the two groups. Secondary analyses indicated that soy protein improved visual memory by 67% but there were no significant between-group differences on other cognitive factors or individual test scores. A 2007 RCT (79 postmenopausal women; mean age 56 years; diets: soy milk (soy milk, 72 mg isoflavones/day), cow's milk, and isoflavone supplement (isoflavone supplement, 70 mg isoflavones/day); 16 weeks) showed that soy milk or soy isoflavone supplements over a 16-week period did not improve or appreciably affect cognitive functioning in healthy, postmenopausal women compared to cow's milk [60]. Also, the soy milk group showed a decline in verbal working memory compared to the cow's milk group.

Dairy Products

Dairy products are shown to have variable effects on age related cognitive performance [61–63]. A 2010 systematic review (3 cross-sectional and 5 prospective studies; 449–4809 subjects; subjects >60 years in prospective studies) found that poorer cognitive performance and an increased risk for vascular dementia were found to be associated with a lower consumption of milk or dairy products [61]. However, the consumption of whole-fat dairy products may be associated with cognitive decline in the elderly. No significant associations were found between milk and yogurt, or cheese consumption and cognitive decline. A 2016 French Supplémentation en Vitamines et Minéraux Antioxydants Study (3076 participants from the general population; mean age 66 years; cognitive assessment; 13 years of follow-up) found no association between total or specific dairy product consumption and working memory [62]. However, higher yogurt consumption was significantly associated with better verbal memory performance. Higher cheese consumption was also significantly associated with better verbal memory performance but this association did not remain significant after adjustment. A 2012 Australian study (38 participants with habitually low dairy intakes (<2 servings/day); 11 men and 27 women; mean age 52 years; mean BMI 31.5; randomised to a high (4 servings/day) or low (1 servings/day) intake of reduced fat dairy; 6 months each diet) showed that spatial working memory performance was significantly improved by 8% following the high dairy diet compared with the low dairy diet [63]. Spatial working memory requires simultaneously storing and manipulating visual-spatial information mediated by the prefrontal cortex.

18.4.2 Beverages

Table 18.5 summarizes the studies associated with polyphenol-rich beverages and alcohol on age-related cognitive performance and dementia [64–83]. Poor cardiovascular health such as endothelial dysfunction or hypertension plays an important role in the development and progression of age related cognitive decline [5–9]. Over the

Table 18.5 Summaries of common polyphenol rich beverages studies in age-related cognitive performance

Objective	Study details	Results
100% Fruit and Vegetable Juices		
Prospective Cohort Studies		
Dai et al. (2006). Assess the effects of consumption of fruit and vegetable juices, as rich sources of polyphenols, in Alzheimer's disease (AD) protection (Kame Project cohort US) [64]	1836 Japanese Americans in King County, Washington, who were dementia-free; mean baseline age 72 years; 54% women; 10 years of follow-up; >80% of subjects drank tea at least once per week; 65% drank 100% fruit or vegetable juices at least once per week; and 20% of subjects possessed one or more ApoE *ε-4* alleles	After adjustment for potential confounders, participants who drank juices ≥3 times per week had a significantly 76% lower risk for AD compared with those who drank juice < once per week. Also, participants who drank juices 1–2 times per week had a 16% lower risk of AD. This inverse association tended to be more pronounced among those with an apolipoprotein E*ε-4* allele and those who were not physically active. Conversely, no association was observed for dietary intake of vitamins E, C, or *β*- carotene or tea consumption
Randomized Controlled Trials (RCTs)		
Kent et al. (2017). Assess whether daily consumption of anthocyanin-rich cherry juice can change cognitive function in older adults with dementia (Australia) [65]	**Single-Blind, Parallel RCT:** 49 subjects with mild-to-moderate dementia; mean age 80 years; 24 women, 25 men; consumption of 200 mL/day of either cherry juice or control juice with negligible anthocyanin content; 12-weeks	Cherry juice improved cognitive function in older adults with Alzheimer's type dementia. Trends were evident, showing improvements in cognitive performance across all tasks with regular cherry juice consumption. Significant improvements in verbal fluency, short-term memory and long-term memory were found in the cherry juice group. Also, cherry juice significantly reduced systolic BP by 4.7 mm Hg compared to the control juice
Alharbi et al. (2016). Investigate if the consumption of flavonoid rich orange juice is associated with acute cognitive benefits in healthy middle-aged men (UK) [66]	**Double-blind, Crossover RCT:** 24 healthy men; mean age 51 years; consumed 240-mL flavonoid rich orange juice (272 mg flavonoids) and a placebo control juice; 2 days separated by a 2-week washout; cognitive function and subjective mood were assessed at baseline (prior to drink consumption) and 2 and 6 h post consumption	Flavonoid rich orange juice was shown to acutely enhance objective and subjective cognition over the course of 6 h in healthy middle-aged adults. The effects on global cognitive performance are summarized in Fig. 18.16
Lamport et al. (2016). Examine the effects of the daily consumption of 100% Concord grape juice (CGJ) for 12 weeks on cognitive function, driving performance, and blood pressure in healthy, middle-aged working mothers (UK) [67]	**Crossover RCT**: 25 healthy mothers of preteen children who were employed for ≥30 h/week; mean age 43 years; consumed 12 ounces (355 mL) of either CGJ (containing 777 mg total polyphenols) or an energy-, taste-, and appearance-matched placebo; daily for 12 weeks; 4-week washout. Verbal and spatial memory, executive function, attention, blood pressure, and mood were assessed at baseline and at 6 and 12 weeks; driving performance assessment in a driving simulator	CGJ was associated with better immediate spatial memory and 2 aspects of driving performance; increased steering accuracy in combination with a faster response time to changes in lead vehicle behavior during car following. The observed effects would account for a reduction in stopping distance of approx 11 m at the speeds driven (40–60 mph; 64–97 km/h), which is an important safety benefit

(continued)

Table 18.5 (continued)

Objective	Study details	Results
Kean et al. (2015). Investigate the effects of flavonoid rich orange juice on cognitive function (US) [68]	**Double-blind, Crossover RCT**: 37 healthy older adults; mean age 67 years; high-flavanoid (305 mg) 100% orange juice and an equicaloric low-flavanoid (37 mg) orange-flavored drink (500 mL) were consumed daily; 8 weeks; 4 weeks washout	In healthy older adults, the daily consumption of flavanoid-rich 100% orange juice significantly improved global cognitive and executive function compared to a low-flavanoid control orange juice after 8 weeks
Bookheimer et al. (2013). Assess the effect of 100% pomegranate juice on cognitive performance (US) [69]	**Double-blind, Parallel RCT:** 32 subjects (28 completers); randomly assigned to drink 8 ounces of either 100% pomegranate juice or a flavor-matched placebo drink; 4 weeks; memory testing, fMRI scans during cognitive tasks, and blood draws for peripheral biomarkers before and after the intervention	Only the pomegranate group showed a significant improvement in the Buschke selective reminding test of verbal memory and a significant increase in plasma trolox-equivalent antioxidant capacity and urolithin α-glucuronide. Also, compared to the placebo group, the pomegranate group had increased f-MRI activity during verbal and visual memory tasks. These results suggest a role for pomegranate juice in augmenting memory function via task-related increases in functional brain activity
Kelly et al. (2013). Evaluate the effects of short-term consumption of nitrate rich beet juice on blood pressure, oxygen uptake kinetics, and muscle and cognitive function in older adults (US) [70]	**Double-blind, crossover RCT:** 12 healthy adults; age range 60–70 years; supplemented their diet with either nitrate-rich concentrated beetroot juice (2 × 70 mL/day, 9.6 mmol/day nitrate) or a nitrate-depleted beetroot juice placebo (2 ×70 mL/day, 0.01 mmol/day nitrates); 3 days	Short-term dietary nitrate intake from beet juice increased plasma nitrate by fourfold and significantly reduced resting blood pressure in normotensive older adults. These results suggest that beet juice may have potential in reducing the risk of hypertension and cardiovascular disease in older adults. The VO2 kinetics was accelerated during treadmill walking, although this did not translate into significant enhanced physical performance and cognitive function
Krikorian et al. (2010). Assess the effect of supplementation with 100% Concord grape juice on memory performance in older adults with early age-related memory decline (US) [71]	**Double-blind, Parallel RCT:** 12 older adults with memory decline but not dementia: mean age 78 years; 8 men and 4 women; 444–621 mL of 100% Concord grape juice/day; 12 week	Concord grape juice significantly improved verbal learning ($p = 0.04$) with non-significant enhancement of verbal and spatial recall. There was no appreciable effect of the intervention on depression symptoms or weight or waist circumference. A small increase in fasting insulin was observed in those that consumed grape juice. These preliminary findings suggest that supplementation with Concord grape juice may help to enhance cognitive function for older adults with early memory decline
Coffee and Tea		
Meta-Analysis and Systematic Review		
Wu et al. (2017). Assess the effects of coffee consumption on dose-response development of cognitive disorders [74]	9 cohort studies; 34,282 participants; baseline age > 60 years; 1.3 to 28 years of follow-up	Coffee consumption exhibited a J-shaped association for incident cognitive disorders (Alzheimers disease, dementia, cognitive decline and impairment). Compared to <1 cup coffee/d, daily consumption of 1–2 cups was associated with a significant 18% lower risk of cognitive disorders, whereas >3 cups of coffee were not significantly different than <1 cup

Table 18.5 (continued)

Objective	Study details	Results
Liu et al. (2017). Evaluate the dose-response relationship of tea consumption and cognitive disorders [75]	17 studies including 6 cohort, 3 case-control and 8 cross-over studies; 48,435 participants; baseline age 50 to 93 years	Tea consumption was inversely and linearly related to risk of cognitive disorders (dementia, cognitive decline and impairment). High tea intake was significantly associated with a significant 27% reduction in cognitive disorder risk with green tea lowering risk by 36% compared to 25% for black tea. The dose response showed a linearly reduced risk of cognitive disorder for tea at 100 ml/d by 6%, at 300 ml/d by 19%, and at 500 ml/d by 29%
Observational Studies		
Gelber et al. (2011). Examine associations of coffee and caffeine intake in midlife with risk of dementia, its neuropathologic correlates, and cognitive impairment (Honolulu-Asia Aging Study; US) [76]	3494 men; mean baseline age 52 years; 25 years of follow-up; 226 cases of dementia and 347 cases of cognitive impairment (multivariate adjusted)	Men with high coffee and caffeine intake in midlife were not associated with cognitive impairment, dementia, or neuropathologic lesions. Also, men in the highest quartile of caffeine intake (≥411.0 mg/day) vs. the lowest quartile (≤137.0 mg/day) had a 55% lower risk of any type of brain lesion (p-trend = .04
Feng et al. (2010). Examine the relationship between tea consumption and cognitive function in older adults (The Singapore Longitudinal Aging Studies) [77]	716 Chinese adults; mean age 65 years; 56% women (multivariate adjusted)	Total tea consumption was independently associated with better performances on global cognition, memory, executive function, and information processing speed. Both black/oolong and green tea consumption were associated with better cognitive performance
Ng et al. (2008). Examine the relation between tea intake and cognitive impairment and decline (The Singapore Longitudinal Aging Studies) [78]	1438 cognitively intact participants in longitudinal analysis; 1–2 years of follow-up (multivariate adjusted)	Total tea intake was significantly associated with a lower prevalence of cognitive impairment, independent of other risk factors. Compared with rare or no tea intake, the risk for cognitive impairment was reduced for low intake by 44%, moderate intake by 55%, and high intake by 63% (p- trend <.001). For cognitive decline, the corresponding risk reductions were 26%, 22% and 43% (p-trend = .042). These effects were most evident for black (fermented) and oolong (semi-fermented) teas, the predominant types consumed by this cohort
Flavanol-rich Cocoa Beverages		
RCTs		
Lamport et al. (2015). Explore the effect of a single acute dose of cocoa flavanols on regional cerebral blood flow (UK) [79]	**Double-blind, Crossover RCT**: 18 subjects; mean age 61 years; 10 men; low (23 mg) or high (494 mg) 330 mL equicaloric flavanol drinks matched for caffeine, theobromine, taste and appearance; pre- and 2 h post-consumption; arterial spin labelling functional magnetic resonance imaging	Significant increases in regional perfusion across the brain were observed following consumption of the high flavanol drink relative to the low flavanol drink, within 2 hours, particularly in the anterior cingulate cortex and the central opercular cortex of the parietal lobe. This increased cerebral blood flow provides a possible acute mechanism by which cocoa flavanols benefit cognitive performance

(continued)

Table 18.5 (continued)

Objective	Study details	Results
Mastroiacovo et al. (2015). Evaluate the effect of cocoa flavanol consumption on cognitive performance in cognitively intact elderly subjects (the Cocoa, Cognition, and Aging Study; Italy) [80]	**Double-blind, Parallel RCT**: 90 older subjects; mean age 70 years; daily a drink containing 993 mg [high cocoa flavanol (HF)], 520 mg [intermediate cocoa flavanol (IF)], or 48 mg [low cocoa flavanol (LF)]; 8 weeks	High cocoa flavanol significantly improved the overall composite cognitive function, z score. Higher cocoa flavanol consumption significantly improved blood pressure and reduced insulin resistance and lipid peroxidation which can be linked to improved cognitive function. Reduction in insulin resistance explained 17% of improvements in composite cognitive performance z score
Sorond et al. (2013). Investigate the relationship between neurovascular coupling measured by Magnetic resonance imaging (MRI) and cognitive function in elderly individuals with vascular risk factors and cocoa consumption (US) [81]	**Double-blind, Parallel RCT:** 60 older subjects; aged 73 years; 2 cups of cocoa daily (flavanol-rich cocoa 609 mg, and flavanol-poor cocoa 13 mg flavanols/serving; 30 days)	Regular high flavanol cocoa beverage intake promoted better neurovascular coupling and greater white matter structural integrity in individuals with baseline impairments with improved neurovascular coupling by 5.6% vs. −2.4% ($p = .001$)

last decade human intervention trials consistently show the potential for a variety of beverages rich in polyphenols to have protective effects on age-related cognitive performance and against the development of neurodegenerative diseases via improving cardiovascular health regulatory mechanisms [64–79]. Alcohol has variable effects on cognitive functions depending on the level of intake and type of alcoholic drink consumed [80–83].

18.4.2.1 100% Juices

Prospective Cohort Study

The US Kame Project cohort (1836 Japanese Americans in King County, Washington, who were dementia-free; mean baseline age 72 years; 54% women; 10 years of follow-up) showed that participants who drank 100% fruit or vegetable juices ≥3 times per week had a significantly 76% lower risk for Alzheimer's disease compared with those who drank 100% juice < once per week [64]. Also, participants who drank 100% juices 1–2 times per week had a 16% lower risk of Alzheimer's disease. This inverse association tended to be more pronounced among those with an apolipoprotein E*ε-4* allele and those who were not physically active.

RCTs

Seven blinded RCTs show the effects of 100% juices on age-related cognitive performance [65–71]. A 2017 parallel RCT (49 subjects with mild-to-moderate dementia; mean age 80 years; 24 women, 25 men; consumption of 200 mL/day of either cherry juice or control juice; 12 weeks) found that cherry juice improved cognitive function in older adults with Alzheimer's type dementia [65]. Significant improvements in verbal fluency, short-term memory and long-term memory were found in the cherry juice group, accompanied by a significant reduction in systolic BP by 4.7 mm Hg compared to the control juice. A 2016 UK crossover RCT (24 healthy men; mean age 51 years; consumed a 240-mL flavonoid rich orange juice (272 mg flavonoids) and a placebo control juice; 2 days; separated by a 2-week wash-out) showed that orange juice improved global cognition within 6 h after consumption (Fig. 18.16) [66]. A 2016 UK cross-over RCT (25 healthy mothers of preteen children who were employed for ≥30 h/week; mean age 43 years; 12 ounces (355 mL) of either 100% Concord grape juice (containing 777 mg total polyphenols) or an energy-, taste-, and appearance-matched placebo; daily for 12 weeks) found that Concord grape juice was associated with better immediate spatial memory and driving performance including steering accuracy in combination with a faster response time to changes in lead following vehicle behavior [67]. Also, concord grape juice consumers had improved car braking reaction time with a reduction in stopping distance of 11 m at the speeds driven (40–60 mph; 64–97 km/h), which is an important safety benefit. A 2015 crossover RCT (37 healthy adults; mean age 67 years; high-flavonoid (305 mg) 100% orange juice and an equicaloric low-flavonoid (37 mg) orange-flavored drink (500 mL) were consumed daily; 8 weeks) showed that daily orange juice consumption significantly improved global cognitive and executive function compared to the low-flavonoid control orange flavored drink after 8 weeks [68]. A 2013 parallel RCT (32 subjects; randomly assigned to drink 8 ounces of either 100% pomegranate juice or a flavor-matched placebo drink; 4 weeks; memory testing, fMRI scans during cognitive tasks) found that the pomegranate group showed a significant improvement in the Buschke selective reminding test of verbal memory and a significant increase in plasma trolox-equivalent antioxidant capacity and urolithin A-glucuronide [69]. Also, the pomegranate group had increased fMRI activity during verbal and visual memory tasks compared to the placebo group, suggesting a role for pomegranate juice in augmenting memory function via task-related increases in functional brain activity. A 2013 crossover RCT (12 healthy adults; age range 60–70 years; supplemented their diet with either nitrate-rich concentrated beetroot juice (2 × 70 mL/day, 9.6 mmol/day nitrate) or a nitrate-depleted beetroot juice placebo (2 × 70 mL/day, 0.01 mmol/day nitrates); 3 days) showed that dietary nitrate intake from beet juice increased plasma nitrate by 4-fold and significantly reduced resting blood pressure in normotensive older adults but this did not translate into significant enhanced improvements in brain metabolism and cognitive function [70]. A 2010 parallel RCT (12 older adults with memory decline but not dementia; mean age 78 years; 8 men and 4 women; 444–621 mL 100% Concord grape juice/day; 12 weeks) found that Concord grape juice significantly improved verbal learning (p = .04) with trends for enhanced verbal and spatial recall suggesting that supplementation with Concord grape juice may

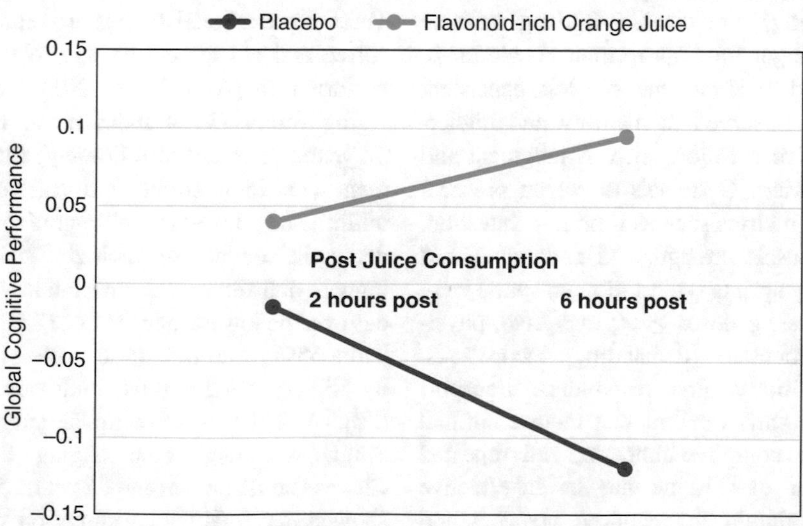

Fig. 18.16 Acute effect of the consumption of high flavonoid orange juice on global cognitive z score in middle-aged men (p = .09) (adapted from [66])

help to enhance cognitive function for older adults with early memory decline [71].

18.4.2.2 Coffee and Tea

Caffeinated beverages, such as coffee and tea are among the most popular beverages in the world. In addition to caffeine they contain polyphenols, chlorogenic acid, theaflavins and other compound that can have direct effects on the brain or influence cardio- and cerebrovascular health to improve cognitive function. Thus, the effects of coffee and tea on cognitive performance and dementia risk is of public health importance. The effects of caffeine have been the most widely evaluated for safety and cognitive function [72]. A 2017 comprehensive systematic review of the potential adverse effects of caffeine consumption found that the evidence generally supports that consumption of up to 400 mg caffeine/day (estimated 4–5 cups of coffee or 5–6 cups of black tea) in healthy adults is not associated with overt, adverse cardiovascular effects, behavioral effects, reproductive and developmental effects, acute effects, or bone status [72]. This review also supports consumption of up to 300 mg caffeine/day in healthy pregnant women as an intake that was generally not found to be associated with adverse reproductive and developmental effects. For optimal cognitive function, caffeine exerts its effects by blocking adenosine receptors [73]. The intake of low (~40 mg) to moderate (~300 mg) caffeine doses showed general improvements in alertness, attention, and reaction time, but less consistent effects were observed in memory and higher-order executive function, such as judgment and decision making. Caffeine's effect on physical performance metrics such as time-to-exhaustion, time-trial, muscle strength and endurance, and high-intensity sprints typical of team sports were evident following doses ≥200 mg. Also, physically and mentally demanding occupations, including military, first responders, transport workers, and shift workers, can require optimal physical and cognitive function, and repeated administration of caffeine may be an effective option to maintain the required physical and cognitive performance.

Meta-analysis and Systematic Review

Two 2017 dose response meta-analyses of observational studies consistently show that coffee and tea improved age related cognitive performance and most common cognitive disorders [74, 75]. For coffee, a dose-response meta-analysis (9 cohort studies; 34,282 participants; 13 to 28 years of follow-up) found a J-shaped association between coffee consumption and the incidence of cognitive disorders (e.g., Alzheimers disease, dementia, cognitive decline or impairment [74]. Compared to < 1 daily cup of coffee, the consumption of 1-2 daily cups was associated with a significant 18% lower risk of cognitive disorders, whereas >4 cups of coffee were not significantly different than <1 cup of coffee. For tea, a dose-response meta-analysis (17 studies including 6 cohort, 3 case-control, and 8 cross-sectional studies; 48,435 participants) found that tea consumption was inversely and linearly associated with the risk of cognitive disorders [75]. The highest tea intake was significantly associated with a 27% lower cognitive disorder risk with green tea lowering risk by 36% compared to 25% for black tea. The dose response analysis for increasing tea intake on reducing cognitive disorder risk at 100 ml/day by 6%, at 300 ml/day by 19% and at 500 ml/day by 29% [75].

Prospective Studies

Three observational studies are representative of coffee and tea effects on age related cognitive performance [76–78]. The 2011 Honolulu-Asia Aging Study (3494 men; mean baseline age 52 years; 25 years of follow-up) found that that men with high coffee and caffeine intake in midlife had a lower risk of cognitive impairment, dementia, or neuropathologic lesions. In the highest quartile of caffeine intake (≥411.0 mg/day) vs. the lowest quartile (≤137.0 mg/day) men had a 55% lower risk of any type of brain lesion by 55% (p-trend = 0.04; multivariate adjusted) [76]. A 2010 cross-sectional analysis of The Singapore Longitudinal Aging Studies (716 Chinese adults; mean age 65 years; 56% women) showed that total tea consumption was independently associated with better performances on the

Min i-Mental State Examination measures of global cognition, memory, executive function, and information processing speed after adjusting for confounding factors [77]. Black/oolong and green tea consumption promoted similar cognitive performance benefits. A 2008 examination of The Singapore Longitudinal Aging Studies (1438 cognitively normal participants in longitudinal analysis; mean baseline age 65 years; 1–2 years of follow-up) showed that total tea intake was significantly associated with a lower prevalence of cognitive impairment, independent of other risk factors. For age-related dementia, low intake significantly reduced risk by 44%, moderate intake by 55%, and high intake by 63% compared to no or rare tea intake [78]. For normal cognitive decline, the corresponding risk reductions for low, moderate and high tea consumption were 26%, 22% and 43% (p-trend = 0.042). These effects were most evident for black (fermented) and oolong (semi-fermented) teas.

18.4.2.3 Flavanol-Rich Cocoa Beverages

RCTs

Three double-blind RCTs are representative of the benefits of flavanol-rich cocoa beverages on age-related cognitive performance [79–81]. A 2015 UK crossover RCT (18 subjects; mean age 61 years; 10 men; pre- and post-consumption of low cocoa flavanol (23 mg) or high cocoa flavanol (494 mg) 330 mL equicaloric flavanol drinks matched for caffeine, theobromine, taste and appearance) found that the high cocoa flavanol drink improved regional cerebral perfusion, especially in the anterior cingulate cortex and the central opercular cortex of the parietal lobe identified by arterial spin labelling functional magnetic resonance imaging within 2 h [79]. This increased cerebral blood flow provides a possible acute mechanism by which cocoa flavanols benefit cognitive performance. Another 2015 RCT (90 older Italian subjects; mean age 70 years; daily drink containing 993 mg [high] cocoa flavanol, 520 mg [intermediate] cocoa flavanol, or 48 mg [low] cocoa flavanol; 8 weeks) showed that the high cocoa flavanol beverage significantly improved the overall composite cognitive function z score as well as significantly improved blood pressure and reduced insulin resistance and lipid peroxidation [80]. A 2013 RCT (60 older US subjects; aged 73 years; 2 cups of cocoa daily (flavanol-rich cocoa 609 mg vs. flavanol-poor cocoa 13 mg flavanols/serving; 30 days) demonstrated that regular high flavanol cocoa beverage intake promoted better neurovascular coupling and greater white matter structural integrity in individuals with baseline impairments [81].

18.4.2.4 Alcohol

Despite chronic excessive alcohol consumption causing progressively increasing neurodegenerative disease risk, a number of studies suggest that low-moderate alcohol consumption, within limits and/or of certain types, may be associated with a decreased cognitive decline and risk of dementia [82]. There are many mechanisms proposed to explain this low to moderate alcohol effect including: (1) the antioxidant properties of the flavonoids in red wine may help prevent the oxidative damage implicated in dementia; (2) by increasing levels of HDL cholesterol and fibrinolytic factors leading to lower platelet aggregation and possibly lower risk of ischemic stroke; and (3) by decreasing cardiovascular risk via the mechanisms described above and possibly enhancing insulin sensitivity or reducing systemic inflammatory response [82]. Table 18.6 summarizes prospective cohort studies on the effects of low to moderate alcohol intake by older adults in cognitive performance and dementia risk [82–88].

Systematic Review and Meta-Analysis

One systematic review and meta-analysis (20 prospective cohort studies, and 3 retrospective matched case-control nested in a cohort; adults >65 years; 1–25 years of follow-up) indicates that intake of small to moderate amounts of alcohol beverage in older adults intake may be protective against dementia by 37% and Alzheimer's disease risk by 43% [82]. The evidence is strongest for red wine consumption but not conclusive.

Table 18.6 Summaries of alcohol beverage studies on age-related cognitive performance

Systematic Review and Meta-Analysis		
Peters et al. (2008). Evaluate the evidence for any relationship between cognitive decline or dementia in the elderly and alcohol consumption [82]	20 prospective cohorts and 3 retrospective matched case-control nested in cohort studies; participants ≥65 years; 1–25 years of follow-up	This meta-analysis suggests that small to moderate amounts of alcohol intake may be protective against dementia by 37% and Alzheimer's disease by 43%. The evidence is strongest for wine consumption but not conclusive
Prospective Studies		
Heymann et al. (2016). Examine the relationship between alcohol, both the amount and type, and cognitive decline in a cohort of Alzheimer's disease patients (US and France) [83]	360 patients with early Alzheimer's disease in New York, Boston, Baltimore and Paris; followed-up biannually for up to 19 years (multivariate adjusted)	Heavy drinkers (8 or more alcoholic drinks/ week) had a faster cognitive decline, deteriorating by 1.85 more points on their global cognitive score annually compared to abstainers ($p = .001$), or 2.44 more points compared to mild-moderate drinkers (1–7 alcoholic drinks/week) ($p = .008$). There was no significant difference when comparing mild-moderate drinkers to abstainers. Increasing standard drinks of hard liquor, but not beer or wine, was also associated with a faster rate of cognitive decline ($\beta = -0.117$ $p = .001$)
Downer et al. (2015). Examine the relationship between midlife and late-life alcohol intake, cognitive functioning, and regional brain volumes among older adults without dementia or a history of abusing alcohol (Framingham Heart Study Offspring Cohort; US) [84]	664 subjects; mean baseline age of 42–75 years; follow-up for 33 years (multivariate adjusted)	Light alcohol consumption during late life is associated with higher episodic memory, but not executive function or global cognition, after controlling for the effects of age, gender, educational attainment, smoking, and *APOE* e4 status. Also, older adults who consumed moderate amounts of alcohol had significantly larger hippocampal volume compared to older adults who did not consume alcohol
Ritchie et al. (2014). Evaluate the effect of alcohol consumption on cognitive function and genetic differences in the ability to metabolize alcohol (Lothian Birth Cohort; UK) [85]	1932 subjects completed the same intelligence test at age 11 and 70 years; alcohol consumption in later life and genotype for a set of four single-nucleotide polymorphisms in 3 alcohol dehydrogenase genes were determined	There was a significant gene × alcohol consumption interaction on lifetime cognitive change ($p = .007$). Subjects with higher genetic ability to process alcohol showed relative improvements in cognitive ability with more consumption, whereas those with low processing capacity showed a negative relationship between cognitive change and higher alcohol consumption. The effect of alcohol consumption on cognitive change appears to depend on genetic differences in the ability to metabolize alcohol
Arntzen et al. (2010). Examine the effect of different alcoholic beverages on cognitive performance in a population based study (Tromso Study; Norway) [86]	5033 stroke-free men and women; 7 years of follow-up; verbal memory, digit-symbol coding test, and tapping test (multivariate adjusted)	Light to moderate wine intake was independently associated with better performance on all cognitive tests in both men and women. There was no consistent association between beer and spirits intake and cognitive performance results. Alcohol abstention was associated with a modest lower cognitive function in women

Table 18.6 (continued)

Systematic Review and Meta-Analysis		
Solfrizzi et al. (2007). Estimate the impact of alcohol consumption on the incidence of mild cognitive impairment (MCI) and its progression to dementia (Italian Longitudinal Study on Aging) [87]	121 MCI patients; aged 65–84 years; 3.5 years of follow-up (multivariate adjusted)	Patients with MCI who consumed up to 1 drink/day had a reduction in the rate of progression to dementia in comparison with patients with MCI who never consumed alcohol. Overall, vs. nondrinkers, patients with MCI who consumed up to 1 drink/day, derived mostly from wine, had a decrease in the rate of progression to dementia by 85%
Stampfer et al. (2005). Examine the effects of moderate alcoholic consumption in women (Nurses' Health Study; US) [88]	12,480 women; mean baseline age 74 years; 2 years of follow-up (multivariate adjusted)	Moderate drinkers (about one drink/day) had better mean cognitive scores than nondrinkers, a reduced risk of general cognitive impairment by 33% and global cognitive score combining the results of all tests by 19%. There were no significant associations between 2 daily drinks and the risk of cognitive impairment or decline vs. non-drinkers. There were no significant risk differences for wine vs. beer

Prospective Studies

Six prospective studies are representative of the effects of alcohol intake on age related cognitive performance [83–88]. A 2016 study (360 patients with early Alzheimers' disease in New York, Boston, Baltimore and Paris; followed-up bi-annually for up to 19 years) found that heavy drinkers (8 or more alcoholic drinks/week) had a faster cognitive decline in their annual global cognitive score compared to abstainers ($p = 0.001$) or mild-moderate drinkers (1–7 alcoholic drinks/week) ($p = 0.008$) [83]. There was no significant difference when comparing mild-moderate drinkers to abstainers. Also, higher consumption of hard liquor, but not beer or wine, was associated with a faster rate of cognitive decline. A 2015 Framingham Heart Study Offspring Cohort (664 subjects; follow-up for 33 years from mean age of 42–75 years) showed that light alcohol consumption during late life is associated with higher multivariate adjusted episodic memory, but not executive function or global cognition [84]. Also, older adults who consumed moderate amounts of alcohol had significantly larger hippocampal volume compared to older adults who did not consume alcohol. The 2014 UK Lothian Birth Cohort (1932 subjects who completed the same intelligence test at age 11 and 70 years; alcohol consumption in later life and genotype determined) found that the effect of alcohol consumption on cognitive change depends on genetic differences in the ability to metabolize alcohol [85]. Subjects with higher genetic ability to process alcohol had relative improvements in cognitive ability with alcohol consumption, whereas those with low processing capacity had a relatively negative effect on cognition with alcohol consumption. A 2010 Norwegian study (5033 adults from the general population; 7 years of follow-up) showed that moderate wine consumption was independently associated with better performance on all cognitive measures in both men and women [86]. The 2007 Italian Longitudinal Study on Aging (121 patients with mild cognitive impairment (MCI); aged 65–84 years; 3.5 years of follow-up) found that patients with MCI who consumed up to 1 drink/day had a reduction in the rate of progression to dementia in comparison with patients with MCI who never consumed alcohol [87]. Overall, compared to non-drinkers, patients with MCI who consumed 1 drink/day, derived mostly from wine, had a decrease in the rate of progression to dementia by 85%. The Nurses' Health Study (12,480 women; mean baseline age 74 years; 2 years of follow-up) showed that moderate drinkers (about one drink/day) had better mean cognitive scores than nondrinkers; moderate drinkers, as compared with nondrinkers had a reduced risk of general cognitive impairment by 33% and global cognitive score combining the results of all tests by 19% (after multivariate adjustment) [88]. There were no significant risk differences for wine vs. beer.

18.4.3 Lutein

Lutein and zeaxanthin are carotenoids that are highly concentrated in human macular pigment in the retina, attenuating blue light exposure, providing protection from photo-oxidation and enhancing visual performance [89]. Recently, interest in lutein has expanded beyond the retina to its possible contributions to brain development and function. Only humans and other primates accumulate lutein within the brain. Recently, lutein has been shown to preferentially accumulate in the human brain and its content in neural tissue has been positively correlated with cognitive performance and reduced risk of dementia. Table 18.7 summarizes RCTs and observational studies on the effects of lutein intake by older adults in cognitive performance and dementia risk [90–99].

18.4.3.1 Randomized Controlled Trials (RCTs)

Two RCTs support the benefits of increased lutein on cognitive performance in humans [90, 91]. A US RCT (39 adults; mean age 63 years; 70% women; daily intake of 1 medium avocado vs. 1 medium potato or 1 cup of chickpeas (control);

Table 18.7 Summary of studies on lutein and age-related cognitive performance and dementia

Objective	Study details	Results
Randomized Controlled Trials (RCT)		
Johnson et al. (2015). Test the effects of daily intake of 1 medium avocado on macular pigment density and cognitive function (US) [90]	**Parallel RCT:** 39 adults mean age 63 years; 70% women; daily intake of 1 medium avocado vs. alternating medium potato or cup of chickpeas (control); on serum lutein levels, macular pigment density and cognition in healthy older adults; serum carotenoids were measured by HPLC; computerized cognitive assessment battery was used for cognition measures; 6 months	At baseline, there were no significant differences between subjects in the avocado and control groups in any of the study measures. At 6 months, serum lutein levels in the avocado group significantly increased from baseline by 20% ($p < .0005$) whereas the potato/chickpea control group increased by 7% ($p < .03$). After 6 months, there was a significant increase in macular pigment density in the avocado group but no change in the control group. In the avocado group the change in macular pigment density was significantly related to an improved spatial working memory ($p < .009$) and problem approaching efficiency ($p < .036$). No significant changes in cognitive function were observed in the control group. These data suggest that an intervention with avocados to increase neural lutein is an effective dietary strategy for cognitive health
Bovier et al. (2014). Evaluate the effect of increased lutein and zeaxanthin on visual processing speed and efficiency in younger adults (US) [91]	**Double-blind Parallel RCT:** 92 young adults; average age 22 years; 36 males and 56 females; 3 interventions: supplements: 20 mg zeaxanthin/day; 26 mg zeaxanthin, 8 mg lutein, 190 mg mixed n-3 fatty acids/day; placebo; 4 months	Significant correlations were found between retinal lutein and zeaxanthin (macular pigment [MP] density) and critical flicker fusion (CFF) thresholds ($p < .01$) and visual motor performance (overall $p < .01$). In general, increasing MP density through supplementation (average increase of about 0.09 log units) resulted in significantly improved visual processing speed
Observational Studies		
Zamroziewicz et al. (2016). Evaluate the effect of serum lutein levels on cognitive performance and intelligence in healthy older adults (cross-sectional study; US) [92]	76 cognitively intact adults; mean age 69 years; 67% women; mean serum lutein 454 pmol/mL (range 120–1328 pmol/mol)	Serum lutein levels were significantly positively associated with gray matter volume of the right para-hippocampal cortex and with crystallized intelligence (the ability to use learned knowledge and experience)

Table 18.7 (continued)

Objective	Study details	Results
Feart et al. (2016). Analyze the relation between plasma carotenoids and the risk of dementia and Alzheimer's disease (Three-City-Bordeaux cohort; French) [93]	1092 nondemented older participants; average baseline age 74 years; average 8.8 years of follow-up; 132 Alzheimers' disease cases	After adjustment for sociodemographic data, diet quality, and clinical variables, including baseline cognitive performances, only higher lutein concentration, considered as a function of plasma lipids, was consistently significantly associated with a decreased risk of all-cause dementia by 20% ($p = .024$) and Alzheimers' disease by 24% ($p = .021$)
Lindbergh et al. (2016). Investigate underlying neural mechanisms for lutein and zeaxanthin using functional magnetic resonance imaging (f-MRI) during cognitive performance (cross-sectional study; US) [94]	43 community-dwelling older adults; mean age 72 years; 58% female; 100% Caucasian); asked to learn and recall pairs of unrelated words in an f MRI-adapted paradigm. Lutein and zeaxanthin levels were measured in retina by macular pigment optical density and serum using validated procedures	This study indicates that higher lutein and zeaxanthin levels, measured both acutely (serum) and acquired (retinal), enhance neural efficiency during verbal learning and memory in older adults. Lutein and zeaxanthin were significantly related to more and efficient blood-oxygen-level-dependent signals in central and parietal operculum cortex, cerebellum and other brain regions
Vishwanathan et al. (2016). Evaluate the relationship between retinal and brain lutein and zeaxanthin in humans (US) [95]	Donated human brain tissue and matched retina for 13 individuals with a mean age at death of 75 years with normal cognitive function or Alzheimer's disease were obtained from the National Disease Research Interchange	Macular pigment carotenoids (lutein, meso-zeaxanthin, and zeaxanthin combined) in the retina were significantly related to the combined concentrations of lutein and zeaxanthin in the occipital cortex. When analyzed separately, only retinal lutein (plus meso-zeaxanthin), not zeaxanthin, was significantly related to lutein in the occipital cortex. No correlations were observed with lutein and zeaxanthin in the hippocampus. Total macular pigment density measured via non-invasive, psychophysical techniques can be used as a biomarker to assess brain lutein and zeaxanthin status in clinical studies
Kelly et al. (2015). Investigate the relationship between macular pigment, serum concentrations of lutein and zeaxanthin, and cognitive function in subjects free of retinal disease with low macular pigment levels (cross-sectional study; Ireland) [96]	105 subjects free of retinal disease with low macular pigment and mean age 47 years; and 121 subjects with age-related macular degeneration (AMD) and mean age 65 years	Significant correlations were evident between macular pigment levels and various measures of cognitive function in both groups ($r = -0.27$–0.26, $p \leq .05$, for all). Both serum lutein and zeaxanthin levels correlated significantly ($r = 0.19$, $p \leq .05$ and $r = 0.20$; $p \leq .05$, respectively) with semantic fluency cognitive scores. For AMD subjects, serum lutein levels also correlated significantly with verbal recognition memory learning slope ($r = 0.20$, $p = .031$)
Renzi et al. (2014). Test whether retinal measures of macular pigment density can be used as a surrogate for brain lutein and zeaxanthin levels related to cognitive function when comparing healthy older adults with mildly cognitively impaired older adults (cross-sectional study; US) [97]	24 subjects with mild cognitive impairment were compared with 24 matched controls; subjects matched with respect to age, BMI, ethnicity, sex, and smoking status; degree of cognitive impairment and cognitive ability was determined via structured clinical interview; macular pigment density was measured psychophysically	In healthy older adults, macular pigment density was significantly related to visual-spatial and constructional abilities ($p = .04$). For subjects with mild cognitive impairment, macular pigment density was broadly and significantly related to cognition including the composite score on the mini-mental state exam, visual-spatial and constructional abilities, language ability, attention, and the total scale on the repeatable battery assessment of neuropsychological status

(continued)

Table 18.7 (continued)

Objective	Study details	Results
Vishwanathan et al. (2014). Determine whether macular pigment density, lutein and zeaxanthin in the macula are related to cognitive function in older adults (cross-sectional study Healthy Aging and Body Composition Study; US) [98]	108 adults, mean age 78 years sampled from the age-related maculopathy ancillary study; serum carotenoids were measured using HPLC; macular pigment density was assessed using heterochromatic flicker photometry; 8 cognitive tests designed to evaluate several cognitive domains including memory and processing speed were administered	Macular pigment density levels were significantly associated with better global cognition, verbal learning and fluency, recall, processing speed and perceptual speed, whereas serum lutein and zeaxanthin were significantly related to only verbal fluency
Johnson et al. (2013). Assess the relationship between serum and brain carotenoids on cognitive performance (cross sectional study; Oldest Old from the Georgia Centenarian Study; US) [99]	Sera from 78 octogenarians and 220 centenarians; brain tissues from 47 centenarian decedents; samples were analyzed for carotenoids, α-tocopherol, and retinol; global cognition, dementia, depression and cognitive domains (memory, processing speed, attention, and executive functioning)	Serum lutein, zeaxanthin, and β-carotene concentrations were most consistently related to better cognition ($p < .05$) in the whole population and in the centenarians. Only serum lutein was significantly related to better cognition in the octogenarians. In the brain, lutein was consistently associated with a range of cognitive measures. There were fewer significant relationships for α-tocopherol. These findings suggest that the status of lutein in the old may especially reflect their cognitive function

6 month-duration) found that serum lutein levels in the avocado group were significantly increased from baseline by 20% compared to an insignificant increase in the control group were by 7% [90]. After 6 months, there was a significant increase in macular pigment density (a biomarker of brain lutein levels) in the avocado group but no change in the control group. In the avocado group the change in macular pigment density was significantly related to an improved spatial working memory and problem approaching efficiency, whereas no significant changes in cognitive function were observed in the control group. These data suggest that an intervention with avocados to increase neural lutein is an effective dietary strategy for cognitive health. Also, a US double-blinded RCT (92 young adults; average age 22 years; 36 males and 56 females; 3 interventions: supplement containing 20 mg zeaxanthin/day; supplement containing 26 mg zeaxanthin, 8 mg lutein, 190 mg mixed n-3 fatty acids/day; and a placebo; 4 months) showed significant correlations between retinal lutein and zeaxanthin macular pigment density and improved visual processing speed [91].

18.4.3.2 Observational Studies

Eight observation studies consistently support the beneficial effects of increased lutein on cognitive performance and reduced Alzheimer's disease risk [92–99]. A 2016 US cross-sectional study (76 cognitively intact adults; mean age 69 years; 67% women) found that serum lutein levels were significantly positively associated with gray matter volume of the right parahippocampal cortex and with crystallized intelligence (the ability to use learned knowledge and experience) [92]. A 2016 French prospective study (1092 nondemented older participants; average baseline age 74 years; average 8.8 years of follow-up) showed that of all the diet quality variables only higher lutein concentration as a function of plasma lipids was consistently significantly associated with a decreased risk of all-cause dementia by 20% and Alzheimers' disease by 24% [93]. Another US cross-sectional study (43 community-dwelling older adults; mean age 72 years; 58% female; 100% Caucasian; asked to learn and recall pairs of unrelated words in an fMRI-adapted paradigm) found that higher lutein and zeaxanthin levels, measured both acutely (serum) and acquired (retinal), enhanced neural efficiency during verbal learning and memory in older adults with improved brain functional signaling efficiency [94]. In a 2016 evaluation of brain and retina tissue from 13 individuals with a mean age at death of 75 years with normal cognitive function or Alzheimer's disease donated from the US National Disease Research Interchange showed that lutein was significantly concentrated in both the brain's occipital cortex and retina macular pigment to confirm use of macular pigment density as a biomarker of brain lutein status in clinical studies [95]. A 2015 Irish cross-sectional study (105 subjects free of retinal disease with low macular pigment; mean age 47 years; 121 subjects with age-related macular degeneration [AMD] and mean age 65 years) found that significant correlations were evident between macular pigment levels and various measures of cognitive function in both groups ($r = -0.27$–0.26, $p \leq 0.05$, for all) and both serum lutein and zeaxanthin levels correlated significantly ($r = 0.19$, $p \leq .05$ and $r = 0.20$; $p \leq .05$, respectively) with semantic fluency cognitive scores [96]. For AMD subjects, serum lutein levels also correlated significantly with verbal recognition memory learning slope ($r = 0.20$, $p = .031$). A 2014 cross-sectional study (24 subjects with mild cognitive impairment were compared with 24 matched controls) showed that macular pigment density was broadly and significantly related to cognition including the composite score on the mini-mental state examination, language ability, attention, and a repeatable assessment of neuropsychological status [97]. The 2014 US Healthy Aging and Body Composition Study (108 adults, mean age 78 years sampled from the agerelated maculopathy ancillary study; serum carotenoids; macular pigment density; eight cognitive tests designed to evaluate several cognitive domains including memory and processing speed) found that macular pigment density was associated with significantly better global cognition, verbal learning and fluency, recall, processing speed and perceptual speed, whereas serum lutein and zeaxanthin were significantly related to only verbal fluency [98]. The US Oldest Old from the Georgia Centenarian Study (78 octogenarians and 220 centenarians; brain tissues from 47 deceased centenarians) showed that serum lutein, zeaxanthin, and β-carotene concentrations were most consistently related to better cognition ($p < 0.05$) in the whole population and in the centenarians whereas only serum lutein was significantly related to better cognition in the octogenarians [99]. These studies indicate that higher serum levels of certain carotenoids may reflect better cognitive function in older age.

18.5 Lifestyle Factors

CVD risk factors such as hypertension, diabetes, and hyperlipidemia increase an individuals' risk for stroke, neurocognitive impairment and dementia [100]. Also, the effects of these CVD risk factors on brain dysfunction are additive. Lifestyle behaviors, including physical activity and healthy dietary habits are recommended to improve CVD risk factors and may aid in the prevention of neurocognitive decline. A US cross-sectional analysis of baseline data from Exercise and Nutritional Interventions for Neurocognitive Health Enhancement (ENLIGHTEN) trial (160 adults with cognitive impairment, without dementia; 67% women; mean age 65 years; completed neurocognitive assessments of executive function, processing speed, and memory; physical activity using accelerometry, aerobic capacity determined by exercise testing, and dietary habits for adherence to the Mediterranean and DASH diets) found that greater aerobic capacity and daily physical activity were associated with better executive functioning, processing speed and verbal memory, DASH diet adherence was associated with better verbal memory whereas higher hs-CRP was associated with poorer executive functioning, processing speed and verbal memory [100]. These findings support the adoption of healthy lifestyle habits to reduce the risk of neurocognitive decline in older adults.

Conclusions

All measures of cognitive performance decline with age, with executive functioning (e.g., working memory, reasoning, task flexibility, problem solving and planning) showing the largest rate of decline with every successive decade of age. There is a considerable degree of heterogeneity in cognitive performance across populations, which can be significantly affected by dietary pattern and specific foods and beverages. In general, following dietary advice for lowering the risk of cardiovascular and metabolic disorders, such as consuming high levels of healthy fats from fish or vegetable oils, non-starchy vegetables, low glycemic index fruits and a diet low in foods with added sugars should be encouraged for cognitive health. There is significant evidence from human studies that low quality diets reduce and high-quality diets enhance global cognitive performance with aging. The MedDiet, DASH diet, and MIND diet (a hybrid of both the MedDiet and DASH diet with an emphasis on specific brain protective foods) are effective in protecting cognitive performance with aging. A number of RCTs and prospective cohort studies support the benefits of high polyphenolic fruits and vegetables, dairy (especially yogurt), 100% juices (polyphenol rich), coffee, tea, flavanol-rich cocoa beverages, and low-moderate wine consumption on improving age-related cognitive performance and reducing risk of dementia, but excessive alcohol consumption can have negative effects on cognitive performance and lead to higher risk of dementia. Lutein has been shown to preferentially accumulate in the human brain and its content in neural tissue as reflected in macular pigment density has been positively correlated with cognitive performance and reduced risk of dementia.

Appendix A: Comparison of Western and Healthy Dietary Patterns per 2000 kcal (Approximated Values)

Components	Western dietary pattern (US)	USDA base pattern	DASH diet pattern	Healthy Mediterranean pattern	Healthy vegetarian pattern (Lact-ovo based)	Vegan pattern
Emphasizes	Refined grains, low fiber foods, red meats, sweets, and solid fats	Vegetables, fruits, whole-grains, and low-fat milk	Potassium rich vegetables, fruits, and low fat milk products	Whole grains, vegetables, fruits, dairy products, olive oil, and moderate wine	Vegetables, fruit, whole-grains, legumes, nuts, seeds, milk products, and soy foods	Plant foods: vegetables, fruits, whole grains, nuts, seeds, and soy foods
Includes	Processed meats, sugar sweetened beverages, and fast foods	Enriched grains, lean meat, fish, nuts, seeds, and vegetable oils	Whole-grains, poultry, fish, nuts, and seeds	Fish, nuts, seeds, and pulses	Eggs, non-dairy milk alternatives, and vegetable oils	Non-dairy milk alternatives
Limits	Fruits and vegetables, and whole-grains	Solid fats and added sugars	Red meats, sweets and sugar-sweetened beverages	Red meats, refined grains, and sweets	No red and white meats, or fish; limited sweets	No animal products
Estimated Nutrients/Components						
Carbohydrates (% Total kcal)	51	51	55	50	54	57
Protein (% Total kcal)	16	17	18	16	14	13
Total fat (% Total kcal)	33	32	27	34	32	30
Saturated fat (% Total kcal)	11	8	6	8	8	7
Unsat. fat (% Total kcal)	22	25	21	24	26	25
Fiber (g)	16	31	29+	31	35+	40+
Potassium (mg)	2800	3350	4400	3350	3300	3650
Vegetable oils (g)	19	27	25	27	19–27	18–27
Sodium (mg)	3600	1790	1100	1690	1400	1225
Added sugar (g)	79 (20 tsp)	32 (8 tsp)	12 (3 tsp)	32 (8 tsp)	32 (8 tsp)	32 (8 tsp)
Plant Food Groups						
Fruit (cup)	≤1.0	2.0	2.5	2.5	2.0	2.0
Vegetables (cup)	≤1.5	2.5	2.1	2.5	2.5	2.5
Whole-grains (oz.)	0.5	3.0	4.0	3.0	3.0	3.0
Legumes (oz.)	–	1.5	0.5	1.5	3.0	3.0+
Nuts/Seeds (oz.)	0.5	0.6	1.0	0.6	1.0	2.0
Soy products (oz.)	0.0	0.5	–	–	1.1	1.5

U.S. Department of Agriculture and U.S. Department of Health and Human Services. Dietary Guidelines for Americans, 2010. 7th Edition, Washington, DC: U.S. Government Printing Office. 2010; Table B2.4; http://www.choosemyplate.gov/ accessed 8.22.2015

U.S. Department of Agriculture, Agriculture Research Service, Nutrient Data Laboratory. 2014. USDA National Nutrient Database for Standard Reference, Release 27. http://www.ars.usda.gov/nutrientdata. Accessed 17 February 2015

Dietary Guidelines Advisory Committee. Scientific Report. Advisory Report to the Secretary of Health and Human Services and the Secretary of Agriculture. Appendix E-3.7: Developing vegetarian and Mediterranean-style food patterns. 2015;1–9

Dietary Guidelines Advisory Committee. Scientific Report. Advisory Report to the Secretary of Health and Human Services and the Secretary of Agriculture. Part D. Chapter 1: Food and nutrient intakes, and health: current status and trends. 2015;1–78

Bhupathiraju SN, Tucker KL. Coronary heart disease prevention: nutrients, foods, and dietary patterns. Clinica Chimica Acta. 2011;412: 1493–1514

Appendix B: Estimated Range of Energy, Fiber, Nutrients and Phytochemicals Composition of Whole Plant Foods/100 g Edible Portion

Components	Whole-grains	Fresh fruit	Dried fruit	Vegetables	Legumes	Nuts/seeds
Nutrients/ Phytochemicals	Wheat, oat, barley, rye, brown rice, whole grain bread, cereal, pasta, rolls and crackers	Apples, pears, bananas, grapes, oranges, blueberries, strawberries, and avocados	Dates, dried figs, apricots, cranberries, raisins and prunes	Potatoes, spinach, carrots, peppers, lettuce, green beans, cabbage, onions, cucumber, cauliflower, mushrooms, and broccoli	Lentils, chickpeas, split peas, black beans, pinto beans, and soy beans	Almonds, Brazil nuts, cashews, hazelnuts, macadamias, pecans, walnuts, peanuts, sunflower seeds, and flaxseed
Energy (kcal)	110–350	30–170	240–310	10–115	85–170	520–700
Protein (g)	2.5–16	0.5–2.0	0.1–3.4	0.2–5.0	5.0–17	7.8–24
Available Carbohydrate (g)	23–77	1.0–25	64–82	0.2–25	10–27	12–33
Fiber (g)	3.5–18	2.0–7.0	5.7–10	1.2–9.5	5.0–11	3.0–27
Total fat (g)	0.9–6.5	0.0–15	0.4–1.4	0.2–1.5	0.2–9.0	46–76
SFA[a] (g)	0.2–1.0	0.0–2.1	0.0	0.0–0.1	0.1–1.3	4.0–12
MUFA[a] (g)	0.2–2.0	0.0–9.8	0.0–0.2	0.1–1.0	0.1–2.0	9.0–60
PUFA[a] (g)	0.3–2.5	0.0–1.8	0.0–0.7	0.0.0.4	0.1–5.0	1.5–47
Folate (μg)	4.0–44	<5.0–61	2–20	8.0–160	50–210	10–230
Tocopherols (mg)	0.1–3.0	0.1–1.0	0.1–4.5	0.0–1.7	0.0–1.0	1.0–35
Potassium (mg)	40–720	60–500	40–1160	100–680	200–520	360–1050
Calcium (mg)	7.0–50	3.0–25	10–160	5.0–200	20–100	20–265
Magnesium (mg)	40–160	3.0–30	5.0–70	3.0–80	40–90	120–400
Phytosterols (mg)	30–90	1.0–83	–	1.0–54	110–120	70–215
Polyphenols (mg)	70–100	50–800	–	24–1250	120–6500	130–1820
Carotenoids (μg)	–	25–6600	1.0–2160	10–20,000	50–600	1.0–1200

[a]SFA (saturated fat), MUFA (monounsaturated fat) and PUFA (polyunsaturated fat)

U.S. Department of Agriculture, Agriculture Research Service, Nutrient Data Laboratory. 2014. USDA National Nutrient Database for Standard Reference, Release 27. http://www.ars.usda.gov/nutrientdata. Accessed 17 February 2015

Ros E, Hu FB. Consumption of plant seeds and cardiovascular health epidemiological and clinical trial evidence. Circulation. 2013;128: 553–565

USDA. What we eat in America, NHANES 2011–2012, individuals 2 years and over (excluding breast-fed children). Available: www.ars.usda.gov/nea/bhnrc/fsrg

Slavin JL, Lloyd B. Health benefits of fruits and vegetables. Adv Nutr. 2012;3:506–516

Rebello CJ, Greenway FL, Finley JW. A review of the nutritional value of legumes and their effects on obesity and its related co-morbidities. Obes Rev. 2014;15:392–407

Gebhardt SE, Thomas RG. Nutritive Value of Foods. 2002; U.S. Department of Agriculture, Agricultural Research Service, Home and Garden Bulletin 72

Holden JM, Eldridge AL, Beecher GR, et al. Carotenoid content of U.S. foods: an update of the database. J Food Comp An. 1999;12:169–196

Lu Q-Y, Zhang Y, Wang Y, et al. California Hass avocado: profiling of carotenoids, tocopherol, fatty acid, and fat content during maturation and from different growing areas. *J* Agric Food Chem. 2009;57(21):10408–10413

Wu X, Beecher GR, Holden JM, et al. Lipophilic and hydrophilic antioxidant capacities of common foods in the United States. J Agric Food Chem. 2004;52:4026–4037

Bhupathiraju SN, Tucker KL. Coronary heart disease prevention: nutrients, foods, and dietary patterns. Clinica Chimica Acta. 2011;412:1493–1514

Dietary Guidelines Advisory Committee. Scientific Report. Advisory Report to the Secretary of Health and Human Services and the Secretary of Agriculture. Part D. Chapter 1: Food and nutrient intakes, and health: current status and trends. 2015;1–78

http://health.gov/dietaryguidelines/2015/guidelines/ Accessed 1.26.2016

References

1. Lipnicki DM, Crawford JD, Dutta R, et al. Age-related cognitive decline and associations with sex, education and apolipoprotein E genotype across ethnocultural groups and geographic regions: a collaborative cohort study. PLoS Med. 2017;14(3):e1002261. https://doi.org/10.1371/journal.pmed.1002261.
2. World Health Organization (WHO). Dementia: a public health priority (2012). World Health Organization Dementia: Fact Sheet No. 362 (2016). http://www.who.int/mediacentr0e/factsheets/fs362/en/. Accessed Apr 2017.
3. Koellhoffer EC, McCullough LD, Ritzel RM. Old maids: aging and its impact on microglia function. Int J Mol Sci. 2017;18:769. https://doi.org/10.3390/ijms18040769.
4. Lopez-Valdes HE, Martinez-Coria H. The role of neuroinflammation in age-related dementias. Rev Inves Clin. 2016;68:40–8.
5. Santo CY, Snyder PJ, Wu W-C, et al. Pathophysiological relationship between Alzheimer's disease, cerebrovascular disease, and cardiovascular risk: a review and synthesis. Alzheimers Dementia (Amst). 2017;7:69–87.
6. Solfrizzi V, Panza F, Frisardi V, et al. Diet and Alzheimer's disease risk factors or prevention: the current evidence. Expert Rev Neurother. 2011;11(5):677–708. https://doi.org/10.1586/ern.11.56.
7. Noble EE, Hau TM, Kanoski SE. Gut to brain dysbiosis: mechanisms linking Western diet consumption, the microbiome, and cognitive impairment. Front Behav Neuorsci. 2017;11:9. https://doi.org/10.3389/fnbah.2017.00009.
8. Wang M, Norman JE, Srinivasan VJ, Rutledge JC. Metabolic, inflammatory, and microvascular determinants of white matter disease and cognitive decline. Am J Neurodegener Dis. 2016;5(5):171–7.
9. Ozawa M, Shipley M, Kivimaki M, et al. Dietary pattern, inflammation and cognitive decline: The Whitehall II prospective cohort study. Clin Nutr. 2017;36:506–12.
10. Pearson KE, Wadley VG, McClure LA, et al. Dietary patterns are associated with cognitive function in the REasons for Geographic and Racial Differences in Stroke (REGARDS) cohort. J Nutr Sci. 2016;5:e38. https://doi.org/10.1017/jns.2016.27.
11. Granic A, Davies K, Adams A, et al. Dietary patterns high in red meat, potato, gravy, and butter are associated with poor cognitive functioning but not with rate of cognitive decline in very old adults. J Nutr. 2016;146:265–74. https://doi.org/10.3945/jn.115.216952.
12. Jacka FN, Cherbuin N, Anstey KJ, et al. Western diet is associated with a smaller hippocampus: a longitudinal investigation. BMC Med. 2015;13:215. https://doi.org/10.1186/s12916-015-0461-x.
13. Shakersaina B, Santonia G, Larssonb SC, et al. Prudent diet may attenuate the adverse effects of Western diet on cognitive decline. Alzheimers Dement. 2016;12(2):100–9. https://doi.org/10.1016/j.jalz.2015.08.002.
14. Tsai HJ. Dietary patterns and cognition decline in Taiwanese aged 65 years and older. Int J Geriatr Psychiatry. 2015;30(5):523–30.
15. Gardener SL, Rainey-Smith SR, Barnes MB, et al. Dietary patterns and cognitive decline in an Australian study of ageing. Mol Psychiatry. 2015;20(7):860–6.
16. Zhu N, Jacobs DR, Meyer KA, et al. Cognitive function in a middle-aged cohort is related to higher quality dietary patterns 5 and 25 years earlier: the CARDIA study. J Nutr Health Aging. 2015;19(1):33–8. https://doi.org/10.1007/s12603-014-0491-7.
17. Ozawa M, Ninomiya T, Ohara T, et al. Dietary patterns and risk of dementia in an elderly Japanese population: The Hisayama Study. Am J Clin Nutr. 2013;97:1076–82.
18. Wengreen HJ, Neilson C, Munger R, Corcoran C. Diet quality is associated with better cognitive test performance among aging men and women. J Nutr. 2009;139:1944–9. https://doi.org/10.3945/jn.109.106427.
19. Attuquayefio T, Stevenson RJ, Oaten MJ, Francis HM. A four-day Western-style dietary intervention causes reductions in hippocampal-dependent learning and memory and interoceptive sensitivity. PLoS One. 2017;12(2):e0172645. https://doi.org/10.1371/journal.pone.0172645.
20. Smyth A, Dehghan M, O'Donnell M, et al. Healthy eating and reduced risk of cognitive decline a cohort from 40 countries. Neurology. 2015;84:2258–65.
21. Masana ME, Koyanagi A, Haro JM, Tyrovolas S. n-3 fatty acids, Mediterranean diet and cognitive function in normal aging: a systematic review. Exp Gerontol. 2017;91:39–50. https://doi.org/10.1016/Jexger.2017o2.008.
22. Wu L, Sun D. Adherence to Mediterranean diet and risk of developing cognitive disorders: an updated systematic review and meta-analysis of prospective cohort studies. Sci Rep. 2017;7:41317. https://doi.org/10.1038/srep41317.
23. Hardman RJ, Kennedy G, Macpherson H, et al. Adherence to a Mediterranean-style diet and effects on cognition in adults: a qualitative evaluation and systematic review of longitudinal and prospective trials. Front Nutr. 2016;3:22. https://doi.org/10.3389/fnut.2016.00022.
24. Petersson SD, Philippou E. Mediterranean diet, cognition function, and dementia: a systematic review of the evidence. Adv Nutr. 2016;7:889–904. https://doi.org/10.3945/an.16.012138.
25. Singh B, Parsaik AK, Mielke MM, et al. Association of Mediterranean diet with mild cognitive impairment and Alzheimer's disease: a systematic review and meta-analysis. J Alzheimers Dis. 2014;39(2):271–82.
26. Lourida I, Soni M, Thompson-Coon J, et al. Mediterranean diet, cognitive function, and dementia. A systematic review. Epidemiology.

2013;24(4):479–89. https://doi.org/10.1097/EDE.0b013e3182944410.

27. Sofi F, Abbate R, Gensini GF, Cesari F. Accruing evidence on benefits of adherence to the Mediterranean diet on health: an updated systematic review and meta-analysis. Am J Clin Nutr. 2010;92:1189–96.
28. Galbete C, Toledo E, Toledo JB, et al. Mediterranean diet and cognitive function: the SUN project. J Nutr Health Aging. 2015;19(3):305–12.
29. Tangney CC, Li H, Wang Y, et al. Relation of DASH- and Mediterranean-like dietary patterns to cognitive decline in older persons. Neurology. 2014;83:1410–6.
30. Samieri C, Okereke OL, Devore EE, et al. Long-term adherence to the Mediterranean diet is associated with overall cognitive status, but not cognitive decline, in women. J Nutr. 2013;143:493–9. https://doi.org/10.3945/jn.112.169896.
31. Wengreen H, Munger RG, Cutler A, et al. Prospective study of Dietary Approaches to Stop Hypertension - and Mediterranean-style dietary patterns and age-related cognitive change: the Cache County Study on memory, health and aging. Am J Clin Nutr. 2013;98:1263–71.
32. Samieri C, Grodstein F, Rosner BA, et al. Mediterranean diet and cognitive function in older age: results from the Women's Health Study. Epidemiology. 2013;24(4):490–9. https://doi.org/10.1097/EDE.0b013e18294a065.
33. Valls-Pedret C, Sala-Vila A, Serra-Mir M, et al. Mediterranean diet and age-related cognitive decline. a randomized clinical trial. JAMA Intern Med. 2015;175(7):1094–103.
34. Martinez-Lapiscina EH, Clavero P, Toledo R, et al. Mediterranean diet improves cognition: the PREDIMED-NAVARRA randomized trial. J Neurol Neurosurg Psychiatry. 2013;84(12):1318–25.
35. Martinez-Lapiscina EH, Clavero P, Toledo E, et al. Virgin olive oil supplementation and long-term cognition: The PREDIMED-Navarra randomized trial. J Nutr Health Aging. 2013;17(6):544–52. https://doi.org/10.1007/s12603-013-0027-6.
36. Valls-Pedret C, Lamuela-Raventos RM, Alexander Medina-Remon A, et al. Polyphenol-rich foods in the Mediterranean diet are associated with better cognitive function in elderly subjects at high cardiovascular risk. J Alzheimers Dis. 2012;29:773–82. https://doi.org/10.3233/JAD-2012-111799.
37. Berendsen AM, Kang JH, van de Rest O, et al. The dietary approaches to stop hypertension diet, cognitive function, and cognitive decline in American older women. J Am Med Dir Assoc. 2017;18(5):427–32. https://doi.org/10.1016/j.jamada.2016.11.026.
38. Haring B, Wu C, Mossavar-Rahmani Y, et al. No association between dietary patterns and risk for cognitive decline in older women with 9-year follow-up: data from the Women's Health Initiative Memory Study. J Acad Nutr Diet. 2016;116:921–30.
39. McEvoy CT, Guyer H, Langa KM, Yaffe K. Neuroprotective diets are associated with better cognitive function: The Health and Retirement Study. J Am Geriatr Soc. 2017. https://doi.org/10.1111/jgs.14922.
40. Morris MC, Tangney CC, Wang Y, et al. MIND diet slows cognitive decline with aging. Alzheimers Dement. 2015;11(9):1015–22. https://doi.org/10.1016/j.jalz.2015.04.011.
41. Morris MC, Tangney CC, Wang Y, et al. MIND diet associated with reduced incidence of Alzheimer's disease. Alzheimers Dement. 2015;11(9):1007–14. https://doi.org/10.1016/j.jalz.2014.11.001.
42. Mannikko R, Komulainen P, Schwab U, et al. The Nordic diet and cognition—The DR's EXTRA Study. Br J Nutr. 2015;114:231–9. https://doi.org/10.1017/S0007114515001890.
43. Berti V, Murray J, Davies M, et al. Nutrient pattern and brain biomarkers of Alzheimer's disease in cognitively normal individuals. J Nutr Health Aging. 2015;19(40):413–23. https://doi.org/10.1007/s12603-014-0534-0.
44. Nurk E, Refsum H, Drevon CA, et al. Cognitive performance among the elderly in relation to the intake of plant foods. The Hordaland Health Study. Br J Nutr. 2010;104:1190–201. https://doi.org/10.1017/S0007114510001807.
45. Lamport DJ, Saunders C, Butler LT, Spencer JPR. Fruits, vegetables, 100% juices, and cognitive function. Nutr Rev. 2014;2(12):774–89.
46. Loef M, Walach H. Fruit, vegetable and prevention of cognitive decline or dementia: a systematic review of cohort studies. J Nutr Health Aging. 2012;16(7):625–30.
47. Devore EE, Kang JH, Breteler MMB. Dietary intake of berries and flavonoids in relation to cognitive decline. Ann Neurol. 2012;72(1):135–43. https://doi.org/10.1002/ana.23594.
48. Chen X, Huang Y, Cheng HG. Lower intake of vegetables and legumes associated with cognitive decline among illiterate elderly Chinese: a 3-year cohort study. J Nutr Health Aging. 2012;16(6):549–52.
49. Nooyens ACJ, Bueno-de-Mesquita HB, van Boxtel MPJ. Fruit and vegetable intake and cognitive decline in middle-aged men and women: the Doetinchem Cohort Study. Br J Nutr. 2011;106:752–61.
50. Peneau S, Galan P, Jeandel C, et al. Fruit and vegetable intake and cognitive function in the SU.VI.MAX 2 prospective study. Am J Clin Nutr. 2011;94:1295–303.
51. Kang JH, Ascherio A, Grodstein F. Fruit and vegetable consumption and cognitive decline in aging women. Ann Neurol. 2005;57(5):713–20.
52. Lee J, Torosyan N, Silverman DH. Examining the impact of grape consumption on brain metabolism and cognitive function in patients with mild decline in cognition: A double-blinded placebo controlled pilot study. Exp Gerontol. 2017;87:121–8. https://doi.org/10.1016/j.exger.2016. 10.004.
53. Neshatdousta S, Saunders C, Castle SM, et al. High-flavonoid intake induces cognitive improvements linked to changes in serum brain-derived neurotrophic factor: two randomised, controlled trials.

Nutr Healthy Aging. 2016;4:81–93. https://doi.org/10.3233/NHA-1615.

54. O'Brien J, Okereke O, Devore E, et al. Long-term intake of nuts in relation to cognitive function in older women. J Nutr Health Aging. 2014;18(5):496–502.
55. Cardoso BR, Apolinário D, da Silva BV, et al. Effects of Brazil nut consumption on selenium status and cognitive performance in older adults with mild cognitive impairment: a randomized controlled pilot trial. Eur J Nutr. 2016;55(1):107–16. https://doi.org/10.1007/s00394-014-0829-2.
56. Sánchez-Villegas A, Galbete C, Martinez-González MA. The effect of the Mediterranean diet on plasma brain-derived neurotrophic factor (BDNF) levels: The PREDIMED-NAVARRA Randomized Trial. Nutr Neurosci. 2011;14(5):195–201.
57. Cheng P-F, Chen J-J, Zhou X-Y, et al. Do soy isoflavones improve cognitive function in postmenopausal women? A meta-analysis. Menopause. 2015;22(2):198–206. https://doi.org/10.1097/gme.0000000000000290.
58. St. John JA, Henderson VW, Hodis HN, et al. Associations of urine excretion of isoflavonoids with cognition in postmenopausal women in the Women's Isoflavone Soy Health Clinical Trial. J Am Geriatr Soc. 2014;62(4):629–35. https://doi.org/10.1111/jgs.12752.
59. Henderson VW, St. John JA, Hodis HN, et al. Long-term soy isoflavone supplementation and cognition in women: a randomized, controlled trial. Neurology. 2012;78:1841–8.
60. Fournier LR, Ryan-Borchers TA, Robison LM, et al. The effects of soy milk and isoflavone supplements on cognitive performance in healthy postmenopausal women. J Nutr Health Aging. 2007;11(2):155–64.
61. Crichton GE, Bryan J, Murphy KJ, Buckley J. Review of dairy consumption and cognitive performance in adults: findings and methodological issues. Dement Geriatr Cogn Disord. 2010;30:352–61. https://doi.org/10.1159/000320987.
62. Kesse-Guyot E, Assmann KE, Andreeva VA, et al. Consumption of dairy products and cognitive functioning: findings from the SU.VI.MAX 2 study. J Nutr Health Aging. 2016;20(2):128–37. https://doi.org/10.1007/s12603-015-0593-x.
63. Crichton GE, Murphy KJ, Howe PRC, et al. Dairy consumption and working memory performance in overweight and obese adults. Appetite. 2012;59:34–40. https://doi.org/10.1016/j.appet.2012.03.019.
64. Dai Q, Borenstein AR, Wu Y, et al. Fruit and vegetable juices and Alzheimer's disease: The Kame Project. Am J Med. 2006;119(9):751–9.
65. Kent K, Charlton K, Roodenrys S, et al. Consumption of anthocyanin-rich cherry juice for 12 weeks improves memory and cognition in older adults with mild-to-moderate dementia. Eur J Nutr. 2017;56(1):333–41. https://doi.org/10.1007/s00394-015-1083-y.
66. Alharbi MH, Lamport DJ, Dodd GF, et al. Flavonoid-rich orange juice is associated with acute improvements in cognitive function in healthy middle-aged males. Eur J Nutr. 2016;55:2021–9. https://doi.org/10.1007/s00394-015-1016-9.
67. Lamport DJ, Lawton CL, Merat N, et al. Concord grape juice, cognitive function, and driving performance: a 12-wk, placebo-controlled, randomized crossover trial in mothers of preteen children. Am J Clin Nutr. 2016;103:775–83. https://doi.org/10.3945/ajcn.115.114553.
68. Kean RJ, Lamport DJ, Dodd GF, et al. Chronic consumption of flavanone-rich orange juice is associated with cognitive benefits: an 8-wk, randomized, double-blind, placebo-controlled trial in healthy older adults. Am J Clin Nutr. 2015;101:506–14.
69. Bookheimer SY, Renner BA, Ekstrom A, et al. Pomegranate juice augments memory and fMRI activity in middle-aged and older adults with mild memory complaints. Evid Based Complement Alternat Med. 2013;946298. https://doi.org/10.1155/2013/946298.
70. Kelly J, Fulford J, Vanhatalo A, et al. Effects of short-term dietary nitrate supplementation on blood pressure, O2 uptake kinetics, and muscle and cognitive function in older adults. Am J Physiol Regul Integr Comp Physiol. 2013;304:R73–83. https://doi.org/10.1152/ajpregu.00406.2012.
71. Krikorian R, Nash TA, Shidler MD, et al. Concord grape juice supplementation improves memory function in older adults with mild cognitive impairment. Br J Nutr. 2010;103:730–4. https://doi.org/10.1017/S0007114509992364.
72. Wikoff D, Welsh BT, Henderson R, et al. Systematic review of the potential adverse effects of caffeine consumption in healthy adults, pregnant women, adolescents, and children. Food Chem Toxicol. 2017:1–64. https://doi.org/10.1016/j.fct.2017.04.002.
73. McLellan TM, Caldwell JA, Lieberman HR. A review of caffeine's effects on cognitive, physical and occupational performance. Neurosci Biobehav Rev. 2016;71:294–312. https://doi.org/10.1016/j.neubiorev.2016.09.01.
74. Wu L, Sun D, He Y. Coffee intake and the incident risk of cognitive disorders: a dose-response meta-analysis of nine prospective cohort studies. Clin Nutr. 2017;36:730–36.
75. Liu X, Du X, Han G, Gao W. Association between tea consumption and risk of cognitive disorders: a dose - response meta-analysis of observational studies. Oncotarget. 2017;8(26):43306–21.
76. Gelber RP, Petrovitch H, Masaki KH, et al. Coffee intake in midlife and risk of dementia and its neuropathologic correlates. J Alzheimers Dis. 2011;23(4):607–15. https://doi.org/10.3233/JAD-2010-101428.
77. Feng L, Gwee X, Kua E-H, Ng T-P. Cognitive function and tea consumption in community dwelling older Chinese in Singapore. J Nutr Health Aging. 2010;14(6):433–8.
78. Ng T-P, Feng L, Niti M, et al. Tea consumption and cognitive impairment and decline in older Chinese adults. Am J Clin Nutr. 2008;88:224–31.

79. Lamport DJ, Pal D, Moutsiana C, et al. The effect of flavanol-rich cocoa on cerebral perfusion in healthy older adults during conscious resting state: a placebo controlled, crossover, acute trial. Psychopharmacology. 2015;232:3227–34. https://doi.org/10.1007/s00213-015-3972-4.
80. Mastroiacovo D, Kwik-Uribe C, Grassi D, et al. Cocoa flavanol consumption improves cognitive function, blood pressure control, and metabolic profile in elderly subjects: the Cocoa, Cognition, and Aging (CoCoA) Study—a randomized controlled trial. Am J Clin Nutr. 2015;101:538–48.
81. Sorond F, Hurwitz S, Salar DH, et al. Neurovascular coupling, cerebral white matter integrity, and response to cocoa in older people. Neurology. 2013;81:904–9.
82. Peters R, Peters J, Warner J, et al. Alcohol, dementia and cognitive decline in the elderly: a systematic review. Age Ageing. 2008;37:505–12. https://doi.org/10.1093/ageing/afn095.
83. Heymann D, Stern Y, Cosentino S, et al. The association between alcohol use and the progression of Alzheimer's disease. Curr Alzheimer Res. 2016;13(12):1356–62.
84. Downer B, Jiang Y, Zanjani F, Fardo D. Effects of alcohol consumption on cognition and regional brain volumes among older adults. Am J Alzheimers Dis Other Demen. 2015;30(4):364–74. https://doi.org/10.1177/1533317514549411.
85. Ritchie SJ, Bates TC, Corley J, et al. Alcohol consumption and lifetime change in cognitive ability: a gene × environment interaction study. Age. 2014;36:1493–502. https://doi.org/10.1007/s11357-014-9638-z.
86. Arntzen SA, Schirmer H, Wilsgaard T, Mathiesen EB. Moderate wine consumption is associated with better cognitive test results; a 7-year follow-up of 5033 subjects in the Tromso Study. Acta Neurol Scand Suppl. 2010;190:23–9. https://doi.org/10.1111/j.1600-0404.2010.01371.x.
87. Solfrizzi V, D'Introno A, Colacicco AM, et al. Alcohol consumption, mild cognitive impairment, and progression to dementia. Neurology. 2007;68:1790–9.
88. Stampfer MJ, Kang JH, Chen J, et al. Effects of moderate alcohol consumption on cognitive function in women. N Engl J Med. 2005;352:245–53.
89. Erdman JW, Smith JW, Kuchan MJ, et al. Lutein and brain function. Foods. 2015;4:547–64. https://doi.org/10.3390/foods4040547.
90. Johnson E, Vishwanathan R, Mohn E, et al. Avocado consumption increases neural lutein and improves cognitive function. FASEB J. 2015; 29(1) Supplement 32.8.
91. Bovier ER, Renzi LM, Hammond BR. A double-blind, placebo-controlled study on the effects of lutein and zeaxanthin on neural processing speed and efficiency. PLoS One. 2014;9:e108178. https://doi.org/10.1371/journal.pone.0108178.
92. Zamroziewicz MK, Paul EJ, Zwilling CE, et al. Para-hippocampal cortex mediates the relationship between lutein and crystallized intelligence in healthy, older adults. Front Aging Neurosci. 2016;8:297. https://doi.org/10.3389/fnagi.2016.00297.
93. Feart C, Letenneur L, Helmer C, et al. Plasma carotenoids are inversely associated with dementia risk in an elderly French cohort. J Gerontol A Biol Sci Med Sci. 2016;71(5):683–8. https://doi.org/10.1093/gerona/glv135.
94. Lindbergh CA, Mewborn CM, Hammond BR, et al. Relationship of lutein and zeaxanthin levels to neurocognitive functioning: an fMRI study of older adults. JINS. 2016;22:1–12. https://doi.org/10.1017/S1355617716000850.
95. Vishwanathan R, Schalch W, Johnson EJ. Macular pigment carotenoids in the retina and occipital cortex are related in humans. Nutr Neurosci. 2016;19(3):95–101. https://doi.org/10.1179/1476830514Y.0000000141.
96. Kelly D, Coen RF, Akuffo KO, et al. Cognitive function and its relationship with macular pigment optical density and serum concentrations of its constituent carotenoids. J Alzheimers Dis. 2015;48:261–77. https://doi.org/10.3233/JAD-150199.
97. Renzi LM, Dengler MJ, Puente A, et al. Relationships between macular pigment optical density and cognitive function in unimpaired and mildly cognitively impaired older adults. Neurobiol Aging. 2014;35:1695–9. https://doi.org/10.1016/j.neurobiolaging.2013.12.024.
98. Vishwanathan R, Iannaccone A, Scott TM, et al. Macular pigment optical density is related to cognitive function in older people. Age Ageing. 2014;43:271–5. https://doi.org/10.1093/ageing/aft210.
99. Johnson EJ, Vishwanathan R, Johnson MA, et al. Relationship between serum and brain carotenoids, α-tocopherol, and retinol concentrations and cognitive performance in the oldest old from the Georgia Centenarian Study. J Aging Res. 2013;2013:951786. https://doi.org/10.1155/2013/951786.
100. Blumenthal JA, Smith PJ, Mabe S, et al. Lifestyle and neurocognition in older adults with cardiovascular risk factors and cognitive impairment. Psychosom Med. 2017;79(6):719–27. https://doi.org/10.1097/PSY.0000000000000474.

Part V

Cancer Prevention and Survival

Dietary Patterns, Whole Plant Foods, Nutrients and Phytochemicals in Colorectal Cancer Prevention and Management

19

Keywords
Colorectal cancer • Colorectal adenomas • Dietary fiber • Antioxidants vitamins • Calcium • Magnesium • Selenium • Folate • Isoflavonoids • Carotenoids • Phenolics • Dietary patterns • Whole plant foods • Fruits • Vegetables • Legumes • Soy products • Whole-grains • Peanuts • Tree nuts • Seeds

Key Points

- Globally colorectal cancer (CRC) rates have doubled since the 1970s and incidence is strongly associated with the Western lifestyle and aging populations.
- As much as 90% of CRC cases may be attributable to dietary factors. A number of nutrients and phytochemicals are considered to be potentially protective against CRC to various degrees including fiber, isoflavones, flavonoids, antioxidant vitamins, carotenoids, folate, calcium, magnesium, and selenium.
- Higher adherence to a Western dietary pattern, which can stimulate a proinflammatory systemic response, can significantly increase risk of colorectal adenomas and CRC, especially in diets high in red or processed meats. In contrast, higher adherence to healthy dietary patterns including the Mediterranean diet (MedDiet), Dietary Approaches to Stop Hypertension (DASH), Healthy Eating Indices, pesco-vegetarian and low inflammatory index diets can significantly reduce risk of colorectal adenoma and CRC.
- Survivors of CRC with high intake of Western dietary patterns had significantly higher odds of CRC mortality and recurrence compared to those consuming healthy diets.
- Dietary patterns rich in fruits, vegetables (including green leafy vegetables, cruciferous and allium vegetables), legumes (including soy), whole-grains (≥3 servings/day) and peanuts may have protective effects against colorectal adenomas and CRC risk.
- Diets rich in dietary fiber have been related to a lower CRC risk due in large part to beneficial effects of butyrate, derived from fiber fermentation by colonic microflora, an inhibitor of colonocyte tumor cell initiation and progression.

M.L. Dreher, *Dietary Patterns and Whole Plant Foods in Aging and Disease*, Nutrition and Health,
https://doi.org/10.1007/978-3-319-59180-3_19

19.1 Introduction

Colorectal cancer (CRC) is among the most common cancers worldwide [1]. CRC rates have doubled since the 1970s and rose by more than 200,000 new cases per year from 1990 to 2012 [1–4]. In 2015, there were 1.7 million new CRC cases globally and 832,000 deaths resulting from CRC. Most cases of CRC are detected in Western countries, but this is changing due to the adoption of Western dietary habits in developing countries over the past few decades [1–4] Incidence is strongly associated with the Western lifestyle and aging populations with 2.4 million new CRC cases projected to be diagnosed in 2035 [2–4]. By gender, CRC is the second most common cancer in women (9.2%) and the third in men (10%). Despite an increasing number of tumors now diagnosed, the CRC mortality rate has decreased because of more appropriate and available information, earlier diagnosis, and improvements in treatment. A recent meta-analysis of 43 studies showed CRC risk was associated with a variety of lifestyle factors including: diet, smoking, alcohol, body fatness, physical activity, medication and/or hormone replacement therapy [5]. As much as 90% of CRC cases appear to be attributable to dietary factors including unhealthy diet, obesity and excessive alcohol intake [6–8]. The 2017 World Cancer Research Fund International Continuous Update Project systematic review and meta-analysis (45 meta-analyses of prospective studies; 15 different foods or food groups; 111 unique cohort studies) found that foods associated with an increased CRC risk were red and processed meat and alcohol and foods associated with a decreased CRC risk were whole grains, vegetables, dairy and fish [9]. Foods not associated with CRC risk were fruits, coffee, tea, poultry, cheese and legumes. Consistent with these findings, the 2017 National Institutes of Health - American Association of Retired Persons (NIH)-AARP) Diet and Health Study (398,458 middle-aged and older adults; 10 years of follow-up) found that among normal-weight and overweight men, CRC risk was 25%-30% lower with high adherence to healthy dietary patterns [10]. High adherence to Western dietary patterns characterized as energy dense, high red/processed meat, salty foods and sweets, and refined grains or higher alcohol consumption are associated with an increased CRC risk, whereas high adherence to a healthy dietary pattern characterized as low to moderate energy dense, high in dietary fiber, fruits and vegetables, legumes, whole-grains, and nuts are associated with decreased CRC risk (Figs. 19.1 and 19.2) [11, 12].

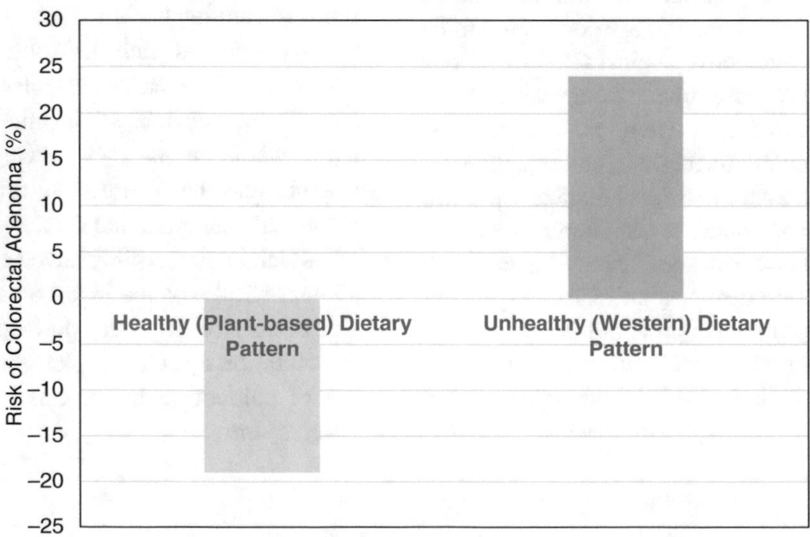

Fig. 19.1 Association between dietary pattern quality and colorectal adenoma risk from a meta-analysis of seven-cohort and five-case-control studies ($p < .004$) (adapted from [11])

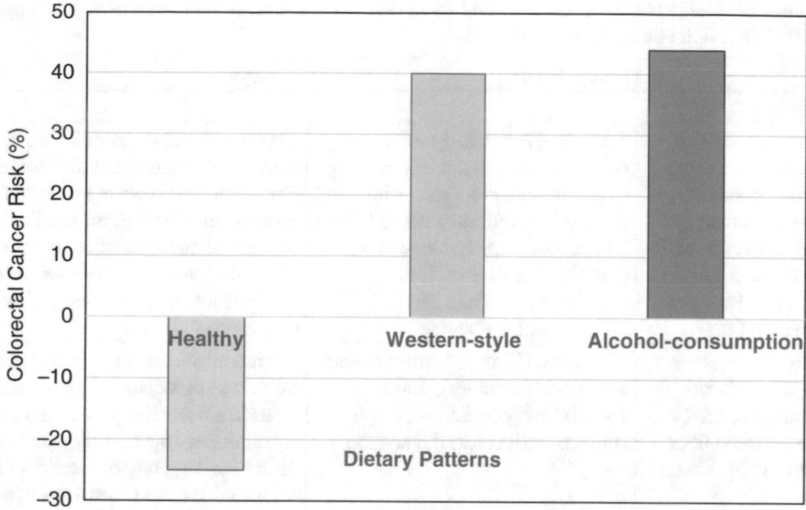

Fig. 19.2 Association between dietary pattern and colorectal cancer risk from a meta-analysis of 40 observational studies (p <.003) (adapted from [12])

An overview of the foods and nutrient composition of the Western and common healthy dietary patterns are provided in Appendix A. The objective of this chapter is to provide a comprehensive review of the effect of dietary patterns and whole (minimally processed) foods, nutrients and phytochemicals on CRC risk.

19.2 Nutrients and Phytochemicals

A number of nutrients and phytochemicals are potentially associated with lower CRC risk to various degrees including by slowing or preventing adenoma-carcinoma progression and protecting normal epithelium cells from acquiring genetic and epigenetic mutations in specific oncogenes or tumor suppressor genes [13–16]. The change from adenoma polyp to adenocarcinomas is usually a slow process over an average period of 10 years. Healthy plant-based dietary patterns rich in fruits, vegetables, legumes, whole-grains, and nuts are important sources of bioactive compounds, which protect against the development of CRC and include fiber, isoflavones, flavonoids, antioxidant vitamins, carotenoids, folate, calcium, magnesium, and selenium. These plant phytochemicals and nutrients may influence a complex array of cancer protective cellular regulatory vprocesses and promote a healthier colonic microbiome ecosystem. Table 19.1 summarizes nutrient and phytochemical systematic reviews and meta- and pooled analyses in CRC and colorectal adenoma risk [17–38].

19.2.1 Dietary Fiber

The fiber protective effects in CRC and colorectal adenoma risk have been extensively evaluated in systematic reviews and meta-and pooled analyses of RCTs and observational studies [17–20]. A 2017 meta-analysis (5 RCTs; 4798 subjects; wheat bran, psyllium, higher fiber diets; 2–8 years) found no statistically significant lowering of adenomatous polyp recurrence or incidence with increased fiber intake; however, the authors concluded that these results should be interpreted with caution, because of the: (1) high subject loss rate to follow-up; (2) issues with dietary compliance; and (3) questions about the reliability of adenomatous polyps as a surrogate biomarker of CRC risk RCTs that are <10 years duration [17]. A 2006 pooled analysis of the Wheat Bran Fiber Trial (WBFT) and Polyp Prevention Trial (PPT) (3209 participants, mean

Table 19.1 Summaries of systematic reviews and meta-and pooled analyses on nutrients and phytochemicals in colorectal cancer (CRC) and colorectal adenoma risk

Objective	Study details	Results
Dietary fiber (fiber)		
Yao et al. (2017) . Assess the effect of fiber on the recurrence of colorectal adenoma in people with a known history of adenomatous polyps and on the incidence of CRC compared to placebo (Cochrane Database Systematic Review) [17]	5 RCTs; 4798 participants, age range 56–66 years; wheat bran, psyllium, or a comprehensive dietary intervention with high fiber whole food sources alone or in combination vs. low-fiber diets, placebo, or a regular diet; 2–8 years of follow-up	This pooled analysis of RCTs showed no statistically significant difference between the fiber-rich intervention and lower fiber control groups. However, these results may be unreliable and should be interpreted cautiously, not only because of the high rate of subjects loss to follow-up and issues with dietary compliance
Ben et al. (2014). Conduct a meta-analysis primarily of case-control studies to analyze the association between fiber intake and risk of colorectal adenoma [18]	20 studies (16 case-control studies and 4 cohort studies); approx. 150,000 subjects and 10,948 subjects with colorectal adenoma	High fiber intake, especially fruit and cereal fiber, was associated with reduced colorectal adenoma risk. The pooled analysis found a significantly inverse colorectal adenoma risk effect per 10 g/day of total fiber by 9%, fruit fiber by 21%, and cereal fiber by 30%. The effects were similar for both early and advanced colorectal adenoma
Aune et al. (2011). Assess the association between and fiber intake and CRC risk from prospective cohort studies (World Cancer Research Fund/ American Institute for Cancer Research Continuous Update Report) [19]	25 prospective cohort studies; 19 were included in the dose-response analyses; 14,514 CRC cases among 1,985,552 subjects; ranges of fiber intake: total fiber (6.3–21.4 g/day), fruit fiber (1.8–15.5 g/day), vegetable fiber (1.9–16.8 g/day), cereal fiber (3.0–16.9 g/day), and legume fiber (1.3–3.8 g/day)	A 10 g/day increase in total and cereal fiber intake was associated with a 10% lower CRC risk with a significant reduction in risk of colon cancer but not rectal cancer. Fruit, vegetable, and legume fiber intake were suggestive for CRC risk reduction but not confirmed.
Jacobs et al. (2006). Determine the pooled effects of increased fiber intake on colorectal adenoma recurrence in men and women from 2 large clinical intervention trials (The Wheat Bran Fiber Trial (WBF) and the Polyp Prevention Trial (PPT); US) [20]	3209 participants combined from 2 RCTs; mean baseline age 64 years; approx. 65% men; analyzed with logistic regression models to examine the effect of a dietary intervention on colorectal adenoma recurrence 1. The WBF trial subjects with recent colorectal adenomas removal were randomly assigned to receive either 13.5 or 2.0 g fiber/ day as a breakfast cereal (wheat bran) supplement for 3-years. 2. The PPT subjects with recent colonic polyp removal were randomized into an intervention diet of decreased fat and increased fiber, fruit, and vegetables or control diet for 4-years	This pooled analysis shows that increased fiber intake was more effective in lowering colorectal adenoma recurrence in men than in women, which may help to explain some of the discrepant results reported from previous trials. For the total pooled population, the adjusted adenoma recurrence risk was insignificantly reduced by 9%. For men, the intervention was associated with statistically significantly reduced risk of recurrence by 19%; for women, no significant association was observed. There was a statistically significant interaction between fiber intake level and sex ($p = .03$)
Soy Isoflavones		
Jiang et al. (2017). Meta-analysis was conducted to quantify the association between isoflavones and CRC risk [21]	5 cohort studies and 5 case-control studies	Case-control studies showed lower CRC risk for isoflavones by 23%, but for cohort studies the pooled CRC risk was reduced by 6%. Dose–response analysis yielded an 8% reduced risk of colorectal neoplasms for every 20 mg/ day increase in isoflavones intake in Asians

Table 19.1 (continued)

Objective	Study details	Results
Yu et al. (2016). Perform a meta-analysis to assess the association between soy isoflavone consumption and CRC risk in humans [22]	17 studies (13 case-control and 4 prospective cohort studies); 273,765 subjects	This analysis found that soy isoflavone consumption reduced CRC risk by 22% (p = .024). Based on subgroup analyses, a significant protective effect was observed with in participants with higher intake of soy foods/products and in Asian populations by 21%
Tse and Eslick (2016). Determine the potential relationship between dietary soy intake and CRC risk with an evaluation of the effects of isoflavone as an active soy constituent [23]	22 case-control and 18 cohort studies; 633,476 participants and 13,639 CRC cases	Although this analysis showed that soy food intake was only associated with a small reduction in CRC risk by 8% (p = .3), subgroup analysis for isoflavone intake suggests a strong inverse association with a significant reduced CRC risk by 24%
Flavonoids (Phenolics)		
Grosso et al (2016). Summarize observational studies on the association between dietary flavonoid intake and cancer risk using meta-analysis [24]	20 studies (9 case-control and 11 cohort studies)	Cohort studies show that flavonoids insignificantly lower CRC risk, while several significant associations were found among case-control studies, including flavonols, quercetin, subclasses of flavanols proanthocyanidins and catechins, and anthocyanins
Jin et al. (2012). Assess the effect of dietary flavonoids on the incidence of colorectal adenoma and CRC (Cochrane Database Systematic Review) [25]	8 studies (5 cohort studies, 2 case-control studies and one RCT); 390,769 participants	Increased intake of flavan-3-ols, epicatechins significantly reduced the risk of both CRC and/or colorectal adenomas. There was medium quality evidence to support that increased intake of procyanidin lowers the incidence of CRC but no significant evidence for anthocyanin intake
Antioxidant vitamins		
Xu et al. (2013). Assess the association between dietary intake of vitamins A, C, and E and the risk of colorectal adenoma, a potential precursor of CRC by meta-analysis [26]	13 studies (12 case–control studies and one nested case–control study); 3832 individuals with colorectal adenoma	In highest vs. lowest analysis, dietary intake of vitamin C reduced the risk of colorectal adenoma by 22% independent of BMI, smoking status, and dietary energy intake (p = .005); with a 9% risk reduction per 100 mg vitamin C. Also, dietary intake of β-carotene was inversely associated with the risk of colorectal adenoma by 53% (p = .009). However, dietary intake of vitamins A and E were insignificantly associated with the risk of colorectal adenoma by 13% each
Pais and Dumitrascu (2013). Estimate the effectiveness of antioxidants on CRC incidence and adenomatous polyp recurrence [27]	20 RCTs: 12 on CRC incidences; 250,676 participants; and eight analyzed colorectal adenoma recurrence; 17,914 participants	Overall antioxidant supplement intake had an insignificant effect on CRC risk or colorectal adenoma recurrence with a pooled reduction by 6% (p = .32). Also, beta carotene was insignificantly associated with CRC risk
Park et al. (2010). Evaluate the associations between intakes of vitamins A, C, and E and risk of colon cancer (the Pooling Project of Prospective Studies of Diet and Cancer) [28]	13 cohort studies; 209,263 men and 466,878 women; 7–20 years of follow-up; 5454 colon cancer cases	Colon cancer risk was significantly reduced by 12% (>4000 vs. ≤1000 μg/day) for vitamin A, 19% (>600 vs. ≤100 mg/day) for vitamin C, and 22% (>200 vs. ≤6 mg/day) for vitamin E. Adjustment for total folate intake attenuated these associations, but the vitamins C and E inverse associations retained their significant lowering effects

(continued)

Table 19.1 (continued)

Objective	Study details	Results
Carotenoids		
Panic et al. (2017). Systematically review the epidemiological evidence for the association between carotenoid intake from natural sources and CRC risk [29]	22 studies (16 case-control studies and 6 cohort studies); 486,393 participants	Cohort studies showed no significant association between intake of specific carotenoids from natural sources, as well as combined carotenoids, and the risk of CRC overall and by anatomic subsite with no evidence of heterogeneity among studies. Case-control studies found insignificant inverse associations with colon cancer incidence for β-carotene by 22%, lycopene by 5%, and lutein/ zeaxanthin by 11%
Mannisto et al. (2006). Analyze the associations between intakes of specific carotenoids (α-carotene, beta-carotene, β-cryptoxanthin, lutein and zeaxanthin, and lycopene) and CRC risk [30]	11 cohort studies (in North America and Europe); 702,647 participants; 6–20 years of follow-up; 7885 CRC cases; carotenoid intakes were estimated from food frequency questionnaires (FFQ) at baseline in each study	Lutein/zeaxanthin (highest vs. lowest quintile of intake) showed a lower pooled multivariate CRC risk by 8% (p-trend = .08). There were no other borderline significant trends for other carotenoids
Folate		
Figueiredo et al. (2011). Assess the effect folic acid intake on the prevention of colonic adenomas by pooled analysis of RCTs [31]	3 large RCTs; 2632 men and women with a history of adenomas; either 0.5 or 1.0 mg/ day of folic acid vs. placebo; mean follow-up of 6–42 months (mean of 31 months)	After 42 months of folic acid use, there was no clear decrease or increase in the occurrence of new adenomas in patients with a history of adenoma. In participants with high alcohol intake, there was a trend for decreasing colorectal adenoma with higher folic acid intake. During the early follow-up reported here, more deaths occurred in the placebo group than in the folic acid group (1.7% vs. 0.5%, p = .002)
Kim et al. (2010). Evaluate the overall and dose effects of folate intake on CRC risk [32]	13 cohort studies; 725,134 participants (229,466 men and 495,668 women); 7–20 years of follow-up; 5720 colon cancer cases	In dose-response analysis, every 100 μg/day increase in total folate intake reduced CRC risk by 2%. Comparing the highest vs. lowest quintile of intake showed reduced pooled risk by 8%. Comparing daily total folate intake of ≥560 mcg vs. <240 mcg, CRC risk was reduced by 13% (p-trend = .009)
Calcium		
Bonovas et al. (2016). Determine the efficacy of calcium supplementation in reducing the recurrence of colorectal adenomas [33]	4 RCTs; daily calcium ranged from 1200 to 2000 mg/day; 36–60 months	Higher calcium intake significantly lowered risk of colonic adenomas by 13% (p < .05) and insignificantly lowered advanced adenomas by 8%
Keum et al. (2015). Evaluate dose-response effects of calcium intake on colorectal adenoma risk [34]	8 prospective studies; 11,005 subjects; total calcium intake ranging from 333 to 2229 mg/day	For total calcium intake, each 300 mg/day reduced adenoma risk by 5%; evidence of nonlinearity was indicated with risk reductions for 1000 mg/day by 8% and for 1450 mg/day by 13% (p-nonlinearity < .01). Calcium intake effects were stronger for high-risk adenomas (≥1 cm in diameter) with 1000 mg calcium/ day reducing risk by 23%

Table 19.1 (continued)

Objective	Study details	Results
Magnesium		
Chen et al. (2012). Assess the association between magnesium intake and CRC risk [35]	8 prospective studies; 338,979 participants; 7.9–28 years of follow-up; 8000 CRC cases	For the highest vs. lowest magnesium intake, the pooled CRC risk was lowered by 11%. For colon cancer, the pooled risk was reduced by 19%. For rectal cancer, the pooled risk was lowered by 6%. In the dose-response analyses, 50 mg magnesium/day lowered colon cancer risk by 7%
Wark et al. (2012). Evaluate the dose-response effect of dietary magnesium on CRC risk [36]	6 prospective cohort studies on CRC; three case-control studies of colorectal adenomas	Each 100-mg/day increase in magnesium intake was associated with 13% lower colorectal adenomas risk and 12% lower CRC risk. Magnesium intake was inversely associated with risk of colorectal adenomas and CRC
Selenium		
Cai et al. (2016). Investigate the association between selenium intake and cancer risk by meta-analysis [37]	10 studies (2 RCTs; 4 cohort studies; 4 case-control studies)	This analysis showed that higher selenium exposure was associated with an insignificantly lower CRC risk by 11% with moderate heterogeneity
Pais and Dumitrascu (2013). Estimate the effectiveness of selenium on CRC incidence and adenomatous polyp recurrence [27]	5 RCTs (3 analyzed CRC incidences and 2 analyzed colorectal adenoma recurrence)	Selenium supplementation was associated with an insignificant lowering of both CRC incidence by 12% ($p = .59$) and colorectal adenoma recurrence by 30% ($p = .16$)
Takata et al. (2012). Evaluate the effect of selenium intake on CRC risk in women in a nested case-control study (Women's Health Initiative (WHI) Observational Study) and meta-analysis of men and women [38]	WHI Observational Study: 804 CRC cases and 805 matched controls; meta-analysis: 12 observational studies and 2 RCTs	Within the WHI, selenium concentrations were relatively high (mean 135.6 mg/L) and were not associated with CRC risk (p-trend = .10). Meta-analysis (highest vs. lowest quantile) showed that increased selenium intake insignificantly reduced CRC risk in women by 3% and in men CRC risk was significantly reduced by 32% ($p = .01$)

baseline age 64 years, 64% men; WBFT: increased wheat bran 13.5 vs. 2.0 g/day from cereal, 3 years; and PPT: diet lower in fat, higher in fiber and fruits and vegetables, 4 years;) showed that men in the study had significantly reduced colon adenoma recurrence risk by 19% whereas no significant association was observed for women (multivariate adjusted) [20]. Using a likelihood-ratio test, a statistically significant interaction between fiber intake and sex was found ($p = .03$). Two systematic reviews and meta-analyses of cohort and case-control studies demonstrate the efficacy of increased fiber intake on CRC risk [18, 19]. A 2014 dose meta-analysis on the effects of fiber intake and colorectal adenomas (16 case-control and 4 cohort studies; 150,000 subjects) found that an increased intake of 10 g fiber significantly reduced colorectal adenomas risk for total fiber by 9%, fruit fiber by 21%, and cereal fiber by 30% [18]. A 2011 dose response meta-analysis affiliated with the World Cancer Research Fund (WCRF) and American Institute for Cancer Research (AICR) Continuous Update Project (19 cohort studies used for dose response analysis; 1,985,552 participants) found a modest, statistically significant fiber dose response for a 10% lower CRC risk per 10 g of total and cereal fiber consumed daily [19].

There are a number of potential fiber related CRC prevention mechanisms. Fiber and fiber metabolites can provide direct protection throughout the colorectal tract by [39–50] including: (1) reducing colorectal exposure to carcinogens by increasing stool weight, decreasing transit time and diluting colonic carcinogenic concentrations, (2) increasing colonic butyrate levels (via fiber fermentation) which is the preferred energy source for colon epithelial cells for optimal barrier protection and anti-inflammatory effects, (3) lowering colonic pH to protect against colonic pathogenic bacterial infections and reduce bacterial enzymes, including 7α-dehydroxylase, which is involved in the formation of secondary bile acids, and other bacterial enzymes known to convert relatively harmless compounds to reactive toxic metabolites and (4) promoting colonic anti-cancer activity by increasing the Warburg effect, arresting the growth of tumors by histone deacetylase (HDAC) inhibitor and anti-inflammatory properties mediated by suppressing the activation of nuclear factor-kB (a transcription factor controlling the expression of genes encoding proinflammatory responses and inflammatory mediators like tumor necrosis factor-α (TNF-α) and nitric oxide) [37–43]. Also, increased fiber intake is associated with lower dietary energy density and metabolizable energy for better weight maintenance, reduced risk of central obesity, and attenuation of colonic microbiota inflammatory activity [45–48].

19.2.2 Soy Isoflavones

Three meta-analyses consistently support CRC risk lowering effects for soy isoflavones by a pooled mean of 23% [21–23]. The association of isoflavones with reduced CRC risk was statistically significant only in case-control studies but not in cohort studies, which are less subject to recall and selection bias. Dose response analysis showed an 8% lower risk of colorectal neoplasms per 20 mg/day increase of isoflavones in Asian populations. The mechanism by which soy isoflavones protect against the development of CRC remains unclear [21, 22]. Isoflavones have similar chemical structure to estrogen, which allows their binding to estrogen receptors with an especially high binding affinity to estrogen receptor β, the predominant estrogen receptor in normal colon mucosa. Though estrogen receptor β progressively decreases with advancing grade and the stage of CRC, dietary isoflavones appear to increase estrogen receptor-*β* expression and exhibit anti-proliferative effects.

19.2.3 Flavonoids (Phenolics)

Whole plant foods, including soy, berries, vegetables, cereals and nuts, as well as tea and coffee are rich in flavonoids or other phenolic compounds [13]. Because most of these plant phenolics are poorly absorbed, they may accumulate in the colon up to the millimolar range and become subjected to conversion by microorganisms into metabolites with potential anti-cancer biological activity. Phenolic compounds in the colon have been found to alter the microbial population by suppressing the growth of *Clostridium* and *Bacteroides* species to promote a healthier microbiota that may promote reduced CRC risk but two meta-analyses of prospective cohorts do not confirm a significant protective role for higher flavonoid intake against CRC risk [24, 25]. Cohort studies show that higher flavonoid intake is not significantly associated with lower CRC and adenomas risk while case-control studies suggest a possible protective CRC role for flavonols, quercetin, subclasses of flavanols proanthocyanidins and epicatechins, and procyanidins.

19.2.4 Antioxidant Vitamins

Antioxidant vitamins A, C, and E, have potent antioxidative and anti-inflammatory properties [6] with the potential to reduce CRC risk by acting as reactive oxygen species scavengers and protecting cells from oxidative stress and inflammation, which can initiate and promote carcinogenesis by inducing gene mutations, DNA damage, genome instability, and cell proliferation. A 2010 meta-analysis of antioxidant vitamins from foods and supplements (10 cohort studies; 209,263 men and 466,878 women; 7–20-years of follow-up) found that the highest intake of antioxidant vitamins C and E lowered CRC risk by 12–22% compared to the lowest intake, after adjusting for total folate intake [28].

A 2013 meta-analysis (13 case-control studies) showed that higher intake of vitamin C significantly reduced the risk of colorectal adenomas by 22%, with a 9% risk reduction per 100 mg vitamin C [26]. Also, higher dietary intake of β-carotene was inversely associated with the risk of colorectal adenomas by 53% ($p = .009$). In contrast, a 2013 meta-analysis of RCTs (12 RCTs on CRC risk; 50,676 subjects; and 8 RCTs on colorectal adenoma recurrence; 7914 subjects) found increased overall antioxidant supplement intake had an insignificant 6% lowering effect on CRC incidence or colorectal adenoma recurrence risk ($p = .32$) [27].

19.2.5 Carotenoids

Carotenoids represent a diverse group of natural pigments present in non-starchy vegetables and fruit. The carotenoids from natural sources can be classified into two groups: hydrocarbons, such as α-carotene, β-carotene, and lycopene; and xanthophylls, such as β-cryptoxanthin, lutein, and zeaxanthin [29]. Several potential mechanisms support protective effects of carotenoids in CRC development by functioning as a provitamin-A and influencing cellular differentiation and proliferation, or by neutralizing free radicals to prevent colorectal colonic cell and tissue damage. A 2017 systematic review and meta-analysis (16 were case-control studies and 6 cohort studies) found no association between the intake of individual and total carotenoids and the risk of CRC overall and by anatomic subsite [29]. One cohort study found for lutein and zeaxanthin (highest vs. lowest quintile of intake) a trend toward reduced CRC risk by 8% (p-trend = .08) [30].

19.2.6 Folate

Since folate (vitamin B-9) is essential for DNA methylation, synthesis, stability, and repair, it has been extensively investigated for its protective role in CRC [6]. The primary sources of folate are from the diet or supplements and by production of folate by colonic bacteria. Folate deficiency results in genomic hypomethylation and defects in DNA synthesis, which may contribute to colonic carcinogenesis. Dietary intake and circulating levels of folate have been inversely associated with CRC and adenoma risk in observational studies with the association being more effective among heavy alcohol consumers because of alcohol's impairment of folate mediated DNA methylation. A 2010 meta-analysis of folate intake effects on CRC risk (13 cohort studies; 725,134 participants; 7–20 years of follow-up) found a significant reduction in CRC risk by 2% per every 100 μg/day increase in total folate intake [31]. Comparing daily total folate intake of ≥560 mcg vs. <240 mcg was associated with a significantly lower CRC risk by 13% (p-trend = .009). However, three large RCTs (2632 men and women with a history of adenomas; either 0.5 or 1.0 mg/day of folic acid or placebo; ≥42 months of follow-up endoscopy) found, after 42 months of folic acid use there was no clear decrease or increase in the occurrence of new adenomas in patients with a history of adenoma [32].

19.2.7 Calcium

Calcium's CRC protective mechanisms include its: (1) involvement in the formation of insoluble soaps with potential carcinogenic free fatty acids and bile acids in the colonic lumen and (2) contribution to the integrity of the intestinal barrier function and homeostasis between the microbiota and their effect on immune response, thought to be mediated by extracellular calcium-sensing receptor signaling [6]. Meta-analysis of both cohort studies and RCTs show that calcium significantly lowers the risk of new or recurrent colorectal adenomas [33, 34]. A pooled analysis of RCTs (four RCTs; calcium 1200–2000 mg/day, 36–60-month duration) found that increased calcium significantly reduced colonic adenomas by 13% ($p < .05$). A dose response meta-analysis (Eight cohort studies; 11,000 subjects) showed that each 300 mg calcium/day lowered adenoma risk by 5% and there were additional protective effects against high-risk adenomas (≥1 cm in diameter) with 1000 mg calcium/day further reducing risk to 23% [34].

19.2.8 Magnesium

Magnesium is an essential mineral, which is most notably present in foods rich in dietary fiber, non-starchy vegetables, fruits, and nuts [35]. Magnesium is required for many physiologic processes that affect CRC risk, including DNA synthesis and repair, glucose metabolism and insulin sensitivity, the regulation of cell proliferation and apoptosis and defense against oxidative stress and inflammatory responses, which may influence colorectal carcinogenesis. Several meta-analyses of cohort studies indicate that increased magnesium intake was inversely associated with risk of colorectal adenomas and CRC [35, 36]. Each 100 mg/day increase in magnesium intake was associated with 13% lower colorectal adenomas risk and 12% lower CRC risk [36].

19.2.9 Selenium

Selenium is not an antioxidant by itself but is required for the anti-oxidative activity of selenoenzymes [6]. There is evidence for a U-shaped relationship between selenium status and protection from cancer, with an optimal circulating level of selenium within the range of 130–150 mcg/L. Several potential anticarcinogenic mechanisms of selenium include: (1) contributing to the antioxidant function of glutathione peroxidases and thioredoxin reductases: (2) association with the regulation of protein folding via the function of the endoplasmic reticulum to influence the process of necrosis and apoptosis of malignant cells; (3) effects on DNA stability. Conversely, the adverse effects of excess selenium intake are possibly increasing risk of diabetes, glaucoma, and dermatologic alterations [6, 37, 38]. Three meta-analysis including both observational studies and RCTs showed that increased selenium insignificantly reduces CRC risk in the total population [27, 37, 38]. One meta-analyses (highest vs. lowest quantile) found that selenium intake was insignificantly associated with reduced CRC risk in women by 3%; however, in men, there was a significant inverse association with a 32% lower risk [38].

19.3 Dietary Patterns

19.3.1 Colorectal Cancer Risk (CRC)

Table 19.2 summarizes seven systematic reviews, meta- or pooled analyses and seven representative prospective cohort studies on the effects of dietary pattern quality and CRC risk [11, 12, 51–62]. Meta-analyses consistently show that dietary pattern quality has a significant effect on colorectal adenomas and CRC risk (Figs. 19.1 and 19.2) [11, 12, 51–55]. A higher adherence score to a Western dietary pattern or proinflammatory diet significantly increased risk of adenomas by 13% a nd CRC risk by 29–65%, especially with high intake of red or processed meats. Higher adherence to healthy dietary patterns including the Mediterranean diet (MedDiet), Dietary Approaches to Stop Hypertension (DASH), Healthy Eating Indices (HEI), vegetarian, and low inflammatory index diets can significantly reduce colorectal adenoma risk by 19% and CRC risk by 8–65%. Among vegetarian diets, the pesco-vegetarian diet was most effective at lowering CRC risk by 33% compared to a non-vegetarian diet [51]. Specific prospective cohort studies show the effects of healthy dietary patterns on colorectal adenoma and CRC risk [56–62]. In postmenopausal women, the HEI-2010 and DASH diet significantly lowered CRC risk by 22–28% [56]. The Adventist Health Study (77,659 subjects; mean 7.3 years of follow-up) found a wide variation of CRC lowering effects for the various types of vegetarian diets compared to non-vegetarians (Fig. 19.3) [58]. The pesco-vegetarian diet reduced CRC risk by 43% vs. 22% for the composite of all vegetarian diets. Vegetarians and 1 day per week meat eaters had 27% lower CRC risk compared to 6–7 day/week meat eaters [57]. The pooled data from the Nurses' Health and Health Professional Follow-up Studies (87,256 women and 45,490 men; up to 26-years of follow-up) found that the

Table 19.2 Summaries of dietary pattern studies in colorectal adenomas and colorectal cancer (CRC) risk

Objective	Study details	Results
Systematic reviews and meta or pooled analyses		
Godos et al. (2016). Evaluate the association between diet quality (plant based dietary patterns vs. meat-based or other Western dietary patterns) and colorectal adenoma risk [11]	7 cohort studies: 94,217 subjects; 3–12 years of follow-up; 7384 colorectal adenoma cases; and 5 case-control studies: 3682 controls and 1578 cases of colorectal adenomas	Higher adherence to healthy dietary patterns was significantly associated with lower risk of colorectal adenomas by 19% and unhealthy dietary patterns had an increased risk by 13% (Fig. 19.1) with no evidence of heterogeneity between type of dietary patterns
Feng et al. (2016). Review the association between dietary patterns and CRC risk [12]	40 observational studies (22 cohort studies, 27 case-control studies, and 1 cross-sectional study)	For the highest vs. lowest adherence to dietary patterns, the 'healthy' pattern was associated with a lower risk for CRC by 25% ($p < .00001$), Western-style pattern increased risk of CRC by 40% ($p < .00001$) and alcohol consumption pattern raised CRC risk by 44% ($p = .003$) (Fig. 19.2)
Godos et al. (2016). Assess the association between vegetarian diets and colorectal cancer risk [51]	4 cohort studies; approx. 642,000 subjects; 7–20 years of follow-up	There was a significantly lower risk of CRC associated with a semi-vegetarian diet by 14% (p-heterogeneity = .82) and a pesco-vegetarian diet by 33% (p-heterogeneity = .46) compared to a non-vegetarian diet
Steck et al. (2015). Examine the effects of index-based dietary patterns on CRC risk (Mediterranean Diet (MedDiet) score, Healthy Eating Index (HEI), and Dietary Inflammatory Index (DII)) [52]	5 case-control studies and seven cohort studies	Comparing highest to lowest score groups, higher MedDiet scores were associated with an 8–54% lower CRC risk, higher HEIs were associated with a 20–56% lower CRC risk. Elevated DII proinflammatory diet scores were associated with a 12–65% higher CRC risk compared with anti-inflammatory rich diets. Low CRC risk diets consisted of higher intake of plant-based foods and lower intake of red or processed meats
Azeem et al. (2015). Assess correlations between various diet types, food or nutrients and colorectal cancer risk among Asian populations [53]	16 observational studies in Asian populations	1. There was a positive (adverse) association between intake of red meats, processed meats, preserved foods, saturated and animal fats, cholesterol, high sugar foods, spicy foods, tubers or refined carbohydrates and CRC risk. 2. There was inverse (protective) association for the intake of calcium/dairy foods, vitamin D, general vegetable/fruit/fiber intake, cruciferous vegetables, soy bean/soy products, selenium, vitamins C, E and B12, lycopene, alpha-carotene, beta-carotene, and folate and CRC risk
Yusof et al. (2012). Identify associations between specific dietary patterns and risk of CRC [54]	Six cohort studies;1.2 million subjects; 5–10-year follow-up	Protective CRC dietary patterns include: healthy and prudent patterns; healthy eating index, alternate healthy eating index, and Mediterranean score and protective foods included: fruits and vegetables, whole-grains, fat reduced diets, dairy, fish, poultry. Elevated CRC risks are shown from Western and traditional meat-eating patterns and foods including: pork processed meat, potatoes, and refined grains
Magalhaes et al. (2012). Evaluate the relationship between dietary patterns and CRC risk [55]	8 prospective cohort studies and 8t case-control studies	1. The healthy pattern, rich in fruit and vegetables, reduced risk of colon cancer by 20% but had no effect on rectal cancer 2. The Western pattern, high in red and processed meats, increased risk of colon cancer by 29% and rectal cancer by 19%

(continued)

Table 19.2 (continued)

Objective	Study details	Results
Specific prospective cohort studies		
Colorectal cancer (CRC) risk		
Vargas et al. (2016). Examine associations between dietary pattern scores and CRC risk (Women's Health Initiative Observational Study; US) [56]	78,273 postmenopausal women; mean baseline age 63 years and BMI 27; mean 12.4-years follow-up; 938 diagnosed with CRC and 238 died from CRC (multivariate adjusted)	Higher adherence to HEI-2010 and DASH dietary recommendations were inversely associated with risk of CRC in this cohort of postmenopausal women by 22–28% lower risk of CRC (highest vs. lowest quintile; $p < .01$). No associations were observed between any diet quality score and CRC specific mortality
Gilsing et al. (2016). Evaluate the effect of vegetarian and low meat diets on CRC risk (Netherlands Cohort Study -Meat Investigation Cohort) [57]	10,210 individuals; 1040 self-defined vegetarians; 20.3-year of follow-up; 437 CRC cases (multivariate adjusted)	Vegetarians and 1 day/week meat eaters showed a modest, borderline significantly decreased CRC risk by approx 27% compared to daily meat eaters. Most of CRC risk lowering was explained by intake of higher intake of fiber and soy products
Orlich et al. (2015). Evaluate the association between vegetarian dietary patterns and CRC incidence (The Adventist Health Study 2; US) [58]	77,659 subjects; mean 7.3 years of follow-up; 380 cases of colon cancer and 110 cases of rectal cancer (multivariate adjusted)	All vegetarians combined vs. non-vegetarians showed reduced risk by 22% for all colorectal cancers, colon cancer by 19% and rectal cancer by 29%; CRC risk was reduced in vegans by 16%, lacto-ovo vegetarians by 18%, pesco-vegetarians by 43% and in semi-vegetarians by 8% compared with nonvegetarians (Fig. 19.3). Effect estimates were similar for men and women and for black and nonblack individuals
Nimptsch et al. (2014). Examine associations between adolescent dietary patterns (derived using factor analysis) and risk of colorectal adenoma in middle adulthood (Nurses' Health Study II; US) [59]	17,221 women completed a retrospective high school food frequency questionnaire in 1998 when they were 34–51 years old, and subsequently underwent an endoscopy by 2007; 1299 women were diagnosed with ≥1 colorectal adenoma (multivariate adjusted)	A higher "prudent" pattern during high school, characterized by high consumption of vegetables, fruit and fish was associated with a significantly lower risk of rectal adenomas by 55% (p-trend = .005), but not colon adenomas. A higher Western dietary pattern during high school, characterized by high consumption of desserts and sweets, snack foods and red and processed meat, was significantly associated with increased risk of rectal adenomas by 78% (p-trend = .005) and advanced adenomas by 58% (p-trend = .08), but not associated with colon or non-advanced adenomas
Fung et al. (2010). Evaluate associations between the Alternate MedDiet (aMed) and the DASH-style diet scores with risk of CRC in middle-aged men and women (Nurses' Health Study and Health Professionals Follow-Up Study; US) [60]	87,256 women and 45,490 men (baseline age 30–55 years for women and baseline age 40–75 years for men) without a history of cancer; up to 26-year follow-up; aMed and DASH scores were calculated up to seven times during follow-up; 1432 cases of incident colorectal cancer among women and 1032 cases in men (multivariate adjusted)	Comparing higher to lower quintiles of the DASH score, the pooled risk was reduced for CRC by 20% (p- trend = .0001) and for colon cancer by 19% (p-trend = .002); higher adherence to the aMed score was associated with borderline significant lower CRC risk by 11% ($p = .06$) (Fig. 19.4)

Table 19.2 (continued)

Objective	Study details	Results
Reedy et al. (2008). Compare healthy dietary indices: Healthy Eating Indices, MedDiet Score, and Recommended Food Score on CRC risk (National Institutes of Health-AARP Diet and Health Study; US) [61]	492,306 subjects; mean baseline age 62 years and BMI 27; 5 years of follow-up, 3110 CRC cases (multivariate adjusted)	For men, there was a significant decreased CRC risk by 25–30% that was comparable across all indexes when comparing the highest vs. lowest quintile scores. For women, a decreased risk was associated with higher adherence to Healthy Eating Indices
Kim et al. (2005). Investigate the associations between dietary patterns and the risk of CRC (Japan Public Health Center-Cohort I) [62]	20,300 men and 21,812 women; three major dietary patterns: traditional, Western and healthy pattern scores; 10-years of follow-up, 370 CRC cases (multivariate adjusted)	The Western dietary pattern increased colon cancer risk by 200% in women. There was no significant association between healthy patterns and increased colon cancer risk in men or women. There was a positive association between a traditional Japanese diet and colon cancer in women but not in men

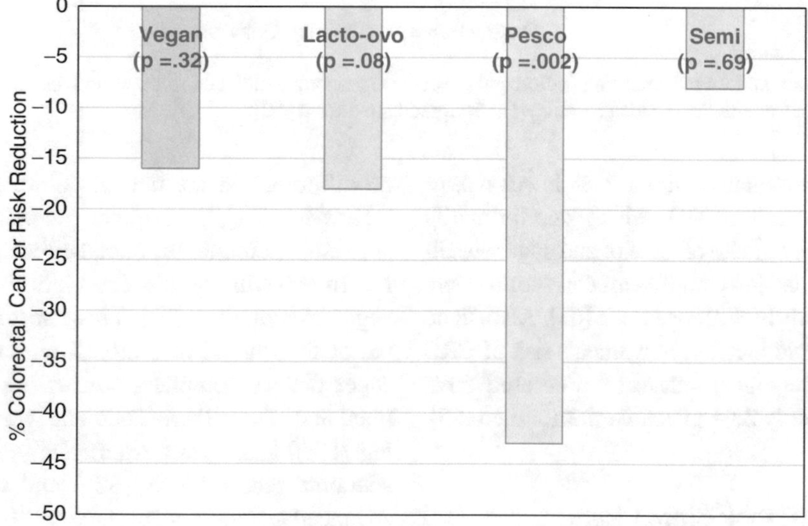

Fig. 19.3 Colorectal cancer risk for various vegetarian diets compared to a non-vegetarian dietary pattern (adapted from [58])

DASH diet was more effective than the MedDiet in reducing CRC risk (Fig. 19.4) [60]. For postmenopausal women, the DASH and Healthy Eating Indices diets were the dietary patterns most effective in lowering CRC risk by 22–28% ($p < .01$) [56, 61]. In women, the higher intake of a Western diet in high school was associated with a 78% increased risk of rectal adenomas ($p < .005$) [59]. In Japanese women, a high Western diet intake was associated with a 3.5-fold increased risk of distal colon cancer [62].

19.3.2 CRC Recurrence or Survival

Table 19.3 summaries four prospective cohort studies on the effects of dietary patterns on CRC recurrence and survival [63–66]. CRC survivors with high intake of Western dietary patterns had significantly increased odds of CRC mortality and recurrence (Fig. 19.5) and a healthy or prudent diet was associated with lower but insignificant odds for CRC mortality or recurrence [66]. In postmenopausal women, higher adherence to Healthy Eating

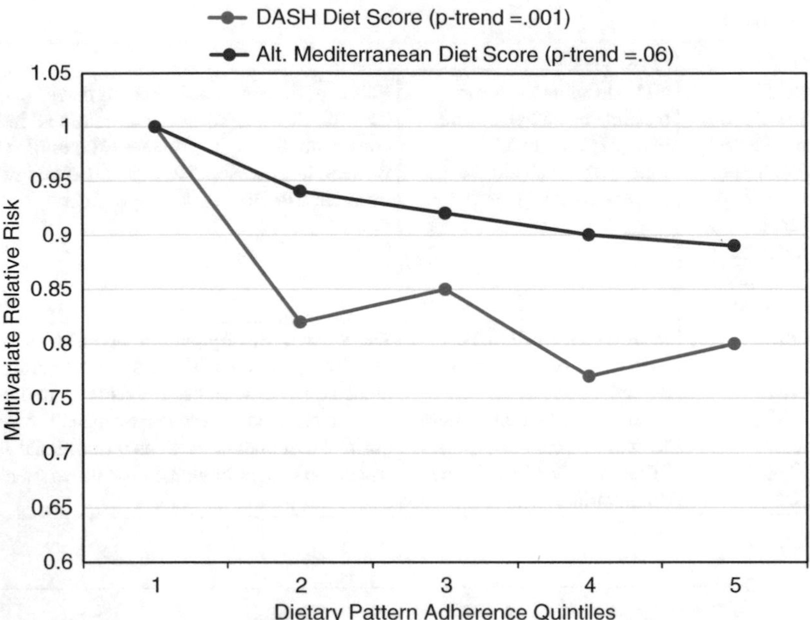

Fig. 19.4 Dietary pattern adherence and colorectal cancer risk in women and men from pooled data from the Nurses' Health Study and Health Professionals Follow-Up Study (adapted from [60])

Indices was associated with a 29% lower risk of mortality (p-trend = .01), which was primarily related to lower intake of alcohol and sugar sweetened beverages [64] and MedDiet scores were associated with 14% reduced risk [63]. Also, there was a three-fold increase in women's risk of CRC mortality with higher intake of processed meat compared to only 22% increased risk for men [65].

19.3.3 CRC Risk Biomarkers

Table 19.4 shows summaries of six RCTs on the effects of dietary patterns on CRC risk biomarkers [67–72]. A crossover RCT comparing the high-fat, low fiber Western diet vs. the traditional high-fiber, low-fat rural African diet over 2 weeks found that the traditional diet improved colonic health by increasing butyrogenic bacteria to increase fecal butyrate concentration and suppressed secondary bile acid formation, which are biomarkers of lower CRC risk [67]. Although the Polyp Prevention Trial (2079 subjects mean baseline age 61 years; 64% men; low fat, high fiber and fruit and vegetables diet vs. usual diet control with minimal guidance for healthy eating) found no difference in the rate of colorectal adenoma recurrence [71], subsequent secondary analyses suggested potential beneficial effects on adenoma recurrence with the low fat, high fiber fruits and vegetables diet [68–70]. These secondary analyses of the Polyp Prevention Trial show that: (1) super dietary compliers consuming about 12 g fiber and about three fruit and vegetable servings/1000 kcals had a significantly lower risk of adenoma recurrence by 32% and multiple and advanced adenoma recurrence by 50% compared to lower compliant controls ($p < .05$) after 4 years [68]; (2) an 8-year follow-up found an insignificant 2% lower colonic adenoma recurrence risk for those consuming higher fruit, vegetable, and fiber dietary patterns vs. the control group [69]; and (3) higher fiber fruit, vegetable, low-fat diets with increased bean intake was inversely associated with the risk of advanced adenoma recurrence by 65% (Fig. 19.6) [70]. A Canadian trial (201 subjects; mean baseline age 58 years; 55% men; 2 years) found that low-fat and high fiber plant food diets reduced adenoma recurrence by 50% along with reduced fecal bile acid concentrations in women but not in men [72]. A 2017 Cochrane systematic review (5 RCTs; 4,798

Table 19.3 Summary of dietary pattern prospective cohort studies in CRC recurrence and survival

Objective	Study details	Results
Jacobs et al. (2016). Investigate the association of four pre- diagnostic a priori diet quality indexes with CRC-specific and all-cause mortality (Multi-ethnic Cohort; US) [63]	>215,000 African-American, Native Hawaiian, Japanese-American, Latino, and white adults living in Hawaii and California; mean age diagnosis 71 years; mean 6-year follow-up; 4204 CRC cases (multivariate adjusted)	A higher alternate Mediterranean Diet score was associated with lower CRC-specific mortality in women by 14% but not in men. Healthy Eating Indices and DASH index were not significantly associated with CRC-specific mortality
Fung et al. (2014). Prospectively examine the association between diet quality scores, dietary patterns and CRC survival (NHS; US) [64]	1201 women diagnosed with stage I–III CRC, median baseline age 66.5 years, BMI 25; median follow-up 11.2 years and median survival 8.0 years; 162 died from CRC (multivariate adjusted)	Only a higher AHEI-2010 score was significantly associated with lower overall mortality by 29% (p-trend = .01) and borderline significantly lower risk of CRC mortality by 28% (p-trend = .07). A sub-component analysis showed that low-moderate alcohol intake and lower intake of sugar sweetened beverages were the primary factors associated with lower CRC risk
Zhu et al. (2013). Examine the association between dietary patterns and CRC disease-free survival (Canada) [65]	529 newly diagnosed CRC patients from Newfoundland; mean baseline age 60 years; 50% women; median 6.4 years of follow-up; 30 cases of CRC cancer recurrence or metastasis (multivariate adjusted)	CRC disease-free survival was significantly decreased among patients with a high processed meat dietary pattern by 82%. No significant associations were observed with the prudent vegetable or the high-sugar patterns and CRC disease-free survival
Meyerhardt et al. (2007). Determine the association of dietary patterns with cancer recurrences and colon cancer recurrence or mortality (US) [66]	1009 patients with stage III colon cancer; median baseline age 60 years; median 5.3 years of follow-up; 324 patients had cancer recurrence, 223 patients died with cancer recurrence (multivariate adjusted)	Patients with high adherence to the Western dietary pattern had significantly increased colon cancer mortality risk by 225% (p-trend <.001) and colon cancer recurrence risk by 185% (p-trend <.001) (Fig. 19.5). In contrast, the prudent dietary patterns were insignificantly associated with cancer recurrence or mortality

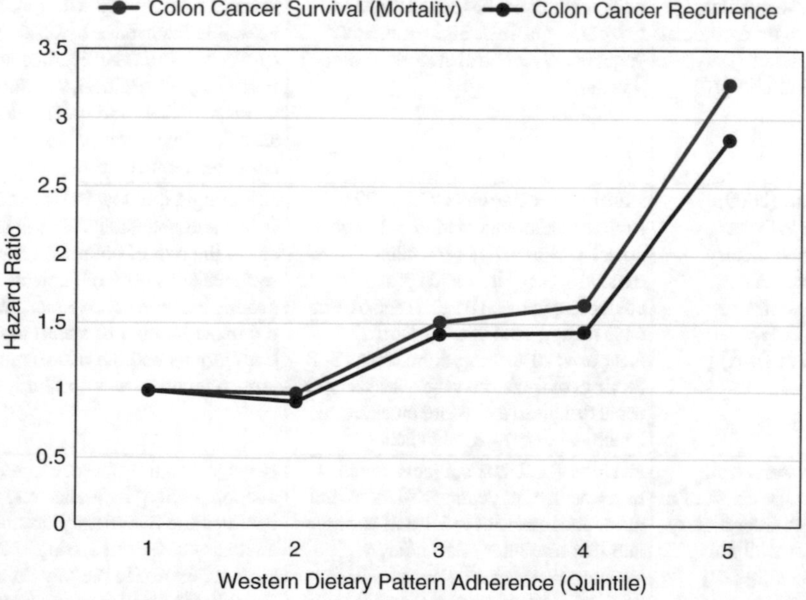

Fig. 19.5 Associations between colon cancer mortality and recurrence with adherence to the Western dietary pattern (p-trend < .001; both) (adapted from [66])

Table 19.4 Summaries of dietary pattern randomized controlled trials (RCTs) in colorectal cancer (CRC) risk biomarkers

Objective	Study details	Results
O'Keefe et al. (2015). Investigate the acute effects of drastic changes in dietary pattern quality in CRC risk (US) [67]	**Crossover RCT:** 20 healthy African Americans and 20 rural Africans; age range 40–65 years; BMI 18–35; 2-weeks; African Americans fed a high-fiber, low-fat African-style diet and rural Africans fed a high-fat, low-fiber Western-style diet, which reversed their usual dietary patterns	African Americans switching to a rural traditional diet had increased saccharolytic fermentation bacteria and fecal butyrate concentrations, and suppressed secondary bile acid synthesis associated with lower CRC risk. The opposite effect was observed in the rural Africans as they switched to an American style Western diet with an increased colon cancer risk profile
Sansbury et al. (2009). Examine the effect of strict adherence to a low-fat, high-fiber, high-fruit and -vegetable intervention on adenoma recurrence risk (Polyp Prevention Trial; US) [68]	**Parallel RCT Secondary Analysis:** 821 subjects completed 4-year follow-up; super compliers (25.6%), inconsistent compliers (44.6%) and poor compliers (29.8%); mean baseline age 61 years; 63% men; BMI 27.5; super compliers averaged baseline intake of 11.7 g/1000 kcal for fiber, and 2.8 servings/1000 kcal of fruit and vegetables	The intervention diet, higher fiber super-compliers had 32% lower fully adjusted risk of adenoma recurrence and 50% lower risk of multiple and advanced adenoma recurrence compared with lower dietary fiber controls ($p < .05$)
Lanza et al. (2007) . Follow a sub-cohort of the original cohort for an additional 4 years to further assess the effect of fruit and vegetables and low-fat diets on recurrence of one or more adenomas (The Polyp Prevention Trial- Continued Follow-up Study; US) [69]	**Parallel RCT Continuation:** 1192 subjects (63% of the original cohort); 801 confirmed colonoscopy reports; mean baseline age 60 years; 66% men; high fiber, high-fruit and -vegetable, and low-fat intervention vs. control; 8-years	This sub-group trial continuation from 4 to 8 years showed an insignificant 2% lower adenoma recurrence risk for the higher fiber, fruit and vegetable and lower fat eating pattern vs. the control group
Lanza et al. (2006). Assess the association between specific fruits, vegetables, and dried pulses on colorectal adenoma recurrence (Polyp Prevention Trial; US) [70]	**Multicenter Parallel RCT:** 1905 subjects; mean baseline age 61 years; 64% men; mean baseline BMI 27.6; low-fat, high-fiber, high-fruit, and vegetable vs. control American diet; 4 years	Higher intake of beans (dietary pulses; median intake 42 vs. 12 g/day) was inversely associated with risk for advanced adenoma recurrence by 65% (p-trend < .001; multivariate adjusted; Fig. 19.6). In addition, vegetables, green beans and peas, and green salad were associated with lower risk for advanced adenoma recurrence
Schatzkin et al. (2000). Investigate the effect of healthy fiber-rich dietary patterns on recurrent colorectal adenomas development (Polyp Prevention Trial; USA) [71]	**Multi-center Parallel RCT:** 2079 subjects; inclusion criteria > = 1 large bowel adenoma removed within 6 months, polyp free colon post colonoscopy; mean baseline age 61 years; 64% males; mean baseline BMI 27.6; diet goals: 20% energy from fat and 5–8 servings of fruits and vegetables daily vs. usual diet given a standard brochure on healthy eating; 4–year duration	Adopting a diet low in fat and high in fiber, fruits, and vegetables did not significantly affect the risk of colorectal adenomas recurrence as 40% of subjects in both groups had at least one recurrent adenoma; the mean number of adenomas was 1.9 in both groups and the rate of recurrence of large adenomas was similar in both groups
McKeown-Eyssen et al. (1994). Assess the effect of a low fat and high fiber dietary pattern on colorectal polyp's recurrence (Canada) [72]	**Parallel RCT:**201 subjects; mean baseline age 58 years; 55% men; diet guidance lower fat to 20% of energy and increase fiber to 50 g/day vs. Western diet; actual diet estimates: 25% vs. 33% of energy from fat and 35 g vs. 16 g fiber/day; 2-year follow-up	No significant difference in recurrence of adenoma polyp incidence rates was found between the two dietary groups. A subgroup analysis conducted among 142 subjects with high adherence to the low-fat and higher fiber diet showed that the women in this group had a 50% reduced risk of adenoma polyp recurrence, associated with reduced fecal bile acids concentration

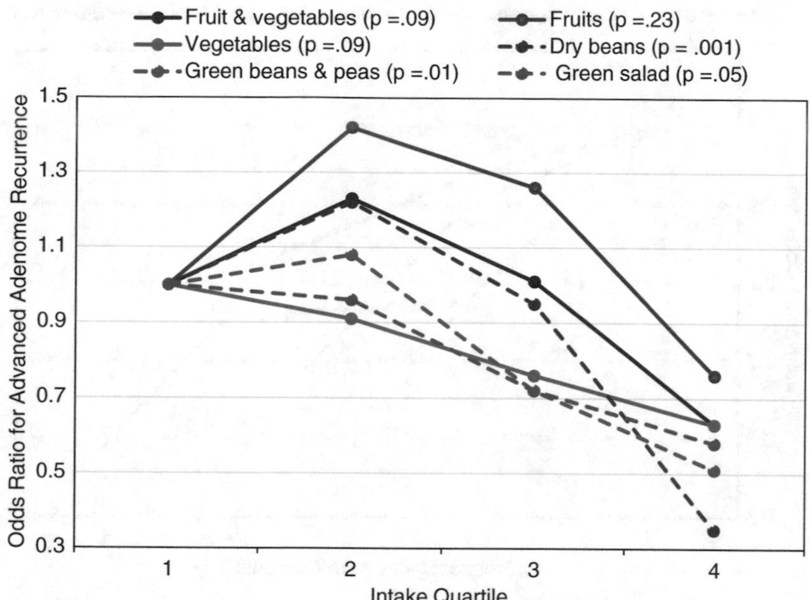

Fig. 19.6 Association between total fruit and vegetables and specific effects of dry edible beans, green beans and peas, and green salad and advanced adenoma recurrence risk from the Polyp Prevention Trial (adapted from [70])

subjects with a history of adenomatous polyps removed prior to the trial; mean baseline age 56 to 66 years; 2-8 years) found fiber-rich dietary patterns supplemented with wheat bran cereals or psyllium insignificantly reduced colorectal adenomas recurrence [73]. However, the Cochrane report authors indicated that these studies should be interpreted with caution because of the high study subject loss to follow-up and adenomatous polyps are a surrogate outcome for CRC that appears to require long-term RCTs to assure more confident conclusions.

19.4 Whole Plant Foods

Healthy diets rich in whole foods such as whole grains, limited intake of meat products, and increasing fruit, vegetable, and legume intake may have CRC protective effects [74, 75]. A 2011 Adventist Health Study (2818 subjects; average 26 years of follow-up) found that high frequency of cooked green vegetables, dried fruit, legumes, and brown rice was associated with a decreased risk of colorectal polyps (Fig. 19.7] [74]. Table 19.5 summarizes the prospective cohort studies on the effects of specific whole plant foods and risk of colorectal adenomas and CRC. An overview of the nutrient and pytochemical composition of whole plant foods are pro vided in Appendix B.

19.4.1 Fruits and Vegetables

There were relatively heterogenous effects of increased fruits and vegetables intake on colorectal adenomas and CRC risk from seven systematic reviews and meta-analyses of cohort and case-control studies [76–82] and eight specific cohort studies in various populations [83–91]

19.4.1.1 Systematic Reviews and Meta-Analyses

Colorectal Adenoma Risk

Two meta-analyses evaluated the effects of fruits and vegetables on colorectal adenomas risk [76, 79]. A 2015 meta-analysis (5 cohort

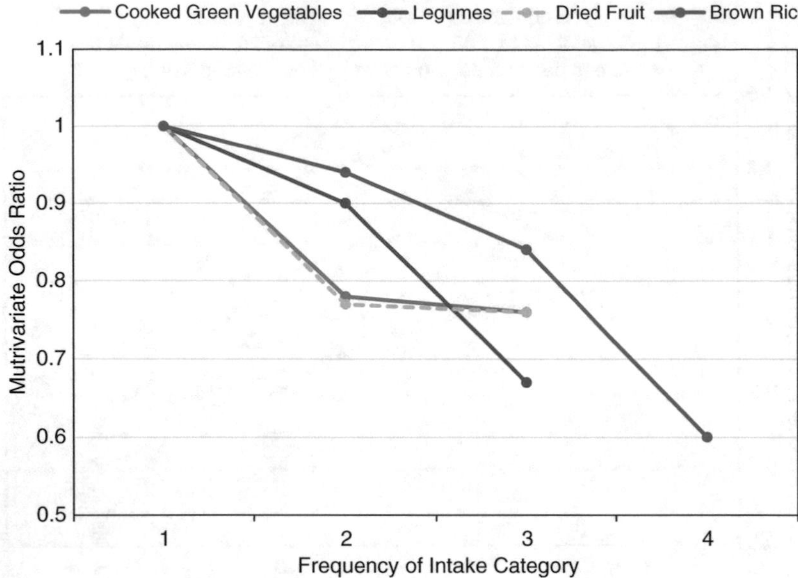

Fig. 19.7 Odds of colon/rectal polyps by specific whole plant foods from The Adventist Health Study ($p < .05$) (adapted from [74])

Table 19.5 Summaries of whole plant foods studies in colorectal cancer (CRC) and colorectal adenoma risk

Objective	Study details	Results
Fruits and vegetables		
Systematic reviews and meta-analysis		
Ben et al. (2015). Evaluate the association between fruit and vegetables and colorectal adenoma risk [76]	5 cohort studies; 126,999 subjects; 2–26-years of follow-up and 17 case-control studies; 11,696 colorectal adenoma cases	Colorectal adenoma risk was reduced with higher intake of vegetables by 9%, combined vegetables and fruits by 18%, and fruits by 21% (Fig. 19.8). Also, a linear dose-response analysis showed reduced risk for each 100-g/day of fruit by 6% and for vegetables by 2%
Kashino et al. (2015). Assess the effects of vegetables on CRC risk among the Japanese population [77]	6 cohort studies; 488,596 subjects; 3602 cases or deaths; and 11 case-control studies	There was insufficient evidence to support an association between intake of vegetables and CRC risk among the Japanese population as there was 0% mean reduced risk in cohort studies and a 25% mean reduced risk in case-control studies
Tse and Eslick (2014). Examine the observational association between cruciferous vegetable intake and risk of developing CRC [78]	11 prospective cohort studies and 18 case-control studies; 5994 CRC cases and 814 colonic adenoma cases	Higher total cruciferous vegetable intake significantly reduced colon cancer risk by 16%; with broccoli lowering risk by 20% (Fig. 19.9). There were insignificant effects of higher cruciferous vegetables intake on colorectal cancer, colonic adenoma and rectal cancer
Turati et al. (2014). Evaluate the effect of allium vegetables on CRC and adenomatous polyps [79]	6 cohort studies and ten case-control studies; 13,333 CRC cases	CRC risk was reduced with high intakes of garlic by 15%, onions by 15% and total allium vegetables by 22%, primarily in case-control studies and with significant heterogeneity. For colorectal adenoma, total allium vegetables reduced risk by 12% with no heterogeneity

Table 19.5 (continued)

Objective	Study details	Results
Wu et al. (2013). Assess the relationship between cruciferous vegetables and CRC risk [80]	11 cohort studies and 24 case-control studies; 1,295,063 subjects; 24,275 CRC cases	Cruciferous vegetables intake had a significantly lower CRC risk by 18% (high vs. low intake). Specific analysis reduced CRC risk for cabbage by 24% and broccoli by 18%. The results from the cohort studies showed borderline statistical significance
Aune et al. (2011). Summarize the CRC risk evidence from cohort studies in categorical, linear, and nonlinear, dose-response meta-analyses [81]	19 cohort studies; >1.5 million participants and 11,800–16,000 cases; 5–15 years of duration	There is a weak and nonlinear inverse association between intake of fruits and vegetables up to 500–600 g/day and CRC risk, with the greatest reduction in risk when increasing intake from very low levels (Fig. 19.10).
Koushik et al. (2007). Examine the associations between fruit and vegetable intakes and risk of colon cancer [82]	14 cohort studies; 756,212 subjects; 6–20 years of follow-up; 5838 colon cancer cases	Total combined fruit and vegetable intakes of ≥800 g/day vs. <200 g/day reduced distal colon cancer risk by 26% (p-trend = .02) and total colon cancer risk by 9% (p-trend = .19). Similar trends were observed for total fruits and total vegetables
Specific prospective cohort studies		
Kunzmann et al. (2016). Evaluate the association between fruit and vegetable intake and the risk of incident and recurrent colorectal adenoma and CRC (Prostate, Lung, Colorectal and Ovarian Cancer (PLCOC) Screening Trial; US) [83]	57,774 individuals; mean age 63 years; median 12.1-year follow-up; 1.004 colorectal adenoma and 738 recurrent adenoma cases; the median dietary intake of fruit and vegetables was 2.4 cups/1000 kcal; 373 g/day (multivariate adjusted)	An inverse dose-response effect was shown between incident and recurrent colorectal adenoma risk and increased total fruit and vegetable intake by 19% (p-trend = .07) with a significant reduced risk of multiple adenomas by 39% (p-trend = .04). Also, higher fruit and vegetable intakes including fruit juice were associated with a borderline reduced CRC risk by 18% (p-trend = .05), with risk reduction increasing to 26% among those with processed meat intake above the median. Higher intake of citrus fruits, melons and berries was associated with a reduced CRC risk by 15% (p-trend = .09)
Leenders et al. (2015). Examine the effects of fruits and vegetables on colon and rectal cancer risk with extended follow-up and variety of intake assessments (EPIC; EU) [84]	40,880 participants; mean baseline age 51 years; 13-year follow-up; 3370 diagnosed colon or rectal cancer cases (multivariate adjusted)	A lower risk of colon cancer was observed with higher intake of fruits and vegetables combined by 13% (p-trend = .02), but no consistent association was observed for separate intake of fruits and vegetables. A high variety of fruits and vegetables consumed was not associated with colon or rectal cancer risk
Aoyama et al. (2014). Evaluate the effect of low intake of vegetables and fruits on CRC risk (Japan Collaborative Cohort Study for Evaluation of Cancer Risk) [85]	45,516 subjects; 58% women; average baseline age 57 years; approx. 20 years of follow-up; 806 CRC cases (multivariate adjusted)	This Japanese population-based cohort study found no significant protective associations between the intake frequency of vegetables or fruits and CRC incidence. These results are consistent with several previous cohort studies in Japanese subjects
Vogtmann et al. (2013). Evaluate the association of fruit and vegetable intake with the risk of colorectal cancer Chinese men (Shanghai Men's Health Study; China) [86]	61,274 men; baseline age 40–70 years; median follow-up of 6.3 years; 398 CRC cases (multivariate adjusted)	High fruit intake was associated with reduced CRC risk by 33% (p-trend =.03), whereas vegetable intake was not significantly associated with risk. In subgroup analyses only fruits and legumes were generally inversely associated with the risk of colon and rectal cancer among middle age and older Chinese men

(continued)

Table 19.5 (continued)

Objective	Study details	Results
Van Duijnhoven et al. (2009). Examine the relationship between self-reported usual consumption of fruit and vegetables and CRC incidence (EPIC; EU) [87]	452,755 subjects; 70% women; 8.8 years of follow-up; 2819 CRC cases (multivariate adjusted)	Higher fruits and vegetables intake was found to significantly reduce CRC risk by 14% (p-trend = .04) and colon cancer by 24% (p-trend < .01). Also, after exclusion of the first 2 years of follow-up, a 100-g increase in consumption fruits and vegetables reduced risk for CRC by 5% (p =.04) and colon cancer by 6% (p = .02)
Nomura et al. (2008). Investigate the association of vegetable and fruit intakes with CRC risk (Multiethnic Cohort Study; US) [88]	85,903 men and 105,108 women; average follow-up of 7.3 years; CRC cases 1138 men and 972 women (multivariate adjusted)	In men, CRC risk was reduced for high intake of fruits and vegetables combined significantly by 26%, for fruit by 20% (p-trend =.09), and for vegetables by 15% 0.85 (p-trend = .05). The inverse associations were stronger for colon than for rectal cancer. In women, none of the associations with vegetables, fruit, or vegetables and fruit combined were significant
Millen et al. (2007). Evaluate effect of fruit, vegetables, or their subgroups on colorectal adenoma incidence (PPCOC Screening Trial; US) [89]	32,470 subjects; 47% women; mean baseline age 63 years; 9 years of follow-up; 3057 cases with at least one distal large bowel adenoma (multivariate adjusted)	Total fruit intake (5.7 vs. 1.2 serving/day) significantly lowered risk of distal adenoma by 25% (Fig. 19.11). Although total vegetable intake was insignificantly associated with colorectal adenoma risk, high intakes of deep-yellow vegetables, dark-green vegetables, and onions and garlic were related to lower colorectal adenoma risk (Fig. 19.12)
Park et al. (2007). Assess the relationship between fruit and vegetable intakes and CRC risk (NIH–AARP Diet and Health Study; US) [90]	488,043 men and women; baseline aged 50–71 years; mean 4.3 years of follow-up; 2972 CRC cases (2048 in men and 924 in women) (multivariate adjusted)	Higher vegetable intake reduced CRC risk by 18% for men (p-trend = .03) but there was an insignificant effect for women. There was an increased CRC risk for very low intake of total fruits and vegetables for men by 26% (p-trend = .006). Among subgroups of vegetables, higher intake of green leafy vegetables was associated with a lower CRC risk for men by 14% (p-trend = .04). Intake of fruits was not related to CRC risk in men or women
Michels et al. (2006). Examine the relationship between fruit and vegetable consumption and the prevalence and incidence of colorectal adenoma (Nurses' Health Study; US) [91]	34,467 women who had undergone colonoscopy or sigmoidoscopy; 19 years of follow-up; 1720 adenomas of the distal colon and rectum cases (multivariate adjusted)	Women consuming ≥5 fruit servings/day had 40% lower risk for developing colorectal adenomas compared with women who consumed only ≤1 fruit servings/day (p-trend = .001). The respective colorectal adenoma risk was reduced by 18% (p-trend = .1) for vegetable consumption
Legumes		
Systematic reviews and meta-analyses		
Total legumes		
Zhu et al. (2015). Investigate the association between dietary legume consumption and risk of CRC [92]	14 cohort studies; 1,903,459 participants; 12,261 CRC cases	Higher legume consumption was associated with a decreased risk of CRC by 9% (p = .01); legume fiber lowered risk by 15% (p = .05). Subgroup analyses indicate that higher legume consumption was inversely associated with CRC risk in Asians by 18% (p <.01) and soybean intake was associated with a decreased risk of CRC by 15% (p = .04)

Table 19.5 (continued)

Objective	Study details	Results
Wang et al. (2013). Assess the association between legume intake and colorectal adenoma risk [93]	Three cohort studies and 11 case control studies; 101,856 participants; 8380 colorectal adenoma cases	Higher intake of legumes was associated with a statistically significant 17% decreased risk of colorectal adenoma. There was no difference between men and women
Soy products		
Tse and Eslick (2016). Determine the association between dietary soy and CRC risk [23]	22 case control and 18 cohort studies; 633,476 subjects; 13,639 CRC cases	Increase in soy foods showed a modest reduced CRC risk by 8% but a subgroup analysis found that the high intake of isoflavones lowered CRC risk by 24% vs. low intake
Yan et al. (2010). Determine the relationship between soy intake and CRC risk [94]	4 cohort studies and 7 case-control studies	Soy foods were associated with a 21% reduction in CRC risk in women ($p = .026$), but not in men
Prospective cohort studies		
Yang et al. (2009). Investigate the effect of soy foods on CRC risk (Shanghai Women's Health Study; China [95])	68,412 women, mean baseline age 52 years; mean 6.4 years of follow-up, 321 CRC cases (multivariate adjusted)	Each 5-g/day intake of soy foods as assessed by dry weight (equivalent to 1 oz. (28.35 g) tofu/day) was associated with an 8% reduced CRC risk. Women in the highest tertile of intake had a reduced CRC risk by 33% compared with those in the lowest tertile (p-trend = .008). This inverse association was primarily confined to post-menopausal women. Similar results were also found for intakes of soy protein and isoflavones
Akhter et al. (2008). Examine the association between soy food intake and CRC risk (Japan Public Health Center-Based Prospective Study) [96]	83,063 Japanese men and women, mean baseline age 57 years; 5 year-follow-up; 886 cases of CRC (291 proximal colon, 286 distal-colon and 277 rectum)	The highest vs. lowest intake of isoflavone, miso soup, and soy food reduced CRC risk in men by approx. 11% ($p < .05$). In women, there was no association observed with CRC risk for any of these soy products or components
Michels et al. (2006). Examine the effect of legume intake on the prevalence and incidence of colorectal adenoma (Nurses' Health Study; US) [91]	34,467 women who had undergone colonoscopy or sigmoidoscopy; 19-year follow-up; 1720 adenomas of the distal colon and rectum cases (multivariate adjusted)	Women who consumed ≥4 servings of legumes/week had a lower colorectal adenoma incidence than women who reported intake of ≤1 serving/week by 33% (p-trend = .005)
Lin et al. (2005). Examined the association between dietary intakes of fruit, vegetables, and fiber and CRC risk in women (Women's Health Study; US) [97]	39,876 healthy women; aged ≥45 years at baseline; average follow-up of 10 years; 223 CRC cases (multivariate adjusted)	Higher intake of legume fiber was associated with a lower CRC risk by 40% (highest vs. lowest quintile; p-trend = .02). One legume serving was associated with reduced CRC risk by 17% (p-trend = .19)
Whole-grains		
Systematic review and meta-analysis		
Aune et al. (2011). Investigate the association between intake of whole grains and CRC risk using dose-response meta-analysis [19]	6 prospective cohort studies; 774,806 participants; 4.5–26-years of follow-up; 7941 CRC cases; total whole grains included whole grain rye breads, other whole grain breads, oatmeal, whole grain cereals, high fiber cereals, brown rice, and porridge; 61–128 g whole-grains/day	The consumption of 3 servings (90 g)/day of whole-grains reduced risk for CRC by 17%, colon cancer by 14% and rectal cancer by 20%

(continued)

Table 19.5 (continued)

Objective	Study details	Results
Haas et al. (2009). Evaluate the effectiveness of whole grain intake on CRC risk [98]	11 cohort studies; 1,719,590 subjects; baseline age 25–76 years; 6–16-years of follow-up; 7745 CRC cases	Increased intake of whole-grains reduced CRC risk in women by 8% and men by 7%; overall lower risk was reduced for colon cancer by 7% and rectal cancer by 11%
Specific prospective cohort studies		
Bakken et al. (2016). Investigate the association between whole-grain bread consumption and CRC incidence among Norwegian women (the Norwegian Women and Cancer Study) [99]	78,254 women; median baseline age 55 years; median 9 years of follow-up; 795 CRC cases (multivariate adjusted)	Higher whole-grain bread intake by Norwegian women was insignificantly associated with reduced CRC risk by 11–14%. A cancer subsite analysis showed higher whole-grain bread intake was weakly associated with a lower risk of proximal colon cancer (p-trend = .09)
Abe et al. (2014). Examine associations between japonica round rice vs. bread, noodles and cereal intake on CRC risk among Japanese adults (the Japan Public Health Center-based prospective Study) [100]	73,501 men and women; average follow-up of 11 years; 1276 CRC cases (multivariate adjusted)	High intake of japonica rice reduced rectal cancer risk in men by 39% (p-trend = .085). No clear patterns of association were found for bread, noodles and cereal intake
Kyra et al. (2013). Investigate the association between whole-grain intake and CRC risk (Scandinavian HELGA cohort) [101]	108,000 Danish, Swedish, and Norwegian subjects; mean baseline age 52 years; median 11 years of follow-up; 1123 CRC cases (multivariate adjusted)	Per 50 g whole-grain products intake, CRC risk was significantly reduced by 6%. Intake of whole-grain wheat was associated with a lower CRC incidence (highest vs. lowest quartile of intake) by 34% but the effect was non-linear (p-trend = .18)
Egeberg et al. (2010). Evaluate the association between intake of total and individual whole-grain products in relation to risk of colon and rectal cancer (Danish Diet, Cancer and Health prospective cohort study) [102]	26,630 men and 29,189 women; mean baseline age 53 years; median 10.6 years of follow-up; 461 colon cancer cases and 283 rectal cancer cases (multivariate adjusted)	Per daily 50 g increment whole grain product intake reduced risk of colon cancer by 15% and rectal cancer by 10% in men. Each 25 g/day of whole-grain bread significantly lowered risk of colon cancer by 11%. For women, no consistent associations between total or individual whole-grains product consumption and colon or rectal cancer risk were observed
Schatzkin et al. (2007) Investigate the relation between fiber and whole-grain food intakes and CRC (National Institutes of Health-AARP Diet and Health Study) [103]	291,988 men and 197,623 women; mean baseline age 63 years; 5-year of follow-up; 2974 CRC cases (multivariate adjusted)	Whole-grain intake was associated with lower CRC risk by 21% for the total cohort (p-trend <.001). In a sub-group analysis, CRC risk was reduced for men by 21% and for women by 13%. The association with whole grain was stronger for rectal than for colon cancer
Larsson et al. (2005). Examine prospectively the association between whole grain consumption and CRC risk in women (Swedish Mammography Cohort) [104]	61,433 women; mean follow-up of 14.8 years; 805 CRC cases (multivariate adjusted)	In women, high intake of whole grains was associated with a lower risk of colon cancer, but not of rectal cancer. Colon cancer risk (≥4.5 vs. <1.5 whole-grain servings/day) was reduced by 33% (p-trend = .06). After excluding cases occurring within the first 2 years of follow-up, the risk was further reduced to 35% (p-trend = .04). Women in the top quintile of cereal fiber intake (>13.6 g/day) had a 27% reduced colon cancer risk (p-trend = .03) compared with those in the lowest quintile (<7.3 g/day)

Table 19.5 (continued)

Objective	Study details	Results
Nuts (including peanuts)		
Yang et al. (2016). Examine the association of long-term nut consumption with CRC risk (Nurses' Health Study; US) [106]	75,680 women; nut intake assessed at baseline and updated every 2–4 years for 30 years; 1503 CRC cases (multivariate adjusted)	CRC risk was reduced for the intake of nuts ≥2 times/week vs. rarely consuming nuts by 14% (p-trend = .04), which was attenuated after further adjusting for BMI and diabetes to 13% (p-trend = .06). No association was observed for peanut butter
Yeh et al. (2006). Examine the relationship of peanut intake and CRC risk (Taiwan community-based cancer screening cohort) [107]	12,026 men and 11,917 women; baseline age 30–65 years; 10 years of follow-up; 107 CRC cases (multivariate adjusted)	CRC risk was reduced for higher peanut intake for men by 27% and for women by 58%
Jenab et al. (2004). Determine the effects of nut and seed intake on CRC risk (EPIC; EU) [108]	478,040 subjects (141,988 men, 336,052 women); 4.8-year follow-up; 1329 CRC cases (multivariate adjusted)	There was no association between higher intake of nuts and seeds and risk of CRC, colon, and rectal cancers in men and women combined. However, a subgroup analysis indicated that higher nut and seed intake in women reduced colon cancer risk by 31% (p-trend = .04)

and 17 case-control studies) found a significant inverse association for increased fruit intake on colorectal adenomas risk by 21% but only 9% for vegetables (higher vs. lower intake; Fig. 19.8); each 100 g/day of total fruit lowered colorectal adenomas risk by 6% compared to only 2% for total vegetables [76]. In a 2014 meta-analysis (six cohort and ten case-controlled studies) total allium vegetables (e.g., garlic and onion) was shown to reduce the incidence of colorectal adenomas by 12% with no heterogeneity [79].

Colorectal Cancer Risk

Five meta-analyses evaluated the effects of fruits and vegetables on CRC risk (Figs. 19.9 and 19.10) [77, 78, 80–82]. A 2011 meta-analysis (19 cohort studies; 1.7 million subjects; 5–15 years of follow-up) showed a weak and nonlinear inverse association between intake of fruits and vegetables in CRC risk with a benefit threshold at between 500 and 600 g/day, with the greatest reduction in risk when increasing intake from very low levels (Fig. 19.10) [81]. A 2007 meta-analysis (14 cohort studies; 746,212 subjects) found that very high combined fruit and vegetable intake (800 g/day) vs. 200 g/day significantly reduced distal colon cancer by 26% with similar trends for fruits and vegetables [82]. Several meta-analyses have observed that increased intake of cruciferous vegetables such as broccoli and cabbage reduce CRC risk, especially for colon cancer (Fig. 19.9) [78, 80]. A 2014 meta-analysis (six cohort and ten case-controlled studies) found for highest vs. lowest intake reduced CRC risk for garlic by 15%, onions by 15% and total allium vegetables by 22% (primarily in response to case-control studies and with significant heterogeneity) [79]. However, a Japanese meta-analysis (6 cohort and 11 case-control studies) showed that there is insufficient evidence supporting a protective effect of increased vegetable intake on CRC risk in a Japanese population [77].

19.4.1.2 Specific Prospective Cohort Studies

US Populations

Five cohort studies evaluated the effect of fruits and vegetables on colorectal adenomas and CRC risk [83, 88–91]. Two prospective analyses from the Prostate, Lung, Colorectal and Ovarian Cancer Screening Trial: (1) a 2016 prospective

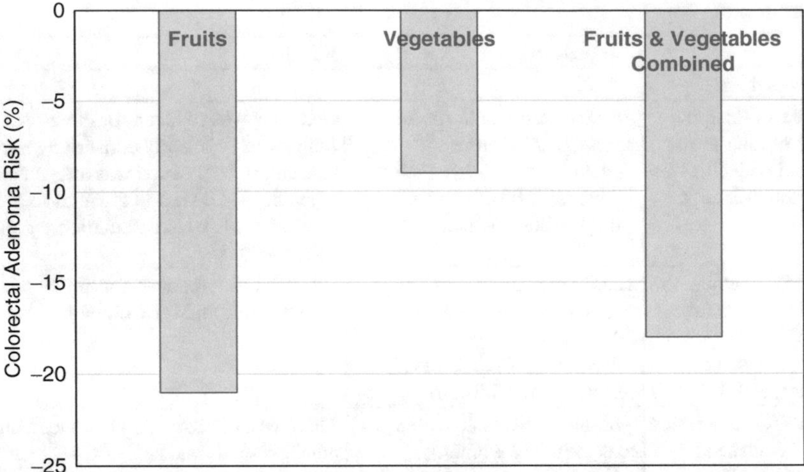

Fig. 19.8 Association between vegetables and fruits intake and colorectal adenoma risk (high vs. low intake) from a meta-analysis (adapted from [76])

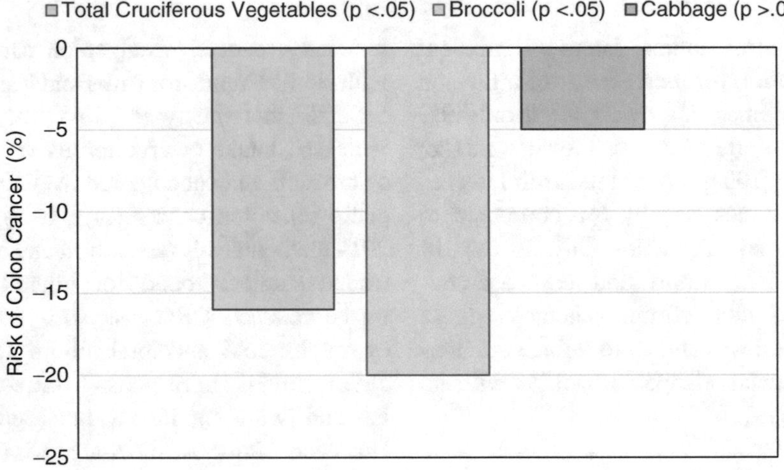

Fig. 19.9 Associations between cruciferous vegetables intake and colon cancer risk based on a meta-analysis (adapted from [78])

analysis (57,774 subjects; 12 years of follow-up) showed an inverse dose-response trend between total fruit and vegetable intake and colorectal adenomas risk (p-trend = .07) and the risk of multiple adenomas was significantly reduced by 39% [83]; and (2) a 2007 analysis (32,470 subjects; 9 years of follow-up) found that total fruit intake (5.7 vs. 1.2 serving/day) significantly lowered risk of distal colon adenoma by 25% (Fig. 19.11) [89]. Although total vegetable intake was insignificantly associated with colorectal adenomas risk, high intakes of deep-yellow vegetables, dark-green vegetables, and onions and garlic were related to lower colorectal adenomas risk (Fig. 19.12) [89]. Also, higher fruit and vegetable intakes including 100% fruit juice were associated with a borderline reduced CRC risk by 18% (p-trend = .05), which was stronger among those with intakes of processed meats above the median by 26% vs. 10% for those with processed meat intakes below median. A 2006 Nurses' Health Study reported that increased total fruit intake (≥5 vs. ≤1 serving(s)/day) significantly reduced colorectal adenomas risk by 40% whereas total

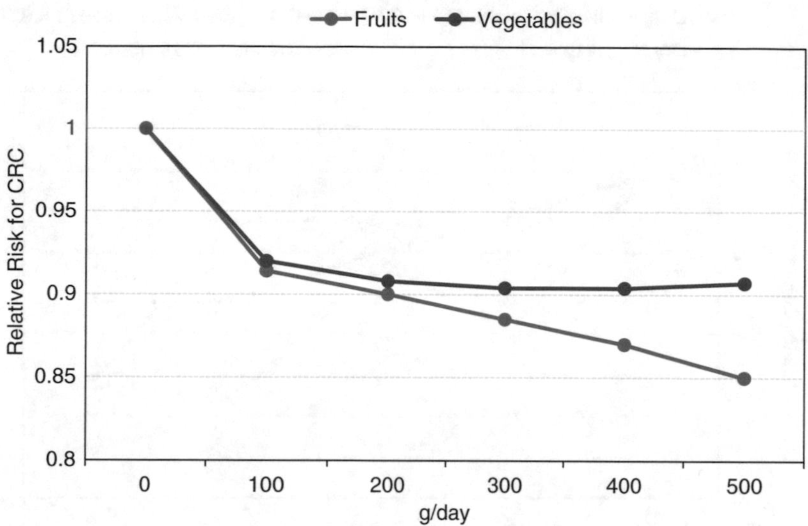

Fig. 19.10 Relationship between fruit and vegetable intake and colorectal cancer (CRC) risk from a meta-analysis of cohort studies (adapted from [81])

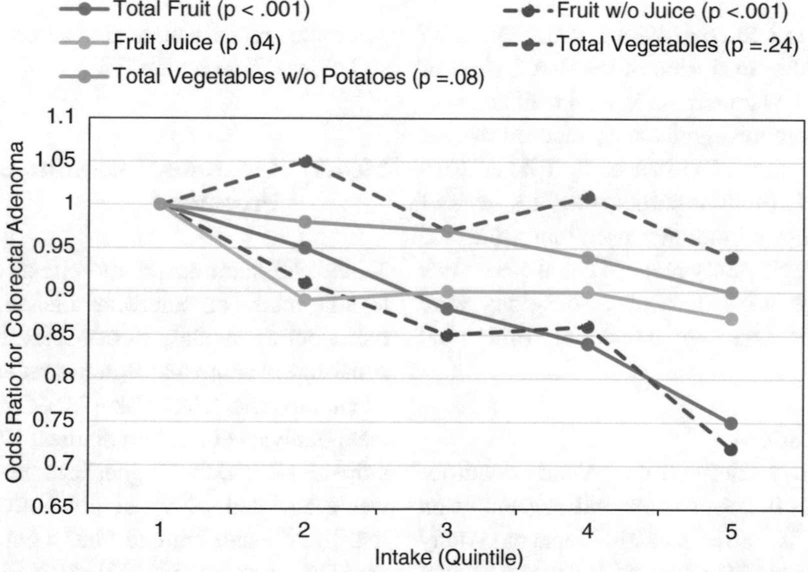

Fig. 19.11 Association between fruits and vegetables and colorectal adenomas from the Prostate, Lung, Colorectal, and Ovarian Cancer Screening Study (adapted from [89])

vegetable intake insignificantly reduced risk by 18% [91]. Two other cohort studies suggest that increased fruit and vegetable intake only significantly reduced CRC risk in men (especially green leafy vegetables) but not in women, which may be related to the amount consumed [88, 90].

EU Populations

Two cohort studies from the EPIC study populations evaluated the effect of fruit and vegetables on CRC risk [84, 87]. A 2009 analysis (452,755 subjects; 8.8 years of follow-up) found that higher total fruits and vegetables intake significantly

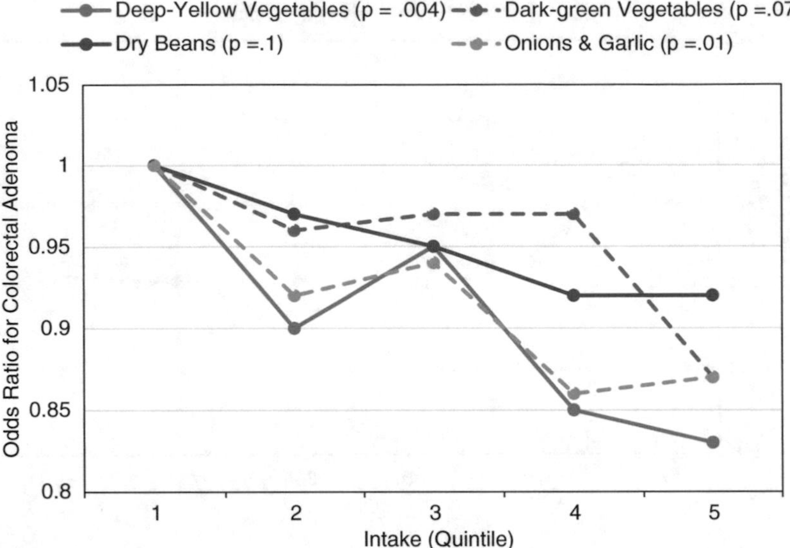

Fig. 19.12 Association between specific vegetables and colorectal adenomas risk from the Prostate, Lung, Colorectal, and Ovarian Cancer Screening Study (adapted from [89])

reduced risk of CRC by 14% and colon cancer by 24%. Also, after exclusion of the first 2 years of follow-up, a 100 g increase in total fruit and vegetable consumption significantly reduced risk for CRC by 5% and colon cancer by 6%. A 2015 EPIC analysis (40,880 participants; 13 years of follow-up) showed that increased total fruits and vegetables significantly reduced colon cancer risk by 13%, but no consistent associations were observed for separate intake of fruits and vegetables.

Asian Populations

Two cohort studies from Asian countries assessed the effects of fruits and vegetables on CRC risk [85, 86]. A 2014 Japanese study (45,516 subject; 20 years of follow-up) found that increased intake of fruits and vegetables was not significantly associated with CRC risk in men or women, which is consistent with other previous Japanese cohort studies [85]. In Chinese men, the Shanghai Men's Health Study (61,274 men; 6.3 years of follow-up) found that increased fruit intake was significantly inversely associated with CRC risk, whereas vegetable intake was not associated with CRC risk except for legumes, which were inversely associated with colon and rectal cancer risk among middle age and older Chinese men [86].

19.4.2 Legumes (including Soy Products)

Table 19.5 summarizes the effects of increased legume intake on colorectal adenomas and CRC risk. Four meta-analyses of observational studies consistently show that legumes reduce colorectal adenomas and CRC risk [23, 92–94]. A 2015 meta-analysis (14 cohort studies; 1,903,459 participants) found that higher legume consumption was associated with a significantly lower CRC risk by 9% and legume fiber significantly lowered CRC risk by 15% [92]. Also, in Asian populations higher legume consumption was associated with significantly reduced CRC risk by 18% and soybean intake was associated with a significantly decreased risk of CRC by 15%. A 2013 meta-analysis (3 cohort and 11 case-control studies; 101,856 subjects) showed that higher legume intake significantly lowered colorectal adenomas risk by 17% for both men and women [93]. A 2010 meta-analysis found that increased soy intake significantly reduced CRC risk only in women by 21% [94], but a 2016 meta-analysis (18 cohort and 22 case-control studies; 633,476 subjects) found a modest reduced CRC risk by 8% in men and women with a higher intake of isoflavones significantly lowering CRC risk by 24% [23]. Two cohort studies in women consistently show that increased intake of legumes or legume fiber reduces both the risk of colorectal adenomas and CRC [91, 97]. The Nurses' Health Study (34,467 women; 19 years of follow-up) showed that women consuming higher legume intake (≥4 vs. ≤1 weekly servings) significantly reduced risk of colorectal adenomas by 33% [91]. Similar findings were observed in the Women's Health Study with higher intake of legume fiber and significantly lower CRC risk [97]. Two cohort studies evaluated the effect of increased soy product intake on CRC risk in Chinese women and in a Japanese population [95, 96]. The Shanghai Women's Health Study (64,412 women; 6.2 years of follow-up) found in women that each 1 oz of tofu was associated with a significant 8% lower CRC risk and the highest tertile of intake was associated with a 33% lower risk [95]. The Japanese Public Health Prospective Study (83,063 subjects; 5 years of follow-up) showed that higher intake of isoflavones, miso soup, and soy food significantly reduced CRC risk in men by 11%, but no association was observed for CRC risk in women [96].

19.4.3 Whole-Grain Products

Table 19.5 summarizes the effects of increased whole-grain intake on CRC risk for observational studies. Two meta-analyses show that higher intake of whole-grains is associated with lower CRC risk [19, 98]. A 2011 meta-analysis (6 cohort studies; 774,806 participants; 4.5–36 years of follow-up) found that three servings daily (90 g/day) of whole-grains reduced risk for CRC by 17%, colon cancer by 14% and rectal cancer by 20% [19]. A 2009 meta-analysis (11 cohort studies; 1,719,590 participants; 6–16-years of follow-up) showed that higher intake of whole-grains reduced CRC risk in women by 8% and men by 7% with an overall population lower risk of colon cancer by 7% and rectal cancer by 11% [98]. Four cohort studies evaluated the CRC protective effect of increased whole-grains consumption in Scandinavian populations [99, 101, 102, 104]. Two cohort studies evaluated the effect of whole-grain intake on both men and women: (1) the 2013 Scandinavian HELGA cohort (108,000 Danish, Swedish, and Norwegian men and women; median 11 years of follow-up) found that per 50 g whole grain products CRC risk was significantly reduced by 6% [101]; and (2) the 2010 Danish Diet, Cancer and Health Study (26,630 men and 29,189 women; median 10.6 years of follow-up) showed that daily 50 g intake of whole grain products was associated with lower risk of colon cancer by 15% and rectal cancer by 10% in men. Higher whole-grain bread was statistically significantly associated with a lower risk of colon cancer with each intake of 25 g/day by 11% [102]. However, for women, no consistent associations between total or individual whole-grains product consumption and colon or rectal cancer risks were observed. Two studies in women showed somewhat conflicting findings: (1) a 2016 Norwegian Women and Cancer Study (78,254 women; 6–16 years of follow-up) showed an insignificant CRC risk reduction by 11–14% for increased whole- grain bread intake [99]; and (2) the Swedish Mammography Cohort (61,433 women; mean follow-up of 14.8 years) found that colon cancer risk was reduced by 33% (p-trend = .06) (≥4.5 vs. <1.5 whole-grain servings/day) [104]. After excluding cases occurring within the first 2 years of follow-up, the risk was further reduced to 35% (p-trend = .04). In a 2014 nested case-control study within the Scandinavian HELGA cohort assessment (450 cases vs. 450 controls), no significant associations were observed across increasing quartiles of whole-grain intake with any subtype of colorectal cancer whereas blood alkylresorcinol concentrations (a biomarker of short and medium term whole-grain intake) were associated with significantly lower distal colon cancer risk by 66% (highest vs. lowest quartiles) [105]. Two cohort studies assessed the effect of increased whole-grain intake on CRC risk [100, 103]. The 2014 Japan Public Health

Centered based Study (73,501 men and women; average follow-up of 11 years) found no clear associations between higher intakes of whole-grains Japonica round and short grain rice, bread, noodle and cereal intake on CRC risk and its subsites in men or women [100]. However, an inverse trend was observed between Japonica rice intake and rectal cancer in men with reduced risk by 39% (p-trend = .085). In the US, the 2007 National Institutes of Health-AARP Diet and Health Study (291,988 men and 197,623; 5 years of follow-up) demonstrated that whole-grain intake was associated with significantly lower CRC risk by 21% for the total cohort; a subgroup analysis indicated that women had a 13% CRC lower risk [103].

19.4.4 Nuts (Including Peanuts)

Table 19.5 summarizes the effects of three prospective cohort studies on the relationship between increased tree nut and peanut intake and CRC risk [106–108]. The US 2016 Nurses' Health Study (75,680 women; 30 years of follow-up) found that the CRC risk was significantly reduced for nuts ≥2 times/week vs. rarely consuming nuts by 14%, which was attenuated after further adjusting for BMI and diabetes to 13% (p-trend = .06) [106]. The Taiwan Community-based Cancer Screening cohort (12,026 men and 11,917 women) showed that increased peanut intake significantly reduced CRC risk in men by 27% and in women by 58% [107]. An EPIC study (478,040 subjects; 4.8 years of follow-up) demonstrated no association between nut and seed intake and CRC risk for men and women combined, but there was a significantly lower risk of colon cancer in women by 31% with increased nut and seed intake [108].

Conclusions

Globally CRC rates have doubled since the 1970s and incidence is strongly associated with the Western lifestyle and aging populations. As much as 90% of CRC cases may be attributable to dietary factors. A number of nutrients and phytochemicals are considered to be potentially protective against CRC to various degrees including fiber, isoflavones, flavonoids, antioxidant vitamins, carotenoids, folate, calcium, magnesium, and selenium. Higher adherence to a Western dietary pattern, which can stimulate a proinflammatory systemic response, can significantly increase risk of colorectal adenomas and CRC, especially in diets high in red or processed meats. In contrast, higher adherence to healthy dietary patterns including the MedDiet, DASH, Healthy Eating Indices, pesco-vegetarian and low inflammatory index diets can significantly reduce risk of colorectal adenoma and CRC. Survivors of CRC with high intake of Western dietary patterns had significantly higher odds of CRC mortality and recurrence compared to those consuming healthy diets. Dietary patterns rich in fruits, vegetables (including green leafy vegetables, cruciferous and allium vegetables), legumes (including soy), whole-grains (≥3 servings/day) and peanuts may have protective effects against colorectal adenomas and CRC risk. Diets rich in dietary fiber have been related to a lower CRC risk due in large part to beneficial effects of butyrate, derived from fiber fermentation by colonic microflora, an inhibitor of colonocyte tumor cell initiation and progression.

Appendix A: Comparison of Western and Healthy Dietary Patterns per 2000 kcals (Approximated Values)

Components	Western Dietary Pattern (US)	USDA Base Pattern	DASH Diet Pattern	Healthy Mediterranean Pattern	Healthy Vegetarian Pattern (Lact-ovo based)	Vegan Pattern
Emphasizes	Refined grains, low fiber foods, red meats, sweets and solid fats	Vegetables, fruits, whole-grains, and low-fat milk	Potassium rich vegetables, fruits a low-fat milk products	Whole grains, vegetables, fruits, dairy products, olive oil, and moderate wine	Vegetables, fruit, whole-grains, legumes, nuts, seeds, milk products and soy foods	Plant foods: vegetables, fruits, whole grains, nuts, seeds and soy foods
Includes	Processed meats, sugar sweetened beverages, and fast foods	Enriched grains, lean meat, fish, nuts, seeds and vegetable oils	Whole-grains, poultry, fish, nuts and seeds	Fish, nuts, seeds, and pulses	Eggs, non-dairy milk alternatives and vegetable oils	Non-dairy milk alternatives
Limits	Fruits and vegetables, whole-grains	Solid fats and added sugars	Red meats, sweets and sugar-sweetened beverages	Red meats, refined grains, and sweets	No red or white meats, or fish; limited sweets	No animal products
Estimated nutrients/components						
Carbohydrates (% Total kcal)	51	51	55	50	54	57
Protein (% Total kcal)	16	17	18	16	14	13
Total fat (% Total kcal)	33	32	27	34	32	30
Saturated fat (% Total kcal)	11	8	6	8	8	7
Unsat. fat (% Total kcal)	22	25	21	24	26	25
Fiber (g)	16	31	29+	31	35+	40+
Potassium (mg)	2800	3350	4400	3350	3300	3650
Vegetable oils (g)	19	27	25	27	19–27	18–27
Sodium (mg)	3600	1790	1100	1690	1400	1225
Added sugar (g)	79 (20 tsp)	32 (8 tsp)	12 (3 tsp)	32 (8 tsp)	32 (8 tsp)	32 (8 tsp)
Plant food groups						
Fruit (cup)	≤1.0	2.0	2.5	2.5	2.0	2.0
Vegetables (cup)	≤1.5	2.5	2.1	2.5	2.5	2.5
Whole-grains (oz.)	0.5	3.0	4.0	3.0	3.0	3.0
Legumes (oz.)	–	1.5	0.5	1.5	3.0	3.0+
Nuts/Seeds (oz.)	0.5	0.6	1.0	0.6	1.0	2.0
Soy products (oz.)	0.0	0.5	–	–	1.1	1.5

U.S. Department of Agriculture and U.S. Department of Health and Human Services. Dietary Guidelines for Americans, 2010. 7th Edition, Washington, DC: U.S. Government Printing Office. 2010; Table B2.4; http://www.choosemyplate.gov/ accessed 8.22.2015.

U.S. Department of Agriculture, Agriculture Research Service, Nutrient Data Laboratory. 2014. USDA National Nutrient Database for Standard Reference, Release 27. http://www.ars. usda.gov./nutrientdata. accessed 17 February 2015.

Dietary Guidelines Advisory Committee. Scientific Report. Advisory Report to the Secretary of Health and Human Services and the Secretary of Agriculture. Appendix E-3.7: Developing vegetarian and Mediterranean-style food patterns.2015;1–9.

Dietary Guidelines Advisory Committee. Scientific Report. Advisory Report to the Secretary of Health and Human Services and the Secretary of Agriculture. Part D. Chapter 1: Food and nutrient intakes, and health: current status and trends. 2015;1–78.

Bhupathiraju SN, Tucker KL. Coronary heart disease prevention: nutrients, foods, and dietary patterns. Clinica Chimica Acta. 2011;412: 1493–1514.

Appendix B: Estimated Range of Energy, Fiber, Nutrients and Phytochemicals Composition of Whole Plant Foods/100 g Edible Portion

Components	Whole-grains	Fresh fruit	Dried fruit	Vegetables	Legumes	Nuts/seeds
Nutrients/ phytochemicals	Wheat, oat, barley, rye, brown rice, whole grain bread, cereal, pasta, rolls and crackers	Apples, pears, bananas, grapes, oranges, blueberries, strawberries, and avocados	Dates, dried figs, apricots, cranberries, raisins and prunes	Potatoes, spinach, carrots, peppers, lettuce, green beans, cabbage, onions, cucumber, cauliflower, mushrooms, and broccoli	Lentils, chickpeas, split peas, black beans, pinto beans, and soy beans	Almonds, Brazil nuts, cashews, hazelnuts, macadamias, pecans, walnuts, peanuts, sunflower seeds, and flaxseed
Energy (kcals)	110–350	30–170	240–310	10–115	85–170	520–700
Protein (g)	2.5–16	0.5–2.0	0.1–3.4	0.2–5.0	5.0–17	7.8-24
Available Carbohydrate (g)	23–77	1.0–25	64–82	0.2–25	10–27	12–33
Fiber (g)	3.5–18	2.0–7.0	5.7–10	1.2–9.5	5.0–11	3.0–27
Total fat (g)	0.9–6.5	0.0–15	0.4–1.4	0.2–1.5	0.2–9.0	46–76
SFA[a] (g)	0.2–1.0	0.0–2.1	0.0	0.0–0.1	0.1–1.3	4.0–12
MUFA[a] (g)	0.2–2.0	0.0–9.8	0.0–0.2	0.1–1.0	0.1–2.0	9.0–60
PUFA[a] (g)	0.3-2.5	0.0–1.8	0.0–0.7	0.0.0.4	0.1–5.0	1.5–47
Folate (µg)	4.0–44	<5.0–61	2–20	8.0–160	50–210	10–230
Tocopherols (mg)	0.1–3.0	0.1–1.0	0.1–4.5	0.0–1.7	0.0–1.0	1.0–35
Potassium (mg)	40–720	60–500	40–1160	100–680	200–520	360–1050
Calcium (mg)	7.0–50	3.0–25	10–160	5.0–200	20–100	20–265
Magnesium (mg)	40–160	3.0–30	5.0–70	3.0–80	40–90	120–400
Phytosterols (mg)	30–90	1.0–83	–	1.0–54	110–120	70–215
Polyphenols (mg)	70–100	50–800	–	24–1250	120–6500	130–1820
Carotenoids (µg)	–	25–6600	1.0–2160	10–20,000	50–600	1.0–1200

[a]SFA (saturated fat), MUFA (monounsaturated fat) and PUFA (polyunsaturated fat)

U.S. Department of Agriculture, Agriculture Research Service, Nutrient Data Laboratory. 2014. USDA National Nutrient Database for Standard Reference, Release 27. http://www.ars. usda.gov./nutrientdata. Accessed 17 February 2015

Ros E, Hu FB. Consumption of plant seeds and cardiovascular health epidemiological and clinical trial evidence. Circulation. 2013;128: 553-565.

USDA. What we eat in America, NHANES 2011-2012, individuals 2 years and over (excluding breast-fed children). Available: www.ars.usda.gov/nea/bhnrc/fsrg.

Slavin JL, Lloyd B. Health benefits of fruits and vegetables. Adv Nutr. 2012; 3:506-516.

Rebello CJ, Greenway FL, Finley JW. A review of the nutritional value of legumes and their effects on obesity and its related co-morbidities. Obes Rev. 2014;15: 392-407.

Gebhardt SE, Thomas RG. Nutritive Value of Foods. 2002; U.S. Department of Agriculture, Agricultural Research Service, Home and Garden Bulletin 72.

Holden JM, Eldridge AL, Beecher GR, et al. Carotenoid content of U.S. foods: An update of the database. J Food Comp An. 1999; 12:169-196.

Lu Q-Y, Zhang Y, Wang Y, et al. California Hass avocado: profiling of carotenoids, tocopherol, fatty acid, and fat content during maturation and from different growing areas. *J* Agric Food Chem. 2009; 57(21):10,408-10,413.

Wu X, Beecher GR, Holden JM, et al. Lipophilic and hydrophilic antioxidant capacities of common foods in the United States. J Agric Food Chem. 2004; 52: 4026-4037.

Bhupathiraju SN, Tucker KL. Coronary heart disease prevention: nutrients, foods, and dietary patterns. Clinica Chimica Acta. 2011;412: 1493-1514.

Dietary Guidelines Advisory Committee. Scientific Report. Advisory Report to the Secretary of Health and Human Services and the Secretary of Agriculture. Part D. Chapter 1: Food and nutrient intakes, and health: current status and trends. 2015;1-78.

http://health.gov/dietary guidelines/2015/guidelines/accessed 1.26.2016.

References

1. Global Burden of Disease Cancer Collaboration. Global, regional, and national cancer incidence, mortality, years of life lost, years lived with disability, and disability-adjusted life-years for 32 cancer groups, 1990 to a systematic analysis for the global burden of disease study. JAMA Oncol. 2015;3(4):524–48. https://doi.org/10.1001/ jamaoncol.2016.5688.
2. Mármol I, Sánchez-de-Diego C, Dieste AP, et al. Colorectal carcinoma: a general overview and future perspectives in colorectal cancer. Int J Mol Sci. 2017;18:197. https://doi.org/10.3390/ ijms1800197.
3. American Cancer Society (ACS). Colorectal cancer facts & figures 2014-2016. Atlanta: American Cancer Society; 2014.
4. World Cancer Research Fund International (WCRF). Colorectal cancer statistics. www.wcrf.org/int/ cancer-facts-figures/data specific-cancer/colorectal cancer-statistics. Accessed 6 May 2015.
5. Bailie L, Loughrey MB, Coleman HG. Lifestyle risk factors for serrated colorectal polyps: a systematic review and meta-analysis. Gastroenterology. 2017;152(1):92–104. https://doi.org/10.1053/j. gastro.2016.09.003.
6. Song M, Garrett WS, Chen AT. Nutrients, foods, and colorectal cancer prevention. Gastroenterology. 2015;148:1244–60.
7. Baena R, Salinas P. Diet and colorectal cancer. Maturitas. 2015;80:258–64.
8. Makarem N, Lin Y, Bandera EV, et al. Concordance with World Cancer Research Fund/American Institute for Cancer Research (WCRF/AICR) guidelines for cancer prevention and obesity-related cancer risk in the Framingham Offspring cohort (1991–2008). Cancer Causes Control. 2015;26(2):277–86. https://doi.org/10.1007/s10552-014-0509.
9. Vieira AR, Abar L, Chan DSM, et al. Foods and beverages and colorectal cancer risk: a systematic review and meta-analysis of cohort studies, an update of the evidence of the WCRF-AICR Continuous Update Project. Annals Oncology. 2017;28:1788–1802.
10. Stone RAT, Waring ME, Cutrona SL, et al. The association of dietary with colorectal cancer among normal weight, overweight and obese men and women: a prospective longitudinal study in the USA. BMJ Open. 2017;7;e015619.
11. Godos J, Bella F, Torrisi A, et al. Dietary patterns and risk of colorectal adenoma: a systematic review and meta-analysis of observational studies. Hum Nutr Diet. 2016;29:757–67. https://doi.org/10.1111/jhn.12395.
12. Feng Y-L, Shua L, Zhenga P-F, et al. Dietary patterns and colorectal cancer risk: a meta-analysis. J Cancer Prev. 2016;26(3):201–11. https://doi.org/10.1097/ CEJ.0000000000000245.
13. MacDonald RS, Wagner K. Influence of dietary phytochemicals and microbiota on colon cancer risk. J Agric Food Chem. 2012;60:6728–35. doi. org/10.1021/jf204230r
14. De Rosa M, Rega D, Costabile V, et al. The biological complexity of colorectal cancer: insights into biomarkers for early detection and personalized care. Ther Adv Gastroenterol. 2016;9(6):861–86. https://doi.org/10.1177/1756283X16659790.
15. Arvelo F, Sojo F, Cotte C. Biology of colorectal cancer. Ecancermedicalscience. 2015;9:520.
16. Brenner H, Kloor M, Pox C. Colorectal cancer. Lancet. 2014;383:1490–502.
17. Yao Y, Suo T, Andersson R, et al. Dietary fibre for the prevention of recurrent colorectal adenomas and carcinomas. Cochrane Database Syst Rev. 2017;1:CD003430. https://doi.org/10.1002/14651858. CD003430.pub2.
18. Ben Q, Sun Y, Chai R, et al. Dietary fiber intake reduces risk for colorectal adenoma: a meta-analysis. Gastroenterology. 2014;146:689–99.
19. Aune D, Chan DSM, Lau R, et al. Dietary fibre, whole grains, and risk of colorectal cancer: systematic review and dose-response meta-analysis of prospective studies. BMJ. 2011;343:d6617.
20. Jacobs ET, Lanza E, Alberts DS, et al. Fiber, sex, and colorectal adenoma: results of a pooled analysis. Am J Clin Nutr. 2006;83:343–9.
21. Jiang R, Botma A, Rudolph A, et al. Phytooestrogens and colorectal cancer risk: a systematic

review and dose–response meta-analysis of observational studies. Br J Nutr. 2017;116:2115–28.
22. Yu Y, Jing X, Li H, et al. Soy isoflavone consumption and colorectal cancer risk: a systematic review and meta-analysis. Sci Rep. 2016;6:25939. https://doi.org/10.1038/srep25939.
23. Tse G, Eslick GD. Soy and isoflavone consumption and risk of gastrointestinal cancer: a systematic review and meta-analysis. Eur J Nutr. 2016;55(1):63–73. https://doi.org/10.1007/s00394-014-0824-7.
24. Grosso G, Godos J, Lamuela-Raventos R, et al. A comprehensive meta-analysis on dietary flavonoid and lignan intake and cancer risk: level of evidence and limitations. Mol Nutr Food Res. 2017;61(4). https://doi.org/10.1002/mnfr.201600930.
25. Jin H, Leng Q, Li C. Dietary flavonoid for preventing colorectal neoplasms. Cochrane Database Syst Rev. 2012;(8):CD009350. doi: 10.1002/14651858. CD009350. pub2.
26. Xu X, Yu E, Liu L, et al. Dietary intake of vitamins A, C, and E and the risk of colorectal adenoma: a meta-analysis of observational studies. Eur J Cancer Prev. 2013;22:529–39.
27. Pais R, Dumitraşcu DL. Do antioxidants prevent colorectal cancer? A meta-analysis. Rom J Intern Med. 2013;51(3-4):152–63.
28. Park Y, Spiegelman D, Hunter DJ, et al. Intakes of vitamins A, C, and E and use of multiple vitamin supplements and risk of colon cancer: a pooled analysis of prospective cohort studies. Cancer Causes Control. 2010;21(11):1745–57. https://doi.org/10.1007/s10552-010-9549-y.
29. Panic N, Nedovic D, Pastorino R, et al. Carotenoid intake from natural sources and colorectal cancer: a systematic review and meta-analysis of epidemiological studies. Eur J Cancer Prev. 2017;26(1):27–37. https://doi.org/10.1097/CEJ.0000000000000251.
30. Mannisto S, Yaun S-S, Hunter DJ, et al. Dietary carotenoids and risk of colorectal cancer in a pooled analysis of 11 cohort studies. Am J Epidemiol. 2007;165:246–55.
31. Kim D-H, Smith-Warner SA, Spiegelman D, et al. Pooled analyses of 13 prospective cohort studies on folate intake and colon cancer. Cancer Causes Control. 2010;21(11):1919–30. https://doi.org/10.1007/s10552-010-9620-8.
32. Figueiredo JC, Mott LA, Giovannucci E, et al. Folic acid and prevention of colorectal adenomas: a combined analysis of randomized clinical trials. Int J Cancer. 2011;129:192–203.
33. Bonovas S, Fiorino G, Lytras T, et al. Calcium supplementation for the prevention of colorectal adenomas: a systematic review and meta-analysis of randomized controlled trials. World J Gastroenterol. 2016;22(18):4594–603. https://doi.org/10.3748/wjg.v22.i18.4594.
34. Keum N, Lee DH, Greenwood DC, et al. Calcium intake and colorectal adenoma risk: dose-response meta-analysis of prospective observational studies. Int J Cancer. 2015;136:1680–7.
35. Chen G-C, Pang Z, Liu Q-F. Magnesium intake and risk of colorectal cancer: a meta-analysis of prospective studies. Eur J Clin Nutr. 2012;66:1182–6. https://doi.org/10.1038/ejcn.2012.135.
36. Wark PA, Lau R, Norat T, Kampman E. Magnesium intake and colorectal tumor risk: a case-control study and meta-analysis. Am J Clin Nutr. 2012;96:622–31.
37. Cai X, Wang C, Yu W, et al. Selenium exposure and cancer risk: an updated meta-analysis and meta-regression. Sci Reports. 2016;6:19213. https://doi.org/10.1038/srep.19213.
38. Takata Y, Kristal AR, King IB, et al. Serum selenium, genetic variation in selenoenzymes, and risk of colorectal cancer: primary analysis from the Women's Health Initiative Observational Study and meta-analysis. Cancer Epidemiol Biomark Prev. 2011;20(9):1822–30.
39. Vipperla K, O'Keefe SJ. Diet, microbiota, and dysbiosis: a 'recipe' for colorectal cancer. Food Funct. 2016;7:1731–40.
40. O'Keefe SJD, Li JV, Lahti L, et al. Fat, fibre and cancer risk in African Americans and rural Africans. Nat Commun. 2015;6:6342. https://doi.org/10.1038/ncomms7342.
41. Borges-Canha M. Role of colonic microbiota in colorectal carcinogenesis: a systematic review. Rev Esp Enferm Dig. 2015;107(11):659–71.
42. Encarnação JC, Abrantes AM, Pires AS, Botelho MF. Revisit dietary fiber on colorectal cancer: butyrate and its role on prevention and treatment. Cancer Metastasis Rev. 2015;34:465–78. https://doi.org/10.1007/s10555-015-9578-9.
43. Kelly CJ, Zheng L, Campbell EL, et al. Crosstalk between microbiota-derived short-chain fatty acids and intestinal epithelial HIF augments tissue barrier function. Cell Host Microbe. 2015;17:662–71.
44. Sebastián C, Mostoslavsky R. Untangling the fiber yarn: butyrate feeds Warburg to suppress colorectal cancer. Cancer Discov. 2014;4(12):1368–70.
45. Keum N, Lee DH, Kim R, et al. Visceral adiposity and colorectal adenomas: dose-response meta-analysis of observational studies. Ann Oncol. 2015;26:1101–9. https://doi.org/10.1093/annonc/mdu563.
46. Riondino S, Roselli M, Palmirotta R, et al. Obesity and colorectal cancer: role of adipokines in tumor initiation and progression. World J Gastroenterol. 2014;20(18):5177–90. https://doi.org/10.3748/wjg.v20.i18.5177.
47. Tucker LA, Thomas KS. Increasing total fiber intake reduces risk of weight and fat gains in women. J Nutr. 2009;139:576–81.
48. Baer DJ, Rumpler WV, Miles CW, Fahey GC Jr. Dietary fiber decreases the metabolizable energy content and nutrient digestibility of mixed diets fed to humans. J Nutr. 1997;127:579–86.

49. Verspreet J, Damen B, Broekaert WF, et al. A critical look at prebiotics within the dietary fiber concept. Annu Rev Food Sci Technol. 2016;7:167–90.
50. Zeng H, Lazarova DL, Bordonaro M. Mechanisms linking dietary fiber, gut microbiota and colon cancer prevention. World J Gastrointest Oncol. 2014;6(2):41–51.
51. Godos J, Bella F, Sciacca S, Galvano F, et al. Vegetarianism and breast, colorectal and prostate cancer risk: an overview and meta-analysis of cohort studies. J Hum Nutr Diet. 2017;30(3):349–59. https://doi.org/10.1111/jhn.12426.
52. Steck SE, Guinter M, Zheng J, Thomson CA. Index-based dietary patterns and colorectal cancer risk: a systematic review. Adv Nutr. 2015;6:763–673.
53. Azeem S, Gillani SW, Siddiqui A, et al. Diet and colorectal cancer risk in Asia—a systematic review. Asian Pac J Cancer Prev. 2015;16(13):5389–96.
54. Yusof AS, Isa ZM, Shah SA. Dietary patterns and risk of colorectal cancer: a systematic review of cohort studies (2000-2011). Asian Pacific J Cancer Prev. 2012;13(9):4713–7. https://doi.org/10.7314/ACJCP.2012.13.9.4713.
55. Magalhaesa B, Peleteiro B, Lunet N. Dietary patterns and colorectal cancer: systematic review and meta-analysis. Eur J Cancer Prev. 2012;21(1):15–23. https://doi.org/10.1097/CEJ.0b013e 3283472241.
56. Vargas AJ, Neuhouser ML, George SM, et al. Diet quality and colorectal cancer risk in the Women's Health Initiative Observational Study. Am J Epidemiol. 2016;184(1):23–32. https://doi.org/10.1093/aje/kwv304.
57. Gilsing AMJ, Schouten LJ, Goldbohm RA, et al. Vegetarianism, low meat consumption and the risk of colorectal cancer in a population based cohort study. Sci Rep. 2015;5:13484. https://doi.org/10.1038/srep13484.
58. Orlich MJ, Singh PN, Sabate J, et al. Vegetarian dietary patterns and the risk of colorectal cancers. JAMA Intern Med. 2015;175(5):767–76. https://doi.org/10.1001/jamainternmed.2015.59.
59. Nimptsch K, Malik VS, Fung TT, et al. Dietary patterns during high school and risk of colorectal adenoma in a cohort of middle-aged women. Int J Cancer. 2014;134:2458–67.
60. Fung TT, FB H, Wu K, et al. The Mediterranean and Dietary Approaches to Stop Hypertension (DASH) diets and colorectal cancer. Am J Clin Nutr. 2010;92(6):1429–35. https://doi.org/10.3945/ajcn.2010.29242.
61. Reedy J, Mitrou PN, Krebs-Smith SM, et al. Index-based dietary patterns and risk of colorectal cancer the NIH-AARP diet and health study. Am J Epidemiol. 2008;168:38–48.
62. Kim MK, Sasaki S, Otani T, et al. Dietary patterns and subsequent colorectal cancer risk by subsite: a prospective cohort study. Int J Cancer. 2005;115:790–8.
63. Jacobs S, Harmon BE, Ollberding NJ, et al. Among 4 diet quality indexes, only the alternate Mediterranean diet score is associated with better colorectal cancer survival and only in African American women in the Multiethnic Cohort. J Nutr. 2016;146:1746–55.
64. Fung TT, Kashambwa R, Sato K, et al. Post diagnosis diet quality and colorectal cancer survival in women. PLoS One. 2014;9(12):e115377. https://doi.org/10.1371/journal.pone.0115377.
65. Zhu Y, Wu H, Wang PP, et al. Dietary patterns and colorectal cancer recurrence and survival: a cohort study. BMJ Open. 2013;3:e002270. https://doi.org/10.1136/bmjopen-2012-.
66. Meyerhardt JA, Niedzwiecki D, Hollis D, et al. Association of dietary patterns with cancer recurrence and survival in patients with stage III colon cancer. JAMA. 2007;298(7):754–64.
67. O'Keefe SJD, Li JV, Lahti L, et al. Fat, fiber and cancer risk in African Americans and rural Africans. Nat Commun. 2015;6:6342. https://doi.org/10.1038/ncomms7342.
68. Sansbury LB, Wanke K, Albert PS, et al. The effect of strict adherence to a high-fiber, high-fruit and -vegetable, and low-fat eating pattern on adenoma recurrence. Am J Epid. 2009;170(5):576–84.
69. Lanza E, Yu B, Murphy G, et al. The Polyp Prevention Trial–Continued Follow-up Study: no effect of a low-fat, high-fiber, high-fruit, and -vegetable diet on adenoma recurrence eight years after randomization. Epidemiol Biomarkers Prev. 2007;16(9):1745–52.
70. Lanza E, Hartman TJ, Albert PS, et al. High dry bean intake and reduced risk of advanced colorectal adenoma recurrence among participants in the polyp prevention trial. J Nutr. 2006;136:1896–903.
71. Schatzkin A, Lanza E, Corle D, et al. Lack of effect of a low-fat, high-fiber diet on the recurrence of colorectal adenomas. Polyp prevention trial study group. N Engl J Med. 2000;342:1149–55.
72. McKeown-Eyssen GE, Bright-See E, Bruce WR, et al. A randomized trial of a low-fat high fibre diet in the recurrence of colorectal polyps. Toronto Polyp Prevention Group. J Clin Epidemiol. 1994;47:525–36.
73. Yao Y, Suo T, Andersson R, et al. Dietary fibre for the prevention of recurrent adenomas and carcinomas. Cochrane Database Syst Rev 2017; CD003430. doi:https://doi.org/10.1002/14651858.CD03430. pub2.
74. Tantamango YM, Knutsen SF, Beeson WL, et al. Foods and food groups associated with the incidence of colorectal polyps: the Adventist Health Study. Nutr Cancer. 2011;63(4):565–72. https://doi.org/10.1080/01635581.2011.55988.
75. Levi F, Pasche C, La Vecchia C, et al. Food groups and colorectal cancer risk. Br J Cancer. 1999;79(7/8):1283–7.
76. Ben Q, Zhong J, Liu J, et al. Association between consumption of fruits and vegetables and risk of colorectal adenoma a PRISMA-compliant meta-analysis of

observational studies. Medicine. 2015;94(42):e1599. https://doi.org/10.1097/MD.000000000000.1599.

77. Kashino I, Mizoue T, Tanaka K, et al. Vegetable consumption and colorectal cancer risk: an evaluation based on a systematic review and meta-analysis among the Japanese population. Jpn J Clin Oncol. 2015;45(10):973–9. https://doi.org/10.1093/jjco/hyv111.
78. Tse G, Eslick GD. Cruciferous vegetables and risk of colorectal neoplasms: a systematic review and meta-analysis. Nutr Cancer. 2014;66(1):128–39. https://doi.org/10.1080/01635581. 2014.852686.
79. Turati F, Guercio V, Pelucchi C, et al. Colorectal cancer and adenomatous polyps in relation to allium vegetables intake: a meta-analysis of observational studies. Mol Nutr Food Res. 2014;58:1907–14. https://doi.org/10.1002/mnfr.201400169.
80. QJ W, Yang Y, Vogtmann E, et al. Cruciferous vegetables intake and the risk of colorectal cancer: a meta-analysis of observational studies. Ann Oncol. 2013;24:1079–87. https://doi.org/10.1093/annonc/mds601.
81. Aune D, Lau R, Chan DSM, et al. Nonlinear reduction in risk for colorectal cancer by fruit and vegetable intake based on meta-analysis of prospective studies. Gastroenterology. 2011;141:106–18.
82. Koushik A, Hunter DJ, Spiegelman D, et al. Fruits, vegetables, and colon cancer risk in a pooled analysis of 14 cohort studies. J Natl Cancer Inst. 2007;99:1471–83.
83. Kunzmann AT, Coleman HG, Huang W-Y, et al. Fruit and vegetable intakes and risk of colorectal cancer and incident and recurrent adenomas in the PLCO cancer screening trial. Int J Cancer. 2016;138:1851–61.
84. Leenders M, Siersema PD, Overvad K, et al. Subtypes of fruit and vegetables, variety in consumption and risk of colon and rectal cancer in the European Prospective Investigation into Cancer and Nutrition. Int J Cancer. 2015;137:2705–14.
85. Aoyama N, Kawado M, Yamada H, et al. Low intake of vegetables and fruits and risk of colorectal cancer: the Japan Collaborative Cohort Study. J Epidemiol. 2014;24(5):353–60.
86. Vogtmann E, Xiang Y-B, Li H-L, et al. Fruit and vegetable intake and the risk of colorectal cancer: results from the Shanghai Men's Health Study. Cancer Causes Control. 2013;24(11):1935–45.
87. van Duijnhoven FJB, Bueno-De-Mesquita HB, Ferrari P, et al. Fruit, vegetables, and colorectal cancer risk: the European Prospective Investigation into Cancer and Nutrition. Am J Clin Nutr. 2009;89:1441–51.
88. Nomura AMY, Wilkens LR, Murphy SP, et al. Association of vegetable, fruit, and grain intakes with colorectal cancer: the Multiethnic Cohort Study. Am J Clin Nutr. 2008;88:730–7.
89. Millen AE, Subar AF, Graubard BI, et al. Fruit and vegetable intake and prevalence of colorectal adenoma in a cancer screening trial. Am J Clin Nutr. 2007;86:1754–64.
90. Park Y, Subar AF, Kipnis V, et al. Fruit and vegetable intakes and risk of colorectal cancer in the NIH–AARP diet and health study. Am J Epidemiol. 2007;166:170–80.
91. Michels KB, Giovannucci E, Chan AT, et al. Fruit and vegetable consumption and colorectal adenomas in the Nurses' Health Study. Cancer Res. 2006;66(7):3942–53.
92. Zhu B, Sun Y, Qi L, et al. Dietary legume consumption reduces risk of colorectal cancer: evidence from a meta-analysis of cohort studies. Sci Rep. 2015;5:8797. https://doi.org/10.1038/srep08797.
93. Wang Y, Wang Z, Fu L, et al. Legume consumption and colorectal adenoma risk: a meta-analysis of observational studies. PLoS One. 2013;8(6):e67335. https://doi.org/10.1371/journal.pone. 0067335.
94. Yan L, Spitznagel EL, Bosland MC. Soy consumption and colorectal cancer risk in humans: a meta-analysis. Cancer Epidemiol Biomark Prev. 2010;19(1):148–58.
95. Yang G, Shu X-O, Li H, et al. Prospective cohort study of soy food intake and colorectal cancer risk in women. Am J Clin Nutr. 2009;89:577–83.
96. Akhter M, Inoue M, Kurahashi N, et al. Dietary soy and isoflavone intake and risk of colorectal cancer in the Japan Public Health Center–Based Prospective Study. Cancer Epidemiol Biomark Prev. 2008;17(8):2128–35.
97. Lin J, Zhang SM, Cook NR, et al. Dietary intakes of fruit, vegetables, and fiber, and risk of colorectal cancer in a prospective cohort of women (United States). Cancer Causes Control. 2005;16:225–33.
98. Haas P, Machado MJ, Anton AA, et al. Effectiveness of whole grain consumption in the prevention of colorectal cancer: meta-analysis of cohort studies. Int J Food Sci Nutr. 2009;60(Suppl. 6):1–13.
99. Bakken T, Braaten T, Olsen A, et al. Consumption of whole-grain bread and risk of colorectal cancer among Norwegian women (the NOWAC Study). Forum Nutr. 2016;8:40. https://doi.org/10.3390/nu8010040.
100. Abe SK, Inoue M, Sawada N, et al. Rice, bread, noodle and cereal intake and colorectal cancer in Japanese men and women: the Japan Public Health Center-based prospective Study (JPHC Study). BJC. 2014;110:1316–21. https://doi.org/10.1038/bjc.2013.799.
101. Kyrø C, Skeie G, Loft S, et al. Intake of whole grains from different cereal and food sources and incidence of colorectal cancer in the Scandinavian HELGA cohort. Cancer Causes Control. 2013;24:1363–74.
102. Egeberg R, Olsen A, Loft S, et al. Intake of wholegrain products and risk of colorectal cancers in the diet, cancer and health cohort study. BJC. 2010;103:730–4.

103. Schatzkin A, Mouw T, Park Y, et al. Dietary fiber and whole-grain consumption in relation to colorectal cancer in the NIH-AARP Diet and Health Study. Am J Clin Nutr. 2007;85:1353–60.
104. Larsson SC, Giovannucci E, Bergkvist L, Wolk A. Whole grain consumption and risk of colorectal cancer: a population-based cohort of 60,000 women. BJC. 2005;92:1803–7.
105. Knudsen MD, Kyrø C, Olsen A, et al. Self-reported whole-grain intake and plasma alkylresorcinol concentrations in combination in relation to the incidence of colorectal cancer. Am J Epidemiol. 2014;179(10):1188–96.
106. Yang M, FB H, Giovannucci EL, et al. Nut consumption and risk of colorectal cancer in women. Eur J Clin Nutr. 2016;70:333–7.
107. Yeh CC, You SL, Chen CJ, Sung FC. Peanut consumption and reduced risk of colorectal cancer in women: a prospective study in Taiwan. World J Gastroenterol. 2006;12(2):222–7.
108. Jenab M, Ferrari P, Slimani N, et al. Association of nut and seed intake with colorectal cancer risk in the European Prospective Investigation into Cancer and Nutrition. Cancer Epidemiol Biomark Prev. 2004;13(10):1595–603.

Dietary Patterns, Whole Plant Foods, Nutrients and Phytochemicals in Breast Cancer Prevention and Management

20

Keywords
Fruits • Vegetables • Soy foods • Whole-grains • Seeds • Dietary fiber • Vitamins • Protein source • Carotenoids • Flavonoids • Isoflavonoids • Lignan • Dietary patterns • Premenopausal • Postmenopausal • Body mass index • Mortality • Estrogen

Key Points

- Dietary choices including: (1) level of adherence to healthy vs Western dietary patterns; (2) high vs low dietary energy density intake; (3) type and level of dietary fat, fiber and protein consumed; (4) adequate vs inadequate intake of calcium, folate and α-tocopherol; (5) type and levels of non-starchy vegetables and fruits containing dietary carotenoids and flavonoids intake; (6) level of phytoestrogen containing legumes and seeds consumed; and (7) higher vs lower intake of alcohol or coffee are examples of dietary factors that may influence breast cancer (BC) risk, recurrence or mortality.
- Biological factors and mechanisms associated with diet and BC risk and survival include: body weight and central adiposity, tumor advancement, systemic and tissue lipid/fatty acid peroxidation and inflammation, epigenetic and transcriptional regulation, hormone levels (e.g., estrogen, insulin, leptin, adiponectin and growth factor cascades), insulin resistance, and various endometabolic and colonic microbiota processes, which can influence BC initiation and progression..
- Lifestyle indicators, which are associated with increased BC risk, recurrence or mortality, especially for postmenopausal women, may include having an overweight or obese BMI, weight gain by over 15 lbs. over 4 years, and physical inactivity. Patients with BC are most often either overweight or obese at diagnosis and obesity increases mortality risk in both pre- and postmenopausal women with BC.
- Meta-analyses reported that healthy dietary patterns reduced overall BC risk, whereas a high consumption of alcohol and a Western diet increased BC risk. Healthy dietary patterns, especially the Mediterranean diet, DASH diet and the vegan diet are effective in reducing BC risk and improving odds for survival. Key adverse dietary components for BC risk and survival include high intake of red and processed meats, high energy dense and high glycemic foods and beverages and >1 alcoholic beverage/day.

M.L. Dreher, *Dietary Patterns and Whole Plant Foods in Aging and Disease*, Nutrition and Health,
https://doi.org/10.1007/978-3-319-59180-3_20

- Highly colored non-starchy vegetables rich in carotenoids and flavonoids have been associated with reduced BC risk, especially in estrogen receptor negative BC. After BC diagnosis, soy foods (>10 mg isoflavones/day or > ½ cup of soy milk or 2 ounces of tofu/day) may help to reduce risk of BC recurrence or mortality in both Asian and Western women.

20.1 Introduction

In women, breast cancer (BC) is the most common cancer worldwide, with an estimated 2.4 million cases in 2015 [1]. Between 2005 and 2015, BC remained the fifth leading global cause of cancer. Overall incident cases have increased by 43% because of population growth (contributing an additional 13%) and aging (contributing 15%). The odds of developing BC between birth and 79 years are 1 in 14 for women globally but these odds increase to 1 in 9 for women in the highest income countries such as in North America, Western Europe, and Australia. The worldwide rise in BC incidence, despite continuous improvements in BC prognosis, is primarily due to longer life expectancy, increased aging populations, and the adoption of Western diets and lifestyles [2, 3]. Hormones such as estrogens, progesterone, insulin, and growth factors, which peak with puberty, pregnancy, and lactation, may influence the lifetime risk of BC because they modulate the structure, growth, and epigenetics of tumor cells. Risk doubles each decade until menopause, when the risk slows down or remains stable, but breast cancer is more common after menopause. In many countries, the 5-year survival rate for women diagnosed with Stage I/II BC (only spread to tissues or nodes under the arm) is 80–90% but if the cancer stage is more advanced (spread to distant lymph nodes or organs) the survival rate falls to about 25%. Breast cancer is a heterogeneous disease with various subtypes [5]. Common BC molecular subtype biological markers, include the presence or absence of estrogen and progesterone receptors, or human epidermal growth factor receptor 2 (HER2). More typically, BC risk and survival is associated with lifestyle, reproductive, and other environmental factors, including aging, early age at menarche, lactation, late menopause, first full-term pregnancy, the use of exogenous hormones (oral contraceptives and combined postmenopausal hormone replacement therapy), alcohol consumption, excess weight, insulin resistance, diet, and physical activity [2–6].

Survival in women diagnosed with early-stage, invasive breast cancer has improved dramatically in the past 25 years [2–7]. This is largely due to the use of evolving pharmacological therapies targeting a reduction in estrogen action and exposure. However, it is estimated that up to 90% of overall cancer risk may be attributable to environmental and lifestyle factors [6]. Women diagnosed with BC often change their eating behavior towards healthier food choices in an attempt to improve their overall health, well-being and survival but they are often unaware of specific and effective dietary guidance [7]. A number of prospective cohort and randomized controlled trials (RCTs) support BC protective benefits of healthy dietary patterns containing fiber and phytochemical rich whole or minimally processed plant foods (whole plant foods), healthy vegetable oils and omega 3 (n-3) fatty acids sources. Also, important is the adherence to a healthy lifestyle and maintaining and achieving a healthy weight which can significantly reduce BC risk, recurrence and improve survival after BC diagnosis compared to Western diets and lifestyles [7–10]. Dietary factors including energy density, type of fat, levels of dietary fiber (fiber), phytoestrogens, carotenoids, flavonoids, type of protein source (red meat vs soy foods), beverages such as alcohol, and others components may play an important role in both promoting and inhibiting BC development. Biological factors and mechanisms associated with diet and BC risk and survival include: body weight and central adiposity, tumor immunity, systemic and tissue lipid/fatty acid peroxidation and inflammation, epigenetic and transcriptional regulation, hormone levels (e.g., estrogen, insulin, leptin, adiponectin and growth factor cascades), insulin resistance, and various endometabolic and colonic microbiota processes, which can influence BC initiation and progression [2–12]. The objective of this chapter is to comprehensively assess the effects of dietary patterns, whole plant foods, nutrients and phytochemicals on BC risk, recurrence and survival.

20.2 Specific Lifestyle, Dietary and Lifecyle Factors

20.2.1 Overview

Lifestyle habits play an important role in BC risk, recurrence and mortality [11–16]. World Cancer Research Fund (WCRF)/American Institute for Cancer Research (AICR) [11, 12] and American Cancer Society (ACS) [13] have developed guidelines, recommending a healthy weight, a diet rich in fiber containing plant foods, and physical activity as important for lowering overall cancer risk, including BC prevention and improved post-diagnosis survival (Table 20.1). For the WCRF/AICR cancer prevention guidelines, the EpiGEICAM case-control study (973 cases of BC and 973 controls from 17 Spanish regions; age range 22–71 years) found a linear association between the degree of diet and lifestyle noncompliance and BC risk [14]. This study found that compared to women who met 6 or more healthy lifestyle recommendations as reference, women meeting <3 recommendations showed a 300+% increased BC risk, especially in postmenopausal women. For premenopausal women, excessive intake of energy dense foods and drinks that promote weight gain increased BC risk by 200+% (p-interaction = 0.014). For postmenopausal women, low intake of healthy fiber-rich plant foods such as fruit, vegetables, whole-grains, and legumes increased BC risk by about 250%. The Women's Health Initiative (65,838 postmenopausal women; mean baseline age 63 years at baseline; mean 12.6 years of follow-up) found that women with the highest ACS guideline scores had significantly lower risk for any cancer by 17%, for BC by 22%, and for colorectal cancer by 52% (Fig. 20.1) and similar risk reductions for cancer mortality (Fig. 20.2) [15]. A multinational European Prospective Investigation into Cancer and Nutrition (EPIC) cohort investigated the effect of a healthy lifestyle index score [HLIS] (5 factors including diet, physical activity, smoking avoidance, alcohol consumption and anthropometry; score range

Table 20.1 Adult guidelines for nutrition and physical activity in cancer prevention

World Cancer Research Fund (WCRF)/American Institute for Cancer Research (AICR) [11, 12]	American Cancer Society (ACS) Guidelines [13]
Maintain a healthy lean body weight without being underweight	Achieve and maintain a healthy lean body weight throughout life
Be physically active for at least 30 min every day	Be as lean as possible throughout life without being underweight
Limit consumption of energy dense foods (particularly processed foods high in added sugar, or low in fiber, or high in fat)	Avoid excess weight gain at all ages. For those who are currently overweight or obese, losing even a small amount of weight has health benefits and is a good place to start
Eat mostly plant foods including a variety of vegetables, fruits, whole grains, and legumes	Engage in regular physical activity and limit consumption of high-calorie foods and beverages as key strategies for maintaining a healthy weight
Limit animal foods such as red and processed meats	Adopt a physically active lifestyle. Adults should engage in at least 150 min of moderate-intensity or 75 min of vigorous-intensity activity weekly spread over the week
Limit alcoholic beverages (2 for men and 1 for women a day)	Limit sedentary behavior such as sitting, lying down, watching television, or other forms of screen-based entertainment. Doing some physical activity above usual activities, no matter what one's level of activity, can have many health benefits
Limit consumption of salty foods and foods processed with salt	Choose foods and beverages in amounts that help achieve and maintain a healthy weight
Meet nutritional needs through diet	Limit consumption of processed meat and red meat
Breastfeed exclusively for up to 6 months	Eat at least 2.5 cups of vegetables and fruits each day
Cancer survivors should follow the recommendations for cancer prevention	Choose whole grains instead of refined grain products
	If you drink alcoholic beverages, limit consumption. Drink no more than 1 drink per day for women or 2 per day for men

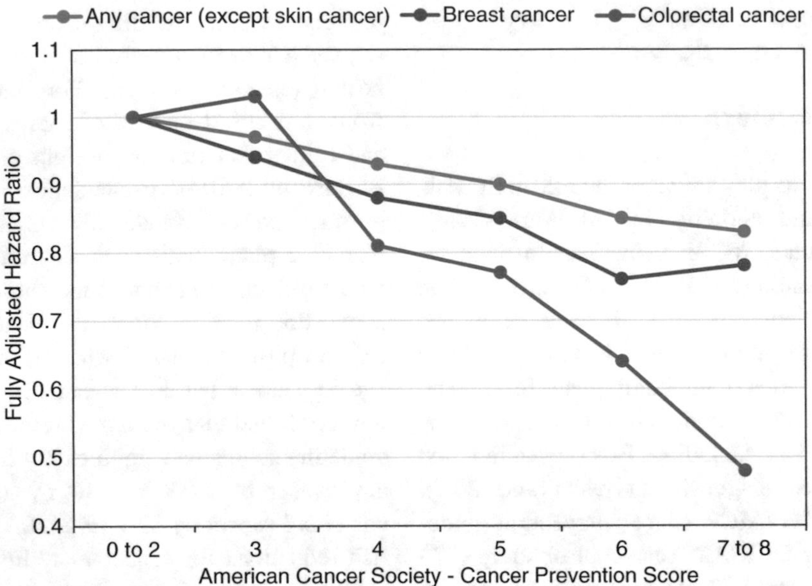

Fig. 20.1 For postmenopausal cancer risk, the effect of American Cancer Society cancer prevention score based on adherence to nutrition and physical activity guidelines from the US Women's Health Initiative (all cancers p < 0.001) (adapted from [15])

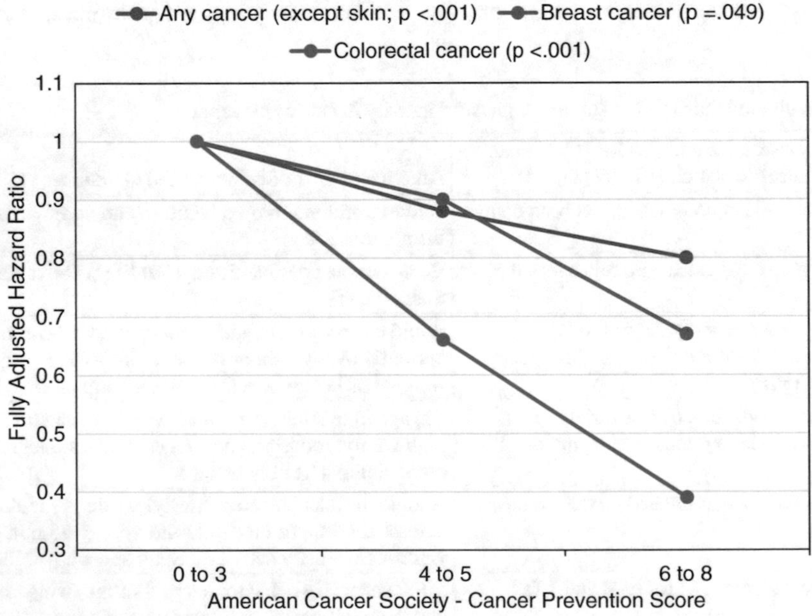

Fig. 20.2 For postmenopausal cancer mortality, the effect of American Cancer Society (ACS) cancer prevention score based on adherence to nutrition and physical activity guidelines from the US Women's Health Initiative (adapted from [15])

of 0–4 for each component with higher values indicating healthier behaviors) on postmenopausal BC risk [16]. This EPIC study (242,918 postmenopausal women; mean baseline age 53 years; median 10.9 years of follow-up) found that each 1 point increase in HLIS lowered BC risk by 3% [16]. The effect of increased HLIS score on BC risk in all women is summarized in Fig. 20.3. Also, the higher specific lifestyle scores are associated with reduced risk of

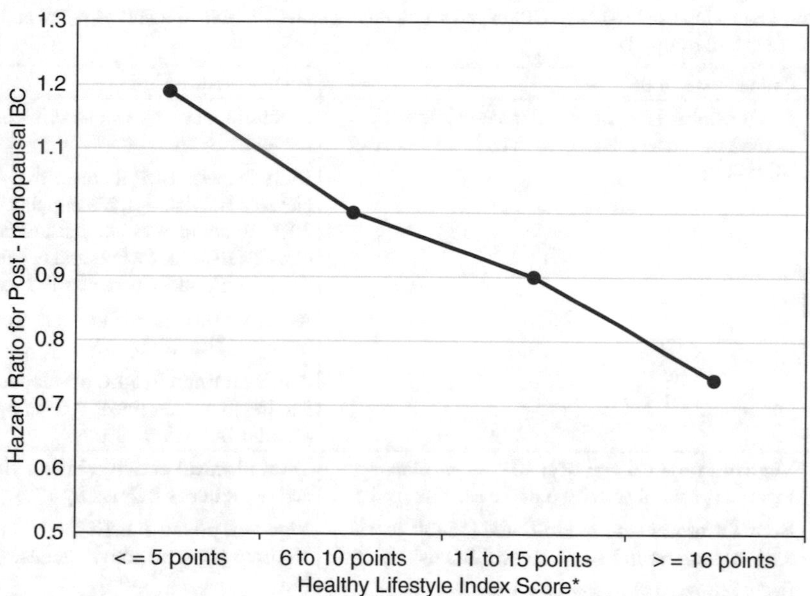

Fig. 20.3 Association between Healthy Lifestyle Index Score (HLIS) and post-menopausal breast cancer (BC) risk from the EPIC cohort study including 242,918 women; median 10.9 years of follow-up (p-trend <0.001; multivariate adjusted) (adapted from [16]). * HLIS was constructed from five factors (diet, physical activity, smoking, alcohol consumption and anthropometry) by assigning scores of 0–4 to categories of each component, for which higher values indicate healthier behaviors

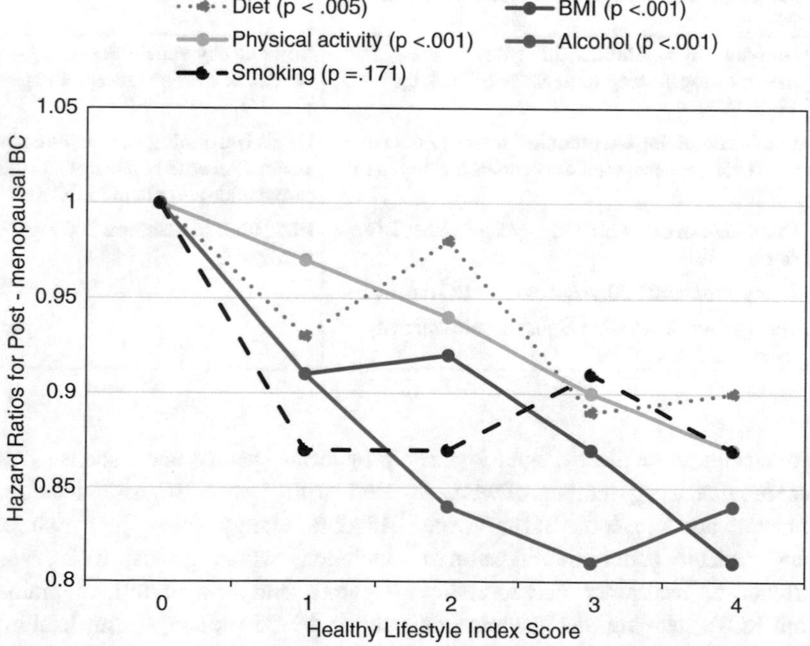

Fig. 20.4 Association between Healthy Lifestyle Index Score (HLIS) and post-menopausal breast cancer (BC) risk from EPIC cohort study including 242,918 women; median 10.9 years of follow-up (adapted from [16])

developing BC among postmenopausal women (Fig. 20.4). Table 20.2 provides a summary of the overall findings on the effects of diet, nutrition, physical activity and BC risk in premenopausal and postmenopausal women based on the 2017 CUP Breast Cancer Systematic Literature Review and the CUP Expert Panel discussions in June 2016 [2].

Table 20.2 Continuous Update Project (CUP) expert panel findings on diet, nutrition and physical activity and breast cancer (BC) risk (adapted from [2])

Evidence	Premenopausal BC	Postmenopausal BC
Convincing	**Adult attained height**: developmental factors leading to greater linear growth by 5 cm increases BC risk by 6%	**Alcoholic beverages:** one drink or 10 g alcohol increases BC risk by 9% **Body fatness**: BMI increase by 5 kg/m^2 elevates BC risk by 12% and mortality risk by 20%, 10 cm increase in waist circumference elevates BC risk by 6%, and 0.1-unit higher waist-to-hip ratio increases BC risk by 10% **Adult weight gain**: 5 kg body weight gain increases BC risk by 6% **Adult attained height**: developmental factors leading to greater linear growth by 5 cm elevates BC risk by 8%
Probable	**Vigorous physical activity:** 30 minutes of daily vigorous physical activity reduces BC risk by 9% **Body fatness in young adulthood (18–30 years):** 5 kg/m^2 increase in BMI decreases BC risk by 18% **Body fatness (before menopause)**: BMI increase by 5 kg/m^2 reduces BC risk by 7%, 10 cm increased in waist circumference by 10 cm or 0.1unit increased waist-to-hip ratio is not associated with BC risk **Alcoholic beverages:** one drink or 10 g alcohol/day increases BC risk by 5%. **Lactation**: 5 months duration reduces BC risk by 2%	**Total physical activity:** higher physical activity reduces BC risk by 13% **Vigorous physical activity:** 30 minutes/day of vigorous physical activity reduces BC risk by 6% **Body fatness in young adulthood (18–30 years):** BMI increase by 5 kg/m^2 decreases BC risk by 18% **Lactation**: 5 months duration reduces BC risk by 2%
Suggestive	**Non-starchy vegetables:** 200 g/day decreases the risk of estrogen receptor negative BC risk by 18–21% **Foods containing carotenoids**: inverse association with beta-carotene, total carotenoids and lutein in BC risk **Diets high in calcium**: 300 mg/day reduces BC risk by 13% **Dairy Products**: 200 g/day reduces BC risk by 5% **Total physical activity:** higher physical activity reduces BC risk by 7%	**Non-starchy vegetables:** 200 g/day decreases the risk of estrogen receptor negative BC by 18–21% **Foods containing carotenoids**: inverse association with beta-carotene, total carotenoids and lutein in BC risk **Diets high in calcium**: 300 mg/day reduces BC risk by 4%

With improvements in medical diagnosis and treatment, there are increasing numbers of women with BC risk factors and long-term BC survivors who are looking at dietary pattern modification to prevent occurrence or recurrence and mortality [17]. Data from RCTs studying diet, exercise, or combined diet and exercise interventions show that the most consistent findings are that reductions in adiposity, and maintaining or gain of skeletal muscle had the most beneficial protective effects on BC outcomes, including survival, risk of recurrence, or biomarkers associated with prognosis. Dietary and exercise patterns associated with lower BC risk include: diets with 45–65% energy from fiber rich carbohydrates including whole grains, fruits, vegetables and legumes and low in refined grains and added sugar; 10–35% energy from healthy dietary fats low in saturated fats; and 10–35% energy from protein which is very low or devoid of processed meats, plus avoiding long periods of physical inactivity and including 150 minutes/week of moderate intensity aerobic activity or 75 minutes/week of vigorous activity and resistance exercise at least

2 days/week [17]. However, the relationship between dietary pattern and BC risk is complex with differences between pre- and postmenopausal women, including estrogen levels, BMI, dietary energy density, diet during adolescence, level of wine or other types of alcoholic beverage, and fiber intake are all examples of factors which can influence the effects of dietary pattern on BC risk, recurrence and survival. Unhealthy dietary patterns and obesity, especially among postmenopausal women, are associated with changes in biomarkers, such as insulin resistance, lipoproteins, estradiol, and micr obiota dysbiosis that are risk factors for BC and cardiovascular diseases [18]. A comparison of Western and Healthy dietary patterns characterizing food components and nutrients are summarized in Appendix A.

20.2.2 Noteworthy Factors

This section highlights some specific factors including elevated BMI in post-menopausal women or after BC diagnosis, ≥15 kg increase in body weight over 4 years, dietary energy density, adolesent and early adulthood diet, and wine and other alcoholic beverages, coffee consumption, and physical activity are related factors that may influence BC risk and survival.

20.2.2.1 Body Mass Index (BMI)

BMI levels outside the normal range in postmenopausal women and after BC diagnosis are associated with increased BC risk, recurrence and mortality [2, 10, 19–21]. A comprehensive systematic review and meta-analysis (82 observational studies; 213,075 BC survivors; 41,477 deaths with 23,182 from BC) demonstrated that higher BMI levels in BC survivors, especially in the obesity range, have unfavorable effects on overall BC risk and survival in both pre- and postmenopausal BC [19]. For each 5 kg/m^2 increment of BMI before, <12 months after, and ≥12 months after diagnosis, there is an increased BC mortality risk observed by 18%, 14%, and 29%, respectively. Another systematic review and meta-analysis (12 observational studies; 23,832 women) found that weight gain of >10% after BC diagnosis is associated with significantly higher all-cause mortality rates by 23% compared with maintaining body weight [20]. In contrast, a 2017 Kaiser Permanente study (12,590 stage I-III breast cancer patients; mean age 59 years) observed that compared to weight maintenance, ≥10% weight losses were associated with worse survival by 163% increase in all-cause mortality [21]. Also, increased waist circumference and waist to hip ratio have been associated with increased BC risk in postmenopausal women [2].

20.2.2.2 Weight Change Across the Lifespan

A review of Nurses' Health Studies findings on BC incidence and survival show a complex relationship between weight change and BC risk across the lifespan [10, 14]. Levels of body fatness in childhood and high BMI at age 18 years are inversely associated with adult plasma insulin-like growth factor 1 (IGF-1) levels, a hormone similar in molecular structure to insulin which plays an important role in childhood growth and continues to have anabolic effects in adults. Although higher BMI at age 18 years was inversely associated with both pre- and postmenopausal BC risk, weight gain after age 18 years was positively associated with risk after menopause, in those who never used hormone therapy (HT). In a subsequent analysis with 26 years of follow-up, it was observed that among women who never used HT, those who had lost more than 10 kilograms after menopause and maintained their weight loss had a lower risk of BC than women with stable weight since menopause. Short-term gain over 4 years by ≥15 lbs. was associated with higher BC risk in premenopausal than postmenopausal women compared to no weight change.

20.2.2.3 Dietary Energy Density

The intake of high dietary energy dense diets is associated with increased BC risk or high dense breast volume [22, 23]. The US Cancer Prevention Study II Nutrition Cohort (56,795 postmenopausal women; 11.7 years of follow-up) showed that high vs low dietary energy density (≥1.7 vs <1.2 kcal/g) significantly increased BC risk by 20% (p-trend = 0.03) independent of hormone receptor status, BMI, age or physical activity level [22]. Also, in premenopausal women each 1 kcal/g increase in dietary energy density is associated with a 26% increase in dense breast volume %, a potential risk factor of BC, after multivariate adjustment (p = 0.01) [23].

20.2.2.4 Adolescence and Early Adulthood

The Nurses' Health Study II found that diet quality during adolescence and early adulthood can influence BC risk in later adulthood [10, 24, 25]. A 2017 Nurses' Health Study (45,204 women; food frequency questionnaire in 1998 about their high school diet (HS-FFQ) and a FFQ in 1991 when they were ages 27–44 years; 22 years of follow-up; 1477 BC cases) found that an adolescent and early adulthood inflammatory dietary pattern characterized by sugar-sweetened and diet soft drinks, refined grains, red and processed meat, and margarine, and low intake of green leafy vegetables, cruciferous vegetables, and coffee, was associated with an increased incidence of premenopausal BC [24]. Women with a high inflammatory pattern score in adolescence and early adulthood had significantly increased risk for premenopausal BC by 35% and by 41% compared with women with healthy low inflammatory diets. This increased risk did not extend to postmenopausal BC and was not significantly different by hormone receptor subtype. A 2016 Nurses' Health Study (45,204 women who completed a 124-item food frequency questionnaire about their high-school diet; 22 years of follow-up; 863 cases of premenopausal BC and 614 cases of postmenopausal BC) showed those consuming the highest quintile of the prudent dietary pattern, characterized by high intake of vegetables, fruits, legumes, fish and poultry, had a 16% lower risk of premenopausal BC (p-trend = 0.07) compared with the lowest quintile [25].

20.2.2.5 Wine and Overall Alcohol Consumption

Low intake of wine or other alcoholic beverages may be protective against BC risk or mortality [26–29]. For wine, a 2016 meta-analysis (8 case-control and 18 cohort studies; 21,149 cases) found a 36% increase in BC risk for highest vs lowest intake with a non-linear dose response showing a protective effect threshold for up-to 1 glass of wine/day above which there was a 0.6% increase in BC risk for each additional g of alcohol/day [26]. A 2008 meta-analysis (dose-response analysis including 4 cohorts and 12 case-control studies) showed that an increase in alcohol consumption of 10 g ethanol/day was associated with statistically significant increased BC risk for hormone receptor positive women by 7–15% [27]. A 2014 meta-analysis (11 case-control studies) found that hormone receptor negative women diagnosed with BC with low to moderate alcohol consumption had a lower risk of BC-specific mortality [28]. The 2016 Danish Diet, Cancer and Health Study (21,523 postmenopausal women; 11 years of follow-up) found that increased alcohol consumption over a 5-year period resulted in increased BC risk and lower coronary heart disease risk compared to stable moderate alcohol intake [29].

20.2.2.6 Coffee

Coffee may impact risk of pre- and post-menopausal BC differently [30–32]. A dose response meta-analysis (37 published observational studies; 966,263 participants; 59,018 BC cases) found a linear dose-response relationship for BC risk with coffee and caffeine, with the risk of BC decreased by 2% (p = 0.05) for every 2 cups/day increment in coffee intake [30]. In subgroup analyses, higher coffee and caffeine intake by postmenopausal women significantly reduced BC risk by 6% and there was a significant 31% lower BC risk for BRCA mutation carriers with higher coffee consumption. A 2015 EPIC study of pre- and postmenopausal women (335,060 women; 11 years of follow-up; 1064 premenopausal BC cases and 9134 postmenopausal cases) found that higher coffee intake was associated with a significant 10% lower BC risk [31]. Caffeinated and decaffeinated coffee were not associated with premenopausal BC risk. A 2008 Nurses' Health Study (85,987 women; 22 years of follow-up; 5272 BC cases) observed no significant association between caffeinated and decaffeinated coffee consumption and BC risk [32]. However, a subgroup analysis showed that postmenopausal women with the highest intake of caffeine-containing beverages had a significant 12% lower BC risk.

20.2.2.7 Physical Activity

Physical inactivity increases postmenopausal and possibly premenopausal BC risk [10, 33]. A 2017 meta-analysis (101 observational studies) found that higher vs. lower levels of moderate-vigorous activity resulted in an approximately 20% lower risk of BC for both pre- and postmenopausal women [33]. Physical activity is postulated to decrease BC risk by lowering ovarian hormone levels. Nurses' Health Study analyses suggest women who reported participating in ≥7 hours of moderate or vigorous physical activity weekly had an 18% lower BC risk [10]. In follow-up analyses, the cumulative and recent physical activity of postmenopausal women were inversely associated with BC risk and among younger women lifetime physical activity was inversely associated with risk of premenopausal BC with a 33% risk reduction, comparing the most- with the least-active women. Also, Nurses Health studies indicate that physical activity is important for survival after breast cancer diagnosis [10]. For improved BC survival, benefits are observed for physical activity equivalent to walking 3–5 h weekly at an average pace or for those who follow the US recommendations of at least 30 min daily of moderate physical activity for at least 5 days weekly, independent of activity level before diagnosis.

20.3 Dietary Patterns

Nine systematic reviews and meta-analyses from observational studies and intervention trials provide insights on associations between diet quality and dietary patterns, and BC risk, recurrence and mortality (Table 20.3) [34–42].

Table 20.3 Summaries of systematic reviews and meta-analyses on dietary quality and dietary pattern studies and breast cancer (BC) risk, recurrence and mortality

Objective	Study details	Results
Systematic reviews and meta- and pooled analyses		
van den Brandt and Schulpen (2017). Investigate the relationship between adherence to the Mediterranean diet (MedDiet) and risk of postmenopausal BC (and estrogen/progesterone receptor subtypes) (The Netherlands Cohort Study and a meta-analysis) [34]	6 cohort studies plus a large cohort (62,573 women; baseline age 55–69 years; mean 20 years of follow-up; alternate MedDiet score excluding alcohol)	MedDiets were associated with lower BC risk for postmenopausal women by 6% and hormone receptor negative BC risk by 23–27% (highest vs. lowest adherence), which is important because of the relatively poor prognosis of these BC subtypes. The large cohort study found that high adherence to the MedDiet (excluding alcohol) lowered risk of estrogen receptor negative BC by 40% (p-trend = 0.032)
Bloomfield et al. (2016). Evaluate the association between the MedDiet with unrestricted fat intake and BC risk and total cancer mortality risk [35]	For total cancer mortality 28 cohort studies (2,262,786 participants; follow-up periods of 4–40 years); for BC incidence (13 observational studies including 3 cohort studies; 7152 subjects); and for Prevencion con Dieta Mediterranea (PREDIMED) RCT (4282 women; baseline age 60–80 years; MedDiets supplemented with extra virgin olive oil or nuts vs guidance for low fat diets; 4.8 years)	This meta-analysis showed that high adherence to MedDiets lowered pooled total cancer mortality by 14% and BC incidence risk by 4% PREDIMED trial found a significant lower BC risk by 57%, CVD events by 29%, and diabetes by 30% in the two higher fat MedDiets combined vs a lower fat control group
Pourmasoumi et al. (2016). Investigate the relationship between the Healthy Eating Index (HEI)/Alternative Healthy Eating Index (AHEI) and BC mortality or survival rates [36]	4 cohort studies; 9819 women; mean baseline age 56 years; mean 7.7 years of follow-up	This analysis showed no significant associations between adherence to these healthy eating indices and risk of BC mortality or survival among postmenopausal women

(continued)

Table 20.3 (continued)

Objective	Study details	Results
Wu et al. (2015). Summarize published Chinese data on the relationship between BC and healthy dietary quality factors [37]	21 case-control studies and 1 cohort study; 23,201 patients: 10,566 in the experimental group and 12,635 in the control group	This analysis showed significant lowering of BC risk with higher intake of vegetables by 23% and fruit and soy foods by 32% each
Xing et al. (2014). Review associations between post-diagnostic healthy low-fat dietary patterns and BC recurrence and all-cause mortality [38]	2 RCTs and one large multi-center prospective cohort study with 9966 BC patients; 5–7.3 years of follow-up	Post-diagnostic healthy "lower-fat dietary pattern" (with emphasis on increased fruit, vegetables and fiber intake) reduced BC recurrence risk by 23% ($p = 0.009$) and all-cause mortality by 17% ($p = 0.05$)
Liu et al. (2014). Evaluate associations between dietary quality factors and BC risk in Chinese women [39]	31 case-control studies and 2 cohort studies; 9299 cases and 11,413 controls	Consumption of both soy and fruit significantly reduced BC risk by 35% ($p < 0.001$) and 34% ($p < 0.001$), respectively. The consumption of vegetables lowered BC risk by 28% with significant heterogeneity
Farsinejad-Marj et al. (2015). Examine the association between MedDiet adherence and BC risk [40]	5 cohort and 3 case-control studies	All pooled results show that MedDiets were inversely associated with BC risk in pre- and postmenopausal women; however, prospective cohort study findings were inconsistent; and case-control study findings generally showed an inverse association between the MedDiet and pre- and postmenopausal BC risk
Albuquerque et al. (2013). Evaluate the association between dietary pattern quality and BC risk [41]	11 cohort studies and 15 case-control studies); 584,437 women; 28,962 BC cases	Dietary patterns characterized by vegetables, fruit, fish, and soy products, as well as dietary patterns designated as traditional MedDiet reduced BC risk whereas alcoholic patterns were associated with increased BC risk. Also, the Western diet was positively associated with BC risk but a majority of the studies had insignificant trends
Brennan et al. (2010). Clarify the relationship between dietary patterns and breast cancer risk [42]	39 case-control and cohort studies including prudent/healthy, Western, and drinker dietary patterns	The pooled higher vs lower adherence to: (1) prudent/healthy dietary patterns lowered BC risk by 11% ($p = 0.02$); (2) drinker dietary pattern cohorts increased BC risk by 21% ($p = 0.01$); and (3) Western/unhealthy dietary patterns increased BC risk by 9% ($p = 0.12$)

20.3.1 Systematic Reviews and Meta-analyses

20.3.1.1 Breast Cancer Risk

Mediterranean diet (MedDiet)

Recently the MedDiet pattern has been shown to be effective in reducing BC risk especially in postmenopausal women [34, 35, 40, 41]. A 2017 meta-analysis (7 cohort studies plus The Netherlands Cohort Study including 62,573 women; baseline age 55–69 years; mean 20 years of follow-up) found that high adherence to a MedDiet lowered BC risk in postmenopausal women [34]. The Netherlands cohort showed a statistically significant inverse association between MedDiet adherence and risk of estrogen receptor negative BC, with a 40% lower risk for high vs. low MedDiet adherence whereas there was a modest inverse trend for estrogen receptor positive or total BC risk (when excluding or limiting alcohol beverage consumption). Also, the meta-analysis found a 6% lower total postmenopausal BC risk for high vs. low MedDiet adherence and a 23–27% lower risk of hormone receptor negative BC, which may have important prevention implications because of the poorer prognosis of receptor negative BC subtypes. A 2016 meta-analysis (28 cohort studies on total cancer risk; >2 million women; 4–40 years of follow-up; 13 observational and 3 cohort studies for BC incidence; and 7152 subjects) found that higher adherence to the MedDiet reduced total cancer mortality by 14% and lowered BC incidence by 4%. The Prevencion con Dieta Mediterranea (PREDIMED) trial (7447 participants/4282 postmenopausal women; MedDiet supplemented with extra-virgin olive oil or tree nuts vs a low-fat control diet; 4.8 years of follow-up) showed that MedDiets reduced common chronic disease with aging including lowering BC risk by 57%, cardiovascular disease by 29% and type 2 diabetes by 30% compared to guidance of low-fat dietary intake [35]. Two other meta-analyses of observational studies also support a modest inverse relationship between the MedDiet and overall BC risk [41, 42].

Healthy vs Western Diets

High adherence to healthy dietary patterns rich in fruits, vegetables, fish and soy products protect against BC risk and adherence to Western dietary patterns tend to increase BC risk [37, 39, 41, 42]. A 2010 meta-analysis (39 case-control and cohort studies) found that healthy dietary patterns significantly reduced overall BC risk by 11%, whereas a high consumption of alcohol significantly increased BC risk by 21% and a Western diet increased BC risk by 9% ($p = 0.12$) [42]. Similar findings were observed in a 2013 meta-analysis (11 cohort studies and 15 case-control studies; 584,437 women) [41]. Two meta-analyses primarily of case-control studies in Chinese women found that diets rich in fruits and vegetables (emphasizing higher fiber intake) and soy products significantly lowered BC risk by approx. 30% [37, 39].

20.3.1.2 Breast Cancer Recurrence and All-Cause Mortality

Several meta-analyses of RCTs and cohort studies support the protective effects of healthy dietary patterns in lowering risk of BC recurrence or mortality [36, 38]. A 2014 meta-analysis (2 RCTs and one large multi-center prospective cohort study with 9966 BC patients; 5–7.3 years of follow-up) found that high adherence to a post-BC diagnostic healthy lower-fat dietary pattern (with emphasis on increased fruit, vegetables and fiber intake) significantly reduced risk of BC recurrence by 23% and all-cause mortality by 17% [38]. However, a meta-analysis (4 cohort studies; 9819 women; mean baseline age 56 years; 7.7 years of follow-up) showed that postmenopausal women with high adherence to the Healthy Eating Indices did not significantly lower BC mortality or increase survival. However, the studies are limited and heterogenous and in need of more and larger studies to confirm [36].

20.3.2 Prospective Cohort Studies

Thirteen cohort studies provide additional insight on the association between diet quality and specific dietary patterns, and BC risk, recurrence, and mortality (Table 20.4) [43–55].

20.3.2.1 Breast Cancer Risk

Western vs Healthy Dietary Patterns

Three prospective cohort studies show that Western diets increase BC risk and a range of healthy dietary patterns decrease BC risk [45, 52, 54]. The 2013 California Teachers Study (91,779 women; mean baseline age 50 years; 14 years of follow-up) found that a plant-based pattern was associated with a significant reduced BC risk by 15% (highest vs lowest intake) and an even greater significant 34% reduced BC risk for hormone receptor negative tumors [45]. In contrast, a high wine dietary pattern was associated with significant increased risk of hormone receptor positive BC risk by 29%. The 2010 UK Women's Cohort Study (35,372 women; mean baseline age 52 years; mean 9 years of follow-up) showed in postmenopausal women significantly lower BC risk dietary with patterns rich in fish by 40% and vegetarian diets by 15% compared to high red meat dietary patterns (Fig. 20.5) [52]. A 2009 French EPIC cohort (65,374 women; mean baseline age 53 years; 9.7 years of follow-up; 2381

Table 20.4 Summaries of prospective cohort studies on dietary quality and dietary patterns and breast cancer (BC) risk, recurrence and mortality

Prospective cohort studies		
Penniecook-Sawyers et al. (2016). Evaluate the association between vegetarian diets and BC risk (Adventist Health Study –2; US) [43]	50,404 women; mean baseline age 63 years; 7.8 years of follow-up; 26,193 vegetarians (multivariate adjusted)	As compared with non-vegetarians, all vegetarians combined had a 3% significant lower BC risk. However, vegans had a 22% lower BC risk (but still non-significant) compared with non-vegetarians (p = 0.09)
Hirko et al. (2016). Examine associations between dietary quality indices and breast cancer risk by molecular subtype among women (Nurses' Health Study (NHS) cohort; US) [44]	100,643 women; mean baseline age 54 years; 22 years of follow-up; 2372 BC cases that could be classified by molecular subtype; dietary quality scores for the alternative Healthy Eating Index (AHEI), alternate Mediterranean diet (aMED), and Dietary Approaches to Stop Hypertension (DASH) dietary patterns (multivariate adjusted)	A higher DASH diet pattern score or adherence was significantly associated with 56% reduced risk of HER2-type BC (p-trend = 0.02), which was primarily associated with increased fruit intake. There were no significant association between the other healthy diets and BC risk
Link et al. (2013). Evaluate dietary patterns and their relation to BC risk in a large cohort of women (California Teachers Study cohort; US) [45]	91,779 women; mean baseline age 50 years; 14 years of follow-up; 4140 BC cases (multivariate adjusted)	High adherence to healthy plant-based dietary patterns was associated with lower BC risk overall by 15% (p-trend = 0.003) and hormone receptor negative tumors by 34% (p-trend = 0.03). Additionally, a dietary pattern with high wine intake was associated with an increased risk of hormone receptor positive tumors by 29%
Couto et al. (2013). Investigate whether adherence to a MedDiet pattern influences BC risk (The Swedish Women's Lifestyle and Health cohort) [46]	44,840 women; baseline age range 30–49 years; 16 years of follow-up on average; 1278 BC cases (multivariate adjusted)	A 2-point increase in MedDiet score was not significantly associated with BC risk for either premenopausal or postmenopausal women
Buckland et al. (2013). Investigate the association between adherence to the alcohol restricted MedDiet and risk of BC (European Prospective Investigation into Cancer and Nutrition cohort study) [47]	335,062 women; 11 years of follow-up; 9009 postmenopausal and 1216 premenopausal first primary invasive BC were identified (multivariate adjusted)	High adherence to an alcohol restricted MedDiet was associated with a lower BC risk for all women by 6% (p = 0.048) and for postmenopausal women by 7% (p = 0.037). For postmenopausal women with hormone receptor negative tumors BC risk was reduced by 20%. In premenopausal women, the MedDiet score was not associated with BC risk
Vrieling et al. (2013). Examine the effect of pre-diagnostic dietary patterns with mortality and BC recurrence in postmenopausal BC survivors (the MARIE study; German) [48]	2522 postmenopausal BC patients; mean 5.5 years of follow-up; 316 deaths occurred, 235 due to BC and 81 due to non-BC causes (multivariate adjusted) Two major dietary patterns were identified: *healthy* (high intakes of vegetables, fruits, vegetable oil, and soups) and *unhealthy* (high intakes of red meat, processed meat, and deep-frying fat)	High adherence to an *unhealthy* dietary pattern was associated with an increased risk of non-BC mortality (highest vs lowest) by 269% (p-trend <0.001) but there were no significant associations with BC-specific mortality and BC recurrence. Adherence to the *healthy* dietary pattern was inversely associated with non-BC mortality by 26% (p-trend = 0.02) and 29% reduced BC recurrence (p-trend = 0.02) in stage I-IIIa patients

Table 20.4 (continued)

Prospective cohort studies		
Izano et al. (2013). Assess the effect of diet quality after BC diagnosis on BC survival (Nurses' Health Study; US) [49]	4103 women with invasive stage I–III BC; median length of follow-up was 112 months and maximum length of follow-up was 277 months; DASH diet score, and the Alternative Healthy Eating Index (AHEI)-2010; 981 women died, 453 BC deaths, 38 BC recurrences and 528 non-BC related deaths (multivariate adjusted)	Highest vs lowest adherence reduced non-BC mortality for the DASH diet by 28% (p-trend = 0.03) and AHEI-2010 diets by 43% (p-trend <0.0001). Diet scores were not significantly associated with BC mortality
Kim et al. (2011). Assess the associations between diet quality and postmenopausal BC survival (Nurses' Health Study; US) [50]	2729 postmenopausal women invasive stage I-III BC; up to 26 years of follow-up; 4 dietary quality scores: Alternative Healthy Eating Index, Diet Quality Index-Revised, Recommended Food Score, and the alternative MedDiet score (multivariate adjusted)	In postmenopausal women with low physical activity, the highest aMedDiet score was associated with lower non-BC mortality risk by 61% (p-trend = 0.0004). No other associations were observed between diet quality indices and either total or non-BC mortality
Fung et al. (2011). Examine the associations of the DASH score and low-carbohydrate diets on the risk of postmenopausal BC (Nurses' Health Study; US) [51]	86,621 women; baseline age 30–55 years; diet quality scores calculated from up to 7 food frequency questionnaires; 26 years of follow-up; 5522 BC cases (multivariate adjusted)	A higher DASH diet score was associated with a 20% reduced risk of estrogen receptor negative BC (p-trend = 0.02), which was largely explained by higher fruits and vegetables intake. Also, a higher vegetable-based, low-carbohydrate-diet score was associated with 19% lower risk of estrogen receptor negative BC (p- trend = 0.03)
Cade et al. (2010). Assess the relationship of 4 common dietary patterns to the risk of BC (UK Women's Cohort Study) [52]	35,372 women; aged between 35 and 69 years (mean baseline age 52 years); dietary patterns based on: fish; red meat intake; and vegetarian intake; mean 9 years of follow-up (multivariate adjusted)	In postmenopausal women, compared to high red meat diets, the higher fish diets significantly reduced BC risk by 40% and the vegetarian diet insignificantly reduced risk by 15% (Fig. 20.5)
Trichopoulou et al. (2010). Evaluate the effect of the traditional MedDiet in a Mediterranean country on BC risk (EPIC; Greece) [53]	14,807 women; average of 9.8 years of follow-up; 240 BC cases (multivariate adjusted)	For all women, every 2 points increase in traditional MedDiet score directionally lowered BC risk by 12%. In a subgroup analysis, postmenopausal women had a significantly lower BC risk by 22% for every 2 points increase in score but there was no effect on BC risk in premenopausal women (Fig. 20.6)
Cottet et al. (2009). Assess the association between postmenopausal dietary patterns and BC risk (EPIC -France) [54]	65,374 women; mean baseline age 53 years; 9.7 years of follow-up; 2381 postmenopausal BC cases (multivariate adjusted)	The MedDiet pattern was associated with lower BC risk by 15% (p-trend = 0.003) and a Western dietary pattern was associated with an increased BC risk by 20% (p-trend <0.007). Adherence to a diet comprising mostly of fruits, vegetables, fish, and olive or sunflower oil, along with avoidance of Western-type foods, may contribute to a substantial reduction in postmenopausal BC risk.

(continued)

Table 20.4 (continued)

Prospective cohort studies		
Kwan et al. (2009). Determine the association of dietary patterns on BC recurrence and mortality of early stage BC survivors (Life After Cancer Epidemiology Study; US) [55]	1901 women diagnosed with early-stage BC; mean baseline age 59 years; 2 dietary patterns were identified: prudent (high intakes of fruits, vegetables, whole grains, and poultry) and Western (high intakes of red and processed meats and refined grains); 6 years of follow-up; 268 BC recurrences and 226 all-cause deaths (multivariate adjusted)	High adherence to the prudent diet was associated with a significantly lower risk of non-BC mortality by 65% whereas high adherence to the Western diet significantly increased risk of non-BC mortality by 115% (Fig. 20.7). Neither dietary pattern was associated with risk of BC recurrence or BC mortality. These findings were independent of physical activity, overweight, or smoking

postmenopausal BC cases) found that Western dietary patterns significantly increased BC risk by 20% and a healthy MedDiet pattern significantly lowered BC risk by 15% [54].

Vegetarian Dietary Patterns

The only prospective study on vegetarian dietary patterns and BC in women is from the Adventist Health Study-2, which has rates of BC that are >20% lower than usual because of very low rates of tobacco and alcohol consumption, a wide diversity of dietary habits and overall good health [43]. Vegetarian diets are classified into four patterns (vegan, lacto-ovo-vegetarian, pesco-vegetarian, and semi-vegetarian). The US Adventist Health Study (50,404 women; mean baseline age 63 years; 7.8 years of follow-up; 26,193 vegetarians) found that compared with non-vegetarians, all vegetarians combined had an insignificantly 3% lower BC risk [43]. However, vegans had a 22% lower BC risk compared with non-vegetarians ($p = 0.09$).

Mediterranean Diet (MedDiet)

Of the four European, prospective cohort studies assessing the effect of adherence to MedDiets on BC risk, three show that higher adherence significantly reduced BC risk and one study found an insignificant effect on BC risk [46, 47, 53, 54]. A 2013 European Prospective Investigation into Cancer and Nutrition (EPIC) study (335,062 women; 11 years of follow-up; 9009 postmenopausal and 1216 premenopausal first primary invasive BC cases) found that high adherence to an alcohol restricted MedDiet significantly lowered BC risk in all women by 6% and in postmenopausal women by 7% compared to low adherence [47]. In postmenopausal hormone receptor negative women, the adherence to an alcohol restricted MedDiet significantly reduced BC risk by 20%. A 2010 Greek EPIC cohort (14,807 women; average of 9.8 years of follow-up) showed a significantly lowered BC risk among postmenopausal women by 22% for every 2 points increase in MedDiet score adherence compared to no effect on BC risk in premenopausal women per 2 point MedDiet score increase (Fig. 20.6) [53]. A 2009 French EPIC cohort (65,374 women; mean baseline age 53 years; 9.7 years of follow-up; 2381 postmenopausal BC cases) found that for postmenopausal women the MedDiet significantly lowered BC risk by 15% and Western dietary patterns significantly increased BC risk by 20% [54]. Adherence to a diet comprising mostly of fruits, vegetables, fish, and olive and sunflower oil, along with minimizing or avoiding Western-type foods, such as processed meats, French fries, appetizers, cakes and pies may contribute to a substantial reduction in postmenopausal BC risk. The 2013 Swedish Women's Lifestyle and Health study (44,840 women; baseline age range 30–49 years; 16 years of follow-up on average) found, in this cohort of relatively young women, that adherence to the MedDiet pattern was not statistically significantly associated with reduced risk of BC overall, especially when alcohol was excluded [46].

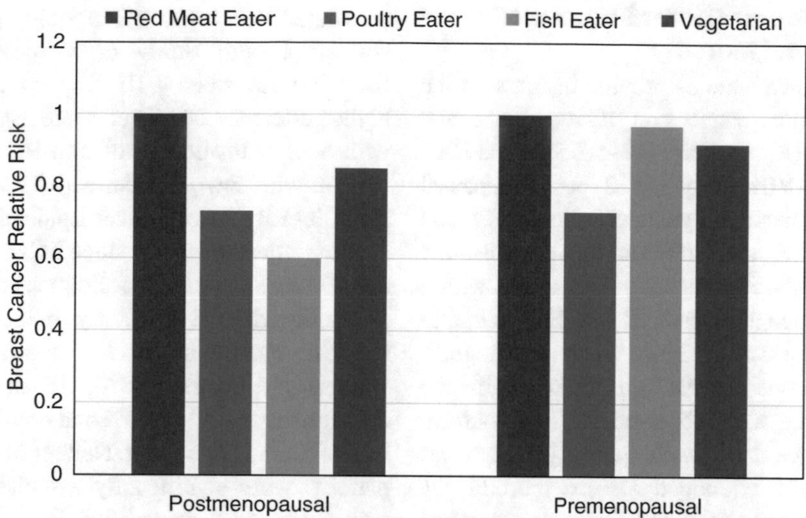

Fig. 20.5 Association between dietary pattern type and postmenopausal vs premenopausal breast cancer (BC) risk from the UK Women's Cohort Study (post-menopausal fish eater risk P < 0.05 after multivariate adjustment) (adapted from [52])

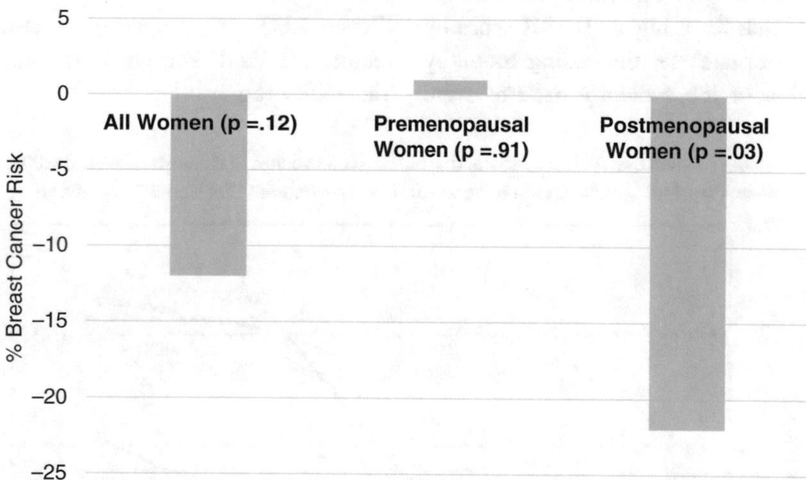

Fig. 20.6 Adherence to the Mediterranean diet (MedDiet) on breast cancer risk from the Greek European Prospective Investigation into Cancer and Nutrition (EPIC) Study (adapted from [53])

Dietary Approaches to Stop Hypertension (DASH) Diet

Two prospective studies observed that high adherence to a DASH dietary pattern can reduce the risk of BC [44, 51]. A 2016 Nurses' Health Study (100,643 women; 22 years of follow-up) observed a significant 56% reduced risk of HER2-type BC among women with a high adherence to the DASH dietary pattern, which was primarily associated with higher fruit intake [44]. Also, a 2011 Nurses' Health Study (86,621 women; baseline age 30–55 years; 26 years of follow-up) observed that a higher DASH score significantly lowered estrogen receptor negative multivariate BC risk by 20% [51].

20.3.2.2 Breast Cancer Recurrence and Morality

Four prospective studies provide insights on the effects of dietary patterns on BC recurrence, and BC and non-BC mortality [48–50, 55]. The 2013 German MARIE study (2522 postmenopausal BC patients; mean 5.5 years of follow-up) found that increasing consumption of an *unhealthy* (Western) dietary pattern was associated with a significant increased risk of non-BC mortality (highest vs lowest) by 269% whereas no significant associations with BC-specific mortality and BC recurrence were observed [48]. In contrast, high adherence to the *healthy* dietary pattern was associated with a reduced non-BC mortality by 26% (highest vs lowest) and 29% reduced risk of BC recurrence in stage I-IIIa patients. A 2013 Nurses' Health Study (4103 women with invasive stage I–III breast cancer; median length of follow-up was 112 months and maximum length of follow-up was 277 months) found a significant lower non-BC risk for a higher DASH score by 28% and an Alternate Healthy Eating Index by 43% but neither of these dietary patterns were associated with lower BC mortality [49]. A 2011 Nurses' Health Study (2729 postmenopausal women with stage I-III BC) observed that a higher alternate MedDiet score was associated with a 61% lower risk of non-BC mortality in women with low physical activity [50]. Finally, the 2009 Life After Cancer Epidemiology Study (1901 women with early stage BC; mean baseline age 59 years; 6 years of follow-up) observed that a healthy diet significantly reduced all-cause mortality by 43% and non-BC mortality by 65%, whereas a Western diet significantly increased all-cause mortality by 53% and non-BC mortality by 115% (Fig. 20.7) [55]. Neither of these dietary patterns were significantly associated with BC recurrence or BC mortality risk.

20.3.3 Randomized Controlled Trials (RCTs)

Eleven RCTs on dietary patterns and BC risk, recurrence and survival are summarized in Table 20.5 [56–66].

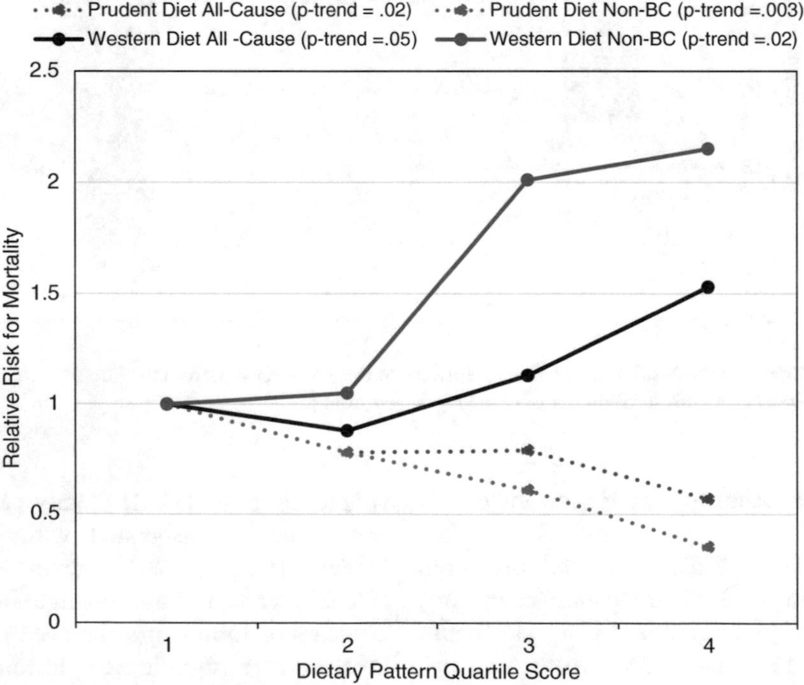

Fig. 20.7 Association between dietary pattern score and all-cause mortality and non-breast cancer (BC) mortality in 1901 postmenopausal women with early stage breast cancer (adapted from [55])

Table 20.5 Summaries of RCTs on dietary patterns and breast cancer (BC) risk recurrence and mortality

Rock et al. (2016). Examine the effects of diet composition on weight loss and BC risk biomarkers [56]	**Parallel RCT**: 245 non-diabetic, overweight/obese women; mean age 50 years; diets: lower fat (20% energy), higher carbohydrate (65% energy); a lower carbohydrate (45% energy), higher fat (35% energy); or a walnut-rich (18% energy) higher fat (35% energy), lower carbohydrate (45% energy); 1 year	All groups had significant mean weight loss after 1 year; the lower fat diet by 9.2%, lower carbohydrate by 6.5%, and walnut-rich diet by 8.2% ($p < 0.0001$). Subgroup analysis showed that insulin sensitive women lost more weight on the lower fat vs. lower carbohydrate group (7.5 kg vs. 4.3 kg; $p = 0.06$), and in the walnut-rich vs. lower carbohydrate group (8.1 kg vs. 4.3 kg; $p = 0.04$). Sex hormone binding globulin, associated with a reduced BC risk, increased within each group except for the lower carbohydrate group ($p < 0.01$). Also, hs-CRP and IL-6 decreased at follow-up in all groups ($p < 0.01$)
Neuhouser et al. (2015). Investigate effect of overweight and obese BMI on BC risk in postmenopausal women (Women's Health Initiative (WHI); US) [57]	**Multi-center Parallel RCT**: 67,142 postmenopausal women aged 50–79 years were enrolled from 1993–1998 with a median of 13 years of follow-up; 40 U.S. clinical centers; 3388 BC cases	Postmenopausal women with overweight and obese BMIs had an increased BC risk compared to normal weight BMI women. Obesity grade 2 and 3 was associated with higher risk for advanced disease including larger tumor size by 112%, positive lymph nodes by 89%, and mortality after BC by 111%. Women with baseline BMI <25 who gained >5% of body weight over the follow-up period had an increased BC risk by 36%
Toledo et al. (2015). Evaluate the effect of 2 interventions with MedDiet vs the advice to follow a low-fat diet (control) on BC incidence (PREDIMED trial; Spain) [58]	**Parallel RCT**: 4282 postmenopausal women; baseline age 68 years; mean BMI 30; < 3% used hormone therapy; median follow-up of 4.8 years; 35 malignant BC cases	The multivariable-adjusted BC risk reduction for the MedDiet with extra-virgin olive oil was 68% ($p = 0.02$) and 41% for the MedDiet with nuts ($p = 0.24$) vs low-fat control. Also, for each additional 5% of energy from extra-virgin olive oil BC risk was reduced by 28%
Martin et al. (2011). Assess the effect of low-fat and high-carbohydrate diets on BC incidence in women at increased risk (Canadian Diet and Breast Cancer Prevention Study) [59]	**Parallel RCT:** 4690 women with elevated mammographic density; mean baseline age 47 years; most were Caucasian and premenopausal at baseline; intervention group received intensive dietary counseling to reduce fat and increase carbohydrate to 65% of calories; average study duration 10 years	The lower dietary fat group (20% energy from fat) had a 19% increased BC risk in women with elevated mammographic breast density compared to a control group (30% energy from fat)

(continued)

Table 20.5 (continued)

Pierce et al. (2009). Secondary analysis of the baseline quartiles of fiber, fiber to fat ratio and vegetable-fruit intake effects in the hot flash negative BC survivor subgroup (Women's Healthy Eating and Living (WHEL) Study; US) [60]	**Multi-center Parallel RCT**: 896 peri and postmenopausal early-stage BC survivors without hot flashes at baseline (1/3 of total trial population); 1 and 4 years; intervention increased servings of vegetables and fruit daily, higher fiber, and lower energy from fat vs 5-a-day diet	The greatest effect on lowering additional BC events occurred among women who were already eating significant amounts of vegetables, fruits, and fiber at baseline rather than the degree of intervention dietary change that was achieved. Hot flash negative BC survivors with the highest of baseline quartiles of fiber, fiber to fat ratio and vegetable-fruit intake had significantly fewer BC recurrence events for 1 and 4 years. For example, after 1 year, the highest baseline fiber consumers (mean 32 g fiber/day) had a 36% lower risk of BC recurrence compared to those with lower fiber intake (mean 12 g/day), which suggests that higher fiber intake may help to attenuate systemic circulating estrogen levels in this peri- and postmenopausal population ($p = 0.02$). After 4-years, there were fewer BC events observed across quartiles of vegetable-fruit and fiber consumption compared to the control group ($p = 0.01$)
Gold et al. (2008). Secondary evaluation of the effect of a low-fat diet high in vegetables, fruit, and fiber on the prognosis of BC survivors with hot flashes or without hot flashes at baseline (WHEL Study; US) [61]	**Multi-center Parallel RCT**: 2967 BC survivors; age 18–70 years; 900 women (30%) in the hot flash-negative group; 7.3-years duration; intervention increased intake of vegetable and fruit servings per day (10 vs 6.5 servings/day), fiber (25.5 vs 19.4 g/day), and reduced percent energy from fat (26.9% vs 31.3%) vs 5-a-day diet	Peri- and postmenopausal women without hot flashes at baseline assigned to the intervention had 31% fewer BC events than those assigned to the 5-a-day control group ($p = 0.02$). These effects may be related to fiber's attenuating effects on circulating estrogen concentrations
Pierce et al. (2007). Assess effects of increased vegetable, fruit, and fiber intake above the 5-a-day recommendations along with reduced fat intake on BC recurrence and all-cause mortality among women with previously treated early stage BC (WHEL; US) [62]	**Multi-center Parallel RCT**: 3088 women; mean baseline age 53 years; mean 7.3-year follow-up; the intervention group achieved and maintained the following dietary changes vs. the 5-a-day fruit and vegetable group through 4 years: higher servings of vegetables by 65%, fruit by 25%, and fiber by 30%, and lower energy intake from fat by 13%	Women in the intervention group had an insignificant lower BC event risk by 4% and lower mortality risk 9% compared to the control group
Prentice et al. (2006). Examine the effects of a healthy low-fat dietary pattern on BC incidence (WHI; US) [63]	**Multi-center Parallel RCT**: 48,835 postmenopausal women, baseline age 50–79 years, without prior breast cancer, including 19% minority race/ethnicity; 40 US clinical sites; intervention diet goals to reduce intake of total fat to 20% of energy and increase intake of vegetables and fruit to at least 5 servings daily and grains to at least 6 servings daily; comparison group participants were not asked to make dietary changes; average duration of 8.1 years	Among postmenopausal women, a low-fat, and higher fruit, vegetable, and whole-grains dietary pattern insignificantly lowered BC risk by 9% compared with women in the control group. Secondary analyses provided greater evidence of BC risk reduction among women having a high-fat diet at baseline

Table 20.5 (continued)

Chlebowski et al. (2006). Evaluate the effect of a healthier dietary intervention significantly lower in dietary fat and energy, and higher in total fiber from fruits and vegetables on prolonged relapse-free survival in women with resected BC (The Women's Intervention Nutrition Study [WINS]; US) [64]	**Phase III Multicenter RCT:** 2437 postmenopausal women with resected, early-stage BC receiving conventional cancer management; median 60-month follow-up; dietary change: fat (33.3 vs 51.3 g/day), daily energy (1460 vs 1531 kcal/day) and total fiber (19.5 vs 17.3 g/day); weight loss 2.3 kg	This dietary intervention rich in fruit and vegetables and lower in dietary fat significantly prolonged BC relapse free survival compared with the control group by 24% ($p = 0.034$). The dietary intervention improved relapse-free survival in women with estrogen receptor negative BC by reducing mortality risk by 42%
Rock et al. (2004). Assess the effects of post-BC diagnosis dietary modifications including increased fruit, vegetables, and fiber on estrogen levels (WHEL study; US) [65]	**Multi-center Parallel RCT**: 291 women with BC history; mean age 55 years; mean BMI 27; dietary goals for the intervention group were increased total fiber, vegetable, and fruit intakes and reduced fat intake; 1 year The intervention group had lower intake of energy from fat (21% vs 28%), higher total fiber intake from fruits and vegetables (29 g/d vs 22 g/day) ($p < 0.001$), and mean weight loss of 1 kg	The higher total fiber intervention group had significantly lower circulatory estradiol concentration after 1 year by 16 pmol/L vs the control group ($p = 0.05$). Change in total fiber (but not fat) intake was significantly and independently related to estradiol levels, which may play a role in lowering the risk of BC recurrence
Rock et al. (2001). Evaluate the effect of a low-fat diet and advice for increased fruits and vegetables on weight change in women after BC diagnosis (WHEL Study; US) [66]	**Multi-center Parallel RCT**: 1010 women with BC history; mean age 54 years; diet intervention was performed by telephone counseling and promoting a low-fat diet that also was high in fiber, vegetables, and fruit intake vs general dietary guidelines to reduce disease risk (control); weight at baseline and 12 months	After 1 year, the general guidance group lost slightly more weight by 0.42 kg compared to the low-fat intervention group. For the total group, body weight was stable in 74% of the subjects with 11% losing weight and 15% gaining weight (which was similar for both groups). The low-fat diet intervention was not associated with significant weight loss in mid-aged women at risk for BC recurrence

20.3.3.1 Breast Cancer Risk, Recurrence and Survival

Obesity

Approximately two-thirds of US and Western countries' women are overweight or obese, placing them at increased risk for postmenopausal BC. A 2015 analysis of the US Women's Health Initiative (WHI) Multicenter Trials (67,142 postmenopausal women aged 50–79 years; median of 13 years of follow-up; 40 U.S. clinical centers; 3388 BC cases) showed that overweight and obese postmenopausal women had an increased BC risk vs normal weight women [57]. Obesity grade 2 + 3 was also associated with significantly higher risk for advanced disease including larger tumor size by 112%, positive lymph nodes by 89%, and mortality after BC by 111%. Women with baseline BMI <25.0 who gained >5% of body weight over the follow-up period had an increased BC risk by 36%, but among women already overweight or obese there was no association of weight change (gain or loss) with BC during follow-up. There was no modification effect of the BMI-BC relationship by postmenopausal hormone therapy and the direction of association across BMI categories was similar for never, past and current hormone therapy use.

Weight Loss

Two RCTs demonstrate that both low-fat and higher fat dietary patterns can promote weight loss, a critical factor in reducing chronic inflammation and BC risk and progression [56, 66]. In both pre- and postmenpausal women (245 non-diabetic, overweight/obese women; mean age 50 years; 3 diets: lower fat diet; a lower carbohydrate diet; or a walnut-rich diet; 1 year) found that all groups had significant mean percent weight loss of 9.2% in the lower fat diet, 6.5% in the lower carbohydrate diet, and 8.2% in the walnut-rich diet at 12 months regardless of dietary fat level [56]. C-reactive protein and interleukin-6 decreased at follow-up in all groups ($p < 0.01$). A 2001 Women's Healthy Eating and Living (WHEL) Trial (1010 women after BC diagnosis; diet intervention was performed by telephone counseling and promoted a low-fat high in fiber, vegetables, and fruit diet vs general health dietary guidance; 12-months) found that the general dietary guidance (without a focus on low-fat) reduced baseline body weight by 0.42 kg more than the healthy low-fat diet intervention [66].

Mediterranean Diet (MedDiet)

A 2015 Spanish PREDIMED Trial (4282 postmenopausal women; baseline age 68 years; mean BMI 30; < 3% used hormone therapy; 2 interventions on MedDiets supplemented with either extra virgin olive oil or mixed nuts compared to advice to follow a low-fat diet (control); median follow-up of 4.8 years) showed that the MedDiet with extra virgin olive oil significantly lowered BC risk by 68% and the MedDiet with nuts lowered BC risk by 41% vs the low-fat control [58]. Also, each additional 5% of energy from extra virgin olive oil reduced BC risk by 28%.

Healthy, Low Fat Diets

Four RCTs show that lower fat diets inconsistently lower BC risk in postmenopausal women and may increase risk, especially in women with elevated mammographic breast density [59, 62–64]. The 2011 Canadian Diet and Breast Cancer Prevention Study (4690 women with elevated mammographic density; mean baseline age 47 years; most were Caucasian and premenopausal at baseline; intervention group received intensive dietary counseling to reduce fat intake to a target of 15% of calories and increase carbohydrate to 65% of calories; average of 10 years of duration) demonstrated that the lower fat diet increased BC risk by 19% in women with elevated mammographic breast density [62]. The 2007 WHEL Trial (3088 women; mean baseline age 53 years; guidance for higher vegetables and fruit, and fiber intake, and lower energy intake from fat vs. the 5-a-day fruit and vegetable control group without guidance for low fat; mean 7.3-years of follow-up) found that women in the intervention group had an insignificant 4% lower BC event risk ($p = 0.63$) and a 9% lower mortality risk ($p = 0.43$) compared to the 5-a-day control group [62]. The US WHI multi-center trial (48,835 postmenopausal women; baseline age 50–79 years; average 8.1 years of follow-up) showed that women consuming a low-fat, healthy fruit, vegetable, and whole-grains rich dietary pattern insignificantly lowered BC risk by 9% compared with those in the control group [63]. Secondary analyses of this trial indicated that women with high-fat diets at baseline had lower BC risk. The 2006 Women's Intervention Nutrition Study (WINS) (2437 women with BC; 60 months) found that lower energy intake (combination of low-dietary fat and higher fiber) and an average weight loss of 2.3 kg significantly improved overall BC survival by 24% and estrogen receptor negative BC risk by 42% compared to the control diet [64].

Menopause Hot Flash Status

Three RCTs indicate that increased fiber intake helps to protect against BC recurrence, especially in women without menopause associated hot flashes [60, 61, 65]. A 2004 WHEL sub-trial (291 women with a history of BC; mean age 55 years; reduced fat, increased fruits and vegetables plus fiber; 1 year) found weight loss of 1 kg vs control diet, and significant reduced estrogen concentrations associated with higher fiber intake [65]. A 2009 secondary analysis of the WHEL Study (896 early stage BC survivors with no hot flashes; 1 and 4 years) found that hot flash negative BC survivors with the highest baseline intake quartiles of fiber, fiber to fat ratio, and vegetable and fruit intake had significantly fewer BC recurrence events after 1 and 4 years [60]. For example, after 1 year, the highest baseline fiber consumer (mean 32 g fiber/day) had a 36% lower risk of BC recurrence compared to those with lower fiber intake (mean 12 g/day), which suggests that higher fiber intake may help to attenuate systemic circulating estrogen levels in peri - and postmenopausal women. Similar findings were observed in another WHEL Study secondary evaluation (2967 BC survivors; 900 hot flash-negative women or 30% of population; 7.3-years duration) which found that peri- and postmenopausal women without hot flashes at baseline assigned to the intervention had significantly fewer BC events by 31% than those assigned to the control group [61].

20.4 Nutrients and Phytochemicals

The nutritional and phytochemical compositions of whole plant foods are summarized in Appendix B. The effects on BC risk with specific bioactive nutritional and phytochemical components of whole plant foods is reviewed in this section.

20.4.1 Dietary Nutrients

The effects of dietary fiber, fat and vitamins on BC risk, recurrence, and survival are summarized in Table 20.6.

20.4.1.1 Dietary Fiber

There are a number of potential biological mechanisms supporting a role for fiber in the prevention, recurrence and survival of BC, especially in postmenopausal women by attenuating systemic estrogen levels, body weight and abdominal fat; and lowering insulin resistance, and circulating C-reactive protein (CRP) (Fig. 20.8) [2, 3, 17]. In postmenopausal women, adequate fiber intake has been hypothesized to protect against BC incidence by decreasing the rate of estrogen (produced from fat cells) recirculation by binding estrogen and increasing its excretion in the feces. The relationship between circulating estrogen levels and BC risk is complex involving BMI, menopausal status, diet during adolescence and estrogen-only hormone replacement therapy. The US Women's Health Trial found that weight loss, especially of abdominal adipose tissue, and healthier dietary patterns with higher fiber to energy intake ratios can lower systemic estrogen and estrogen metabolites levels in postmenopausal women to lower BC risk [18]. The Finnish Diabetes Prevention Trial (522 obese adults; mean baseline age 55 years and BMI 31; 2/3 women; 3 years) found that high fiber, lower fat and lower energy density diets are significant predictors of weight loss (Fig. 20.9) [67]. Fiber intake is a major short-fall 'nutrient', especially in highly developed countries such as the US with high energy dense diets where <5% of the populations consume adequate fiber with the mean fiber intake at only about half of the recommended level [68, 69]. The systematic reviews and meta-analyses and prospective cohort studies on the effects of increased fiber intake on BC risk, recurrence and survival are summarized in Table 20.6 [70–83].

Systematic Reviews and Meta- and Pooled Analyses

Several meta-analyses of prospective studies and RCTs generally demonstrate that increased fiber intake has a role in reducing BC risk [70–73]. A 2016 meta-analysis (20 cohort and 4 case-control studies; 3,662,421 participants; 51,939 BC cases; 1–20-year follow-up) showed that in postmenopausal women the highest total fiber intake significantly reduced BC risk by 12% compared to the lowest intake [70]. Three meta-analyses of prospective studies show a clear inverse association between increased fiber intake and BC risk with 10 g of total fiber significantly reducing BC risk by 4–7% [70, 72, 73]. For fiber-sub-types, the dose-response analyses per 10 g show a lower BC risk for soluble fiber by 9%, for insoluble fiber by 5%, and for fruit and cereal fiber by 4–5% [72]. The BC risk reducing effects were only significant in studies with higher total fiber intake increased by ≥13–15 g/day vs

Table 20.6 Summaries of dietary fiber, fat, protein, folate and antioxidant vitamin studies on breast cancer (BC) risk, recurrence and mortality

Objective	Study details	Results
Dietary fiber		
Systematic reviews and meta- and pooled analyses		
Chen et al. (2016). Update previous meta-analysis on the effectiveness of total fiber intake on BC risk [70]	20 cohort and 4 case-control studies up to March 2016; 3,662,421 participants; 51,939 cases; US, Canada, Europe, China, and Malaysia; 1–20-year follow-up	Highest vs lowest total fiber intake significantly reduced BC risk by 12%, particularly in postmenopausal women (p = 0.027). Dose-response analysis found that every 10-g total fiber intake was associated with a 4% reduction in BC risk (p < 0.002)
Xing et al. (2014). Evaluate the pooled association between diets lower in fat, and higher in fruits, vegetables, and fiber and breast cancer (BC) recurrence and survival by meta-analysis [71]	2 RCTs: 5525 women wit h BC (1) Women's Intervention Nutrition Study (WINS); 2437 women; median 60 months of duration and (2) Women's Healthy Eating and Living (WHEL) study; 3088 women; mean 7.3 years; plus, Collaborative Women's Longevity Study, a large multi-center prospective cohort study with 4441 BC patients for 5.5-year follow-up	This meta-analysis of the pooled data from 2 large RCTs and one large prospective study found that post-diagnostic diets lower in fat, and higher in fruits and vegetables and fiber reduced the risk of BC recurrence by 23% (p = 0.009) and BC related mortality by 17% (p = 0.05)
Aune et al. (2012). Assess the pooled association between total fiber and specific fiber source intake and BC risk by systematic review and dose-response meta-analysis [72]	16 cohort studies, 500,000–1,000,000 participants; 15,000–26,000 BC cases up to August 2011	This analysis found an overall 7% lower BC risk for higher total fiber intake but significant risk reduction was only observed among studies with an increased intake of fiber by 15.8 g or mean total fiber intake of 29.4 g/day. Dose-response analyses showed per 10 g lowered BC risk for total fiber by 5%, soluble fiber by 9%, insoluble fiber by 5%, fruit fiber by 5%, and cereal fiber by 4% but only 1% for vegetable fiber
Dong et al. (2011). Examine the association between total fiber intake and risk of BC by conducting a meta-analysis of prospective cohort studies [73]	10 cohort studies through January 2011; 712,195 participants; 16,848 BC cases; North America, Europe, and China; studies with both premenopausal women, postmenopausal women, both; follow-up period ranged from 4.3–18 years, with a median of 8 years	For all women, increasing total fiber intake by15 g/day significant lowered BC risk by 11%. Dose-response analysis found a significant 7% reduction in BC risk for every 10 g/day increment of fiber intake (p-trend = 0.004) based on 6 of the studies with no evidence of heterogeneity
Prospective Studies		
Farvid et al. (2016). Evaluate fiber intake during adolescence and early adulthood in relation to BC risk (The Nurses' Health Study II; US) [74]	90,534 women; mean baseline age 36.4 years; 20 year-follow-up; 2833women were diagnosed with BC; 44,263 of these women had data on adolescent fiber intake; 1118 women were diagnosed with BC (multivariate adjusted)	Higher fiber intake during adolescence and early adulthood may be especially important in reducing BC risk (Fig. 20.10). Higher total fiber intake in adolescence and early adult life reduced BC risk by 25% (p-trend = 0.004). Higher total fiber intake during adolescence was associated with a 16% lower BC risk (p-trend = 0.04). Among all women, higher total fiber intake in early adulthood significantly lowered BC risk by 19% (p-trend = 0.002); higher intakes of soluble fiber lowered risk by14% (p-trend = 0.02) and insoluble fiber reduced risk by 20% (p-trend <0.001)

Table 20.6 (continued)

Objective	Study details	Results
Chhim et al. (2015). Investigate whether fiber intake modulates the association between alcohol intake and hormone dependent BC risk (Supplémentation en Vitamines et Minéraux Antioxydants study; France) [75]	3771 women; completed at least 6 valid 24-h dietary records during the first 2 years of follow-up; median 12 years of follow-up; 158 BC cases confirmed (multivariate adjusted)	The combination of high alcohol consumption and low fiber intake acted synergistically to increase hormone dependent BC risk and the effects on BC risk when stratified by median intake is summarized in Fig. 20.11
Ferrari et al. (2013). Investigate associations between total fiber and its main food sources (vegetables, fruit, cereals, and legumes) and BC risk (The European Prospective Investigation into Cancer and Nutrition [EPIC]) [76]	334,849 women; mean baseline age approx. 50 years (range 35–70 years); tumor subtypes: hormone receptor positive and negative tumors; median follow-up 11.5 years; 11,576 invasive BC cases (multivariate adjusted)	Diets rich in total fiber and, particularly, vegetable fiber modestly and significantly reduced BC risk, independently of menopausal status. Total fiber was inversely associated with BC risk by 7% for each 10-g total fiber intake. In premenopausal women, there was a significant 34% lower risk (p-trend = 0.02) for those consuming both high-fiber (>26 g/day) and low-fat (< 63 g/day) diets compared with high-fat (>89 g/day) and low-fiber (< 18 g/day) diets but this interaction between fiber and fat intake was not significant in post-menopausal women. For vegetable fiber (excluding potatoes, legumes, soy and tomato products), BC risk was reduced by 15% for each 5 g/day intake (p-trend = 0.01), independent of menopausal status or hormone receptor status
Park et al. (2009). Examine the relation of fiber intake to BC risk by hormone receptor status and histologic type among post-menopausal women (National Institutes of Health-AARP Diet and Health Study; US) [77]	185,598 postmenpausal women; mean age: 62 years; average of 7-year follow-up; 5461 BC cases were identified, of which 3341 cases had hormone dependent BC (multivariate adjusted)	Fiber was associated with preventing BC through non-estrogen pathways among post-menopausal women. Higher total fiber intake was associated with a 13% lower BC risk (p-trend = 0.02). The association was stronger for hormone negative tumors with lower risk by 44% (p-trend = 0.008) than for hormone positive tumors with a lower risk by 5% (p-trend = 0.47). Fruit was the most effective fiber source in reducing BC risk. Soluble fiber intake was inversely associated with BC by 17% (p-trend = 0.02). Total fiber effect on lowering the risk of BC was independent of the level of dietary fat intake (p = 0.08)
Cade et al. (2007). Evaluate associations between total fiber and fiber source on BC risk in a cohort including large numbers of vegetarians (The UK Women's Cohort Study) [78]	35,792 women (17,781 post-menopausal women and 15,951 pre-menopausal women at baseline; mean baseline age 52 years (mean 45 years premenopausal and 59 years menopausal); 18% vegetarian; 10-year follow-up; cases of invasive BC (350 post-menopausal and 257 pre-menopausal) (multivariate adjusted)	In older premenopausal women, higher total fiber intake significantly lowered BC risk by 52% (p-trend = 0.01; ≥ 30 g vs < 20 g/day). Also, higher cereal fiber reduced BC risk by 41% (p-trend = 0.05; ≥ 13 g/day vs < 4 g/day) and fruit fiber had a borderline inverse BC risk lowering effect by 19% (p-trend = 0.09; ≥ 6 g/day vs < 2 g/day). No significant BC lowering effects were seen for post-menopausal women

(continued)

Table 20.6 (continued)

Objective	Study details	Results
Mattisson et al. (2004). Investigate the associations between intakes of plant foods, fiber and dietary fat and BC risk (The Malmo¨ Diet and Cancer cohort; Sweden) [79]	11,726 postmenopausal women; 342 BC cases; 11-year follow-up (multivariate adjusted)	This study supports the hypothesis that dietary patterns high in fiber and low/moderate in fat are associated with lower risk of post-menopausal BC. High fiber intakes were associated with a lower risk of postmenopausal BC by 42% (25.9 vs 12.5 g/day; p-trend = 0.056; multivariate adjusted). A significant interaction (p = 0.049) was found between fiber- and fat-tertiles with higher fiber and lower-fat dietary patterns having the optimal impact for reducing post-menopausal BC risk
Holmes et al. (2004). Evaluate the association of total fiber, fiber fractions, carbohydrate, glycemic index, and glycemic load with the risk of BC (Nurses' Health Study; US) [80]	88,678 participants; mean age 56.5 years at assessment; 68% post-menopausal and 38% on hormone replacement; 18-year follow-up; 4092 BC cases (multivariate adjusted)	This study found no overall significant association between the midlife intake of total fiber (25 g/day vs 12 g total fiber/day (mean intake 18.1 g/day) on BC risk. However, these findings do not exclude the possibility that diets including a very high intake of fiber (>30 g/day) may reduce BC risk. In postmenopausal women, there was a positive association between glycemic index and BC risk by 15% (p-trend = 0.02) with a stronger association among women whose BMI was <25 with doubling of risk to 28% (p-trend = 0.003). For specific fiber types, higher fruit fiber had a moderate trend toward reduced BC risk by 8% (p = 0.08)
Terry et al. (2002). Examine the association between total dietary fiber and dietary fiber fractions, and BC risk (Canadian National Breast Screening Study) [81]	89,835 women ages 40–59 years; 16.2-year follow-up; 2536 BC cases were diagnosed; self-completed questionnaire regarding diet and physical activity (multivariate adjusted)	Total fiber (26 g/day vs 15 g/day) and specific fiber fractions or types appear to be weakly associated with reduced BC risk. Higher total fiber intake insignificantly lowered BC risk by 8% (p = 0.16). There were similar insignificant risk reductions for intakes of specific fiber fractions, including soluble and insoluble fiber, fiber from cereals, fruit, and vegetables
Willett et al. (1992). Evaluate the hypothesis that dietary fat increases and fiber decreases BC risk (Nurses' Health Study; US) [82]	89,494 women; 34–59 years of age; 8-year followed up; 1439 incident cases of BC, including 774 among postmenopausal women (multivariate adjusted)	Total fiber intake (≥ 22 g/day vs ≤ 11 g/day; mean intake 17 g/day) did not protect against BC risk in pre- or postmenopausal women (p = 0.62). However, this study cannot exclude the possibility that higher total fiber intake or that some specific fraction may lower BC risk. Also, this study did not find an adverse effect of high levels of dietary fat on BC risk
Dietary fat and fat subtypes		
Systematic reviews and meta-analyses		
Brennan et al. (2017). Clarify the association between dietary total fat and saturated fat on BC mortality [83]	15 prospective cohort studies	There was no difference in BC specific mortality or all-cause mortality for women in the highest vs the lowest category of total fat intake. However, BC specific mortality was 51% higher for women in the highest vs the lowest intake of saturated fat
Cao et al. (2016). Evaluate the effect of total dietary fat and serum fatty acids on BC risk [84]	For total dietary fat: 24 cohort studies; 1,387,366 subjects and 38,262 BC cases; for individual fatty acids: 7 cohort study articles; 3511 subjects; 1334 BC cases	Total dietary fat (highest vs. lowest category) was associated with a 10% increase in BC risk, which was insignificant after adjusting for traditional BC risk factors. No significant association was observed between animal fat, vegetable fat, saturated fatty acids, monounsaturated fatty acids, polyunsaturated fatty acids, n-3 PUFA, n-6 PUFA, eicosapentaenoic acid, docosahexaenoic acid, alpha-linolenic acid, oleic acid, linoleic acid and arachidonic acid and BC risk

Table 20.6 (continued)

Objective	Study details	Results
Xia et al. (2015). Determine quantitative relationship between dietary saturated fat intake and BC risk [85]	52 studies (24 cohort studies and 28 case-control studies); > 50,000 women diagnosed with BC	High intake of saturated fat increased BC risk by 18% in case-control studies and 4% in cohort studies vs lower intake. A subgroup analysis of case-control studies found significant positive associations between higher saturated fat intake and BC risk in Asians by 17%, Caucasians by 19%, and postmenopausal women by 33%
Xin et al. (2015). Investigate the association of high vegetable oils consumption and breast cancer risk, and evaluate the dose–response relationship [86]	5 prospective cohort studies and 11 retrospective case-control studies; > 150,000 women; 11,161 BC events	Higher consumption of total vegetable oils reduced BC risk by 12%, and dose-response analyses showed that each 10-g vegetable oil/day insignificantly lowered BC risk by 2%. However, higher olive oil intake significantly reduced BC risk by 24%
Yang et al. (2014). Ascertain the relationship between n-3/n-6 ratio and BC risk [87]	6 prospective nested case-control and 5 cohort studies; 274,135 women; 8331 BC events; across different countries	Women with higher dietary ratio of n-3/n-6 PUFAs had a significantly lower risk of BC by 10%. One USA study with higher ratio of n-3/n-6 in serum phospholipids showed significantly lowered BC risk by 27% (p-trend = 0.004)
Prospective cohort studies		
Farvid et al. (2014). Examine the association between fat intake and BC incidence (Nurses' Health Study II; US) [88]	88,804 women; baseline age 26–45 years; 20 years of follow-up; 2830 BC cases (multivariate adjusted)	Higher total fat intake was not associated with BC risk overall except for a positive association observed between animal fat intake and BC risk by 18% (p-trend = 0.01). This positive association with animal fat intake was seen among premenopausal women, but not among postmenopausal women. Also, any associations between BC risk and saturated fat, monounsaturated fat and animal fat, were attenuated and non-significant after adjustment for red meat intake. Other types of fat were not significantly associated with BC risk
Boeke et al. (2014). Evaluate intakes of total fat, specific types of fat, and cholesterol prior to diagnosis in relation to lethal BC risk (Nurses' Health Study II; US) [89]	88,804 women; baseline age 26–45 years; 20 years of follow-up; 9979 invasive breast cancer cases developed, of which 1529 went on to become lethal (multivariate adjusted)	Higher total fat intake was associated with a slightly lower BC mortality risk by 15% (p-trend = 0.05). Specific types of fat were generally not associated with BC mortality risk
Sieri et al. (2008). Investigate the association between fat consumption and BC risk (European Prospective Investigation into Cancer and Nutrition [EPIC]) [90]	319,826 women; baseline age 20–70 years; mean of 8.8 years of follow-up; 7119 women developed BC (multivariate adjusted)	In all women, high saturated fat intake increased BC risk by 13% vs lowest intake (p-trend = 0.038). Also, in postmenopausal women, high saturated fat intake increased BC risk by 21% for nonusers of hormone therapy (p-trend = 0.044)
Chajes et al. (2008). Assess the effect of trans vs oleic monounsaturated fat intake and BC risk (EPIC -France) [91]	19,934 women; mean baseline age 57 years; 7 years of follow-up; 363 BC cases (multivariate adjusted)	High intake of industrial type trans-fat or serum trans fatty acids increased postmenopausal BC risk by 75% (p-trend = 0.018). cis-Monounsaturated fatty acids were unrelated to BC risk

(continued)

Table 20.6 (continued)

Objective	Study details	Results
Holmes et al. (1999). Determine whether intake of fat and fatty acids are associated with BC risk (Nurses' Health Study; US) [92]	88,795 women; baseline age 30–55 years; 14 years of follow-up; 2956 BC cases (multivariate adjusted)	Compared to women consuming 30.1–35% energy from fat, those consuming ≤20% of energy from fat had a 15% higher BC risk (p-trend = 0.03). A dose-response assessment found that a 5% increase in total fat energy or specific fatty acid were not significantly associated with BC risk except for trans-fat (from industrial processing) with each 1% energy intake increasing BC risk by 9% in post-menopausal women. Also, each 5% total fat replacement of carbohydrate reduced BC risk by 4%
Protein source		
Wu et al. (2016). Conduct a meta-analysis to assess the association between protein source and BC risk [93]	46 prospective cohort studies	Higher total red meat, fresh red meat, and processed meat intake may be risk factors for breast cancer, whereas higher soy food and skim milk intake may reduce BC risk (Fig. 20.12). In dose-response analysis BC risk decreased by 9% for soy food, by 4% for skim milk, and 10% for yogurt, and increased by 9% for processed meat and by 7% for total red meat
Farvid et al. (2014). Investigate the association between dietary protein sources in early adulthood and BC risk (Nurses' Health Study II; US) [94]	88,803 women; 20 years of follow-up; 2830 BC cases (multivariate adjusted)	Higher intake of total red meat was associated with an increased overall BC risk by 22% (p-trend = 0.01). However, higher intakes of poultry, fish, eggs, legumes, and nuts were not related to BC risk overall. When the association was evaluated by menopausal status, higher intake of poultry was associated with a lower BC risk in postmenopausal women by 27% (p-trend = 0.02), but not in premenopausal women with a 7% lower risk (p-trend = 0.60). In estimating the effects of exchanging different protein sources, substituting one serving/day of legumes for a daily serving of red meat lowered BC risk by 15% among all women and 19% lower risk among premenopausal women. Also, substituting one serving/day of poultry for one serving/day of red meat was associated with a 17% lower BC risk and a 24% lower postmenopausal BC risk. Also, substituting one serving/day of combined legumes, nuts, poultry, and fish for one serving/day of red meat was associated with a 14% lower risk of BC risk overall
Dietary Folate intake		
Zhang et al. (2014). Assess the dose response association between folate and BC risk [95]	14 prospective cohort studies; 677,858 women	Dose-response analysis showed a nonlinear relationship as a potential J-shaped correlation between folate intake and BC risk (p = 0.007). The analysis revealed that a daily folate intake of 200–320 mg was associated with a lower breast cancer risk, but BC risk increased significantly with a daily folate intake >400 mg
Dietary antioxidant vitamins		
Hu et al. (2015). Meta-analysis and regression to assess the association between plasma retinol, vitamin A, C and α-tocopherol levels, and BC risk [96]	40 studies including 28 case-control studies and 12 nested case–control studies	There was a significant increased BC risk for women with the lowest plasma α-tocopherol 5.74–9.16 μmol/L and a significantly lower BC risk for higher plasma vitamin C levels only in case-control studies. However, there was no significant association between plasma retinol and BC risk

Table 20.6 (continued)

Objective	Study details	Results
Hu et al. (2011). Meta-analysis and regression evaluation of the association between intake of retinol, vitamins A, C and E dietary intake, and BC risk and estimate their dose-response effects [97]	51 studies (3 RCTs, 9 cohort studies; 2 nested case-control studies, and 36 case-control studies)	Higher total vitamin A and retinol intake could significantly lower BC risk by 17%. Although the dietary vitamin E, and total vitamin E intake reduced BC risk significantly when data from all studies were pooled, the results became insignificant when data from cohort studies were analyzed. No significant dose-response relationship was observed for the higher intake of these vitamins and reduced BC risk
Vitamin D Intake and Blood 25-hydroxyvitamin D [25(OH)D]		
Kim and Je et al. (2014). Assess the association between vitamin D intake and blood 25(OH)D on BC risk or mortality [98]	30 prospective studies	Overall there was an insignificant, weak inverse association between vitamin D intake or blood 25(OH)D levels and BC risk. However, among BC patients high blood 25(OH)D levels were significantly associated with a 42% lower risk of BC mortality. There was no significant heterogeneity among the studies
Calcium		
Meta-analyses		
Hidayat et al. (2016). Investigate the association of serum calcium and BC risk [99]	11 cohort studies; 872,895 participants; 26,606 BC cases	Higher calcium intake reduced overall BC risk by 8% with moderate heterogeneity (p = 0.026). In the subgroup analysis, premenopausal BC risk was reduced by 25% compared to 6% for postmenopausal BC. Dose-response analysis revealed that each 300 mg/day increase in calcium intake was associated with reduced BC risk for premenopausal women by 8% and postmenopausal BC by 2%

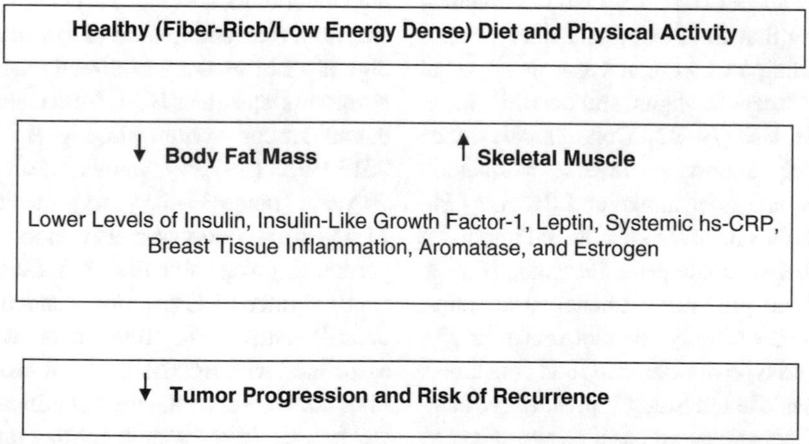

Fig. 20.8 Potential mechanisms by which high adherence to a healthy fiber-rich dietary pattern and appropriate levels physical activity routines on lowering breast cancer risk and recurrence (adapted from [17])

control diets or total fiber intake ≥25 g/day [72, 73]. A pooled analysis (5525 women in the Women's Intervention Nutrition Study, median 60 months of duration; the Women's Healthy Eating and Living study, mean 7.3 years duration; and the Collaborative Women's Longevity Study, 4441 BC patients, 5.5-year follow-up) found that post-diagnostic diets lower in fat, and higher in fruits and vegetables and fiber significantly reduced the risk of BC recurrence by 23% and BC-related mortality by 17% [71].

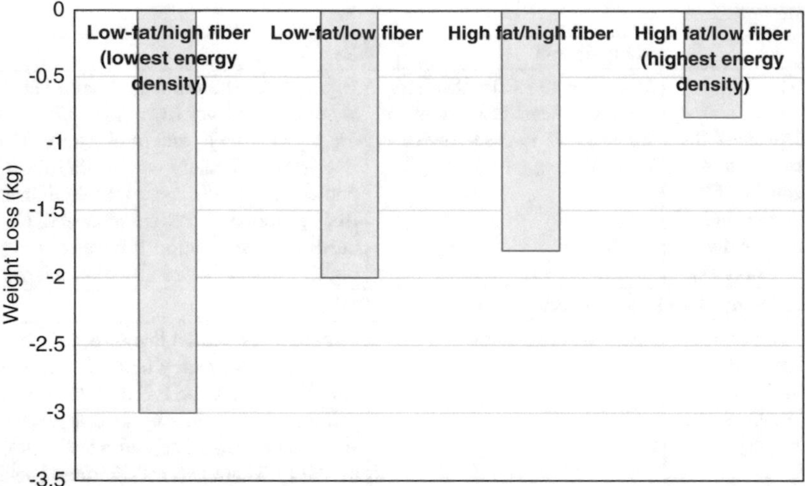

Fig. 20.9 Effect of dietary fiber and fat intake on energy density and weight loss in overweight and obese adults over 3 years (adjusted for age, sex, baseline weight, baseline fiber and fat intake, and baseline and follow-up physical activity) (adapted from [67])

Prospective Cohort Studies

Nine prospective studies summarize the effect of increased dietary fiber intake on BC risk [74–82]. Although the pre-2005 cohort studies generally observed a weak or insignificant association between fiber and BC risk, they did not preclude the possibility that fiber or certain fiber components, depending on a women's age, menopausal or hormone receptor status and/or BMI level, may affect BC risk [79–82]. Cohort studies since 2005 generally report an inverse association between adequate fiber intake and BC risk [74–78]. These studies have also uncovered important interactions between adequate fiber intake during adolescence and pre- vs postmenopausal status, estrogen receptor affinity, alcohol intake or glycemic load and type of fiber-rich food consumed. A 2016 Nurses' Health Study II prospective analysis (90,534 women; mean baseline age 36 years; 20 year-follow-up; 2833 women were diagnosed with BC; 44,263 of these women had data on adolescent fiber intake) found that higher fiber intake during adolescence and early adulthood may be especially important in reducing BC risk (Fig. 20.10) [74]. Higher total fiber intake in adolescence and early adult life significantly reduced BC risk by 25%. A 2015 analysis of the French Supplémentation en Vitamines et Minéraux Antioxydants study (3771 women; completed at least 6 valid 24-h dietary records during the first 2 years of follow-up; median 12-year follow-up) showed that increased fiber intake is protective against the increased BC risk associated with high alcohol intake (Fig. 20.11) [75]. In stratified analyses, the combination of low fiber intake and high alcohol intake was directly associated with hormone-dependent BC risk increase by 1.5-fold but not among women with higher fiber intake. A 2013 EPIC (334,849 women; mean baseline age 50 years (range 35–70 years); median follow-up 11.5 years) found that diets rich in total fiber and particularly vegetable fiber modestly and significantly reduced BC risk, independently of menopausal status [76]. Total fiber was inversely associated with BC risk by 7% for each 10-g total fiber intake. Vegetable fiber significantly lowered BC risk by 15% for each 5 g/day intake, excluding potatoes, legumes, soy and tomato products, independent of menopausal status. A 2009 National Institutes of Health-AARP Diet and Health Study (185,598 postmenpausal women; mean baseline age 62 years; average of 7-year follow-up) showed that fiber can play a role in preventing BC through non-estrogen pathways among post-menopausal women [77]. Higher total fiber intake was inversely associated with a

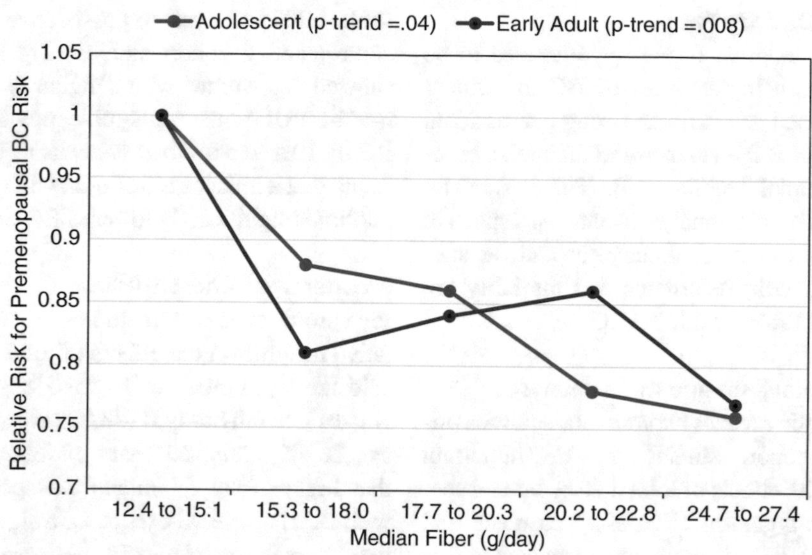

Fig. 20.10 Associations between adolescent and early adulthood fiber intake and breast cancer (BC) risk premenopausal adult women from Nurses' Health Study II (multivariate adjusted) (adapted from [74])

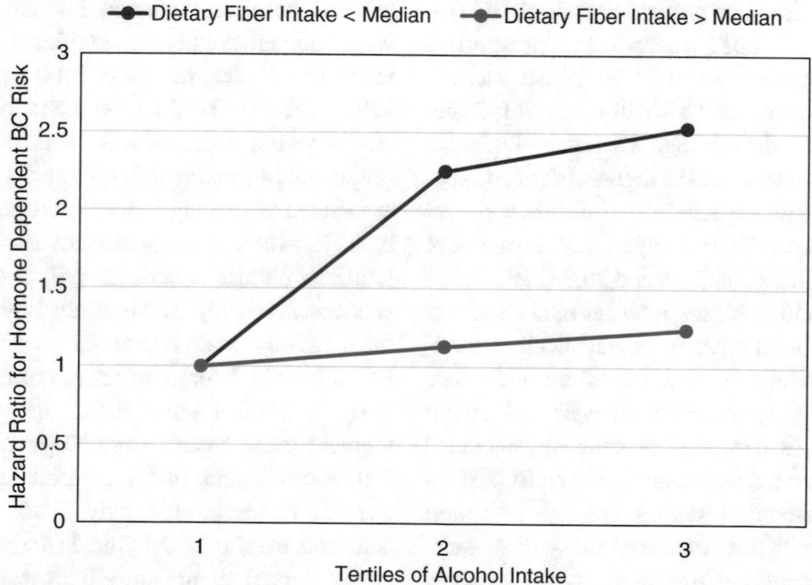

Fig. 20.11 Associations between tertiles of alcohol intake and hormone dependent breast cancer (BC) risk stratified by median dietary fiber intake (p-interaction = 0.01) (adapted from [75])

13% lower BC risk. The association was stronger for hormone negative tumors with lower risk by 44% (p-trend = 0.008) than for hormone positive tumors with a lower risk by 5% (p-trend = 0.47). Subgroup analysis found that: (1) fruit was the most effective fiber source in reducing BC risk; (2) soluble fiber was inversely associated with BC by 17%; and (3) total fiber effects on lowering the risk of BC was independent of the level of dietary fat intake.

20.4.1.2 Dietary Fat

Dietary fat intake was long hypothesized to be associated with higher rates of BC in affluent countries, based primarily on strong international correlations of BC incidence and fat intake, especially in animal studies [10]. The systematic reviews and meta-analyses and prospective cohort studies on total dietary fat and fat subtypes on BC risk, recurrence and mortality are summarized Table 20.6 [83–92].

Systematic Reviews and Meta-Analyses

Five systematic reviews and/or meta-analyses primarily of cohort studies provide important insights on the effects of total dietary fat and specific fat sub-types on BC risk, recurrence and mortality [83–87]. These analyses indicated that total dietary fat intake is less important than the type of fat consumed, with lower intake of saturated fat and higher n-3 to n-6 ratio or higher marine n-3 PUFA being the most effective dietary fat considerations for protecting against BC risk or mortality. A 2017 analysis (15 prospective studies) concluded that total fat intake was not significantly associated with all-cause or BC specific mortality whereas higher saturated fat intake was associated with a 51% higher risk of BC specific mortality, especially in postmenopausal women [83]. A 2016 analysis (24 prospective studies; 1,387,366 subjects and 38,262 BC cases) found that neither higher total fat intake nor any specific fatty acid types were statistically significantly associated with BC risk, after multivariate adjustments [84]. A 2015 analysis (24 cohort studies and 28 case-control studies) concluded that high saturated fat intake increased BC risk by 18% in case-control studies and 4% in cohort studies [85]. In the case-control studies, there were significant positive associations between higher saturated fat intake and BC risk in postmenopausal women by 33%, whereas there was no association between higher dietary saturated fat intake and BC risk among premenopausal women in any studies. A 2015 analysis (5 prospective and 11 case-control studies) found that higher vegetable oil intake reduced BC risk by 12% and higher olive oil appears to have a BC protective effect with a reduced BC risk by 24% [86]. A 2014 analysis (6 prospective nested case-control and 5 cohort studies; 274,135 women) showed that women with a higher dietary ratio of n-3/n-6 PUFAs have a significantly lower risk of BC by 10% and a subset analysis of USA women found that a higher ratio of n-3/n-6 in serum phospholipids significantly lowered BC risk 27% [87].

Prospective Cohort Studies

Five prospective cohort studies provide representative insights on the effects of total fat and fatty acid sub-types intake on BC risk [88–92]. A 2014 Nurses' Health Study II (88,804 women; baseline age 26–45 years; 20 years of follow-up) found that higher total fat intake was not associated with BC risk overall except for a significant positive association observed between animal fat intake and BC risk overall by 18% [88]. This positive association with animal fat intake was seen among premenopausal women, but not among postmenopausal women. Also, any associations between saturated fat and animal fat, were attenuated and non-significant after adjustment for red meat intake. A 2008 analysis of the EPIC cohort (319,826 women; baseline age 20–70 years; mean of 8.8 years of follow-up) found that in women high saturated fat intake was associated with a significant increase in BC risk by 13%, whereas no significant association with total, monounsaturated, or polyunsaturated fat was observed [90]. In this study, higher saturated fat intake by postmenopausal women increased BC risk by 21% for nonusers of hormone therapy. Also, a 2008 French EPIC analysis (19,934 women; mean baseline age 57 years; 7 years of follow-up) found that increased intake of the trans-monounsaturated fatty acids (palmitoleic acid and elaidic acid found in industrially processed foods) significantly increased BC risk in postmenopausal women by 75% [91]. A 1999 Nurses' Health Study (88,795 women; baseline age 30–55 years; 14 years) showed that a 5% increase in total fat energy or specific fatty acid was not significantly associated with BC risk except for trans-fat (from industrial processing) which with each 1% energy intake increased BC risk by 9% in post-menopausal women [92]. A 5% increase in total fat as a substitute for carbohydrate reduced BC risk by 4%. There is little support for lower total fat intake or specific fatty acids being associated with BC risk, expect possibly for industrial trans or saturated fat.

20.4.1.3 Dietary Protein Source

Protein is important in the maintenance of human tissues and the regulation of various physiological functions, which may influence BC risk [93, 94]. A 2016 dose response meta-analysis (46 prospective cohort studies) found each serving of various protein sources can significantly effect BC risk (Fig. 20.12) [93]. A 2014 Nurses' Health Study II analysis (88,803 women; 20 years of follow-up) found that higher intake of total red meat was associated with a significant increased overall BC risk by 22% [94]. However, higher intakes of poultry, fish, eggs, legumes, and nuts were not related to BC risk overall. When the association was evaluated by menopausal status, higher intake of poultry was associated with a significantly lower BC risk in postmenopausal women by 27%, but not in premenopausal women with a 7% lower risk (p-trend = 0.60). In estimating the effects of exchanging different protein sources, substituting one serving/day of legumes for one serving/day of red meat was associated with a 15% lower BC risk among all women and a 19% lower risk among premenopausal women. Also, substituting one serving/day of combined legumes, nuts, poultry, and fish for one serving/day of red meat was associated with a 14% lower risk of BC risk overall.

20.4.1.4 Dietary Folate Intake

Previous observational studies regarding the existence of an association between folate intake and BC risk have been inconsistent [95]. A 2014 dose-response meta-analysis (14 prospective cohort studies; 677,858 women) showed a non-linear relationship between folate intake and the risk of breast cancer, and discovered a potential J-shaped correlation between folate intake and BC risk [96]. This analysis also revealed that a daily folate intake of 200–320 mg was associated with a lower breast cancer risk, but BC risk increased significantly with a daily folate intake >400 mg [95].

20.4.1.5 Antioxidant Vitamins

Retinol, vitamins A, C and E are hypothesized to reduce BC risk due to their roles in the regulation of cell growth, differentiation and apoptosis (retinol, vitamin A) and enhancing immune function, anti-inflammation and antioxidant

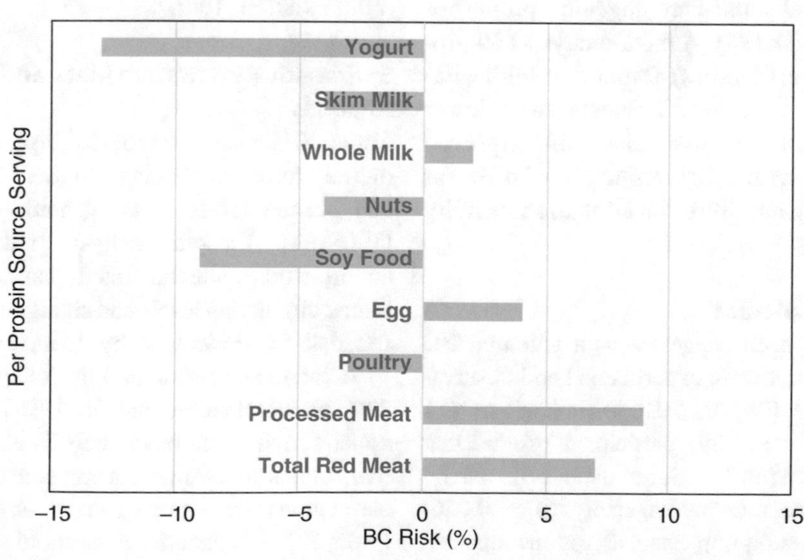

Fig. 20.12 Association between protein source (per serving) and breast cancer (BC) risk from a meta-analysis of 46 prospective studies (adapted from [93])

activities (vitamin C and E) but experimental and epidemiologic studies have yielded conflicting results on the relationship between dietary antioxidant vitamins and BC risk [96, 97]. A 2015 meta-analysis of plasma retinol, vitamins A, C and α-tocopherol levels, and BC risk (40 studies including 28 case-control studies and 12 nested case-control studies) showed no significant association between plasma retinol and BC risk but a significant increased BC risk for women with the lowest plasma α-tocopherol [96]. Also, there was a significant negative association between plasma vitamin C and BC risk only in case-control studies but not for other vitamins. A 2011 meta-analysis intake of retinol, vitamin A, C and E levels and BC risk (3 RCTs, 9 cohort studies; 2 nested case-control studies, and 36 case-control studies) showed that higher total vitamin A and retinol intake could significantly lower BC risk by 17% [97]. Although dietary vitamin E reduced BC risk significantly when data from all studies were pooled, the results became insignificant when data from cohort studies were analyzed.

20.4.1.6 Vitamin D and Blood 25-Hydroxyvitamin D [25(OH)D]

Experimental studies suggest that vitamin D has potential anti-carcinogenic properties against BC risk [98]. A meta-analysis (30 prospective cohort studies) found that high vitamin D status is weakly associated with lower BC risk but strongly associated with improved BC survival with a risk reduction of 42% for BC mortality and 39% for all-cause mortality [98].

20.4.1.7 Calcium

Calcium has been suggested as a potential BC protective factor from experimental and observational studies [99]. A 2016 meta-analysis (11 cohort studies; 872,895 participants) found that higher calcium intake reduced overall BC risk by 8% with moderate heterogeneity ($p = 0.026$) [99]. In the subgroup analysis, premenopausal BC risk was reduced by 25% compared to 6% for postmenopausal BC. Dose-response analysis showed that each 300 mg/day increase in calcium intake was associated with a lower BC risk in premenopausal women by 8% and postmenopausal women by 2%.

20.4.2 Phytochemicals

The effects of phytochemicals found in fruits, vegetables, dietary pulses, soy, nuts and seeds including carotenoids, flavonoids, and phytoestrogens (isoflavonoids and lignans) on BC risk, recurrence, and survival are summarized in Table 20.7.

20.4.2.1 Carotenoids

Carotenoids are naturally occurring richly colored pigments providing the yellow, orange, and red colors of many fruits and vegetables, which can act as a biomarker of their intake. α-Carotene, β-carotene, β-cryptoxanthin, lutein, zeaxanthin, and lycopene are the most prevalent, comprising 90% of circulating carotenoids. They are believed to be anticarcinogenic, with possible biologic activities including antioxidation, enhanced gap-junction intercellular communication, immunoenhancement, inhibition of tumorigenesis and malignant transformation, and metabolism to retinoids, which in turn contributes to cellular differentiation [100].

Systematic Reviews and Meta-and Pooled Analyses

Three 2012 analyses provide important insights on the protective effects of higher dietary intake and plasma levels of carotenoids on BC risk [100–102]. A pooled analysis of 8 prospective cohort studies demonstrated that women with higher circulating levels had significantly reduced BC risk for α-carotene by 13%, β-carotene by 17%, lutein and zeaxanthin by 16%, lycopene by 22%, and total carotenoids by 19% [100]. A systematic review and meta-analysis of 25 prospective studies found that plasma concentrations of carotenoids are more strongly associated with lower BC risk than are carotenoids assessed by dietary questionnaires [101]. Only dietary intake of β-carotene was significantly associated with a reduced BC risk by 5% per 5000 mg/day. In contrast, plasma concentration measures showed significantly lower BC risk for total carotenoids, β-carotene, α-carotene, and lutein by 18–32%. A dose-response meta-analysis of carotenoid dietary intake (24 case-control studies, one nested case-control study and 6 cohort studies) reported that higher intake of dietary α-carotene significantly reduced BC risk by 9% and dietary β-carotene intake reduced the risk by 6% when

Table 20.7 Summary of phytochemicals studies on breast cancer (BC) risk, recurrence, and mortality

Carotenoids		
Systematic review and meta- and pooled analyses		
Eliassen et al. (2012). Examine associations between circulating carotenoids and BC risk [100]	8 cohort studies; 3055 cases and 3956 controls	Women with higher circulating levels of α-carotene, β-carotene, lutein and zeaxanthin, lycopene, and total carotenoids may be at reduced BC risk. Statistically significant inverse associations (highest vs lowest quintile) with BC risk were found with α-carotene by 13%, β-carotene by 17%, lutein and zeaxanthin by 16%, lycopene by 22%, and total carotenoids by 19%
Aune et al. (2012). Systematic review and meta-analysis of prospective studies of dietary intake and blood concentrations of carotenoids and BC risk [101]	25 prospective cohort studies	Of the 6 carotenoids assessed by dietary intake questionaires, only β-carotene was significantly associated with a reduced BC risk by 5% per 5000 mg/day. In contrast, blood concentration measures showed lower BC risk for total carotenoids by 22% per 100 μg/dL, β-carotene by 26% per 50 μg/dL, α-carotene by 18% per 10 μg/dL, and for lutein by 32% per 25 μg dL. Blood concentrations of carotenoids are more strongly associated with lower BC risk than are carotenoids assessed by dietary questionnaires
Hu et al. (2012). Comprehensively summarize the associations between carotenoids and BC risk and quantitatively estimate their dose–response relationships [102]	24 case-control studies, 1 nested case-control study and 6 cohort studies	Comparing the highest with the lowest intake: dietary α-carotene intake significantly reduced BC risk by 9.0% ($p = 0.01$) and dietary β-carotene intake reduced the risk by 6.0% ($p = 0.05$) when data from cohort studies were pooled. Total α-carotene intake had the strongest association with reducing BC risk. There were no significant associations between dietary intake of β-cryptoxanthin, lutein/zeaxanthin, or lycopene and BC risk
Prospective cohort or nested case-control studies		
Eliassen et al. (2015). Examine the timing of carotenoid exposure and association with BC risk, recurrence and mortality (Nurses' Health Study; US) [103]	32,826 women donated blood samples; > 20 years of follow-up; 2767 BC cases were diagnosed and matched with control subjects (multivariate adjusted)	Higher concentrations of α and β-carotenes lycopene, and total carotenoids were associated with 18–28% statistical significant lower risks of BC (p-trend <0.001). Plasma carotenoid concentrations were strongly inversely associated with BC recurrence and mortality with higher β-carotene intake reducing risk by 68% (p-trend <0.001)
Boeke et al. (2014). Examine adolescent carotenoid intake in relation to benign breast disease (BBD) in young women (Growing Up Today Study cohort; US) [104]	6593 adolescent girls; baseline age 12 years; 10–12 years of follow-up; intakes of α-carotene, β-carotene, β-cryptoxanthin, lutein/zeaxanthin, and lycopene from food-frequency questionnaires (multivariate adjusted)	β-Carotene intake was inversely associated with BBD; comparing the highest to lowest quartile, the multivariate-adjusted odds for BBD were reduced by 42% (p-trend = 0.03). α-carotene and lutein/zeaxanthin were also inversely associated with BBD, but the associations were not statistically significant

(continued)

Table 20.7 (continued)

RCT		
Rock et al. (2005). Examine the relationship between plasma carotenoid concentration, as a biomarker of vegetable and fruit intake, and risk for a new BC event in a cohort of women with a history of early-stage breast cancer (Women's Healthy Eating and Living Study; US) [105]	1551 women previously treated for BC were randomly assigned to the control or a higher fruit and vegetable diet intervention trial arm; mean dietary carotenoid intake in this cohort was 14 mg/day; 7-years; 205 women had recurrent BC	Women in the highest quartile of plasma total carotenoid concentration had significantly reduced risk for new BC events by 43%, after controlling for covariates influencing BC prognosis
Flavonoids		
Systematic reviews and meta-analysis		
Hui et al. (2013). Examine the association between flavonoids, each flavonoid subclass (except isoflavones) and BC risk by conducting a meta-analysis [106]	12 studies (6 cohort and 6 case-control); 9513 cases and 181,906 controls Common flavonoids foods and beverages, include onions, broccoli, tea, aromatic herbs, celery, chamomile tea, cocoa, red wine, grapes, apples, green tea, oranges, berries and black currants	The risk of BC was significantly decreased in women with high intake of flavonols by 12% and flavones by 17% compared with a low intake of flavonols and flavones. No significant association was found for flavan-3-ols, flavanones, anthocyanins or total flavonoids, which lowered BC risk by 2–7%. When studies were stratified by menopausal status significant lower BC was observed only in post-menopausal women
Phytoestrogens (Isoflavonoids and Lignans)		
Systematic review and meta-analyses		
Isoflavonoids		
Chen et al. (2014). Explore the soy isoflavone-breast cancer association stratified by menopausal status [107]	10 cohort studies and 21 case-control studies	In Asian countries, higher soy isoflavone intake significantly lowered BC risk by 41% in both pre- and post-menopausal women. However, in Western countries, soy isoflavone intake had a marginally significant protective BC risk lowering effect only for postmenopausal women by 8%
Xie et al. (2013). Examine the association between isoflavones intake and BC risk by meta-analysis [108]	22 studies (7 cohort and 15 case-control designs); menopausal status in 14 studies; 9 studies from Asian populations and 5 studies from Western populations	Higher isoflavone intake significantly reduced the BC risk in Asian women by 32% compared to an insignificant reduction of 2% in Western women. Further analysis found that the intake of isoflavones reduced BC risk by 54% in postmenopausal Asian women and 37% in premenopausal women. The observed insignificant effect of soy intake in studies of Western women appears to be primarily due to the relatively lower intake of soy isoflavones in general
Dong and Qin (2011). Examine the association of soy isoflavones consumption and risk of BC incidence or recurrence, by conducting a meta-analysis of prospective studies [109]	14 cohort studies of BC incidence (369,934 participants and 5828 BC cases) and 4 cohort studies of BC recurrence (9656 BC patients and 1226 recurrent cases)	Higher soy isoflavones consumption was associated with 11% lower overall BC risk. A significant protective effect of soy isoflavones was only observed in studies conducted with Asian women with a lower BC risk of 24%. In Western women, the BC risk was only reduced by 3%. Also, soy isoflavones intake were associated with lower overall BC recurrence risk by 16%

Table 20.7 (continued)

Lignans		
Seibold et al. (2014). Meta-analysis on the effect of lignans on post-menopausal BC risk and mortality [110] Major dietary sources of lignans are flax, sunflower, pumpkin seeds and fiber-rich cereal.	6 prospective studies; 5–10 years of follow-up	Higher lignan intake by BC patients was significantly associated with lower mortality risk for all-cause by 43% and BC by 46%. Also, high enterolactone concentrations per 10 nmol/L were significantly associated with lower mortality for all-cause and BC by 6% for both
Buck et al. (2010). Conduct a meta-analysis on the association of lignan intake and BC risk [111]	11 prospective studies and 10 case-control studies	Lignan exposure was associated with an insignificant 8% lower overall BC risk, whereas in postmenopausal women, high lignan intake was associated with a significant 14% reduced BC risk

data from cohort studies were pooled but dietary intake of β-cryptoxanthin, lutein/zeaxanthin, or lycopene did not show reduced BC risk [102].

Prospective Cohort or Nested Case-Control Studies

Two studies are representative of the prospective studies on the effects of carotenoids on BC risk recurrence, mortality [103, 104]. A 2015 Nurses' Health Study (32,826 women; > 20 years of follow-up) found that higher plasma concentrations of a α and β-carotenes, lycopene, and total carotenoids were associated with 18–28% statistically significantly lower BC risk [103]. Plasma carotenoid concentrations were strongly inversely associated with BC recurrence and mortality with higher β-carotene intake reducing risk by 68%. The 2014 Growing Up Today Study (6593 adolescent girls; baseline age 12 years; 10–12 years of follow-up) showed that higher dietary β-carotene int ake reduced the risk of benign breast disease by 42%; α-carotene and lutein/zeaxanthin showed insignificant reduced BC risk trends [104].

Randomized Controlled Trial (RCT)

A 2005 analysis of the Women's Healthy Eating and Living Study (1551 women previously treated for BC who were randomly assigned to higher fruit and vegetable diets vs control; 7 years) found that women in the highest quartile of plasma total carotenoid concentration had significantly reduced risk for a new BC event by 43% after controlling for covariates influencing BC prognosis [105].

20.4.2.2 Flavonoids

Flavonoids are a large family of polyphenolic plant compounds, which may have biological effects related to their ability to modulate a number of cell-signaling cascades with antiinflammatory, anti-thrombogenic, antidiabetic, anticancer, and neuroprotective activities [106]. Common flavonoid rich foods, include onions, broccoli, aromatic herbs, celery, cocoa, red grapes, apples, oranges and other citrus fruits, berries, and black currants. A 2013 meta-analysis (6 cohort and 6 case-control) showed that BC risk was significantly decreased in women with high intake of flavonols by 12% and flavones by 17% but no significant association was found for flavan-3-ols, flavanones, anthocyanins or total flavonoids intake which showed a 2–7% lower BC risk [106]. Higher flavonoid intake only significantly reduced BC risk in post-menopausal women.

20.4.2.3 Phytoestrogens

Soy Isoflavonoids

Isoflavones are the major flavonoids found in legumes, particularly soybeans [107, 108]. Soy isoflavones are known to have weak estrogenic activity due to their structural similarity with 17-β-estradiol. Estrogens are signaling molecules that exert their effects by binding to estrogen receptors within cells. Soy isoflavones can preferentially bind to estrogen receptor-β mimicking the effects of estrogen in some tissues and blocking the effects of estrogen in others. Three systematic reviews and meta-analyses provide an overview on soy isoflavonoids and BC risk

[107–109]. A 2014 analysis (35 cohort and case-control studies) found that higher soy isoflavone intake by both pre- and post-menopausal Asian women significantly lowered BC risk by 41% whereas in Western women increased soy isoflavone intake marginally lowered risk by 8% [107]. A 2013 analysis (7 cohort and 15 case-control studies) found that higher isoflavone intake significantly reduced the BC risk in post-menopausal Asian women by 54% and in pre-menopausal women by 37% compared to an insignificant reduction of 2% in Western women [108]. A 2011 analysis (14 cohort studies of BC incidence; 369,934 participants; and 4 cohort studies of BC recurrence; 9656 BC patients) concluded that in all women higher isoflavones consumption lowered BC risk by 11% and in Asian women higher isoflavones lowered risk by 24% compared to 3% in Western women [109]. Also, higher soy isoflavones intake lowered BC recurrence risk by 16% in all women studies. The general lack of significant effect of isoflavones on BC risk in the studies of Western women may be due to the relatively lower frequency or level of isoflavone intake, as there is little evidence that Asian women respond differently to soy isoflavones than non-Asian women.

20.4.2.4 Lignans

Plant lignans are found in seeds (sunflower, pumpkin, sesame, flaxseeds), whole-grain cereals and (fiber-rich) vegetables [110]. They are metabolized by the colonic microbiota to the biologically active forms enterolactone and enterodiol. Because of structural similarities, lignans can bind to estrogen receptors and thus exert both estrogenic and anti-estrogenic effects. Enterolactone, a lignan metabolite, has been positively correlated with sex hormone binding globulin, which may lead to lower concentrations of circulating sex hormones by binding free estradiol. Two systematic reviews and meta-analyses provide an overview on lignans and BC risk and mortality [110, 111]. A 2014 analysis (6 prospective studies; 5–10 years of follow-up) found that higher lignin intake significantly lowered risk of mortality for all-cause by 43% and BC risk by 46%. Also, high blood enterolactone concentrations per 10 nmol/L were significantly associated with lower all-cause mortality by 6%, and BC-specific for all-cause mortality by 6% [110]. A 2010 analysis (11 prospective studies and 10 case-control studies) showed that higher lignan intake was associated with a significant 14% lower overall BC risk in postmenopausal women [111].

20.5 Whole (Minimally Processed) Plant Foods

20.5.1 Fruits and Vegetables

Fruits and vegetables contain numerous nutrients and phytochemicals which may reduce BC risk, including fiber which can bind estrogens during enterohepatic circulation, and a range of antioxidants such as carotenoids, flavonoids, and vitamins, which can prevent oxidative damage [112]. Table 20.8 summarizes the effect of fruits and vegetable studies on BC risk, recurrence and survival [112–121].

20.5.1.1 Systematic Reviews and Meta- and Pooled Analyses

Five systematic reviews and meta- and pooled analyses provide important insights into the effect of fruits and vegetables on BC risk, recurrence and mortality [112–116]. A 2017 analysis (9 cohort studies and 1 RCT; a total of 31,210 BC cases; median follow-up of 6.6 years) showed a borderline inverse association between pre-diagnostic intake of fruit, and improved odds of overall BC survival by 17%. Whereas intake of vegetables was not significantly associated with survival with improved survival odds of 4% [112]. No significant association was found between intake of vegetables and fruits and breast cancer-specific mortality after BC-diagnoses. Also, intake of cruciferous vegetables was not found to be protective against BC-specific mortality. Another 2017 analysis (12 cohort studies; 41,185 participants; follow-up ranged from 3 to 18 years) found no significant associations between fruit and vegetable intake (fruits and vegetables combined,

Table 20.8 Summaries of fruit and vegetables studies on breast cancer (BC) risk, recurrence and survival

Objective	Study details	Results
Systematic reviews and meta- and pooled analyses		
He et al. (2017). Conduct a meta-analysis investigating the association between consumption of vegetables and fruits and BC survival [112]	9 cohort studies and 1 RCT; 31,210 BC cases; median follow-up of 6.6 years	There was a borderline significant inverse association for pre-diagnostic intake of fruits and 17% improved odds of BC survival, whereas intake of vegetables was not significantly associated with BC survival with improved odds of 4% [108]. No significant association was found between intake of vegetables and fruits and BC-specific mortality. Also, intake of cruciferous vegetables was not protective against BC-specific mortality. Finally, increased post-diagnostic intake of vegetables and fruits was not significantly associated with better odds of BC survival
Peng et al. (2017). Evaluate the overall effect of fruit and vegetable intake on the prognosis of breast cancer [113]	12 cohort studies; 41,185 participants; length of follow-up ranged from 3 to 18 years	Comparing the highest with the lowest intake, the risk for all-cause mortality was reduced for intake of total vegetables by 4%, for cruciferous vegetables by 1%, and fruits by 12%. BC-specific mortality risk was insignificant for fruit and vegetable intake; total vegetable intake reduced risk of BC recurrence by 11% and cruciferous vegetables reduced BC recurrence by 2%. No significant associations were found between fruit and vegetable intake (fruits and vegetables combined, total vegetable intake, cruciferous vegetable intake and fruit intake) and BC prognosis (all-cause mortality, BC-specific mortality and BC recurrence)
Jung et al. (2013). Assess the association between fruit and vegetable intake and risk of estrogen receptor negative BC risk (Pooling Project of Prospective Studies of Diet and Cancer; US) [114]	20 prospective studies; follow-up of 11–20 years; 34,526 BC cases identified among a total of 993,466 women; receptor status information was available for 24,673 BC patients	Total fruit and vegetable intake was statistically significantly inversely associated with risk of estrogen receptor negative BC but not with the risk of BC overall or estrogen receptor positive BC tumors. The inverse association for estrogen receptor negative tumors was observed primarily for vegetable consumption. The pooled lower BC risk comparing the highest vs lowest quintile of total vegetable consumption was 18% for estrogen receptor negative BC (p-trend <0.001). Higher total fruit consumption was non-statistically significantly associated with lower risk of estrogen receptor negative BC by 6%
Aune et al. (2012). Clarify the association between fruit and vegetable intake and breast cancer risk [115]	15 prospective studies; 5 European, 7 North America and 3 Asia studies	High intake of fruits and fruits and vegetables combined, but not vegetables, is associated with modest but significant reductions in breast cancer risk for the highest versus the lowest intake by 11% for fruit and vegetables combined, 8% for fruits and 1% for vegetables (including starchy vegetables). In dose-response analyses, per 200 g/d reduced risk by 4% for fruit and vegetables combined, 5% for fruits and 0% for vegetables

(continued)

Table 20.8 (continued)

Objective	Study details	Results
Smith-Warner et al. (2001). Examine the association between breast cancer and total and specific fruit and vegetable group intakes [116]	8 prospective studies; 351,825 women; 7377 BC cases	For comparisons of the highest vs lowest quartiles of intake (pooled multivariate), insignificant associations with lower BC risks were observed for total fruits 7% (p-trend = 0.08), total vegetables by 4% (p-trend = 0.54), and total fruits and vegetables by 7% (p-trend = 0.12)
Prospective cohort studies		
Farvid et al. (2016). Evaluate the association between fruit and vegetable intake during adolescence and early adulthood and BC risk (Nurses' Health Study II; US) [117]	90,476 premenopausal women; aged 27–44 years who completed a questionnaire on diet in 1991 and 44,223 of those women who completed a questionnaire about their diet during adolescence in 1998; 22 years of follow-up; 3235 BC cases (multivariate adjusted)	Total fruit intake during adolescence was associated with a significantly lower BC risk by 25% (median intake 2.9 servings/day vs 0.5 serving/day). Higher early adulthood intake of fruits and vegetables rich in α carotene (yellow-orange vegetables such as carrots, sweet potatoes, pumpkin, winter squash and dark-green vegetables such as broccoli, green beans, green peas, spinach, and avocado) was associated with lower risk of premenopausal BC by 18% (median intake 0.5 serving/day vs median intake 0.03 serving/day). For individual fruits and vegetables, greater consumption significantly reduced BC risk (per 2 servings/week) for apples by 7%, bananas by 9%, and grapes by19% during adolescence and oranges by 7% and kale by 30% during early adulthood The association with adolescent fruit intake was stronger for both estrogen and progesterone receptor negative cancers than for the positive counterparts
Emaus et al. (2016). Investigate the association between vegetable and fruit intake and steroid hormone receptor–defined BC risk (European Prospective Investigation into Cancer and Nutrition [EPIC] study) [118]	335,054 women; mean age 51 years; median 11.5 years of follow-up; 10,197 BC cases (multivariate adjusted)	Higher vegetable intake was associated with a 13% lower overall BC risk vs low vegetable intake. The inverse association was most apparent for hormone receptor negative BC with lower risk by 26% (highest vs lowest intake; multivariate p-trend = 0.03). Fruit intake was not significantly associated with total and hormone receptor–defined BC risk
Fung et al. (2013). Examine the associations of specific fruits and vegetables on risk of estrogen receptor negative BC risk in postmenopausal women (Nurses' Health Study; US) [119]	75,929 women; baseline aged 38–63 years; followed for up to 24 years; 792 incident cases of estrogen receptor negative post-menopausal BC (multivariate adjusted)	For every 2 servings/week consumption of total berries BC risk was reduced by 18% (p = 0.01) and for ≥1 serving week of blueberries by 31% (p = 0.02) compared with non-consumers. Also, consuming ≥2 servings of peaches/nectarines/week lowered BC risk by 41% (p = 0.02). Risk of estrogen receptor negative BC was not associated with intakes of other specific fruits or vegetables (Fig. 20.13)

Table 20.8 (continued)

Objective	Study details	Results
Bao et al. (2012). Evaluate associations of fruits, vegetables and animal foods with BC risk (Shanghai Breast Cancer Study; China) [120]	3443 BC cases and 3474 healthy controls; 6 years of follow-up (multivariate adjusted)	Total vegetable intake was inversely related to BC risk with a 20% reduction for the highest quintile (p- trend = 0.02; multivariate adjusted). Significantly reduced BC risk between 16 and 24% was shown for high intake of allium vegetables, fresh legumes, citrus fruits and Rosaceae fruits, but inconsistent associations were observed for total fruit intake. Elevated risk was observed for all types of meat and fish intake, while intakes of eggs and milk were associated with a decreased risk of breast cancer
Masala et al. (2012) Evaluate the relationship between vegetables and fruit consumption, overall and by specific types, and BC risk (Italian section of the EPIC study; Mediterranean population) [121]	31,510 women; baseline age range 34–64 years; 45% post-menopausal; median 11 years of follow-up; 1072 BC cases (multivariate adjusted)	There was an inverse association between all "vegetables" and BC with a highest vs lowest intake reducing risk by 35% (p-trend = 0.03). For vegetable sub-types, there was an inverse association between leafy green vegetables, fruiting vegetables (e.g., peppers or eggplant) and raw tomatoes and BC risk (Fig. 20.14). However, there was no protective association observed for fruit overall or its subtypes

total vegetable intake, cruciferous vegetable intake and fruit intake) and BC prognosis (all-cause mortality, BC-specific mortality and BC recurrence) [113]. A 2013 Pooling Project of Prospective Studies of Diet and Cancer analysis (20 prospective studies; 993,466 women; follow-up of 11–20 years) showed that increased total fruit and vegetable intake was statistically significantly inversely associated with risk of estrogen receptor negative BC but not with the risk of BC overall or estrogen receptor positive BC tumors [114]. The inverse association for estrogen receptor negative tumors was observed primarily for vegetable consumption. Higher total vegetable intake was associated with a significant 18% lower risk for estrogen receptor negative BC but higher total fruit consumption was associated with an insignificant 6% lower risk of estrogen receptor negative BC. A 2012 dose-response analysis (15 prospective studies) found that higher intake of fruits, and fruit and vegetables combined, but not vegetables, was associated with modest but significant reductions in BC risk for the highest versus the lowest intake by 11% for fruit and vegetables combined, 8% for fruit and 1% for vegetables (including starchy vegetables) [115]. In dose-response analyses, per 200 g/day showed reduced BC risk for fruit and vegetables combined by 4%, fruit by 5%, and vegetables by 0%. An earlier 2001 analysis (8 prospective studies; 351,825 women; 7377 BC cases) showed highest vs lowest quartiles of fruit and vegetable intake (pooled multivariate) had insignificant associations with lower BC risks (total fruits 7%, total vegetables by 4%, and total fruits and vegetables by 7%) [116].

20.5.1.2 Prospective Cohort Studies

Five prospective cohort studies provide more details of the effects of specific fruits and vegetables and their dose-response effects on BC risk [117–121]. A 2016 Nurses' Health Study II analysis (90,476 premenopausal women; aged

27–44 years; 44,223 of those women completed a questionnaire about their diet during adolescence in 1998; 22 years of follow-up) found that total fruit intake during adolescence was associated with a significantly lower BC risk by 25% (median intake 2.9 servings/day vs 0.5 serving/day) [117]. Higher early adulthood intake of fruits and vegetables rich in α carotene (yellow-orange vegetables such as carrots, sweet potatoes, pumpkin, winter squash and dark-green vegetables such as broccoli, green beans, green peas, spinach, and avocado) was associated with lower risk of premenopausal BC by 18% (median intake 0.5 serving/day vs median intake 0.03 serving/day). For individual fruits and vegetables, greater consumption significantly reduced BC risk (per 2 servings/week) for apples by 7%, bananas by 9%, and grapes by19% during adolescence and oranges by 7% and kale by 30% during early adulthood. A 2016 EPIC analysis (335,054 women; mean age 51 years; median 11.5 years of follow-up) showed that higher vegetable intake had a 13% lower (mainly hormone receptor–negative) BC risk [118]. An inverse association for vegetable intake was most apparent for hormone receptor negative BC with a significant 26% lower BC risk (highest vs lowest intake; multivariate adjusted) but the effect of fruit intake on BC risk was not significantly associated with total and hormone receptor BC risk. A 2013 Nurses' Health Study analysis (75,929 women; baseline aged 38–63 years; followed for up to 24 years) found that estrogen receptor negative BC risk was significantly reduced per 2 servings/week of total berries, peaches and nectarines and ≥1 serving week of blueberries (Fig. 20.13) [119]. A 2012 Shanghai Breast Cancer Study analysis (3443 BC cases and 3474 healthy controls; 6 years of follow-up) showed that total vegetable intake was inversely related to BC risk with a 20% reduction for the highest quintile of intake [120]. Significant reduced BC risk of between 16 and 24% was shown for high intake of allium vegetables, fresh legumes, citrus fruits and Rosaceae fruits (apples, pears, berries) but inconsistent associations were observed for total fruit intake. A 2012 Italian EPIC analysis (31,510 women; baseline age range 34–64 years; 45% post-menopausal; median 11 years of follow-up) found an inverse association between all

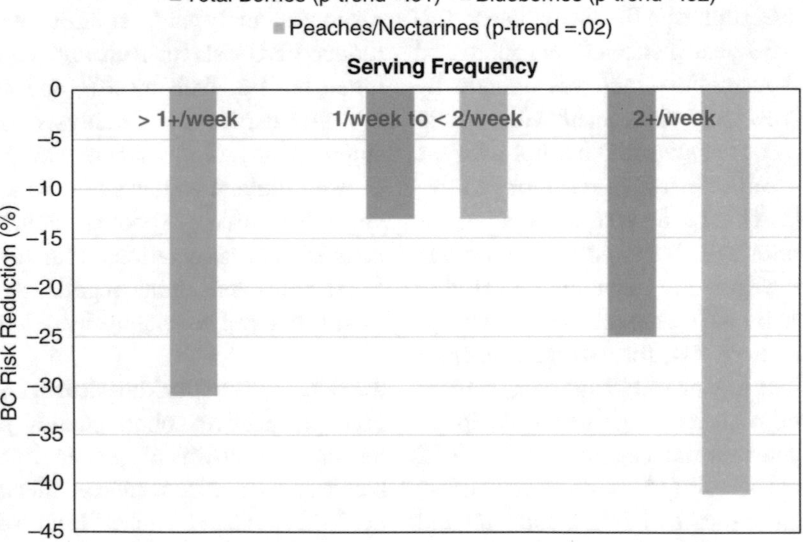

Fig. 20.13 Association between specific fruits and breast cancer (BC) risk in estrogen negative post-menopausal women from the Nurses' Health Study (adapted from [119])

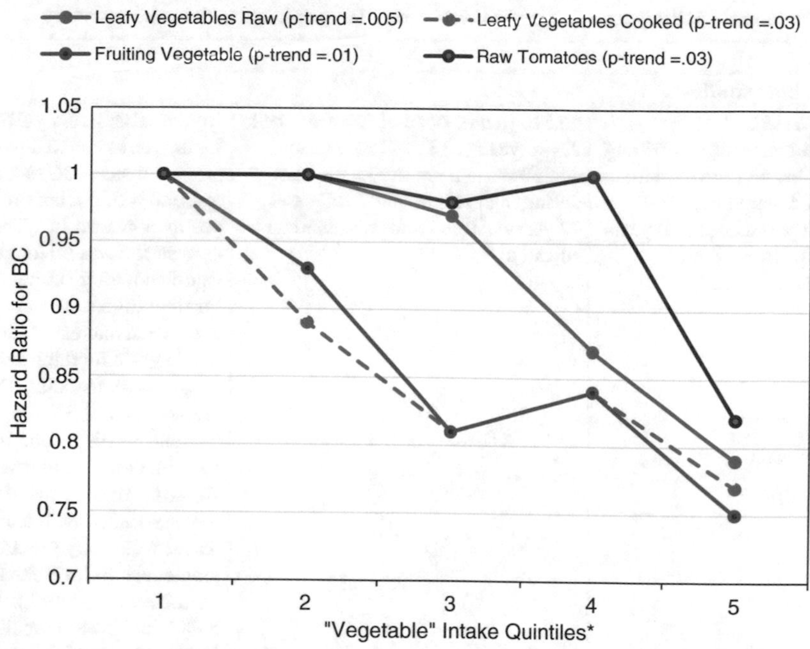

Fig. 20.14 Association between specific vegetables and breast cancer (BC) risk (adapted from [121]). * leafy vegetables raw intake range 6–32 g/day; leafy vegetables cooked intake range 5–25 g/day; fruiting (peppers/eggplant) vegetable intake range 15–57 g/day; rae tomatoes 14–76 g/day

vegetables and BC risk with a significant 35% reduction for highest vs lowest intake [121]. For sub-types of vegetables, there was an inverse association between BC risk and leafy green vegetables, fruiting vegetables (e.g., peppers or eggplant) and raw tomatoes (Fig. 20.14), but there was no protective association observed for fruit overall or its subtypes.

20.5.2 Whole Grains

Whole-grains, are rich sources of fiber, micronutrients and phytochemicals that may influence breast cancer risk. Table 20.9 summarizes the findings of two prospective cohort whole-grain studies on BC risk [122, 123]. A 2016 Nurses' Health Study II analysis (90,516 premenopausal women; aged 27–44 years; 3235 BC cases and 44,263 women reported their diet during high school, 1347 BC cases; 22 years of follow-up) found that adult intake of whole-grain foods was associated with significantly lower premenopausal BC risk by 18%, but not postmenopausal BC risk [122]. This association was no longer significant after further adjustment for fiber intake. The average of adolescent and early adulthood whole grain food intake was suggestively associated with lower premenopausal BC risk by 26% (p-trend = 0.09). Adult consumption of brown rice was associated with lower BC risk for all women by 6% and for premenopausal women by 9% (per each 2 servings/week). Adult white bread intake was associated with increased overall BC risk by 2% (per each 2 servings/week). Whole-grain pasta intake was inversely associated with overall BC risk. These results suggest that high whole-grain food intake may be associated with lower BC risk before menopause. A 2009 Danish Diet, Cancer and Health Cohort study analysis (25,278 postmenopausal women; mean follow-up of 9.6 years) showed in postmenopausal women that higher intake of whole grain products was not significantly associated

Table 20.9 Whole-grain and soy food studies on breast cancer (BC) risk, recurrence and mortality

Whole-grains		
Prospective cohort studies		
Farvid et al. (2016). Evaluate individual grain-containing foods and whole and refined grain intake during adolescence, early adulthood, and premenopausal years in relation to BC risk (Nurses' Health Study II; US) [122]	90,516 premenopausal women; aged 27–44 years; 3235 BC cases and 44,263 women reported their diet during high school, 1347 BC cases; 22 years of follow-up (multivariate adjusted)	Higher adult intake of whole grain foods was associated with lower premenopausal BC risk by 18% (p-trend = 0.03), but not postmenopausal BC. This association was no longer significant after further adjustment for fiber intake. The average of adolescent and early adulthood whole grain food intake was suggestively associated with lower premenopausal BC risk by 26% (p-trend = 0.09). Total refined grain food intake was not associated with BC risk. Adult brown rice intake was associated with lower BC risk for all women by 6% and for premenopausal women by 9% (per each 2 servings/week). Adult white bread intake was associated with increased overall BC risk (per each 2 servings/week by 2%). Whole grain pasta intake was inversely associated with overall BC risk. These results suggest that high whole grain food intake may be associated with lower BC risk before menopause
Egeberg et al. (2009). Investigate the association between intake of whole grain products and BC risk by hormone receptor status (Danish Diet, Cancer and Health Cohort study; Denmark) [123]	25,278 postmenopausal women; mean follow-up of 9.6 years; 978 BC cases (multivariate adjusted)	In postmenopausal women, higher intake of whole grain products was not significantly associated with a lower BC risk. Intake of rye bread, oatmeal and whole grain bread was not associated with BC risk
Soy Foods		
Systematic reviews and meta-analyses		
Wu et al. (2015). Assess the effect of diet on BC risk in Chinese women [37]	15 case-control studies; 11,283 Chinese women: 4602 in the experimental group and 6681 in the control group	Higher intake of soy foods significantly lowered BC risk by 32% (p = 0.02)
Nagata et al. (2014). Review epidemiological studies of soy intake and breast cancer among Japanese women [124]	5 cohort studies and 6 case-control studies	The association between soy foods and BC risk in Japanese women is inconsistent. Only 2 of the 5 cohort studies associated soy foods with a significantly lower risk of BC in postmenopausal women. In the case-control studies only 2 of 6 studies reported a significantly reduced BC risk

Table 20.9 (continued)

Chi et al. (2013). Evaluate the associations between soy food intake after cancer diagnosis with breast cancer survival [125]	5 cohort studies; 11,206 patients	Higher soy food intake after BC diagnosis was associated with better survival, reduced mortality by 15% and recurrence by 21%. Subgroup analysis of estrogen receptor status showed that higher soy food intake was associated with reduced mortality in both estrogen receptor negative and positive patients by 25% and 28%, respectively, in both premenopausal and postmenopausal women. Also, higher soy food intake was associated with reduced BC recurrence in estrogen receptor negative and positive by 36% and 33%, respectively, and in postmenopausal patients by 33%
Zhong and Zhang (2012). Explore the association of soy food intake and BC risk by meta-analysis [126]	23 case-control and 1 cohort studies	The pooled analysis of all studies showed that the highest intake of soy foods reduced BC risk by 14% vs the lowest intake. The protective effect was only observed in case-control studies. Also, the protective effect of soy foods was only observed in Asian women with a reduced BC risk of 24% compared to no association with Western women. In Asian women, the cohort studies found lower BC risk by 19% in post-menopausal women
Trock et al. (2006). Meta-analysis of soy intake and BC risk [127]	12 case-control and 6 cohort or nested case-control studies	Among all Asian and Western women, higher soy intake was modestly associated with reduced BC risk by 14%. When analyzed by soy protein intake (grams/day), there was statistically significantly association with lower BC risk by 6% only among premenopausal women
Prospective cohort studies		
Nechuta et al. (2012). Evaluate the association between postdiagnosis soy food consumption and breast cancer outcomes among US and Chinese women (After Breast Cancer Pooling Project) [128]	9514 BC survivors; mean baseline age 54 years; mean follow-up of 7.4 years; 1171 total deaths (881 from BC) and 1348 recurrences; soy isoflavone intake (mg/day) was measured with validated food-frequency questionnaires (multivariate adjusted)	Despite large differences in soy isoflavone intake by country, isoflavone consumption was inversely associated with BC recurrence, among both US and Chinese women, regardless of whether data were analyzed separately by country or combined. The consumption of ≥10 mg isoflavones/day from soy foods was associated with reduced risk of all-cause mortality by 13%, breast cancer-specific mortality by 17% and a statistically significantly reduced risk of recurrence by 25%

(continued)

Table 20.9 (continued)

Caan et al. (2011). Examine the Women's Healthy Eating and Living (WHEL) study population for the effect of soy intake on BC prognosis [129]	3088 early stage BC survivors; followed for a median of 7.3 years; soy food isoflavone intakes were measured post-diagnosis by using a food frequency questionnaire (multivariate adjusted)	Overall mortality risk was inversely associated with isoflavone intake (p-trend = 0.02). Women at the highest levels of isoflavone intake (>16.3 mg isoflavones, equivalent to ≥ one-half cup soymilk or 2-oz. tofu each day) had a 54% lower total mortality risk compared with the lowest quintile of soy intake but there was an insignificant 22% lowering of BC recurrence (p-trend = 0.47)
Shu et al. (2009). Evaluate the association of soy food intake after diagnosis of BC with total mortality and BC recurrence (Shanghai Breast Cancer Survival Study; China) [130]	5042 female BC survivors; mean age 53 years; median follow-up of 3.9 years; 444 deaths and 534 relapses (multivariate adjusted)	Higher soy food intake, as measured either by soy protein or soy isoflavone intake, lowered total mortality and BC recurrence by 33% vs lower intake

with a lower BC risk. Intake of rye bread, oatmeal and whole grain bread was not associated with BC risk [123].

20.5.3 Soy Foods

Soy food might have potential BC inhibitory effects as it is a rich source of isoflavones and a healthy protein source as well as having a range of other nutrients and phytochemicals associated with reduced BC risk [37]. Table 20.9 summarizes systematic reviews and meta-analyses, and representative prospective cohort studies on the effects of soy foods on BC risk, recurrence and mortality [37, 124–130].

20.5.3.1 Systematic Review and Meta-Analyses

Five systematic reviews and meta-analyses provide important insights on the associations between soy foods and BC risk and mortality. A 2015 analysis of studies of Chinese women (15 case-control studies; 11,283 women) showed higher intake of soy foods significantly lowered BC risk by 32% [37]. A 2014 analysis of studies of Japanese women (5 cohort studies and 6 case-control studies) found inconsistent results with only 2 of the 5 cohort studies and 2 of 6 case-control studies significantly associated with lower risk of BC in postmenopausal women [124]. A 2013 analysis (5 cohort studies; 11,206 patients) found that higher soy food intake after BC diagnosis was associated with better survival; reduced BC mortality by 15% and reduced BC recurrence by 21% [125]. Subgroup analysis of estrogen receptor status showed that soy food intake was associated with reduced mortality in both estrogen receptor negative and positive patients in both pre- and postmenopausal women. A 2012 analysis (23 case-control studies and 1 cohort study) found that soy foods intake was inversely associated with BC risk with a 14% reduction (highest vs lowest intake) [126]. Also, the protective effect of soy foods was only observed in Asian women with a reduced BC risk of 24% compared to no association with Western women. In Asian women, the one cohort study found that higher soy foods intake reduced BC risk by 19% in postmenopausal women. A 2006 meta-analysis (12 case-control and 6 cohort or nested case - control studies) showed that high soy intake was modestly associated with reduced BC risk by 14% among all women [127]. When exposure was analyzed by soy protein intake in grams/day, there was a statistically significant lower BC risk by 6% among premenopausal women.

20.5.3.2 Prospective Cohort Studies

Three prospective studies provide representative insights into the effects of soy foods on BC risk and recurrence [128–130]. A 2012 analysis of After Breast Cancer Pooling Project of Chinese and US women (9514 BC survivors; mean baseline age 54 years; mean follow-up of 7.4 years) showed that despite large differences in soy isoflavone intake by country, isoflavone consumption was inversely associated with BC recurrence among both US and Chinese women, regardless of whether data were analyzed separately by country or combined [128]. The consumption of ≥10 mg isoflavones/day from soy foods was associated with a nonsignificant reduced risk of all-cause mortality by 13%, breast cancer-specific mortality by 17% and a statistically significant reduced risk of recurrence by 25%. A 2011 prospective examination of the Women's Healthy Eating and Living (WHEL) study population (3088 early stage BC survivors; followed for a median of 7.3 years) showed that overall mortality risk was inversely associated with isoflavone intake [129]. Women at the highest levels of isoflavone intake (>16.3 mg isoflavones, equivalent to ≥ one-half cup soymilk or 2-ounces of tofu each day) had a significant 54% reduction in BC mortality risk compared with those in the lowest quintile of soy intake. A 2009 analysis of the Shanghai Breast Cancer Survival Study (5042 BC survivors; mean age 53 years; median follow-up of 3.9 years) showed that soy food intake, as measured either by soy protein or soy isoflavone intake, was inversely associated with BC mortality and recurrence with a 33% reduction (highest vs lowest intake) [130].

Conclusions

Dietary choices including: (1) level of adherence to healthy vs Western dietary patterns; (2) high vs low dietary energy density intake; (3) type and level of dietary fat, fiber and protein consumed; (4) adequate vs inadequate intake of calcium, folate and α-tocopherol; (5) type and levels of non-starchy vegetables and fruits containing dietary carotenoids and flavonoids intake; (6) level of phytoestrogen containing legumes and seeds consumed; and (7) higher vs lower intake of alcohol or coffee are examples of dietary factors that may influence breast cancer (BC) risk, recurrence or mortality. Biological factors and mechanisms associated with diet and BC risk and survival include: body weight and central adiposity, tumor advancement, systemic and tissue li pid/fatty acid peroxidation and inflammation, epigenetic and transcriptional regulation, hormone levels (e.g., estrogen, insulin, leptin, adiponectin and growth factor cascades), insulin resistance, and various endometabolic and colonic microbiota processes, which can influence BC initiation and progression. Lifestyle indicators, which are associated with increased BC risk, recurrence or mortality, especially for postmenopausal women, may include having an overweight or obese BMI, weight gain by over 15 lbs over 4 years, and physical inactivity. Patients with BC are most often either overweight or obese at diagnosis and obesity increases mortality risk in both pre- and postmenopausal women with BC. Meta-analyses reported that healthy dietary patterns reduced overall BC risk, whereas a high consumption of alcohol and a Western diet increased BC risk. Healthy dietary patterns, especially the Mediterranean diet, DASH diet and the vegan diet are effective in reducing BC risk and improving odds for survival. Highly colored non-starchy vegetables rich in carotenoids and flavonoids have been significantly associated with reduced BC risk especially in estrogen receptor negative BC. Key adverse dietary components for BC risk and survival include high intake of red and processed meats, high energy dense and high glycemic foods and beverages and >1 alcoholic beverage/day. After BC diagnosis, soy foods (>10 mg isoflavones/day or > ½ cup of soy milk or 2 ounces of tofu/day) may help to reduce BC recurrence or mortality in both Asian and Western women.

Appendix A: Comparison of Western and Healthy Dietary Patterns per 2000 kcal (Approximated Values)

Components	Western Dietary Pattern (US)	USDA Base Pattern	DASH Diet Pattern	Healthy Mediterranean Pattern	Healthy Vegetarian Pattern (Lact-ovo based)	Vegan Pattern
Emphasizes	Refined grains, low fiber foods, red meats, sweets, and solid fats	Vegetables, fruits, whole-grains, and low-fat milk	Potassium rich vegetables, fruits, and low fat milk products	Whole grains, vegetables, fruits, dairy products, olive oil, and moderate wine	Vegetables, fruit, whole-grains, legumes, nuts, seeds, milk products, and soy foods	Plant foods: vegetables, fruits, whole grains, nuts, seeds, and soy foods
Includes	Processed meats, sugar sweetened beverages, and fast foods	Enriched grains, lean meat, fish, nuts, seeds, and vegetable oils	Whole-grains, poultry, fish, nuts, and seeds	Fish, nuts, seeds, and pulses	Eggs, non-dairy milk alternatives, and vegetable oils	Non-dairy milk alternatives
Limits	Fruits and vegetables, and whole-grains	Solid fats and added sugars	Red meats, sweets and sugar-sweetened beverages	Red meats, refined grains, and sweets	No red or white meats, or fish; limited sweets	No animal products
Estimated nutrients/components						
Carbohydrates (% Total kcal)	51	51	55	50	54	57
Protein (% Total kcal)	16	17	18	16	14	13
Total fat (% Total kcal)	33	32	27	34	32	30
Saturated fat (% Total kcal)	11	8	6	8	8	7
Unsat. fat (% Total kcal)	22	25	21	24	26	25
Fiber (g)	16	31	29+	31	35+	40+
Potassium (mg)	2800	3350	4400	3350	3300	3650
Vegetable oils (g)	19	27	25	27	19–27	18–27
Sodium (mg)	3600	1790	1100	1690	1400	1225
Added sugar (g)	79 (20 tsp)	32 (8 tsp)	12 (3 tsp)	32 (8 tsp)	32 (8 tsp)	32 (8 tsp)
Plant food groups						
Fruit (cup)	≤1.0	2.0	2.5	2.5	2.0	2.0
Vegetables (cup)	≤1.5	2.5	2.1	2.5	2.5	2.5
Whole-grains (oz.)	0.5	3.0	4.0	3.0	3.0	3.0
Legumes (oz.)	–	1.5	0.5	1.5	3.0	3.0+
Nuts/Seeds (oz.)	0.5	0.6	1.0	0.6	1.0	2.0
Soy products (oz.)	0.0	0.5	–	–	1.1	1.5

U.S. Department of Agriculture and U.S. Department of Health and Human Services. Dietary Guidelines for Americans, 2010. 7th Edition, Washington, DC: U.S. Government Printing Office. 2010; Table B2.4; http://www.choosemyplate.gov/ accessed 8.22.2015

U.S. Department of Agriculture, Agriculture Research Service, Nutrient Data Laboratory. 2014. USDA National Nutrient Database for Standard Reference, Release 27. http://www.ars.usda.gov/nutrientdata. Accessed 17 February 2015

Dietary Guidelines Advisory Committee. Scientific Report. Advisory Report to the Secretary of Health and Human Services and the Secretary of Agriculture. Appendix E-3.7: Developing vegetarian and Mediterranean-style food patterns.2015;1–9

Dietary Guidelines Advisory Committee. Scientific Report. Advisory Report to the Secretary of Health and Human Services and the Secretary of Agriculture. Part D. Chapter 1: Food and nutrient intakes, and health: current status and trends. 2015;1–78

Bhupathiraju SN, Tucker KL. Coronary heart disease prevention: nutrients, foods, and dietary patterns. Clinica Chimica Acta. 2011;412: 1493–1514

Appendix B: Estimated Range of Energy, Fiber, Nutrients and Phytochemicals Composition of Whole Plant Foods/100 g Edible Portion

Components	Whole-grains	Fresh fruit	Dried fruit	Vegetables	Legumes	Nuts/seeds
Nutrients/ Phytochemicals	Wheat, oat, barley, rye, brown rice, whole grain bread, cereal, pasta, rolls and crackers	Apples, pears, bananas, grapes, oranges, blueberries, strawberries, and avocados	Dates, dried figs, apricots, cranberries, raisins and prunes	Potatoes, spinach, carrots, peppers, lettuce, green beans, cabbage, onions, cucumber, cauliflower, mushrooms, and broccoli	Lentils, chickpeas, split peas, black beans, pinto beans, and soy beans	Almonds, Brazil nuts, cashews, hazelnuts, macadamias, pecans, walnuts, peanuts, sunflower seeds, and flaxseed
Energy (kcals)	110–350	30–170	240–310	10–115	85–170	520–700
Protein (g)	2.5–16	0.5–2.0	0.1–3.4	0.2–5.0	5.0–17	7.8–24
Available Carbohydrate (g)	23–77	1.0–25	64–82	0.2–25	10–27	12–33
Fiber (g)	3.5–18	2.0–7.0	5.7–10	1.2–9.5	5.0–11	3.0–27
Total fat (g)	0.9–6.5	0.0–15	0.4–1.4	0.2–1.5	0.2–9.0	46–76
SFA[a] (g)	0.2–1.0	0.0–2.1	0.0	0.0–0.1	0.1–1.3	4.0–12
MUFA[a] (g)	0.2–2.0	0.0–9.8	0.0–0.2	0.1–1.0	0.1–2.0	9.0–60
PUFA[a] (g)	0.3–2.5	0.0–1.8	0.0–0.7	0.0.0.4	0.1–5.0	1.5–47
Folate (ug)	4.0–44	<5.0–61	2–20	8.0–160	50–210	10–230
Tocopherols (mg)	0.1–3.0	0.1–1.0	0.1–4.5	0.0–1.7	0.0–1.0	1.0–35
Potassium (mg)	40–720	60–500	40–1160	100–680	200–520	360–1050
Calcium (mg)	7.0–50	3.0–25	10–160	5.0–200	20–100	20–265
Magnesium (mg)	40–160	3.0–30	5.0–70	3.0–80	40–90	120–400
Phytosterols (mg)	30–90	1.0–83	–	1.0–54	110–120	70–215
Polyphenols (mg)	70–100	50–800	–	24–1250	120–6500	130–1820
Carotenoids (ug)	–	25–6600	1.0–2160	10–20,000	50–600	1.0–1200

U.S. Department of Agriculture, Agriculture Research Service, Nutrient Data Laboratory. 2014. USDA National Nutrient Database for Standard Reference, Release 27. http://www.ars. usda.gov./nutrientdata. Accessed 17 February 2015

Ros E, Hu FB. Consumption of plant seeds and cardiovascular health epidemiological and clinical trial evidence. Circulation. 2013;128: 553–565

USDA. What we eat in America, NHANES 2011–2012, individuals 2 years and over (excluding breast-fed children). Available: www.ars.usda.gov/nea/bhnrc/fsrg

Slavin JL, Lloyd B. Health benefits of fruits and vegetables. Adv Nutr. 2012; 3:506–516

Rebello CJ, Greenway FL, Finley JW. A review of the nutritional value of legumes and their effects on obesity and its related co-morbidities. Obes Rev. 2014;15: 392–407
Gebhardt SE, Thomas RG. Nutritive Value of Foods. 2002; U.S. Department of Agriculture, Agricultural Research Service, Home and Garden Bulletin 72
Holden JM, Eldridge AL, Beecher GR, et al. Carotenoid content of U.S. foods: An update of the database. J Food Comp An. 1999; 12:169–196
Lu Q-Y, Zhang Y, Wang Y, et al. California Hass avocado: profiling of carotenoids, tocopherol, fatty acid, and fat content during maturation and from different growing areas. *J* Agric Food Chem. 2009; 57(21):10408–10413
Wu X, Beecher GR, Holden JM, et al. Lipophilic and hydrophilic antioxidant capacities of common foods in the United States. J Agric Food Chem. 2004; 52: 4026–4037
Bhupathiraju SN, Tucker KL. Coronary heart disease prevention: nutrients, foods, and dietary patterns. Clinica Chimica Acta. 2011;412: 1493–1514
Dietary Guidelines Advisory Committee. Scientific Report. Advisory Report to the Secretary of Health and Human Services and the Secretary of Agriculture. Part D. Chapter 1: Food and nutrient intakes, and health: current status and trends. 2015;1–78
http://health.gov/dietaryguidelines/2015/guidelines/ accessed 1.26.2016

[a]SFA (saturated fat), MUFA (monounsaturated fat) and PUFA (polyunsaturated fat)

References

1. Global Burden of Disease Cancer Collaboration. Global, regional, and national cancer incidence, mortality, years of life lost, years lived with disability, and disability-adjusted life-years for 32 cancer groups, 1990 to 2015. A systematic analysis for the Global Burden of Disease Study. JAMA Oncol. 2017;3(4):524–48. https://doi.org/10.1001/jamaoncol.2016.5688.
2. World Cancer Research Fund/American Institute for Cancer Research. Continuous Update Project Report. Diet, nutrition, physical activity, and breast cancer. 2017. wcrf.org/breast-cancer.
3. World Cancer Research Fund International/American Institute for Cancer Research. Continuous Update Project Report: diet, nutrition, physical activity, and breast cancer survivors. 2014.
4. Rossi RE, Pericleous M, Mandair D, Whyand TME. The role of dietary factors in prevention and progression of breast cancer. Anticancer Res. 2014;34: 6861–76.
5. American Cancer Society. Breast cancer facts & figures 2013–2014. Atlanta: American Cancer Society, Inc; 2013.
6. Anand P, Kunnumakkara AB, Sundaram C, et al. Cancer is a preventable disease that requires major lifestyle changes. Pharm Res. 2008;25:2097–116. https://doi.org/10.1007/s11095-008-9661-9.
7. Thomson CA, Thompson PA. Dietary patterns, risk and prognosis of breast cancer. Future Oncol. 2009;5(8):1257–69. https://doi.org/10.2217/fon.09.86.
8. Harmon BE, Boushey CJ, Shvetsov YB, et al. Associations of key diet-quality indexes with mortality in the Multiethnic Cohort: the Dietary Patterns Methods Project. Am J Clin Nutr. 2015;101(3):587–97. https://doi.org/10.3945/ajcn.114. 090688.
9. Schwingshackl L, Hoffmann G. Diet quality as assessed by the healthy eating index, the alternate healthy eating index, the dietary approaches to stop hypertension score, and health outcomes: a systematic review and meta-analysis of cohort studies. J Acad Nutr Diet. 2015;115(5):780–800.e5. https://doi.org/10.1016/j.jand.2014.12.009.
10. Rice MS, Eliassen AH, Hankinson SE, et al. Breast cancer research in the Nurses' Health Studies: exposures across the life course. Am J Public Health. 2016;106:1592–8. https://doi.org/10.2105/AJPH.2016.303325.
11. World Cancer Research Fund/American Institute for Cancer Research. Food, nutrition, physical activity, and the prevention of cancer: a global perspective; 2007. p. 289–95.
12. American Institute for Cancer Research. Recommendations for cancer prevention. www.aicr.org/reduce-your-risk/recommendations-for-cancer-prevention/recommendations. Accessed 17 May 2015.
13. Kushi LH, Doyle C, McCullough M, et al. American Cancer Society guidelines on nutrition and physical activity for cancer prevention: reducing the risk of cancer with healthy food choices and physical activity. CA Cancer J Clin. 2012;62(1):30–67.
14. Castelló A, Martín M, Ruiz A, et al. Lower breast cancer risk among women following the World Cancer Research Fund and American Institute for Cancer Research lifestyle recommendations: EpiGEICAM Case-Control Study. PLoS One. 2015;10(5):e0126096. https://doi.org/10.1371/journal.pone.0126096.
15. Thomson CA, McCullough MJ, Wertheim BC, et al. Nutrition and physical activity cancer prevention guidelines, cancer risk, and mortality in the Women's Health Initiative. Cancer Prev Res. 2014;7(1):42–53.
16. McKenzie F, Ferrari P, Freisling H, et al. Healthy lifestyle and risk of breast cancer among postmenopausal women in the European Prospective Investigation into Cancer and Nutrition cohort study. Int J Cancer. 2015;136:2640–8.
17. Dieli-Conwright CM, Lee K, Kiwata JL. Reducing the risk of breast cancer recurrence: an evaluation

of the effects and mechanisms of diet and exercise. Curr Breast Cancer Rep. 2016;8:139–50. https://doi.org/10.1007/s12609-016-218-3.

18. Bhargava A. Fiber intakes and anthropometric measures are predictors of circulating hormone, triglyceride, and cholesterol concentrations in the Women's Health Trial. J Nutr. 2006;136:2249–54.
19. Chan DSM, Vieira AR, Aune D, et al. Body mass index and survival in women with breast cancer-systematic literature review and meta-analysis of 82 follow-up studies. Ann Oncol. 2014;25:1901–14. https://doi.org/10.1093/annonc/mdu042.
20. Playdon MC, Bracken MB, Sanft TB, et al. Weight gain after breast cancer diagnosis and all-cause mortality: systematic review and meta-analysis. J Natl Cancer Inst. 2015;107(120):djv275. https://doi.org/10.1093/jnci/djv275.
21. Cespedes Feliciano EM, Kroenke CH, Bradshaw PT, et al. Postdiagnosis weight change and survival following a diagnosis of early-stage breast cancer. Cancer Epidemiol Biomark Prev. 2017;26(1):44–50. https://doi.org/10.1158/1055-9965.EPI-16-0150.
22. Hartman TJ, Gapstur SM, Gaudet MM, et al. Dietary energy density and postmenopausal breast cancer incidence in the Cancer Prevention Study II Nutrition Cohort. J Nutr. 2016;146:2045–50.
23. Jones JA, Hartman TJ, Klifa CJ, et al. Dietary energy density is positively associated with breast density among young women. J Acad Nutr Diet. 2015;115(3):353–9. https://doi.org/10.1016/j.jand.2014.08.015.
24. Harris HR, Willett WC, Vaidya RL, Michels KB. An adolescent and early adulthood dietary pattern associated with inflammation and the incidence of breast cancer. Cancer Res. 2017;77(5):1179–87. https://doi.org/10.1158/0008-5472.CAN-16-2273.
25. Harris HR, Willett WC, Vaidya RL, Michels KB. Adolescent dietary patterns and premenopausal breast cancer incidence. Carcinogenesis. 2016;37(4):376–84. https://doi.org/10.1093/carcin/bgw023.
26. Chen J-Y, Zhu H-C, Guo Q, et al. Dose-dependent association between wine drinking and breast cancer risk- meta-analysis findings. Asian Pac J Cancer Prev. 17(30):1221–33. https://doi.org/10.7314/APJCP.2016.17.3.1221.
27. Suzuki R, Orsini N, Mignone L, et al. Alcohol intake and risk of breast cancer defined by estrogen and progesterone receptor status—a meta-analysis of epidemiological studies. Int J Cancer. 2008;122:1832–41. https://doi.org/10.1002/ijc.23184.
28. Ali AMG, Schmidt MK, Bolla MK, et al. Alcohol consumption and survival after a breast cancer diagnosis: a literature -based meta-analysis and collaborative analysis of data for 29,239 cases. Cancer Epidemiol Biomark Prev. 2014;23(6):934–45. https://doi.org/10.1158/1055-9965.EPI-13-0901.
29. Dam MK, Hvidtfeldt UA, Tjonneland A, et al. Five-year change in alcohol intake and risk of breast cancer and coronary heart disease among postmenopausal women: prospective cohort study. BMJ. 2016;353:i2314. https://doi.org/10.1113/bmj.i2314.
30. Jiang W, Wu Y, Jiang X. Coffee and caffeine intake and breast cancer risk: an updated dose-response meta-analysis of 37 published studies. Gynecol Oncol. 2013;129(3):620–9. https://doi.org/10.1016/j.ygyno.2013.03.014.
31. Bhoo-Pathy N, Peeters PHM, Uiterwaal CSPM, et al. Coffee and tea consumption and risk of pre- and postmenopausal breast cancer in the European Prospective Investigation into Cancer and Nutrition (EPIC) cohort study. Breast Cancer Res. 2015;17:15. https://doi.org/10.1186/s13058-015-0521-3.
32. Ganmaa D, Willett WC, Li TY, et al. Coffee, tea, caffeine and risk of breast cancer: A 22-year follow-up. In J Cancer. 2008;122:2071–6.
33. Neilson HK, Farris MS, Stone CR, et al. Moderate-vigorous recreational physical activity and breast cancer risk, stratified by menopause status: a systematic review and meta-analysis. Menopause. 2017;24(3):322–44. https://doi.org/10.1097/GME.0000000000000745.
34. van den Brandt PA, Schulpen M. Mediterranean diet adherence and risk of postmenopausal breast cancer: results of a cohort study and meta-analysis. Int J Cancer. 2017;140:2220–31.
35. Bloomfield HE, Koeller E, Greer N, et al. Effects on health outcomes of a Mediterranean diet with no restriction on fat intake. A systematic review and meta-analysis. Ann Intern Med. 2016;165(7):491–500. https://doi.org/10.7326/M16-0361.
36. Pourmasoumi M, Karimbeiki R, Vosoughi N, et al. Healthy eating index/alternative healthy eating index and breast cancer mortality and survival: a systematic review and meta-analysis. Asia Pac J Oncol Nurs. 2016;3:297–305. https://doi.org/10.4103/2347-5625.189819.
37. Wu Y-C, Zheng D, Sun JJ, et al. Meta-analysis of studies on breast cancer risk and diet in Chinese women. Int J Clin Exp Med. 2015;8(1):73–85.
38. Xing M-Y, Xu S-Z, Shen P. Effect of low-fat diet on breast cancer survival: a meta-analysis. Asia Pac J Cancer Prev. 2014;15:1141–4. https://doi.org/10.7314/APJCP.2014.15.3.1141.
39. Liu X-O, Huang Y-B, Gao Y, et al. Association between dietary factors and breast cancer risk among Chinese females: systematic review and meta-analysis. Asian Pac J Cancer Prev. 2015;15(3):1291–8. https://doi.org/10.7314/APJCP.2014.15.3.1291.
40. Farsinejad-Marj M, Talebi S, Ghiyasvand R, Miraghajani M. Adherence to Mediterranean diet and risk of breast cancer in premenopausal and postmenopausal women. Arch Iran Med. 2015;18(11):786–92.
41. Albuquerque RCR, Baltar VT, Marchioni DML. Breast cancer and dietary patterns: a systematic review. Nutr Rev. 2013;72(1):1–17.
42. Brennan SF, Cantwell MM, Cardwell CR, et al. Dietary patterns and breast cancer risk: a systematic review and meta-analysis. Am J Clin Nutr. 2010;91:1294–302.

43. Penniecook-Sawyers JA, Jaceldo-Siegl K, Fan J, et al. Vegetarian dietary patterns and the risk of breast cancer in a low-risk population. Br J Nutr. 2016;115(10):1790–7. https://doi.org/10.1017/S0007114516000751.
44. Hirko KA, Willett WC, Hankinson SE, et al. Healthy dietary patterns and risk of breast cancer by molecular subtype. Breast Cancer Res. 2016;155(3):579–88. https://doi.org/10.1007/s10549-016-3706-2.
45. Link LB, Canchola AJ, Bernstein L, et al. Dietary patterns and breast cancer risk in the California Teachers Study cohort. Am J Clin Nutr. 2013;98:1524–32.
46. Couto E, Sandin S, Lof M, et al. Mediterranean dietary pattern and risk of breast cancer. PLoS One. 2013;8(2):e55374. https://doi.org/10.1371/journal.pone.0055374.
47. Buckland G, Travier N, Cottet V, et al. Adherence to the Mediterranean diet and risk of breast cancer in the European Prospective Investigation into Cancer and Nutrition cohort study. Int J Cancer. 2013;132:2918–27.
48. Vrieling A, Buck K, Seibold P, et al. Dietary patterns and survival in German postmenopausal breast cancer survivors. Br J Cancer. 2013;108:188–92. https://doi.org/10.1038/bjc.2012.521.
49. Izano MA, Fung TT, Chiuve SS, et al. Are diet quality after breast cancer diagnosis associated with improved breast cancer survival? Nutr Cancer. 2013;65(6):820–6. https://doi.org/10.1080/01635581.2013.804939.
50. Kim HER, Willett WC, Fung T, et al. Diet quality indices and postmenopausal breast cancer survival. Nutr Cancer. 2011;63(3):381–8. https://doi.org/10.1080/01635581.2011.535963.
51. Fung TT, Hu FB, Hankinson SE, et al. Low carbohydrate diets, dietary approaches to stop hypertension diets, and the risk of postmenopausal breast cancer. Am J Epidemiol. 2011;174(6):652–60. https://doi.org/10.1093/aje/kwr148.
52. Cade JE, Taylor EF, Burley VJ, Greenwood DC. Common dietary patterns and risk of breast cancer: analysis from the United Kingdom Women's Cohort Study. Nutr Cancer. 2010;62(3):300–6. https://doi.org/10.1080/01635580903441246.
53. Trichopoulou A, Bamia C, Lagiou P, Trichopoulos D. Conformity to traditional Mediterranean diet and breast cancer risk in the Greek EPIC (European Prospective Investigation into Cancer and Nutrition) cohort. Am J Clin Nutr. 2010;92:620–5.
54. Cottet V, Touvier M, Fournier A, et al. Postmenopausal breast cancer risk and dietary patterns in the E3N-EPIC Prospective Cohort Study. Am J Epidemiol. 2009;170:1257–67. https://doi.org/10.1093/aje/kwp257.
55. Kwan ML, Welzien E, Kushi LH, et al. Dietary patterns and breast cancer recurrence and survival among women with early-stage breast cancer. J Clin Oncol. 2009;27:919–26. https://doi.org/10.1200/JCO.2008.19.4035.
56. Rock CL, Flatt SW, Pakiz B, et al. Effects of diet composition on weight loss, metabolic factors and biomarkers in a 1-year weight loss intervention in obese women examined by baseline insulin resistance status. Metabolism. 2016;65(11):1605–13. https://doi.org/10.1016/j.metabol. 2016.07.008.
57. Neuhouser ML, Aragaki AK, Prentice RL, et al. Overweight, Obesity and Postmenopausal Invasive Breast Cancer Risk. JAMA Oncol. 2015;1(5):611–21. https://doi.org/10.1001/jamaoncol. 2015.1546.
58. Toledo E, Salas-Salvadó J, Donat-Vargas C, et al. Mediterranean diet and invasive breast cancer risk among women at high cardiovascular risk in the PREDIMED trial. A randomized clinical trial. JAMA Intern Med. 2015;175(11):1752–60. https://doi.org/10.1001/jamainternmed.2015.4838.
59. Martin LJ, Li Q, Melnichouk O, et al. A randomized trial of dietary intervention for breast cancer prevention. Cancer Res. 2011;71(1):123–33. https://doi.org/10.1158/0008-5472.CAN-10-1436.
60. Pierce JP, Natarajan L, Caan BJ, et al. Dietary change and reduced breast cancer events among women without hot flashes after treatment of early-stage breast cancer: subgroup analysis of the Women's Healthy Eating and Living Study. Am J Clin Nutr. 2009;89(suppl):1565S–71S.
61. Gold EB, Pierce JP, Natarajan L, et al. Dietary pattern influences breast cancer prognosis in women without hot flashes: The Women's Healthy Eating and Living Trial. J Clin Oncol. 2008;27:352–9.
62. Pierce JP, Natarajan L, Caan BJ, et al. Influence of a diet very high in vegetables, fruit, and fiber and low in fat on prognosis following treatment for breast cancer: the Women's Healthy Eating and Living (WHEL) randomized trial. JAMA. 2007;298:289–98.
63. Prentice RL, Caan B, Chlebowski RT, et al. Low-fat dietary pattern and risk of invasive breast cancer The Women's Health Initiative Randomized Controlled Dietary Modification Trial. JAMA. 2006;295(6):629–42.
64. Chlebowski R, Blackburn GL, Thomson CA, et al. Dietary fat reduction and breast cancer outcome: interim efficacy results for the Women's Intervention Nutrition Study (WINS). J Natl Cancer Inst. 2006;98:1767–76.
65. Rock CL, Flatt SW, Thomson CA, et al. Effects of a high-fiber, low-fat diet intervention on serum concentrations of reproductive steroid hormones in women with a history of breast cancer. J Clin Oncol. 2004;22(12):2379–87.
66. Rock CL, Thomson C, Caan BJ, et al. Reduction in fat intake is not associated with weight loss in most women after breast cancer diagnosis: evidence from a randomized controlled trial. Cancer. 2001;91:25–34.
67. Lindstrom J, Peltonen M, Eriksson JG, et al. High-fibre, low-fat diet predicts long-term weight loss and decreased type 2 diabetes risk: the Finnish Diabetes Prevention Study. Diabetologia. 2006;49:912–20. https://doi.org/10.1007/s00125-006-0198-3.

68. Dahl WJ, Stewart ML. Position of the Academy of Nutrition and Dietetics: health implications of dietary fiber. J Acad Nutr Diet. 2015;115:1861–70.
69. Hoy MK, Goldman JD. Fiber intake in the US population. What we eat in America, NHANES 2009–2010. Food Surveys Research Group. 2014; Dietary Data Brief No 12:1–6.
70. Chen S, Chen Y, Ma S, et al. Dietary fibre intake and risk of breast cancer: a systematic review and meta-analysis of epidemiological studies. Oncotarget. 2016;7(49):80980–9.
71. Xing M-Y, Xu S-Z, Shen P. Effect of low-fat diet on breast cancer survival: a meta-analysis. Asian Pac J Cancer Prev. 2014;15(3):1141–4. https://doi.org/10.7314/APJCP.2014.15.3.1141.
72. Aune D, Chan DSM, Greenwood DC, et al. Dietary fiber and breast cancer risk: a systematic review and meta-analysis of prospective studies. Ann Oncol. 2012;23:1394–402.
73. Dong J-Y, He K, Wang P, Qin L-Q. Dietary fiber intake and risk of breast cancer: a meta-analysis of prospective cohort studies. Am J Clin Nutr. 2011;94:900–5.
74. Farvid MS, Eliassen H, Cho E, et al. Dietary fiber intake in young adults and breast cancer risk. Pediatrics. 2016;137(3):e20151226. https://doi.org/10.1542/peds.2015-1226.
75. Chhim A-S, Fassier P, Latino-Martel P, et al. Prospective association between alcohol intake and hormone dependent cancer risk: modulation by dietary fiber intake. Am J Clin Nutr. 2015;102(2):182–9. 10.39445/ajcn.114.098418.
76. Ferrari P, Rinaldi S, Jenab M, et al. Dietary fiber intake and risk of hormonal receptor–defined breast cancer in the European Prospective Investigation into Cancer and Nutrition Study. Am J Clin Nutr. 2013;97:344–53.
77. Park Y, Brinton LA, Subar AF, et al. Dietary fiber intake and risk of breast cancer in postmenopausal women: the National Institutes of Health-AARP Diet and Health Study. Am J Clin Nutr. 2009;90:664–71.
78. Cade JE, Burley VJ, Greenwood DC. Dietary fibre and risk of breast cancer in the UK Women's Cohort Study. Int J Epidemiol. 2007;36:431–8.
79. Mattisson I, Wirfalt E, Johansson U, et al. Intakes of plant foods, fibre and fat and risk of breast cancer—a prospective study in the Malmo¨ Diet and Cancer cohort. Br J Cancer. 2004;90:122–7.
80. Holmes MD, Liu S, Hankinson SE, et al. Dietary carbohydrates, fiber, and breast cancer risk. Am J Epidemiol. 2004;159:732–9.
81. Terry P, Jain M, Miller AB, et al. No association among total dietary fiber, fiber fractions, and risk of breast cancer. Cancer Epidemiol Biomark Prev. 2002;11:1507–8.
82. Willett WC, Hunter DJ, Stampfer MJ, et al. Dietary fat and fiber in relation to risk of breast cancer an 8-year follow-up. JAMA. 1992;268:2037–44.
83. Brennan SF, Woodside JV, Lunny PM, et al. Dietary fat and breast cancer mortality: a systematic review and meta-analysis. Crit Rev Food Sci Nutr. 2017;57(10):1999–2008.https://doi.org/10.1080/10408398.2012.724481.
84. Cao Y, Hou L, Wang W. Dietary total fat and fatty acids intake, serum fatty acids and risk of breast cancer: a meta-analysis of prospective cohort studies. Int J Cancer. 2016;138:1894–904. https://doi.org/10.1002/ijc.29938.
85. Xia H, Ma S, Wang S, Sun G. Meta-analysis of saturated fatty acid intake and breast cancer risk. Medicine. 2015;94(52):e2391. https://doi.org/10.1097/MD0000000000002391.
86. Xin Y, Li X-Y, Wan L-X, Huang T. Vegetable oil intake and breast cancer risk: a meta-analysis. Asian Pac J Cancer Prev. 2015;16(12):5125–1535. https://doi.org/10.7314/APJCP.2015.16.12.5125.
87. Yang B, Ren X-L, Fu Y-Q, et al. Ratio of n-3/n-6 PUFA and risk of breast cancer: a meta-analysis of 274,135 adult females from 11 independent prospective studies. BMC Cancer. 2014;14:105.
88. Farvid MS, Cho E, Chen WY, et al. Premenopausal dietary fat in relation to pre- and postmenopausal breast cancer. Breast Cancer Res Treat. 2014;145:255–5. https://doi.org/10.1007/s10549-014-2895-9.
89. Boeke CE, Eliassen AH, Chen WY, et al. Dietary fat intake in relation to lethal breast cancer in two large prospective cohort studies. Breast Cancer Res Treat. 2014;146(2):383–92. https://doi.org/10.1007/s10549-014-3005-8.
90. Sieri S, Krogh V, Ferrari P, et al. Dietary fat and breast cancer risk in the European Prospective Investigation into Cancer and Nutrition. Am J Clin Nutr. 2008;88:1304–12.
91. Chajes V, Thiebaut ACM, Rotival M, et al. Association between serum trans-monounsaturated fatty acids and breast cancer risk in the E3N-EPIC Study. Am J Epidemiol. 2008;167:1312–20. https://doi.org/10.1093/aje/kwn069.
92. Holmes MD, Hunter DJ, Colditz GA, et al. Association of dietary intake of fat and fatty acids with risk of breast cancer. JAMA. 1999;281:914–20.
93. Farvid MS, Cho E, Chen WY, et al. Dietary protein sources in early adulthood and breast cancer incidence: prospective cohort study. BMJ. 2014;348:g3437. https://doi.org/10.1136/bmj.g3437.
94. Wu J, Zeng R, Huang J, et al. Dietary protein sources and incidence of breast cancer: a dose-response meta-analysis of prospective studies. Forum Nutr. 2016;8:730. https://doi.org/10.3390/nu8110730.
95. Zhang Y-F, Shi W-W, Gao H-F, et al. Folate intake and the risk of breast cancer: a dose-response meta-analysis of prospective studies. PLoS One. 2014;9(6):e100044. https://doi.org/10.1371/journal.pone.0100044.
96. Hu F, Wu Z, Li G, et al. The plasma level of retinol, vitamins A, C and α-tocopherol could reduce breast cancer risk? A meta-analysis and meta-regression. J Cancer Res Clin Oncol. 2015;141:601–14. https://doi.org/10.1007/s00432-014-1852-7.

97. Hu F, Jiang C, Baina WY, et al. Retinol, vitamins A, C and E and breast cancer risk: a meta-analysis and meta-regression. Cancer Causes Control. 2011;22:1383–96. https://doi.org/10.1007/s10552-011-9811-y.
98. Kim Y, Je Y. Vitamin D intake, blood 25(OH)D levels, and breast cancer risk or mortality: a meta-analysis. Br J Cancer. 2014;110:2772–84. https://doi.org/10.1038/bjc.2014.175.
99. Hidayat K, Chen G-C, Zhang R, et al. Calcium intake and breast cancer risk: meta-analysis of prospective cohort studies. Br J Nutr. 2016;116:158–66. https://doi.org/10.1017/S0007114516001768.
100. Eliassen AH, Hendrickson SJ, Brinton LA, et al. Circulating carotenoids and risk of breast cancer: pooled analysis of eight prospective studies. J Natl Cancer Inst. 2012;104:1905–16. https://doi.org/10.1093/jnci/djs461.
101. Aune D, Chan DSM, Vieira AR, et al. Dietary compared with blood concentrations of carotenoids and breast cancer risk: a systematic review and meta-analysis of prospective studies. Am J Clin Nutr. 2012;96:356–73. https://doi.org/10.3945/ajcn.112.034165.
102. Hu F, Yi BW, Zhang W, et al. Carotenoids and breast cancer risk: a meta-analysis and meta regression. Breast Cancer Res Treat. 2012;131:239–53. https://doi.org/10.1007/s10549-011-1723-8.
103. Eliassen AH, Liao X, Rosner B, et al. Plasma carotenoids and risk of breast cancer over 20 y of follow-up. Am J Clin Nutr. 2015;101:1197–205. https://doi.org/10.3956/ajcn.114.105080.
104. Boeke CE, Tamini RM, Berkey CS, et al. Adolescent carotenoid intake and benign breast disease. Pediatrics. 2014;133:e1292–8. https://doi.org/10.1542/peds.2013-3844.
105. Rock CL, Flatt SW, Natarajan L, et al. Plasma carotenoids and recurrence-free survival in women with a history of breast cancer. J Clin Oncol. 2005;23:6631–8. https://doi.org/10.1200/JCO.2005.19.505.
106. Hui C, Qi X, Qianyong Z, et al. Flavonoids, flavonoid subclasses and breast cancer risk: a meta-analysis of epidemiologic studies. PLoS One. 2013;8(1):e54318. https://doi.org/10.1371/journal.pone.0054318.
107. Chen M, Rao Y, Zheng Y, et al. Association between soy isoflavone intake and breast cancer risk for pre- and post-menopausal women: a meta-analysis of epidemiological studies. PLoS One. 2014;9(2):e89288. https://doi.org/10.1371/journal.pone.0089288.
108. Xie Q, Chen M-L, Qin Y, et al. Isoflavone consumption and risk of breast cancer: a dose-response meta-analysis of observational studies. Asia Pac J Clin Nutr. 2013;22(1):118–27. https://doi.org/10.6133/apjcn.2013.22.1.16.
109. Dong J-Y, Qin L-Q. Soy isoflavones consumption and risk of breast cancer incidence or recurrence: a meta-analysis of prospective studies. Breast Cancer Res Treat. 2011;125:315–23. https://doi.org/10.1007/s10549-010-1270-8.
110. Seibold P, Vrieling A, Johnson TS, et al. Enterolactone concentrations and prognosis after postmenopausal breast cancer: assessment of effect modification and meta-analysis. Int J Cancer. 2014;135:923–33. https://doi.org/10.1002/ijc.28729.
111. Buck K, Zaineddin AK, Vrieling A, et al. Meta-analyses of lignans and enterolignans in relation to breast cancer risk. Am J Clin Nutr. 2010;92:141–53. https://doi.org/10.3945/ajcn.2009.28573.
112. He J, Gu Y, Zhang S. Consumption of vegetables and fruits and breast cancer survival: a systematic review and meta-analysis. Sci Rep. 2017;7:599. https://doi.org/10.1038/s41598-017-00635-5.
113. Peng C, Luo W-P, Zhang C-X. Fruit and vegetable intake and breast cancer prognosis: a meta-analysis of prospective cohort studies. Br J Nutr. 2017;117:737–49. https://doi.org/10.1017/S0007114517000423.
114. Jung S, Spiegelman D, Baglietto L, et al. Fruit and vegetable intake and risk of breast cancer by hormone receptor status. J Natl Cancer Inst. 2013;105:219–36. https://doi.org/10.1093/jnci/djs635.
115. Aune D, Chan DSM, Vieira AR, et al. Fruits, vegetables and breast cancer risk: a systematic review and meta-analysis of prospective studies. Breast Cancer Res Treat. 2012;134(2):479–93.
116. Smith-Warner SA, Spiegelman D, Yaun SS, et al. Intake of fruits and vegetables and risk of breast cancer: a pooled analysis of cohort studies. JAMA. 2001;285:769–76.
117. Farvid MS, Chen WY, Michels KB, et al. Fruit and vegetable consumption in adolescence and early adulthood and risk of breast cancer: population based cohort study. BMJ. 2016;353:i2343. https://doi.org/10.1136/bmj.i2343.
118. Emaus MJ, Peeters PHM, Bakker MF, et al. Vegetable and fruit consumption and the risk of hormone receptor–defined breast cancer in the EPIC cohort. Am J Clin Nutr. 2016;103:168–77.
119. Fung TT, Chiuve SE, Willett WC, et al. Intake of specific fruits and vegetables in relation to risk of estrogen receptor-negative breast cancer among postmenopausal women. Breast Cancer Res Treat. 2013;138(3):925–30. https://doi.org/10.1007/s10549-013-2484-3.
120. Bao P-P, Shu X-O, Zheng Y, et al. Fruit, vegetable, and animal food intake and breast cancer risk by hormone receptor status. Nutr Cancer. 2012;64(6):806–19.
121. Masala G, Assedi M, Bendinelli B, et al. Fruit and vegetables consumption and breast cancer risk: the EPIC Italy study. Breast Cancer Res Treat. 2012;132:1127–36. https://doi.org/10.1007/s10549-011-1939-7.
122. Farvid MS, Cho E, Eliassen AH, et al. Lifetime grain consumption and breast cancer risk. Breast Cancer Res Treat. 2016;159(2):335–45. https://doi.org/10.1007/s10549-016-3910-0.
123. Egeberg R, Olsen A, Loft S, et al. Intake of whole grain products and risk of breast cancer by hormone

receptor status and histology among postmenopausal women. Int J Cancer. 2009;124:745–50. https://doi.org/10.1002/ijc.23992.

124. Nagata C, Mizoue T, Tanaka K, et al. Soy intake and breast cancer risk: an evaluation based on a systematic review of epidemiologic evidence among the Japanese population. Jpn J Clin Oncol. 2014;44(3):282–95. https://doi.org/10.1093/jjco/hyt203.
125. Chi F, Wu R, Zeng Y-C, et al. Post-diagnosis soy food intake and breast cancer survival: a meta-analysis of cohort studies. Asian Pac J Cancer Prev. 2013;14(4):2407–12.
126. Zhong X, Zhang C. Soy food intake and breast cancer risk: a meta-analysis. Wei Sheng Yan Jiu. 2012;41(4):670–6.
127. Trock BJ, Hilakivi-Clarke L, Clarke R. Meta-analysis of soy intake and breast cancer risk. J Natl Cancer Inst. 2006;98(7):459–71.
128. Nechuta SJ, Caan BJ, Chen WY, et al. Soy food intake after diagnosis of breast cancer and survival: an in-depth analysis of combined evidence from cohort studies of US and Chinese women. Am J Clin Nutr. 2012;96:123–32. https://doi.org/10.3945/ajcn.112.035972.
129. Caan BJ, Natarajan L, Parker B, et al. Soy food consumption and breast cancer prognosis. Cancer Epidemiol Biomark Prev. 2011;20(5):854–8. https://doi.org/10.1158/1055-9965.EPI-10-1041.
130. Shu XO, Zheng Y, Cai H, et al. Soy food intake and breast cancer survival. JAMA. 2009;302(22):2437–43. https://doi.org/10.1001/jama.2009.1783.

Index

A
Adenoma recurrence, 531
Age related dementia, 466, 472, 478–481, 483, 490–492, 496–499, 501, 504, 505
  beverages, 492
    alcohol, 499, 501
    caffeinated, 498
    flavanol-rich cocoa beverages, 499
    100% juices, 496, 497
  diet quality, 467, 471
  foods sources, 483
    fruits and vegetables, 483, 490
    nuts, 490
    soy *vs*. milk protein, 491, 492
    whole grains, 490
  healthy dietary patterns, 471
    DASH diets, 481
    MedDiet, 472, 478–480
    MIND diet, 481
    Nordic diet, 483
  lifestyle factors, 505
  lutein, 501
    observation studies, 504, 505
    RCTs, 501, 504
  pathological mechanisms, 466
Age-related cognitive performance, 468–470, 473–477, 484–489, 493–496, 500–504
Age-related macular degeneration (AMD), 504
Aging related diseases, 4, 6
Alcohol consumption
  prospective studies, 499, 501
  systematic review and meta-analysis, 499
Aldosterone, 370
All-cause mortality, 567
Alternate Healthy Eating Index (AHEI), 40, 258, 264
Alzheimer's disease, 477, 482
American Heart Association's (AHA) healthy dietary criteria, 314
Ancestral fiber-rich whole foods diets, 213
Anthocyanins, 493
Antioxidant vitamins, 522
Apolipoprotein E (Apo-E), 466
Australian Blue Mountains Eye Study, 34, 35, 41

B
Beverages, 492, 496
  alcohol, 420
  coffee, 420
  flavanol-rich cocoa beverages, 499
  100% juices, 496
  RCTs, 496–498
  sugar and sweetened soda, 420
Biological age, 4
Blood 25-hydroxyvitamin D [25(OH)D], 577
Blood pressure (BP), 370, 390, 398–401, 448
  DASH diet *vs*. Western-type diet, 378
  fruit juice, 401, 402
  fruits and vegetables
    intake, 398, 401
    RCTs, 399–400
  healthy dietary pattern mechanisms, 380
  healthy lifestyle factors, 371
  hypocaloric DASH-type *vs*. low fat weight-loss diet, 377
  soy milk/cow's milk-based diet, 403
  whole *vs*. refined grains, 395
  whole-grain RCTs, 393–395
Body mass index (BMI), 557
  all-cause mortality risk, 9
  body composition, 10
  disability at retirement, 11
Body weight, 370
Brain-derived neurotrophic factor (BDNF), 491
Breast cancer (BC), 552, 556
  lifestyle factors, 552
  molecular subtype biological markers, 552
  2017 World Cancer Research Fund International/American Institute of Cancer Research Continuous Update (CUP) Project Report, 556
Breast cancer risk, 566, 569–571
  healthy *vs*. Western diets, 561
  MedDiet pattern, 559
  RCTs, 566
    body weight, 566
    healthy, low fat diets, 570
    MedDiet, 570

M.L. Dreher, *Dietary Patterns and Whole Plant Foods in Aging and Disease*, Nutrition and Health,
https://doi.org/10.1007/978-3-319-59180-3

Breast cancer risk, (*cont.*)
menopause hot flash status, 570, 571
weight loss, 569
recurrence/mortality, 560–564
British Whitehall II study, 35, 42

C

Caffeinated beverages, 498
Calcium meta-analyses, 577
Calcium, CRC, 523
Canadian cost-of-illness analysis, 130
Cancer prevention, adult guidelines, 553
Cardiometabolic deaths, 336
Cardiovascular disease (CVD), 351, 370, 390, 396, 449
Carotenoids, 523, 582
cohort studies, 585
RCTs, 585
systematic reviews and meta-analyses, 582, 583
Celiac disease, 168
Central obesity, 8, 10
Childhood constipation, 146
Chinese Longitudinal Healthy Longevity Survey, 35
Chronic constipation, 146
Chronic kidney disease (CKD), 414, 418–425
abdominal obesity, 414
dietary factors, 419
dietary fiber, 416, 417
dietary patterns, 420
cohort studies, 423, 424
nutritional guidelines, 425
RCTs, 425
dose-response relationship, 416
fiber intake/day, 418
food ingredients
beverages, 420
minerals, 419
healthy diets, 415
lifestyle, 415
MedDiet, 424
protein source, 415–417
systemic inflammation, 420
Western dietary patterns, 414
whole plant foods
fruits and vegetables, 419
whole grains, 418
Chronic Renal Insufficiency Cohort (CRIC), 415
Chronological age, 4
Clostridium difficile infections, 120–127
Coffee, 558
Cohort studies, BC risk
DASH diet, 566
MedDiet, 564, 565
recurrence/mortality, 566
vegetarian dietary patterns, 564
Western *vs*. healthy dietary patterns, 561, 564
Colonic microbiota, 118–120
bacteroides-related bacteria, 118
butyrate-producing bacteria, 118
dysbiosis, 118
fiber intake, 118, 119
fiber-rich dietary patterns (*see* Fiber-rich dietary patterns)
human biological functions, 118
lifestyle factors, 118, 119
proteobacteria, 118, 119
Colorectal adenoma, 516, 518–521, 540
dietary pattern studies, 525–527
systematic reviews and meta-analyses, 531
vegetables and fruits intake, 538
whole plant foods, 532–537
Colorectal cancer (CRC), 516–524, 528, 531, 537–542
dietary pattern studies, 524–527
nutrients and phytochemicals, 516
cohort studies, 521
mechanisms, 521–524
systematic reviews and meta pooled analyses, 517
RCTs, 517, 530
recurrence/survival, 527, 529
specific prospective cohort studies, 524, 527, 541
Asian populations, 540, 541
EU populations, 539
legumes, 540
nuts (peanuts), 542
risk biomarkers, 528, 531
Scandinavian populations, 541, 542
US populations, 537, 538, 541
systematic reviews and meta-analyses, 524, 537, 540, 541
colorectal adenoma risk, 531
vegetarian diets *vs*. non-vegetarian dietary pattern, 527
whole plant foods, 531–537
fruits and vegetables, 531
Constipation, 148–161
Academy of Nutrition and Dietetics recommendations, 146
American Academy of Pediatrics recommendations, 146
American College of Gastroenterology recommendations, 146
American Medical Association recommendations, 146
causes, 146
childhood constipation, 146
chronic constipation, 146
definition, 147
European Food Safety Authority recommendations, 146
fecal bulking index and total fiber content, 149
fiber laxation mechanisms, 147, 148
fiber-rich dietary patterns
breads, 157, 158
breakfast cereals, 157
cereal brans, 152, 153
cereal sources, 149–156
chicory inulin, 155, 160, 161
dose response RCT, 156

fecal bulking index and total fiber content, 148
food ingredient intervention trials, 150–155
kiwi fruit, 153, 154, 159
oat bran, 158
Pajala porridge, 157
plant cell walls, 148
plant foods, 151
polydextrose, 154, 159, 160
prebiotics, 148, 156–158
prunes, 153, 156, 158
psyllium, 155, 156, 160
soluble corn fiber, 154, 160
synbiotics, 156
systematic reviews, 149
wheat bran, 148
whole fruits and vegetables *vs*. fruit and vegetable juices, 153, 158
Coronary artery disease (CAD), 356, 360
Coronary artery risk development in young adults (CARDIA), 470
Coronary heart disease (CHD), 318–327, 337, 350, 370, 440
AHA healthy dietary criteria, 314
ancient *vs*. modern grain effect, 344
DASH diet
prospective cohort studies, 323–325
RCTs, 324–327
death rates, 314
dietary carbohydrates *vs*. dietary fat, 328–330
Elderly Dietary Index, 327, 328
foods *vs*. beverages, 337
fruits and vegetables studies, 346–349
healthy behaviors, 336
Healthy Eating Index, 314, 315
healthy lifestyles, 314
healthy *vs*. Western dietary patterns, 315–318, 330, 331
ideal healthy diet, 314
MedDiet
dietary patterns, 318
prospective studies, 318–322
RCTs, 320–324
non-soy legumes studies, 353–354
nuts and seeds studies, 356–359
soy product studies, 354–355
suboptimal diet quality, 314
vegetarian dietary patterns, 327
whole-grain studies, 339–342
C-reactive protein (CRP), 338, 351, 571

D

Dairy products, 492
Dementia, 466, 467
Diabesity, 14
Diet plans, 18
Dietary antioxidant vitamins, 576
Dietary approaches to stop hypertension (DASH), 36, 201, 202, 204, 323–327, 373, 376, 382, 433, 438–440, 481, 524, 566
blood pressure, 374–375
CHD (*see* Coronary heart disease (CHD))
dietary patterns, 372
full-fat/low-fat dairy foods, 376
NAFLD, 305, 306
obesity, 201, 202, 204, 210
observational studies, 373
RCTs, 373
meta-analyses, 373, 376
type 2 diabetes prevention and management, 271, 272
Dietary energy density, 416, 558
Dietary fat, 572–577
Dietary fiber, 416, 417, 517, 572–578
Dietary folate intake, 576
Dietary nutrients, 571, 577–580
antioxidant vitamins, 581
blood 25-hydroxyvitamin D [25(OH)D], 582
calcium, 582
dietary fat
cohort studies, 580
systematic reviews and meta-analyses, 579, 580
dietary fiber, 571
cohort studies, 577, 578
meta-analyses, 571, 577
folate intake, 581
protein source, 581
vitamin D, 582
Dietary patterns (DP), 28, 371, 420, 423, 424, 470, 471, 556–559
chronic disease risk, 36–40
cohort studies
meta-analysis, 423
prospective studies, 423, 424
dietary quality score, 28
dietary rules, 29
healthy dietary patterns, 28, 34–36
lifestyle factors, 557
adolescence and early adulthood, 558
beverages, 558, 559
BMI, 557
dietary energy density, 558
physical activity, 559
weight change across lifespan, 557
meta-analyses, 30
mortality risk, 30–35
nutrient-dense diets, 28
nutritional guidelines, 425
pooled prospective data analyses, 30
RCTs, 425
telomere length, 49–51
Western dietary pattern (*see* Western dietary patterns)
Dietary protein sources, 415, 416, 456, 458, 459, 572–577
legumes, 457, 458
nuts and peanuts
cohort studies, 459
meta-analyses, 458
Dietary pulses/total legumes, 459

Diverticular disease, 178–186
alcoholic beverages, 177, 178
coffee, 177
complications, 166, 167
diarrhea predominate IBS, 167
dietary patterns and foods, 176, 177
fiber mechanisms
body weight regulation, 185, 186
colonic health, 184, 185
fiber-rich dietary patterns
hospital admission/death risk, 180, 181
intervention trials, 180, 183, 184
non-vegetarian *vs.* vegetarian diets, 180, 182
observational studies, 178–180
quality score and risk, 180, 181
total fiber intake, 180, 182
FODMAPs highly fermentable fiber, 178
FODMAPs intake, 167
meta-analysis, 167
NIDDK recommendations, 178
nuts and seeds, 176–178
symptoms, 167

E
Elderly Dietary Index, 327, 328
Elevated blood pressure, 391
End stage renal disease (ESRD), 414, 420
Energy dense diets, 196
Estimated baseline glomerular filtration rate (eGFR), 416
European Prospective Investigation into Cancer and Nutrition (EPIC), 455, 553
Exercise and Nutritional Interventions for Neurocognitive Health Enhancement (ENLIGHTEN), 505

F
Fasting lipid profiles, 351
Fermentable oligosaccharides, disaccharides, monosaccharides and polyols (FODMAPs) diets, 169, 170, 173–177
diverticular disease, 167, 178
IBS, 168
colonic related health concerns, 173
low FODMAPs diet *vs.* high diets & traditional IBS dietary guidance, 174, 176, 177
observational studies, 173
potential food sources, 170, 174
RCTs, 173–176
Fiber biological mechanisms, 224
colonic effects, 224
eating and digestion rates, 223
energy density, 222
fiber and healthy dietary pattern mechanisms, 222, 223
postprandial satiety signaling, 223, 224
satiety and energy metabolism, 224, 225
Fiber-rich dietary patterns, 213–220, 226, 227, 577
Canadian cost-of-illness analysis, 130
Clostridium difficile colonic infections, 125, 127
colorectal cancer, 127, 128
fecal short-chain fatty acids (SCFAs), 120, 125
fruits and vegetables, 120
healthy aging, 130
hs-C-reactive protein (hs-CRP) levels, 130, 131
inflammatory bowel disease, 127
meta-analysis, 130
metabolic syndrome, 129, 130
microbiota composition and frailty, 132–135
mortality risk, 130, 131
obesity
fiber intake and adult obesity risk, 213, 215
high fiber foods ranking, 219, 226, 227
observational studies, 214–217
pre-agricultural *vs.* present day Western dietary pattern, 213, 214
RCTs, 215, 218–220
observational studies, 120–123
pig-human colonic model, 120, 126
premature death, 130
RCTs, 120, 123, 124
type 2 diabetes, 129
vegetarian *vs.* omnivore dietary patterns, 120, 126
weight control, 127–129
Western and healthy dietary patterns, 120, 136
whole-grains, 120, 124, 125
Finnish nutritional guidelines, 15
Finnish prospective study, 11
Flavanol-rich cocoa beverages, 499
Flavonoids, 499, 522, 584, 585
Flaxseeds, 405
Folate (vitamin B-9), 523, 572–577
Foods sources, 483, 487, 490
fruits and vegetables, 483
cohort studies, 487
RCTs, 490
systematic reviews, 483
French SU.VI.MAX study, 18
Fruits and vegetables, 74–89, 344, 345, 396, 419, 587–589
chronic disease risk
breast cancer, 79, 84
colorectal cancer, 79, 83
CVD, 74–81
diabetes, 78, 82, 83
hypertension and blood pressure, 76, 77, 80–82
ischemic stroke, 77, 78, 82
cohort studies, 345, 349
meta-analyses, 345
flavonoids, 70
healthy aging
age related cognitive performance, 84–88
general aging and frailty, 86–89
mortality risk, 70–74
RCTs, 349
USDA MyPlate educational concept, 70
Fruit juices, 401

H
Healthy aging, 130, 396
  body weight, 16, 17
  dietary patterns, 17–19
  Finnish nutritional guidelines, 15
  healthy lifestyles, 15
  physical activity, 19
Healthy dietary patterns, 197–214, 225, 226, 471
  age-related cognitive performance, 44–49
  all-cause mortality risk, 36
  Alzheimer's disease, 44–49
  DASH and Nordic diets, 39
  diet quality score, 41, 43
  fiber-rich dietary patterns, 120, 136
  frailty risk, 42, 44
  healthy aging and frailty, 41, 42
  ideal aging, 42, 44
  MedDiet, 472
  non-US cohorts study, 34
  obesity
    common dietary patterns, 197, 225, 226
    DASH dietary pattern, 201, 202, 204
    MedDiet, 200, 201, 203, 204
    overall diet quality, 198–204
    vegetarian dietary pattern, 202, 205
  RCTs
    DASH diet, 208, 210
    MedDiet, 205–211
    Nordic diet, 208, 210–213
    vegetarian diets, 209, 212, 214
  US cohorts studies, 36
  Western dietary pattern, 38
    diet modifications, 28, 29
Healthy Eating Index, 314, 315
Healthy lifestyle factors, 19–22
Healthy Lifestyle Index Score (HLIS), 555
Healthy Nordic diet, 439
Healthy Nordic food index, 441
Healthy vegan dietary patterns, 433
Healthy *vs.* Western diets, 433, 561
Helsinki Businessmen Study, 17
Hemorrhagic stroke, 431, 448
Histone deacetylase (HDAC), 522
Honolulu Heart Program/Honolulu Asia Aging Study, 16
Hormone therapy (HT), 557–558
100% juices, 496
Hypertension, 370, 372, 373, 376, 377, 381, 382, 390, 396, 397
  cohort studies, 392
  dietary patterns, 371
    DASH, 372, 373, 376
    guidelines, 381
    MedDiet, 377, 381
    Nordic diet, 381
    potential mechanisms, 382
    vegetarian diets, 381, 382
  fruits and vegetables, 396
    cohort studies, 396
    meta-analyses, 396, 397
  healthy dietary pattern mechanisms, 380
  legumes, 402
  non-soy legumes, 402
  RCTs, 392, 396
  refined-grain intake, 393
  soy foods, 403
  whole plant foods, 390
Hypocaloric diets, 196

I
Insulin-like growth factor 1 (IGF-1), 557
International Study on Macro/Micronutrients and Blood Pressure (INTERMAP), 397–398
Irritable bowel syndrome (IBS), 166, 168–170, 173, 186, 187
  celiac disease, 168
  dietary fiber
    high fiber whole/minimally processed plant foods, 186, 187
    psyllium, 169, 170, 173
    RCTs, 170
    sub-type, 169, 170
    wheat bran, 169, 170, 173
  diverticular disease (*see* Diverticular disease)
  fiber intake, 168
  FODMAP diets (*see* Fermentable oligosaccharides, disaccharides, monosaccharides and polyols (FODMAPs) diets)
  foods and drinks, 167
  pathogenesis, 166
  pathophysiology, 168, 169
  postprandial worsening symptoms, 168
  subtypes, 166
  symptoms, 166
Ischemic heart disease (IHD), 344
Ischemic stroke, 431, 448
  fruits and vegetables, subtypes, 454
  whole, refined and total grain intake, 451
Isoflavone-rich isolated soy protein (soy protein), 491, 492
Isoflavonoids, 584
Isolated fiber ingredients, 219–222

L
Lacto-ovo-vegetarian, 433
Legumes, 349, 350, 402, 457, 540
  age-related cognitive function, 93, 96
  breast cancer risk, 93, 95
  cardiometabolic and type 2 diabetes risk management, 91, 92, 94, 95
  colorectal cancer risk, 92, 95
  CVD and stroke risk, 89–94
  mortality risk, 89, 90
  non-soy legumes, 350, 351
  soy products, 351, 356, 458
Life's Simple 7, 432, 433
Life-sustaining processes, 4

Lignans, 585, 586
Low-density lipoprotein- cholesterol (LDL-C), 336, 338
Lutein, 501
observation studies, 504
RCTs, 501, 504

M

Macular pigment density, 504, 505
Magnesium, CRC, 523
Mediterranean diet (MedDiet), 18, 36, 47, 48, 205–207, 209–211, 266–271, 318–323, 377, 378, 380, 382, 424, 426, 433, 435–438, 479–481, 524, 559, 564
all-cause mortality, 20
Alzheimer's disease, 47
blood pressure, 379–380
CHD (*see* Coronary heart disease (CHD))
cognitive disorders, 47
cohort studies, 478, 479
meta-analysis, 30, 47
NAFLD, 304, 305
obesity, 200, 201, 203, 204
observational studies, 377
protective effects, 44–48
RCTs, 378, 479, 480
high fiber-rich MedDiet, 207, 209, 211
hypocaloric MedDiet, 207, 209, 211
meta-analyses, 205, 206, 378, 380
non-energy restricted MedDiet, 207, 209, 210
systematic reviews, 205, 206
unrestricted MedDiet, 205, 206, 210
score, 35
systematic reviews and meta-analyses, 472, 478
type 2 diabetes prevention and management
meta-analyses, 266–269
representative studies, 266–271
Mediterranean-DASH diet intervention for neurodegenerative delay (MIND), 481, 482
Merck Manual primary strategies, 8
Meta-analyses, BC risk, 559, 561
healthy *vs*. Western diets, 561
MedDiet pattern, 559
recurrence/mortality, 561
Metabolic dysfunction, 8
Metabolic syndrome, 14
Microalbuminuria, 425
Microbiota ecosystem, 406
Mild cognitive impairment (MCI), 490
Minerals
magnesium, 420
phosphorus-containing ingredients, 420
sodium, 419
Mini–Mental State Examination (MMSE), 466
Monounsaturated fatty acids (MUFAs), 296, 376, 404, 459
MyPlate method, 259
MyPlate visual educational tool, 234

N

National Institute of Diabetes and Digestive and Kidney Diseases (NIDDK) recommendations, 178
National Institutes of Health (NIH)-AARP Diet and Health Study, 60
Nonalcoholic fatty liver disease (NAFLD), 296–304, 307, 308
body weight and central adiposity, 294, 295
carotenoids, 298, 299
clinical risk factors, 292
coffee, 298
DASH, 305, 306
de novo lipogenesis, 293
definition, 292
dietary patterns
dietary pattern quality, 299–304
energy restricted/weight loss diets, 299, 300
low-carbohydrate diets, 299, 300
Western and healthy dietary patterns, 307, 308
dietary tips, 292
fiber-rich whole plant foods
body weight and central obesity control, 296, 297
systemic inflammation and insulin resistance attenuation, 297, 298
flavonoids, 299
fructose intake, 293
habitual diet, 292
Iranian case control study, 292
mean liver fat, 294
MedDiet, 304, 305
metabolic dysfunctions, 292
MUFAs, 296
NASH, 292
omega-3 fatty acids, 295, 296
pathogenesis, 292, 293
prevalence, 292
prevention and management, 292
risk factors, 293
soy based diet, 299
SREBF1, 293
vitamin E, 298
Nonalcoholic steatohepatitis (NASH), 292
Non-*APOE* ε4 allele, 466
Non-soy legumes
cohort studies, 350, 402
RCTs, 351, 402
Nordic diet, 208, 210, 212, 213, 381, 382, 483
Nordic food index, 274, 275
Nurses' Health Study, 10, 11, 17, 34
Nutrition science, 29
Nuts, 96–106
almonds, 96
cardiometabolic disease and type 2 diabetes biomarkers
age-related cognitive function, 102, 105
intervention trials, 101, 102, 104, 105
systematic review and meta-analyses, 100, 101, 104
telomeres, 102, 105, 106

chronic disease risk, 97–100, 103, 104
mortality risk
prospective cohort studies, 96–103
randomized controlled trial, 103
and peanuts, 458
and seeds, 359, 360, 404

O
Obesity, 8, 197–213, 234
definition, 196
dietary approaches, weight loss, 197
healthy dietary patterns (*see* Healthy dietary patterns)
hypocaloric diet plan, 197
long-term weight loss maintenance, 234
metabolic regulatory processes, 196, 234
thermogenesis, 196
weight and body composition regulation (*see* Whole plant foods)
weight maintenance determinants, 196
weight regain metabolic processes, 196
Omega-3 fatty acids, 295
Osteoarthritis Initiative study, 11

P
Phenolics. *See* Flavonoids
Physical and physiological changes of aging, 4, 5
Physically active lifestyle, 19
Physicians' Health Study, 34
Phytochemicals, 582–585
carotenoids, 582
flavonoids, 585
Phytoestrogens, 584
lignans, 586
soy isoflavonoids, 585, 586
Plant based diet, 18
Polyphenols, 480
Polyunsaturated fatty acids (PUFAs), 404
Post-menopausal breast cancer, 555
cancer mortality, 554
vs. pre-menopausal breast cancer, 565
Post-menopausal women, stroke mortality, 449
Prediabetes, 14, 15
Prevencion con Dieta Mediterranea (PREDIMED), 36, 380, 559
Proteobacteria, 118, 119, 129
Public health policies, 4

R
Randomized controlled trials (RCTs), 341, 356, 392, 396, 437, 467, 552, 556, 567–569
body weight, 566
carotenoids, 585
CRC risk, 530
flaxseeds, 405
healthy, low fat diets, 570
MedDiet, 479, 480, 570
menopause hot flash status, 570, 571
meta-analyses of, 561
nuts intake, 404
sesame seeds, 405
weight loss, 569
REasons for Geographic and Racial Differences in Stroke (REGARDS), 435, 470
Renin-angiotensin aldosterone system (RAAS), 370

S
Sarcopenia, 15
Scandinavian HELGA cohort studies, 62
Sedentary lifestyle, 13
Selenium, CRC, 524
Sesame seeds, 405
Short chain fatty acids (SCFAs), 390
Soy foods, 458
cohort studies, 352, 594, 595
observational studies, 403
RCTs, 352, 403
systematic reviews and meta-analyses, 594
Soy isoflavonoids, 522, 586
Soy *vs.* milk protein, 491
Sterol regulatory element-binding transcription factor 1 (SREBF1), 293
Stroke, 431, 433–435, 437–439, 448, 449, 452, 455, 456, 458, 459
dietary patterns, 433
cohort studies, 433–435, 437, 438
DASH diet, 438, 439
healthy Nordic diet, 439
RCTs, 437
specific studies, 435
dose-response analysis, 455
foods and beverages, 448
fruits and vegetables, 452–454
healthy *vs.* Western diets, 433, 434
MedDiet, 435–437
modifiable risk factors, 432, 433
risk in US women, 435
whole-and refined-grain intake, 450–451
whole plant foods, 448
dietary protein sources, 456, 458, 459
fruits and vegetables, 449, 452, 455
whole-grains, 449

T
Thermogenesis, 196
Total legume/dietary pulse, 458
Triglycerides (TG), 342
2017 World Cancer Research Fund International/ American Institute of Cancer Research Continuous Update (CUP) Project Report, 556

Type 2 diabetes, 14–15
diet quality
AHEI, 259–264
healthy and unhealthy dietary patterns, 264, 265
plant-based dietary indices, 264
prospective cohort studies, 261–263, 265
RCT, 263, 266
risk decreasing *vs*. increasing foods, 259, 263
systematic reviews and pooled/meta-analyses, 259–265
dietary patterns, 258
fiber-rich foods, 283
general guidance, 258
MedDiet (*see* Mediterranean diet (MedDiet))
moderate *vs*. high carbohydrate diet, 271, 272
mortality rates, 258
MyPlate method, 259
Nordic food index, 274, 275
Nurses' Health Studies, 259
PREDIMED intervention, 282
prevalence rate, 258
prevention and management, 259–271, 276–282
adult-onset diabetes, 258
AHEI, 258
anti-inflammatory and anti-oxidant dietary patterns, 282
DASH diet, 271, 272
risk assessment model, 258
vegetarian diets, 271–274
Western and healthy dietary patterns, 259, 284
whole body inflammatory homeostasis, 282
whole plant foods
fruits and vegetables, 276, 278–280
legumes, 276, 281
pulse consumption, 276
tree nuts and flaxseeds, 281, 282
US dietary guidelines, 276
whole-grains, 276–278

U
Unhealthy aging phenotypes
metabolic syndrome, 14
prediabetes, 14, 15
sarcopenia, 15
type 2 diabetes, 14–15
Unhealthy/premature aging, 8
US dietary guidelines, 58
US National Health and Nutrition Examination Surveys (NHANES), 336
US NIH-AARP Diet and Health Study, 62
US Nurses' Health and Health Professionals Follow-Up studies, 60

V
Vegetarian dietary patterns, 202, 564
Vegetarian diets, 381, 382
hypertension risk *vs*. omnivore diet, 382
Vitamin D intake, 577

W
Warburg effect, 522
Western dietary patterns, 12, 13, 466, 467, 472
diet modifications, 28, 29
fiber-rich dietary patterns, 120, 136
vs. healthy dietary patterns, 38, 52, 53, 383, 384, 441, 543, 564, 596
vs. high-fiber, 528
Nurses' Health Study, 34
Physicians' Health Study, 34
risk factors, 28
Whole grains, 418, 490
Whole plant foods, 59, 60, 70, 89, 96, 234, 241–247, 249–251, 276–282, 336, 448, 531, 544, 571, 578–582, 585, 586
biological mechanisms, 58
dietary nutrients, 571
antioxidant vitamins, 581
calcium, 582
dietary fat, 579, 580
dietary fiber, 571, 578
dietary protein source, 581
folate intake, 581
vitamin D, 582
energy, fiber, nutrients and phytochemicals composition, 252, 253
fruits and vegetables, 419, 449, 452, 455, 531, 586, 590
advantages, 241
Dietary Guidelines for Americans recommendations, 241 (*see* Fruits and vegetables)
prospective cohort studies, 242, 243, 245–247
RCTs, 243, 244, 247
systematic reviews and meta-analyses, 241–245
general recommendations, 58
legumes, 248, 249 (*see* Legumes)
nutrient and phytochemical compositions, 58, 106, 107
nuts (*see* Nuts)
phytochemicals, 582
carotenoids, 582, 585
flavonoids, 585
phytoestrogens, 585, 586
protein foods, 247, 248
soy food, 594, 595
specific whole/processed plant food choices, 234, 235
sub-optimal dietary intake, 59, 60
total and specific nuts
almonds, 249–251
Atwater energy tables, 249
meta-analysis, 249
prospective cohort studies, 249, 250
walnuts, 251
type 2 diabetes prevention and management (*see* Type 2 diabetes)
type 2 diabetes risk, 58, 59
Whole-grains, 63–70, 276–278, 337, 338, 343, 449, 591, 592
American intake, 60

brown *vs.* white rice, 237, 240
CHD, 338
chronic disease risk
colorectal cancer, 66, 68
CVD, 63, 64, 66
hypertension/BP, 63–67
ischemic stroke, 65, 67
microbiota, 68, 69
type 2 diabetes, 65, 67, 68
visceral fat, 69, 70
cohort studies, 338, 342
meta-analyses, 338
components, 391
CRC risk, 541
dietary patterns, 59
disease specific mortality risk, 60–63
energy-restricted dietary intervention, 237, 240
examples, 59
meta-analyses, 60
myocardial infarction (MI), 343
National Institutes of Health (NIH)-AARP Diet and Health Study, 60
oat ready-to-eat, 240, 241
observational studies, 235–237
periodontal disease, 69, 70
RCTs, 237–241, 342, 343
vs. refined grain products, 235
Scandinavian HELGA cohort studies, 62
type 2 diabetes prevention and management
RCTs, 277, 278
representative cohort studies, 277
systematic reviews and meta-analyses, 276, 277
US dietary guidelines, 235
US NIH-AARP Diet and Health Study, 62
US Nurses' Health and the Health Professionals Follow-Up studies, 60
Wine/alcoholic beverages, 558
Women's Healthy Eating and Living (WHEL), 570

Z
Zeaxanthin, 501

Printed in the United States
By Bookmasters